Applied Pathophysiology

A Conceptual Approach to the Mechanisms of Disease

Applied Pathophysiology

A Conceptual Approach to the Mechanisms of Disease

Third Edition

Carie A. Braun, PhD, RN
Professor of Nursing
College of St. Benedict/St. John's University
St. Joseph, Minnesota

Cindy M. Anderson, PhD, RN, WHNP-BC, ANEF, FAHA, FNAP, FAAN
Associate Professor
College of Nursing
The Ohio State University
Columbus, Ohio

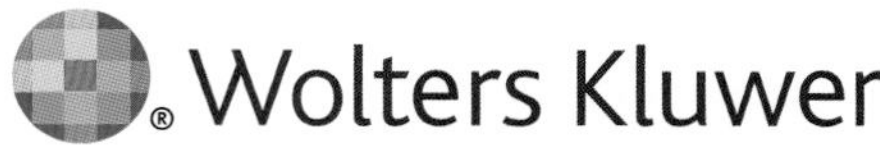

Philadelphia • Baltimore • New York • London
Buenos Aires • Hong Kong • Sydney • Tokyo

Acquisitions Editor: Jay Campbell
Product Development Editor: Linda G. Francis
Production Project Manager: David Orzechowski
Marketing Manager: Leah Thomson
Design Coordinator: Holly McLaughlin
*Prepress Vendor:*S4Carlisle Publishing Services

3rd Edition

9 8 7 6 5 4 3 2

Printed in China

Library of Congress Cataloging-in-Publication Data
Names: Braun, Carie Ann, author. | Anderson, Cindy Miller, author.
Title: Applied pathophysiology : a conceptual approach to the mechanisms of disease / Carie A. Braun, Cindy M. Anderson.
Other titles: Pathophysiology
Description: Third edition. | Philadelphia : Wolters Kluwer Health, [2017] | Preceded by Pathophysiology / Carie A. Braun, Cindy M. Anderson. 2nd ed. c2011. | Includes bibliographical references and index.
Identifiers: LCCN 2016023449 | ISBN 9781496335869
Subjects: | MESH: Pathology | Physiology | Physiological Phenomena
Classification: LCC RB113 | NLM QZ 4 | DDC 616.07—dc23 LC record available at https://lccn.loc.gov/2016023449

LWW.com

CCS0718

This edition is dedicated to my colleagues at the College of St. Benedict/St. John's University who provided the encouragement and time for this edition to become a reality.

—Carie A. Braun

To my students who provide a constant source of enthusiasm and motivation; to my husband, Kevin, and daughters, Rachel, Amy, and Michelle, who provide unconditional support, motivation, and love; and to my friends and colleagues, especially Marena, for their consistent encouragement.

—Cindy M. Anderson

Preface

This third edition comes at a time when conceptual curricula and concept-based learning are gaining a strong foothold. Should the student learn through a body-systems approach or a conceptual altered functional approach? This text teaches pathophysiology through the lens of body function concepts and what happens when function is altered through injury or disease. The text then illustrates these concepts through select diseases, or clinical models. By explaining the core concepts of altered human function, students can apply a deeper understanding to a range of diseases, rather than trying to memorize facts about specific conditions. Because students learn through application, they learn to think about pathophysiology as in a clinical setting, by working from symptoms to the cause, rather than the other way around.

At its core, this edition continues to emphasize student learning, application of knowledge, active learning strategies, critical thinking, and evidence-based practice through the many features and learning resources that accompany this text. We are excited for the opportunity to share this learning tool and continue to welcome your valuable feedback!

Learning Resources

The supplemental material that accompanies this book provides numerous online opportunities for students to reinforce their learning.

Students can also purchase the study guide, a supplement tailored specifically to the approach and content of Pathophysiology. It contains test-taking strategies, concept-mapping exercises, case studies, and quiz questions to further ensure comprehension.

Instructors' resources are available at the Website (http://connection.lww.com/BraunAnderson). Included in the instructors' resources are the following valuable assets:

- PowerPoint presentations by chapter
- Test generator
- Image bank
- Additional case studies
- Answers to chapter exercises
- Additional learning activities
- Conversion tools

Detailed lesson plans are also available to help instructors transition from a standard body-systems approach to the conceptual approach presented here.

Applied Pathophysiology: A Conceptual Approach to the Mechanisms of Disease represents a paradigm shift in thinking and learning about pathophysiology focused on functional alterations in health. Learning pathophysiology can be fascinating and challenging at the same time. The goal of this text is to focus on the fascinating.

User's Guide

In today's health care careers, a thorough understanding of pathophysiology is more important than ever. *Applied Pathophysiology: A Conceptual Approach to the Mechanisms of Disease* not only provides the conceptual knowledge you will need, but also teaches you how to apply it. This User's Guide introduces you to the features and tools of this innovative textbook. Each feature is specifically designed to enhance your learning experience, preparing you for a successful career as a health professional.

Take a few minutes to look through the text and get acquainted with its organization. The table of contents of Applied Pathophysiology: A Conceptual Approach to the Mechanisms of Disease is structured around concepts of altered human function. The categories, devised by a group of educators, were selected by analyzing and clustering human health conditions with high prevalence, incidence, and severity. Clusters were formed by looking at the common impacts and ultimate results of different groups of diseases on the human body.

This novel approach shows you how diseases are rarely confined to one body system and challenges you to build on previously gained knowledge. An integrative study at the end of the book emphasizes the practical nature of the material by helping you apply the complex pathophysiologic concepts that you have learned to a common condition—diabetes mellitus.

Next, take a look at the chapters themselves. We have included some important tools to help you learn about pathophysiology and apply your new knowledge:

LEARNING OBJECTIVES →

Highlight important concepts—helping you organize and prioritize learning.

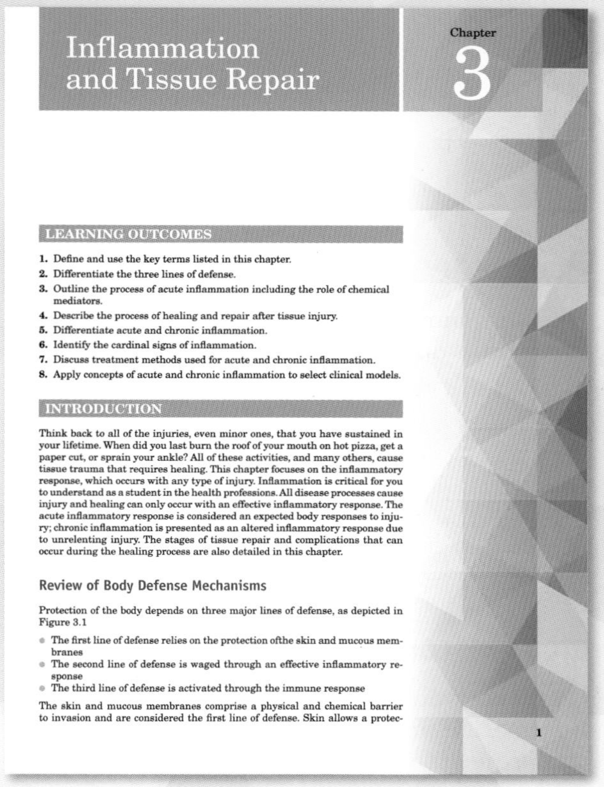

Inflammation and Tissue Repair

Chapter 3

LEARNING OUTCOMES

1. Define and use the key terms listed in this chapter.
2. Differentiate the three lines of defense.
3. Outline the process of acute inflammation including the role of chemical mediators.
4. Describe the process of healing and repair after tissue injury.
5. Differentiate acute and chronic inflammation.
6. Identify the cardinal signs of inflammation.
7. Discuss treatment methods used for acute and chronic inflammation.
8. Apply concepts of acute and chronic inflammation to select clinical models.

INTRODUCTION

Think back to all of the injuries, even minor ones, that you have sustained in your lifetime. When did you last burn the roof of your mouth on hot pizza, get a paper cut, or sprain your ankle? All of these activities, and many others, cause tissue trauma that requires healing. This chapter focuses on the inflammatory response, which occurs with any type of injury. Inflammation is critical for you to understand as a student in the health professions. All disease processes cause injury and healing can only occur with an effective inflammatory response. The acute inflammatory response is considered an expected body responses to injury; chronic inflammation is presented as an altered inflammatory response due to unrelenting injury. The stages of tissue repair and complications that can occur during the healing process are also detailed in this chapter.

Review of Body Defense Mechanisms

Protection of the body depends on three major lines of defense, as depicted in Figure 3.1

- The first line of defense relies on the protection ofthe skin and mucous membranes
- The second line of defense is waged through an effective inflammatory response
- The third line of defense is activated through the immune response

The skin and mucous membranes comprise a physical and chemical barrier to invasion and are considered the first line of defense. Skin allows a protec-

1

CONCEPT MAPS

Visually illustrate the important interrelationships of key concepts.

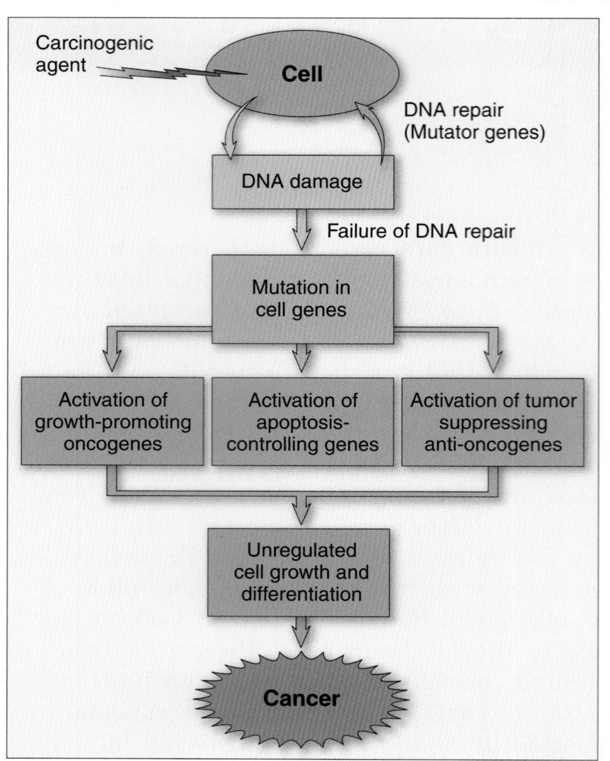

Figure 7.2. Concept map. The genomic mechanisms of cancer. (Modified from Porth CM. *Essentials of Pathophysiology: Concepts of Altered Health States*. Philadelphia, PA: Lippincott Williams & Wilkins; 2003, with permission.)

FROM THE LAB

Explain common laboratory procedures and results.

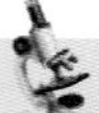

FROM THE LAB

C-reactive protein (CRP) and the erythrocyte sedimentation rate (ESR) are two nonspecific tests of inflammation. Elevations in either test will signify inflammation is present, but neither will identify the exact source or location of the inflammation. CRP is often the preferred test for acute inflammation. CRP signifies the presence of a specific protein triggered by plasma protein systems during the inflammatory process. The erythrocyte sedimentation rate (also referred to as a sed rate) is a nonspecific method of testing for inflammation. During the inflammatory process, the coagulation cascade results in increased circulating levels of fibrinogen, which causes cells to stick together. When measured in a tube in the lab, red blood cells (RBCs) exposed to the inflammatory process will fall faster and will clump together. The ESR test then measures (in mm/hr) the level of RBC stacking.[2]

STOP AND CONSIDER

Challenge you to think beyond the information presented in the textbook as you proceed through the chapter.

Stop and Consider

What lines of defense are you enhancing by putting on an antibiotic ointment and covering a laceration with a band-aid?

SUMMARY

Provide a concise review of the chapter, highlighting the key points you should understand after reading the chapter.

SUMMARY

- Inflammation is required for tissue healing and occurs in response to tissue injury.
- Inflammatory mediators, under the direction of the three plasma protein systems, regulate the inflammatory response.
- Inflammatory mediators elicit vascular and cellular responses characterized by vasodilation, increased capillary permeability, chemotaxis, cellular adherence, and cellular migration.
- Phagocytic cells (neutrophils and later macrophages) taxi to the site to engulf and destroy harmful substances.
- Removal of the injury will direct resolution of the acute inflammatory response.

CASE STUDIES

Case studies and related questions help you build critical thinking skills and apply the chapter material to real-world clinical scenarios. You are encouraged to search the Internet for relevant journal articles and Websites to confirm your predictions.

CASE STUDY 3.1

A friend has disclosed that she has been having problems with heartburn. She has been told that she has gastroesophageal reflux disease (GERD), in which stomach acid backs up into the esophagus causing esophagitis. Think about which clinical model is most related to this process. From your reading related to cellular injury and adaptations as well as inflammation, answer the following questions:

1. What anatomic problem most likely leads to gastroesophageal reflux?
2. What is the injury in gastroesophageal reflux?
3. What would the acute inflammatory response look like?
4. Why might this condition become a chronic problem?
5. What pathophysiologic changes would most like- ...flux? ...nifesta-

PRACTICE EXAM QUESTIONS

Provide practice and review for the types of questions to expect on an exam.

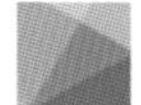

PRACTICE EXAM QUESTIONS

1. You get a paper cut and experience pain at the site. This response is related to:
   a. Increased perfusion at the site
   b. Increased exudate and chemical mediators at the site
   c. Bacteria that have entered the wound
   d. Vasoconstriction at the site

2. Inflammation is ultimately needed to:
   a. Increase inflammatory mediators at the site to vasoconstrict the area
   b. Increase platelets at the site for clotting
   c. Restore functional cells
   d. Prepare the site for healing

3. A wound is 6 cm × 6 cm × 4 cm. A wound with these dimensions needs to heal through:
   a. Secondary intention
   b. Primary intention
   c. Tertiary intention
   d. Scar tissue formation

DISCUSSION AND APPLICATION

Help you gauge your understanding of what you have learned.

DISCUSSION AND APPLICATION

1. What did I know about inflammation and tissue repair prior to today?
2. What body processes are affected by inflammation? What are the expected functions of those processes? How does inflammation impact those processes?
3. What are the potential etiologies for inflammation? How does inflammation develop?
4. Who is most at risk for developing inflammation? How can inflammation be prevented?
5. What are the human differences that affect the etiology, risk, or course of inflammation?
6. What clinical manifestations are expected during inflammation?
7. What special diagnostic tests are useful in determining the diagnosis and course of inflammation?

BONUS WEBSITE

Inside the front cover of your textbook, you will find your personal access code. Use it to log on to thePoint—the companion Website for this textbook. The Website includes the following features to help you reinforce and review your knowledge:

- Pathophysiology animations
- A quiz bank of additional review questions to help you study for exams

Visit http://thePoint.lww.com/activate to kick-start your pathophysiology success today!

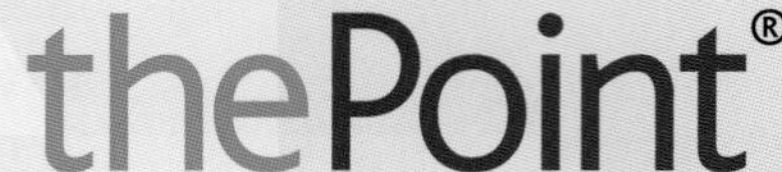

As you can see, all the chapter features are designed to hone critical thinking skills and judgment, build clinical proficiency, and promote comprehension and retention of the material by applying pathophysiologic knowledge, rather than merely memorizing facts and figures.

Reviewers

The publisher and authors gratefully acknowledge the many professionals who shared their expertise and assisted in developing this textbook, helping us refine our plan, appropriately targeting our marketing efforts, and setting the stage for subsequent editions. We are grateful to the following reviewers:

Jeanne Calvert, MS
Associate Professor, Biology
University of St. Francis
Ft. Wayne, Indiana

Karen Chandra, RN, MSN, MBA
Nursing Department
Harper College
Palatine, Illinois

Thomas Chartrand, DC
Associate Lecturer
Clinical Lab Sciences
University of Wisconsin
Milwaukee, Wisconsin

William Hill
Anishinabek Educational Institute
North Bay, Ontario

Kathleen Holbrook, BS
Director
A & H Training Corp.
Latham, New York

Joseph Inungu, MD, PhD
Professor
School of Health Sciences
Central Michigan University
Mt. Pleasant, Michigan

John Knesel
Associate Professor, Biology
University of Louisiana
Monroe, Louisiana

Lori Knight, CCHRA(C)
Instructor
Health Information Services Program
SIAST, Regina
Saskatchewan, Canada

Jeffrey Kushner
Associate Professor
Department of Integrated Science and Technology
James Madison University
Harrisonburg, Virginia

Treena Lemay, BScN
Professor
Health and Community Studies
Algonquin College
Pembroke, Ontario, Canada

Vikki McCleary, PhD
Assistant Professor
Physician Assistant Program
School of Medicine & Health Sciences
University of North Dakota
Grand Forks, North Dakota

Irene L. E. Mueller, EdD
HIA Program Director and Assistant Professor
Health Sciences
Western Carolina University
Cullowhee, North Carolina

Stephanie Olsen
Instructor, Health Information
SAIT Polytechnic
Calgary, Alberta

David Reff, BS, DDS
Program Director
Dental Assisting and Dental Hygiene
Apollo College
Boise, Idaho

Kristine Scordo, PhD, RN, CS, ACNP
Director
Acute Care Nurse Practitioner Program
Wright State University
Dayton, Ohio

Rachel Smetanka, PhD
Assistant Professor, Biology
Southern Utah University
Cedar City, Utah

J. Steve Smith, MD
Professor
Medical Technology Program
University of West Florida
Pensacola, Florida

Catherine Thompson, PhD, MS, PT
Assistant Professor, PT Education
Rockhurst University
Kansas City, Missouri

David Weissman, MD
Associate Professor, Pathology
Robert Wood Johnson Medical School
New Brunswick, New Jersey

Jean Zorko, MS
Assistant Professor
Stark State College of Technology
Canton, Ohio

Acknowledgments

I acknowledge the team at Lippincott Williams & Wilkins for believing in a conceptual approach way before it was vogue.

—Carie A. Braun

I acknowledge the help and direction provided by the staff at Lippincott Williams & Wilkins.

—Cindy M. Anderson

Contents

3. Inflammation and Tissue Repair 34

14. Altered Reproductive Function 340

Introduction to Pathophysiology

Chapter
1

LEARNING OUTCOMES

1. Define and use the key terms listed in this chapter.
2. Discuss the value of prerequisite science courses as a foundation for learning pathophysiology.
3. Differentiate individual versus population-focused care.
4. State and give examples of the three levels of prevention upon which interventions are based.
5. Describe the relevance of gender, age, race, ethnicity, locale, and socioeconomic status to pathophysiology.
6. Explain the significance of evidence-based practice to pathophysiology.

INTRODUCTION

Defining Pathophysiology

What is pathophysiology? **Pathophysiology** is the study of the functional changes that occur in the body as a result of an injury, disorder, or disease. Applying pathophysiology combines what we know about **pathology**, the study of changes in cells and tissues as a result of injury or disease, and **physiology**, the mechanisms of human body functioning. Pathophysiology is often referred to as a study of the mechanisms of disease.

When you study pathophysiology, you must recognize the interdependence of altered structure and function. **Structure** is how the human body is put together, including the component parts and location of those parts. This is often learned in a course in human anatomy. **Function** is concerned with how these component parts operate together. This is most often discovered in a course in human physiology. In addition, preparation in other health science topics such as human biology, microbiology, and chemistry is helpful. Pathophysiology builds on previous learning and applies that learning to discern what happens to both structure and function in the human body in the face of injury, disorder, and disease.

Understanding Pathophysiology

PATHOGENESIS

The first step to understanding pathophysiology is to recognize and use key terms appropriately. First, consider the onset of the disease. **Disease** is the functional impairment of cells, tissues, organs, or organ systems. In this text, the term *disease* is often used broadly to include injuries, disorders, illnesses, and even **syndromes**, defined as a specific condition with a recognizable, predictable pattern. The origination and development at the point of disease onset is referred to as its **pathogenesis**, literally the disease beginning. The pathogenesis encompasses when the disease process first begins to the point when the disease presents itself. For example, in diabetes mellitus, pancreatic beta islet cell destruction can begin years before the onset of diabetes. The pathogenesis is concerned with factors at the onset of pancreatic beta islet cell destruction, the progression of cell destruction, and the point of developing signs of diabetes mellitus. Although we may not know what exactly triggered the original beta islet cell destruction, we can still understand the pathogenesis by studying cellular and tissue changes in those who develop the disease. Many times this occurs in individuals with specific **risk factors**, or vulnerabilities. An example of a set of risk factors for coronary artery disease is provided in Box 1.1. Modifiable risk factors are those that can be changed by the individual. For example, dietary intake, weight, and smoking are risk factors that are modifiable, whereas genetic composition or gender is not. The goal in studying pathogenesis is often to prevent disease from occurring. When prevention is not possible, understanding the pathogenesis can facilitate early diagnosis and intervention to avoid complications and improve quality of life.

ETIOLOGY

At the very beginning of the disease process, there is an **etiology**, or precise cause of disease. Sometimes the etiology is identifiable, as with the inhalation of a viral microorganism that causes influenza in the airways. In this case, the etiology is traced to a specific **pathogen**, or disease-causing microorganism. Sometimes the etiology is unknown or **multifactorial** (having more than one genetic and/or environmental causing events), such as with cardiovascular disease or cancer. When there is no known etiology, the disease is termed **idiopathic**.

Box 1.1 Examples of Risk Factors

The presence of one or more of these select risk factors increases a person's chances for developing coronary artery disease:

- Elevated blood cholesterol level
- Elevated blood pressure
- Cigarette smoking
- Family history/genetic predisposition
- Obesity
- Sedentary lifestyle

Nosocomial disease is the result of exposure to infection in the health care environment. For example, a nosocomial illness is one where a child gets varicella (chicken pox) while being a patient in the hospital. The child did not have varicella when admitted, but was exposed during hospitalization and contracted the disease. Health care professionals have an important obligation to prevent the spread of disease in the health care setting through appropriate hand hygiene and infection control measures. **Iatrogenic** diseases are those that are the inadvertent result of medical treatment. For example, a patient who develops a urinary tract infection from the placement of a urinary catheter has an iatrogenic disease.

Stop and Consider

Would you consider iatrogenic and nosocomial diseases to be medical errors?

CLINICAL MANIFESTATIONS

Clinical manifestations are the presenting signs and symptoms of the disease. More specifically, the **signs** of a disease are the observable or measurable expressions. For example, in herpes simplex (a cold sore), a sign would be redness with raised, clear, fluid-filled vesicles on the individual's lip. The signs are considered as the **objective** manifestations that can be seen or measured by the health care professional. The **symptoms** are indicators that are reported by the ill individual and are considered the **subjective** manifestations because they are not directly observable by the practitioner. Symptoms of herpes may include tingling or discomfort at the site of the vesicles or a feeling of lethargy, or tiredness. These symptoms are difficult for the health care provider to observe or to measure. In addition, patients may describe **precipitating factors**, or triggers, that promote the onset of clinical manifestations. Examples of precipitating factors that promote shortness of breath and coughing in asthma are listed in Box 1.2.

Box 1.2 Examples of Precipitating Factors

Individuals with asthma often report one or more of these precipitating factors that lead to an asthma exacerbation:

- Exercise
- Cold weather
- Upper respiratory infection
- Stress
- Dust/dust mites
- Pollen
- Animal dander
- Mold

Signs and symptoms can be local or systemic. **Local** refers to those manifestations that are found directly at the site of disease and are confined to that specific area. Examples of local manifestations are confined redness, swelling, bruising, or pain. **Systemic** manifestations present throughout the body and are not confined to one area, such as with fever, lethargy, generalized body aching, or high blood pressure. Timing is also important in classifying disease processes and clinical manifestations. **Acute** manifestations or acute diseases are those that begin abruptly and last a few days to a few months. The common cold is a good example of an acute disease. There is a noticeable onset, the disease lasts 10 to 14 days, and there is complete resolution. **Chronic** diseases, however, generally last longer than 6 months and are **insidious**, or gradual, in onset. With chronic disease, the person can have **remissions**, or symptom-free periods, and **exacerbations**, the flaring of symptoms. **Subacute** is a term used to describe diseases that fall somewhere between acute and chronic in duration and severity.

Some conditions are completely **asymptomatic**; that is, the person does not have any noticeable symptoms even though diagnostic tests may indicate that the disease is present. Screening tests, such as Pap smears, breast mammograms, or blood pressure measurements, are invaluable for detecting diseases that are asymptomatic.

DIAGNOSIS AND TREATMENT

Health care providers cluster the presenting clinical manifestations, laboratory, and diagnostic tests to determine a **diagnosis**, or label, for the disease. A recognizable cluster of clinical manifestations can be diagnosed as a syndrome, such as with Down syndrome. You are probably very familiar with many different medical diagnoses and syndromes. The clinical models in this text use the medical diagnosis to identify the various conditions. Some health professionals use different diagnostic categories to describe disease processes. For example, nursing professionals use nursing diagnoses to describe the human response to illness, such as altered fluid balance and ineffective airway clearance. Depending on the health profession that you are studying, you may find there are other terms used to diagnose your patients.

The **prognosis** for a patient is the forecast or prediction of how the individual will proceed through the disease process. An excellent prognosis indicates that the individual will most likely recover completely. A poor prognosis signifies increasing risk for **morbidity**, a negative outcome with disease complications that impact the quality of life, and possibly **mortality**, or death. Prognosis is often based on health statistics across populations where the rates of survival and outcomes of others with similar diseases help predict the individual patient's outcome.

The treatment of disease is dependent upon the etiology and clinical manifestations. Treatment is aimed at eliminating or reducing the cause of disease and thereby eliminating or reducing the clinical manifestations. For example, in a burn injury, treatment is aimed at removing the source of the burn and then cooling the skin and protecting the body from infection. Each chapter will highlight pharmacologic, or drug, interventions used to treat disease. Figure 1.1 details the relationships between many of these terms.

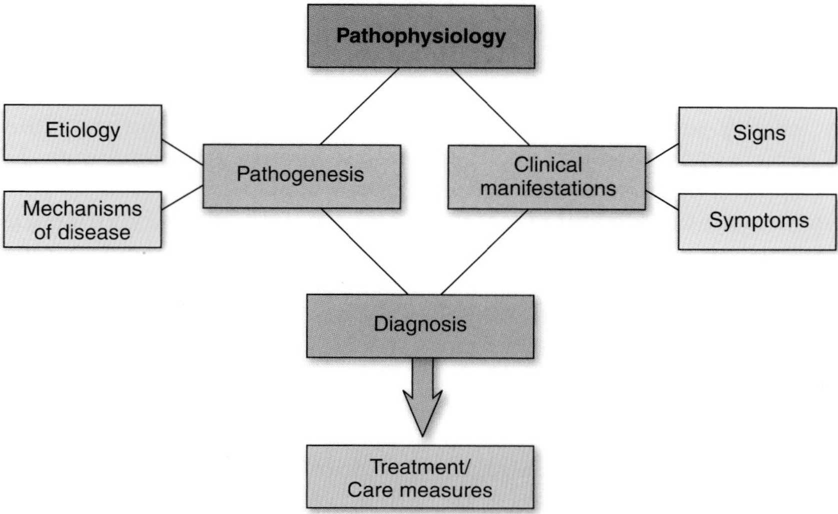

Figure 1.1. Concept map. Pathophysiology terms.

Applying Pathophysiology

INDIVIDUAL HEALTH

You will undoubtedly spend much of your health professional career caring for individuals. In whatever setting you choose to practice, the focus must be on the whole person, defined by that individual's perception of health and illness. **Health**, defined as the perceived wholeness of body, mind, and spirit, and **illness**, a state that results in suffering or distress, are on a dynamic continuum. The continuum implies that individuals perceive themselves to be anywhere along the line of "extremely healthy" to "extremely ill." There are varying degrees of health and varying degrees of illness. Dynamic means the patient's perceptions of how healthy or ill he or she is can change from day to day, month to month, or year to year. Effective communication with your patients can determine where they perceive themselves along this continuum and how you can best help them maintain or return to optimal health.

Stop and Consider
Are you healthy or ill? How do you know? What characteristics describe someone who is healthy? When does a person often become labeled as ill? Think about a situation where a person was diagnosed with an illness but considered themselves to be healthy. How about when a person does not have a diagnosis but considers themselves to be ill?

In other science coursework, you have probably talked about the concept of homeostasis. **Homeostasis** is a dynamic balance in the body marked by the appropriate and effective response to stimuli, thereby keeping the body in a steady state. Although it often happens at a cellular level, homeostasis is an important body goal and is often reflected in the patient's perception of the health–illness continuum. Throughout this text you will develop a greater appreciation for the response systems in the body that allow homeostasis to continue. You will also learn what happens when stressors present excessive and insurmountable challenges to homeostasis.

An important thing to keep in mind when caring for individual patients is that people should not be defined by their pathophysiology. Calling a patient by his or her disease state ignores the holistic physical, spiritual, emotional, and psychological components that comprise all of us. Health professionals should avoid calling patients "diabetics" or "the skull fracture in room 202" and replace these labels with "the woman with diabetes" or "the patient in room 202 with a skull fracture." After all, if the overall goal is high-quality holistic health care, this can begin only in a genuinely caring environment (Fig. 1.2).

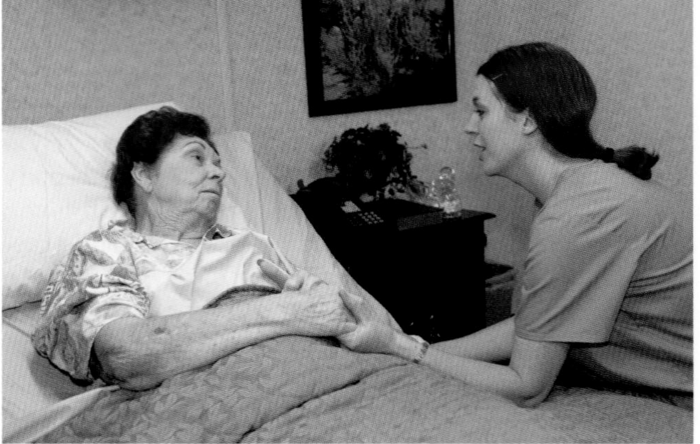

Figure 1.2. People first. A practitioner listens to a patient. The focus needs to be on the *patient;* the health problem is always secondary. (From Carter PJ, Lewsen S. *Lippincott's Textbook for Nursing Assistants: A Humanistic Approach to Caregiving*. Philadelphia, PA: Lippincott Williams & Wilkins; 2005.)

POPULATION HEALTH

Your role as a health professional also requires that you consider the health of populations. Focusing on **epidemiology**, the study of disease in populations, has many advantages such as:

1. Recognition of where a disease is most widespread
2. Recognition of who is most affected by the disease
3. Discovering why the disease is presenting in that population
4. Discovering how to reduce the spread of disease, reduce morbidity, or eradicate the disease in that population

Health statistics are an important aspect of population-focused health care. **Incidence** is the rate of occurrence of a disease at any given time. Incidence represents the probability that a disease will occur in a certain population. For example, the incidence of Down syndrome, or the chance that one will be born with Down syndrome, is approximately 1 in 691.[1] **Prevalence** is the number or percentage of a population that is affected by a particular disease at a given time. As an example of prevalence, 400,000 people in the United States are currently living with Down syndrome.[1]

When the incidence and prevalence of a disease are predictable and stable, this is termed **endemic**. A dramatic increase in disease incidence in a population is called an **epidemic** and represents a rate considerably above the endemic rate. When an epidemic spreads across continents, the disease is considered to be a **pandemic**. The World Health Organization (WHO) is an important epidemiology resource and provides a yearly guide to health statistics for its member states. The annual World Health Reports detail mortality and life expectancy rates across the globe and provide incidence and prevalence statistics for numerous diseases. For example, in the 2014 update, the 10 leading causes of death worldwide were listed as ischemic heart disease, stroke, chronic obstructive pulmonary disease, lower respiratory infections, lung cancer, HIV/AIDS, diarrheal diseases, diabetes, injury, and hypertensive heart disease.[2] Decreasing the incidence and prevalence of these conditions can have the greatest impact on the health of populations around the world.

Stop and Consider
Look for current reports related to health. What epidemic conditions are currently present in your geographic area? What is being reported around the world? Do you notice any pandemic condition reports?

DISEASE PREVENTION

Prevention of disease is a critical role for the health professions. Disease prevention is most often discussed in three levels: primary, secondary, and tertiary.

1. **Primary prevention:** Primary prevention prohibits a disease condition from occurring. An example is wearing a bike helmet to prevent a head injury.
2. **Secondary prevention:** Secondary prevention is the early detection of disease through screening and early treatment. An example is performing breast or testicular self-examination every month for early cancer detection.
3. **Tertiary prevention:** Tertiary prevention is rehabilitation of a patient after detection of disease. Tertiary prevention focuses on preventing complications or progression of the condition; for example, applying physical therapy and occupational therapy interventions to improve gross and fine motor function after a stroke.

Stop and Consider
What activities do you participate in that would count as primary prevention? How about secondary prevention? Identify other examples of tertiary prevention.

Evidence-Based Practice

Evidence-based practice is a way of caring for others that is cognizant of the most current research and knowledge in the health professions. The Research Notes feature of this text highlights some of the current research on the various pathophysiologic concepts and diseases. However, evidence-based practice goes beyond one piece of research and encompasses the totality of what is known through research and the knowledge and practices of clinical experts.

Health professionals must be prepared to work effectively with people of all races and cultures. This requires a conscientious respect for human health variations. Evidence-based practice and epidemiology provide a framework for determining those most likely to be afflicted with certain diseases based on gender, age, race, locale, socioeconomic factors, or ethnicity. Recognizing differences based on these factors will help promote effective prevention measures. Health professionals must always balance what is known from an epidemiologic standpoint with what is unique to each human based on his or her life situation, avoid stereotyping, and be ready to identify and assist all patients in promoting health.

Pathophysiology is arguably one of the most important subjects that you will ever study as a student in the health professions. Your patients will rely on you to recognize health problems and act accordingly. Decisions about pharmacologic treatments, surgical interventions, health promotion measures, nutritional interventions, and even genetic counseling are dependent upon your learning in this course.

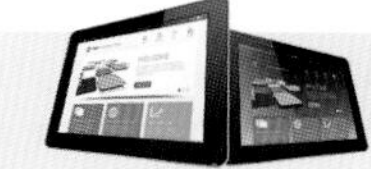

RESEARCH NOTES

The Human Genome Project, completed in 2003, determined DNA sequence patterns among diverse populations in order to identify "DNA regions" associated with complex diseases, such as cancer, diabetes, heart disease, and certain types of mental illness. Current research has taken this idea a step further in discovering that DNA sequencing is not the only determinant of health and disease.[3] Epigenetics is the study of genetic control by factors other than a person's DNA sequence. Epigenetics controls the "on" and "off" switch of genes and which proteins are transcribed. This growing body of research will provide additional clues to the human and environmental factors that increase the risk and development of disease.

Functional Concepts of Altered Health

The information contained in this book represents a journey into the world of conceptual learning. A **concept** is a general idea that can be applied to similar

Box 1.3 Functional Concepts of Altered Health

Basic alterations in cells and tissues
Inflammation
Immunity
Infection
Genetic and developmental disorders
Altered cellular proliferation and differentiation
Altered fluid/electrolyte and acid/base balance
Altered neuronal transmission
Altered mood and behavior
Altered sensory function and pain perception
Altered hormonal/metabolic processes
Altered reproductive function
Altered ventilation and diffusion
Altered tissue perfusion
Altered nutrition
Altered elimination
Degenerative changes in aging

situations. In other words, a conceptual approach in pathophysiology clusters current knowledge about human health and disease and organizes that knowledge into meaningful and useful ideas. These ideas are referred to as functional alterations in health. Box 1.3 lists the select functional alterations upon which this text is based.

A conceptual approach dictates learning general disease processes and then applying these processes to specific conditions. It is impossible to detail every disease condition. A conceptual approach supplies you with the tools to be more effective at figuring out what is known and how this applies to that which is unknown. The effective application of that knowledge to the health care setting is the destination.

SUMMARY

- Pathophysiology is the study of the mechanisms of disease and focuses on the physiology of altered health states; specifically, the functional changes that accompany a particular injury, syndrome, or disease.
- Those studying pathophysiology are concerned with the etiology, pathogenesis, and clinical manifestations of disease; this involves the analysis of cellular, tissue, organ, and body system changes that occur in a disease state.
- Health professionals cluster signs and symptoms (also called clinical manifestations) to formulate a diagnosis, or label, for the disease condition. Appropriate interventions can then be applied, with respect to human diversity, to provide high-quality health care and to promote optimal health outcomes.
- Epidemiology is a science that deals with the study of disease trends in populations; epidemiologists identify the incidence and prevalence of diseases worldwide, including the presence of endemic, epidemic, and pandemic conditions. A major goal of understanding disease is to effectively apply the three levels of prevention whenever possible.

CASE STUDY 1.1

Kim is a 10-year-old girl who presents to the urgent care clinic with a 14-day history of nasal stuffiness, copious amounts of green nasal drainage, fever, generalized headache ("my whole head hurts"), facial pain above and below the eyes, and fatigue. Kim reports that her younger sister recently had a "bad cold"; no one else in the family is currently ill. Kim's medical history is significant for seasonal allergies, usually flaring up this time of the year. Kim has been using her antihistamine medication to block the seasonal allergies, but this treatment has not been effective. Kim's mother reports that Kim is "constantly stressed out and puts way too much pressure on herself." Kim says that her biggest concern is missing the school musical; she is the lead and the opening production is in 2 days. Upon physical examination, Kim has an oral temperature of 100.4°F. The practitioner taps gently above and below Kim's eyes; her sinuses are tender when touched. The lymph glands along her neck are enlarged and tender. Kim undergoes sinus radiographs (X-rays). The radiographs indicate fluid accumulation in the frontal and maxillary sinuses. Kim is diagnosed with sinusitis, related to a persistent upper respiratory infection. Kim is prescribed a 3-week course of antibiotics to treat the sinus infection.

1. Would you define Kim as healthy or ill? Explain.
2. What risk factors does Kim have that could have led to the development of the sinusitis?
3. What is the etiology of Kim's sinusitis? Would the sinusitis be considered either nosocomial or iatrogenic? Explain.
4. Identify the symptoms that Kim reports.
5. Identify the signs leading to the diagnosis of sinusitis.
6. How would you categorize this illness: acute or chronic? Explain.
7. Which of the manifestations are local and which are systemic?
8. What is the prognosis for Kim?
9. What aspects related to human diversity and disease would be important to consider with regard to Kim?

10. What additional dimensions of the health history would you need to explore to provide holistic health care?

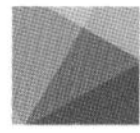

CASE STUDY 1.2

Jay is a public health worker and is charged with developing an immunization tracking program for residents of his county aged birth to 21 years. Jay is primarily interested in measles vaccination rates. There has been a major increase in measles diagnoses in young children and adolescents from the years 2010 to 2015 (10 cases in the county in 2010 up to 20 cases in 2015). The current chance of county residents being diagnosed with measles before the age of 21 is 1 in 200,000. Jay is interested in understanding why this increase occurred over such a short period of time.

1. Explain how you can look at this scenario from both an individual perspective and a population perspective.
2. What level of prevention is indicated in the case study? How could the other levels of prevention be represented within this scenario?
3. What is the incidence and prevalence of measles in this case study? Would this situation be considered endemic, epidemic, or pandemic? Explain.
4. What are some of the possible explanations for the major increase in measles cases?
5. What could be some of the ways to track immunizations within the county system?
6. Explain how evidence-based practice would have a role in Jay's work.

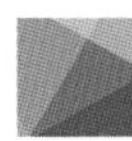

PRACTICE EXAM QUESTIONS

1. You are expecting your first child and are told that the child has a 1 in 800 chance of being born with a congenital anomaly. This statistic refers to the:
   a. Incidence
   b. Prevalence
   c. Epidemic
   d. Diagnosis

2. You decide that it has been too long since your last physical examination, so you schedule an appointment for a routine health screening. You have a blood cholesterol level checked and it is within the expected range. This activity represents which level of prevention?
   a. Primary prevention
   b. Secondary prevention
   c. Tertiary prevention
   d. None of these

3. At your health screening, you describe the following: achiness, lethargy, and vague abdominal discomfort. These are categorized as:
   a. Local manifestations
   b. Systemic manifestations
   c. Signs
   d. Symptoms

4. The study of functional alterations in human health because of an injury, disease, or syndrome describes which of the following?
   a. Pathology
   b. Pathophysiology
   c. Physiology
   d. Morphology

5. A patient wants to know what has caused his illness. This information is termed the:
   a. Etiology
   b. Pathogenesis
   c. Epidemiology
   d. Nosocomia

6. Joe has many risk factors for the development of lung cancer. Which of these is NOT modifiable?
   a. Smoking
   b. Family history of lung cancer
   c. Working in an asbestos-filled area
   d. Poor nutritional intake

7. Which of the following terms indicates the dynamic steady state that the body strives to achieve every day?
   a. Homeostasis
   b. Mortality
   c. Morbidity
   d. Health

8. Which of the following contributes to evidence-based practice and high-quality patient care?
   a. Primary research
   b. Clinical expertise
   c. Meta-analysis studies
   d. All of these contribute

9. Cancer is on the rise across the globe. Which term describes this phenomenon?
   a. Epidemic
   b. Endemic
   c. Pandemic
   d. Morbidity

10. Your grandmother is diagnosed with congestive heart failure and is told that she has 6 months to live. This prediction is referred to as her:
    a. Prognosis
    b. Diagnosis
    c. Morbidity rate
    d. Prevalence

DISCUSSION AND APPLICATION

1. What did I know about pathophysiology prior to today?
2. How does the study of pathophysiology build on what I have learned in previous courses?
3. How can I use what I have learned?

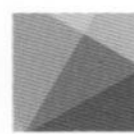

RESOURCES

World Health Organization Health Statistics:
http://www.who.int

Healthy People 2020 outlines the health goals for the United States:
http://www.healthypeople.gov

United States National Health Statistics:
http://www.cdc.gov/nchs/

Canadian Health Statistics:
http://www.statcan.gc.ca

References

1. National Down Syndrome Society. About Down syndrome: Down syndrome fact sheet. http://www.ndss.org. Accessed September 10, 2015.
2. World Health Organization. World health statistics 2015. http://www.who.int/mediacentre/factsheets/fs310/en/. Accessed September 10, 2015.
3. Simmons D. Epigenetic influence and disease. *Nat Educ.* 2008;1(1):6.

Find additional resources for this chapter at http:thePoint.lww.com thePoint®

Altered Cells and Tissues

Chapter

2

LEARNING OUTCOMES

1. Define and use the key terms listed in this chapter.
2. Discuss the changes in cells and tissues after injury.
3. Compare and contrast cellular structural adaptations to injury.
4. Identify maladaptive cellular responses to injury.
5. Recognize health conditions that can precipitate maladaptive cellular responses.
6. Describe diagnostic tests and potential treatment strategies relevant to cellular and tissue alterations.
7. Apply cellular adaptations and maladaptations to select clinical models.

INTRODUCTION

When considering health and disease, what comes to mind first? The answer may be organs and organ systems. **Organs**, fully differentiated body parts with specialized functions, are more familiar and are used more often in discussion about health and disease. Although most people can describe a heart, brain, or liver, it is harder to describe the tissues and cells that determine organ structure and function. **Tissues** are groups of similar cell types that combine to form a specific function. Like organs, the four major tissue types in the body (epithelium [skin], connective tissue [including blood, bone, and cartilage], muscle, and nerve) are familiar. **Cells**, the basic units that make up tissues, are the sites where changes in structure and function lead to symptoms and diseases in individuals. This chapter discusses the responses of cellular structure and function caused by stress, injury, or damage. Many of the concepts introduced here are expanded in subsequent chapters. Developing an understanding of these responses will help the student to translate these adaptations to the signs and symptoms of disease states that result from cellular injury.

Module 1 Review of Cellular Structure and Function

The cell is the smallest independent unit of the living individual. The structural components of the cell and the function of its components contribute to the integrity of the cell and the individual. Consequently, cell damage or injury can affect the functioning of organs, body systems, and overall health.

Cellular Components

The component parts of the cell in a human (eukaryote) provide structure and determine functional capacity. Physiologic functioning at the cellular level is critical to proper functioning of tissues and organs and to the health of the individual.

CELLULAR MEMBRANE

Each cell is surrounded by a **plasma membrane**, which protects the cell by creating a barrier that separates the intracellular components from the extracellular environment surrounding it. The plasma membrane represents an organized structure composed of lipids, carbohydrates, and proteins arranged in a **bilayer** (two layers). The lipid bilayers are mainly made up of **phospholipids** (phosphate [PO_4^-] bound to lipid). The phosphate connected to the lipid structure is known as the "head." The lipid structure is known as the "tail" because of its shape. The heads are polar or **hydrophilic** (having affinity to water). The lipid tails, composed of fatty acid chains, are nonpolar or **hydrophobic** (lacking an affinity to water). Two of these lipid layers align so that the nonpolar tail portions are intertwined and the polar heads line both the outer and inner surface of the cell. **Glycolipids** (carbohydrate bound to lipid) also make up the lipid bilayer, but are present in smaller numbers than phospholipids. The barrier created by the hydrophobic lipid bilayer prevents the unintentional passage of water-based substances across the hydrophilic cell surface. The cell membrane allows for transfer of ions and molecules into and out of the cell for homeostasis, containment of the essential organelles and structures inside the cell, and communication of cellular signals between the cell and the external environment.

Proteins are often suspended in the plasma membrane, acting as receptors that bind substances, including hormones. Proteins that pass through the entire membrane are known as **transmembrane proteins**, allowing communication and transport between the extracellular and intracellular environments. **Integral proteins** are a specific type of transmembrane protein that, because of the tight binding to lipid tails, becomes part of the membrane itself. Integral proteins often form channels that allow for the transport of ions (atom with an electrical charge) across the plasma membrane. Peripheral proteins do not pass through the entire membrane, projecting into either the intracellular or the extracellular environment. Because peripheral proteins do not pass through the entire membrane, they are not involved in transport functions. Figure 2.1 shows the structure of the lipid bilayer and proteins of the plasma membrane.

CYTOPLASM AND ORGANELLES

The cytoplasm contains the organelle structures essential for cellular survival. **Cytoplasm**, a colloidal substance surrounding the cell nucleus, is composed of water, proteins, fats, electrolytes, glycogen, and

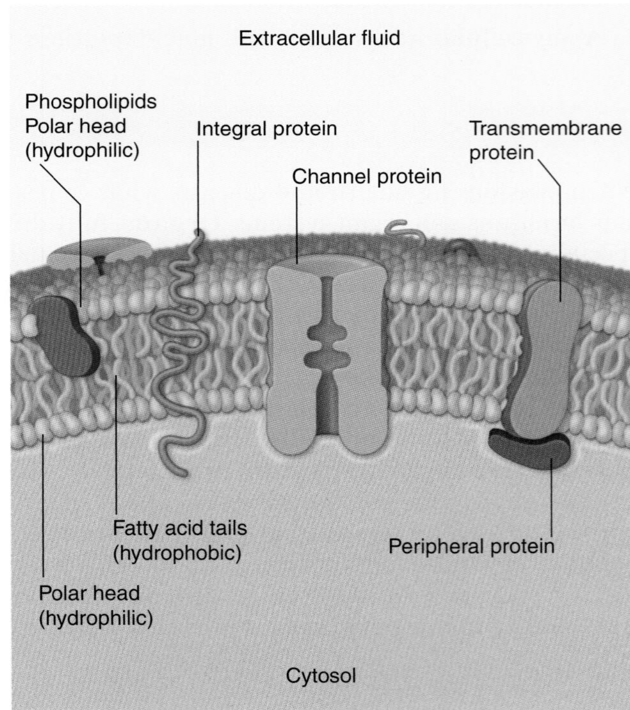

Figure 2.1. Structure of the plasma membrane. The structure of the plasma membrane shows the arrangement of polar heads in contact with both the extracellular fluid and cytosol, and the nonpolar tails forming the center of the lipid bilayer. The embedded membrane proteins, including channel, transmembrane, peripheral and integral proteins, are shown related to their relationship with the plasma membrane.

pigments. **Organelles** are structures within a cell that perform a distinct function; these structures include the following:

- **Endoplasmic reticulum**
  - A complex network of tubules, producing proteins and fats
  - Important in the regulation of ions within the cell
  - Types
    - Rough
      - Synthesis of proteins via bound ribosomes
      - Production of lysosomal enzymes (acid hydrolases)
    - Smooth
      - Synthesis of lipids, lipoproteins, and steroid hormones
      - Regulation of intracellular calcium
- **Golgi apparatus**
  - Membranous structure
  - Prepares substances produced by the endoplasmic reticulum for secretion out of the cell
- **Lysosome**
  - Small sacs surrounded by membrane
  - Digests cellular debris with hydrolytic enzymes
  - Important in the metabolism of particular substances
- **Peroxisomes**
  - Membrane-enclosed sacs smaller than lysozymes
  - Contain enzymes called oxidases that neutralize **oxygen free radicals** (atoms carrying an unpaired electron and no charge)
  - Promote survival of the cell by neutralizing harmful substances potentially damaging to the cell
- **Proteasomes**
  - Large organelles that recognize abnormally folded or formed proteins
  - Involved in **proteolysis** (breakdown of protein)
- **Mitochondria**
  - Site of aerobic (oxygen dependent) cellular respiration
  - Principal producer of cellular energy source, **adenosine triphosphate (ATP)**
  - Contain the cytochrome enzymes of terminal electron transport necessary for the production of ATP

Enclosed by a structure called a nuclear envelope, the **nucleus** of the cell contains **deoxyribonucleic acid (DNA)**, heredity material carrying the cell's genetic instructions that is copied in cellular reproduction (Chapter 6). Each cell contains 23 pairs of **chromosomes**, coiled structures of tightly packed **chromatin** (DNA, histone and nonhistone proteins), forming an individual's genetic code. The **genes**, individual units of inheritance, are pieces of DNA arranged along the chromosome. Genes determine the code for production of specific proteins that determine characteristics or functions. The membrane surrounding the nucleus contains "pores," providing access for protein products to move from the nucleus to the cytoplasm of the cells.

CYTOSKELETON

The **cytoskeleton** comprises tubule and filament structures that contribute to cell shape, movement, and intracellular transport. The main cytoskeleton components include:

- Microtubules
  - Thin protein structures composed of tubulin
- Microfilaments
  - Thin
    - Comprise the protein actin
  - Intermediate
    - Comprise filaments with diameter sized between thin and thick filaments
  - Thick
    - Comprise the protein myosin

Cellular Function

Functions common to many cell types include:

- Transportation
- Ingestion
- Secretion
- Respiration
- Communication
- Reproduction

Specialized cellular function is determined by cell type. Examples of specialized functions of cells are movement in muscle cells and conduction in nerve cells.

CELLULAR MECHANISMS OF TRANSPORTATION

The semipermeable character of the cell membrane allows for the transport of some substances but acts as a barrier to others. For cells to obtain the nutrients and other substances needed for survival, they must develop functional mechanisms for the passage of substances through the cell membrane. The movement of substances is often classified according to the amount of energy required in the act of transport.

Passive Transport

Substances may enter the cell passively, meaning that no energy is required by this process. **Diffusion**, or movement of particles from an area of higher concentration to lower concentration (**concentration gradient**), is an example of passive transport. Electrical charge in particles can also promote movement across the cell membrane. Particles become uniformly distributed, achieving a state of equilibrium. Small particles and lipid-soluble gases, including carbon dioxide and oxygen, are common examples of substances involved in this type of transport. The ability and rate of particles to diffuse through the membrane are affected by the particle size and by the size of the **membrane pore**, the membrane passage between the extracellular and intracellular environment.

Membranes may be impermeable to particles, but most allow movement of water (Chapter 8). **Osmosis** is the process by which water passively moves across the semipermeable cell membrane. A concentration gradient promotes movement of water from areas of high concentration to low concentration. The pressure generated by this process is known as **osmotic pressure**.

The movement of some substances across the cell membrane requires **facilitated diffusion,** aided by the use of transport proteins. Although facilitated diffusion is not energy-dependent, substances are unable to independently cross the membrane because of their large size or hydrophilic characteristics that require transport proteins to promote passage. Glucose is an example of a large substance needing transport proteins to allow movement across the cell membrane. Facilitated diffusion is also important in the movement of ions through channels of integral proteins, bypassing the lipid-soluble portion of the cell membrane. Ion channels allow passage of specific substances and are often classified according to the type of triggers that prompt opening and closing. Categories of ion channels include:

- Leak channels: open without need for stimulation
- Gated channels: open and close in response to stimuli
  - Voltage-gated; stimulated by change in **membrane potential** (electrical charge inside a cell membrane in relation to the surrounding extracellular fluid)
  - Ligand-gated; stimulated by receptor–ligand binding (substance binding to the receptor)
  - Mechanically gated; stimulated by vibration, stretching, and pressure

Active Transport

Active transport requires energy when transporting particles across the cell membrane. Diffusion moves particles passively along the concentration gradient, whereas active transport moves particles against the concentration or the electrochemical gradient. A common example of the active transport mechanism is the movement of sodium out of the cell across the

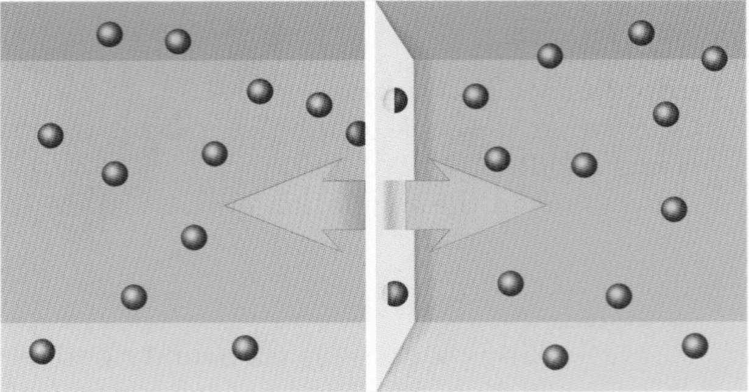

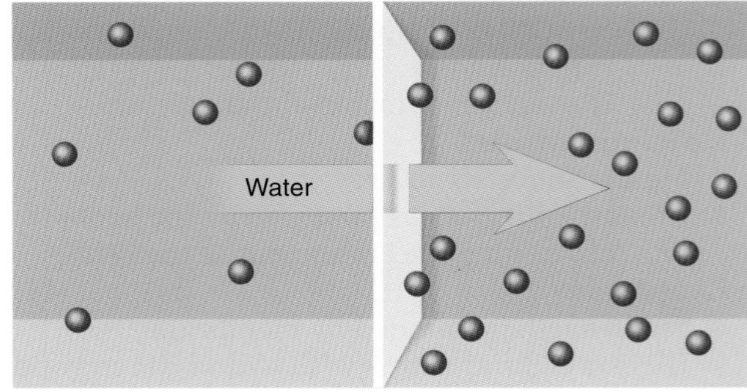

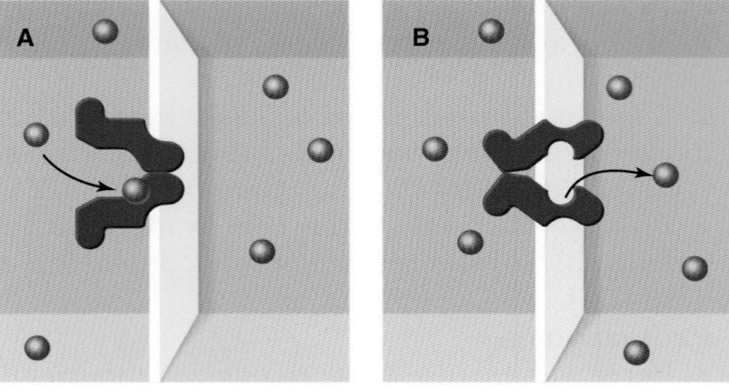

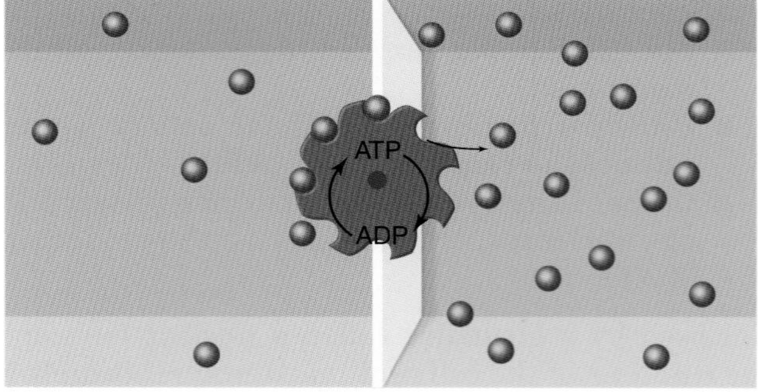

Figure 2.2. Mechanisms of cellular membrane transport. **A:** Particles move across the semipermeable membrane to achieve equal distribution during diffusion. **B:** Water flow is regulated by osmotically active particles in osmosis. **C:** Transport proteins are required for particles to move across the membrane in facilitated diffusion. **D:** ATP drives movement of particles across the membrane in active transport.

membrane with the assistance of the sodium-potassium (Na^+/K^+)-ATPase pump. Energy is required for transport because the concentration of sodium outside the cell is far greater than inside the cell. This pump also moves extracellular potassium across a large concentration gradient to the intracellular space. This process requires the direct use of energy in the form of ATP, also known as **primary active transport**. When movement of a second substance depends on energy derived from the active transport of the primary substance, the process is known as **secondary active transport**. Systems in which substances are transported in the same direction are known as **cotransport** or **symport**. Movement of substances in opposite directions is considered **countertransport** or **antiport** movement. Figure 2.2 describes mechanisms of cellular membrane transport.

INGESTION

The cellular plasma membrane serves an important function as a barrier to the external environment; however, specific processes allow the cell to **ingest** substances necessary for its own use into the cytoplasm. **Endocytosis** is the process used to transport large substances into cells. Two categories of endocytosis are pinocytosis and phagocytosis. **Pinocytosis** is the ATP-requiring process of ingesting contents of small liquid-containing vesicles. **Phagocytosis** is the process of ingesting large particles such as cells, bacteria, and damaged cellular components, resulting in the release of **oxygen free radicals**. Phagocytosis is critical in the defense of the body from foreign invaders (Chapter 4). Any alteration in the ability of the cell to ingest substances required for survival or in the demand on cells to ingest substances can result in the cellular foundation of disease.

SECRETION

The Golgi apparatus works with the endoplasmic reticulum to package products into vesicles, then directs their delivery within the cell and outside the cell, also known as **secretion** (extracellular release of products). The vesicles move from the Golgi into the cytoplasm and then out of the cell via the cell membrane, a process known as **exocytosis**. The Golgi apparatus contains enzymes that attach sugars to proteins, forming large glycoproteins. Lysosomes are formed by the Golgi apparatus and are responsible for digestive functions within the cell. Substances such as proteins, carbohydrates, damaged cellular structures, and pathogens are broken down for removal or recycling by hydrolytic enzymes, called acid hydrolases, contained within the lysosomes. Figure 2.3 illustrates the concepts of endocytosis and exocytosis.

RESPIRATION

The cell's survival depends on the availability of ATP produced by cellular respiration as a source of energy for all cellular functions. Cellular **respiration** is a series of metabolic processes that transforms fuel molecules into energy (in the form of ATP) and waste products. **Anaerobic respiration** is the process of ATP production that occurs without oxygen. The chemical reactions of oxidation and reduction between oxygen and nutrient products such as glucose

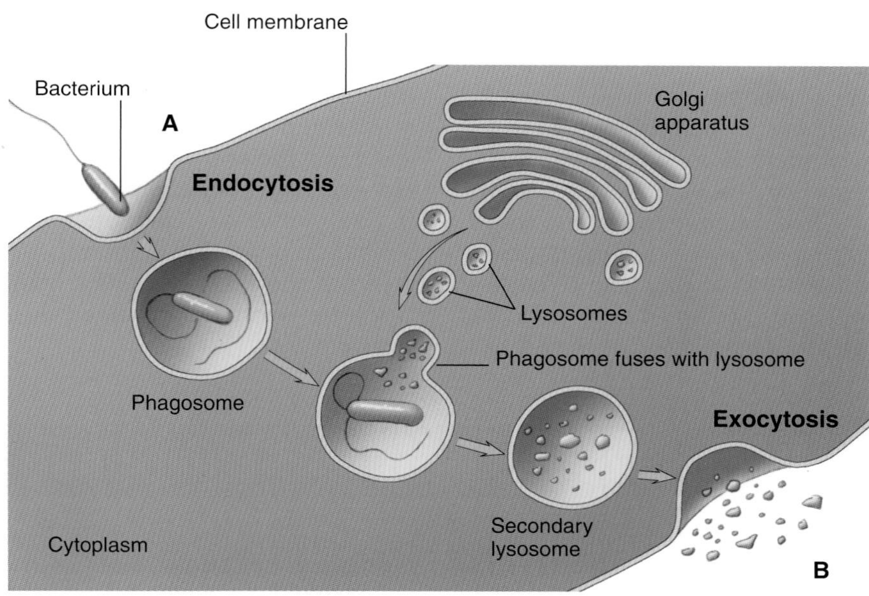

Figure 2.3. Vesicular transport. **A:** Objects enter the cell by the process of endocytosis. **B:** Vesicles bind to the plasma membrane and release their contents through a process called exocytosis. (From Premkumar K. *The Massage Connection: Anatomy and Physiology*. Baltimore, MD: Lippincott Williams & Wilkins; 2004.)

is called **aerobic respiration**. **Glycolysis**, the process of breaking down glucose in the cytosol of the cell, occurs in the absence of oxygen and is completed outside of the mitochondria. Anaerobic glycolysis reaction produces a small amount of ATP (two molecules for each molecule of glucose metabolized) and chemical products, including pyruvate. The **citric acid cycle** breaks down sugars, fats, and proteins to produce products used for energy production in the mitochondria. Together with oxygen, glycolytic and citric acid cycle byproducts enter into the metabolic pathways in the mitochondria and result in energy production through oxidative phosphorylation, a process known as aerobic respiration. These aerobic pathways produce a total of 30 to 38 molecules of ATP for each molecule of glucose metabolized. The waste products produced in aerobic respiration include carbon dioxide, water, and heat, all readily excreted.

COMMUNICATION

The proteins required for cell function are a product of the cell itself, produced by genes in response to cellular needs. These products include proteins used for cell structure and cell function, and enzymes used to stimulate chemical reactions. Impaired proteolytic enzyme activity, often a result of a genetic mutation, has been linked to the development of disease, including diabetes, cataracts, multiple sclerosis, and Duchenne muscular dystrophy.[1] **Feedback mechanisms** regulate gene activation to tightly control the production of proteins and to prevent cell damage caused by overproduction or underproduction.

Optimal function of tissues requires cell-to-cell communication. The message, or signal, transmitted from one cell to another cell influences cellular behavior and plays a role in determining function. The target cell is able to communicate through a special protein known as a **receptor**. Receptors can be present on the cell membrane (membrane bound) or within the cell (intracellular). Signaling molecules, or **ligands**, bind to receptors in a specific way, similar to a key turning a lock. When a ligand binds to a receptor, the target cell begins the process of communication known as **signal transduction**. The tightness, or strength of binding, is also referred to as **binding affinity**. The binding of an extracellular ligand to a membrane-bound receptor begins a cascade of signaling events that alters cell behavior. For a ligand to bind to an intracellular receptor, it must be able to diffuse across the plasma membrane and enter the cell.

A ligand binding to receptors that results in signal transduction with a local effect is known as **paracrine signaling**. The ligands involved in paracrine signaling (**local mediators**) exert a rapid local response. A wider range of impact occurs when signal transduction affects cell behavior within the entire organism (**endocrine signaling**). The ligands involved in endocrine signaling are called **hormones**. Hormones can influence cell behavior on a larger scale. Because of the dependence on the required processes and blood flow needed to carry the hormones through the body where they can bind with receptors, this pathway is often slower and lasts longer than paracrine signaling. Hormone influences in the body are discussed in detail in Chapter 13.

REPRODUCTION

Reproduction of cells is another function operating under genetic control. Genes control the growth of cells, timing of the division of cells, and differentiation of cells. The rate of cell growth is specific to each cell type and is regulated to meet the constantly changing needs of the individual. Cell size is determined primarily by the amount of functional DNA in the cell. Without DNA reproduction, cells can grow only to a particular size before they stop growing.

Cell division occurs at different times depending on the cell type and on the signals sent to the cell for division. **Proliferation** is the increase in cell number. **Differentiation**, or changes in physical and functional properties of cells, directs the cell to develop into specific cell types. As all cells contain identical genetic material, this process explains why one cell contributes to the development of one tissue while another can develop into a different tissue. This process occurs by the repression of certain genes in a cell and the expression of others in the same cell. Alterations in the proliferation and differentiation of cells are described in detail in Chapter 7. To see a video demonstrating the cell cycle, visit http://thePoint.lww.com, using the scratch-off code on the inside front cover.

thePoint®

Module 2 Cellular Adaptation and Response to Stress

Cells are consistently challenged with stressors that can lead to altered function. Cellular structures must adapt their function when faced with damage and injury for the cell to survive. Potentially damaging conditions faced by cells include changes in oxygenation, temperature, molecular toxins, and electrolytes. The two responses of the cell to these stressors are **adaptation** or **death**. Mechanisms

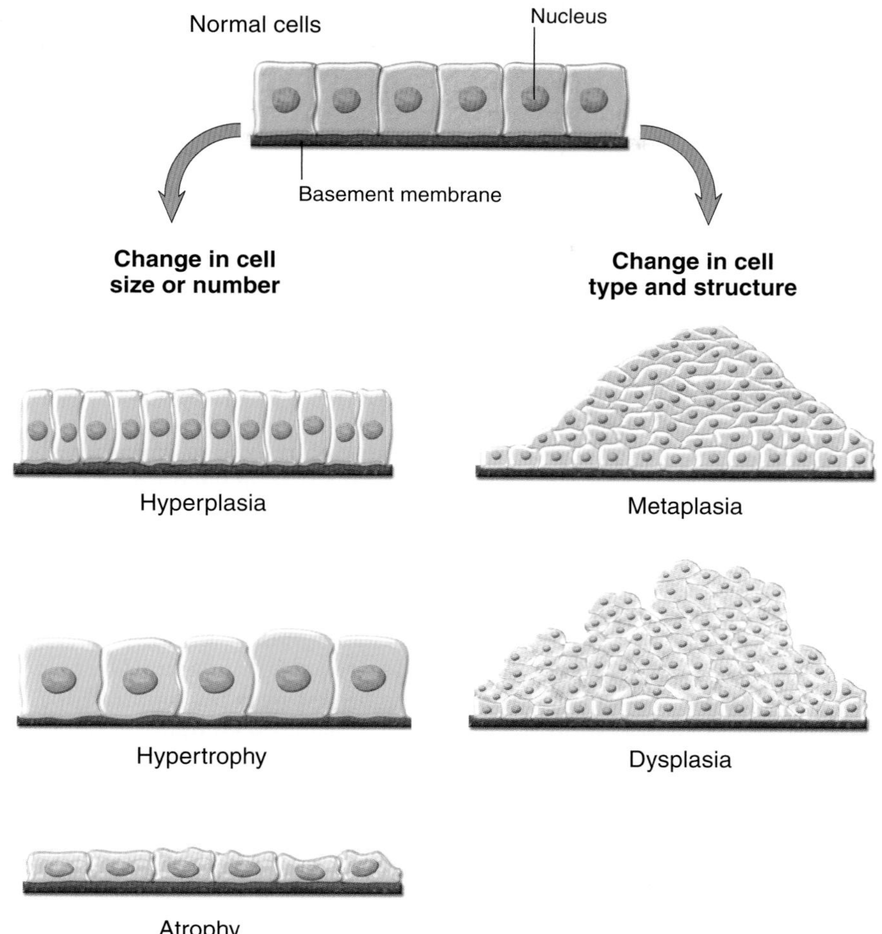

Figure 2.4. Adaptive cell changes. Normal cells adapt to stress by altering size, number, or type/structure. (Courtesy Anatomical Chart Company.)

that promote cellular adaptation result from signals that cause changes in gene function. The ways in which these cells respond form the cellular basis of disease (Fig. 2.4). Cellular responses include changes in size, number, and structure.

Stop and Consider
What would happen if cells did not have the ability to adapt to stressors? What are the implications in health and disease?

Atrophy

Atrophy is the decrease in the size of a cell and can occur for several reasons. A decrease in the functional demand on a cell prompts a decrease in cell size. This type of decrease often occurs when a limb is immobilized in a cast and active muscle movement is impaired. The lack of muscle movement reduces demand on muscle cells, leading to decreased cell size. Muscle cell atrophy causes reduction in the muscle itself due to the large numbers of cells affected. A decreased oxygen supply to the cell, or **ischemia**, can also contribute to a decrease in cell size. Ischemia can occur secondary to a blockage in the arterial blood supply, which reduces the delivery of oxygen. Although cells may have the ability to adapt to a chronically reduced oxygen supply via atrophy, a complete lack of oxygenation is more likely to result in irreversible cell death.

Many cells depend on specialized signals to maintain function. Atrophy is often the response of these cells when signals are removed. The sources of these signals are often hormones, which target specific cell types. A similar event occurs when neural signals are removed from cells dependent on them for normal functioning. Chronic nutritional deprivation and the process of aging also result in decreased cell size, which translates into decreased organ size. Atrophy also can occur as a response to the removal of hormonal signals that stimulate growth, resulting in **involution**, or decreased size, of tissues and organs. Atrophy may result in the manifestation of clinical signs and symptoms stemming from the decrease in size and function of the organ involved.

Spinal muscular atrophy is an example of an atrophic condition. Spinal muscle atrophy results from disuse caused by impaired neural innervation to muscle tissue. Signals to muscle cells are decreased because of loss of motor neuron cells of the brain or spinal cord. The decreased stimulation of muscle cells because of loss of neural signaling causes atrophy, resulting in weakness of voluntary muscles. The loss of function associated with the atrophic cell and tissue changes highlights many conditions characterized by atrophy.

Hypertrophy

Hypertrophy is an increase in cell size. Cells often respond with hypertrophy from an increase in **trophic**, or growth, signals. Signals stimulating an increase in sex hormones are responsible for the development of hypertrophied reproductive cells during puberty as well as in the breast cells during pregnancy that allow mothers to make and deliver breast milk. Increased demand can also contribute to hypertrophy. Strength-building exercise often results in an increase in muscle cell size and muscle mass.

Hypertrophy of the adenoid tissue is a common and familiar condition. **Adenoid hypertrophy** is caused by enlargement of lymphoepithelial adenoid tissue in the back of the nasal area and can result in obstruction of the nasal passage. The increased functional demand required of the lymph tissue in filtering out infectious agents in the upper respiratory tract can lead to an increase in lymphoid and epithelial cell size. The most common effects of adenoid hypertrophy are snoring, bad breath, and stuffy nose. More serious consequences of adenoid hypertrophy can affect respiratory function, with manifestations of sleep apnea, pulmonary hypertension, or heart failure.

Hyperplasia

Hyperplasia is an increase in the number of cells. Like hypertrophy, hyperplasia can also be caused by hormone signaling and an increase in workload. Because some of the same conditions cause both hyperplasia and hypertrophy, they are often seen together. For example, the uterus responds to the increase in hormone levels of estrogen during monthly menstrual cycles by increasing the number of cells in the uterus. Also, when people are exposed to high altitudes, adaptation to this stressor includes an increased production of red blood cells to maximize the hemoglobin oxygen-carrying ability. This "increased workload" to oxygenate, stresses the cell to produce this adaptation.

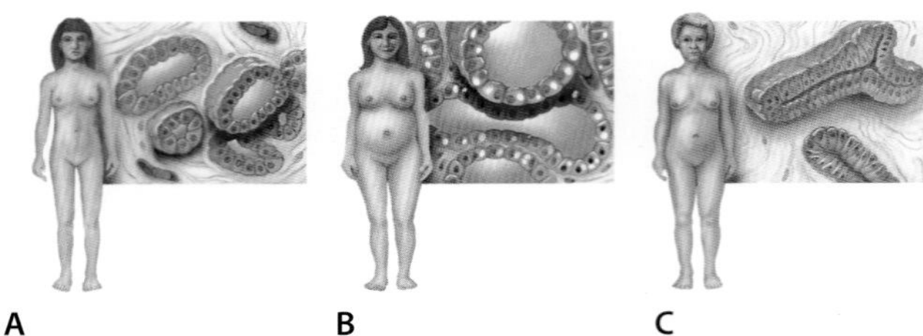

Figure 2.5. Breast tissue adaptation to trophic signals. **A:** Puberty (hyperplasia). **B:** Pregnancy (hypertrophy). **C:** Menopause (atrophy). (Courtesy Anatomical Chart Company.)

Adaptation of cells and tissues to hormonal signals is a dynamic process. One cell or tissue type can undergo a series of adaptations in response to varied signals over a lifetime. This process is clearly illustrated in the adaptations of the ductal tissue of the breast over a woman's lifetime, as in Figure 2.5. The hormonal changes of puberty induce hyperplastic changes in the breast, noted by increased size of the functional lobular and ductal tissue. Hormones secreted during pregnancy promote hypertrophic changes in breast tissue to support production and delivery of breast milk. When hormone production drops during menopause, atrophic changes associated with decreased breast size are noted. These changes result from the intensity of trophic signals induced by the hormones, which promote the genetic basis of these adaptations.

Metaplasia

Metaplasia refers to the changing of one cell type to another. This is one way that cells can adapt to a persistent stressor. In the case of a person with gastroesophageal reflux disease (GERD), the cells of the esophagus are exposed to the damaging acidic contents of the stomach. Over time, these cells often change from a squamous epithelium cell type to a glandular cell type in response to the stressor. A similar situation occurs when cells that line the bronchial tubes of the lungs are exposed to cigarette smoke over a period of time. This exposure leads to cell adaptation to this stressor by the development of squamous metaplasia, in which the columnar cells turn into squamous cells in the cell's attempt to survive the exposure to toxins (Fig. 2.6). When the stressor that caused these cell changes is removed, cells often return to their normal state. In the presence of a persistent stressor, cells may develop responses that lead to pathologic changes.

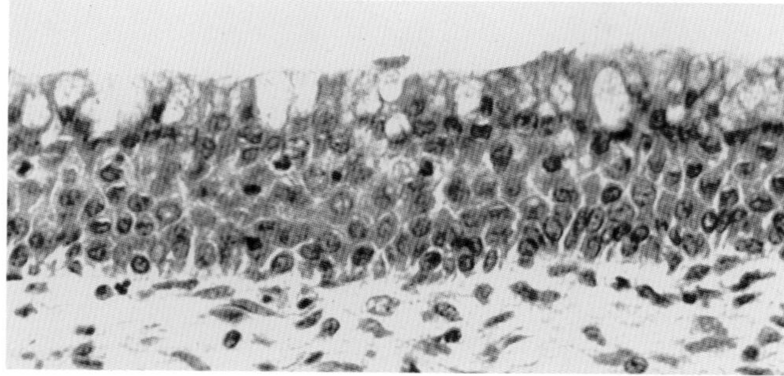

Figure 2.6. Squamous metaplasia in the transformation zone. The proliferating cells displace the glandular epithelium. The metaplastic cells mature into glycogen-rich squamous cells. (From Rubin E, Farber JL. *Pathology*. 4th ed. Philadelphia, PA: Lippincott Williams & Wilkins; 2005.)

Dysplasia

Dysplasia refers to the actual change in cell size, shape, uniformity, arrangement, and structure. As with metaplasia, dysplasia is often a cell's response to a chronic and persistent stressor and is likely to resolve when the stressor is removed. Dysplasia is caused by abnormal differentiation of dividing cells and is considered a problem in regulating cell growth. When cell reproduction occurs, the DNA may be reproduced with **mutations**, or changes in the genetic material that makes up the chromosomes. These mutations are often repeated as more cells divide and proliferate. Although these cells are not cancerous, they may appear as an early change that can progress to cancer. Figure 2.7 depicts the progression from normal cells (Figure 2.7A) to mild dysplasia (Figure 2.7B) to severe dysplasia (Figure 2.7C).

Bronchopulmonary dysplasia (BPD) is a condition in which stressors prompt cellular alterations that lead to chronic, irreversible tissue changes. Some infants require high concentrations of oxygen and mechanical ventilation at birth, often because of respiratory distress and the inability to maintain adequate levels of tissue oxygenation. BPD is associated with prolonged supplemental oxygen concentrations greater than that in room air (21%) during the early newborn period of life. The bronchial and alveolar tissues of the lungs become thickened, reducing the ability to take air into the lungs, oxygenate tissues throughout the body, and excrete waste products, including carbon dioxide. The damage is the likely result of the combination of cellular stressors and the susceptibility to damage in the developmentally immature lung tissue.

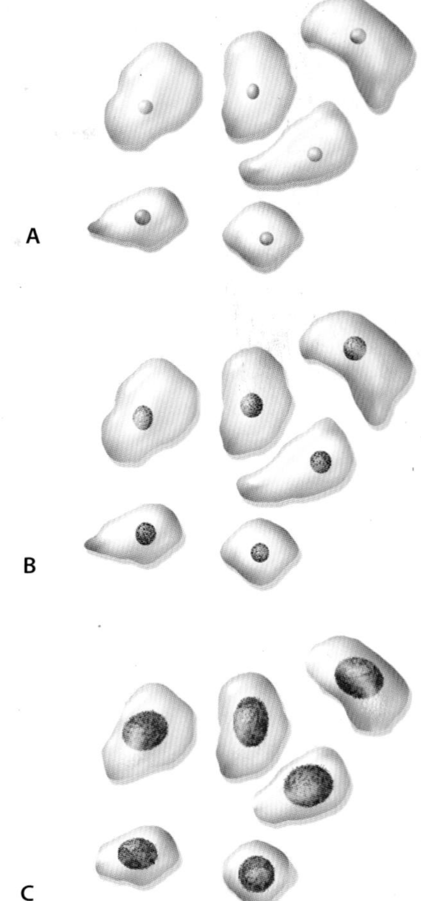

Figure 2.7. Cellular changes in dysplasia. **A:** Large squamous cells with small nuclei. **B:** Nucleus increasing in size and darkening in color. **C:** Markedly enlarged and darkened nucleus with abnormal chromatin. (Courtesy Anatomical Chart Company.)

Stop and Consider

What are the common characteristics of the different mechanisms of cellular adaptation? What are the differences?

Module 3 Cellular Injury and Death

As discussed earlier in the chapter, in the process of cellular adaptation, exposure to stressors can cause changes in both cell structure and function. Many of the adaptations that cells make allow the cell to survive. If the stressor is too great or lasts too long, the cell may lose its ability to adapt, resulting in death. Conditions such as ischemia can be overcome if the exposure is not too great and does not last too long. Other conditions, such as oxidative stress, radiation, chemicals, and pathogens (bacteria and viruses) can cause cell injury, followed by cell death if the damage is too great.

Mechanisms of Cell Death

The changes in cell and organelle structure and function prevent the cell from returning to a normal condition. Cellular damage that overwhelms the capability for recovery results in cellular death. The two major ways in which cells die are by the processes of apoptosis and necrosis.

APOPTOSIS

Apoptosis can be both a physiologic and a pathologic cell response to cellular signals. Apoptosis is often referred to as "cellular suicide." It is programmed cell death prompted by a genetic signal and is designed to replace old cells with new. Cells are programmed for death for many reasons, including damaged genetic material or mutation, old age of the cell, and an attempt to decrease the actual number of cells. Death occurs in the cell because of enzyme reactions in the cell that change the structure, and therefore function, of the organelles and other cell components.

This process is common during the development of the embryo when cells grow and develop into well-defined organs and systems. Embryonic hands begin as outgrowths in the shape of buds, progressing to webbed, flattened, paddle shapes by the fifth week of development. Cartilage and bone development is followed by bone ossification during the seventh week, along with the transformation of the webbed hand into digits through the process of apoptosis by the eighth week. Alterations in this process of apoptosis during embryologic development can lead to the manifestation known as **syndactyly**, the fusion or incomplete separation of digit soft tissue.

NECROSIS

Necrosis, another mechanism of cell death, is different from apoptosis. Cell death by necrosis is a disorderly process associated with inflammation (see Chapter 3). **Necrosis** is death of cells related to cell injury. Injury causes damage to cellular structures, including the mitochondria, depleting ATP. Without ATP to energize cellular processes, organelles and cells swell, disrupting the plasma cell membrane barrier. The loss of the cell membrane barrier allows the spilling out of the cell contents from within the cell. Enzymes are released that dissolve the cell components, which in turn trigger white blood cells to respond and digest the cellular debris through phagocytosis. The result is local inflammation and death of cells. When overgrowth of infectious agents is combined with decreased blood flow, necrosis can occur (Fig. 2.8).

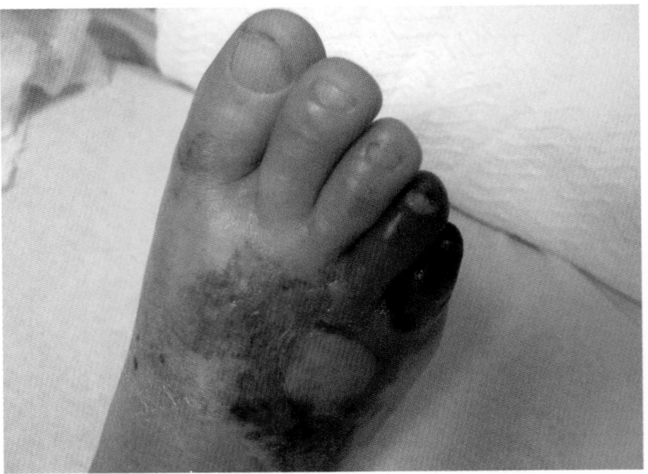

Figure 2.8. Necrosis. Diabetic foot with necrosis of the digits. (Image provided by Stedman's.)

Causes of Cell Injury and Death

Injury to cells stems from a variety of sources of stress (Fig. 2.9). Infection from bacteria, virus, protozoa, or fungi can initiate damage to cells (Chapter 5). Physical injury from mechanical, thermal, or chemical sources can cause damage to the structure of a cell and affect cell function. **Mechanical injury** can be caused by impact of a body part causing direct injury, such as falling off a skateboard or a bike. **Thermal injury** is caused by extremes of temperature, as occurs with burns and frostbite. Toxins can also cause harm to cells. These toxins can be **endogenous** (from within the body system). For example, when a person has an allergic reaction, toxins are released from within the body, which cause cell damage and associated symptoms (Chapter 4). Toxins can also be **exogenous** (from the external environment). A common exogenous toxin is alcohol, which can damage the cells of the liver with prolonged exposure. Damage to cells can also result from **deficit injury**, in which the cell is deprived of oxygenation, hydration, and nutrition. This is commonly seen in conditions of ischemia (see Chapter 16), severe malnutrition, and eating disorders such as anorexia nervosa (Chapter 17).

It may be helpful to remember the common causes of cell injury and death with the acronym TIPS:

- *T*oxins (chemical, pathogenic)
- *I*nfections
- *P*hysical injury (mechanical, chemical, thermal)
- *S*erum deficit injury (nutrition, hydration, oxygenation)

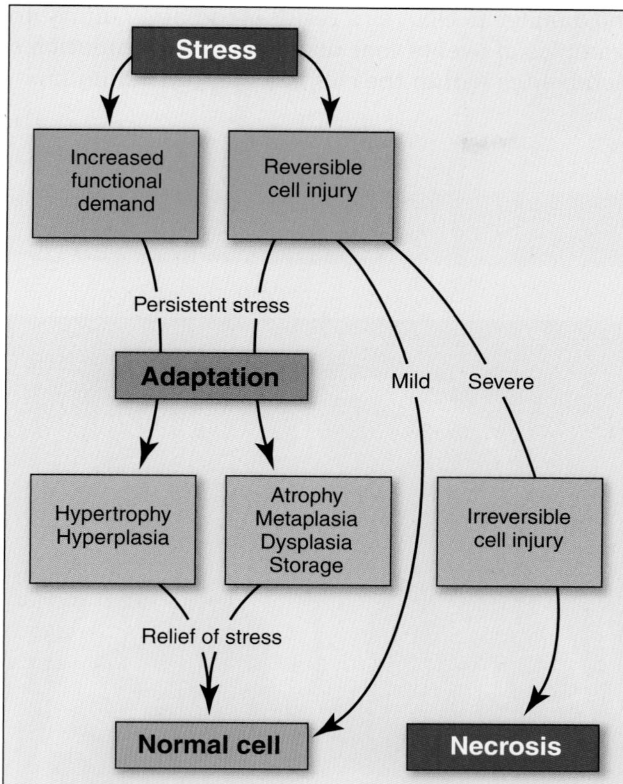

Figure 2.9. Cellular response to stress. (Modified from Rubin E, Farber JL. *Pathology*. 4th ed. Philadelphia, PA: Lippincott Williams & Wilkins; 2005.)

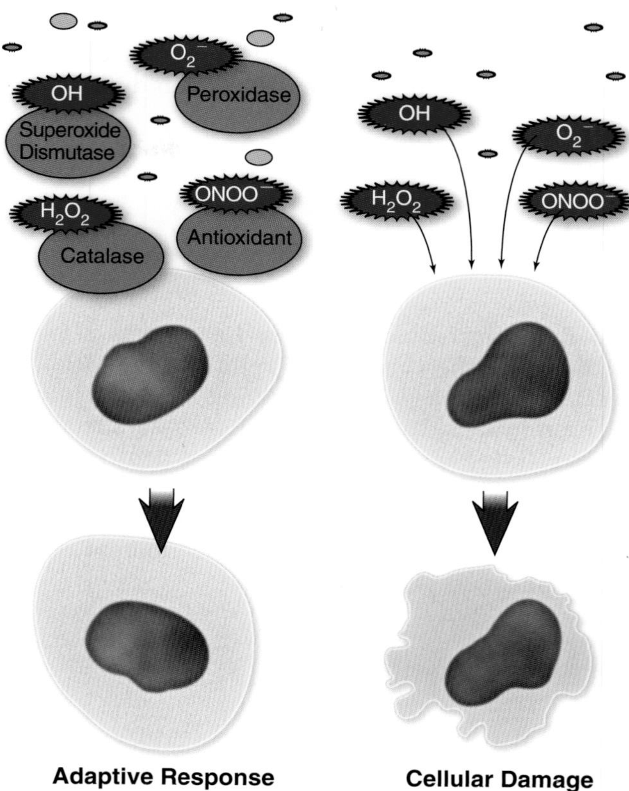

Figure 2.10. Cellular response to oxidative stress. Oxidative stress occurs as a result of increased reactive oxygen species (ROS), decreasing antioxidants or inability to neutralize or repair damage caused by ROS with ROS scavengers.

Cells can be damaged in a variety of ways that result in injury or death. Oxidative stress can be increased by many conditions, including biologic aging, infection, inflammation, ischemia, radiation, and use of chemicals and drugs. Oxidative stress involves exposure of cells to **reactive oxygen species (ROS)**, toxic oxygen molecules or radicals that are formed by the reaction between oxygen (O_2) and water (H_2O) during mitochondrial respiration. ROS species include superoxide (O_2^-), hydrogen peroxide (H_2O_2), the hydroxyl radical (OH), and peroxynitrite ($ONOO^-$). Cell damage can result from too many ROS or not enough available enzymes, including catalase, to convert these radicals to less harmful substances. Cellular damage resulting from ROS is known as **free radical injury**. ROS produces damage to cells, often by targeting DNA. Injury by ROS exposure has been implicated in many disease conditions, including heart disease, diabetes, cancer, and others. ROS scavengers, such as catalase, peroxidase, superoxide dismutase, and antioxidants, can work with detoxifying enzymes to limit cell damage (Fig. 2.10). The use of antioxidants, such as vitamin E, may reduce oxidative stress for many disease conditions.[2,3]

Stop and Consider

Hydrogen peroxide (H_2O_2) is familiar to most people as a product to be used on cuts and scrapes. The solution that can be bought at the local grocery store contains 3% of H_2O_2, with the remaining 97% of the solution made up of water. When the solution is applied to a cut or scrape, the combination of H_2O_2 combines with the enzyme catalase, which is released from the damaged cells and blood. Catalase causes a chemical reaction, converting hydrogen peroxide into water (H_2O) and oxygen (O_2). The evidence of this reaction is the foam that is produced when the hydrogen peroxide is applied to the injury, releasing the oxygen gas.

$$H_2O_2 \xrightarrow{catalase} H_2O + O_2$$

Catalase works the same way in the cells of the body to scavenge ROS, minimizing oxidative damage.

http://science.howstuffworks.com/question115.htm

Damage to cells can result in disruption of metabolic processes that can prove fatal. The imbalance of electrolytes, ischemia caused by oxygen deprivation, and damage to DNA as a result of radiation injury are examples of events that may lead to accumulation of metabolites within the cell, causing further injury.

Module 4 Clinical Models

The following clinical models have been selected to illustrate the concepts of cellular adaptation in health and disease. While reading the descriptions of these models, think about the stressors that can cause cellular adaptation, injury, and death and the responses of the cells to the stressors. Consider the concepts of cellular adaptation as they apply to the specific conditions to assist in the understanding and application of these concepts.

Cerebral Atrophy

Cerebral atrophy is a common feature of many diseases that affect the brain rather than a disease. Cerebral atrophy describes the reduction in size of the cells in the cerebrum of the brain. The progressive reduction in the size of the neurons leads to the reduction in the brain tissue itself. Neurons are the functional cells in brain tissue and are responsible for conducting neural impulses within the brain and to other areas of the body. Many neurologic diseases are associated with loss of neuronal function due to atrophy, several of which are included as clinical models in this text (Fig. 2.11).

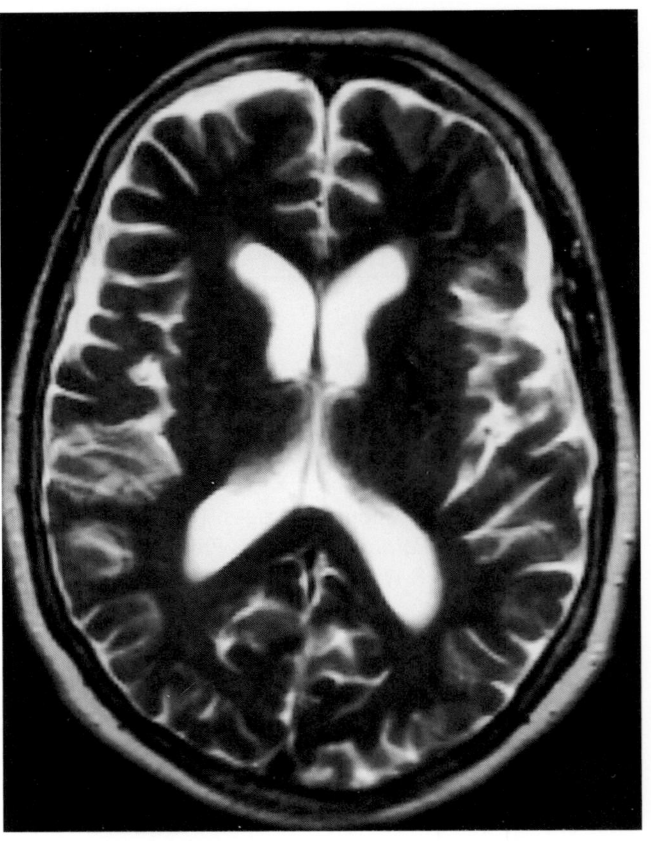

Figure 2.11. Cerebral atrophy. MRI of the brain shows enlargement of the ventricles and deepening of the sulci, evidence of cerebral atrophy.

PATHOPHYSIOLOGY

Cerebral atrophy may be either a cause or consequence of a neurologic disorder. Decreased stimulation resulting from reduction in physical and intellectual activities may lead to atrophy of brain structures.[4,5] Individuals with low levels of B vitamins may experience increased brain atrophy, an example of deficit injury.[6] Cerebral atrophy can result from mechanical injury (traumatic brain injury) or injury due to toxins (encephalitis), leading to loss of neurologic cells, tissue, and associated functions.

Destruction of neurons and the loss of neurotransmitter production in one part of the brain may lead to atrophy of neurons in another region because of lack of stimulation. Conditions leading to reduced perfusion to the brain increase the risk of injury due to a deficit in oxygen and nutrient delivery. Neurotoxic injury resulting from ischemia, hyperthermia, inflammation, or trauma may exceed the ability of the neuron to recover, leading to neuronal death. Subcortical ischemic vascular disease reduces perfusion to the brain, with affected individuals manifesting decreased psychomotor speed, executive control, and global cognitive function.[7] Brain atrophy in multiple sclerosis is characterized by a loss of gray and white brain matter, leading to the manifestations involving motor defects and cognitive impairment.[8] As neurons decrease in size, their physical relationship with other neurons changes. The close connections between neurons are required for effective communication; as neurons atrophy, communication is further impaired as the distance between neurons increases. Because neurons are not able to replicate, death leads to permanent loss of cells and function.

CLINICAL MANIFESTATIONS

The manifestations of cerebral atrophy can be focal (localized to a particular region) or global (affecting the entire brain). Neurons in each area of the brain provide specific functions (see Chapter 10). As neurons atrophy, the function associated with those neurons becomes altered. Neuronal atrophy in the frontal and temporal lobes of the brain leads to cognitive impairment. Alzheimer's disease, a condition affecting memory and comprehension, is associated with atrophy of the hippocampus and cerebral cortex.[9] Movement disorders result from neuronal atrophy in the basal ganglia, responsible for production of the neurotransmitter dopamine required for motor function.

The pattern of brain atrophy contributes to a wide range of manifestations related to degree of atrophy. Cerebral palsy is a condition that occurs because of neuronal insult during a critical time in brain development, during the prenatal, perinatal, or postnatal periods. Manifestations vary from mild to severe and may involve motor skills, coordination, and balance and seizure activity, reflecting the involved areas of the brain.

DIAGNOSIS

Brain atrophy is a pathologic finding related to a significant range of neurologic diseases. The first step in diagnosis is designed to determine underlying pathology in order to identify the specific condition and initiate appropriate treatment. Early diagnosis is critical in neurologic disease associated with brain atrophy because of the limited ability to restore function that has been lost by the time the diagnosis is made.

A careful history that includes signs and symptoms, including onset, duration, and severity, is the first step in the diagnostic process. The early manifestations of brain atrophy may be difficult to identify at first because of the slow and subtle development of signs. The signs of brain atrophy may be first observed by others rather than the affected individual who may be unable or unwilling to disclose symptoms. Physical exam is needed to define specific neurologic defects, which in turn is needed for actual diagnosis. Specific measures of brain atrophy include brain imaging to measure tissue loss. Functional imaging may include positron emission tomography (PET) and single photon emission computed tomography (SPECT) which, combined with CT and magnetic resonance imaging (MRI) techniques, have become increasingly common and are used in determination of location and severity of atrophy.[8] Together, the strategies of history, physical exam, and imaging techniques aid in the diagnosis, prognosis, and treatment of conditions associated with brain atrophy.

TREATMENT

Treatment of individuals with brain atrophy is targeted toward prevention or slowing of continued pathology. When neurons are atrophied and damaged, recovery is severely limited because of the inability of neurons to replicate. Supportive care assists individuals in completing activities of daily living. Physical, speech, or occupational therapy is critical to promotion of optimal function. Pharmacologic therapies may be instituted to address impairment in neurologic signal transmission. Treatment is individualized based on the specific diagnosis and the type of brain atrophy involved, with a goal of maximizing function and minimizing continued pathology.

Stop and Consider
Why does age and developmental maturity affect the degree of brain atrophy that can be expected?

Cardiac Hypertrophy

Myocardial cells, or cardiac myocytes, differ from other cells because they do not continually divide and replace themselves. After the first 4 weeks of life, growth of the heart is achieved by hypertrophy of existing cardiac myocytes. Injury to these cells often results in permanent damage and chronic cardiac disease. **Cardiac hypertrophy**, or hypertrophic cardiomyopathy, is a disease of cardiac muscle that results from excessive workload and functional demand. The most common cause of sudden unexpected cardiac death in young individuals, primary hypertrophic cardiomyopathy, is most common among individuals less than 30 years of age.[11] The most common cause of secondary cardiac hypertrophy is increased blood pressure, imposing additional workload on the ventricle.

PATHOPHYSIOLOGY

Primary hypertrophic cardiomyopathy, without a specifically known cause, is often a result of an inherited non–sex-linked genetic autosomal-dominant trait. Secondary hypertrophy is often caused by an underlying condition that causes an increase in ventricle workload. Hypertrophy can occur in the right ventricle because of increased pressure in the pulmonary circulation or in the left ventricle due to increased pressure in the systemic circulation, as in hypertension. In systemic hypertension, the left ventricle of the heart may be forced to pump harder because of an increase in outflow pressure from a stiff aortic valve or increased pressure in the aorta. The left ventricle is the main pump of the heart, moving blood received from the lungs into the aorta, providing oxygen rich arterial circulation to the body. Impaired pumping in the left ventricle leads to decreased arterial output from the heart and congestion or backflow of blood into the left atrium and the pulmonary circulation. Perfusion to the heart muscle itself is also affected, reducing delivery of oxygen to the myocytes and other cardiac cells. In left ventricular hypertrophy, the wall of the left ventricle, responsible for the pumping of blood out of the aorta into the systemic circulation, becomes thickened and stiff as a result of the increase in myocardial cell size. The muscle becomes less effective at contracting despite the increased size of the myocardial cells. The lack of **compliance**, or stiffness, of the ventricle may prevent adequate filling and therefore may lower cardiac output. This rigidity of the ventricle combined with smaller chamber size eventually leads to "pump failure" and cardiac decompensation. This condition exemplifies the way in which increased workload produces a biochemical signal that causes a genetic response resulting in hypertrophy. Figure 2.12 illustrates hypertrophy of the left ventricle.

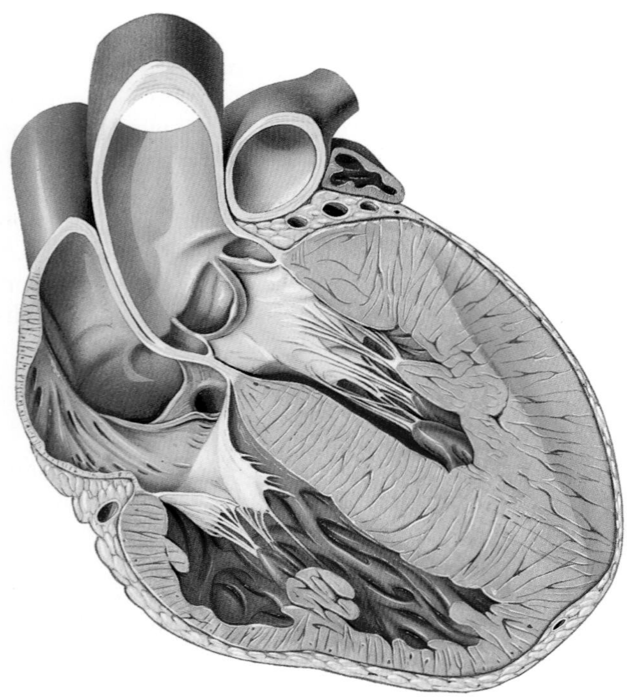

Figure 2.12. Hypertrophy of the left ventricle caused by hypertension. (Courtesy Anatomical Chart Company.)

CLINICAL MANIFESTATIONS

The evidence of cardiac hypertrophy is variable in its expression. Some individuals do not develop symptoms, and others develop manifestations that severely limit function. Massive ventricular hypertrophy leads to the clinical manifestations of this condition. Symptoms of pump failure are based on its severity and can include shortness of breath, chest pain, and **syncope** (fainting). Syncope is of particular concern because its manifestation is a marker for sudden death. Cardiac hypertrophy can also lead to irregular heart rate and rhythm. As the cardiac myocytes enlarge, the physical relationship of cardiac conducting cells becomes altered, disrupting electrical signaling in the heart tissue.

DIAGNOSIS

Preclinical diagnosis in primary cardiac hypertrophy can be achieved by genetic testing when a family history of the condition exists. For those identified with the associated genetic mutation, the earliest identification of manifestations of disease is paramount. In those with secondary cardiac hypertrophy, treatment of the underlying cause is critical to management of the progression of pathology. Secondary cardiac hypertrophy is often the result of high blood pressure or disease of the heart valves. Routine screening to determine blood pressure, exercise tolerance, and the presence of ventricular arrhythmia can be done periodically to identify impaired cardiovascular function. Screening techniques can include:

- Electrocardiogram (EKG): evaluates electrical activity of the heart
  - 12-lead EKG: identifies electrical defects while at rest
  - Ambulatory Holter EKG: identifies arrhythmias during activities of daily living
- Two-dimensional echocardiogram: ultrasound measurement of ventricle dimensions, heart valves, and blood vessels (aorta, pulmonary artery)
- Exercise stress testing: determine cardiovascular response to exercise

On physical examination, a heart murmur during cardiac contraction is often heard. Resting left ventricular outflow obstruction requires increased ventricular work to move blood out and is associated with high blood pressure, diagnosed when systolic pressure gradient across the aortic heart valve reaches 30 mm Hg; it is considered moderate to severe when systolic pressure gradient reaches 50 mm Hg or exceeds 75 mm Hg, respectively. Obstruction of left ventricular outflow is often manifested by arrhythmia of the atria, bradyarrhythmia (abnormally slow heart rate), systolic ejection murmur, or abnormal peripheral vascular response.

TREATMENT

Treatment strategies target symptom relief and prevention of sudden cardiac death. Primary cardiac hypertrophy should be treated at the earliest manifestation of disease. The secondary form of cardiac hypertrophy can be improved if the condition and the factors causing it are identified and treated before the cells undergo permanent damage. Treatment is geared toward relaxation of the ventricle and relief of the outflow obstruction that is increasing the ventricular workload. An example of this is use of antihypertensive medications to lower the resistance against which the left ventricle must pump when the hypertrophy is caused by underlying hypertension.

Treatment includes pharmacologic management with drugs designed to relieve the resistance against which the left ventricle must pump. Treatment may also lead to regression of the left ventricular hypertrophy. Angiotensin II receptor blockers (ARBs) are the drugs of choice, followed by calcium channel blockers and angiotensin converting enzyme (ACE) inhibitors, for effective treatment of left ventricular muscle mass.[12] Surgery to reduce left ventricular muscle mass or to repair heart valves may be needed, but complications from this treatment are significant. An alternative to surgery, alcohol ablation of the septum, causes necrosis of the interventricular septum by the injection of alcohol into a small arterial branch leading to the muscle source.[13] Activity restrictions may be required to minimize the risk of sudden cardiac death, especially for young athletes involved in strenuous activities.

Stop and Consider
What is the benefit of causing necrosis of the interventricular septum in the treatment of cardiac hypertrophy?

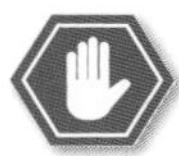

Stop and Consider
The effect of cardiac hypertrophy involving the left ventricle was described in this clinical model. What would happen if hypertrophy involved the right ventricle?

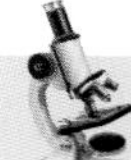

FROM THE LAB

At the cellular level, cardiac hypertrophy is associated with disorganization of myocardial cell pattern and arrangement, leading to impaired cardiac muscle contraction. Several genetic mutations have been identified in familial hypertrophic cardiomyopathy that result in alterations in proteins necessary for cardiac muscle contraction. Testing for familial hypertrophic cardiomyopathy is done by analyzing DNA from a blood sample to identify mutations in genes that are known to be associated with the condition. Most commonly involved genes produce myosin (MYH7, MYBPC) and troponin (TNNT2, TNNI3), critical elements for contraction of cardiac muscle. The abnormal proteins cannot function appropriately and contribute to the hypertrophic changes. Cells seen under a microscope are disordered, lacking the normal parallel alignment necessary to produce normal electrical conduction and contraction.

Acromegaly

Acromegaly is a condition of hyperplasia prompted by hormone stimulation of excessive growth. The condition is derived from the Greek words for extremities (acro) and enlargement (megaly). The term acromegaly provides an accurate description of the most common clinical manifestations—abnormal growth of the hands and feet.

PATHOPHYSIOLOGY

A form of hyperpituitarism, secretion of excessive growth hormone from the pituitary gland and secondary increase in **insulin-like growth factor 1 (IGF-1)** results in exaggerated skeletal and organ growth occurring after **epiphyseal**, or long bone ossification site, closure. The hypothalamus secretes two hormones that regulate growth hormone secretion by the pituitary. Hypothalamic secretion of somatostatin has an inhibitory effect on the pituitary, decreasing secretion of pituitary growth hormone. The stimulation of pituitary growth hormone secretion is induced by hypothalamic production of growth hormone releasing hormone (GHRH). Growth hormone binds to its receptor and begins signaling events in the cell, which induces a genetic response involving cell-cycle control. This event stimulates **proliferation**, or rapid reproduction of cells, which leads to hyperplasia. The secretion of growth hormone stimulates the production of IGF-1 in the liver. The actions of IGF-1 promote growth in bones, cartilage, soft tissues, and organs. Normally, this increase in IGF-1 along with other regulatory hormones signals the pituitary to reduce the production of growth hormone via the influence of somatostatin (Fig. 2.13). When this negative feedback loop fails, growth hormone secretion continues in an unregulated fashion. In more than 90% of these individuals, the oversecretion of growth hormone can be attributed to the presence of a benign pituitary tumor called an adenoma.

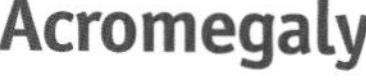

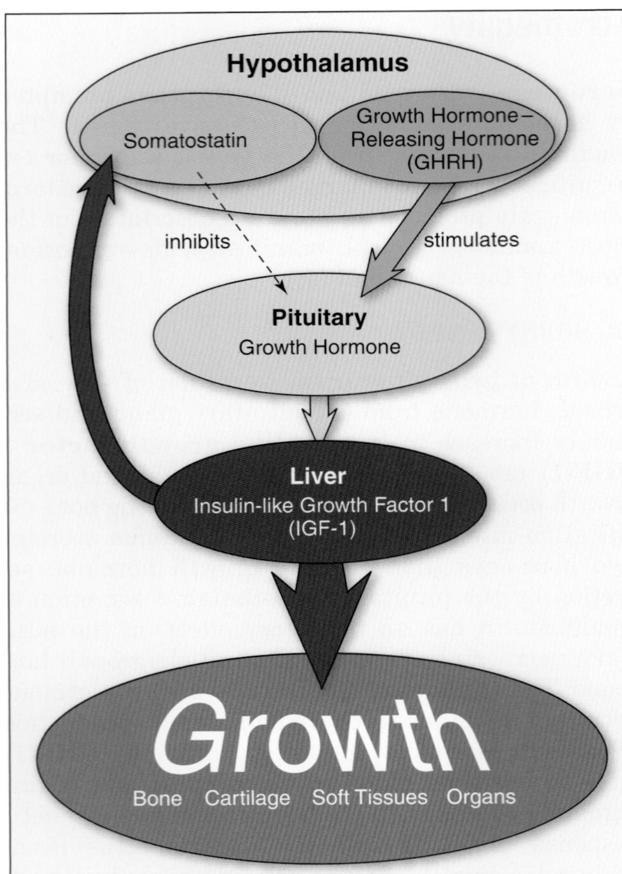

Figure 2.13. Feedback mechanism for growth stimulation. Regulation of growth hormone by growth hormone-releasing hormone (GHRH) promotes growth through the action of insulin-like growth factor 1 (IGF-1). Increases in IGF-1 trigger an increase in somatostatin to inhibit growth. Dysregulation can result in gigantism or acromegaly.

Acromegaly is often confused with a similar condition known as **gigantism,** also a condition of hyperplasia characterized by excessive growth. The difference between this condition and acromegaly is the timing of growth hormone excess. In gigantism, growth hormone excess occurs prior to the closure of the epiphyseal growth plates of the long bones. For this reason, gigantism affects infants and children, increasing their height up to three times of the expected height for their age.

CLINICAL MANIFESTATIONS

Symptoms of acromegaly are related to excessive growth. Manifestations of acromegaly can include:

- Soft tissue swelling (difficulty getting rings on and off)
- Enlarged hands and feet
- Altered facial features
    - Prominence of jaw, brow, and nasal bone
    - Enlargement of tongue and lips
    - Increased spacing between teeth
- Pain and numbness in hands
- Deepening voice
- Snoring
- Skin changes
    - Coarse hair growth
    - Oily appearance
    - Sweating
    - Body odor
    - Development of skin tags
- Altered reproductive functioning
    - Menstrual cycle alterations (women)
    - Impotence (men)
    - Breast discharge

Objective symptoms of skeletal growth include increased size of hands and feet, facial brow, jaw, and nasal bone, as well as increased spacing of teeth. Arthritis and carpal tunnel syndrome may also result from overgrowth of bone, cartilage, and soft tissue. Hyperplasia of the cells of sinuses and vocal cords may lead to a deepened voice and upper airway obstruction. Excessive sweating and skin odor may result from glandular hyperplasia. Skin may become thick and oily and develop skin tags. Menstrual disorders in women and sexual dysfunction in men may occur. Enlargement of organs, including liver, spleen, kidneys, and heart, may also result from hyperplasia and lead to serious health consequences, including sleep apnea, type 2 diabetes, colon cancer, and cardiovascular disease. Acromegaly can induce both hyperplastic and hypertrophic changes in cardiovascular tissue. The hyperplastic cardiac changes in acromegaly eventually lead to cardiac hypertrophy and possibly heart failure if left untreated.[15] Suppression of growth hormone and IGF-1 can reverse these changes, decreasing left ventricular mass and restoring cardiac function, highlighting the cells' adaptive responses. Figure 2.14 illustrates the clinical manifestations of acromegaly in men and women.

Acromegaly resulting from pituitary adenoma causes manifestations related to physical pressure on surrounding structures as the adenoma increases in size. Pressure on brain tissues affects associated nerves, leading to the development of headaches and impaired vision. The function of the pituitary itself can be altered because of adenoma compression, resulting in altered production of other pituitary hormones and contributing to the reproductive manifestations of acromegaly.

DIAGNOSIS

The diagnosis of this condition may be delayed because of the slow and insidious onset of clinical

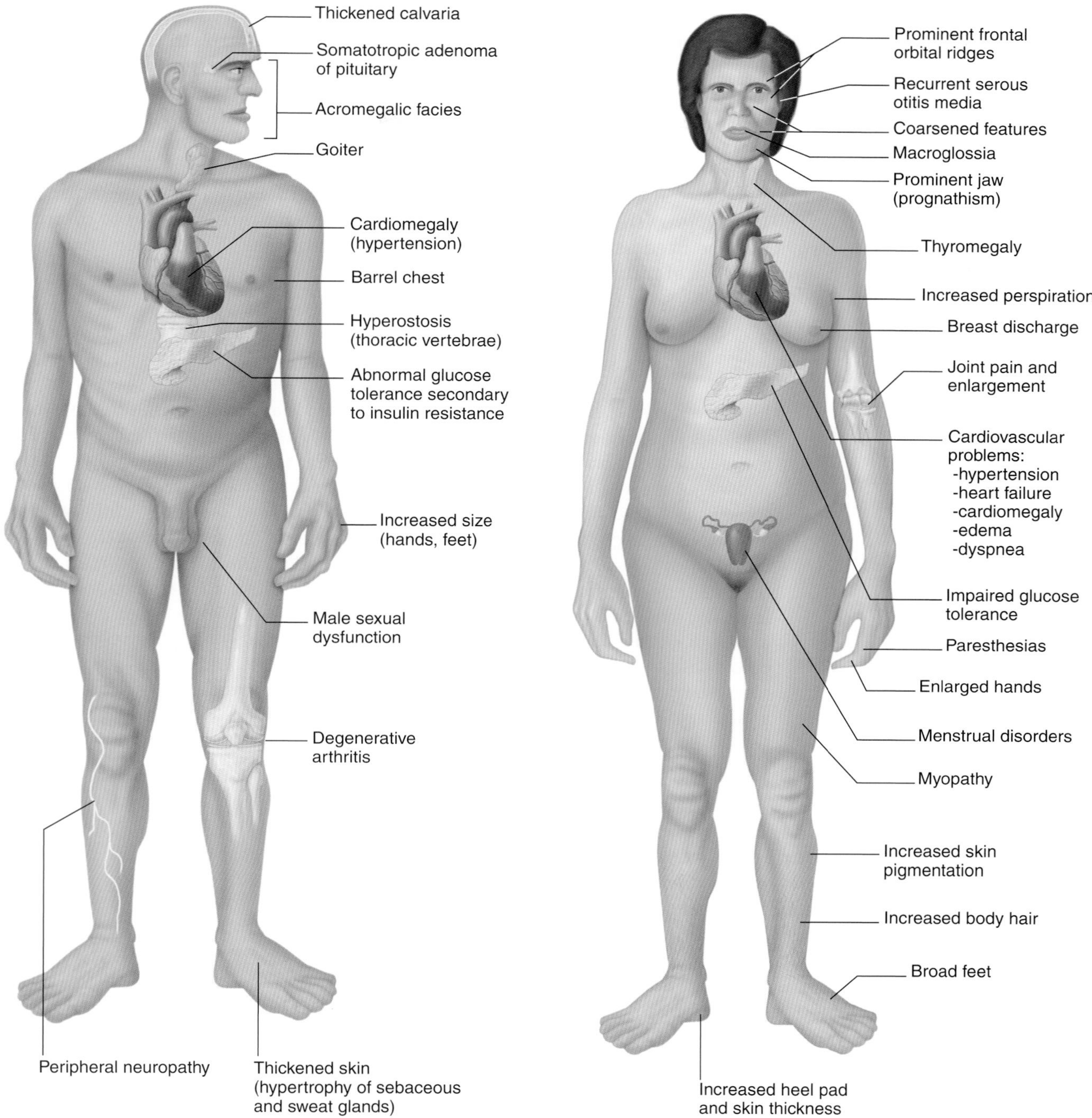

Figure 2.14. Clinical manifestations of acromegaly. Excessive growth from acromegaly causes hyperplasia and multiple clinical manifestations in both men **(A)** and women **(B)**.

manifestations. Confirmation of the diagnosis of acromegaly depends on elevated levels of IGF-1 in the blood followed by measurement of growth hormone. A specific method of growth hormone measurement and follow-up is required to obtain accurate and reliable results (see From the Lab, below). Once acromegaly is diagnosed, the next step is to determine whether the cause is related to pituitary adenoma. The presence of a pituitary adenoma can be diagnosed with imaging techniques including MRI.

TREATMENT

Treatment is designed to reduce the overproduction of IGF-1 and growth hormone to reverse or reduce the effects of acromegaly. The chronic effects can be halted if the condition is identified early in its course before permanent cell injury occurs. Treatment options include:

- Drug therapy
- Radiation therapy
- Surgical removal of adenoma

Pharmacologic management of acromegaly is directed toward reduction in pituitary growth hormone secretion or action. Drugs may be used as sole therapy or as a means to reduce the size of pituitary adenoma, improving prognosis for successful surgical removal. Drugs may also be used as adjuvant therapy after surgical removal of the adenoma, when complete cure is not attained. Three classes of drugs are the main agents for treatment of acromegaly: somatostatin analogs, dopamine agonists, and growth hormone antagonists. Somatostatin analogs work through inhibition of growth hormone secretion, similar to endogenous somatostatin. An additional benefit of somatostatin analog therapy is reduction in pituitary adenoma size. The somatostatin analog octreotide induces an inhibitory effect on the pituitary, reducing growth hormone and IGF-1 secretion, with long-acting release formulations allowing for less frequent dosing (once per month). Dopamine agonists are a second treatment choice, though less effective than the somatostatin analogs. The dopamine agonist cabergoline is the drug of choice, acting at the level of the pituitary to reduce growth hormone and subsequent IGF-1 secretion. Growth hormone antagonist pegvisomant binds to growth hormone receptors, blocking endogenous growth hormone and related growth hormone effects.

Radiation can be used as the primary treatment or in combination with pharmacologic and/or surgical management. Radiation of the pituitary is designed to promote cell death in the adenoma. Complications can include extension of the area of cell death that include healthy pituitary tissue, leading to subnormal secretion of other hormones, in addition to growth hormone.

Surgical removal of the pituitary adenoma is also an effective management strategy. Prognosis is best when the adenoma is small, termed a microadenoma (less than 1 cm). Prognosis for successful surgery includes a primary tumor of less than 10 mm in diameter and a preoperative growth hormone blood level of less than 40 ng/mL. Large tumors may require reduction in size using pharmacologic therapies prior to surgical intervention. Transsphenoidal hypophysectomy, a technique for adenoma removal through an incision in the nose, immediately reduces symptoms attributed to both excessive hormonal stimulation of growth and those related to compression of surrounding tissues. Even after successful surgery, follow-up for recurrence is necessary.

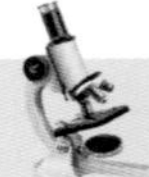

FROM THE LAB

IGF-1 levels in the blood are stable and therefore provide an accurate result to support the diagnosis of acromegaly.[17] Growth hormone levels can be measured in the blood, but are not reliable based on a single measurement because of the typical variations in secretion throughout the day. Measurement of growth hormone is most accurate when measured as a component of a glucose tolerance test as growth hormone secretion is influenced by blood glucose levels. Under physiologic conditions, growth hormone levels decrease when blood glucose levels rise via negative feedback regulation. Growth hormone levels can be tested after a glucose tolerance test to determine if there is an alteration in negative feedback, indicating pathologic secretion of growth hormone. Within 2 hours of ingestion of 75 g of glucose, growth hormone is suppressed to less than 1 ng/mL under physiologic conditions. An elevated growth hormone level 1 hour after the glucose ingestion indicates that glucose did not suppress growth hormone secretion, leading to the diagnosis of acromegaly.[14]

Stop and Consider

Why does growth hormone excess in children produce manifestations that are different than those in adults?

Cervical Metaplasia and Dysplasia

Cervical development is a dynamic process, evolving throughout the reproductive lifetime. The cells of the cervix respond to the hormonal environment, promoting adaptive and maladaptive responses.

PATHOPHYSIOLOGY

The epithelial cells of the cervix are arranged in a multilayer organization much like that of the skin. Actively dividing cells are located along the basal layer and are not usually found at the surface layer. The cervix is made up of two distinct cell types: squamous epithelium and columnar (glandular) epithelium (Fig. 2.15). **Squamous epithelium**, the cell type lining the outside of the cervix and the vagina, is apparent on physical examination when the cervix is visualized. **Columnar epithelium** is the cell type lining the **endocervical canal**, the area

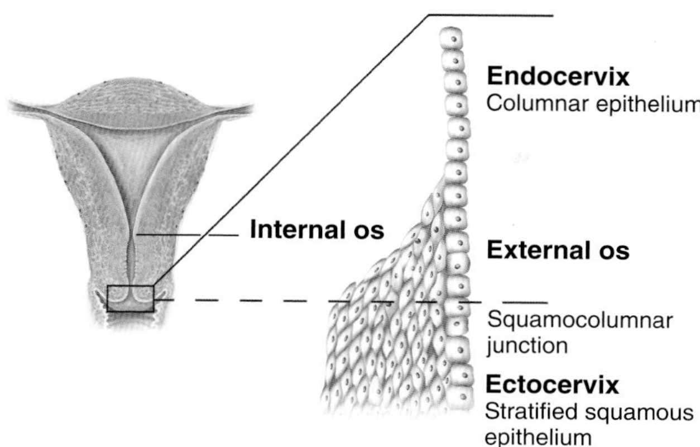

Figure 2.15. Cell types comprising the transformation zone. The endocervix is lined by columnar epithelium. The ectocervix is lined with stratified squamous epithelium. The squamocolumnar junction marks the merging point of these two epithelial cell types. (Courtesy Anatomical Chart Company.)

between the external and internal cervical os. This cell type provides secretions that plug the canal with mucus and protect the uterus from pathogens that can ascend from the vagina.

The location at which these two cell types merge is known as the **squamocolumnar junction**. This area is dynamic throughout a woman's reproductive life, migrating and changing location on the cervix in response to stimuli, including hormones and pH. The area comprising the merging of these cell types is called the **transformation zone** (Fig. 2.16). As the transformation zone migrates from inside the endocervical canal to the outside of the cervix, or **ectocervix**, it can often be visualized on physical examination. High estrogen levels, as experienced in the luteal phase of the menstrual cycle and during pregnancy, promote the gradual transition of squamous epithelium to columnar epithelium. Low estrogen levels, as occur in menopause, cause the squamo-columnar junction to recede into the endocervical canal where it can no longer be visualized on physical examination. The adaptations that these cell types undergo are examples of metaplasia—the cellular response of changing from one type to another in the face of an environmental stressor.

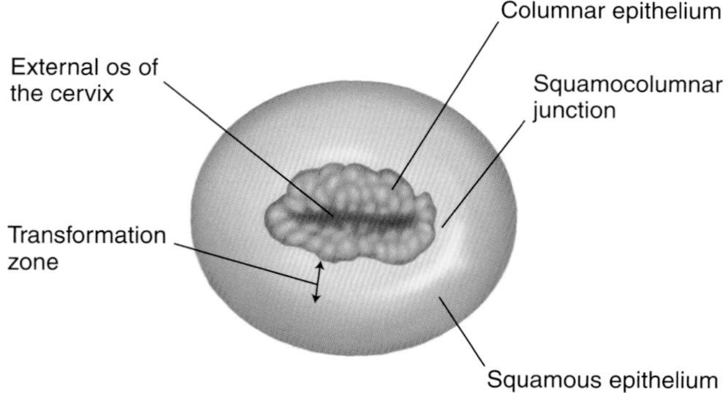

Figure 2.16. Transformation zone of the external cervical os. The transformation zone comprises the area distal to the squamocolumnar junction and is the site of squamous metaplasia. (From Bickley LS, Szilagyi P. *Bates' Guide to Physical Examination and History Taking*. 8th ed. Philadelphia, PA: Lippincott Williams & Wilkins; 2003.)

Although the metaplastic changes of the cervix are not pathologic, the squamous epithelial cell component of the transformation zone is vulnerable to stressors, which may cause the cells injury or damage. The epithelium can be injured by several factors, including chronic infection, irritation, and trauma. The transformation zone represents the most likely site for the cellular response of dysplasia. Cells altered with dysplastic changes are characterized by an abnormal growth and a disordered process of differentiation (dividing cells are not confined to the basal layer). Dysplastic cells are sloughed off the cervical surface prematurely and are often immature.

Changes in cellular structures, particularly in the nucleus, are apparent in dysplastic cervical cells. Alterations in the **chromatin**, genetic material of compressed DNA, are responsible for the darkened appearance of the cell nucleus and the abnormal differentiation of dividing cells. Cervical dysplasia is considered to be a precancerous condition. If identified and treated early, the damaged cervical cells can be replaced by normal cells, leading to full recovery. If left untreated, the cells may recover spontaneously or may progress into **malignancy** or cancer.

CLINICAL MANIFESTATIONS

There are no signs and symptoms of cervical dysplasia, emphasizing the importance of routine cervical cytologic screening for early detection. The presence of risk factors for cervical dysplasia should be considered when determining screening type and frequency. Risk factors include:

1. Early onset sexual activity
2. Multiple (more than three) sexual partners
3. Exposure to human papilloma virus
4. Smoking

The **human papilloma virus (HPV)** is implicated as a common factor in the development of cervical dysplasia.[16,17] HPV enters the host cell and can be integrated into its genome. The changes in the DNA are translated into unregulated cellular reproduction and can potentially result in cancer, although not all strains of the virus are considered to be potentially **oncogenic** (cancer causing).

Stop and Consider

Can the prevalence of high-risk types of HPV vary geographically? Why is it important to determine the most common types of high-risk HPV in a particular region or geographic area?

DIAGNOSIS

Identification of cervical dysplasia is achieved through both screening and diagnostic testing.

Screening Tests

Routine screening of cervical cells is done to identify characteristics of cells. Cells from the ectocervix, ideally from the more vulnerable transformation zone, and from the endocervical canal are obtained for microscopic evaluation. Metaplastic and dysplastic changes can be determined with this screening method.[18,19] In addition to identification of cellular changes, some screening tests can determine whether an oncogenic form of HPV is present by DNA analysis. The results of these tests are used to determine treatment and follow-up plans (Table 2.1).

The Papanicolaou (Pap) smear, named for the originator Dr. George Papanicolaou, has been the primary method of cervical screening since the early 1940s. Cells from the ectocervix and endocervix are collected during a pelvic examination. Placement of a speculum into the vagina allows viewing of the cervix. A collecting device, often referred to as a spatula, is placed on the transformation zone of the ectocervix, and superficial cells are collected by rotating the collection device. Cells from the endocervix are also collected during this procedure. In a conventional Pap smear, the cells are placed (smeared) on a glass slide and preserved with fixative for subsequent examination by a cytotechnologist or a pathologist. Cells collected from the cervix can also be placed in a vial of preservative solution for analysis using a newer method of Pap smear analysis, liquid-based Pap testing. The liquid-based method of analysis is used for determination of cervical cell infection with oncogenic HPV subtypes.

Recommendations for screening of US women at low risk for cervical dysplasia include:

- Initial screening at age 21
- Screening women aged 21 to 29 years with Pap test alone at intervals of every 3 years
- Pap test and HPV co-testing every 5 years in women ≥30 and <65 years of age

Among older women who have risk factors (prior abnormal Pap test, smoking history, previous HPV-related disease, or new partners) or were inadequately screened, Pap test every 2 to 3 years or co-testing every 5 years is recommended. Women with HIV infection or who are immunocompromised have limited ability to clear HPV infection and therefore should be screened more aggressively for cervical dysplasia.

The results of the Pap smear screening are used in consideration of management and treatment strategies. Results of Pap screenings are reported using the Bethesda System as follows:

- Negative for intraepithelial lesion or malignancy
  - No signs of cancer or precancerous changes
- Epithelial cell abnormalities
  - Atypical squamous cells of undetermined significance (ASC-US)
  - Atypical squamous cells, cannot rule out high-grade squamous intraepithelial cell lesion (ASC-H)
  - Low-grade squamous intraepithelial lesion (LGSIL)
  - High-grade squamous intraepithelial lesion (HGSIL)
  - Squamous cell carcinoma

Table 2.1 Laboratory and Diagnostic Tests Used With Cervical Dysplasia

Lab or Diagnostic Test	Purpose of the Test	Procedure
Physical examination	Visual evaluation of cervix	Speculum examination of the ectocervix to detect transformation zone and general appearance
Cervical sampling	Obtaining a specimen for cytologic evaluation	Pap smear requiring the use of a spatula for ectocervical sample and a cytobrush for endocervical sample or liquid sampling also capable of determining human papilloma virus (HPV) type
Cervical assessment	Evaluation of the cervix and endocervical canal for evidence of dysplasia	Examination of the cervix with a colposcope; sampling of endocervical canal and biopsy of all lesions suspected of dysplasia
Diagnostic excisional procedure	Provide histologic sample of the transformation zone and endocervical canal for evaluation	Laser conization, cold-knife conization, loop electrosurgical excision (LEEP), and loop electrosurgical conization comprise the surgical procedures employed to obtain specimens

- Glandular cell abnormalities
  - Atypical endocervical or endometrial cells
  - Atypical, favor neoplastic
  - Endocervical adenocarcinoma in situ (AIS)
  - Adenocarcinoma

Identification of high-risk HPV strains provides further information for determining treatment approaches. Analysis of cells for the presence and strain of HPV DNA indicates infection with the virus and identifies the risk status for the presence of oncogenic HPV subtypes.

Diagnostic Tests

Diagnostic testing is performed based on cellular screening tests. Evaluation of tissue is completed to obtain an accurate diagnosis and to form the basis of treatment. One of the most common diagnostic tests is the colposcopy. Colposcopy allows a more careful visual observation of cervical changes and serves as a guide for biopsy site selection. An outpatient procedure, colposcopy is similar to a Pap smear in the approach of visualization of the cervix using a speculum. Rather than viewing the cervix with the naked eye, the tissue is magnified by a colposcope, a binocular-like device placed about 30 cm outside the opening of the vagina. An acetic acid solution is applied to the cervix, which causes areas to turn white (aceto–white), suggestive of dysplasia. Small, 1/8-inch tissue sections (punch biopsies) are taken from the whitened areas and sent to pathology for analysis. Further tissue is collected by endocervical curettage, providing a tissue sample from the endocervix. A narrow instrument (curette) is passed into the endocervix to obtain the sample, providing tissue for accurate diagnosis.

Biopsy results are reported as cervical intraepithelial neoplasia (CIN) of varying severity (CIN 1, mild dysplasia; CIN 2, moderate dysplasia; CIN 3, severe dysplasia), carcinoma in situ, squamous cell carcinoma (invasive cancer of squamous cells), and adenocarcinoma (invasive cancer of glandular cells).

Persistent infection with HPV types 16 and 18 is most commonly associated with cervical cancer, responsible of approximately 70% of cases.[16] HPV types 31, 33, 45, 52, and 58 are also implicated in development of cervical cancer, accounting for approximately an additional 19% of cases. Noncarcinogenic genital warts are associated with HPV types 6 and 11. Vaccine development against pathogenic HPV types includes the quadrivalent vaccine Gardasil, which targets four HPV subtypes 6, 11, 16, and 18. Gardasil 9 extends protection to nine HPV subtypes, including 6, 11, 16, 18, 31, 33, 45, 52, and 58. The bivalent Cervarix targets the two most common oncogenic HPV subtypes 16 and 18. Vaccine effectiveness is greatest when administered prior to HPV infection, that is, prior to initiating sex. Routine immunization is recommended for girls and boys aged 11 to 12 years but can be initiated as early as age 9. For those not vaccinated at these early ages, catch-up immunization is recommended for those aged 13 to 26 years. Vaccine administration includes three doses over a minimum of 24 weeks.[18]

TREATMENT

Treatment to remove superficial cells (ablative) is an option for women with CIN in the absence of glandular cell involvement or invasive squamous cell disease. Cryosurgery, a form of cold therapy that destroys mildly dysplastic cells, is a common ablative therapy for cervical dysplasia. Liquid nitrogen is applied to the dysplastic cells on the ectocervix, identified by colposcopy via a probe placed in the desired area. CO_2 laser ablation is accomplished by directing a laser toward the cervical lesion under colposcopic guidance, destroying the tissue by vaporization. Heat ablation methods include cold coagulation and electrocoagulation diathermy ablation, with variations in temperature and time of treatment associated with depth of cervical tissue destruction. In cases of carcinoma, a hysterectomy may be indicated.

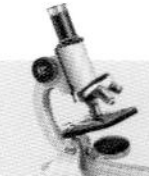

FROM THE LAB

Interpretation of traditional Pap smears with cells viewed in a slide preparation is limited by the quality of the collection. Cells may be placed too thickly on the slide, obscuring some of the cells from view. Other cell types, such as bacteria, yeast, and blood cells, can also prevent adequate viewing of the cervical cells of interest. Liquid-based preparations, also known as liquid-based cytology, allow the cells collected to be placed in a fixative filled vial rather than on a slide. One advantage of this method is the ability of the cytotechnologist or pathologist to view cells more clearly. Cells of interest can be analyzed more easily because of removal of mucus, bacteria, yeast, and other cells. An additional benefit provided by liquid-based Pap preparations includes the ability to screen for oncogenic HPV subtypes.

Environmental Toxin Injury and Cardiovascular Disease

Results from numerous studies worldwide have provided an important link between exposure to airborne environmental toxins and pollution with the development of cardiovascular disease. Air pollution is an important environmental toxin associated with cardiovascular disease, containing particulate matter, carbon monoxide, nitrogen oxides, sulfur dioxide, ozone, and lead. Fine particles in air pollution are associated with an increase in mortality and with the development of cardiovascular disease caused by inflammation, atherosclerosis, and altered cardiac function. The evidence is so strong that the American Heart Association includes air pollution as a known risk factor for cardiovascular disease.[20]

Cigarette smoking is one of the most common environmental pollutants known to cause cellular damage. Cigarette smoke contains cancer-causing chemicals (formaldehyde, benzene), toxic metals (lead, arsenic), and poisonous gases (carbon monoxide, hydrogen cyanide). These toxic substances promote the development of physical cellular injury and contribute to disease and illness.[21]

PATHOPHYSIOLOGY

The toxins in cigarette smoke are present in both **mainstream** (active) and **sidestream** (passive or secondhand) smoke. When the toxin-containing smoke enters the lung, the free radicals (O_2^-, H_2O_2, and $ONOO^-$) promote the development of oxidative stress. This results in inflammation, release of cytokines, vascular dysfunction, and altered gene activation and contributes to the development of atherosclerosis. The resulting cellular damage increases an individual's risk of developing coronary heart disease.[22] Studies have demonstrated that even small exposures to these toxins can cause a significant increase in cardiovascular disease.[23]

CLINICAL MANIFESTATIONS

The manifestations of exposure to firsthand and secondhand smoke reflect the overall effects of pathology on the entire body. From cellular dysfunction to organ involvement, smoking affects nearly all body systems. According to a report by the US Surgeon General,[24] the following findings represent the consequences of smoking on health:

- There is a causal relationship between exposure to secondhand smoke and increased risk of stroke.
- Smoking is the leading cause of premature death in the United States.
- More than 20 million premature deaths in the last five decades were due to smoking and exposure to secondhand smoke.

Health consequences of smoking include aortic aneurysm, acute myeloid leukemia, cataract, cancer (cervical, kidney, pancreatic, stomach, bladder, esophageal, laryngeal, lung, oral, and throat), pneumonia, periodontitis, chronic lung diseases, coronary heart and cardiovascular diseases (including ischemic stroke), reproductive effects, and sudden infant death syndrome.[25]

DIAGNOSIS

Smoking serves as both a causative and additive factor in cardiovascular disease.[26] History may reveal poor exercise tolerance because of impaired ability of the heart or blood vessels to meet the increased demands of activity. Dyspnea is a frequent complaint that may indicate either an underlying cardiovascular or a pulmonary condition. Cool, pale, and painful extremities may indicate the presence of a clot or the presence of peripheral vascular disease. Physical examination may reveal increased blood pressure and heart rate, and decreased cardiac output, and coronary blood flow. Laboratory studies may indicate markers of cardiovascular disease, including decreased high-density lipoprotein (HDL) and increased low-density lipoprotein (LDL).

TREATMENT

Smoking cessation is the first step in the prevention of further complications. Smoking cessation is a challenge for many individuals. Steps recommended for successful cessation include:

- Set a quit date
- Address barriers
- Consider treatment options of behavioral counseling and medication
- Learn new skills and behaviors
- Be prepared for relapse or difficult situations

Nicotine replacement therapy is designed to relieve nicotine withdrawal symptoms. The combination of delivery systems that include the long-acting patch with

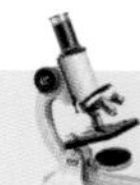

FROM THE LAB

Cotinine, a nicotine metabolite, can be measured in the blood, urine, or saliva. Cotinine levels can provide an objective measurement of exposure to active or passive smoke. After smoking cessation, it can take up to 2 weeks for cotinine levels to reach nonsmoking levels in blood and several weeks in urine. Since the early 1990s, cotinine levels in nonsmokers have decreased by more than 70% in adults, 58% in children, and 55% in adolescents, indicating lowered environmental smoke exposure.[27]

a short-acting method such as lozenge, gum, inhaler, or nasal spray is considered first-line treatment. Another pharmacologic treatment targets the nicotinic receptor agonist varenicline, reducing nicotine withdrawal symptoms as well as blocking the rewarding aspects of smoking. Bupropion, a norepinephrine/dopamine reuptake inhibitor is another pharmacologic option for use in smoking cessation. Although some smoking-related damage may be reversible, treatment of the persistent health consequences of smoking is disease specific and may be required long term.

Stop and Consider
Who is most at risk for illness related to secondhand smoke? What increases vulnerability to disease?

SUMMARY

- Cellular homeostasis depends on the proper functioning of cellular components, with direct effects on tissues and organs.
- Cellular adaptations to stress, injury, and damage form the basis of all disease.
- Alterations in cell size (atrophy and hypertrophy), cell number (hyperplasia), and cell structure (metaplasia and dysplasia) cause changes in tissue function and impact the entire person.
- Most cellular adaptations are necessary for cell survival.
- When damage exceeds the ability of the cell to adapt to a stressor, cell death by apoptosis or necrosis results.
- The clinical models presented in this chapter illustrate the applications of the concepts of cellular adaptation, including atrophy, hypertrophy, hyperplasia, metaplasia, dysplasia, apoptosis, and necrosis.

CASE STUDY 2.1

You are spending the winter skiing high in the mountains of Colorado. You notice that exertion while skiing makes you tired and that you do not have as much energy as you did before staying in the mountains. You realize you are feeling this way because your body cannot take in as much oxygen at the higher altitude. One long-term adaptation your body must make is to increase the production of red blood cells to better oxygenate your tissues and cells. Based on the information in this chapter and on additional readings, answer the following questions:

1. What is the most likely stressor that will cause your cells to adapt?
2. What adaptations are your cells likely to make to respond to the stressor?
3. What is the potential outcome if your cells are unable to adapt?
4. What lab tests can be used to identify the expected adaptations?
5. Can any treatments be used to support your body's adaptation?

Log onto the Internet. Search for a relevant journal article or Web site that details oxygenation at higher altitude to confirm your predictions.

CASE STUDY 2.2

A 56-year-old man arrived in the emergency room, complaining of chest pain. After evaluation, it was decided that he needed a coronary angiogram to determine if there were areas of blockage causing ischemia. One day after the angiogram, his renal function began to deteriorate. He was diagnosed with contrast-induced nephropathy.

1. What is contrast-induced nephropathy?
2. What is the epidemiology of contrast-induced nephropathy?
3. What is the etiology of contrast-induced nephropathy?
4. What adaptations are your cells likely to make to respond to the stressor?
5. How does the cellular injury manifest?
6. What can be done to prevent or treat nephrotoxic cellular injury in contrast-induced nephropathy?

Log onto the Internet. Search for a relevant journal article or Web site that details cellular injury and adaptation resulting from contrast-induced nephropathy to confirm your predictions.

PRACTICE EXAM QUESTIONS

1. The organelle that is involved in cellular respiration and is linked to the development of oxidative stress is known as the:
   a. Endoplasmic reticulum
   b. Golgi apparatus
   c. Lysosome
   d. Mitochondria

2. Cells develop into tissues with specialized structure and function through the process of:
   a. Differentiation
   b. Proliferation
   c. Endocytosis
   d. Exocytosis

3. The cell's typical response to a decrease in trophic signal is:
   a. Atrophy
   b. Hypertrophy
   c. Hyperplasia
   d. Phagocytosis

4. Cell death by necrosis is:
   a. The cell's way of replacing aged cells with new cells
   b. Also known as programmed cell death
   c. Often a response to inflammation
   d. Commonly seen during the period of embryo development

5. You are caring for a female patient who has reported a noticeable decrease in breast size and muscle mass. Which of the following conditions and causes is the most likely explanation?
   a. Puberty
   b. Pregnancy
   c. Menopause
   d. Acromegaly

6. The changes seen in cells adapting to stressors that promote metaplasia:
   a. Are irreversible
   b. Can result in cancer
   c. Change from one cell type to another
   d. Show abnormal differentiation

7. Cellular atrophy results in
   a. Increase in tissue volume due to increase in cell number
   b. Increase in tissue volume due to increase in cell size
   c. Decrease in tissue volume due to decrease in cell size
   d. No change in tissue volume

8. Treatment of chronic conditions associated with cerebral atrophy
   a. Are effective at restoring neuronal function
   b. Are targeted toward slowing neuronal injury and atrophy
   c. Are best initiated when advanced signs and symptoms are evident
   d. Are not indicated

9. Which of the following hormones is secreted from the anterior pituitary?
   a. Growth hormone
   b. Somatostatin
   c. Growth hormone releasing hormone
   d. Insulin-like growth factor 1

10. Which one of the following is a diagnostic test for cervical dysplasia?
   a. Liquid-based Pap cytology
   b. Conventional Pap cytology
   c. Cervical punch biopsy
   d. HPV testing

11. Which of the following reactive oxygen species is scavenged by catalase?
   a. Hydroxyl radical
   b. Peroxynitrite
   c. Superoxide
   d. Hydrogen peroxide

12. Which of the following terms describes cells that are enlarged, with darkened nuclei and abnormal chromatin
   a. Hyperplastic
   b. Dysplastic
   c. Metaplastic
   d. Aplastic

DISCUSSION AND APPLICATION

1. What did I know about basic alterations in cells and tissues before today?
2. What body processes are affected by altered cellular and tissue adaptation? How do cellular and tissue adaptations impact those processes?
3. What are the potential etiologies for altered cellular and tissue adaptation? How do cellular and tissue adaptations develop?
4. Who is most at risk for developing altered cellular and tissue adaptation? How can these alterations be prevented?
5. What are the human differences that affect the etiology, risk, or course of altered cellular and tissue adaptation?
6. What clinical manifestations are expected in the course of altered cellular and tissue adaptation?
7. What special diagnostic tests help to determine the diagnosis and course of altered cellular and tissue adaptation?
8. What are the goals of care for individuals with altered cellular and tissue adaptation?
9. How does the concept of altered cellular and tissue adaptation build on what I have learned in the previous chapter and in the previous courses?
10. How can I use what I have learned?

RESOURCES

American Heart Association. Diseases and conditions: cardiomyopathy: http://www.heart.org/HEARTORG/Conditions/More/Cardiomyopathy_UCM_444459_SubHomePage.jsp Retrieved March 7, 2016.

Centers for Disease Control and Prevention. Second National Report on Human Exposure to Environmental Chemicals:
http://www.cdc.gov/exposurereport
Retrieved March 7, 2016.

National Institute of Diabetes and Digestive and Kidney Diseases. Acromegaly:
http://endocrine.niddk.nih.gov/pubs/acro/acro.htm
Retrieved March 7, 2016.

National Institute of Neurological Disorders and Stroke. Cerebral atrophy:
http://www.ninds.nih.gov/disorders/cerebral_atrophy/cerebral_atrophy.htm
Retrieved March 7, 2016.

Ries LAG, Eisner MP, Kosary CL, et al. SEER Cancer Statistics Review, 1975–2005. Bethesda, MD: National Cancer Institute:
http://seer.cancer.gov/csr/1975_2005/
Retrieved March 7, 2016.

References

1. Zatz M, Starling A. Calpains and disease. *N Engl J Med*. 2005;352(23):2413–2423.
2. Gaziano JM. Vitamin E and cardiovascular disease: observational studies. *Ann N Y Acad Sci*. 2004;1031:280–291.
3. Stone WL, Krishnan K, Campbell SE, et al. Tocopherols and the treatment of colon cancer. *Ann N Y Acad Sci*. 2004;1031:223–233.
4. Colcombe SJ, Erickson KI, Scalf PE, et al. Aerobic exercise training increases brain volume in aging humans. *J Gerontol A Biol Sci Med Sci*. 2006;61:1166–1170.
5. Gordon BA, Rykhlevskaia EI, Brumback CR, et al. Neuroanatomical correlates of aging, cardiopulmonary fitness level, and education. *Psychophysiology*. 2008;45:825–838.
6. Erickson KI, Suever BL, Prakash RS, et al. Greater intake of vitamins B_6 and B_{12} spares gray matter in healthy elderly: a voxel-based morphometry study. *Brain Res*. 2008;1199:20–26.
7. Apostolova LG, Thompson PM. Mapping progressive brain structural changes in early Alzheimer's disease and mild cognitive impairment. *Neuropsychologia*. 2008;46:1597–1612.
8. Jokinen H, Kalska H, Ylikoski R. Longitudinal cognitive decline in subcortical ischemic vascular disease—the LADIS study. *Cerebrovasc Dis*. 2009;27:384–391.
9. Grassiot B, Desgranges B, Eustache F, et al. Quantification and clinical relevance of brain atrophy in multiple sclerosis: a review. *J Neurol*. 2009;256(9):1397–1412.
10. Maron BJ, Ackerman MJ, Nishimura RA, et al. Task force 4: HCM and other cardiomyopathies, mitral valve prolapse, myocarditis, and Marfan syndrome. *J Am Coll Cardiol*. 2005;45(8):1340–1345.
11. Lipshultz SE, Sleeper LA, Towbin JA, et al. The incidence of pediatric cardiomyopathy in two regions of the United States. *N Engl J Med*. 2003;348(17):1647–1655.
12. Klingbell AU, Schneider M, Martus P, et al. A meta-analysis of the effects of treatment on left ventricular mass in essential hypertension. *Am J Med*. 2003;115(1):41–46.
13. Noble S, Sigwart U. Therapeutic management of hypertrophic cardiomyopathy: alcohol septal ablation or surgical myomectomy? *Expert Rev Cardiovasc Ther*. 2014;12(9):1041–1044.
14. Minuto F, Resmini E, Boschetti M, et al. Assessment of disease activity in acromegaly by means of a single blood sample: comparison of the 120th minute postglucose value with spontaneous GH secretion and with the IGF system. *Clin Endocrinol (Oxf)*. 2004;61(1):138–144.
15. Vitale G, Pivonello R, Lombardi G, et al. Cardiovascular complications in acromegaly. *Minerva Endocrinol*. 2004;29(3):77–88.
16. Muñoz N, Bosch X, de Sanjosé S, et al. Epidemiologic classification of human papillomavirus types associated with cervical cancer. *N Engl J Med*. 2003;348;518–527.
17. Matsukura T, Sugase M. Human papillomavirus genomes in squamous cell carcinomas of the uterine cervix. *Virology*. 2004;324(2):439–449.
18. Workowski KA, Bolan GA. Sexually transmitted diseases treatment guidelines, 2015. *MMWR Recomm Rep*. 2015;64(RR3):1–137.
19. Wright TC Jr, Cox JT, Massad LS, et al. 2001 Consensus guidelines for the management of women with cervical cytological abnormalities. *JAMA*. 2002;287(16):2120–2129.
20. Brook RD, Raiagopaian S, Pope CA, et al. Particulate matter air pollution and cardiovascular disease: an update to the scientific statement from the American Heart Association. *Circulation*. 2010;121(21):2331–2378.
21. Ambrose JA, Barua RS. The pathophysiology of cigarette smoking and cardiovascular disease: an update. *J Am Coll Cardiol*. 2004;43(10):1731–1737.
22. Whincup PH, Gilg JA, Emberson JR, et al. Passive smoking and risk of coronary heart disease and stroke: prospective study with cotinine measurement. *BMJ*. 2004;329(7459):200–205.
23. Pechacek TF, Babb S. How acute and reversible are the cardiovascular risks of secondhand smoke? *BMJ*. 2004;328(7446):980–983.
24. U.S. Department of Health and Human Services. *The Health Consequences of Smoking—50 Years of Progress: A Report of the Surgeon General, 2014*. Rockville, MD: U.S. Department of Health and Human Services, Centers for Disease Control and Prevention, National Center for Chronic Disease Prevention and Health Promotion, Office of Smoking and Health; 2014.
25. Pope CA III, Burnett RT, Thurston GD, et al. Cardiovascular mortality and long-term exposure to particulate air pollution: epidemiological evidence of general pathophysiological pathways of disease. *Circulation*. 2004;109(1):71–77.
26. Liu Y, Goodson JM, Zhang B. Air pollution and adverse cardiac remodeling: clinical effects and basic mechanisms. *Front Physiol*. 2015;6:162. http://dx.doi.org/10.3389/fphys.2015.00162. Accessed June 20, 2015.
27. Center for Disease Control and Prevention. *CDC's Second National Report on Human Exposure to Environmental Chemicals: Spotlight on Cotinine*. Rockville, MD: U.S. Department of Health and Human Services; 2003.

Chapter

3 Inflammation and Tissue Repair

LEARNING OUTCOMES

1. Define and use the key terms listed in this chapter.
2. Differentiate the three lines of defense.
3. Outline the process of acute inflammation, including the role of chemical mediators.
4. Describe the process of healing and repair after tissue injury.
5. Differentiate acute and chronic inflammation.
6. Identify the cardinal signs of inflammation.
7. Discuss treatment methods used for acute and chronic inflammation.
8. Apply concepts of acute and chronic inflammation to select clinical models.

INTRODUCTION

Think back to all of the injuries, even minor ones, that you have sustained in your lifetime. When did you last burn the roof of your mouth on hot pizza, get a paper cut, or sprain your ankle? All of these activities, and many others, cause tissue trauma that requires healing. This chapter focuses on the inflammatory response, which occurs with any type of injury. Inflammation is critical for you to understand as a student in the health professions. All disease processes cause injury, and healing can occur only with an effective inflammatory response. The *acute* inflammatory response is considered an expected body response to injury; *chronic* inflammation is presented as an altered inflammatory response because of unrelenting injury. The stages of tissue repair and complications that can occur during the healing process are also detailed in this chapter.

Review of Body Defense Mechanisms

Protection of the body depends on three major lines of defense, as depicted in Figure 3.1:

- The first line of defense relies on the protection of the skin and mucous membranes.
- The second line of defense is waged through an effective inflammatory response.
- The third line of defense is activated through the immune response.

The skin and mucous membranes comprise a physical and chemical barrier to invasion and are considered the first line of defense. Skin allows a protective

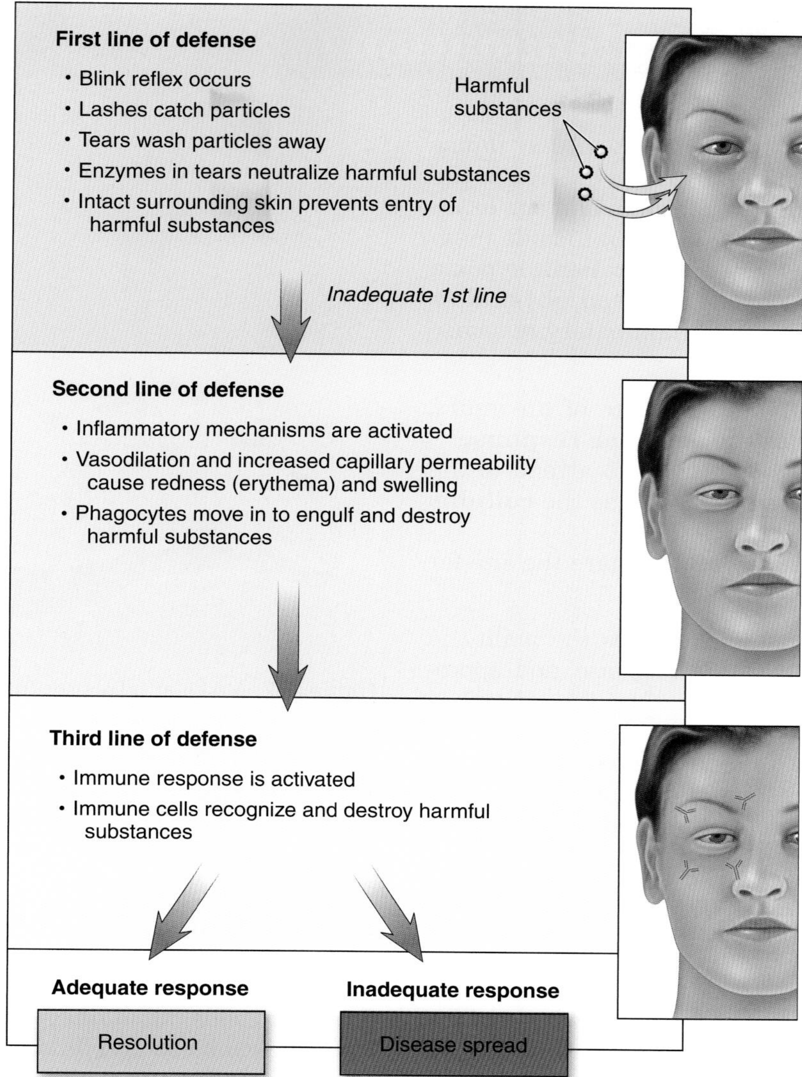

Figure 3.1. Lines of defense.

physical barrier against harmful substances in the external environment. Areas not covered by skin are protected by chemically coated mucous membranes that help to neutralize or destroy many harmful invaders. Tears and saliva are examples of enzyme-filled fluids that bathe mucous membranes and offer essential protection to the eyes and oral cavity. Breaks in the skin and mucous membranes or loss of protective fluids allow microorganisms and other harmful agents to enter the body and threaten homeostasis.

Stop and Consider
What can you do to improve or strengthen your first line of defense?

The second line of defense, or inflammatory response, is activated when the first line of defense is inadequate. The inflammatory response is nonspecific; that is, the process of waging an inflammatory response is identical regardless of the cause of injury. The **immune response** is considered to be the third line of defense. The immune response wages a specific defense depending on the type of invader; this is the focus of Chapter 4.

Stop and Consider
What lines of defense are you enhancing by putting on an antibiotic ointment and covering a laceration with a Band-Aid?

Module 1 Acute Inflammation

Acute inflammation is triggered by tissue injury and is essential for healing. **Injury** is defined in the broadest sense to include any form of damage or alteration to cells or tissues. Injury can include invasion by microorganisms, cellular mutations, hypoxia or anoxia, nutritional deficiencies, and physical or chemical damage. The acute inflammatory response has three major goals:

1. To increase blood flow to the site of an injury, which is referred to as the **vascular response**
2. To alert the products of healing to attend to the site of injury, which is referred to as the **cellular response**
3. To remove injured tissue and prepare the site for repair and healing

The process of inflammation requires the ability to recognize the injury, activate a response, and appropriately shut down the response when the injury has passed. The result is tissue repair, regeneration, or the formation of scar tissue. To see a video on acute inflammation, visit http://thePoint.lww.com, using the scratch-off code on the inside front cover. thePoint®

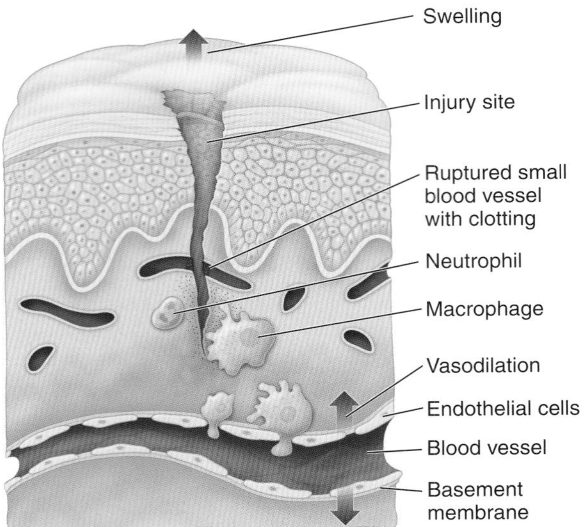

Figure 3.2. Vascular response. Inflammation causes widening of endothelial cell junctions and vasodilation. (Modified from Werner R, Benjamin BE. *A Massage Therapist's Guide to Pathology*. 3rd ed. Baltimore, MD: Lippincott Williams & Wilkins; 2005, with permission.)

Vascular Response

Tissue injury requires a response at the level of the blood vessel near the site of the injury. Put simply, clotting must occur. If the blood vessels are considered roads, injury requires that the roads be widened and expanded to allow for emergency vehicles to get to the scene of the accident. The objective is to attract sufficient products of clotting and healing to the site of injury and to prevent infection.

Anatomically, the structure of the blood vessels must change to accommodate this increase in emergency vehicle traffic.

- The blood vessels **dilate**, or widen, to accommodate increased blood flow to the site of injury.
- The lining of the blood vessel becomes more **permeable**, or loosens to allow cells to easily move from the vessel into the injured tissue.

Loosening of the blood vessel must occur with the basement membrane of the blood vessel and adjacent endothelial cells (Fig. 3.2). **Endothelial cells** form a tight junction within the inner lining of the blood and lymphatic vessels and the heart. Endothelial cells are connected to the basement membrane. The **basement membrane** is the outer membrane of the vessels, which separates the vessel from the tissues of the body. The vessel walls are needed to confine blood cells and plasma, but with injury, they must be loosened to allow for movement of healing fluids and cells into damaged tissues.

Increased blood and fluid are needed at the site of the injury for two reasons:

1. Blood is composed of cells active in **phagocytosis**, the process of engulfing and removing harmful agents, as well as cells essential in promoting healing and developing an immune response.
2. Increased fluid dilutes harmful substances at the site of the injury.

Inspection of a scraped knee after a bike accident will show a layer of watery fluid that seeps from the wound. **Exudate**, the watery fluid that accumulates at the site of injury, has a high protein and leukocyte concentration. This is a sure sign that the vessels have become more permeable and that cells active in phagocytosis are present and ready to fend off microorganisms. Healing can then begin.

This whole process is orchestrated through the work of potent chemicals, referred to as inflammatory mediators. **Inflammatory mediators**, specifically vasoactive inflammatory mediators, facilitate the process of widening and loosening the blood vessels at the site of injury. Inflammatory mediators are

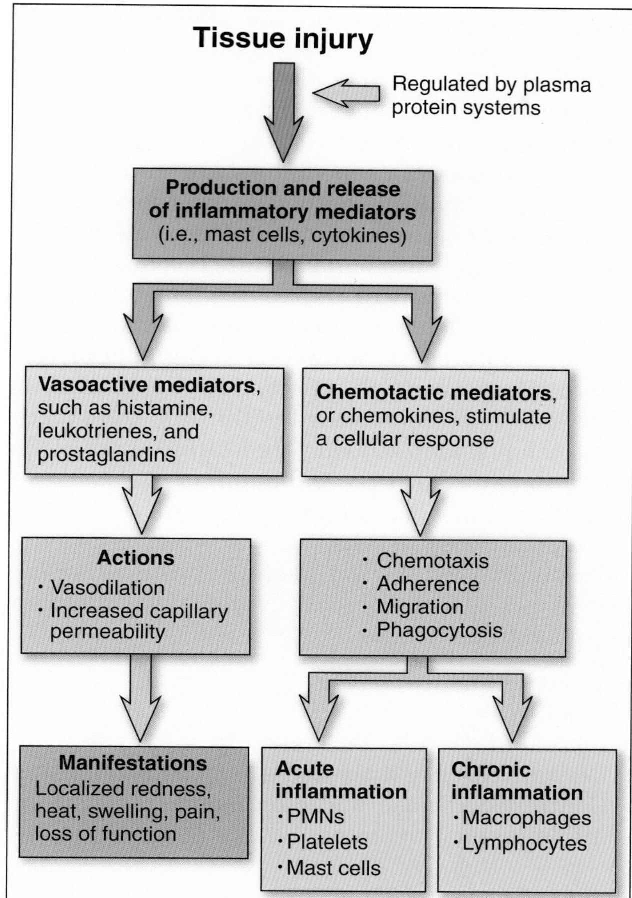

Figure 3.3. Concept map. An overview of the importance of chemical mediators in the vascular and cellular responses of inflammation. PMNs, polymorphonuclear neutrophils. (Modified from Rubin E, Farber JL. *Pathology*. 4th ed. Philadelphia, PA: Lippincott Williams & Wilkins; 2005, with permission.)

located in the blood plasma and in many cells, including platelets, mast cells, basophils, neutrophils, endothelial cells, monocytes, and macrophages. The location of inflammatory mediators is important; these substances must be constantly ready to respond to injury anywhere in the body. Figure 3.3 illustrates the major roles of the inflammatory mediators in the inflammatory process. Refer to this figure frequently as you move through this chapter.

INFLAMMATORY MEDIATORS WITHIN CELLS

As mentioned, some inflammatory mediators are formed within the blood plasma and some are formed within cells. Within cells, most of these inflammatory mediators are generated in the cell plasma membrane or are made up of proteins within the cell. Most commonly, it is the white blood cells (WBCs) that produce and release inflammatory mediators; platelets, endothelial cells, and injured tissue cells are also potential sources. The generation and activation of inflammatory mediators is a complex process. Try not to get overwhelmed. In this section, focus on the key inflammatory cells, where they are located, examples of inflammatory mediators released from those cells, and what their role is in the inflammatory process.

Inflammatory Mediators Within White Blood Cells

The **mast cell** is an important inflammatory mediator. Mast cells are leukocytes (WBCs) that are housed throughout the connective tissues of the body and near all blood vessels. The placement of the mast cell allows for a rapid response directly at the site of the injury. Mast cells are similar to having emergency first responders trained in all neighborhoods. They are right there on the scene. The mast cell is responsible for the production and immediate release of inflammatory mediators through a process of **degranulation**, the mast cell breaks apart and releases inflammatory mediators in the form of extracellular granules (grain-like particles). The **basophil**, a WBC that also contains granules, functions in the same manner. Examples of inflammatory mediators released by mast cells include histamine, leukotrienes, and prostaglandins.

Stop and Consider

Where have you heard the names of the various inflammatory mediators listed above? What do you already know about these inflammatory mediators?

Signals to trigger, enhance, and discontinue the inflammatory response are also generated within other WBCs, such as lymphocytes and monocytes/macrophages. For example, **cytokines** are more than a hundred distinct cell proteins most often found within WBCs that have a vital role in regulating inflammation; they are active from the onset of vasodilation and increased vascular permeability to the resolution of the inflammatory response. Each of the different cytokines is released from a specific cell and serves a specific purpose. For example, cytokines released from lymphocytes are called lymphokines. Those released from monocytes or macrophages are called monokines. Other examples of cytokines include interleukins, growth factors, interferons, and chemokines. Now try not to hyperventilate here. The main point is that potent inflammatory mediators are released from a variety of WBCs in order to effectively orchestrate the inflammatory process.

Inflammatory Mediators Within Platelets

Platelets are also active in generating and releasing inflammatory mediators to promote vasodilation, clotting, attraction of WBCs, and healing of injured tissues. Serotonin is one example of an inflammatory mediator found in platelets. Serotonin causes vasodilation and increased vascular permeability, allowing cells of healing to arrive quickly to the site of injury. Histamine, which functions similarly to serotonin, is found in both WBCs and platelets.

Inflammatory Mediators Within Endothelial or Injured Tissue Cells

Inflammatory mediators can also be released from endothelial cells or injured tissue cells. For example, **platelet-activating factor** is a complex lipid stored in cell membranes, including those of endothelial cells that line blood vessels, and in many other types of cells that can become injured. Platelet-activating factor is a potent inflammatory mediator that has a key role in promoting vessel vasodilation, clotting, and attracting infection-fighting WBCs to the site of injury.

Another example is arachidonic acid. **Arachidonic acid** is a substance derived from the plasma membrane of an injured cell, which generates various inflammatory mediators through a complex chemical conversion. Inflammatory mediators associated with arachidonic acid include prostaglandins, lipoxins, leukotrienes, and thromboxane. These inflammatory mediators are active in the processes of vasodilation and vasoconstriction, increasing vascular permeability, bronchodilation and bronchoconstriction, and attraction of leukocytes. Corticosteroids are a highly effective group of anti-inflammatory drugs that work to block the production of arachidonic acid, thereby decreasing the inflammatory response. Corticosteroids also have a role on inhibiting the immune response, as discussed in Chapter 4.

Stop and Consider
Why would you want to block the production of arachidonic acid and inhibit the work of the inflammatory mediators?

INFLAMMATORY MEDIATORS WITHIN PLASMA

Inflammatory mediators can also circulate continuously within blood plasma. This is usually accomplished through the work of three major interrelated pathways. These pathways are responsible for the activation and deactivation of inflammatory mediators that circulate in the plasma. Table 3.1 summarizes these three pathways.

Multiple sources and pathways to induce and suppress inflammation are necessary because the inflammatory response *must occur* to heal tissues, and the inflammatory mediators are so *potent and powerful* that multiple pathways are needed to regulate these substances. Impaired activation of inflammation can lead to inadequate blood flow to the injured area. This will impair healing by limiting phagocytosis, clot formation, and repair of injured tissues. Impaired inhibition of inflammation can lead to an uncontrolled inflammatory response, the depletion of proteins needed within the three pathways (complement, clotting, and kinin). Loss of the ability to shut down the inflammatory response effectively can also lead to **autoimmunity**, a self-attack against body tissues.

To summarize, the initial steps in the inflammatory response influenced by vasoactive inflammatory mediators include:

- Tissue injury
- Blood vessel vasodilation
- Increased vascular permeability
- Clotting cascade activated
- Continued release and circulation of vasoactive inflammatory mediators

Cellular Response

After the vessels are dilated and permeable, the cells essential for healing are needed at the site of injury. As with the vascular response, the cellular response

Table 3.1 Continuously Circulating and Interrelated Plasma Systems That Regulate Inflammation

System	Key Characteristics
Complement	Several proteins that comprise 10%–15% of plasma; produced in liver
	Triggered by the presence of microorganisms
	Once triggered, activates a cascade of inflammatory mediators
	Primary role to destroy and remove microorganisms to prevent infection through **opsonization** (making bacteria vulnerable to phagocytosis) and cell **lysis** (destruction)
Clotting	Promotes coagulation through a cascade of clotting factors
	Suppresses coagulation when clotting is complete
	Various clotting factors produce and release inflammatory mediators
Kinin	Source of highly potent vasoactive inflammatory mediators
	Amplify the inflammatory response by triggering other inflammatory mediators

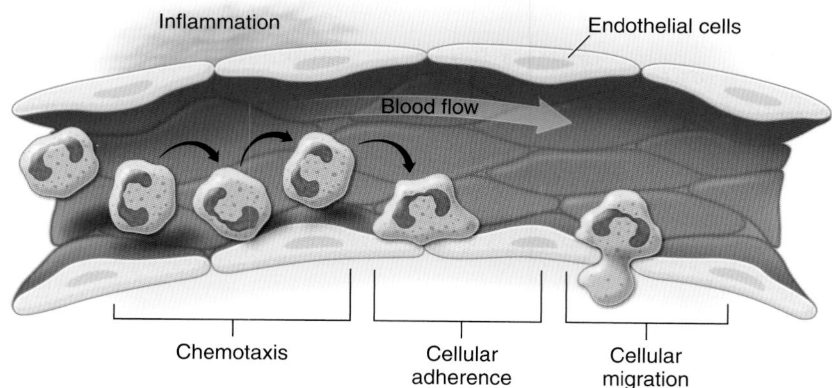

Figure 3.4. Cellular response: chemotaxis, adherence, and migration. (Modified from Rubin E, Farber JL. *Pathology*. 4th ed. Philadelphia, PA: Lippincott Williams & Wilkins; 2005, with permission.)

is regulated by inflammatory mediators. Three steps are needed for a successful cellular response: (1) chemotaxis, (2) cellular adherence, and (3) cellular migration (Fig. 3.4).

Chemotaxis is a process of moving certain cells to the site of injury. Specific inflammatory mediators, referred to as **chemotactic factors**, are activated, which attract specific types of cells. The neutrophil chemotactic factor attracts neutrophils. The eosinophil chemotactic factor attracts eosinophils, and so forth.

Table 3.2 Cells Active in the Cellular Response

Cell	Role
Leukocytes (WBCs)	Phagocytosis; removal of dead tissue
Neutrophils	A type of WBC; earliest phagocytic responders
Macrophages	A type of WBC; large, long-lived phagocytes associated with a prolonged (chronic) inflammatory response; monocytes are immature macrophages
Erythrocyte (red blood cells)	Carry oxygen to tissues
Platelets	Trap harmful substances; stop bleeding; form structural origin of repair

WBC, white blood cell.

Blood cells are constantly moving through the vascular system. Attraction and binding, or cellular **adherence**, is another step essential for effective phagocytosis. Cellular adherence is regulated by:

- Inflammatory mediators, specifically, chemotactic factors released by endothelial cells
- Receptors that bind leukocytes to the surface of endothelial cells near the site of injury

Cellular migration is the third essential step in the cellular response. The cellular response depends on the ability of cells, primarily leukocytes, erythrocytes, and platelets, to migrate, or move across, endothelial cells and get to the exact site of the injury. In the process of **diapedesis**, cells can move between and through endothelial junctions. The role of the major cells activated in the cellular response is summarized in Table 3.2. Leukocyte is a global term for many different types of WBCs, including neutrophils, monocytes, macrophages, mast cells, basophils, and T and B lymphocytes. Because there is extensive crossover of cellular activity between the inflammatory response, immune response, and the subsequent development of infection, this discussion of the cells will continue into the next two chapters and beyond.

During phagocytosis, inflammatory cells release inflammatory mediators to attract more neutrophils. The neutrophil itself also releases potent inflammatory mediators as it works to engulf and digest impaired tissue. During this aggressive process, unaffected, healthy tissue is also destroyed. Tissue destruction is minimized by the work of inhibitor proteins in the plasma-derived complement, clotting, and kinin systems.

GENERAL MANIFESTATIONS

The local manifestations of acute inflammation are often referred to as the **cardinal signs**. These signs include **erythema** (redness), heat, swelling, pain, and loss of function. **Lymphadenitis**, or enlargement and inflammation of the nearby lymph nodes, can occur as a function of filtering or draining harmful substances at the injury site. Local manifestations with rationales are presented in Table 3.3. These manifestations are primarily related to vasodilation and fluid accumulation in the tissues as a result of the activation of inflammatory mediators.

Table 3.3 Local Manifestations of Acute Inflammation

Manifestation	Rationale
Redness (erythema)	Vasodilation; increased blood flow to the injured area
Heat	Vasodilation; increased blood flow to the injured area
Incapacitation	Loss of function is related to tissue damage from injury, pain, and swelling at the site
Pain	Increased vascular permeability and accumulation of fluid causes compression in the tissues; inflammatory mediators can also directly elicit a pain response
Exudate and edema	Extracellular fluid accumulation often in tissues because of increased vascular permeability

Systemic manifestations related to the inflammatory response include fever, leukocytosis, and a higher percentage of circulating plasma proteins. **Pyrexia**, or fever (an elevated core body temperature), is a result of inflammatory mediators acting directly on the hypothalamus. The hypothalamus is responsible for controlling body temperature. An elevated body temperature stimulates phagocytosis and can also inhibit the growth of certain microorganisms. **Leukocytosis** is an elevation in WBCs, or leukocytes, with a count usually above 10,000/mm^3. Typically, the individual has a WBC count of 5,000 to 10,000/mm^3. All laboratory information is approximate because variability in laboratory ranges exists among various populations and sources. Leukocytosis demonstrates the increased circulation of WBCs to aid in healing. Plasma proteins are also increased as a result of the three plasma protein systems discussed previously. These proteins are called acute-phase reactants and can be measured through the use of laboratory tests, such as C-reactive protein (CRP). Common blood tests used to detect inflammation are presented in Table 3.4.

Stop and Consider

What does an elevation in leukocytes, erythrocyte sedimentation rate (ESR), or CRP levels tell you about the *location* of acute or chronic inflammation?

TREATMENT

The inflammatory response has multiple components and is often considered "overzealous," which explains the efforts of the booming pharmaceutical industry to find effective anti-inflammatory drugs. Damage to healthy surrounding tissue is a common occurrence in the acute inflammatory response. Therefore, the initial treatment principles for acute inflammation are to:

1. Reduce blood flow to the local area
2. Decrease swelling
3. Block the action of various inflammatory mediators
4. Decrease pain

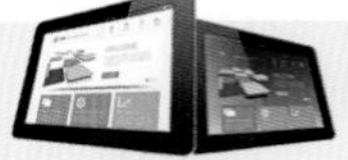

RESEARCH NOTES

In a recent issue of Inflammation Research, scientists are uncovering new ways of thinking about pharmacologic treatment for inflammation. Current therapy targets one aspect of the inflammatory process (e.g., blocking the production of arachidonic acid). Emerging research is demonstrating a significant value of designer drugs created to target several aspects of tissue repair. Such drugs combine actions of multiple cells and chemicals to regulate the complex metabolic and immune pathways underlying inflammation. The authors note, "addressing multiple targets of inflammation holistically, in moderation, is probably a more evolutionarily viable strategy, as compared to current therapy, which addresses drug targets in isolation."[1]

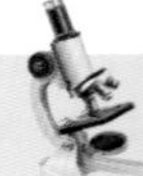

FROM THE LAB

CRP and the erythrocyte sedimentation rate (ESR) are two nonspecific tests of inflammation. Elevations in either test will signify inflammation is present, but neither will identify the exact source or location of the inflammation. CRP is often the preferred test for acute inflammation. CRP signifies the presence of a specific protein triggered by plasma protein systems during the inflammatory process. The erythrocyte sedimentation rate (also referred to as a sed rate) is a nonspecific method of testing for inflammation. During the inflammatory process, the coagulation cascade results in increased circulating levels of fibrinogen, which causes cells to stick together. When measured in a tube in the lab, red blood cells (RBCs) exposed to the inflammatory process will fall faster and will clump together. The ESR test then measures (in mm/hr) the level of RBC stacking.[2]

Table 3.4 Common Blood Tests Used to Detect Acute Inflammation

Blood Test	Reference Values	Changes With Inflammation
White blood cell count	5,000–10,000 cells/mm^3	Circulating white blood cells are increased, often above 10,000/mm^3
White blood cell differential	Neutrophils, 45%–75% Bands (immature neutrophils), 0%–5% Eosinophils, 0%–8% Basophils, 0%–3% Lymphocytes, 16%–46% Monocytes, 4%–11%	Measures proportion of each of the five types of white blood cells; the proportion of immature neutrophils (bands) is increased in comparison to other white blood cell types
Erythrocyte sedimentation rate	0–17 mm/hr for men 1–25 mm/hr for women 44–114 mm/hr in pregnancy 1–13 mm/hr for children	Detects red blood cell clumping or stacking as a result of increased fibrinogen levels; levels increase, often above 100 mm/hr for those with inflammation
C-reactive protein	Routine CRP <10 mg/L High sensitivity CRP, 0.1–3.8 mg/L	>10 mg/L indicates significant inflammatory disease
Complement activity	Total complement, 63–145 U/mL C3 (comprises 70% of total protein in the complement system), 80–184 mg/dL	Elevated in inflammation signifying the activation of complement; over time may decrease, indicating that complement factors are exhausted
Prothrombin time	Measured in time to coagulate, approximately 11.2–13.2 seconds	Increased prothrombin levels result in a reduced time to coagulate
Fibrinogen	175–400 mg/dL	Elevated during inflammation to promote coagulation

CRP, C-reactive protein.

The goal of treatment is to minimize damage to healthy, unaffected tissue and promote rapid healing. Pharmacologic, or drug treatments for inflammation most commonly block the action of inflammatory mediators, thereby reducing the swelling, pain, redness, and warmth typical of inflammation. Table 3.5 illustrates the actions of common pharmacologic treatments for inflammation. Nonpharmacologic treatments for inflammation initially include rest, ice, compression, and elevation. Once the initial treatment has been employed, resolution may improve with the application of warmth/heat and increased movement. As with all health conditions, optimal fluid and nutritional intake is needed to facilitate healing.

Stop and Consider

The RICE (rest, ice, compression, elevation) protocol is employed frequently in acute injury to minimize the effects of inflammation. How does each of these components reduce inflammation?

RESOLUTION OF ACUTE INFLAMMATION

The acute inflammatory response is self-limited. Once the offending agent has been destroyed and removed, feedback systems regulated by the three plasma protein systems (clotting, complement, and kinin), along with the relevant inflammatory mediators, deactivate the inflammatory response, allowing the tissue to heal.

Table 3.5 Common Pharmacologic Agents Used to Treat Inflammation

Pharmacologic Agent	Action
Aspirin	Inhibits the conversion of arachidonic acid to prostaglandins to suppress inflammation, reduce pain, and reduce fever
Nonsteroidal anti-inflammatory drugs	Similar to aspirin; inhibit the anti-inflammatory conversion of arachidonic acid to prostaglandins (NSAIDs) Examples: ibuprofen, naproxen
Glucocorticoids	Act through several mechanisms to interrupt the inflammatory process: inhibit synthesis of chemical mediators and reduce swelling, warmth, redness, and pain; suppress infiltration of phagocytes and avert tissue damage from release of lytic (cell-destroying) enzymes; suppress lymphocyte proliferation; and reduce immune component of inflammation. Example: prednisone

NSAIDs, nonsteroidal anti-inflammatory drugs.

Module 2 Healing and Tissue Repair

Tissue repair is similar to home repair. If a home is damaged, the destroyed area needs to be sealed off to prevent further exposure to the external environment. Then a process can begin to clear the debris, rebuild the walls and roof, and restore the interior working contents of the home, such as the electrical system, appliances, or heating system. Likewise, the goal of tissue healing and repair is to seal the wound, clear the debris, and restore the structural and functional integrity of the injured area. This process is often divided into three phases: the inflammatory phase, the proliferative phase, and the remodeling phase. Within these phases, structural supports must be rebuilt and functional cells and tissues regenerated or replaced (Fig. 3.5).

The construction workers of tissue repair fit into the following categories:

- Clotting (coagulation) factors to stop bleeding and form a fibrin clot
- Inflammatory mediators to promote chemotaxis to the affected area
- Proteinases (enzymes) to degrade dead tissue
- Proteinase inhibitors to prevent healthy tissue breakdown
- Matrix, or structural, proteins to rebuild architectural supports
- Molecule receptors to attract cells needed to form a structural matrix
- Adhesion molecules to provide "stickiness" to these cells
- Growth factors to promote regeneration of new cells and tissues

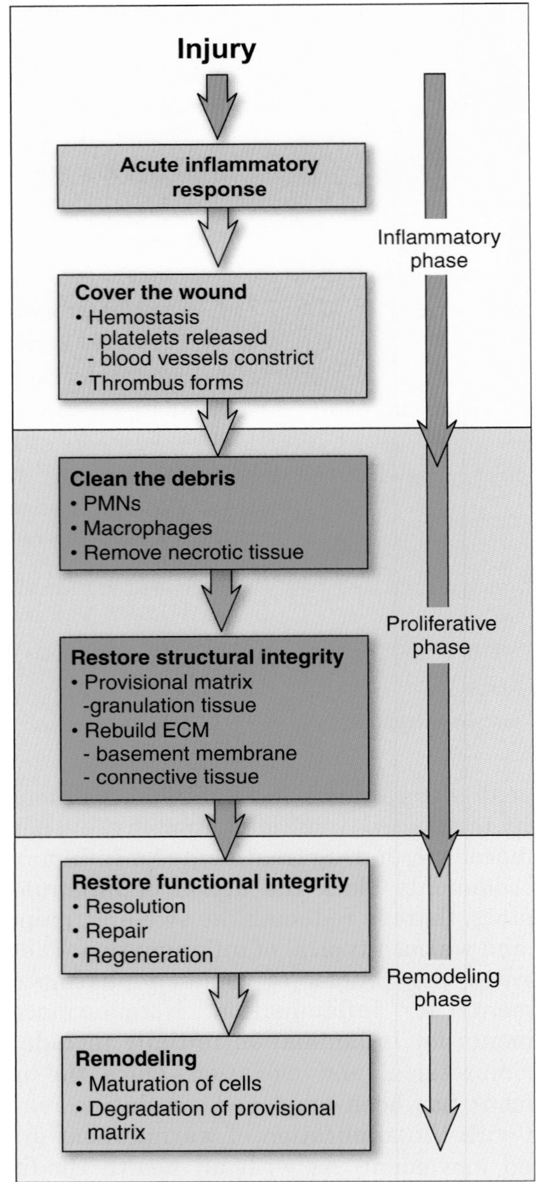

Figure 3.5. Concept map. Phases of healing and tissue repair. ECM, extracellular matrix; PMNs, polymorphonuclear neutrophils.

Sealing the Wound

Inflammatory mediators released from platelets and other cells constrict blood vessels and form a clot at the site. A protective scab is formed from dried blood and exudate. This protective clot and subsequent scab is also called a **thrombus**. The role of the thrombus is to form a physical barrier to prevent additional harmful substances from entering the wound. This covering also prevents the loss of plasma. Epithelial (skin) cells regenerate under the thrombus. Once reepithelialization is complete, enzymes degrade the scab. To see a video on hemostasis, visit thePoint® http://thePoint.lww.com.

Stop and Consider
Why is it not a good idea to pick off a scab before a wound has healed?

Clearing the Debris

Chemical mediators activate neutrophils to move into the injured area and begin the work of healing. The inflammatory response activates neutrophils and later macrophages to engulf, digest, and remove harmful substances and debris. The process of healing cannot begin until the necrotic cells and tissues are removed.

Restoring Structural Integrity

Restoring structural integrity depends on the delicate balance of tissue destruction and construction. Tissue lysis, or breakdown and removal, is accomplished through the work of enzymes that are needed to rid the body of the damaged tissue. Growth factors and matrix proteins are responsible for rebuilding the **extracellular matrix** (ECM), the layers of architectural structures that support the cells.

Extracellular matrices include the basement membrane and connective tissue layers. The basement membrane serves to:

1. Provide a supportive architectural structure
2. Support **reepithelialization**, or the movement of epithelial cells to form a covering over the wound
3. Store growth factors
4. Restore neuromuscular function
5. Support the development of **parenchymal** tissues, that is, those tissues made up of cells with a specific function (such as neurons, myocardial cells, and epithelial cells)

The basement membrane is reproduced by endothelial, epithelial, muscle, adipose (fat), and Schwann (nerve fiber) cells. The basement membrane must be restored before reepithelialization can occur. Extensive damage to the basement membrane is a hindrance to reepithelialization because the basement membrane must be replaced first.

Another structural ECM is connective tissue (Fig. 3.6). The connective tissue layer is composed primarily of collagen, elastin, and glycoproteins. This layer is also referred to as stromal or interstitial tissue. The connective tissue layer provides storage of proteins, an exchange medium between proteins and other cells, and architectural support and physical protection from trauma by resisting stretching or compressing of tissues. Cells such as fibroblasts, adipose cells, endothelial cells, osteocytes, and chondrocytes stimulate the replacement of connective tissue.

Fibroblasts are important cells that produce and replace the connective tissue layer. Fibroblasts are stimulated by macrophages. The fibroblast moves into the area to support the constructive phase of wound healing. Fibroblasts actively manufacture and secrete collagen. **Collagen** helps to fill in the gaps left after the removal of damaged tissues. Excess collagen production leads to tissue fibrosis and can result in scarring at the site of injury.

The connective tissue layer is also composed of elastin and glycoproteins. **Elastin** allows stretching and recoil of tissue. Elastin is resistant to damage, but is also slow and difficult to replace. Damaged

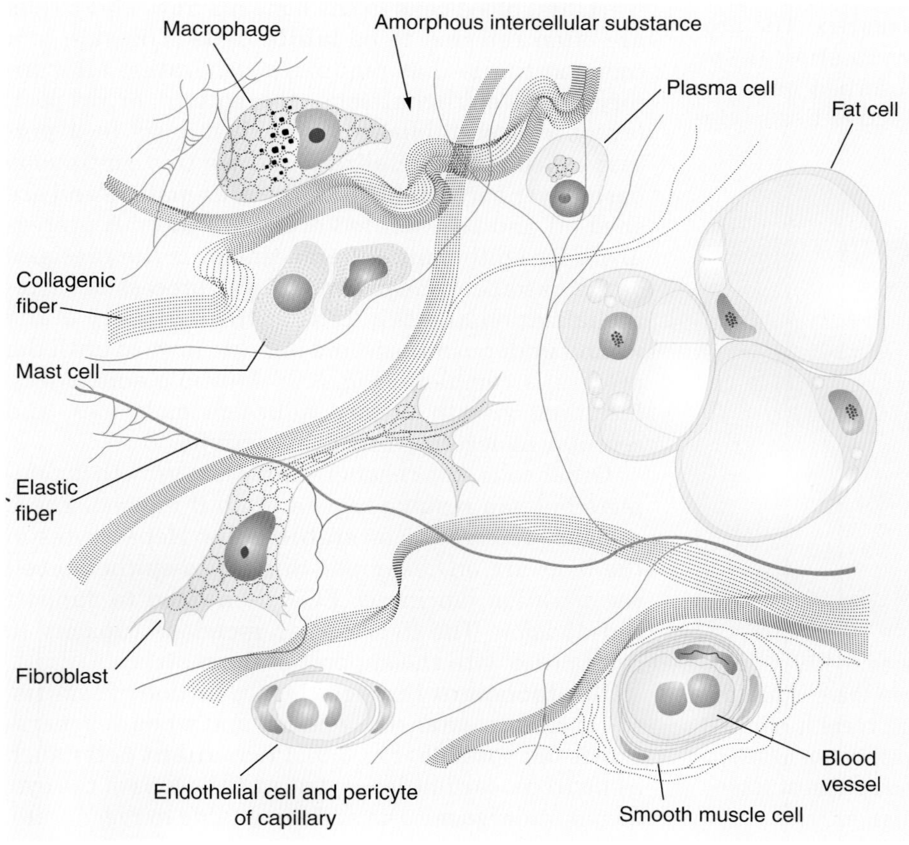

Figure 3.6. Diagram of cells that may be seen in loose connective tissue. The cells lie in the extracellular matrix that is bathed in tissue fluid that originates in capillaries. (From Cormack DH. *Ham's Histology*. 9th ed. Philadelphia, PA: J. B. Lippincott; 1987, with permission.)

tissue is often less flexible after injury. Glycoproteins are essential within the basement membrane and connective tissue layer. **Glycoproteins** regulate cell movement across the matrix, provide a place for attachment of the cells to the matrix, and prompt the cells to function.

Basement membranes and connective tissue layers are continuously present and must be replaced to support architectural structure and tissue function. A third, temporary ECM also forms in response to injury. This temporary matrix, called a **provisional matrix**, promotes healing by decreasing blood and fluid loss at the site and attracting and supporting fibroblasts, endothelial cells, and epidermal (skin) cells. When an injury occurs, increased vascular permeability allows proteins from the plasma to move to the site and form this provisional protective layer.

Macrophage activity converts this provisional matrix into **granulation tissue** (Fig. 3.7). Granulation tissue is connective tissue characterized by extensive macrophages and fibroblasts, and the promotion of **angiogenesis**, or the generation of new blood vessels, at the site. The generation of blood vessels, particularly capillaries, at the site is needed for oxygen/carbon dioxide exchange and to provide other nutrients to the newly developing tissue. Granulation tissue is most noted for the presence of an extensive network of capillaries. As the wound heals, granulation tissue loses the excessive capillary network and retains only that needed to support the final connective tissue matrix. The provisional matrix and specialized granulation tissue are no longer needed and are reabsorbed once the wound is healed and the final connective tissue matrix is in place.

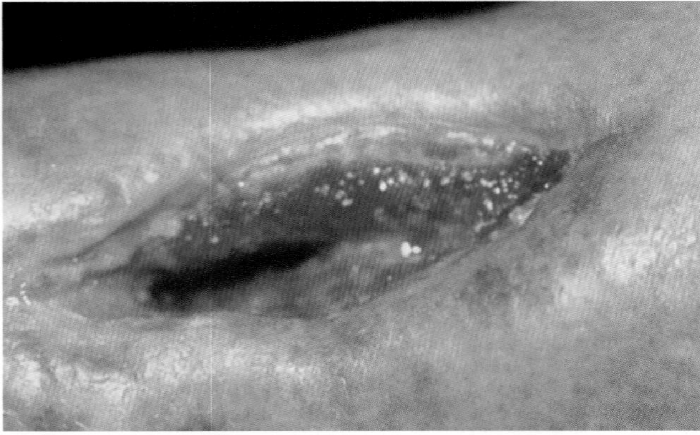

Figure 3.7. Epithelial resurfacing. Note epithelial resurfacing at superior aspect of wound, where there is healthy granulation tissue. At the inferior aspect, there is minimal epithelial resurfacing because of poor quality granulation. At the left side of the wound, there is no epithelial resurfacing because there is no granulation tissue.

Restoring Functional Integrity

A major goal in healing is to restore the functional integrity of parenchymal tissues. Parenchymal tissues are those that perform a specific body function, such as neuronal (brain) tissue, epithelial (skin) tissue, cardiac myocyte (heart) tissue, or hepatocyte (liver) tissue. Without restoring functional integrity, even minor injuries would be problematic. Restoring functional integrity can be accomplished by one of three processes:

1. Resolution
2. Regeneration
3. Replacement. To see a video on wound healing, visit http://thePoint.lww.com thePoint®

Resolution is healing in response to mild injury with minimal disruption to cells, such as with a small superficial scratch or mild sunburn. The epithelial cells basically slough and regenerate without incident. Resolution is like "business as usual." Healing is rapid.

Regeneration of parenchymal tissues can occur only in those cells that undergo mitotic division. This is accomplished through (1) **proliferation** (growth and reproduction), (2) **differentiation** (cells mature and become more specialized), or (3) **diapedesis** (migration of nearby cells). Some cells constantly regenerate through mitosis, particularly epithelial cells of the skin, gastrointestinal tract, and urinary tract, and blood cells in the bone marrow. These cells are often referred to as **labile cells**. The skin is a common tissue that requires regeneration after injury. Basal epithelial cells (the bottom, or deepest, layer) are reestablished through mitosis in a process called reepithelialization. Once this continuous basal layer is reestablished, the cells mature and are shed off and regenerated every few days. A prerequisite for epithelial cell replacement is the presence of the basement membrane. In the process of reepithelialization, the skin cells at the periphery of the wound undergo mitosis and migrate inward until the process is complete (Fig. 3.8). Multiple substances, including growth factors, adhesion molecules, and receptor molecules, direct this activity.

Other cells stop regenerating when growth is complete but can resume regeneration if injured. These cells are referred to as **stable cells**. Hepatocytes in the liver are one example. Similar to epithelial cell regeneration, an intact ECM is needed to support cell division. The liver has tremendous capacity to regenerate with the support of the matrix.

Replacement through the production of scar tissue occurs in extensive wounds and when regeneration is not possible (Fig. 3.9). **Permanent cells**, such as neurons, cardiac myocytes, and the lens of the eye, do not undergo mitosis and are unable to regenerate.

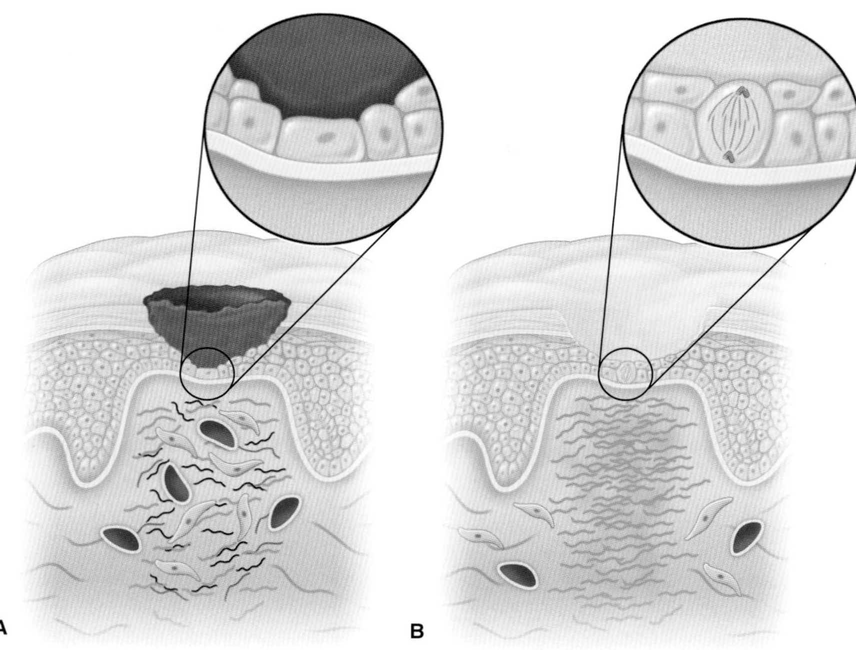

Figure 3.8. Regeneration and migration of epidermal cells. **A:** The migration of epidermal cells, sustained by the mitotic activity of neighboring cells, fills the wound gap and displaces the scab. **B:** The gap created by the wound has been repaired. The mitotic activity of the epidermal cells will restore the epidermal thickness. (Modified from Rubin E, Farber JL. *Pathology*. 4th ed. Philadelphia, PA: Lippincott Williams & Wilkins; 2005, with permission.)

When permanent cells are damaged, the functional tissue is replaced with connective tissue. For example, if neuronal tissue of the brain is destroyed by a brain tumor, the neurons do not regenerate, and the damaged area of the brain does not function as it had prior to the injury. Connective tissue, or scar tissue, can also replace labile or stable cells if the injury and subsequent damage is extensive. For example, in a severe burn that covers a large area of the body, connective scar tissue will replace the epithelial tissues of the skin. The scar tissue fills in the gap but does not function as the parenchymal tissue.

Conditions That Promote Wound Healing

Wound healing requires certain conditions. Promotion of wound healing depends primarily on adequacy of the vascular and cellular inflammatory responses, reformation of the ECM (including collagen deposition), and regeneration of those cells capable of mitosis.

These processes are enhanced and supported by an adequate dietary intake of water, proteins, carbohydrates, fats, vitamins, and minerals. The most beneficial of these nutrients are proteins and vitamins, particularly vitamins A and C. Proteins are needed during every phase of repair, including ECM regeneration and angiogenesis. Vitamins A and C are needed for reepithelialization and collagen synthesis. Adequate blood flow is also needed to transport inflammatory cells and products of healing to the injured site and to oxygenate cells and tissues.

Stop and Consider
What did you eat and drink yesterday? What nutrients did you consume that would promote wound healing?

Healing by Intention

Wounds that are smaller with approximated wound edges will heal much more quickly and easily than wounds that are large and craterlike. Approximated wound edges are those that are "lined up" or close together, such as that which occurs with a paper cut or a surgical incision. These wounds heal by **primary intention**. When healing occurs by primary intention, the wound is basically closed with all areas of the wound connecting and healing simultaneously. The risk for infection is reduced and scarring is minimal.

Larger, open, craterlike wounds must heal by **secondary intention**. These wounds heal from the bottom up. The process is much slower and more involved than the primary intention process. Healing by secondary intention results in a greater risk for infection and scarring. Figure 3.10 compares healing by primary intention with healing by secondary intention.

Stop and Consider
How does the concept of healing by primary or secondary intention compare to the body's three lines of defense?

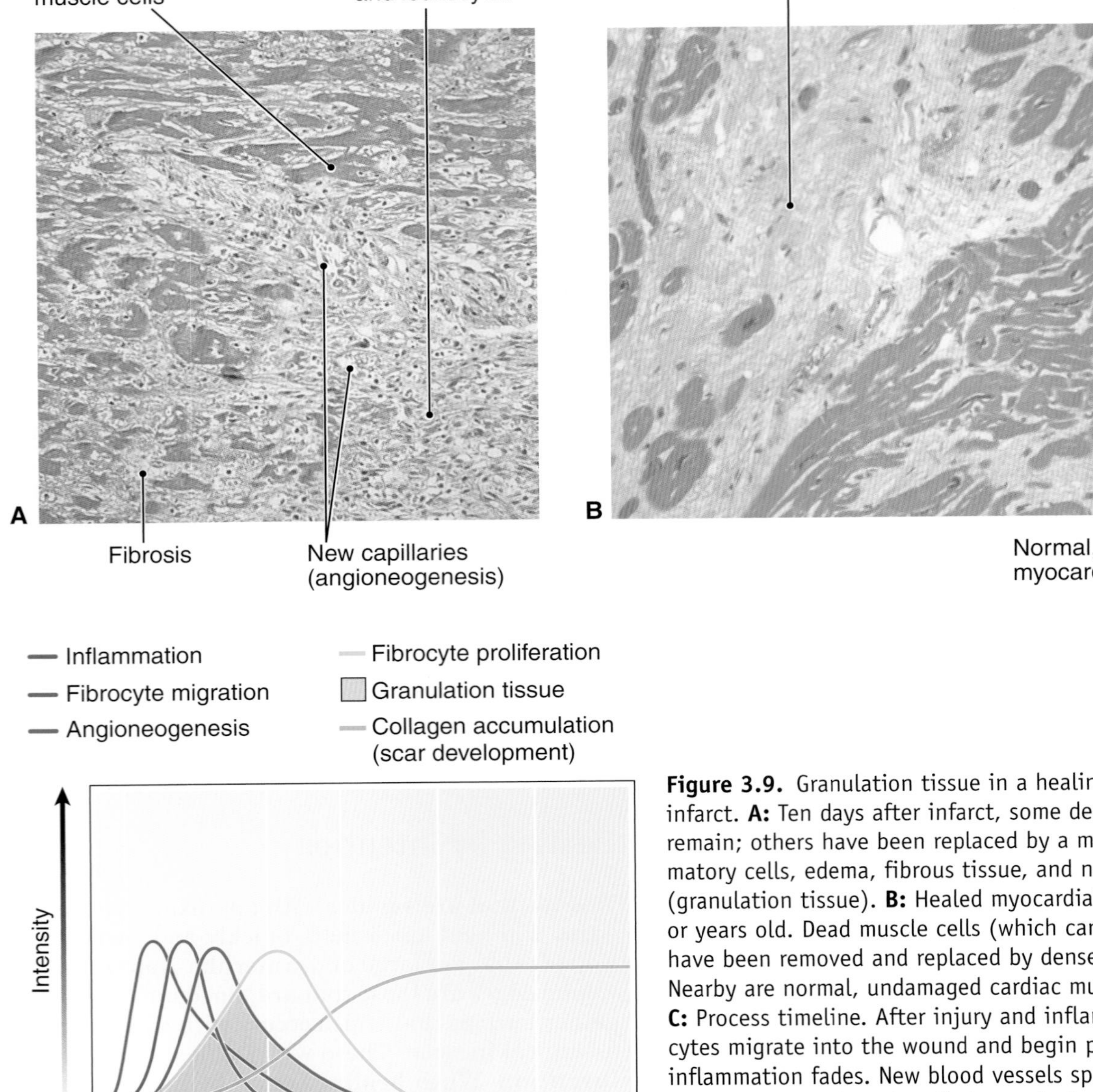

Figure 3.9. Granulation tissue in a healing myocardial infarct. **A:** Ten days after infarct, some dead muscle cells remain; others have been replaced by a mixture of inflammatory cells, edema, fibrous tissue, and new blood vessels (granulation tissue). **B:** Healed myocardial infarct, months or years old. Dead muscle cells (which cannot regenerate) have been removed and replaced by dense scar tissue. Nearby are normal, undamaged cardiac muscle cells. **C:** Process timeline. After injury and inflammation, fibrocytes migrate into the wound and begin proliferating as inflammation fades. New blood vessels sprout and form a rich fibrovascular mix called granulation tissue, which fades as collagen deposited by fibrocytes accumulates as a scar.

COMPLICATIONS OF HEALING AND TISSUE REPAIR

Impaired wound healing can occur at any point in the process of closing the wound, clearing the debris, and restoring structural and functional integrity. Primary factors that impact wound healing are an ineffective inflammatory response, inadequate immune response, inadequate nutritional status, and poor tissue perfusion. Common complications of wound healing include:

- Infection
- Ulceration
- Dehiscence
- Keloid development
- Adhesions

Infection (Chapter 5) refers to invasion by microorganisms. Destroying the first line of defense, along with many other factors, such as a poor inflammatory and immune response, will promote infection and ultimately impair wound healing. As mentioned, tissue healing also requires adequate **perfusion** (passage of oxygenated blood) to the site. Poor perfusion can lead to ulceration. **Ulcers** are circumscribed, open, craterlike lesion of the skin or mucous membranes. These areas are necrotic and

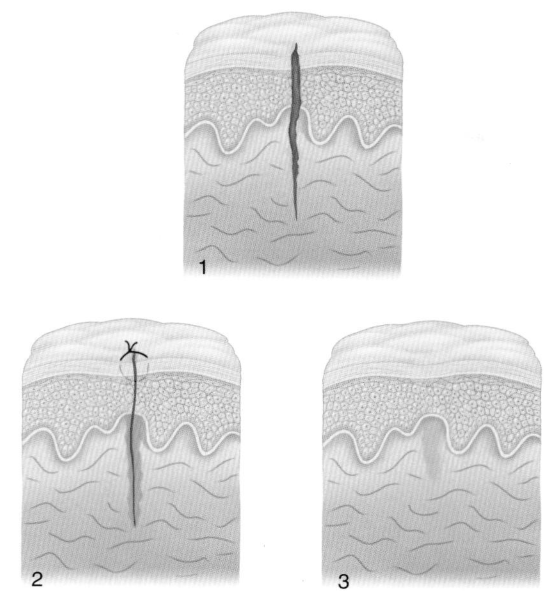

A Healing by primary intention (wounds with approximated edges)

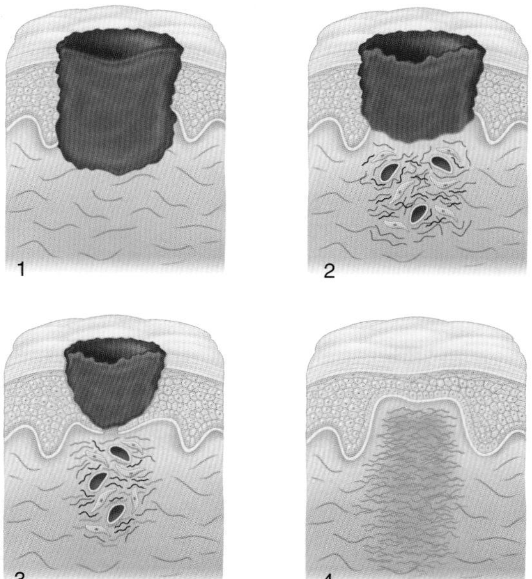

B Healing by secondary intention (wounds with separated edges)

Figure 3.10. Comparison of healing by primary versus secondary intention. **A:** Healing by primary intention. **A1:** A wound with closely approximated edges and minimal tissue loss. **A2:** Such a wound requires minimal cell proliferation and neovascularization to heal. **A3:** The result is a small scar. **B:** Healing by secondary intention. **B1:** A wound in which the edges are far apart with substantial tissue loss. **B2:** This wound requires extensive cell proliferation and granulation tissue to heal. **B3:** The wound is reepithelialized from the margins, and collagen fibers are deposited into the granulation tissue. **B4:** Granulation tissue is eventually reabsorbed and replaced by a large scar. (Modified from Rubin E, Farber JL. *Pathology*. 4th ed. Philadelphia, PA: Lippincott Williams & Wilkins; 2005, with permission.)

open to further invasion by microorganisms. Ulcers are often resistant to healing because of the lack of perfusion to the site and persistent habitation by microorganisms. Ulcers are a common complication of gastritis, one of the clinical models in this chapter.

Wound **dehiscence** is a problem of deficient scar formation, in which the wound splits or bursts open, often at a suture line. Wound separation, like ulceration, opens the area to invasion by microorganisms. This is a possible complication early after surgery because of mechanical stresses put on the wound during movement or coughing. Poor development of the ECM and ineffective or inadequate collagen is often the cause of wound dehiscence later in the recovery period.

Keloid development is the opposite of dehiscence. **Keloids** are hypertrophic scars that result from excessive collagen production at the site of injury (Fig. 3.11). Keloids occur with higher frequency in those with deeply pigmented skin and tend to develop in those between the ages of 10 and 30 years with a familial disposition to developing keloids. Keloids are often seen only as a cosmetic problem, but these large areas of scarring represent ineffective healing at the site. Attempts at removal of the keloid often result in another keloid forming in the same location.

Adhesions are also a problem with collagen deposition. Collagen fibers can develop and form adhesions with injuries located in or nearby serous (watery) body cavities, such as the peritoneum (inner lining of the abdomen). **Adhesions** are fibrous connections between serous cavities and nearby tissues, which do not allow the surrounding tissues to move freely. Abdominal surgery presents an increased risk for adhesion development. The collagen fibers connect to organs within the peritoneum, such as the bowel, bladder, and ovaries. Adhesions restrict free movement of the organ and cause pain and loss of organ function.

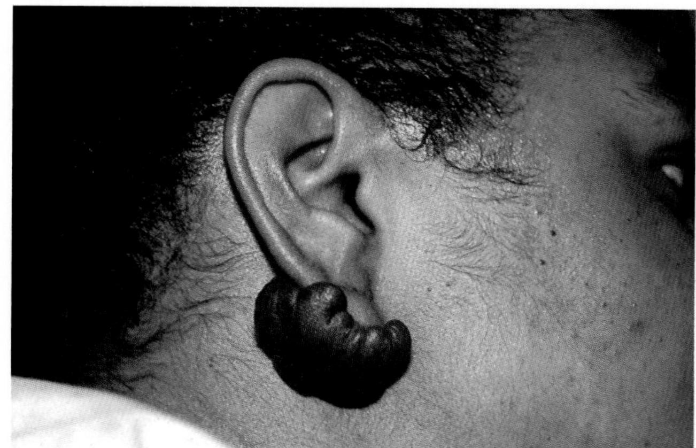

Figure 3.11. Keloid. This woman developed a keloid as a reaction to having her earlobe pierced. (Modified from Rubin E, Farber JL. *Pathology*. 4th ed. Philadelphia, PA: Lippincott Williams & Wilkins; 2005, with permission.)

Module 3 Chronic Inflammation

Chronic inflammation represents a persistent or recurrent state of inflammation lasting several weeks or longer. This state occurs when the acute inflammatory and immune responses are unsuccessful. Chronic inflammation can be related to an unrelenting injury, persistent infectious process, or an autoimmune condition. Autoimmunity occurs when the immune system identifies self-cells as "foreign" and attacks these cells (Chapter 4). Often, injuries or infections that cause chronic inflammation are subtle and slow-growing. Chronic inflammation differs from acute inflammation in many ways, as illustrated in Table 3.6.

Table 3.6 Comparison of Acute and Chronic Inflammation

Characteristic	Acute Inflammation	Chronic Inflammation
Time	Resolution within a few weeks	Present for a prolonged period of time, usually greater than 6 months
Chief phagocytic cells	Neutrophils	Monocytes Macrophages Lymphocytes
Restoration	Minimal scarring	Marked by fibrosis, scarring, or granuloma formation

Cells of Chronic Inflammation

Cellular activity is notably different between acute and chronic inflammation. The longer-lasting activity of monocytes, macrophages, and lymphocytes is more prominent in chronic inflammation. Monocytes circulate in the blood to the site of injury and mature into macrophages in the tissues. As monocytes mature into macrophages, they produce **proteinases** and fibroblasts. Proteinases are enzymes that destroy elastin and other tissue components. These enzymes help to break down dead tissue; unfortunately, these enzymes do not discriminate. Proteinase activity is responsible for ongoing tissue destruction at and surrounding the site of the persistent injury. Fibroblasts are also active in chronic inflammation. Fibroblasts are responsible for collagen development, which contributes to the extensive scarring characteristic of chronic inflammation. Scarring leads to permanent loss of function and deformity of the tissue or organ.

Granuloma Formation

In some cases, chronic inflammation results in **granuloma** formation (Fig. 3.12). Granulomas are nodular inflammatory lesions that encase harmful substances. Granuloma formation is also regulated by macrophages. Granulomas typically form when the injury is too difficult to control by the usual inflammatory and immune mechanisms, such as with foreign bodies or certain microorganisms. One classic example of a microorganism that results in granuloma formation is *Mycobacterium tuberculosis*, the bacteria responsible for tuberculosis infection (Chapter 5).

By forming granulomas, macrophages protect healthy, unaffected surrounding tissue from further damage. Macrophages adapt into **giant cells** or **epithelioid cells**. Giant cells are phagocytes that can engulf particles much larger than the typical macrophage. Epithelioid cells gather and contain smaller substances by forming a wall, or fibrotic granuloma, around the affected area. Inside the wall, macrophages are busy phagocytizing harmful substances. As a result, necrosis fills the inside of the granuloma. Gradually, the necrosis diffuses through the granuloma wall and a fibrotic capsule remains.

GENERAL MANIFESTATIONS

The general manifestations of chronic inflammation can be similar to those of acute inflammation during a flare-up of symptoms, such as redness, heat, pain, swelling, and loss of function. These symptoms may lead to scarring in the affected area or granuloma formation, as discussed earlier. Other systemic manifestations associated with chronic inflammation may include fever, malaise, anemia, fatigue, anorexia, weight loss, or weakness. Remission of the chronic inflammation can occur in some conditions; during these times, the patient will have no symptoms.

TREATMENT

The treatment of chronic inflammation is aimed at removing the source of injury if possible and managing symptoms. Long-term use of anti-inflammatory, analgesic, or immune-modifying

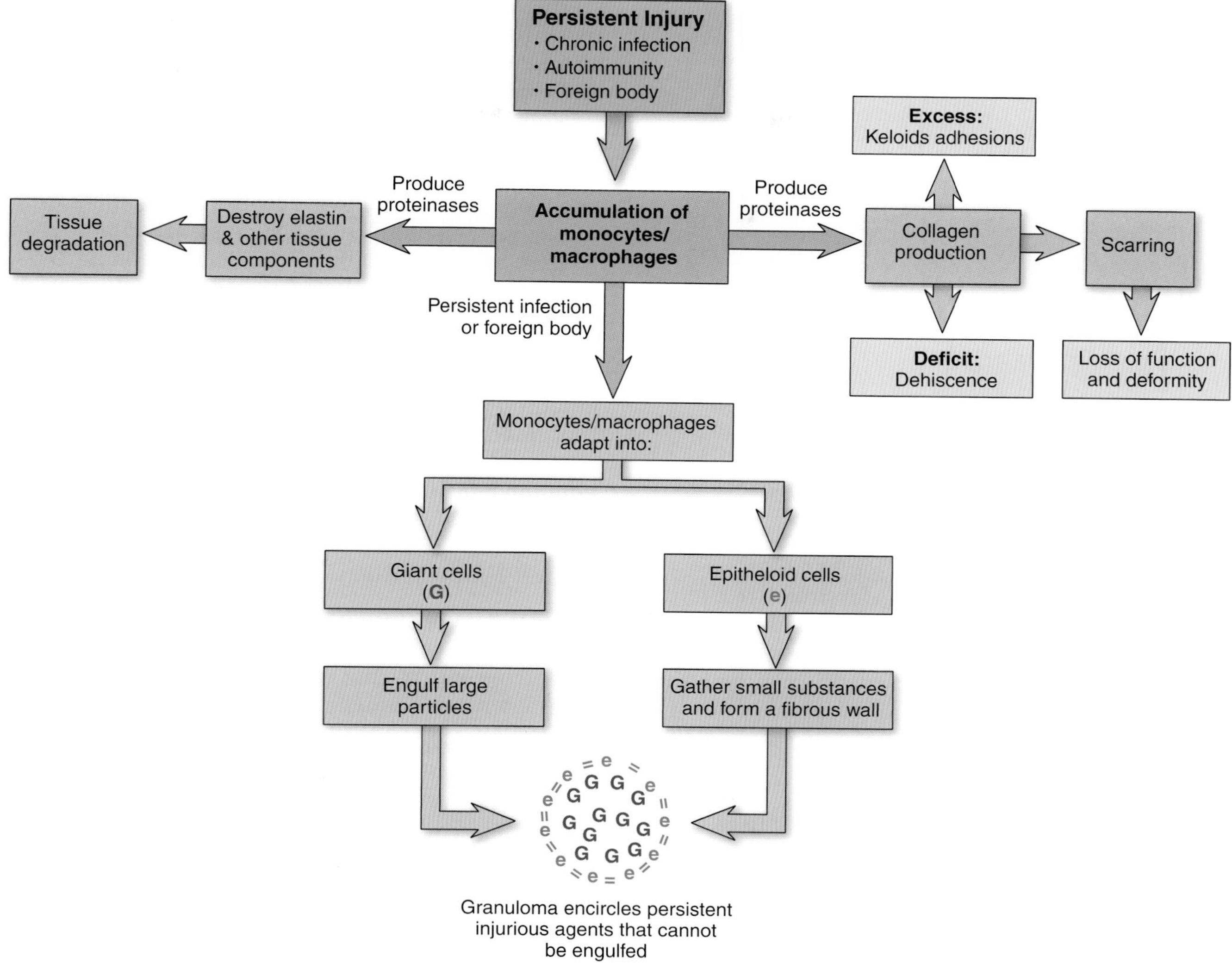

Figure 3.12. Concept map. The process of chronic inflammation leading to granuloma formation.

drugs is often needed. Chronic infections as a source of chronic inflammation would be treated with antimicrobial drugs (Chapter 5). Nonpharmacologic treatments are important as well, such as the use of heat or cold, immobilization, dietary changes, exercise/physical therapy, and rest. Complementary therapies, such as homeopathic preparations, acupuncture, and guided imagery, should also be explored with patients and monitored for safety and effectiveness.

Module 4 Applied Pathophysiology Clinical Models

The following clinical models have been selected to aid in the understanding and application of inflammatory processes. When reading about the clinical models, visualize the process of acute versus chronic inflammation and healing and note the commonalities and unique features of each model.

Sinusitis

Sinusitis, also known as rhinosinusitis, refers to symptomatic inflammation of the paranasal sinuses and nasal cavity. About 1 in 8 US adults have sinusitis, resulting in more than 20% of antibiotic

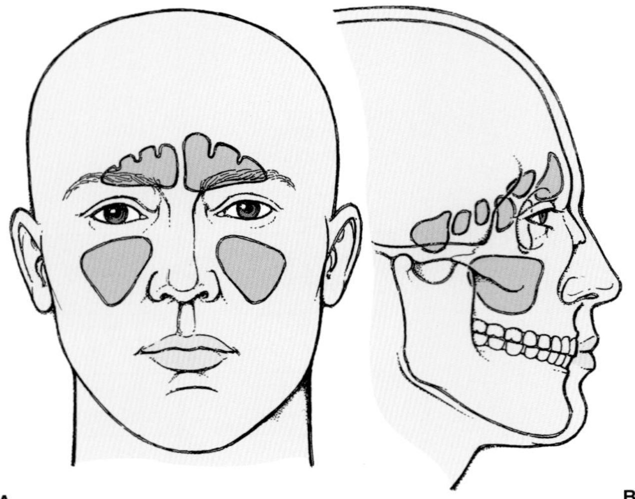

Figure 3.13. Paranasal sinuses: anterior **(A)** and lateral **(B)** views of head.

prescriptions.[3] Children average around 6 to 8 upper respiratory tract infections (the common cold) per year, with around 10% of these further complicated by acute bacterial sinusitis. Sinusitis can be either acute or chronic.

FUNCTIONS OF THE SINUSES

Figure 3.13 depicts the paranasal sinuses, open spaces lined with protective mucosa, composed of ciliated, pseudostratified columnar epithelial cells interspersed with goblet cells. Goblet cells are responsible for secreting mucins, which is the main component of mucus. The main function of sinuses is to produce mucus that moisturizes and protects the inside of the nose. Although the nasal cavity is usually colonized with bacteria, the sinuses are most often sterile.

ACUTE SINUSITIS

Acute sinusitis is inflammation of the lining of the paranasal sinuses lasting 4 to 8 weeks. Subacute sinusitis lasts 8 to 12 weeks. Recurrent acute sinusitis occurs when the patient has up to four episodes per year, with the sinus inflammation resolving completely between episodes.

Pathophysiology

Sinuses produce secretions, which normally flow in one direction toward the ostia. The ostia provide outflow of the drainage and prevent backflow and contamination of the sinuses. If the ostia and outflow of mucus are blocked, most often because of allergy, viruses, or some other form of irritation, this can result in sinusitis. Secondly, as the nasal cavity is not sterile, impaired clearance of the mucus by protective cilia or altered mucus quality or quantity can also lead to sinusitis. Patients with cystic fibrosis and chronic respiratory allergies are at higher risk for sinusitis because of chronic nasal inflammation, changes in mucus, and mucociliary clearance issues.

The primary etiology for acute sinusitis is viral infections transmitted via respiratory droplets from person to person. The most frequently implicated viruses are rhinovirus, adenovirus, coronaviruses, parainfluenza, and the influenza A and B viruses. The presence of bacterial sinusitis is often a complication of overwhelming viral infection, which has caused increased mucus secretion, obstruction, and impaired mucociliary clearance. Other conditions that predispose to bacterial infection include respiratory allergy, facial injury, dental infections, or immunodeficiency/immunosuppression. On rare occasions, sinusitis can be the result of fungal invasion.

Clinical Manifestations

Clinical manifestations for acute sinusitis are related to the congestion of sinuses with excessive, obstructed mucus and inflammation. These clinical manifestations include:

- Facial pain over the sinus regions of the face increasing with straining or bending down (can be unilateral)
- Fever
- Nasal congestion and/or excessive nasal discharge and postnasal drainage
- Persistent cough
- Fatigue

Diagnostic Criteria

The diagnosis of acute sinusitis is often made through physical examination, revealing the clinical manifestations above, following an upper respiratory infection that has lasted greater than 10 days. General laboratory tests for inflammation or infection, such as ESR, CRP, and WBC counts, can be used, but are nonspecific.

Sinus radiographs may be helpful when the diagnosis is in question. X-rays reveal opaque, mucus-filled, thickened sinuses (Fig. 3.14).

Treatment

The primary goal of treatment is to eliminate the infection and care for the symptoms of sinusitis. Approximately 40% of acute sinusitis cases resolve spontaneously without antibiotics.[3] However, for patients without spontaneous resolution, appropriate antibiotics are needed for 14 to 21 days. Antihistamine (in respiratory allergy) and decongestant medications may be helpful. Nasal sprays that promote

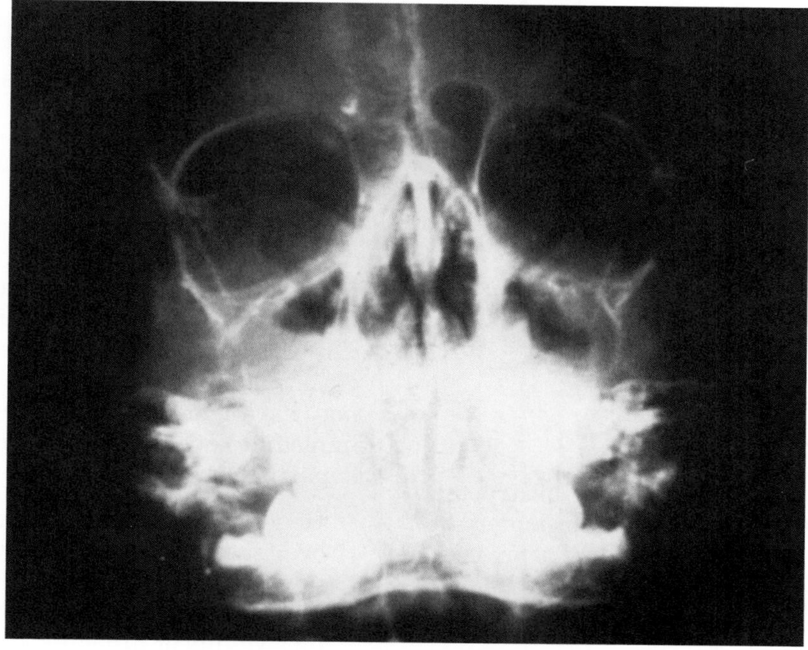

Figure 3.14. Maxillary sinusitis. This radiograph demonstrates bilateral maxillary sinusitis. There is an air–fluid level present in the right maxillary sinus and an example of mucosal swelling demonstrated in the left maxillary sinus.

vasoconstriction, such as oxymetazoline hydrochloride, should be used only up to 5 days. Otherwise, the patient could experience rebound nasal congestion and swelling.

Further evaluation is warranted if the clinical manifestations of sinusitis persist beyond antibiotic treatment or if there are episodes of recurrence. If antibiotic therapy has failed and thick, purulent sinus secretions persist, sinuses can be more aggressively treated surgically.

Chronic Sinusitis

Chronic sinusitis is a persistent low-grade inflammation of the paranasal sinuses lasting over 12 weeks with or without flares of acute sinusitis. Chronic sinusitis can occur with or without nasal polyps or as an allergic or fungal disease. Risk factors include[4]:

- Anatomic abnormalities of the ostiomeatal complex (e.g., septal deviation)
- Allergic rhinitis
- Aspirin sensitivity
- Asthma
- Nasal polyps
- Nonallergic rhinitis (e.g., vasomotor rhinitis, cocaine abuse)
- Defects in mucociliary clearance
- Nasotracheal intubation
- Nasogastric intubation
- Hormonal (e.g., puberty, pregnancy, oral contraception)
- Obstruction by tumor
- Immunodeficiency
- Cystic fibrosis
- Primary ciliary dyskinesia, Kartagener syndrome
- Wegener granulomatosis
- Repeated viral upper respiratory tract infections
- Smoking
- Environmental irritants and pollutants
- Periodontitis/significant dental disease

Similar to acute sinusitis, chronic sinusitis often begins as stasis of secretions inside the sinuses, which can be triggered by obstruction of the ostia or mucosal edema. Most cases of chronic sinusitis are due to acute sinusitis that either is untreated or does not respond to treatment.

PATHOPHYSIOLOGY

Currently, chronic sinusitis is thought to be a multifactorial inflammatory disease combining environmental factors, such as persistent infection or allergens, with genetic factors, such as metabolic abnormalities or immune deficiencies. These multifactorial triggers or risk factors, when present, disrupt mucociliary clearance and result in mucus stagnation, creating an environment conducive to bacterial growth and chronic inflammation in the sinuses.

CLINICAL MANIFESTATIONS

In contrast to acute sinusitis where facial pain and fever are common manifestations, chronic sinusitis is much more insidious in its onset. The common clinical manifestations include:

- Nasal congestion
- Nasal and postnasal discharge
- Sore throat
- Foul breath, unpleasant taste
- Low-grade fever
- Fatigue, anorexia
- Chronic cough
- **Hyposmia**, the reduced ability to smell
- Facial fullness, discomfort, pain, and headache (with polyps)

DIAGNOSTIC CRITERIA

Diagnosis is based on a persistence of obstructed and mucus-filled sinuses over 12 weeks or longer. At least two of the following symptoms must be present:

- Anterior or posterior mucopurulent drainage
- Nasal obstruction
- Facial pain, pressure, fullness
- Hyposmia

These must be accompanied by the presence of chronic inflammation, resulting in at least one of the following:

- Purulent mucus or edema in the middle meatus or ethmoid region
- Polyps in the nasal cavity or middle meatus

The above findings are confirmed by the presence of mucosal thickening, changes to the surrounding bones, and/or changes in air–fluid levels visualized via CT scan.

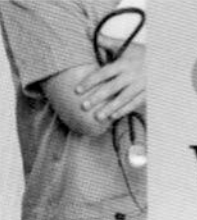

CLINICAL PRACTICE

When to Seek Medical Care

Clinicians should advise patients to call a doctor when experiencing pain or pressure in the upper face accompanied by nasal congestion or discharge, postnasal drip, fever for several days, or ongoing bad breath unrelated to dental problems. If left untreated, complications of sinusitis can occur that may lead to severe medical conditions. If you have the following symptoms, you may have a medical emergency and should seek immediate evaluation in a hospital's emergency department:

- Headache and fever with soft tissue swelling over the frontal sinus may indicate an infection of the frontal bone.
- Severe pain when moving the eye, fever, eyelid swelling or drooping, or vision changes due to infection in the eye socket as a result of ethmoid sinusitis; permanent blindness can result.
- Severe pain in the eye, one or both dilated pupils, fever, eyelid swelling, or vision changes can also be related to a blood clot in the sinuses.
- Personality changes, headache, neck stiffness, high fever, altered consciousness, visual problems, or seizures are signs that the sinusitis has penetrated the meninges of the central nervous systems (meningitis), which is a medical emergency.

TREATMENT

The goals of treatment are to reduce mucosal swelling, promote sinus drainage, and clear any infections that may be present. This often means that the patient will need a combination of glucocorticoids (oral or topical through a nasal spray), antibiotics, and nasal saline irrigation. If these treatments are ineffective, a referral to an otolaryngologist for consideration of sinus surgery is warranted. If the chronic disease is severe, if there are orbital or intracranial complications, or if the patient is immunocompromised, hospitalization is required.

Burn Injuries

Every year in the United States, burns cause 2 million injuries, with over 5,000 of these resulting in death.[5] The most common causes include fire/flame exposure (46%), scalding (32%), hot object contact (8%), electrical burns (4%), and chemical burns (3%). Burn injuries cause an inflammatory response locally and can have major systematic effects as well.

FUNCTIONS OF THE SKIN

The skin serves as an important barrier between the body and the external environment. It is composed of the dermis, which is a dense, irregular connective tissue, and the epidermis, a layer of epithelial tissue. The epidermis and dermis are separated by the basement membrane. The skin protects internal structures from invasion by infectious or harmful agents and mechanical damage. The skin prevents dehydration, regulates body temperature, and produces vitamin D. Understanding the vital function of the skin is important because loss of function is a critical manifestation of inflammatory processes.

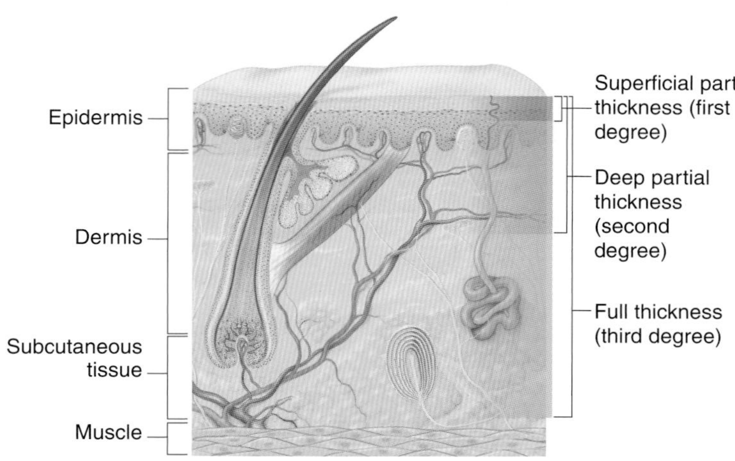

Figure 3.15. Classification of burns by depth of injury. Superficial partial-thickness burns enter the epidermis. Deep partial-thickness burns penetrate the epidermis and dermal layers. Full-thickness burns penetrate all skin layers and can progress to underlying structures as well. (Courtesy Anatomical Chart Company.)

BURNS

Pathophysiology

Burns can result from thermal injury, electrical injury, caustic chemical injury, radiation exposure, or inhalation of noxious fumes. In thermal injuries, higher temperature and increased length of heat exposure increase the severity of the burn. Temperatures above 45°C (113°F) cause proteins to denature, and irreversible cellular damage occurs. The extent of damage from chemical injuries depends on the toxicity of the chemical, location of exposure (particularly in the eyes, respiratory tract, or gastrointestinal tract), and length of exposure. Electrical injuries follow the path of least resistance in the body, that is, along tissue, fluids, blood vessels, and nerves. Serious electrical trauma results from the electrical current passing through vital organs, nerves, and blood vessels. Electrical currents can disrupt cardiac conduction and cause immediate death.

With all burns, the injury triggers an acute inflammatory response. The extent and nature of the inflammation, along with corresponding clinical manifestations, diagnostic criteria, and treatment, primarily depend on the surface area that is affected as well as the depth of the burn injury (Fig. 3.15).

Superficial partial-thickness burns, also known as first-degree burns, damage the epidermis. Mild sunburn is one example. This radiation-induced injury triggers vasodilation of the dermal blood vessels and increased capillary permeability, causing erythema, pain, and swelling of affected areas. Superficial partial-thickness burns do not result in cell necrosis or scarring. The ECM generally remains intact, allowing uneventful healing of superficial partial-thickness burns as endothelial and epithelial cells rapidly regenerate. Healing occurs within a week.

Deep partial-thickness burns, also known as second-degree burns, damage epidermal skin layers and penetrate some dermal skin layers. Scalding with hot liquids, more severe sunburn, mild to moderate chemical burns, or flash flame exposure can lead to deep partial-thickness burns. Epidermal and dermal layers separate, fluid accumulates between these layers, and blisters form (Fig. 3.16). A loss of function of the skin as the first line of defense allows microorganisms to invade the tissue. If necrosis occurs in the upper epidermal cell layers but the basal cell layer remains intact, scarring is avoided. More commonly, however, necrosis results in both epidermal and upper dermal layers. Collagen fills in the gaps left after the removal of damaged tissues. Excess collagen production often leads to tissue fibrosis and scarring at the burn site. The process of healing occurs within approximately 2 to 4 weeks.

Full-thickness burns, also known as third-degree burns, damage the epidermis and dermis and can penetrate subcutaneous layers as well. Contact

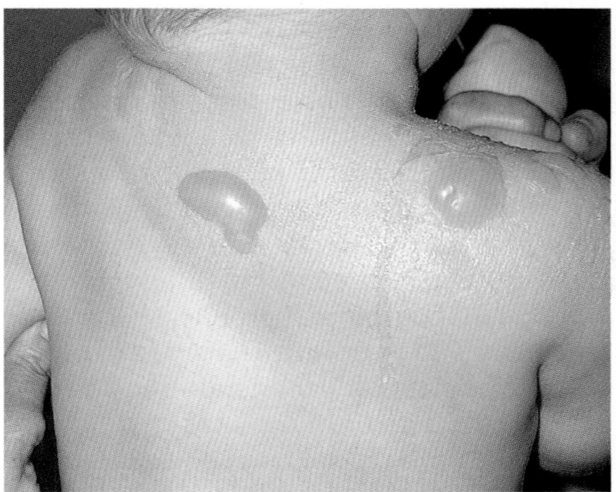

Figure 3.16. Deep partial-thickness (second-degree) sunburn. Epidermal and dermal layers separate, fluid accumulates between the layers, and blisters form. (From Fleisher GR, Ludwig S, Baskin MN. *Atlas of Pediatric Emergency Medicine*. Philadelphia, PA: Lippincott Williams & Wilkins; 2004, with permission.)

with extremely hot objects, exposure to a flame, electrical exposures, and caustic chemicals are likely to result in full-thickness burns. The severity depends on the temperature or type of chemical and the length of exposure. Destruction of blood vessels is also common as heat cauterizes the vessels. The healing of full-thickness burns is challenged by extensive loss of elastin, replacement of skin cells with collagen, and invasion by microorganisms. Regeneration of epithelial cells is impaired because of destruction of the ECM. Scarring is often extensive. Loss of elasticity is evidenced by **contractures**, areas of thick, shortened, and rigid tissue.

Stop and Consider

Hematocrit is a laboratory test that indicates the percentage of RBCs in a designated volume of blood. Would an individual with partial-thickness and full-thickness burns covering 20% body surface area have a decrease or increase in this laboratory value? What would be the impact of this change?

The loss of skin function results in multiple potential complications, particularly in severe burn injuries, defined as full-thickness burns covering greater than 20% of the adult body surface area, including:

1. Body fluid shifts that cause impaired blood circulation, edema, and dehydration
2. Microorganism invasion that leads to infection
3. Overwhelming metabolic demands that increase the risk for malnutrition
4. Problems with temperature regulation

In widespread inflammation, impaired blood circulation and cellular dehydration can result as fluids shift from cells and blood vessels into the tissues (edema). This is due to massive capillary permeability and direct damage to blood vessels at the site of the burn injury (Fig. 3.17). In patients with full-thickness burns, water loss is extensive: Approximately 0.3 mL of body water per square centimeter is lost per day. When full-thickness burns cover 70% of the body, extensive fluid shifts out of the blood vessels and swells into the tissues, resulting in severe hypovolemia (low fluid volume in the blood vessels). The blood becomes viscous (thick), heat converts RBCs from a concave to a spherical shape, and the flow of blood is altered. At the local site of the burn, **thrombi**, or clots, can develop, oxygenated blood flow is restricted, and necrosis can develop as the burned tissue becomes hypoxic. An inadequate amount of blood in the circulation leads to **shock**, a state of inadequate perfusion (oxygenated blood flow) to peripheral tissues. Poor perfusion is particularly problematic in vital organs, which require a constant flow of oxygen to survive. In partial-thickness burns, capillary permeability is

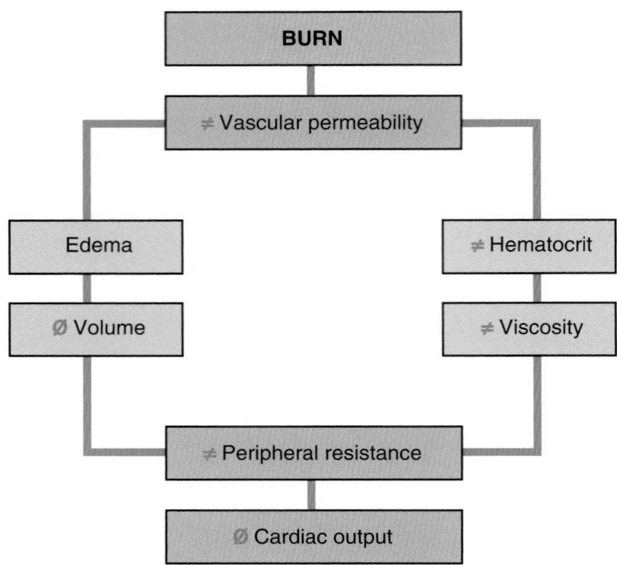

Figure 3.17. Hemodynamic changes in burn injury. (From Nettina S. *The Lippincott Manual of Nursing Practice*. 7th ed. Philadelphia, PA: Lippincott Williams & Wilkins; 2001, with permission.)

restored after 24 to 48 hours and interstitial fluid shifts decrease after this time. This allows the volume of fluid in the blood vessels needed for optimal circulation.

The loss of skin function as a result of burn injuries also allows for ready access for microorganisms and stresses the metabolic and reparative processes of the body. Burns covering a larger surface area pose a greater risk for the development of **sepsis**, which is a bacterial infection of the blood, and septic shock. In full-thickness burns, dead tissue and exudate convert into an **eschar**, which is a thick, coagulated crust. The eschar must be surgically removed to prevent extensive microorganism growth. Energy, protein, and oxygen use are also increased because of the extensive reparative processes required in substantial burn injuries. If these increasing needs are not met, tissue hypoxia, tissue wasting, and infection are the potential results.

CLINICAL MANIFESTATIONS

Clinical manifestations primarily depend on the depth of the burn injury. Superficial partial-thickness burns result in erythema, warmth, pain, swelling, and loss of function of affected areas. Deep partial-thickness burns lead to blistering, along with erythema, warmth, pain, edema, and **serous exudate**, which is a clear fluid that seeps out of the tissues. Erythema, eschar formation, edema, and exudate characterize full-thickness burns. Full-thickness burns destroy nerve endings, sweat glands, and hair follicles. Destruction of nerve endings

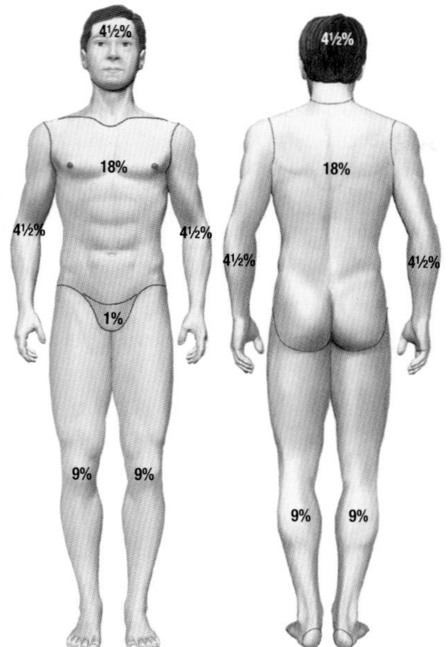

Figure 3.18. Rule of nines. Estimating the extent of burns in adults. (Courtesy Anatomical Chart Company.)

inhibits the pain response in areas where the burn has penetrated all skin layers. The individual with a full-thickness burn is not pain free, however. Areas of deep and superficial thickness burns, like a bull's eye, often surround full-thickness burns. Pain is notable in these surrounding tissues.

DIAGNOSTIC CRITERIA

Wound depths (superficial, deep partial, or full thickness) are classified according to the affected tissue layers. Surface area is also a significant variable in determining the diagnosis and treatment of a burn injury. Calculation of adult body surface area is aided using the "rule of nines" depicted in Figure 3.18. For children under 5 years, body proportions do not match that of the adult. For example, although the trunk and arms are similar in proportion to the adult, the infant's head and neck make up 18% of total body surface area, and each lower extremity accounts for 14%. Health care professionals who treat childhood burns should refer to a "modified rule of nines" appropriate for the specific age of the child.

Estimation of the rule of nines, along with a determination of the thickness of the burn, allows the health professional to determine the severity of the injury and direct treatment. The American Burn Association has published criteria for distinguishing minor, moderate, and major burns (Table 3.7).

TREATMENT

Initial treatment for minor and moderate burns requires removing the source of injury and stopping the burning process. Chemical burns should be flushed with copious amounts of water. In minor burns, the wound is cleansed with tepid sterile saline (cool but not cold) or water. In some cases, the wound is covered with an antimicrobial ointment and dressed with fine-mesh gauze. Dressings are usually changed every 1 to 2 days. Frequent (daily) dressing changes aid in **debridement**, which is a process of mechanically removing debris, including necrotic tissue, from the wound. Analgesics can be used to treat pain.

Moderate and major burns require emergency medical attention. Also, burns larger than the palm of the hand or those that involve the face, hands, feet, or genital areas require specialized intervention in a burn treatment center. Treatment for moderate and major burns, as with other emergencies, focuses on the airway, breathing, and circulation. Once these are stabilized, administration of intravenous fluids is instituted to replace water and sodium losses. Administering fluids helps to restore the circulating blood volume and improves perfusion of vital organs. Because metabolic demands increase significantly with the stress of a burn injury, nutrition support in the form of increased calories and protein is needed. Analgesics and antibiotics are also used to treat pain and infection. Protective isolation measures are often instituted to protect the patient from contact with microorganisms as much as possible.

Wound management for major burns involves cleansing with sterile saline while wearing powder-free gloves (powder will irritate the burn wound), removing blisters or necrotic tissue as appropriate, covering the wound with a sterile

Table 3.7 American Burn Association (ABA) Burn Severity Grading Scale

	Minor[a]	Moderate	Major
Partial-thickness	<10% TBSA	10%–20% TBSA	>20% TBSA
Full-thickness			All
Treatment	Usually treated at home	Admission to hospital; may require specialized burn center treatment	Admission to specialized burn center

[a]Minor burns exclude any burn involving the face, hands, feet, and perineum; also exclude electrical burns, inhalation injuries, or other trauma.
ALL, acute lymphocytic leukemia; TBSA, total body surface area.
http://www.ameriburn.org/BurnCenterReferralCriteria.pdf

dressing, and preventing infection. Hydrotherapy, which involves soaking in a tub or showering once or twice per day, is used to cleanse the wound by removing dead tissue and exudate. Full-thickness burns are unable to undergo reepithelialization and require surgical excision and grafting to close the wound. Skin grafting is a process of using self or donor tissue to cover and protect the exposed area. This transplanted epithelial tissue supports cellular regeneration, decreases invasion by microorganisms, and minimizes scarring. Long-term rehabilitation (tertiary prevention) involves prevention of complications such as scar formation, contractures, deformity, and chronic pain. Treatment may also involve psychosocial support because those with burn injuries may experience depression or other psychologic sequelae.

Arthritis

Arthritis is a general term for degeneration or inflammation of the joints and refers to a group of diseases of varying pathogenesis. Inflammatory arthritis is usually a result of chronic infections, autoimmune conditions, or other chronic irritants in the joint capsule. Rheumatoid arthritis, a systemic autoimmune disease leading to chronic inflammation of synovial tissue, is the selected clinical model.

FUNCTIONS OF SYNOVIAL JOINTS

The primary function of joints is skeletal stability and mobility. Synovial joints, particularly those in the knees, wrists, hands, fingers, and feet, are highly mobile and common targets for inflammation. Synovial joints are also highly vascular. The two-layer synovial membrane lines the joint capsule. One layer is composed of connective tissue, elastin, adipocytes, fibroblasts, macrophages, and mast cells. The second layer is a row of synovial cells, which are capable of phagocytosis and secreting synovial fluid. Synovial fluid nourishes, cushions, and protects the joint from microorganisms. Synovial cells are labile cells, which can quickly regenerate.

Between the bone and synovial membrane is cartilage. Cartilage is composed of chondrocytes, collagen, water, and protein glycans. Collagen forms an ECM, which attaches bone to the cartilage. Cartilage is needed to distribute body weight and to decrease joint friction. Cartilage must be replaced by collagen if damaged; chondrocytes do not regenerate.

RHEUMATOID ARTHRITIS

Rheumatoid arthritis (RA) is a systemic autoimmune disease characterized by chronic inflammation and hyperplasia of the synovial membranes with increased synovial exudate, leading to swelling and thickening of the synovial membranes, joint erosion, and pain. The onset of disease occurs typically between the ages of 36 and 50 years. RA affects 0.8% of adults worldwide. Females are affected three times more often than males, and the rate of comorbidities is high with depression, asthma, and cardiovascular problems being the most common comorbid conditions.[6]

Pathophysiology

Although the exact cause of RA is unknown, the etiology is likely a combination of:

- Genetic susceptibility
- An immune triggering event
- The subsequent development of autoimmunity against synovial cells

The triggering injury in RA that leads to inflammation is difficult to pinpoint and is often never determined. Despite the lack of an identifiable trigger, autoimmunity plays a key role. $CD4^+$ helper T cells have been implicated as activating the inflammatory response along with the release of cytokines. Lymphocytes and plasma cells then form antibodies in the synovial membrane and cartilage. The antibodies are formed against specific antigens. The antibodies actually see other antibodies within the body as foreign (see From the Lab).

In RA, the antigens and antibodies form complexes, called immune complexes. These immune complexes are found in the synovium of most individuals diagnosed with RA. These antigen–antibody complexes trigger the complement system, thereby stimulating an exaggerated inflammatory response.

The inflammatory response is marked by excess production and release of inflammatory mediators. These inflammatory mediators act on the vasculature of the joints to cause increased vasodilation and capillary permeability. The joint becomes erythematous, warm, swollen, painful, and difficult to move. Exudate accumulates in the synovium. Neutrophils

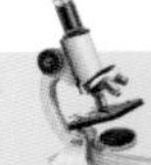

FROM THE LAB

Rheumatoid factor (RF), a substance that can be found in the blood, synovial fluid, and synovial membranes, signifies that antibodies (IgM, IgG, or IgA) are acting against other antibodies (mainly IgG). RF is present in the vast majority of patients who have RA and can also be found in a variety of other conditions. The presence of RF in RA often signifies more severe disease.

and macrophages move into the site to defend against harmful substances. This process, while necessary, also promotes the production of destructive tissue enzymes. Synovial cells adapt by rapidly regenerating. The synovium, after the initial bout of inflammation, is altered and causes the following changes:

1. Mild edema
2. Accumulation of the cells of chronic inflammation (macrophages, plasma cells, and lymphocytes)
3. Acceleration of angiogenesis
4. Accumulation of fibrin
5. Synovial cells continue to undergo reactive hyperplasia

These initial synovial changes usually demonstrate minimal damage to the joints.

Exacerbations of the disease progressively damage affected joints through pannus formation, cartilage erosion, fibrosis, and joint fixation and deformity (Fig. 3.19). **Pannus** is granulation tissue that forms over the inflamed synovium and cartilage as a result of accelerated angiogenesis. Pannus is filled with synovial cells, which undergo hyperplasia and migrate, along with the pannus, over the cartilage. The pannus and synovial cells are joined by mast cells, lymphocytes, and macrophage giant cells. These cells further exacerbate inflammation and tissue destruction. Pannus separates the cartilage from synovium, thereby depriving the cartilage of nutrients. The pannus also produces enzymes that break down the cartilage and can erode the adjacent bone as well. These erosions are irreversible. Fibroblasts work to form and replace the connective tissue layer by producing and secreting collagen. Collagen fills in the gaps that remain after tissue damage. As a result, fibrosis forms in the joint capsule. Fibrosis impairs joint mobility and can result in a debilitating fixation of the joint, a condition termed **ankylosis**. Limited joint movement decreases the workload of surrounding muscle tissue, leading to muscle tissue atrophy. Inflammatory cells can also irritate surrounding muscle tissue, resulting in muscle spasms.

CLINICAL MANIFESTATIONS

The severity of RA can range from mild to debilitating. Involvement is characteristically symmetric and can involve any number of joints, producing erythema, pain, swelling, warmth, and decreased mobility. Malalignment or deviation of symmetrical joints is a common clinical manifestation of long-standing RA (Fig. 3.20). Malalignment is caused by a combination of cartilage and bone erosion, fibrosis, ankylosis, muscle spasms, and muscle atrophy. Pain and stiffness is often most notable upon rising in the morning and after periods of immobility.

Common systemic manifestations during disease exacerbations are low-grade fever, fatigue, anorexia, weight loss, and weakness. Chronic pain can also lead to isolation and depression. Manifestations of long-standing RA can also be found outside of the joint capsule. Granulomas, called nodules, can form on blood vessels throughout the body. Vasculitis, an inflammatory condition involving small- and medium-sized arteries, may also occur in those with long-standing disease.

DIAGNOSTIC CRITERIA

No definitive test exists to diagnose RA. Diagnosis is based on history and physical examination (during which stiffness and pain in symmetrical joints is

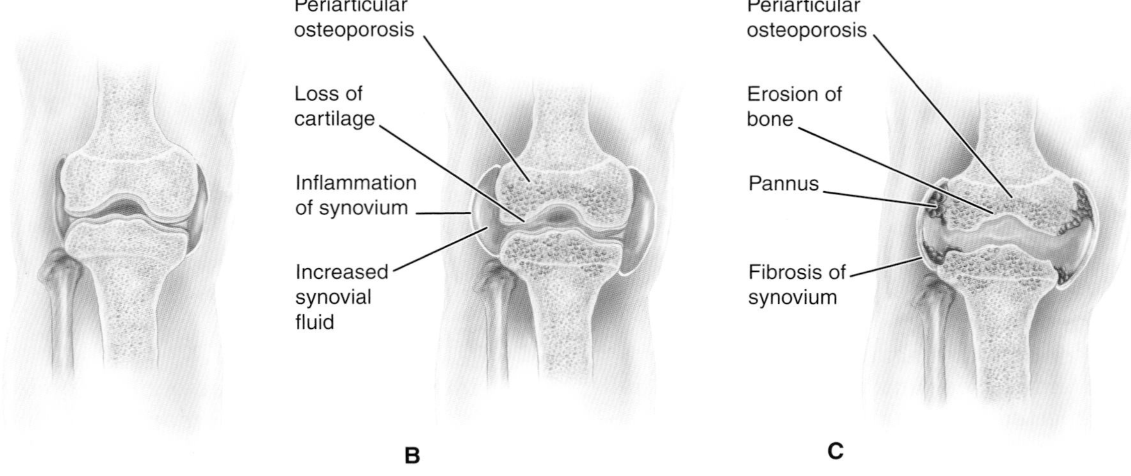

Figure 3.19. Normal joint **(A)**; early rheumatoid arthritis with fluid accumulation and synovial swelling **(B)**; late rheumatoid arthritis with pannus formation, eroded articular cartilage, and joint space narrowing **(C)**.

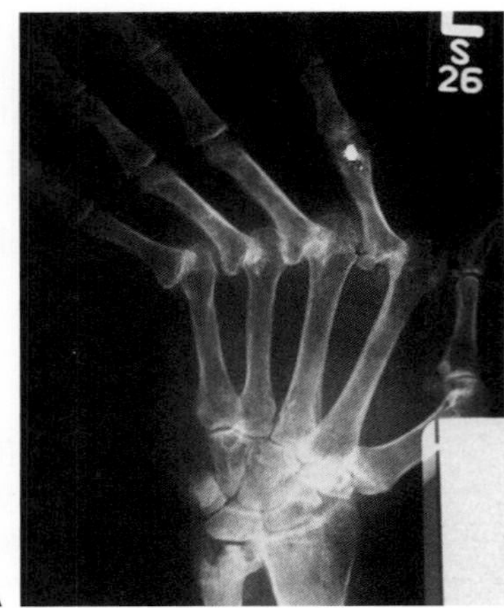

A

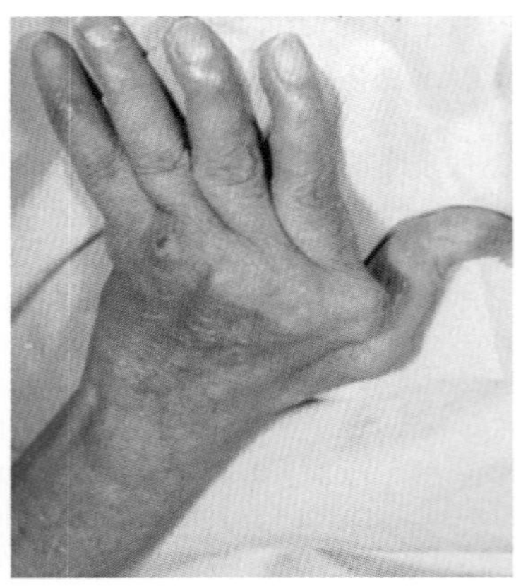

B

Figure 3.20. Deviation of joints in rheumatoid arthritis, as shown in a radiograph **(A)** and a photograph **(B)**. (**A:** Reprinted with permission from Harris JH Jr, Harris WH, Novelline RA. *The Radiology of Emergency Medicine*. 3rd ed. Baltimore, MD: Williams & Wilkins; 1993:440; **B:** Reprinted with permission from Smeltzer SC, Bare BG. *Textbook of Medical–Surgical Nursing*. 10th ed. Philadelphia, PA: Lippincott Williams & Wilkins; 2003, with permission.)

demonstrated), and it may involve several diagnostic tests. Test results that increase the likelihood of RA as the diagnosis include:

1. An elevated serum ESR
2. An elevated serum CRP level
3. The presence of RF significant for antibodies against IgG
4. A positive antinuclear antibody (ANA) assay indicating suspected autoimmune disease
5. The presence of inflammatory products in a synovial joint fluid analysis
6. Visualization with a radiograph demonstrating joint damage

RA presents a diagnostic challenge because multiple autoantibodies are known to be associated with this disease. Many of these tests are nonspecific and indicate the presence of an inflammatory or autoimmune process but do not directly point to RA as the cause. Each test also has a risk of false-positive (positive result without the disease) or false-negative (negative result with the disease) results. RF appears to have the greatest advantage in diagnosing early RA compared with multiple other autoantibody tests; however, it is unlikely that a single antigen is involved in the development of RA. The diagnostic challenge can lead to frustration for the patient and health care professional and may lead to a delay in treatment.

TREATMENT

Treatment of RA involves a careful balance of pharmacologic and nonpharmacologic treatment strategies. Medications employed include anti-inflammatory drugs, immunosuppressive drugs, and medications that otherwise induce remission. Nonpharmacologic strategies involve the balance of activity and rest, physical therapy exercises to promote joint mobility, and the use of splints and other devices that allow the joints to rest and help to prevent deformities. Heat or cold therapy can be helpful. In some cases, synovectomy or total joint replacement surgery may be needed to reduce pain and deformity.

Gastritis

Gastritis refers to inflammation of the lining of the stomach, or gastric mucosa, thereby impairing gastric function. Gastritis can be both acute and chronic.

RESEARCH NOTES

Current research is uncovering connections between RA and a number of other chronic conditions, such as cancer, cardiovascular disease, and diabetes. In a recent study, a significant increase in cardiovascular disease was noted in patients with RA who had more acute flares than those who spent more time in remission. The researchers concluded that tight inflammation control and improved flare management are critical to decreasing the cumulative cardiovascular burden of RA.[7]

FUNCTIONS OF THE STOMACH

The stomach functions as an organ of protection, digestion, and absorption, primarily absorbing water and alcohol. Stomach acid forms a first line of defense by destroying many types of microorganisms and other harmful substances on contact. During the digestive process, foods and liquids are mixed

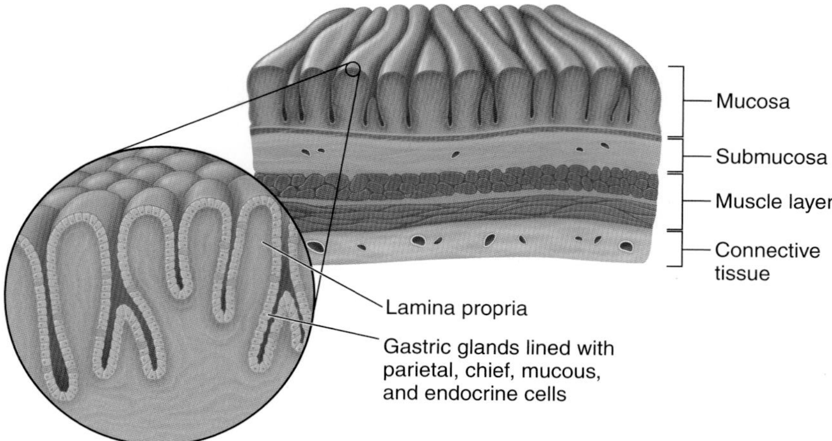

Figure 3.21. Gastric lining. The lining of the stomach contains four types of glandular epithelial cells: mucous, parietal, chief, and endocrine.

with gastric secretions, composed of mucus, acid, enzymes, hormones, and intrinsic factor (IF). Secretion of these substances is accomplished through the work of gastric glands lined by specialized epithelial cells (Fig. 3.21).

Epithelial cells form a tight connection. This connection is an important source of protection from the corrosive effects of gastric acid. Prostaglandins also play a key role in maintaining the integrity of the gastric mucosa through the stimulation of a protective mucus barrier.

Stop and Consider

Explain how anti-inflammatory drugs that inhibit prostaglandins can cause or further exacerbate gastritis.

The surface mucus barrier is highly vascular and dependent on a rich blood supply to support gastric function. Restriction or loss of perfusion to this layer can be a cause of gastritis. For example, altered perfusion can occur in the case of shock when blood is shunted to vital organs and not to the stomach, causing the protective mucus barrier to form ulcers and perforate.

Acute Gastritis

Acute gastritis refers to inflammation in the gastric mucosa most often caused by the ingestion of irritants such as aspirin, alcohol, or certain microorganisms. Acute gastritis typically occurs over a short period and is considered reversible when the causative agent is removed. Although gastritis is often associated with having too much stomach acid, the role of gastric acid hypersecretion is unclear.

PATHOPHYSIOLOGY

The gastric mucosa is accustomed to and functions best in the acidic environment of the stomach. Exposure to gastric irritants inhibits the production of gastric mucosa and makes the mucosa more vulnerable to acidic stomach contents. This leads to an acute inflammatory response ranging from mild erythema to erosion and gastric perforation (Fig. 3.22). Epithelial cells become necrotic. The underlying gastric tissue is eroded. Hemorrhaging often occurs. Gastric acid is allowed to escape the confines of the gastric mucosa and corrode nearby tissues. Perforation may occur in severe cases.

Perforating Ulcer

Penetration of wall creating a passage for gastric acids, other fluids and air to enter adjacent spaces of the body

Exudate

Granulation tissue

Figure 3.22. Gastric perforation as a result of acute gastritis.

CLINICAL MANIFESTATIONS

Clinical manifestations are dependent on the severity and range from mild to severe abdominal pain, which can be accompanied by indigestion (heartburn), loss of appetite, nausea, vomiting, and hiccups. **Hematemesis**, or vomiting blood, can occur. Anemia may result from mild gastric hemorrhage. Severe hemorrhage and perforation is quickly followed by shock and is a medical emergency.

DIAGNOSTIC CRITERIA

The patient history often reveals aspirin or other nonsteroidal anti-inflammatory drug use, excessive alcohol intake, recent contaminated food intake, or conditions causing ischemia of the gastric mucosa. The physical examination may reveal abdominal tenderness. Direct visualization of the stomach with an endoscope is needed to visualize ulcers in the mucosa, and a stool analysis may show occult blood in the fecal material. Hemoglobin or hematocrit levels provide information about anemia.

TREATMENT

Treatment begins with removal of the gastric irritant. Medications are then needed temporarily to buffer gastric acid or decrease gastric acid production. The healing of gastritis and gastric ulceration depends on regeneration of the epithelial cells that line the gastric mucosa. Most acute gastritis improves rapidly when the irritant is removed and treatment is initiated.

Chronic Gastritis: Infection

Chronic gastritis is related to an unrelenting injury, such as with chronic infection or autoimmunity. Chronic gastritis due to *Helicobacter pylori* is an example caused by chronic infection. *H. pylori* infection is most prevalent in Asia and in developing countries with poor sanitation. About half of the world's population is infected.

PATHOPHYSIOLOGY

H. pylori is a gram-negative proteobacterium that is passed from person to person through infected saliva and stool. The microorganism is ingested and multiplies on the epithelial surface cells and mucus barrier. *H. pylori* produces enzymes that neutralize gastric acid, and the microorganism is able to survive. The microorganisms then produce toxins that can destroy the mucosal barrier (Fig. 3.23).

In response to the microorganism-induced injury, inflammatory mediators trigger an intense inflammatory response. Phagocytes work to engulf, destroy, and remove these aggressive microorganisms. Neutrophils migrate to the lamina propria and gastric epithelium to phagocytize the bacteria. As the infection becomes chronic, macrophages and T and B lymphocytes move in an attempt to rid the body of the offending bacteria. *H. pylori* tends to remain contained within the mucosal barrier and surface epithelial cells, and unlike acute gastritis, there are no erosions of the gastric mucosa. Instead, epithelial cells and mucosal glands atrophy. Eventually, the chronic inflammatory response wanes. The mucosal lining of the stomach remains thin, and gastric acid production and secretion is impaired.

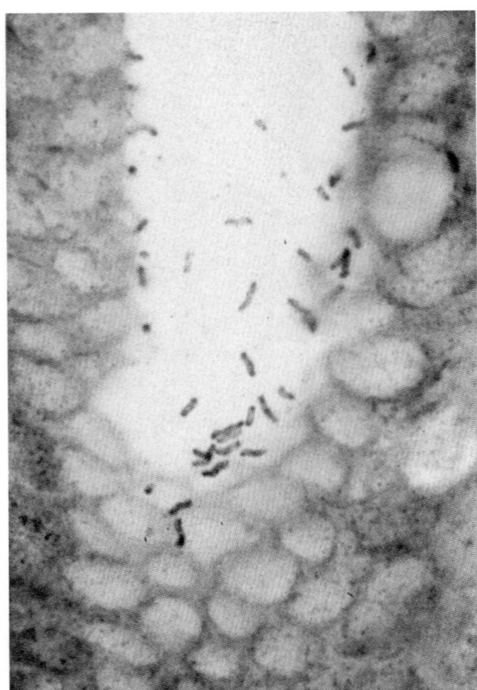

Figure 3.23. Infective gastritis. *H. pylori* appears as small curved rods on the surface of the gastric mucosa. (From Rubin E, Farber JL. *Pathology*. 3rd ed. Philadelphia, PA: Lippincott-Raven; 1999:687, with permission.)

CLINICAL MANIFESTATIONS

Dyspepsia, a vague epigastric discomfort associated with nausea and heartburn, is a possible clinical manifestation. Some patients may experience a loss of appetite or vomiting. Most infected people, however, are asymptomatic carriers.

DIAGNOSTIC CRITERIA

Diagnosis of chronic gastritis caused by *H. pylori* infection is accomplished through direct endoscopic visualization and biopsy of gastric tissue. A breath test can be used to measure the presence of an enzyme given off when the bacterium converts urea to carbon dioxide in the lungs. Protein antibodies against *H. pylori* may also be detected in the blood, indicating past or present infection with the bacteria.

TREATMENT

Because *H. pylori* is buried deep in the stomach mucosa, multiple antibiotics are needed to treat this infection along with proton pump inhibitors or bismuth, which have antimicrobial properties and raise gastric pH. Over time, certain strains of *H. pylori* can lead to chronic ulcers and gastric cancer.

Chronic Gastritis: Autoimmune

Chronic gastritis can also result from autoimmune processes. Although more rare than other forms of chronic gastritis, antibodies are produced against gastric parietal cells or IF.

PATHOPHYSIOLOGY

Parietal cells secrete hydrochloric acid. When antibodies are formed against parietal cells, gastric acid secretion is impaired. Intrinsic factor is needed for intestinal absorption of B_{12}. When antibodies are formed against IF, absorption of B_{12} is impaired. B_{12} is a critical vitamin that promotes DNA synthesis in RBCs. Impaired DNA synthesis in RBCs leads to a marked decrease in RBCs and low hemoglobin levels. This condition is known as pernicious anemia. Chronic inflammation related to autoimmunity allows T cells to infiltrate the gastric mucosa, destroying epithelial cells and causing gastric atrophy.

CLINICAL MANIFESTATIONS

Autoimmune gastritis can be asymptomatic. The presence of pernicious anemia may be the first clue that chronic gastritis is present. Manifestations of anemia include weakness, light-headedness, pale mucous membranes, and fatigue. Clinical manifestations can also include dyspepsia, vague abdominal pain, nausea, vomiting, and anorexia.

DIAGNOSTIC CRITERIA

Diagnosis of autoimmune gastritis can be determined only with histologic examination of the gastric mucosa. Several biopsy samples are obtained and analyzed for atrophic changes in the cells. Antiparietal or anti-IF antibodies may present in a blood sample, which indicate an autoimmune process against the parietal cells or IF. Because autoimmunity against IF impairs B_{12} absorption, a low B_{12} level will be noted in the blood.

TREATMENT

Treatment is aimed at blocking the autoimmune attack against the parietal cells. The administration of B_{12} intramuscular injections monthly is needed to facilitate absorption of this important vitamin. Similar to *H. pylori*, autoimmune gastritis can lead to gastric cancer.

Pancreatitis

Pancreatitis refers to inflammation of the pancreas, resulting in destruction of the pancreas by pancreatic enzymes. Pancreatitis can be both acute and chronic.

FUNCTIONS OF THE PANCREAS

The pancreas is both an endocrine and exocrine gland located in the upper posterior abdomen on the patient's left side. The endocrine pancreas (about 20% of the gland) produces insulin; the exocrine pancreas (80% of the gland) produces and secretes digestive enzymes. These digestive enzymes are essential for the metabolism of carbohydrates, fats, and proteins.

Digestive enzymes are produced within the acinar cells of the pancreas, are stored in zymogens, and are released into the pancreatic duct and to the small intestine, where digestion can then occur. In a process of negative feedback, the secretion of pancreatic enzymes is reduced when digestion is complete. Disruption of this protective process triggers pancreatic enzymes to become activated and self-destruct through autodigestion.

Acute Pancreatitis

PATHOPHYSIOLOGY

Acute pancreatitis may occur when there is an injury to the acinar cells, zymogen, pancreatic duct, or protective digestive feedback mechanisms in the exocrine pancreas. Common causes include duct blockage by gallstones or excessive alcohol use (Fig. 3.24). In about 10% of cases, the cause is unknown.[8] Alcohol is a major cause of pancreatic autodigestion by triggering:

- Intracellular accumulation of digestive enzymes
- Premature enzyme activation and release
- Increased permeability of ductules and easy passage of enzymes to the parenchyma
- Increased protein content of pancreatic secretions and creation of protein plugs

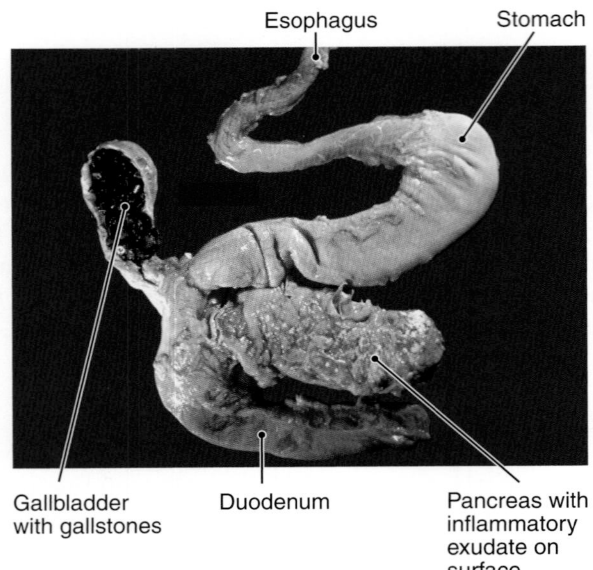

Figure 3.24. Acute pancreatitis as a result of gall stone obstruction.

The injury triggers blockage of enzymatic pathways, the activation of trypsin and the zymogen, spilling of secretory enzymes, and ultimately inflammation. Neutrophils, tumor necrosis factor, and interleukins (early responders) and macrophages (later) mediate the inflammatory response. Consistent with the inflammatory cascade, there is increased vascular permeability in the pancreas, leading to edema. This condition is referred to as acute edematous pancreatitis. Later, hemorrhage and necrosis ensue, leading to a state of hemorrhagic or necrotizing pancreatitis with eventual granuloma or abscess formation. In severe cases, necrosis is widespread, and there is organ dysfunction and potentially systemic multiorgan failure.

CLINICAL MANIFESTATIONS

Clinical manifestations are related to the inflammatory response occurring in the pancreas and its resulting pain and digestive impact. These manifestations include:

- Upper abdominal pain of sudden onset, growing in intensity, and leading to a dull, steady ache often radiating to the back
- Nausea, vomiting, anorexia, and/or diarrhea

DIAGNOSTIC CRITERIA

Diagnosing acute pancreatitis is generally achieved through the history and physical examination, noting the presence of clinical manifestations above. Laboratory testing is implemented to aid in the diagnosis. Tests for complete blood count, ESR, and CRP levels may give clues to the presence of inflammation. Specific laboratory tests include measuring:

- **Serum amylase and lipase:** Levels of these enzymes are typically elevated in acute pancreatitis. Both are digestive enzymes (amylase breaks down carbohydrates and lipase breaks down fats) that are excessively released with inflammation of the pancreas.
- **Serum alkaline phosphatase, total bilirubin, aspartate aminotransferase (AST), and alanine aminotransferase (ALT):** These are liver enzymes, which are likely to be elevated in cases of pancreatitis caused by gallstones.

When the diagnosis is in doubt or the symptoms are severe, imaging studies, such as ultrasound, CT, or MRI, are needed to aid in determining the location and potentially the cause of the pancreatic injury.

TREATMENT

Treatment aims to eliminate the cause of pancreatic injury if at all possible and to care for the symptoms. Patients should receive aggressive IV hydration in the first 24 hours. In mild pancreatitis with no nausea or vomiting, patients can continue oral feeding. Otherwise, all patients must be NPO (nothing by mouth). Analgesics should be administered to manage pain. Surgical removal of gallstones is warranted if they are present.

Patients with severe pancreatitis, often defined as a CRP level above 10 mg/dL along with severe symptoms and potential for negative sequelae, should be hospitalized in the intensive care unit to prevent complications of shock, renal failure, or systemic multiorgan failure. Ranson's Criteria for Pancreatitis Mortality[9] is a tool that helps to determine the patient's prognosis based on WBC count, age, AST level, hematocrit, blood urea nitrogen level, fluid requirements, and other indicators. Intensive treatment is successful if the patient has no pain, is able to take in adequate nutrition, and has experienced no complications.

Chronic Pancreatitis

Chronic pancreatitis is an ongoing inflammatory process of the pancreas, characterized by irreversible cellular and tissue changes. Chronic pancreatitis differs from acute pancreatitis in duration, and its impact on both the endocrine and exocrine functions of the pancreas. The most common causes are chronic alcohol abuse (60% to 70%), autoimmune or hereditary disease (10%), and in 20% of cases the cause is unknown.[10]

PATHOPHYSIOLOGY

As described above, alcohol has an effect on the pancreas, whereas enzymes and protein accumulation cause the pancreatic ducts to become obstructed. Obstruction leads to ischemia. The acinar cells become atrophic and fibrotic, leading to loss of function. When alcohol abuse is chronic, the demands of metabolizing alcohol lead to oxidative stress, which promotes further cellular injury and organ damage.

Autoimmunity (Chapter 4) can occur against the pancreas, resulting in chronic pancreatitis. The etiology is often undetermined; however, as a result of high levels of circulating autoantibodies, there is diffuse enlargement of the pancreas and narrowing of the ducts. Certain autoimmune disorders, which disrupt metabolic processes, have also been associated with chronic pancreatitis. One major example is renal tubular acidosis (Chapter 9), a condition of excess acid accumulation in the body due to a failure of the kidneys to appropriately acidify urine. Cystic fibrosis (Chapter 15) is an example of a genetic condition that can promote chronic pancreatic inflammation. Recurrent acute pancreatitis can also promote a state of fibrosis and necrosis characteristic of chronic pancreatitis. Whatever the etiology, the pathophysiology is based on the fibrotic changes of the pancreas due to the presence of chronic inflammatory cells and fibroblast proliferation.

CLINICAL MANIFESTATIONS

Typically, a patient with chronic pancreatitis has severe intermittent episodes of abdominal pain (mid or upper right-sided, radiating to the back) lasting several hours and at unpredictable intervals. The development of disease has likely begun several months to years before the onset of symptoms. Diarrhea, steatorrhea (fatty stools), and weight loss can also occur as a result of damage to the digestive functions of the exocrine pancreas; however, this occurs only after 90% of the pancreas has been destroyed.

DIAGNOSTIC CRITERIA

Endoscopic retrograde cholangiopancreatography (ERCP) is considered the gold standard for diagnosing chronic pancreatitis (Fig. 3.25). In ERCP, the stomach and duodenum are visualized through an endoscope and then a radiographic contrast dye is injected into the ducts of the biliary tree and pancreas so that the obstructed pancreatic pathways can be seen on radiographs. Serum amylase and lipase (described above) may be elevated in acute exacerbations of disease, but over time the levels are normal to low because of fibrotic changes in the pancreas and loss of function, whereas enzymes can no longer be concentrated. Although expensive and invasive, direct aspiration of the pancreatic duct or the duodenum, where the pancreas deposits enzymes, can be tested to determine levels of pancreatic bicarbonate and enzymes that have been secreted.

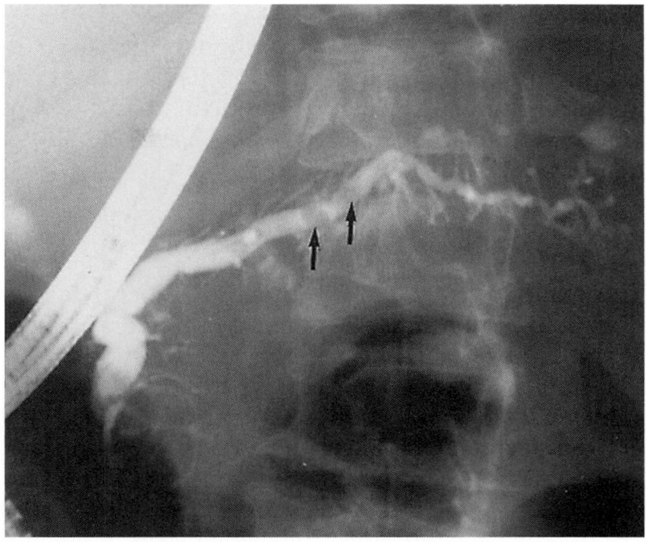

Figure 3.25. Endoscopic retrograde cholangiopancreatography (ERCP) illustrates moderate dilation of the main pancreatic duct and ectasia of the secondary ducts associated with moderately advanced chronic pancreatitis. Arrows indicate intraductal pancreatic stones.

TREATMENT

Treatment for chronic pancreatitis is based on the cause and focused on healing:

- Pain management
- Behavior modification to promote a healthy lifestyle: alcohol cessation, smoking cessation, exercise, quality nutrition
- Surgical intervention to correct cyst, abscess, obstruction, or fistula formation

Inflammatory Bowel Disease

Inflammatory bowel disease (IBD) refers to chronic inflammatory processes most commonly in the small and large intestine, but it can occur anywhere along the gastrointestinal tract from the mouth to the anus. The most common forms of IBD include Crohn disease and ulcerative colitis.

The incidence of IBD is highest in developed countries, where persons in colder climates and urban areas have an increased risk. The American Jewish population has a four to five times greater prevalence than in other groups. Among those of European descent in the United States, the prevalence of ulcerative colitis is estimated at 116 per 100,000 people, and this is slightly increased at 133 per 100,000 people for Crohn disease. The risk appears similar for African Americans but is lower for Asian Americans and Hispanic Americans. Males and females are equally affected.[11]

FUNCTIONS OF THE SMALL INTESTINE

The small intestine is composed of several layers (Fig. 3.26). From inner to outer, these layers consist of the mucosa, submucosa, muscularis, and serosa. The innermost mucosal tissue is composed of three sublayers: mucous columnar epithelium, lamina propria (connective tissue), and the thin muscularis layer. The mucous epithelium layer lines the villi, which provide a large surface area. These villi are lined with columnar cells, which secrete mucus, enzymes, and hormones. The submucosa is a thick connective tissue layer that houses nerves, small glands, and blood vessels.

The primary functions of the small intestine are digestion and absorption. Enzymes secreted by villi promote digestion. Vitamins, minerals, fats, carbohydrates, proteins, water, and electrolytes, such as sodium and potassium, are absorbed through columnar epithelium of the intestinal mucosa. The lamina propria houses infection-fighting macrophages, plasma cells, and lymphocytes. Replacement of columnar epithelial cells is rapid, primarily because of the presence of the crypts of Lieberkühn. These pit-like depressions store cells that can quickly differentiate into replacement cells. The rate of production and differentiation of epithelial cells is increased with injury, thereby promoting healing and repair.

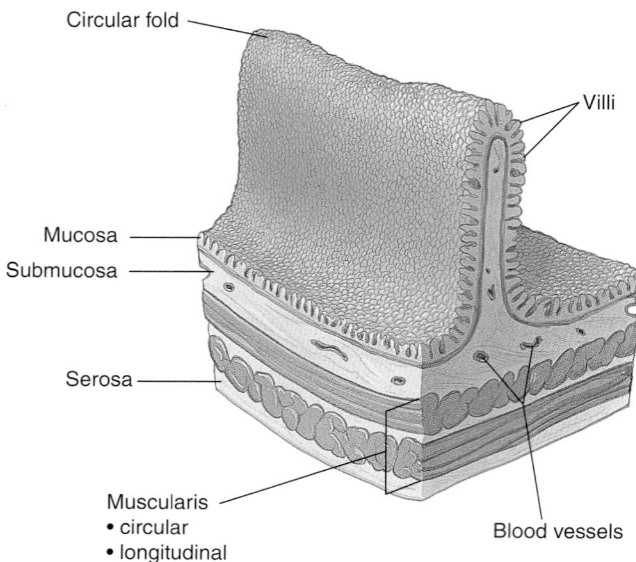

Figure 3.26. Wall of small intestine.

Crohn Disease

Crohn disease is selected as a clinical model to demonstrate chronic inflammatory process in the small intestine. It is recurrent and characterized by a granulomatous inflammatory process. Although Crohn disease can be found anywhere along the gastrointestinal tract, the small intestine and ascending colon, particularly the submucosal layers, are most often affected.

PATHOPHYSIOLOGY

The exact cause of Crohn disease is unknown. Consistent with many other chronic inflammatory conditions, autoimmunity and genetic etiologies have been suggested. Family history does play a role: Those with a family history of bowel inflammation are more likely to develop Crohn disease. Environmental factors, such as smoking, diet, or microorganisms, may trigger the condition as well. As with all conditions, Crohn disease has varying levels of disease severity.

As mentioned, chronic inflammation occurs in patchy segments (called "skip lesion") of the intestine and penetrates all layers of those segments. Between affected areas of intestine is unaffected, noninflamed bowel tissue. Inflammation begins in the mucosa and submucosa. Increased permeability and vascularity contributes to edema and fibrosis. Macrophages, plasma cells, and lymphocytes are released in response to inflammatory mediators. Granulomas develop to wall off affected areas.

As the affected bowel segments become further inflamed, interior surfaces thicken because of excessive edema, fibrosis, and granuloma formation (Fig. 3.27). The thickening of the bowel can lead to total bowel obstruction. Ingested food is unable to move through the digestive tract, which is a life-threatening emergency. Although thickening and granuloma formation are most characteristic of Crohn disease, ulcers can form in the intestinal mucosa. These ulcers can become deep and penetrate through bowel layers, forming a fistula. A **fistula** is an abnormal track or passage that forms between two segments of bowel or other epithelial tissue. At the base of a fistula, an **abscess**, or pocket of purulent (containing pus) exudate, is likely to develop. External surfaces can also be affected by the chronic inflammatory response. Outer surfaces can stick to other sections of bowel and form adhesions, further limiting bowel function.

Destruction of the mucosa and submucosa leads to damage to the villi and crypts. This damage impairs absorptive and epithelial regenerative functions within the affected areas. Malnutrition from the inability to properly absorb nutrients further

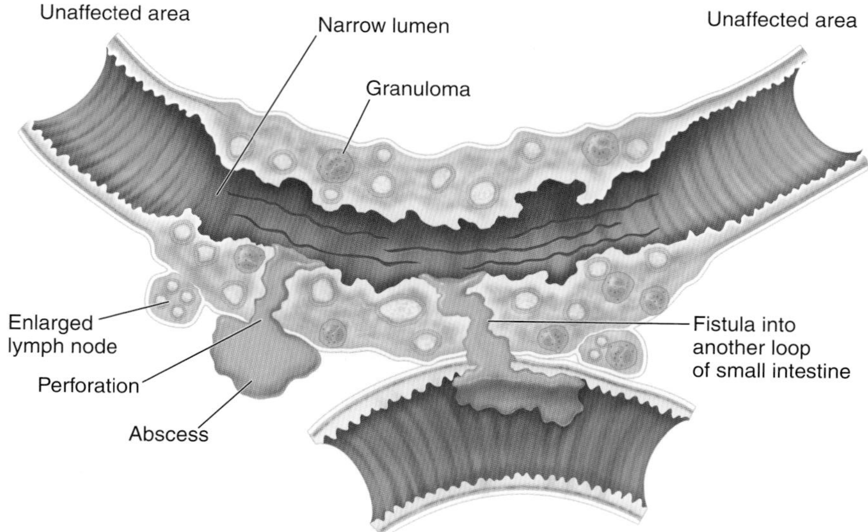

Figure 3.27. Major features of Crohn disease. (Modified from Rubin E, Farber JL. *Pathology*. 4th ed. Philadelphia, PA: Lippincott Williams & Wilkins; 2005, with permission.)

exacerbates problems with healing. The most severe complication is massive infection and shock from total bowel obstruction and perforation.

CLINICAL MANIFESTATIONS

Clinical manifestations are related to rapid stool transit time, intestinal edema and fibrosis, and loss of absorptive function that results from bowel inflammation during periods of exacerbation. Symptoms depend on the location of the affected areas. Abdominal pain, intermittent nonbloody diarrhea, malnutrition, and **occult**, or hidden, blood in the stool are possible clinical manifestations. Nonbloody diarrhea often indicates greater involvement in the submucosal layer as compared to the mucosal layers. If the colon mucosal layer is involved, diarrhea may contain mucus, blood, or pus. Abdominal pain is often relieved with defecation. Systemic manifestations are also common with Crohn disease and can include fever, weight loss, and fatigue. Anemia is often present when there is chronic blood loss through the gastrointestinal tract.

DIAGNOSTIC CRITERIA

Diagnosis of Crohn disease is based on the patient history, physical examination, and diagnostic tests. Direct visualization with an endoscope (sigmoidoscopy) or with radiographs shows a cobblestone pattern to the mucosa with alternating affected and unaffected areas of inflammation. Complications, such as abscesses or fistulas, can also be detected through radiographs or CT scan. Stool cultures may be needed to rule out infectious processes.

TREATMENT

Treatment is symptomatic. Medications that suppress the inflammatory and immune responses are most often used. Dietary changes are required, and foods that irritate the bowel, such as spicy foods, should be avoided. Individuals with Crohn disease need a diet high in calories and protein, and low in fat and fiber during exacerbations. Surgical intervention may be needed to remove damaged bowel or to repair fistulas. Those with Crohn disease are at increased risk of small intestine and colorectal cancer.

FUNCTIONS OF THE LARGE INTESTINE

The anatomy of the large intestine is similar to the small intestine, with the notable absence of villi in the large intestine. Columnar epithelial cells and mucus-secreting cells make up the mucosa of the large intestine. The major function of the large intestine is to absorb water and electrolytes.

Ulcerative Colitis

Ulcerative colitis is selected as a chronic inflammatory condition of the colon. Ulcerative colitis is found exclusively in the large intestine and does not affect other areas of the gastrointestinal tract (Fig. 3.28). It most often affects the mucosal layer but can extend into the submucosa.

PATHOPHYSIOLOGY

The exact cause of ulcerative colitis is not known. Autoimmunity has been implicated because antibodies

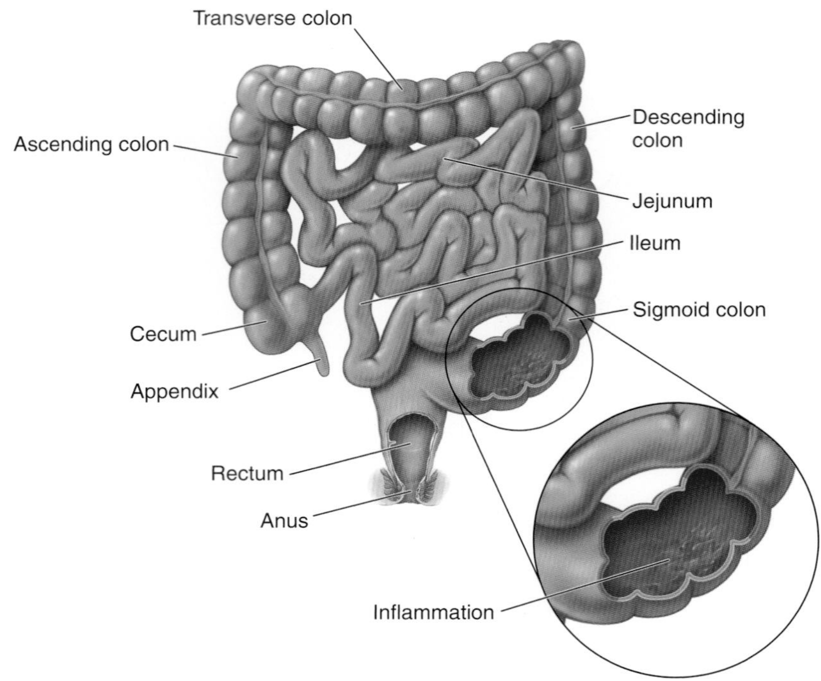

Figure 3.28. Ulcerative colitis. Chronic inflammation associated with ulcerative colitis is found exclusively in the large intestine.

to epithelial cells in the colon have been found in some individuals with ulcerative colitis. Ulcerative colitis typically begins in the distal region of the rectum and extends up the descending colon. The area of inflammation often remains on the surface of the mucosa and is continuous; ulcerative colitis does not skip any areas of the colon along the way (Fig. 3.29).

With ulcerative colitis, inflammation invades the superficial mucosa and causes **friability**, a state where tissue readily bleeds. The mucosa becomes erythematous and granular. Hemorrhagic lesions in the crypts of Lieberkühn, highly characteristic of ulcerative colitis, can form into abscesses. Extensive exudate is present early in the process, and necrosis and ulceration are common. Inflammatory processes promote the development of pseudopolyps. Over time, epithelial cells of the mucosa begin to atrophy. Metaplasia can occur. Those with long-standing ulcerative colitis demonstrate a higher risk for colorectal cancer than those with Crohn disease. Other potential complications include obstruction, perforation, and massive hemorrhage. Table 3.8 and Figure 3.30 compare pathophysiologic differences with Crohn disease and ulcerative colitis.

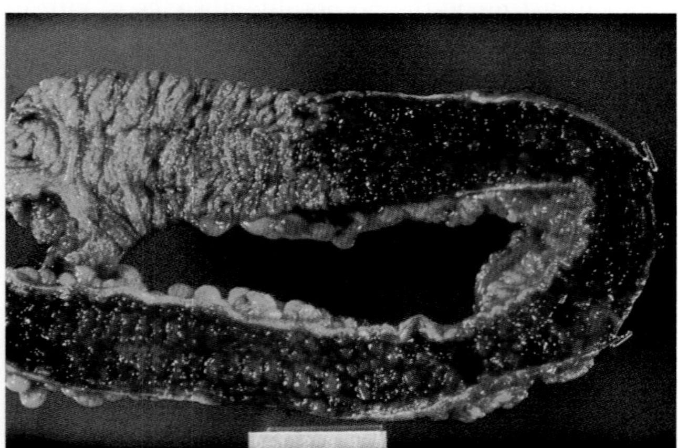

Figure 3.29. Ulcerative colitis. Prominent erythema and ulceration of the colon begin in the ascending colon and are most severe in the rectosigmoid area. (From Ruben E, Farber JL. *Pathology*. 3rd ed. Philadelphia, PA: Lippincott-Raven; 1999:731, with permission.)

CLINICAL MANIFESTATIONS

Clinical manifestations are related to large intestine irritability and friability. Diarrhea, often with rectal bleeding, is the most common clinical manifestation. Abdominal pain, fever, weakness, fatigue, and anemia can also occur. Functional losses with ulcerative colitis are related to the extent of inflammation; impaired water and electrolyte absorption are notable with extensive disease.

DIAGNOSTIC CRITERIA

Ulcerative colitis is diagnosed through endoscopy, which shows mucosal erythema. Radiographs can detect colonic dilation, ulcers, perforation, or

Table 3.8 Comparison of Crohn Disease and Ulcerative Colitis

	Crohn Disease	Ulcerative Colitis
Location	Small intestine and ascending colon	Descending colon
Pattern	Skip lesions	Continuous
Depth	Primarily submucosal	Primarily mucosal
Diarrhea	Watery	Bloody
Abdominal pain	Yes	Yes
Bowel obstruction	Common	Uncommon
Cancer risk	Increased	Higher risk than with Crohn's

obstruction. Severity is based on the number of bowel movements with rectal bleeding and the presence of systemic manifestations:

- Mild = fewer than four bowel movements per day; no systemic manifestations
- Moderate = greater than four bowel movements per day; no systemic manifestations
- Severe = greater than four bowel movements per day with systemic manifestations and low blood albumin (protein) levels

TREATMENT

Treatment is symptomatic. Anti-inflammatory, antidiarrheal, and immunosuppressive medications are sometimes used. A healthy diet and adequate fluid intake are recommended. Avoidance of certain foods such as milk, caffeine, or spicy foods may be recommended. Surgery may be needed if medical therapies are ineffective, or if perforation or obstruction occurs.

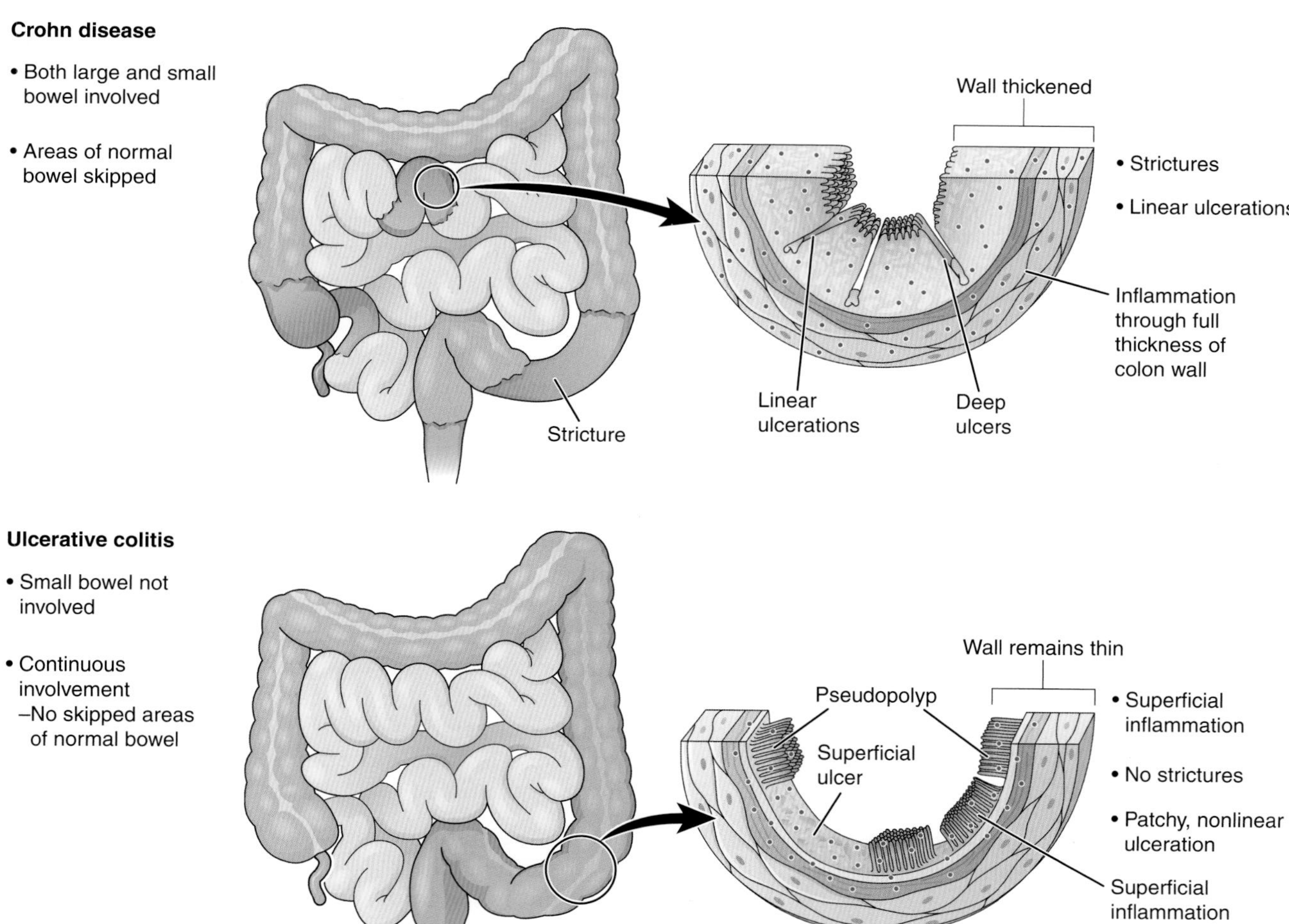

Figure 3.30. Crohn disease and ulcerative colitis. The two drawings illustrate critical differences in how the two diseases affect the gastrointestinal tract.

SUMMARY

- Inflammation is required for tissue healing and occurs in response to tissue injury.
- Inflammatory mediators, under the direction of the three plasma protein systems, regulate the inflammatory response.
- Inflammatory mediators elicit vascular and cellular responses characterized by vasodilation, increased capillary permeability, chemotaxis, cellular adherence, and cellular migration.
- Phagocytic cells (neutrophils and later macrophages) taxi to the site to engulf and destroy harmful substances.
- Removal of the injury will direct resolution of the acute inflammatory response.
- Tissue healing is a multistep process that involves covering the wound, clearing the debris, and restoring structural and functional integrity.
- The results of the inflammatory response are to repair, regenerate, or replace damaged tissue.
- Persistent injury, such as with chronic infection or autoimmune conditions, results in chronic inflammation.
- Chronic inflammation differs from acute inflammation in the types of prominent cells and in the tissue repair process. Macrophages and fibroblasts are much more prominent, resulting in increased tissue destruction, fibrosis, scarring, and granuloma formation.
- Chronic inflammatory outcomes contribute to poor wound healing. Other complications of wound healing include infection, ulcers, wound dehiscence, keloid formation, and adhesions.

CASE STUDY 3.1

A friend has disclosed that she has been having problems with heartburn. She has been told that she has gastroesophageal reflux disease (GERD), in which stomach acid backs up into the esophagus, causing esophagitis. Think about which clinical model is most related to this process. From your reading related to cellular injury and adaptations as well as inflammation, answer the following questions:

1. What anatomic problem most likely leads to gastroesophageal reflux?
2. What is the injury in gastroesophageal reflux?
3. What would the acute inflammatory response look like?
4. Why might this condition become a chronic problem?
5. What pathophysiologic changes would most likely occur with chronic gastroesophageal reflux?
6. What would you expect for clinical manifestations?
7. What diagnostic tests might be used?
8. What treatment measures would you anticipate?

Log on to the Internet, using the search words "gastroesophageal reflux." Search for relevant journal articles or Web sites that detail this condition, and confirm your predictions.

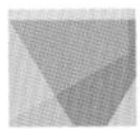

CASE STUDY 3.2

Jason is a long-distance runner. He is in the clinic today complaining of heel pain and tightness along the back of his foot and ankle. He has been recently running indoors on the treadmill as the weather has been too cold to run outside. He is diagnosed with Achilles tendonitis. From your reading related to cellular injury and adaptations as well as inflammation, answer the following questions:

1. What anatomic problem most likely leads to tendonitis?
2. What is the injury in tendonitis?
3. What would the acute inflammatory response look like?
4. Why might this condition become a chronic problem?
5. What pathophysiologic changes would most likely occur with tendonitis?
6. What would you expect for clinical manifestations?
7. What diagnostic tests might be used?
8. What treatment measures would you anticipate?

Log on to the Internet, using the search words "tendonitis." Search for relevant journal articles or Web sites that detail this condition, and confirm your predictions.

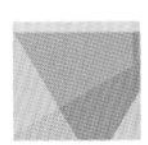

CASE STUDY 3.3

Melanie has had a recent cold with symptoms of runny nose, sneezing, coughing, congestion, and malaise. Today, she is concerned that she has a sharp pain in her chest. She goes to see her health care provider, and is diagnosed with costochondritis, an inflammation in the cartilage between the ribs. From your reading related to cellular injury and adaptations as well as inflammation, answer the following questions:

1. What anatomic problem most likely leads to costochondritis?
2. What is the injury in costochondritis?
3. What would the acute inflammatory response look like?
4. Why might this condition become a chronic problem?

5. What pathophysiologic changes would most likely occur with costochondritis?
6. What would you expect for clinical manifestations?
7. What diagnostic tests might be used?
8. What treatment measures would you anticipate?

Log on to the Internet, using the search words "costochondritis." Search for relevant journal articles or Web sites that detail this condition, and confirm your predictions.

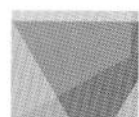

PRACTICE EXAM QUESTIONS

1. You get a paper cut and experience pain at the site. This response is related to:
   a. Increased perfusion at the site
   b. Increased exudate and chemical mediators at the site
   c. Bacteria that have entered the wound
   d. Vasoconstriction at the site

2. Inflammation is ultimately needed to:
   a. Increase inflammatory mediators at the site to vasoconstrict the area
   b. Increase platelets at the site for clotting
   c. Restore functional cells
   d. Prepare the site for healing

3. A wound is 6 cm × 6 cm × 4 cm. A wound with these dimensions needs to heal through:
   a. Secondary intention
   b. Primary intention
   c. Tertiary intention
   d. Scar tissue formation

4. A major difference between the acute and chronic inflammatory response is that in chronic inflammation:
   a. Inflammatory mediators are released
   b. Neutrophils are much more prominent
   c. Granulomas form around certain invaders
   d. Granulation tissue is present

5. Which is not a local manifestation of acute inflammation?
   a. Edema
   b. Redness
   c. Loss of function
   d. Leukocytosis

6. Depth of injury is important to determine with burns. You are in the sun too long without sunscreen and develop redness and blistering on your face, chest, and back. What depth of burn did you experience?
   a. Superficial partial-thickness burn
   b. Deep partial-thickness burn
   c. Full-thickness burn
   d. Dermal thickness burn

7. The hospitalized burn patient wants to know why you need to remove his dressings every day. It is painful and he wants to avoid uncovering his burn injury. You explain that removing the dressings promotes:
   a. Debridement
   b. Infection
   c. Skin function
   d. Drying the exudate

8. What is the one definitive test to diagnose rheumatoid arthritis?
   a. A positive rheumatoid factor (RF)
   b. An elevated erythrocyte sedimentation rate (ESR)
   c. A positive antinuclear antibody (ANA)
   d. One test is not definitive

9. Which of the following is the most common cause of acute gastritis?
   a. Poor gastric perfusion
   b. Too much stomach acid
   c. Ingestion of aspirin, alcohol, or other chemicals
   d. *H. pylori* infection

10. Why is Crohn disease more likely to cause intestinal obstruction than ulcerative colitis?
    a. Crohn disease is located in the small intestine.
    b. Crohn disease causes granulomas to form in the submucosal layer.
    c. Crohn disease causes abdominal pain and watery diarrhea.
    d. Crohn disease is exacerbated by certain foods, such as spicy foods.

11. A patient is taking an anti-inflammatory drug for rheumatoid arthritis. What is the most likely action for this drug?
    a. Blocks the chemical mediators of inflammation
    b. Enhances the body's immune system
    c. Increases blood flow to the tissues
    d. Decreases scar formation

12. Which of the following is the most common cause of acute pancreatitis?
    a. Cancer
    b. Autoimmunity
    c. Excess alcohol intake
    d. Cystic fibrosis

13. Rheumatoid arthritis results in joint immobility as a result of:
a. Synovial fluid loss
b. Pannus formation
c. Rheumatoid factor
d. Joint deviation

14. Which of the following meals would you recommend to a patient with a wound to promote healing?
a. Eggs and orange juice
b. Spaghetti and garlic toast
c. Steak and potatoes
d. Tomato soup and grilled cheese

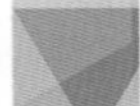

DISCUSSION AND APPLICATION

1. What did I know about inflammation and tissue repair prior to today?
2. What body processes are affected by inflammation? What are the expected functions of those processes? How does inflammation impact those processes?
3. What are the potential etiologies for inflammation? How does inflammation develop?
4. Who is most at risk for developing inflammation? How can inflammation be prevented?
5. What are the human differences that affect the etiology, risk, or course of inflammation?
6. What clinical manifestations are expected during inflammation?
7. What special diagnostic tests are useful in determining the diagnosis and course of inflammation?
8. What are the goals of care for individuals with inflammation?
9. How does the concept of inflammation build on what I have learned in the previous chapters and in previous courses?
10. How can I use what I have learned?

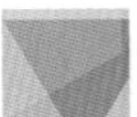

RESOURCES

Inflammation Research Foundation:
http://www.inflammationresearchfoundation.org/

American Burn Association:
http://www.ameriburn.org/

E-medicine:
http://emedicine.medscape.com/

References

1. Geetha M, Unnikrishnan M. Multi-target drugs to address multiple checkpoints in complex inflammatory pathologies: evolutionary cues for novel "first in class" anti-inflammatory drug candidates. *Inflamm Res*. 2015;64:747–752.
2. Corbett J. *Laboratory Tests and Diagnostic Procedures With Nursing Diagnoses*. 8th ed. Upper Saddle River, NJ: Prentice Hall; 2012.
3. Brook I. Acute sinusitis. 2015. http://emedicine.medscape.com/article/232670-overview
4. Brook I. Chronic sinusitis. 2015. http://emedicine.medscape.com/article/232791-overview
5. American Burn Association. Burn incident fact sheet. http://www.ameriburn.org/resources_factsheet.php. Accessed January 10, 2015.
6. Dougados M, Soubrier M, Antunez A, et al. Prevalence of comorbidities in rheumatoid arthritis and evaluation of their monitoring: results of an international, cross-sectional study (COMORA). *Ann Rheum Dis*. 2014;73:62–68.
7. Myasoedova E, Chandran A, Ilhan B, et al. The role of rheumatoid arthritis (RA) flare and cumulative burden of RA severity in the risk of cardiovascular disease. *Ann Rheum Dis*. doi:10.1136/annrheumdis-2014-206411.
8. Gardner T. Acute pancreatitis. 2015. http://emedicine.medscape.com/article/181364-overview
9. Ranson JH. Etiological and prognostic factors in human acute pancreatitis: a review. *Am J Gastroenterol*. 1982;77:633–638.
10. Huffman JL. Chronic pancreatitis. 2015. http://emedicine.medscape.com/article/181554-overview
11. Rowe WA. Inflammatory bowel disease. 2015. http://emedicine.medscape.com/article/179037-overview

Find additional resources for this chapter at http:thePoint.lww.com thePoint®

Altered Immunity

Chapter

4

LEARNING OUTCOMES

1. Define and use the key terms listed in this chapter.
2. Describe the function of the cellular components (lymphocytes, macrophages, and antigen-presenting cells) in adaptive immune defense process.
3. Differentiate between the innate and adaptive immune responses.
4. Define the processes of primary and secondary antibody responses in the development of immunity.
5. Outline the similarities and differences between the types of T lymphocytes active in cell-mediated immunity.
6. Predict the potential alterations in immune responses resulting from dysfunction in the immunoglobulins IgA, IgD, IgE, IgG, and IgM.
7. Compare and contrast the process of altering immune function associated with host defense failure, hypersensitivity, autoimmunity, and alloimmunity.
8. Recognize the interactions between cell-mediated and humoral immune responses necessary for mounting an effective immune response.
9. Apply concepts of altered immune function to select clinical models.

INTRODUCTION

People live in a world in which there is a constant risk of harmful substances entering their bodies. Even when asleep, the body's defenses are protecting against overwhelming infection. These defenses are provided by the coordination of the many components that make up the immune system. The first line of defense, the skin and mucous membranes, and the second line of defense, the inflammatory response, were reviewed in detail in Chapter 3. The innate immune response is rapid and nonspecific, involving inflammatory response processes. The adaptive immune response, the third line of defense, allows the body to seek out and destroy new and old foreign invaders and is the focus of the discussion in this chapter. The adaptive immune response is targeted and specific, involving two primary processes: cell-mediated immunity and humoral immunity.

This chapter provides a brief review of normal function, followed by the pathophysiology of alterations in immune function. Examples of conditions with pathogenesis resulting from altered immunity will highlight the application of concepts of altered immune responses. Developing an understanding of these responses will help to translate the signs and symptoms of disease states that result from maladaptive immune responses. Application of these concepts will form the basis for diagnosis, prevention, and treatment of a variety of conditions associated with altered immunity.

Module 1 Review of Immune Function

The process by which the body recognizes foreign substances and neutralizes them to prevent damage is known as **immunity**. Adaptive immune defense is characterized by:

- **Specificity:** The immune cells seek out and destroy targeted foreign invaders.
- **Memory:** The immune cells produce substances that remember and more easily destroy return offenders.

thePoint® To see a video on the immune response, visit http://thePoint.lww.com. **Immunology** is the study of the structure and function of the immune system, as well as the phenomena of immunity, induced sensitivity, and allergy. The immune system response, referred to as adaptive immunity, is stimulated when specialized cells come in contact with an **antigen**, a substance that induces a state of sensitivity or an immune response. Typically, the antigen is foreign and recognized as "nonself," prompting an immune response that spares "self" body cells. The adaptive immune response is initiated by two main components: the type of antigen presented to the cells and the type of cells to which the antigen is presented. The processes of cell-mediated and humoral immunity work together in the destruction of specifically targeted cells. The adaptive immune response involves central and peripheral immune structures, as well as primary and accessory cellular components, in the development of specific immune responses, summarized in Table 4.1. The cells and

Table 4.1 Function of Immune Defense Components

Component	Location and/or Function
Central Immune Structures: Immune Cell Production and Maturation	
Bone marrow	Production of lymphocytes
	Maturation of B lymphocytes
Thymus	Gland located in the mediastinum
	Differentiation and maturation of lymphocytes
Peripheral Immune Structures: Process Antigen and Promote Association With Mature Immune Cells	
Lymph nodes	Rounded masses of lymphatic tissue
	Spread out along lymphatic vessels
	Contain many lymphocytes, which filter the lymphatic fluid
Spleen	Site of lymphocyte migration
Lymphoid mucosal tissue (tonsils, Peyer patches, appendix)	Site of lymphocyte aggregation
Primary Cellular Components	
T lymphocytes	Matured in thymus
	Essential in adaptive cell-mediated immunity
	Destruction of cellular antigens
	Promote antibody production by B lymphocytes
	Account for 60% of blood lymphocytes
B lymphocytes	Matured in bone marrow
	Essential in mediating adaptive humoral immunity
	Production of antibodies/immunoglobulins
	Account for 10%–20% of blood lymphocytes
Accessory Cellular Components	
Macrophage	Essential in mediating innate immunity
Neutrophil	Bind invading microbes to cell surface receptors
Dendritic cells	Process and present antigen to T and B lymphocytes, stimulating adaptive immune response
	Phagocytosis to prevent colonization, entry, and spread of microbes

organs of the body work in exquisite harmony to protect the body against bacteria, parasites, viruses, and allergens in well-defined processes.

Cellular Components of Immunity

Many of the cell types involved in immune response were first introduced in Chapter 3 because some of the same cells are involved in the inflammatory response. The initial, rapid response to foreign invaders is known as the innate immune response, a nonspecific response associated with inflammation.

The cellular components involved in innate immunity are also important in adaptive immunity as they are able to process the foreign antigens through phagocytosis and then present them to the cells involved in adaptive immunity. This step is essential for the recognition of foreign antigens by adaptive immunity cells. Cellular components of immune defense are illustrated in Figure 4.1.

IMMUNE CELL ORIGIN

The immune cells of adaptive immunity have a common origin in the pluripotent hematopoietic stem cells. Originating in the bone marrow, the pluripotent hematopoietic stem cells produce two precursor cell types: the **lymphoid progenitor** and the **myeloid progenitor**. Natural killer cells, T lymphocytes and B lymphocytes, are derived from the lymphoid progenitor cells. The myeloid progenitor cells produce other types of cells through the granulocyte/macrophage progenitor. These cells include the monocytes, dendritic cells, granulocytes, and mast cells.

Lymphoid Progenitor Cells

White blood cells (WBCs), also known as leukocytes, are the basic functional units of the immune system. Lymphocytes account for 25% to 35% of the leukocytes circulating in the blood, although 99% of lymphocytes are located in the lymph fluid. Three major categories of WBCs are derived from the lymphoid progenitor cells and play an essential role in immune function. These cell types include:

1. T lymphocytes
2. B lymphocytes
3. Natural killer cells

The **T lymphocytes** mature and fully differentiate in the *thymus*. T lymphocytes require contact with an antigen that signals the T lymphocytes to proliferate and differentiate into the following classifications of cells:

- **Cytotoxic T lymphocytes:** direct destruction of antigen-carrying cells

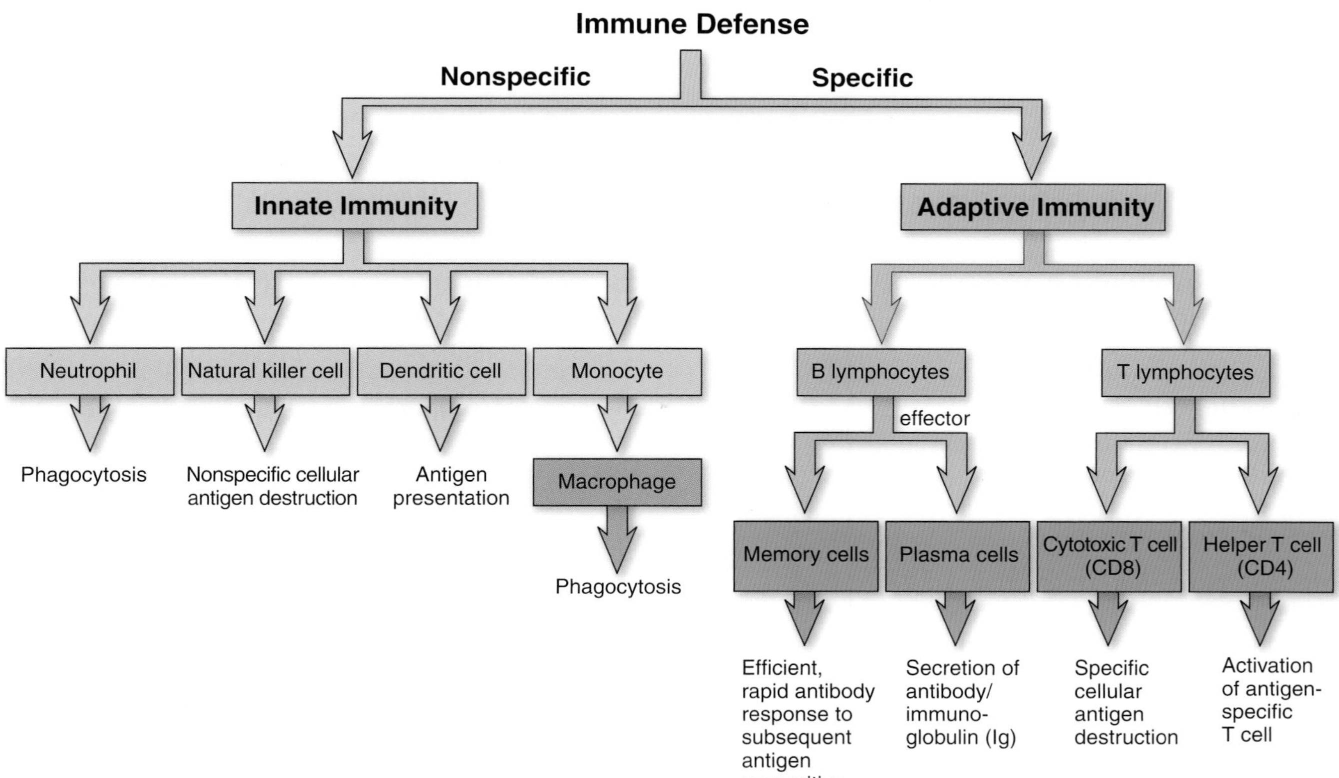

Figure 4.1. Concept map. Cellular components involved in immune defense.

- **Helper T lymphocytes:** enhance humoral and cell-mediated responses of the immune system
- **Suppressor T lymphocytes:** inhibit humoral and cell-mediated responses

The cytotoxic T lymphocyte attacks tumor cells and cells infected with viruses, while the helper T lymphocyte activates other cells needed for an appropriate immune response. Suppressor T lymphocytes provide a balance, limiting immune responses. Each T lymphocyte has a unique receptor, or **T-cell receptor (TCR)**, which is able to bind to antigens, promoting a specific immune response.

B lymphocytes develop in the *bone marrow.* B lymphocytes migrate from the bone marrow to the peripheral lymphoid tissues, where they become activated after contact with an antigen. Binding of the antigen with the B lymphocyte stimulates differentiation of B lymphocytes into antibody-secreting plasma cells. The B lymphocytes recognize specific antigens because of the **B-cell receptor**, or **BCR**, bound to the cell membrane of the B lymphocytes. The uniqueness of antigen–BCR binding contributes to the specificity of the adaptive immune response. After antigen–BCR binding, the B lymphocytes differentiate into plasma cells, which proliferate and begin to produce and secrete large quanitities of antibodies that target the specific antigen bound to the BCR. Antibodies are released from the membranes of plasma cells. The secreted antibody is known as **immunoglobulin**, or **Ig**. The main classes of immunoglobulins include IgA, IgG, IgM, IgD, and IgE (Table 4.2). These antibodies are designed to detect and bind to *specific* antigens, each playing a different role in the immune response.

Natural killer (NK) cells are large, granular lymphocytes. NK cells are active in innate immunity. NK cells circulate until they come in contact with cells they can recognize as a threat, such as virally infected cells or tumor cells. NK cells exert their cytotoxic effect through attack and killing of targeted cells.

Myeloid Progenitor Cells

Myeloid progenitor cells produce granulocytes and monocytes, which are leukocytes essential to immune function. Granulocytes, named for the cytoplasmic granules common to all types, are phagocytic cells. Monocytes are also phagocytic cells, able to engulf larger quantities of debris than granulocytes.

The **granulocytes**, also known as polymorphonuclear (PMN) leukocytes, include neutrophils, eosinophils, and basophils. Although these cells do not live long, their production can be dramatically increased when stimulated. **Neutrophils** are present in the greatest number and are most important in the rapid response to bacterial infection. Neutrophils are phagocytes that are the first responders in the inflammatory response. **Eosinophils** offer the greatest protection against parasites, whereas **basophils** complement the actions of mast cells, important in the establishment of allergic reactions.

Monocytes are large, mononuclear leukocytes, representing 3% to 7% of the total number of circulating leukocytes.[1] Circulating monocytes become activated when in contact with an antigen, prompting differentiation into **macrophages** and movement out of the circulation into the tissues. The antigen-carrying cell is ingested by the macrophage, where it undergoes phagocytosis. During the processing of the antigen, macrophages display antigen markers on the cell surface where they can be recognized by the receptors on T and B lymphocytes. Macrophages are known by different cell names that are determined by the location of tissues where they reside. These cell types include:

- Histiocytes (loose connective tissue)
- Microglial cells (brain)
- Kupffer cells (liver)

Table 4.2 Primary Role of Immunoglobulin Classes

Immunoglobulin	% of Total	Characteristics
IgA	15	Concentrated in bodily secretions such as breast milk, tears, and saliva Protection of mucous membrane–lined structures
IgG	75	Most common circulating antibody Produced in primary and secondary immune responses Activates complement Antibody activity against toxins, viruses, and bacteria Passive immunity in newborns via placental transfer
IgM	10	First immunoglobulin to proliferate in immune response Bound to B lymphocytes Activates complement
IgD	0.2	Bound to and activates B cells
IgE	0.004	Bound to mast cells in skin and mucous membranes Stimulates mast cell release of histamine in allergic immune response, leading to inflammation

Dendritic cells are critical to the processing and display of antigens to T lymphocytes. Mature dendritic cells take up antigens when they are encountered in the circulation. **Langerhans cells**, immature dendritic cells in the skin, carry surface receptors for immunoglobulin and complement, important in the immune response.

Lymphatics

The lymphatic system is composed of central and peripheral organs and is important in the establishment of the immune response. Lymphocytes are produced and differentiated in the central organs, bone marrow, and thymus. The **peripheral organs** serve as sites for maintenance of the lymphocytes and are the organs in which immune responses are often initiated. These organs include the spleen, lymph nodes, and other lymphoid mucosal tissue, such as tonsils and the appendix. The **lymphatic system** circulates the lymphocytes in lymph fluid. **Lymph fluid** is a filtration product of extracellular fluid from tissues and is returned to blood. **Lymph nodes** are joined segments of lymphatic vessels. The vessels of the lymphatic system work in concert with the blood vessels to promote an effective immune response (Fig. 4.2).

The lymphatic system traps antigen captured by cells of the immune system. This process allows the antigen to be presented to immune cells and stimulates the immune response. The lymph also serves to maintain signals to the **naïve lymphocytes**, or those that have not yet encountered an antigen, enabling them to survive. The absence of such a signal results in apoptosis, or programmed death, of cells, as discussed in Chapter 2. This process is essential to the regulation of the number and type of circulating lymphocytes.

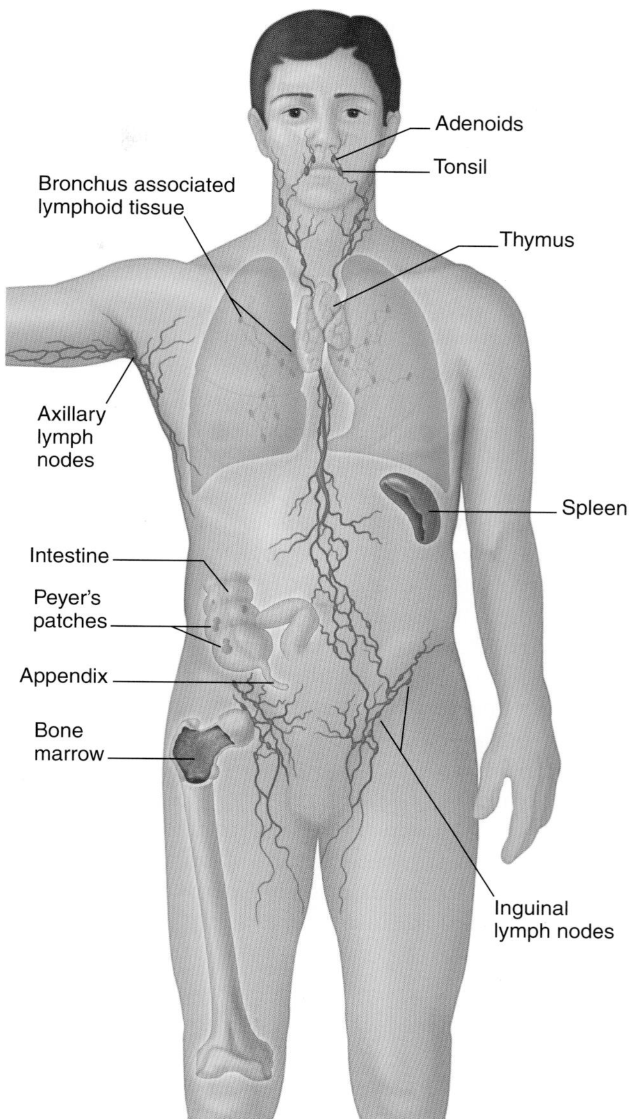

Figure 4.2. Structures of the lymphatic system.

Stop and Consider
When increased lymphocyte production is stimulated, these additional cells travel to the lymph nodes. How could you determine if this was occurring with a physical examination? What signs and symptoms might a person have if this occurs?

Immune Processes

The immune response is vital to an individual's survival. As a result, the immune system involves processes that are both redundant and complementary to one another. The two distinct and specialized processes of immunity are adaptive immunity and innate immunity. **Innate immunity** is the first responder to insult. This immune response is rapid and can be initiated by many different pathogens, without requiring prior exposure. **Adaptive immunity**, humoral and cell-mediated, occurs over a lifetime, promoting the body's ability to adapt to the threat of reinfection.

INNATE IMMUNITY

Macrophages, neutrophils, and dendritic cells are the primary cell types involved in innate immunity. The cells of the innate immune system are the rapid responders to organisms that pose a threat of infection. In addition, these cells work in harmony with the adaptive immune system to initiate and direct continued protection from infection. The functions of the innate immune system include:

- Prevention of microbe colonization
- Prevention of microbe entry
- Prevention of microbe spread

The first exposure to a microorganism initiates an immune response through detection of foreign antigens, as discussed in Chapter 3. An inflammatory response is then initiated. The receptors on the surface of macrophages recognize components common to bacterial, viral, fungal, and parasitic organisms. The inflammatory response initiates the phagocytic process and stimulates the release of chemical mediators with specific purposes. This rapid, early response of the innate immune system is critical to the defense against infection, and it may be adequate to control infection without further action.

Dendritic cells located in the tissues are primarily responsible for presenting the antigen and phagocytosis, which is stimulated in the same manner as macrophages and neutrophils. Dendritic cells are especially important in recognizing hidden antigens. Certain pathogens conceal themselves in envelopes but can be shown to lymphocytes after ingestion by dendritic cells. For this reason, mature dendritic cells are also known as **antigen-presenting cells**. They assist in the recognition of particles that are not part of the individual, or are **nonself**. The innate immune system initiates the activity of the adaptive immune system by this process of recognition of nonself.

ADAPTIVE IMMUNITY

B and T lymphocytes and dendritic cells are the primary cell types involved in adaptive immunity. The adaptive immune system is stimulated by phagocytosis and activation of antigen-presenting cells. Key properties of the adaptive immune system include:

- **Specificity:** targeted response to a distinct antigen
- **Diversity:** recognition of a wide variety of antigens
- **Memory:** rapid and robust response to previously recognized antigens
- **Self and nonself recognition:** ability to distinguish between antigens on body cells and foreign antigens

Adaptive immunity is characterized by a slower response to the introduction of microorganisms than that of the innate immune system. When an organism is reintroduced, immune memory leads to a more rapid and intense immune response. Immunity can be acquired in different ways:

- Active
  - Development of antibodies in response to an antigen
  - Achieved through actually having a specific disease or vaccine immunization against a particular disease
- Passive
  - Immunity transfer from host to recipient
  - Achieved via mother to infant transfer via placenta or breast milk or injection with high concentrations of antibody, such as immune gamma globulin

The adaptive immune system, including humoral and cell-mediated immunity, provides essential defense against specific antigens.

Humoral Immunity

Antibodies, essential components of adaptive immunity, were first identified in the plasma, or humor, as it once was known. The term **humoral immunity** refers to adaptive immunity–involving antibodies. **Antibodies** are immunoglobulins that react with an antigen in a specific way. Immunoglobulins are composed of two regions. The **constant region** forms the base of the Y-shaped antibody and is the most stable component. The two **variable regions** are structured to allow binding to specific antigens. IgG is the most abundant class of immunoglobulin. Because of its size and shape, IgG is able to enter body tissues from body fluids. IgG is the only immunoglobulin that is able to cross the placenta, providing passive immunity to the developing fetus. IgA provides passive immunity from mother to newborn through breast milk, transferring essential immune defense prior to the development of an adequate immune response in the infant. IgM is the initial circulating antibody produced in response to antigen challenge and the first to be produced by the newborn. Located on the B lymphocyte cell membrane, IgD is involved in the binding of antigen and stimulation of differentiation of B lymphocytes into plasma cells. IgE on the cell surfaces of mast cells and basophils leads to cellular degranulation upon antigen binding, triggering the release of chemical mediators involved with inflammation and allergies.

Each B lymphocyte carries a single, specific receptor that recognizes a unique antigen pattern. When an antigen is recognized by the BCR, B lymphocyte activation is initiated, causing proliferation and differentiation of targeted B lymphocytes into **effector cells** (plasma cells that secrete antibodies). The process of activation and differentiation of naïve lymphocytes into effector cells takes approximately 4 to 5 days. Most of these effector cells undergo apoptosis (programmed cell death) after the end of their

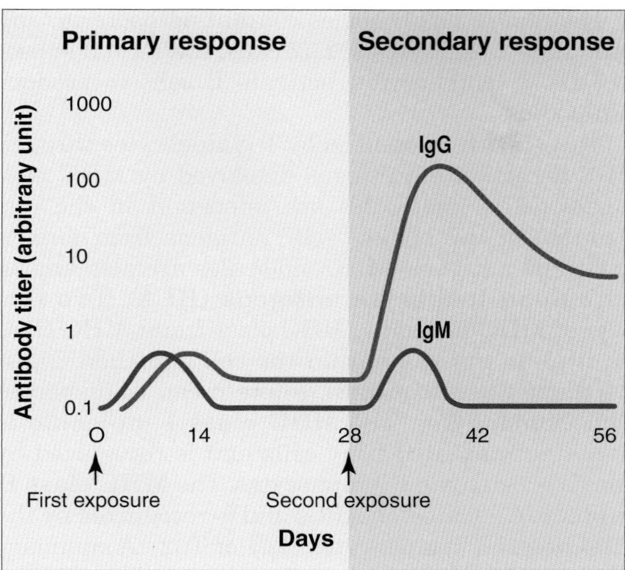

Figure 4.3. Primary and secondary antibody responses. The level of antibodies in the primary and secondary responses to a specific antigen. (From Premkumar K. *The Massage Connection: Anatomy and Physiology*. Baltimore, MD: Lippincott Williams & Wilkins; 2004.)

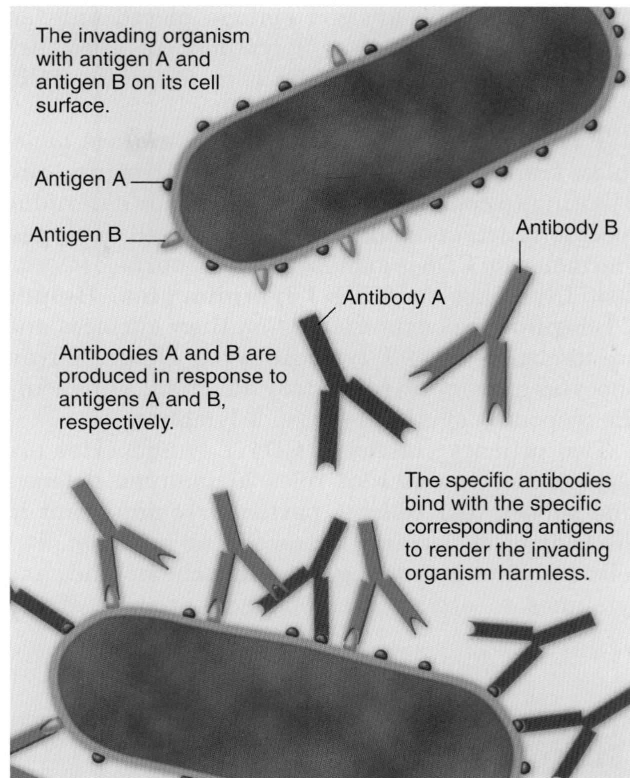

Figure 4.4. Specificity of antigen–antibody binding. Antibodies bind with specific antigens, stimulating clonal expansion, the proliferation of antigen-specific lymphocytes capable of mounting an immune response.

lifespan, although some continue to exist after the antigen is eliminated. These remaining cells are then known as **memory cells**, an important component of **immunologic memory**. These memory cells respond much more rapidly when reexposed to the same antigen, dramatically shortening and intensifying the immunologic response (Fig. 4.3). This process is accomplished through the secretion of higher levels of antibodies and those that bind with higher affinity to the antigens.

Clones of the B lymphocytes carrying cell surface receptors for specific antigens (**clonal selection**) respond by differentiating into plasma cells capable of secreting large quantities of single specificity antibody (**clonal expansion**), the result of antigen occupying the specific BCR (Fig. 4.4). In this way, the humoral immune response can generate a defense that recognizes and targets distinct antigens in a specific manner.

Antibodies protect cells from pathogens in three major ways:

1. The binding of the antigen to the antibody, which prevents the antigen from infecting cells (**neutralization**). The antigen–antibody complex is removed by agglutination (clumping together) or precipitation (falling out of solution).
2. The promotion of phagocytosis and destruction of the pathogen through the phagocyte's ability to recognize the constant region of the antibody that is bound to or coating the antigen (**opsonization**)
3. The activation of complement, which supplements that of the innate system, further enhancing the actions of the antibodies

Cell-Mediated Immunity

Cytotoxic T lymphocytes are the primary immune cells involved in **cell-mediated immunity**, a component of the adaptive immune response. Cell-mediated immunity results in the recognition and destruction of cells carrying non–self-antigens. Cytotoxic T lymphocytes detect pathogens inside the cell where they cannot be recognized by antibodies. Cells infected with viruses displayed on the cell surface are recognized by cytotoxic T lymphocytes. The cytotoxic T lymphocytes kill the cells before viral replication is complete, thereby controlling the further spread of infection. The specificity of T-lymphocyte recognition of foreign antigens involves cell surface markers on antigen-presenting cells (APCs) and infected body cells known as major histocompatibility complex (MHC) molecules, lymphocyte identification by membrane molecules known as clusters of differentiation (CD) and TCRs with specific antigen binding sites. In short, the antigen is processed by an APC, with the antigen epitope placed onto an MHC on the APC surface. T lymphocytes recognize and bind processed antigens with a specific TCR, leading to death of the affected cell.

T lymphocytes display membrane surface molecules, known as **clusters of differentiation**, contributing to cell specificity. CD molecules determine specific functions and responses of T-cell subtypes. The molecule CD8 is expressed on the surface of cytotoxic T lymphocytes (**CD8 T lymphocytes**). **Helper T lymphocytes** express CD4 on their surfaces and are known as **CD4 T lymphocytes**. Helper T lymphocytes provide a regulatory function, enhancing the responses of other types of T lymphocytes.

Two primary classes of CD4 T lymphocytes are responsible for different roles in immune defense. One subset, **T_H1** cells, is particularly important in the control of bacterial intracellular infection. T_H1 cells activate macrophages, secrete chemokines and cytokines to attract macrophages, promote fusion of lysosomes with vesicles containing bacteria, and stimulate phagocytosis. **T_H2** cells, the second subset of CD4 T lymphocytes, activate B cells to produce antibodies.

Targets are recognized by T lymphocytes through TCR detection of antigens displayed by MHC molecules. MHC molecules are important in the recognition of the body's "self" antigens from foreign "nonself" antigens. MHC molecules are also known as **human leukocyte antigens (HLA)**. Two subsets of MHC molecule, MHC class I and MHC class II, trap an antigen within the cell and then transport it to the cell surface, where it can be displayed to T lymphocytes. The **MHC class I molecule** is found on nucleated body cells and is recognized by the CD8 cytotoxic T lymphocytes. The **MHC class II molecule** is found on APCs and is recognized by the CD4 helper T lymphocytes (T_H1 or T_H2). A summary of the steps involved in activation of the adaptive immune system is depicted in Figure 4.5.

Module 2 Process of Altering Immune Function

Daily defense against infection requires interplay between the immune system processes. Failure of even one immune system component can result in catastrophic consequences, presenting a significant risk for disease and death. Altered immunity can result from:

- **Failure of host defense mechanisms:** the impaired ability to mount an immune defense
- **Hypersensitivity:** inappropriate excessive immune responses
- **Autoimmunity:** inappropriate response to "self"
- **Alloimmunity:** reactions directed at tissue antigens from other individuals of the same species

Host Defense Failure

Failure of the **host** (the person on which the pathogen lives) to defend against infection occurs in a variety of ways. Pathogens can trick the immune system, evading the normal signal that stimulates a defense response. The ability of pathogens to multiply in the host cell and spread to others is essential to continued propagation. A "successful" pathogen is one that grows without alerting the immune system to mount a response and is replicated without causing immediate harm to the host. For example, if a virus is too vigorous and kills the host cell, the virus will not be able to multiply.

One of the most effective methods used by pathogens to evade detection from the immune system is called **antigenic variation**. Many pathogens have multiple variations of antigens, making recognition by T and B lymphocytes potentially difficult. Even though the body may have been previously infected by one variant of the pathogen and was able to mount an effective immune response, a variation in the same pathogen will appear new. The pathogen may not be recognized and therefore does not stimulate the immune "memory." Antigenic variation explains the potential of reinfection by a pathogen with a slightly different antigenic epitope. Variations in antigens can also occur because of genetic mutations. Mutated antigens are genetically different enough to prevent identification as a previously recognized pathogen, preventing the mounting of a rapid antibody response. Health concerns resulting from antigenic variation occur each year as influenza (flu) season approaches. Because of frequent genetic mutations, new strains of the influenza virus develop that are capable of escaping detection by the immune system.

Stop and Consider

People can suffer from the same illness, such as a cold, many times. What is a possible explanation for this?

Viruses can evade detection by the immune system by going into **latency**, or a period of inactivity.

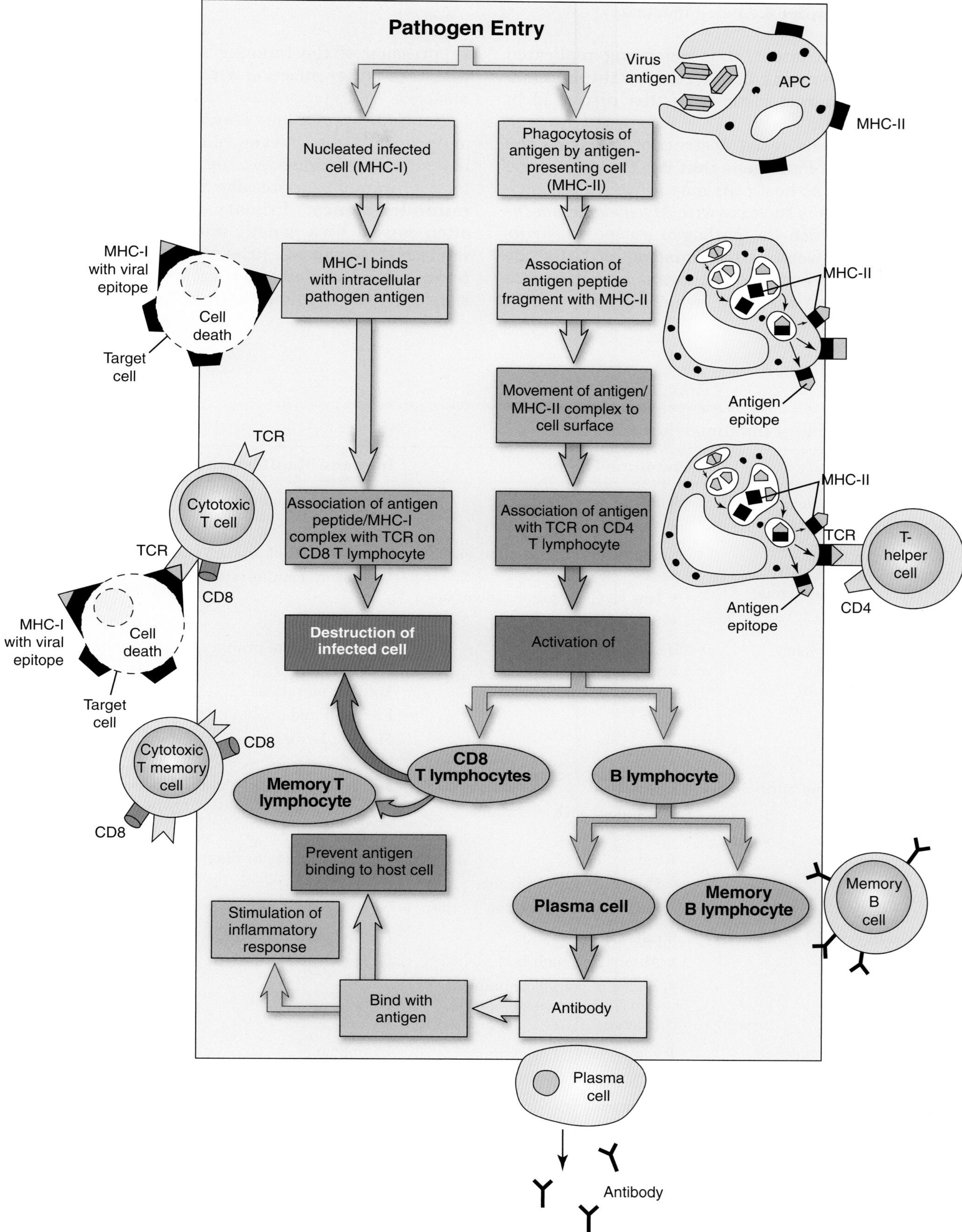

Figure 4.5. Activation of the adaptive immune system. Adaptive immunity is activated on pathogen recognition, stimulating cell-mediated and humoral immunity. Cell-mediated immunity is activated when the major histocompatibility complex (MHC) I/antigen complex binds to the T-cell receptor (TCR) on cytotoxic (CD8) T lymphocytes. Humoral immunity is activated on association of the MHC II/antigen complex with the TCR on helper (CD4) T lymphocytes. B lymphocyte effector plasma cells produce antigen-specific antibodies that prevent antigen binding to the host cell and stimulate the inflammatory response.

When a virus is latent, it is not being replicated and therefore remains undetected by the immune system. This characteristic is further discussed in Chapter 5.

Some pathogens resist destruction by using the immune system. Pathogens that use the cells of the immune system as host cells may prevent their own destruction. This is the case with *Mycobacterium tuberculosis*, in which the pathogen escapes destruction by the lysosome, which instead protects the pathogen. However, some pathogens can stimulate a strong immune response, which then promotes suppression of the immune system. This is sometimes seen after infection with the virus that causes measles.

Immunosuppression resulting from inhibition or incapacitation of even one immune component has significant consequences. The most significant form of immunosuppression is that caused by **immunodeficiency**. Primary immunodeficiency is often caused by a genetic mutation, impairing immune responsiveness. Primary immunodeficiency is frequently identified when recurrent, severe infections are seen in young children. Table 4.3 describes

Table 4.3 Primary Immunodeficiencies

Condition	Immune Deficit	Immune Manifestation
X-linked agammaglobulinemia (Bruton's disease)	B cell • Absent to few B cells	No antibody production
Common variable immune deficiency (CVID) (hypogammaglobulinemia)	Normal B-cell number, but impaired function • Low levels of gamma globulins • Low levels of IgA	Common form of primary immunodeficiency Variable in manifestations
Selective IgA deficiency	B cell • Low levels of IgA	Common form of primary immunodeficiency (1:300) Mild presentation Frequent and unusual infections May not be diagnosed until third or fourth decade
Severe combined immune deficiency	T and B cell • Complete lack of immune defense	Most rare (1:500,000) multiple forms associated with decreased NK cells, circulating T cells, and serum Ig
DiGeorge anomaly	T cell • Underdeveloped thymus • Decrease in circulating T cells	Frequent infections diagnosed soon after birth
X-linked hyper-IgM syndrome	B cell • Absent IgA, high IgM • T cells impaired communication for Ig type switching to B cells	Neutropenia, opportunistic infections GI and liver dysfunction
Wiskott-Aldrich syndrome	T and B cell • Progressive disease in T cells • Decreased IgM	Lymphoma Eczema Autoimmune disease
Ataxia-telangiectasia	T and B cell • Decreased IgA, IgG • Decreased circulating T cells • Immature thymus	Malignancies of the lymphoid tissues X-ray sensitivity
Chronic granulomatous disease	• Impaired phagocytosis • Inability to produce compounds for oxygen transport	Recurrent, severe bacterial and fungal infections

GI, gastrointestinal; NK, natural killer.

common forms of primary immunodeficiency. Immunodeficiency that is a result of another disease is known as secondary immunodeficiency. These deficiencies can involve:

- Defective humoral function
- Deficient phagocyte numbers and functional ability
- Altered T-lymphocyte signaling
- Altered cytokine production and function

The absence of an adequate immune response may lead to overwhelming infection.

Stop and Consider

Some immunodeficiency diseases primarily affect one cell type. What part of the immune defense would be affected if the number of neutrophils was decreased? What would occur with a decrease in the number of macrophages? What would occur with a decrease in the number of plasma cells?

Hypersensitivity

Disorders that result from excessive immune responses to allergens are known as hypersensitivity reactions. **Allergens** are antigens commonly considered to be harmless, unlike the pathogenic organisms discussed previously. The response to these allergens is inappropriate, ranging in severity from mild to severe, and it can be potentially life threatening. The allergens may be environmental, such as pollen, dust, or food products (e.g., nuts), or they may be certain proteins or components found in drugs. In other words, potential allergens are things encountered as a part of daily life.

Allergic reactions to insect stings, primarily honeybees, yellow jackets, hornets, wasps, and fire ants, cause cutaneous reactions (swelling, itching, redness), with the potential for severe systemic reaction. The location of insects causing allergic reactions varies throughout regions of the United States, with yellow jackets prominent in the northern region, wasps in the southwest, and fire ants in the southeast. Food allergies affect both children and adults, with incidence declining with advancing age.[1] In children, food allergy prevalence rose from 3.4% to 5.1% over the last decade, with more than 90% of food allergies due to milk, eggs, wheat, soy, peanuts, and tree nuts. Among adults, peanuts, tree nuts, fish, and shellfish are the most common culprits. Allergies to penicillin are commonly reported, although only a minority of individuals indicating a penicillin allergy have a positive skin test documenting an IgE response to the drug. If a true allergy to penicillin is documented, other "cillin" drugs (i.e., penicillin, ampicillin, and amoxicillin) should be avoided as well, such as the cephalosporin class drugs. These drugs contain a common structure, the beta lactam ring, that can stimulate the allergic response. Hypersensitivity disorders are classified based on four major types of reactions, described in Table 4.4.

Symptoms of allergy result from tissue injury and can vary depending on the route and the "dose" of the allergen exposure. Allergen exposure can occur through inhalation, ingestion, injection, or physical contact. Symptoms can be local (itching and irritation at the point of contact) or systemic (difficulty breathing and oxygenating, as occurs in asthma or anaphylaxis).

Special testing to determine specific allergens capable of stimulating hypersensitivity reactions can be completed. Several methods may be used, including:

- Scratch/prick skin test
  - A small amount of a suspected allergen is placed on the skin, followed by scratching or pricking the skin, introducing the allergen to the skin surface. An allergen is identified when a local hypersensitivity reaction occurs.
- Intradermal skin test
  - The allergen is injected under the skin, followed by observation of a local hypersensitivity reaction.

Table 4.4 Types of Hypersensitivity Reactions

Category	Etiology	Activated Immune Cells	Injury
Type I, immediate hypersensitivity reaction	IgE-mediated	Helper T (T_H2) Mast cells Basophils	Allergic reaction: local (atopic) inflammation; system (anaphylactic) life threatening
Type II, antibody-mediated reaction	IgG- or IgM-mediated	Macrophage	Reaction against normal "self" antigens; opsonization and lysis of cells
Type III, immune complex–mediated reaction	IgG- and IgM-mediated	Complement Neutrophils	Deposition of insoluble antigen–antibody complex
Type IV, cell-mediated hypersensitivity reaction	T-cell-mediated	CD8 T lymphocytes CD4 T_H1 lymphocytes	Inflammatory response leading to cell lysis

- Skin patch test
  - The allergen is placed in a liquid solution on a pad secured to skin, followed by observation of a local hypersensitivity reaction in 24 to 72 hours.
- Measurement of serum IgE
  - Hypersensitivity reaction is determined by the amount of specific IgE antibodies in the blood.
- Elimination diet
  - Suspected food allergens are eliminated, followed by reintroduction and observation of hypersensitivity reaction.

Allergy testing involves exposure of an individual to a potential allergen. Severe reactions can result, requiring testing to be completed under close medical supervision. Allergy testing is an effective method to determine specific allergenic substances. This information can be used to inform individuals of substances to avoid, if possible, and to prevent and treat hypersensitivity reactions.

TYPE I OR IMMEDIATE HYPERSENSITIVITY REACTION

Immediate hypersensitivity reactions are also known as IgE-mediated hypersensitivity responses to antigen challenges. Initial exposure to an allergen in a vulnerable individual stimulates the production of **IgE**, an immunoglobulin important in the development of protective immunity. Allergy is most often caused by inhaled allergens taken in at low doses. These small, dry allergens dissolve and become soluble when they come in contact with mucous membranes. Dendritic cells are activated by these allergens. Dendritic cells then travel to the lymph nodes where they present the allergens to naïve T lymphocytes, promoting their differentiation into T_H2 cells. Specific chemical signals can cause B lymphocytes to produce IgE antibodies in place of other types of antibodies. IgE produced by the plasma cells within inflamed tissue binds with high affinity to receptors on mast cells and basophils. When IgE encounters and binds an allergen, mast cells and basophils degranulate, release chemical mediators and cause injury to cells, producing the symptoms associated with allergy. Lipid products from cell membranes, including leukotrienes and prostaglandins, are also released in this process. Repeated exposure to the same allergen produces an IgE-mediated hypersensitivity response that is responsible for a range of symptoms, some of which can be life threatening. Type I hypersensitivity reaction is an example of a pathophysiologic exaggeration of a defensive immune response (Fig. 4.6).

Immediate hypersensitivity reactions are initiated within minutes of allergen exposure. Some hypersensitivity reactions, including asthma, are known to have symptoms associated with two separate response stages. The symptoms associated with stage 1 are related to mast cell degranulation followed by the release of chemical mediators. They include vasodilation and nonvascular smooth muscle

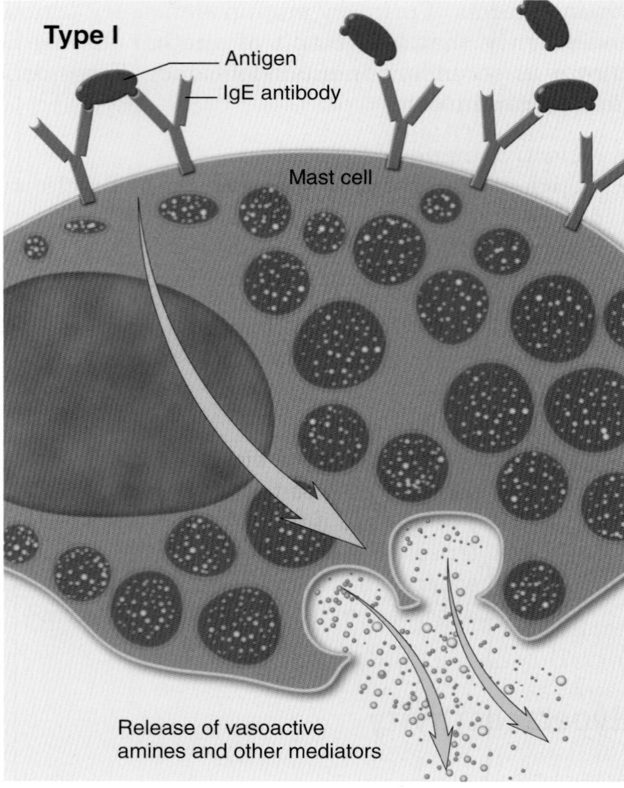

Figure 4.6. Type I immediate hypersensitivity reaction. Antigen–IgE antibody binding induces release of chemical mediators from mast cells.

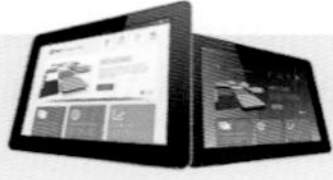

RESEARCH NOTES

Immunotherapy for the treatment of hypersensitivity reactions resulting from insect stings has been used to improve prognosis. While effective in reducing the manifestations of type I hypersensitivity responses, venom immunotherapy (VIT) is also associated with adverse systemic effects. In a clinical trial, the use of purified and nonpurified formulations of VIT and the association with adverse systemic effects were investigated. The use of purified VIT extract reduced the incidence of severe local and systemic reactions, providing evidence of improvement in treatment options in individuals with hypersensitivity to insect stings.[2]

contraction that lasts approximately 1 hour. The second stage follows in approximately 2 to 8 hours and results in symptoms associated with the lipid mediators released from the plasma membrane of degranulated cells. These symptoms are similar to those in stage 1 but last longer. In addition, recruitment of eosinophils and leukocytes results in an inflammatory response in the affected tissues.

Not everyone develops hypersensitivity reactions after allergen exposure. People who develop symptoms after exposure to a wide number of commonly encountered allergens are described as **atopic**, which means that IgE responses are stimulated from exposure to these typically benign substances. Many allergies are familial, meaning they are genetic tendencies that are passed on from one generation to another. Avoidance of potential allergens may prevent the development of atopy, especially early in development.

Systemic manifestations of type I immediate hypersensitivity reactions are potentially life threatening. **Anaphylaxis** represents an extremely serious response to type I immediate hypersensitivity reaction. It is characterized by edema and vasodilation and leads to hypotension. Anaphylaxis is discussed in detail in Module 4: Clinical Models.

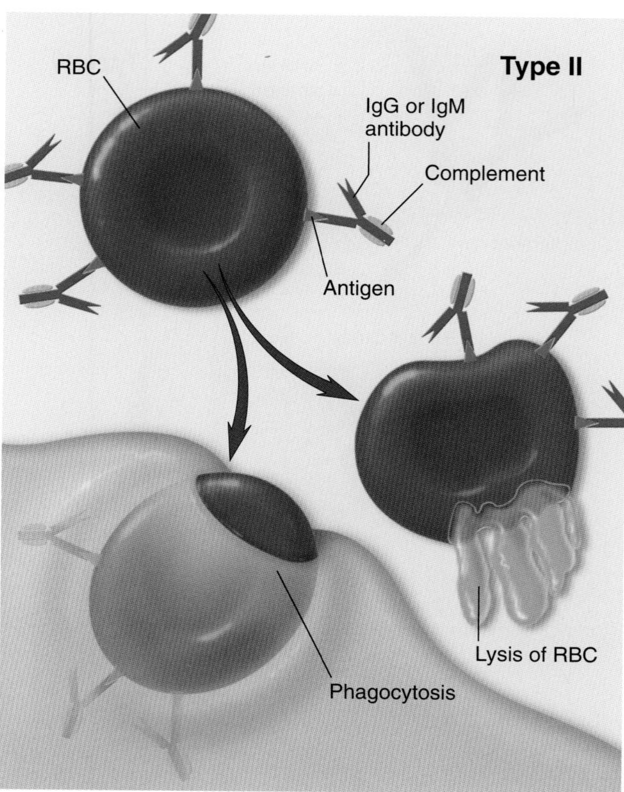

Figure 4.7. Type II antibody-mediated hypersensitivity reaction. Cell-bound antigen binds to IgG or IgM antibodies, leading to a cytotoxic reaction. RBC, red blood cell.

TYPE II ANTIBODY-MEDIATED REACTIONS

Antibody-mediated reactions are the result of mistaken identity. Usually harmless substances are identified as harmful; an immune response is mounted that results in cell damage. The reaction in type II hypersensitivity is tissue specific, usually involving destruction of a target cell by antibody binding to antigen on the cell surface. Cell destruction and tissue damage often result from harm inflicted by macrophage phagocytosis and complement-mediated effects. This is a direct response resulting from an antigen–antibody reaction.

Responses of these types are seen in certain drug reactions, blood transfusion reactions, Graves disease, and hemolytic disease of the newborn. Often, the affected cells include blood cells. When the antibody binds to the antigen on the cell, the cell is lysed and destroyed. This results in disease related to the loss of these cells and includes anemia (decreased red blood cells [RBCs]), thrombocytopenia (decreased platelets), and leukopenia (decreased WBCs). Symptoms are related to the degree of loss of these blood cell types (Fig. 4.7).

Treatment for this type of reaction involves removal of the antigen causing the reaction. When a drug is involved, the administration of the drug is halted to prevent further immune-mediated cellular damage. Avoidance of the antigen is recommended to prevent subsequent, increasingly serious reactions. This drug information is requested and marked prominently on medical records to prevent inadvertent administration in the future. When a patient's treatment involves blood replacement with transfusion, a lab procedure called blood typing and cross-matching is done on recipients to allow matching with donor blood. If a reaction occurs inadvertently during transfusion, the administration of blood is immediately halted. A similar condition known as Rh isoimmunization, the result of exposure to the Rh antigen in a naïve individual, is covered in greater detail in the clinical model section of this chapter.

TYPE III IMMUNE COMPLEX–MEDIATED REACTION

Cellular and tissue damage caused by type III reactions are the indirect result of complement activation stimulated by the deposition of insoluble antigen–antibody complexes. Immune complex activation of complement results in widespread damage from several mechanisms. Altered blood flow, vascular permeability, and the response of inflammatory cells result in damage to blood vessels and organs, including kidney glomeruli, small blood vessels in the skin, and the synovial lining of joints. The

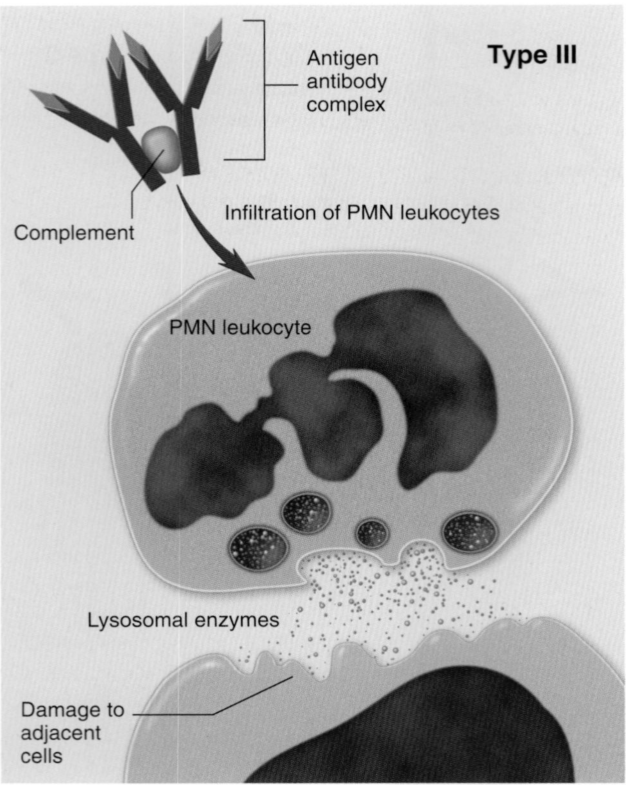

Figure 4.8. Type III immune complex–mediated reaction. Type III reactions are the result of the formation and deposition of immune complexes in tissues, causing acute inflammation polymorphonuclear neutrophil (PMN).

deposition of antigen–antibody complexes triggers the inflammatory immune response of complement activation and recruitment of inflammatory cells (Fig. 4.8). This response was originally seen in individuals who received horse antisera, once used as a treatment for tetanus. These individuals developed a condition referred to as **serum sickness** and responded with local symptoms of itching and rash at the injection site as well as systemic symptoms of edema and fever approximately 7 days after antisera injection. These symptoms resulted from antigen–antibody complex deposition in blood vessels and tissue, prompting complement activation and an inflammatory response.

When the location of this complex-mediated immune response is in the skin, the resulting area of localized tissue necrosis is referred to as an **Arthus reaction**. Although the initial exposure results in symptoms that resolve with time, subsequent exposure can cause a more serious response, sometimes resulting in death. Conditions most commonly associated with this response include the autoimmune diseases of systemic lupus erythematosus (SLE) and rheumatoid arthritis (as discussed in Chapter 3). The administration of certain drugs, including anti-lymphocyte globulin (an immunosuppressive agent used in transplant patients) and streptokinase (thrombolytic agent used with patients having a myocardial infarction), can also stimulate this response.

TYPE IV CELL-MEDIATED HYPERSENSITIVITY REACTION

The heightened immune responses in type IV reactions are caused by T-lymphocyte-mediated reactions rather than antigen–antibody reactions. Two types of these reactions are distinguished by different mechanisms and associated response times. They include direct cell-mediated cytotoxicity and delayed type hypersensitivity reactions.

In **direct cell-mediated toxicity**, damage occurs in cells and tissues as a direct response to CD8 cytotoxic T-lymphocyte destruction of cells with recognized antigens. CD8 cytotoxic T lymphocytes attack all infected cells with recognized antigens, whether the antigen is harmful or not. This response can actually be more harmful than the damage inflicted by the pathogen, as in the case of some forms of hepatitis, in which liver damage is primarily caused by the cell-mediated toxicity rather than by the virus itself.

Delayed hypersensitivity reactions are mediated by antigen-specific T lymphocyte. T lymphocytes respond to antigens presented to them, as described in the earlier discussion of their normal role in immune response. Often, these responses occur on the skin and are mediated by APCs and CD4 helper T lymphocytes of the T_H1 type. Antigens more likely to cause this reaction are small, can penetrate the skin, and can stimulate itching. These antigens react with "self" proteins and create complexes that can bind to MHC molecules seen as foreign by T lymphocytes, stimulating an immune response (Fig. 4.9).

The two phases of delayed hypersensitivity reaction are sensitization and elicitation. The **sensitization phase** begins when the antigen crosses the skin, the first line of defense. Antigens are taken up by Langerhans' cells and transported to the lymph nodes. Once in the lymph nodes, these cells develop into mature dendritic cells, which are able to present antigens to helper T lymphocytes and activate them. Memory cells are produced and become localized in the dermis.

During the **elicitation phase**, the memory T lymphocytes in the dermis are stimulated by a subsequent exposure to the specific antigen. Cytokines and chemokines are released, stimulating the attraction of macrophages and additional T lymphocytes to the area. This results in a visible local reaction at the site of antigen entry. Blood vessel permeability

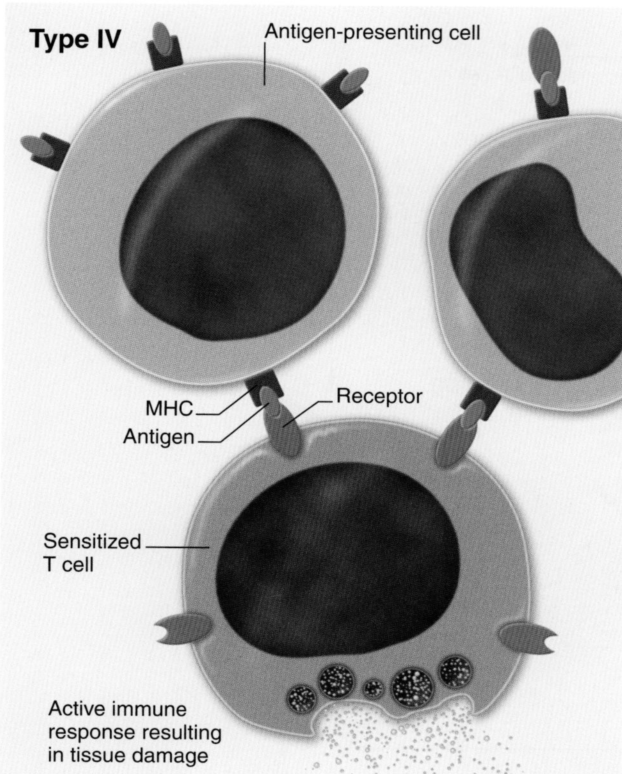

Figure 4.9. Type IV T-cell-mediated delayed hypersensitivity reaction. Type IV reactions occur 1 to 3 days after antigen exposure, resulting in erythema and itching. MHC, major histocompatibility complex.

is increased, leading to swelling. The T-cell-mediated response takes between 24 and 72 hours. This condition is often referred to as contact dermatitis. It can also be initiated by the injection of an antigen to determine an individual's prior exposure to *M. tuberculosis*, commonly referred to as a tuberculin or Mantoux test. Reactions from poison ivy are also the result of type IV hypersensitivity reactions.

Autoimmunity

One of the critical functions of the immune system is to distinguish "self" from "nonself." When this recognition fails or is not controlled, severe **autoimmune** (directed at an individual's own tissues) disease can develop. The two major ways in which this occurs are by specific recognition of "self" antigens and by overzealous responses to chronic infection. The acute autoimmune response can convert to a chronic response if the involved antigen is not adequately cleared or if a positive feedback loop develops in response to the inflammatory process, as described in Chapter 3.

Autoimmune disease can be directed at specific organs, as seen in type II hypersensitivity reactions, or it can have a systemic or whole body effect, as seen in type III hypersensitivity reactions. For example, in Graves disease, the organ affected is the thyroid gland, and antibodies are specifically directed against the thyroid itself (Fig. 4.10). In contrast, SLE is characterized by antibodies formed against proteins found in cells throughout the body, causing systemic disease. We will discuss the specific pathology related to autoimmunity seen in SLE in Module 4, later in this chapter.

Failure in the development of self-tolerance may occur at various steps of immune development. Situations that can trigger autoimmunity include:

- Inadequate elimination of self-reactive lymphocytes in central lymphoid tissues
- Altered **lymphocyte ignorance** (converting lymphocytes from nonresponsive to self-reactive)
- Stimuli, such as infection, overriding the nonresponsive nature of naïve T lymphocytes
- Impaired T-lymphocyte inactivation (prolonged or irreversible)
- Failure to recognize antigen due to MHC–antigen complex interaction
- Release of antigens sequestered during development
- Close resemblance between foreign and self-antigen, also known as **molecular mimicry**
- Inappropriate activation of TCRs by superantigens

A **familial tendency**, or propagation of autoimmunity among family members, is a common trait in autoimmune disease. Both genetic predisposition and environmental factors appear to promote the development of disease. Although a few types of autoimmune disease are caused by an alteration in a single gene, most involve many genes (most of which are unknown), making identifying a responsible target and determining an effective treatment difficult. Drugs and chemical toxins can also precipitate the development of autoimmunity, although the exact mechanism involved is unclear.

Although difficult, treatment and prevention of autoimmunity continue to be areas of intense interest. The development of newer techniques and increased knowledge of the science of immunology have been instrumental in promoting recent advances to develop effective clinical treatments. The study of T-cell-mediated responses has uncovered the existence of suppressor cells, also known as **regulatory T cells**. These cells, as their name implies, are able to suppress autoreactive lymphocytes and regulate the immune response. Isolation of these specialized T lymphocytes and the administration of them to individuals are future potential therapeutic strateies for those diagnosed with autoimmune disease.

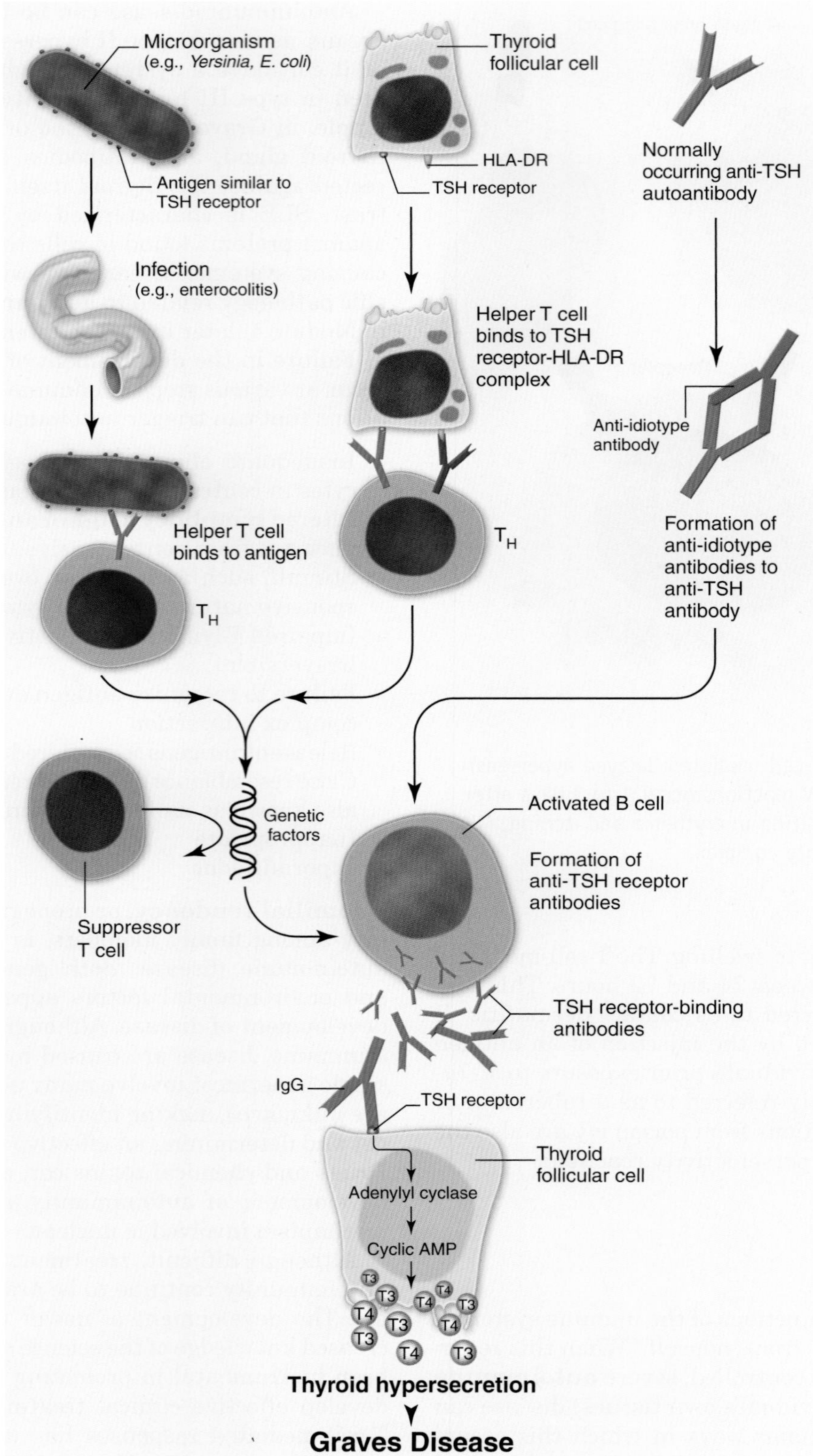

Figure 4.10. Possible mechanisms of organ-specific autoimmune disease: Graves disease. This figure depicts three possible pathways by which B cells are activated to produce anti-TSH receptor antibodies. These antibodies stimulate thyroid cells to secrete T3 and T4. Indirect pathways shown to the left and middle involve activation of helper T cells along with genetic factors that inhibit suppressor T cells. The pathway on the right shows antibodies against anti-TSH antibodies cross-reacting with the TSH receptor. HLA-DR, human leukocyte antigen-D related. (Modified from Rubin E, Farber JL. *Pathology*. 4th ed. Philadelphia, PA: Lippincott Williams & Wilkins; 2005.)

Alloimmunity

Alloimmunity occurs when an immune response is stimulated in response to the presence of cells from another individual of the same species. Alloimmunity can occur after allograft (transplantation of body tissues) or allotransfusion (transfusion of body fluids, such as blood or plasma).

GRAFT REJECTION

Grafts (unattached tissues or organs used for implantation) are commonly used in the treatment of disease. The acceptance of grafted tissue donated from one individual to another depends on the matching of MHC molecules. MHC molecules are **polymorphic** (occurring in more than one form) and **polygenic** (containing several MHC class I and II genes). These two characteristics make matching the MHC molecules challenging. The likelihood of a match increases when both donor and recipient are related, but even then matching is not guaranteed. Grafts from different sites on the same person (**autograft**) or from genetically identical individuals/monozygotic twins (**syngeneic**) are fully accepted; however, a graft between unrelated individuals (**allograft**) is often rejected after 10 to 13 days without drugs to control immune response.

Stop and Consider
Why is there less chance of rejection when a transplant occurs between identical twins? Is the chance of rejection the same if the twins are fraternal (not identical)?

Adaptive immune responses mediated by T lymphocytes (CD4 and CD8) are responsible for rejection of grafted tissue due to the recognition of **alloantigens** (proteins that vary between individuals) as foreign. When APCs from the donor leave the graft site and travel via the lymphatic system, host T lymphocytes are activated. These activated T lymphocytes travel back to the graft and attack the alloantigens, destroying the grafted tissue.

The presence of **alloantibodies** (antibodies produced against alloantigens) can contribute to the rapid rejection of grafts, known as **hyperacute graft rejection**. These antibodies recognize and attack antigens on endothelial cells lining blood vessels, stimulating both the complement and clotting cascades. Vessels become **occluded**, or blocked, preventing perfusion and resulting in cell and tissue death to the affected site. This is often seen in **blood transfusion**, the most common form of tissue transplant. The antibodies in the recipient interact with antigens from the donor leading to systemic effects, because blood type antibodies can bind to all tissue types. This issue can be avoided by ensuring that the recipient's blood type is the same as the donor (determined by **blood typing**) and that the recipient has no antibodies that are able to react with the WBCs of the donor (determined by **cross-matching**).

GRAFT VERSUS HOST DISEASE

Graft versus host disease (GVHD) presents a contrast to graft rejection. The most common condition resulting in GVHD is the transplantation of **hematopoietic stem cells**, or cells that can differentiate into healthy blood cells. This treatment is often used to fight bone marrow cancers such as leukemia or to cure immunodeficiencies. Transplantation of hematopoietic stem cells can result in an individual's ability to produce normal, healthy blood cells in place of the deficient or damaged cells that result in disease. For transplantation to be successful, the diseased recipient bone marrow must first be destroyed. Donor stem cells may then be transplanted. GVHD occurs when the T lymphocytes of the donor recognize the recipient's body as being different or foreign. Donor-immunocompetent T lymphocytes (CD4 and CD8) detect antigens in the recipient's tissue and mount an attack. The immunocompromised recipient tissue cannot mount a defense against the attack, which results in a type IV hypersensitivity reaction. This disease, which can be fatal, is characterized by rash, diarrhea, and liver disease.

Module 3 Immune Response Manipulation

As previously discussed, many diseases are the result of an immune response that fails to distinguish "nonself" from "self" antigens. When this occurs, the immune response is then directed toward "self" and serves as the basis for chronic inflammation, which leads to cellular alterations and injury. As the understanding of the mechanisms regulating immune function grows, these discoveries can be used to manipulate the immune system favorably. Many treatment strategies are based on interference with the responses seen in autoimmunity and hypersensitivity. Exploitation of these mechanisms may also play a significant role in the treatment of disease.

Treatment of Maladaptive Immune Responses

Immune responses can be inappropriate or exaggerated as is the case in allergy, autoimmune disease, and tissue rejection. Control of unwanted immune responses decreases the signs and symptoms associated with illness and disease. Suppression of the immune system, which also suppresses the inappropriate immune response, is the goal of treatment. This general response carries with it the risks associated with immunosuppression, particularly the increased risk of opportunistic infection (see Chapter 5).

A number of classes of drugs are used to regulate immune responses, and each target a particular mechanism. The first class is anti-inflammatory drugs, usually in the corticosteroid family. One of the most common of these drugs is prednisone. Prednisone is a synthetic analog of **cortisol**, the hormone synthesized in the adrenal cortex (see Chapter 11). Prednisone has a body-wide effect typically seen with hormones because almost all body cells carry the receptor for cortisol. When the intracellular receptor binds with prednisone, a signaling cascade is initiated that regulates the **transcription** (transfer of genetic information) of a large number of genes. The amount of prednisone taken for treatment translates into blood levels much higher, or **supraphysiologic**, compared with that found with the normal secretion of cortisol. This causes an exaggerated cellular response with both beneficial and potentially harmful results. The beneficial effects are the desired outcomes of treatment and include anti-inflammatory effects as a result of immune response suppression. The adverse effects are wide-ranging because of the body-wide responses induced; these effects include elevated blood sugar, loss of bone mineral, thinning of skin, weight gain, altered fat deposition, and fluid retention. A delicate balance to create the desired effect and minimize adverse effects is necessary for optimal treatment outcome.

Stop and Consider

The adrenal gland stops producing cortisol during prednisone treatment. Why does this happen? What are the special considerations made when prednisone treatment is no longer needed?

A second class of drugs commonly employed in regulation of immune response is cytotoxic drugs. Commonly used drugs in this family include methotrexate, azathioprine, mycophenolate, and cyclophosphamide. A common mechanism among these drugs includes interferance with DNA synthesis in dividing cells. Rapidly dividing cells are most sensitive to the effects of this mechanism and include the cells of the bone marrow (lymphocytes, RBCs, and platelets), the cells lining mucosal membranes of the gastrointestinal tract, the cells of a developing fetus, and hair follicle cells. The proposed target in this method of treatment is dividing lymphocytes, with the desired outcome of decreased immune function. As a result of the nonspecific nature of the drugs, their use is associated with significant adverse effects. High doses of these toxic drugs are used when the treatment goal is elimination of all dividing lymphocytes. These patients then require bone marrow transplant to resume production of necessary blood cells. Lower doses, commonly accompanied by anti-inflammatory drugs, are used to manage unwanted immune responses.

Bacterial and fungal derivative drugs are a third class of drugs used to regulate immune function. These drugs alter signal transduction pathways in T lymphocytes, reducing inflammation by alteration of the reproductive cell cycle. Commonly used drugs in this family include cyclosporine A, tacrolimus, and rapamycin. Predominantly used in transplant patients, these drugs prevent tissue rejection by binding to a group of intracellular proteins. These proteins then form complexes that alter signal transduction pathways used in the proliferation of T lymphocytes and the clonal expansion of activated T lymphocytes. Because each of these drugs has a specifically targeted mechanism of action in the signal pathway, they are often used in combination. Another class of drugs target cytokine activity, limiting immune responses. These drugs are designed to interfere with the binding of the cytokine tumor necrosis factor-alpha (TNF-alpha) to its receptor, reducing inflammation. Interferons also reduce inflammation and are used in the treatment of the autoimmune condition multiple sclerosis (Chapter 9).

Ideally, drugs specifically targeting the mechanism of chronic inflammation resulting from inappropriate immune responses will be developed. The optimal treatment effect of regulating inappropriate immune responses and maintaining functional responses is the objective in the management of related diseases. The use of this biologic therapy is ongoing clinically to specify targets in the signal transduction pathway.

Immune Response in Disease Management

Using the body's own immune system to attack pathologic cells is another mechanism by which the immune system can be exploited to achieve a positive outcome. Cancer, a disease resulting from uncontrolled proliferation of a single transformed cell, is a central target for this type of strategy. Pathophysiologic processes associated with cancer are discussed in detail in Chapter 7. Development of a drug that can promote the ability of the immune system to distinguish normal cells from transformed cancer cells would be a useful treatment strategy. The desired outcome is the recognition and destruction of cancer cells while avoiding the destruction of normal cells, thereby preserving immune function and minimizing adverse effects.

Immune Response in the Prevention of Disease

Vaccines work by stimulating immunity through exposure to an antigen. This immune response is designed to reactivate quickly when reexposure to the antigen occurs, the result of immunologic memory. Early vaccination technique was attempted to prevent smallpox by using a small amount of actual pathogen to stimulate immunity. However, the safety of this technique was not ensured—some people actually contracted the illness and died. Later, the use of vaccines made from pathogen analogs derived from other species was effective in stimulating immunity and was a much safer alternative. For vaccines to be effective, the following requirements must be met:

- Vaccines must be safe and must avoid the development of actual disease.
- Vaccines must protect against illness caused by live pathogens.
- Vaccines must provide long-lasting protection.
- Vaccines must stimulate antibody production and T-cell-mediated immunity.
- Vaccines must be accessible and affordable.
- Vaccines must have minimal side effects.

Modern vaccination techniques include the use of **attenuated** (reduced ability to cause disease) or killed organisms. In some cases, **conjugated vaccines,** which promote activation of more than one cell type, are necessary to stimulate an adequate immune response to a specific pathogen. The use of adjuvants, or substances that increase immune response to antigens, is sometimes necessary for stimulation of protective immune responses.

Stop and Consider
Many vaccines are available to protect against common diseases and conditions. What are some reasons why people do not get immunized?

Module 4 Clinical Models

The following clinical models have been selected to illustrate the concepts of altered immunity. As you read the descriptions that follow, think about the concepts of altered immune function as they apply to the specific conditions to help understand and apply these concepts to the models.

Immune Maladaptation: AIDS

AIDS is a condition representative of altered host defense. It is a secondary immunodeficiency caused by infection with the **human immunodeficiency virus (HIV)**. HIV is an enveloped retrovirus that infects CD4 helper T lymphocytes, dendritic cells, and macrophages. Symptoms of acute HIV infection include vague flulike complaints associated with the activation of CD8 cytotoxic T lymphocytes and CD4 T_H1 lymphocytes. Initially, this response works to control infection by killing HIV-infected cells, followed by antibody production against the virus. The hallmark of AIDS is the loss of cell-mediated and humoral immunity due to the loss of CD4 T_H1 lymphocytes.

Sub-Saharan Africa has been particularly affected by the HIV epidemic. According to UNAIDS, a joint United Nations and World Health Organization program on HIV/AIDS, 25.8 million people were living with HIV in Sub-Saharan Africa in 2014, accounting for approximately 70% of new HIV infections worldwide.[3] In the United States, approximately 50,000 people are infected with HIV annually. Youth aged 13 to 24 years account for 26% of new HIV infections. Men who have sex with men are at highest risk. There are 1.2 million individuals aged 13 and older living with HIV, with males representing 74% of cases among adolescents and adults.[4] Among young adults aged 20 to 24 in the United States, almost 10,000 men and women were living with AIDS at the end of 2006.[5] In North America, AIDS continues to disporportionately affect African Americans and Aboriginal people in the United States and Canada, respectively.[6]

PATHOPHYSIOLOGY

HIV is transmitted by sexual contact, blood contamination, and perinatally between individuals. Infection with HIV occurs across mucosal surfaces covered with stratified squamous epithelium, including the vagina, cervix, and anus. Cell targets of HIV infection include dendritic cells, macrophages, and CD4 helper T lymphocytes. Dendritic cells bind HIV and transport it to the lymphoid tissues where it encounters the CD4 helper T lymphocytes. When the virus enters the host cell, the viral RNA is transcribed into complementary DNA, which is then integrated into the host cell, stimulating replication of this provirus. The virus undergoes rapid replication, associated with the generation of many viral mutations. These mutations are numerous and can occur within a day, promoting the development of antigenic variation. Viral drug resistance develops rapidly, requiring the use of combination therapy.

CLINICAL MANIFESTATIONS

Initial infection with HIV is asymptomatic. The time period between initial infection and symptom development is typically 2 to 4 weeks but can extend to a period of several months. Early symptoms of acute HIV infection, also known as acute retroviral syndrome, are generalized and typically include fever, lymphadenopathy, sore throat, skin rash, joint and muscle pain along with headache. As the disease progresses, the CD4 helper T-lymphocyte number gradually declines, promoting significant immunosuppression. The loss of CD4 T lymphocytes is caused by the killing of infected cells by viruses, the apoptosis (programmed cell death) of infected cells, and the killing of CD4 helper T lymphocytes by CD8 cytotoxic T lymphocytes. Cell-mediated immunity is lost when the CD4 helper T-lymphocyte level is too low, contributing to the risk of opportunistic infection. Resistance is lost to many common pathogens, including the fungi *Candida*. Activation of latent viruses may occur, promoting symptoms and disease. Kaposi sarcoma, a tumor of endothelial cells, and non-Hodgkins lymphoma are AIDS-defining cancers of decreasing prevalence after widespread antiretroviral therapy (ART) adoption. HIV-infected individuals with lowered immune function are at risk for pneumonia though the incidence of *Pneumocystis carinii (jiroveci) pneumonia* has decreased significantly since adoption of ART. Lowered immune function in HIV-infected individuals increases risk for non–AIDS-defining cancers and bacterial forms of pneumonia seen in the general population. Metabolic complications (including dyslipidemia, diabetes mellitus, bone disease), certain non–AIDS-defining cancers, and coinfections are also linked with HIV infection. Hematologic, renal, and hepatic toxicities are complications of HIV infection and treatment. Neurocognitive impairment, anxiety, and depression are more common among individuals infected with HIV. Figure 4.11 shows many of the conditions experienced by patients with immunosuppression due to AIDS.

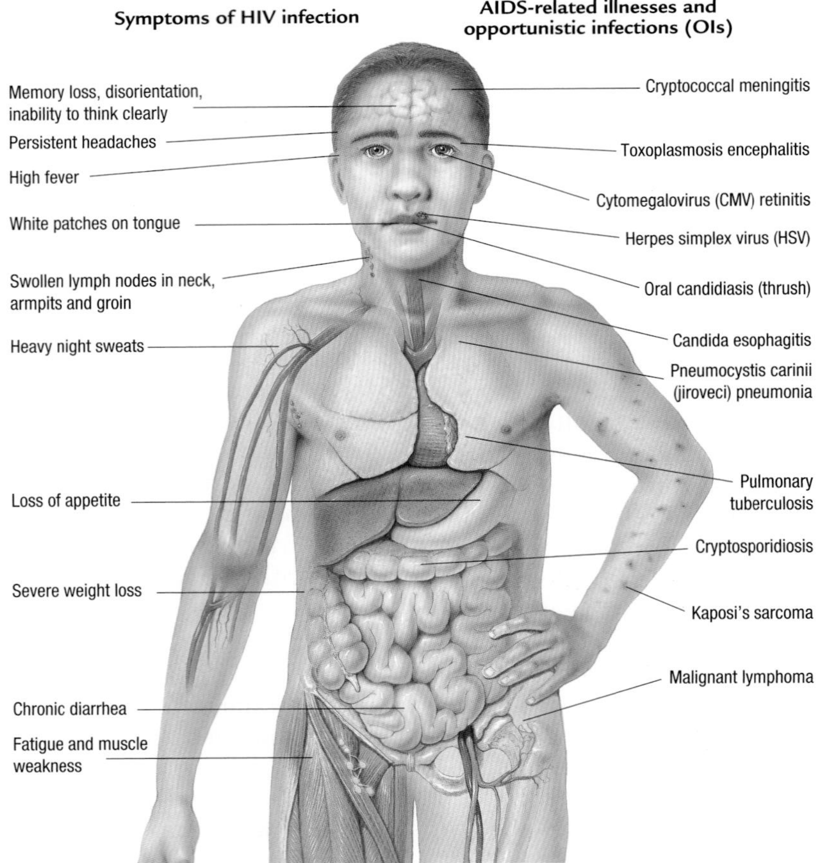

Figure 4.11. Manifestations of HIV infection and AIDS. (Courtesy Anatomical Chart Company.)

These conditions are normally controlled or prevented by CD4 helper T-lymphocyte-stimulated cell-mediated immunity, lost when CD4 host T-lymphocyte numbers are significantly decreased.

Stop and Consider
Why are immunosuppressed patients at greater risk for cancer?

DIAGNOSTIC CRITERIA

Recommendations for HIV screening from the Centers for Disease Control and Prevention (CDC) include routine initial screening in individuals aged 13 to 64 years. Annual repeat screening is advised for all those at high risk for HIV infection.[6] Individuals at risk for infection (i.e., intravenous drug users, diagnosis with a sexually transmitted disease, diagnosis/treatment for hepatitis or tuberculosis, sex with someone HIV positive or HIV status unknown) should be screened. The criteria used in the diagnosis of HIV infection is often based on initial tests that identify HIV viral load (HIV RNA), HIV-1 antigen (p24) and HIV-1 and HIV-2 antibody (immunoassay). It takes most people about 3 months from time of exposure to develop antibodies to HIV. This occurrence is known as **seroconversion**. People are usually asymptomatic at this time and can unknowingly infect others with the virus.

Progression of HIV infection is based on laboratory criteria and on signs and symptoms of immunosuppression. Later complications related to immunosuppression include infection with candidiasis, cytomegalovirus, mycobacterium, toxoplasmosis, *Pneumocystis carinii (jiroveci) pneumonia*, movement disorders, dementia, non-Hodgkin lymphoma, or Kaposi sarcoma of the skin and mucous membranes. The CDC classifies the stages of HIV infection based on CD4 T-lymphocyte counts for surveillance purposes.[7] Stages of infection among those ≥6 years of age include stage 0 (early HIV infection based on a negative HIV test result within 6 months of a confirmed positive result), stage 1 (≥500 cells/µL), stage 2 (200 to 499 cells/µL), and stage 3 (<200 cells/µL). When an individual meets the criteria for stage 3, that is consistent with AIDS. Worsening disease and immune status are correlated with a progressively decreased number of CD4 helper T lymphocytes.

TREATMENT

Prevention from HIV exposure is a critical first step in avoiding HIV infection. For individuals at high risk, preexposure prophylaxis (PrEP) includes daily antiretroviral medication coupled with other preventive strategies (e.g., condoms), which can be used to reduce the risk of HIV infection. Postexposure prophylaxis (PEP) includes the initiation of 2 to 3 antiretroviral medications as soon as possible, but no more than 3 days, after HIV exposure and should be continued for 28 days. Recommended treatment of HIV is the use of ART. Initiation of ART in early HIV infection is associated with suppression of HIV viral load, improved CD4 T-lymphocyte counts, and markers of immune function.

The goals of ART include:

- Maximal and long-lasting viral load suppression
- Restoration or preservation of immune function
- Reduction in morbidity and mortality related to HIV

Because of the ability of the HIV retrovirus to evade the immune system by mutating into different forms, resistance to drug therapy is a primary concern. Testing of drug resistance to determine the effectiveness of antiretroviral drug virus replication inhibition is necessary for the selection of the most effective multidrug antiviral medication regimens. Specific drugs included in ART are designed to delay disease progression by suppressing viral replication and addressing the issues of increasing drug resistance.[8] These drugs can be categorized into classes known as nucleoside and nucleotide analog reverse transcriptase inhibitors (NRTIs), nonnucleotide reverse transcriptase inhibitors (NNRTIs), protease inhibitors (PIs), and integrase strand transfer inhibitors (INSTIs). Although the use of ART has increased effectiveness over monotherapy or combined two-drug therapy, significant barriers contribute to failed treatment regimens. To increase the patient's willingness and ability to use these drugs, ongoing counseling and assistance with problem areas are critical to successful treatment. More information about specific strategies can be found in the guidelines for counseling by the CDC listed in the resource section at the end of this chapter.

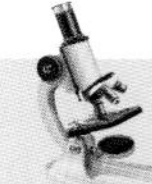

FROM THE LAB

Diagnosis of HIV infection is made by the detection of the presence of HIV antibodies. A screening test known as immunoassay detects the HIV antibody. Body fluid samples (saliva, blood, or urine) may be tested. A positive screening test is not diagnostic of HIV infection and requires a confirmatory test. Other tests that can confirm HIV infection include tests that detect the HIV antigen. The amount of HIV in the blood can be determined by a test for viral load. The competency of the immune system can be determined by measurement of the CD4 T-lymphocyte cell count.

Stop and Consider
What special considerations must a person with AIDS take to limit illness caused by immunosuppression? What considerations must others make to protect a person with AIDS?

Immune Maladaptation: Anaphylactic Reaction

This clinical model represents a systemic response to a type I hypersensitivity reaction. Anaphylaxis can occur from exposure to drugs, environmental compounds, insect venom or stings, or food products that stimulate an exaggerated immune response. Reexposure to an allergen is responsible for triggering this IgE-mediated event. The induced systemic response produces a hypersensitivity reaction affecting many organ systems, which is potentially fatal without treatment.

PATHOPHYSIOLOGY

Exposure to an allergen in an individual previously sensitized by that allergen stimulates the classical allergic hypersensitivity response of degranulation of mast cells and basophils. The IgE bound to receptors on these cells induces the release of chemical mediators when binding with the allergen occurs (Fig. 4.12). The reaction occurs locally but is spread beyond the site of allergen entry by the bloodstream. Vascular smooth muscle dilates, bronchial smooth muscle constricts, and vascular permeability increases, accounting for the clinical manifestations seen in this condition. These effects are potentially fatal without intervention and supportive care.

CLINICAL MANIFESTATIONS

The clinical manifestations stimulated by anaphylactic reaction are determined by the amount of antigen-specific IgE present, the dose of the antigen, and the route of antigen transmission. A biphasic (two-phase) response results from the release of chemical mediators, including histamine, prostaglandins and leukotrienes (bronchoconstriction), and cytokines (increased IgE production and inflammation). The initial response occurs within minutes to a few hours and includes severe **bronchospasm** (contraction of the smooth muscle in the bronchi and bronchioles of the lungs, decreasing airway size and making it difficult to breathe), skin flushing, **urticaria** (itching), and **angioedema** (sudden subcutaneous edema). The first phase is a response to short-acting chemical mediators, and the second phase of this reaction is caused by longer-acting substances occurring approximately 4 hours after the first phase reaction. During the second phase, severe bronchospasm recurs and is often accompanied by severe hypotension and edema. Immediate evaluation and treatment of these manifestations must be instituted because of the emergency nature of anaphylaxis. Severe reactions can result in anoxia and death.

Stop and Consider
Why don't all people stung by insects develop systemic symptoms of anaphylaxis?

DIAGNOSTIC CRITERIA

Diagnosis is based on symptoms and history. Symptoms of acute onset of illness after antigen/allergen exposure involving skin (hives, itch, flush) and mucous membranes (swelling of lips/tongue), respiratory compromise (wheeze, bronchospasm, and increased work of breathing) and drop in blood pressure (possibly associated with fainting or incontinence), and gastrointestinal symptoms (abdominal cramping/vomiting) are criteria for anaphylaxis diagnosis. People on multiple drugs and people suffering from insect sting, atopy, or food allergy are especially susceptible. Testing to determine the responsible antigen can be done to educate the patient about specific allergens to avoid or to provide the basis of future treatment. Prognosis is based on the severity of symptoms and the time it takes to provide treatment for acute symptoms.

TREATMENT

Removal of anaphylaxis trigger, if possible, is the first step in management. Initial treatment is designed to treat symptoms and limit inflammation. Immediate administration of epinephrine to relax bronchial smooth muscle, reform endothelial tight cell junctions in blood vessels, and control cardiovascular effects is the first line of treatment. Inhaled bronchodilators may also assist in the treatment of bronchospasm. Airway management, including the use of supplemental oxygen, are important in promoting oxygen delivery to cells and tissues. Antihistamines may help reduce the symptoms stimulated by histamine release, such as itching and increased vessel permeability. Fluids may be provided to restore intravascular volume. If the initial treatment is delayed, the prognosis worsens. The symptoms associated with the second phase are much more difficult to treat and may require intubation and mechanical ventilation to provide oxygenation.

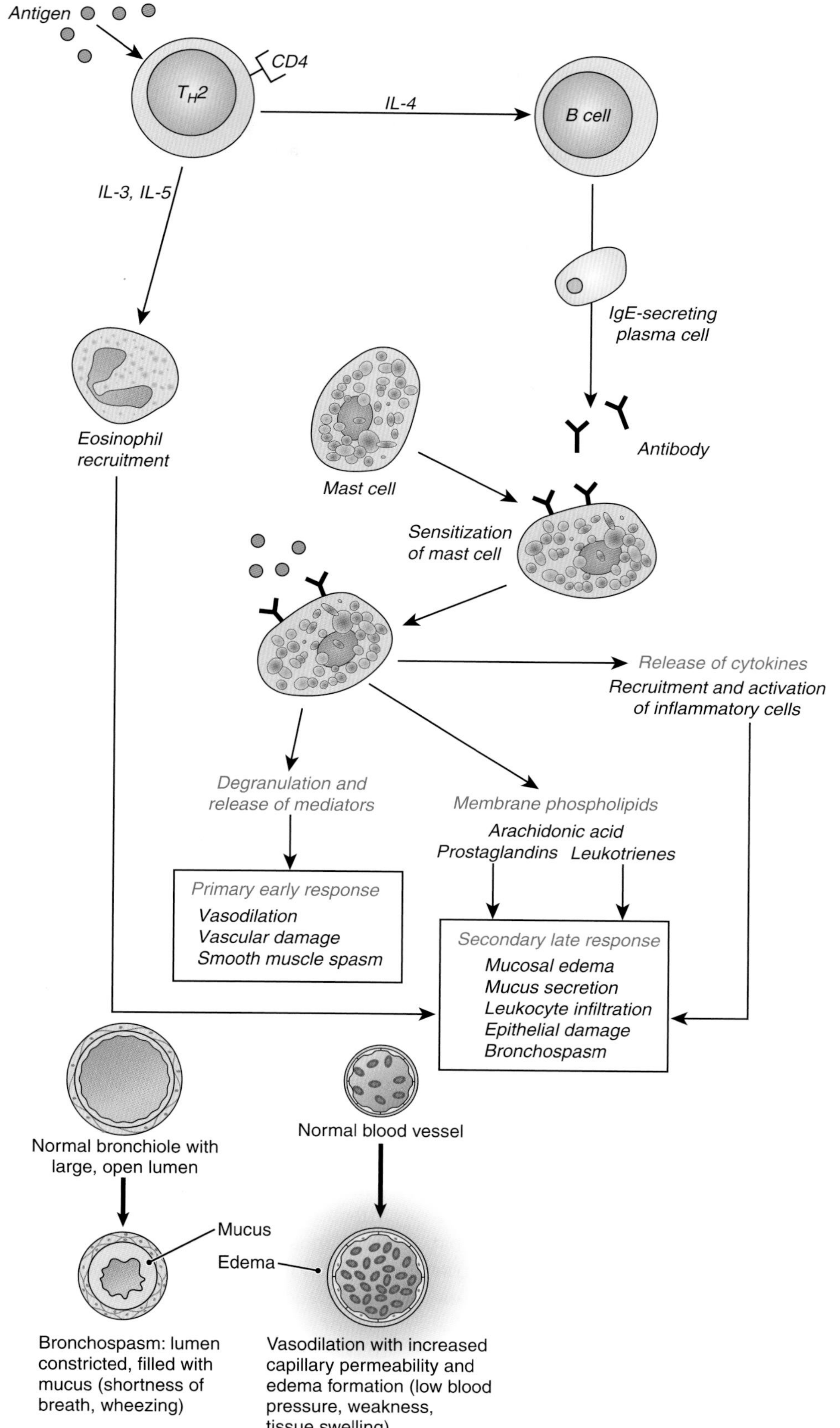

Figure 4.12. IgE-mediated response in anaphylactic reaction. Allergen triggers B lymphocyte differentiation into IgE-secreting plasma cell, stimulated by an activated type II helper T lymphocyte (T_H2). IgE attaches to the mast cell. When the allergen reappears, it binds to the mast cell-bound IgE and triggers mast cell degranulation, releasing chemical mediators that stimulate primary early response manifestations. Secondary late response manifestations are the result of lipid mediators released from phospholipids in the destructed cell membrane and recruitment of eosinophils by T_H2 lymphocytes.

Long-term treatments include desensitization and signaling pathway blockade of effectors. The goal of desensitization is to:

1. Switch the IgE response to an IgG response
2. Bind the allergen and prevent stimulation of IgE-mediated responses by skin injection of allergen in progressively larger doses
3. Change the helper T-lymphocyte effectors from T_H2 to T_H1 cells to downregulate the IgE response

Blockade of signaling pathways of mediators stimulating hypersensitivity responses, including cytokines, is another potential long-term treatment.

Immune Maladaptation: Systemic Lupus Erythematosus

Systemic lupus erythematosus (SLE) is an example of a type III hypersensitivity reaction. SLE is considered an autoimmune disease and features responses from both the innate and humoral immune systems. The chronic nature of this disease is a result of persistent antigen-promoting complex deposition and inflammation. Autoantibodies are targeted against the self-antigenic components of the cell membrane (antiphospholipid), cytoplasm (anticytoplasmic), and cell nucleus (antinuclear), including the DNA. Binding of antigen with these antibodies stimulates activation of the complement system and accumulation of immune complexes. The location of these complexes and the organs that are involved determine the symptoms of the disease (Fig. 4.13). Because the involved antigens are present in all of the cells, SLE is a chronic, systemic disease that can potentially damage a wide range of cell types and locations.

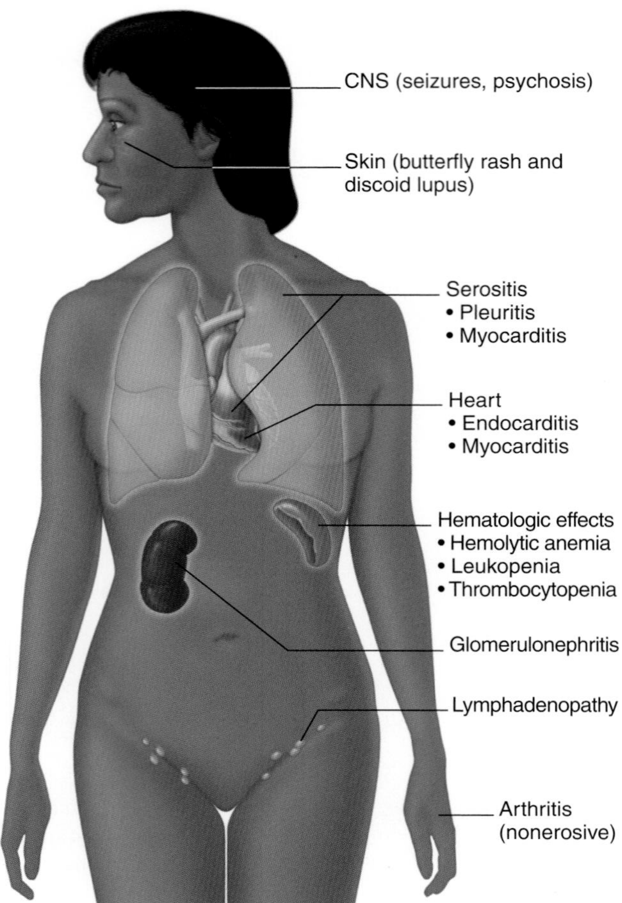

Figure 4.13. Complications of systemic lupus erythematosus. CNS, central nervous system.

PATHOPHYSIOLOGY

The exact events that stimulate the development of SLE are not fully known. A genetic or familial tendency combined with hormonal and environmental influences seems to make a person more susceptible to developing the disease (Fig. 4.14). SLE, most commonly found in women, tends to run a course with exacerbations (disease flare-ups) and **quiescence** (decreased symptoms). The MHC and HLA systems appear to be involved in the development of autoimmune activity, triggered by an unknown event, perhaps infection or another pathologic process. A breakdown in self-tolerance results in the stimulation of APCs, the evasion of normal immune response by molecular mimicry, or the alteration of antigens that make them unable to be recognized as "self." The ability to remove cells that recognize "self" by apoptosis is altered. The result is the activation of the B lymphocytes to develop autoantibodies and cytotoxic T lymphocytes, which then promote inflammation and complex deposition in susceptible organs of the body, causing permanent organ damage.

CLINICAL MANIFESTATIONS

Clinical signs and symptoms develop in the organs affected by the pathology associated with SLE. Organs most commonly affected include the skin, kidney, and musculoskeletal system. In addition, people diagnosed with lupus may develop neurologic, pulmonary, and cardiac disease. Typical manifestations in SLE include:

- Joint pain and swelling
- Skin rashes
- Fatigue
- Pericardial effusion (swelling around the heart)
- Pleural effusion (swelling around the lungs)

These systemic clinical manifestations contribute to the diagnosis of the disease and can also provide

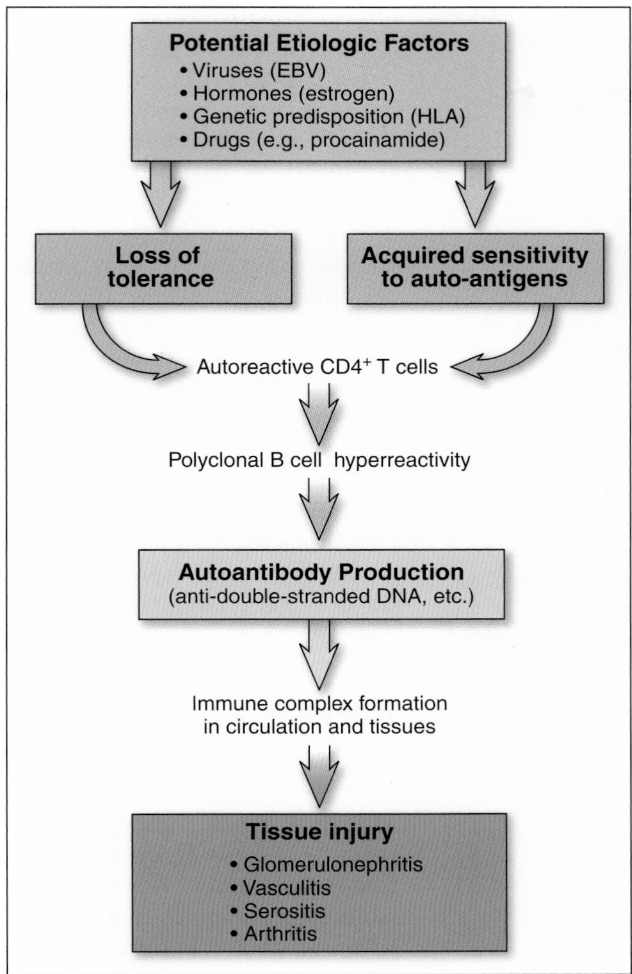

Figure 4.14. Pathogenesis of systemic lupus erythematosus. EBV, Epstein–Barr virus; HLA, human leukocyte antigen. (From Rubin E, Farber JL. *Pathology*. 4th ed. Philadelphia, PA: Lippincott Williams & Wilkins; 2005.)

valuable information about the activity of the disease and effectiveness of treatment strategies.

DIAGNOSTIC CRITERIA

Diagnosis of SLE is determined by a combination of subjective symptoms, objective physical findings, and laboratory values. Criteria for use in classifying SLE patients for inclusion in clinical and research studies have been established by the American College of Rheumatology (ACR).[9] Although not intended for diagnostic purposes, these criteria are often used for that purpose. Eleven criteria are outlined by the ACR, four of which must be present to obtain a diagnosis of SLE. These criteria include:

1. Rash
   a. Butterfly rash over cheeks (**malar**) (Fig. 4.15)

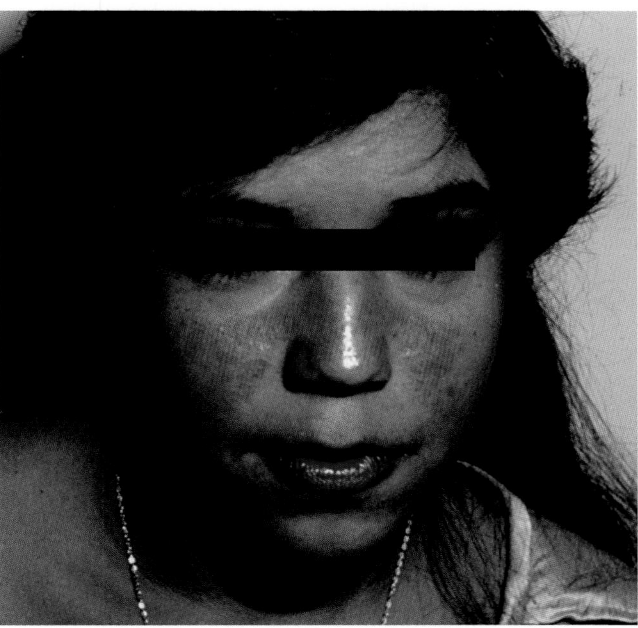

Figure 4.15. Malar (butterfly) rash in systemic lupus erythematosus. (From Goodheart HP. *Goodheart's Photoguide of Common Skin Disorders*. 2nd ed. Philadelphia, PA: Lippincott Williams & Wilkins; 2003.)

   b. Red, raised, **discoid** (round) rash, sometimes with scaling or plugged follicles
   c. Sensitivity to the sun resulting in rash (**photosensitivity**)
2. **Ulcers**, or open areas, in the mouth or nasopharynx
3. Arthritis, associated with tenderness, swelling, or fluid buildup (as seen in RA) in at least two peripheral joints
4. **Pleuritis** (inflammation of the lining of the lungs or pleural cavity) or **pericarditis** (inflammation of the lining of the heart)
5. **Proteinuria** (protein in the urine) greater than 5 g/dL or +3 on a dip stick, or **cellular casts** (compacted collection of protein, cells, and debris that are formed in kidney tubules) suggesting renal involvement
6. Seizures or psychosis, suggesting neurologic involvement
7. Anemia, leukopenia, or **thrombocytopenia** (abnormally low number of platelets), suggesting hematologic involvement
8. Lab values including anti-DNA antibody, anti-Sm (antibody to Smith nuclear antigen), or a false-positive test for syphilis
9. Abnormal antinuclear antibody (ANA)

The criteria reinforce the importance of looking at the entire person, rather than just a lab test, to identify the disease and illness accurately. The entire clinical picture is necessary to provide proper treatment and care for a specialized condition.

Table 4.5 Treatment Options for Systemic Lupus Erythematosus

Drug	Desired Effect	Adverse Effect
Salicylates	Anti-inflammatory	GI bleeding and upset
NSAIDs	Anti-inflammatory	GI bleeding and upset
Glucocorticoids	Anti-inflammatory	Hypertension Hyperglycemia Hyperlipidemia Hypokalemia Osteoporosis Infection Fluid retention Weight gain
Hydroxychloroquine	Immunosuppression	Macular damage Photosensitivity Rash
Azathioprine	Immunosuppression	Myelosuppression (anemia, thrombocytopenia) Hepatotoxicity
Cyclophosphamide	Immunosuppression	Myelosuppression Malignancy Infection Cystitis Infertility
Methotrexate	Immunosuppression	Myelosuppression Hepatotoxicity Pulmonary disease

GI, gastrointestinal; NSAIDs, nonsteroidal anti-inflammatory drugs.

TREATMENT

Treatment for SLE varies among individuals. Considerations for treatment include clinical manifestations, duration of desired treatment, and toleration of associated side effects. Early treatment is essential to minimize morbidity and mortality, although this must be balanced with the significant risk of adverse effects from the treatments themselves, including the development of atherosclerotic heart disease, osteoporosis, hypertension, diabetes, infection, and even death (Table 4.5).

Initially, pharmacologic management may involve nonsteroidal anti-inflammatory drugs (NSAIDs), although ultimately it often involves the use of corticosteroids for symptom control and anti-inflammatory effects. The disease is often managed with other drugs designed to delay the progress and resulting damage, including disease-modifying anti-rheumatoid drugs (DMARD) as are used in RA. The antimalarial drug Plaquenil may be used to slow disease progress. In more aggressive cases, immunosuppressant drugs, including cyclophosphamide, rituxamid, and mycophenolate, may be necessary. Providing appropriate drug treatment to prevent damage while simultaneously decreasing potentially damaging side effects is difficult and often requires care planned by a rheumatologist who specializes in these types of conditions.

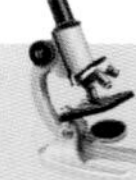

FROM THE LAB

Lab tests used to diagnose SLE are designed to detect the antibodies directed against cell components in the cytoplasm and nucleus. These include antinuclear antibodies (ANA) and extractable nuclear antigens (ENA), a group of several cellular proteins and antibodies that include antibodies to Smith antigen (anti-Sm). Once SLE is diagnosed, laboratory tests used to evaluate disease activity and prognosis include measurement of anti-dsDNA (anti-double stranded DNA, detecting antibodies against DNA) and complement (C3 and C4). Future work in determining more specific and sensitive biomarkers of SLE includes evaluation of the products of complement activation and inhibition, cytokines (including the interleukins and TNF-alpha), circulating immune complexes (CICs), measurement of the number of abnormal T-cell types by cell surface marker (i.e., CD4, CD8), and markers of B-cell activation.

Immune Maladaptation: Rh Isoimmunization

This clinical model represents a type II cytotoxic antibody-mediated reaction. Rh isoimmunization is a direct antigen–antibody hypersensitivity reaction between a mother and her fetus. The damage that results from this reaction includes cell destruction of the antigen targets, which are the fetal RBCs. This condition, known as **hemolytic** (destruction of blood cells) disease of the fetus and newborn, is a result of this blood cell destruction.

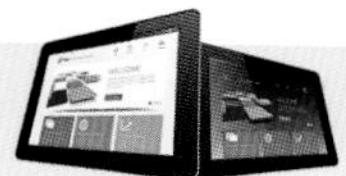

RESEARCH NOTES

Currently, a great deal of research is being conducted that focuses on the development of a pharmacologic treatment for SLE that is both effective and has minimal side effects. Increasingly refined approaches are being investigated to achieve maximum benefit and improve treatment outcome. A treatment approach in individuals with significant renal involvement based on histologic characteristics has the potential to reduce drug dosage and duration of use. In lupus nephritis, the site of accumulation of immunoglobulins in the renal glomeruli, the specificity of the immunoglobulins to antigens and the inflammation induced upon antigen–antibody complex deposition are factors that may be used to determine optimal therapy for this serious manifestation of SLE.[10]

PATHOPHYSIOLOGY

Hemolytic disease of the fetus and newborn is caused by maternal alloantibodies, which target paternally inherited antigens. Many antigens can be targeted in this disease, but the antigen usually involved is D (Rho), one of the primary antigens responsible for the determination of Rh-positive blood type. If a person is D antigen positive, he or she is identified as being Rh-positive; a person without the D antigen is known as Rh-negative.

A fetus often has a different R factor from the mother. This does not usually cause any immune response because each has a separate circulation not designed to mix. Maternal blood circulates through the maternal portion of the **placenta,** a specialized organ sustaining the fetus, by providing oxygenation, nutrition, endocrine, and excretion functions. The chorionic villi contain fetal capillaries that allow exchange of substances between mother and fetus across a membrane, without the actual mixing of maternal and fetal circulations. Most substances in the maternal and fetal circulations, with the exception of high molecular weight compounds, can cross the placental membrane using a variety of transport mechanisms. These transport mechanisms include passive diffusion, facilitated diffusion, and active transport. If the mother has not had prior exposure to the D antigen and therefore no production of antibodies against it, the mother is unable to stimulate an immune response to an antigen it cannot recognize in the separate fetal circulation.

If fetal blood enters the maternal circulation unintentionally, fetal D antigen on the fetal RBCs can pass into the maternal blood supply. In a D antigen naïve Rh-negative individual, the D antigen is recognized as foreign, stimulating an antibody response against the antigen. Though IgG has the ability to cross the placenta to reach the target of the D antigen on RBCs in the fetal circulation, the response of maternal primary antibody production is slow and therefore does not severely affect the fetus. Once antibodies are produced, the mother is then "sensitized" against the antigen and is able to mount a rapid, robust immune response if the antigen presents itself to the maternal system in the future because of immulogic memory.

If the Rh-negative mother becomes pregnant again with an Rh-positive fetus, maternal anti-D IgG will cross the placenta into the fetal circulation. Maternal anti-D IgG will recognize and target the D antigen-bearing fetal RBCs for destruction. The memory cells, a component of the humoral immunologic memory response, respond rapidly and are able to produce increased levels of antibodies with a higher affinity to the fetal D antigen. The transplacental passage of maternal antibody (IgG) into the fetus results in RBC destruction and the condition known as hemolytic anemia (Fig. 4.16).

CLINICAL MANIFESTATIONS

Fetuses suffering from Rh isoimmunization are at increased risk for the development of anemia, hydrops (accumulation of edema), and death. Severe hemolysis of fetal RBCs can be worsened by increased erythropoiesis, resulting in the production of large numbers of immature nucleated erythrocytes, known as erythroblastosis fetalis. Destruction of RBCs allows the release of cellular components, some of which can produce additional pathology. One of the components of the breakdown of hemoglobin in RBCs is bilirubin. Bilirubin, in its unconjugated form, is lipid soluble, a characteristic that prevents excretion of this potentially toxic substance. After birth, infants may have a newborn course complicated by kernicterus (unconjugated bilirubin deposits in the basal ganglia of the brain), lethargy, hearing loss, cerebral palsy, and learning problems.

DIAGNOSTIC CRITERIA

Identification of a mother at risk for sensitization and those who are sensitized is completed as a component of routine prenatal care. Maternal blood is screened to determine whether the mother is Rh-positive or -negative as the initial step in identifying risk. In addition, a screen for antibodies to the D antigen is completed to identify whether the mother is already sensitized.

Fetal blood type and Rh are not determined in routine pregnancies because that would require

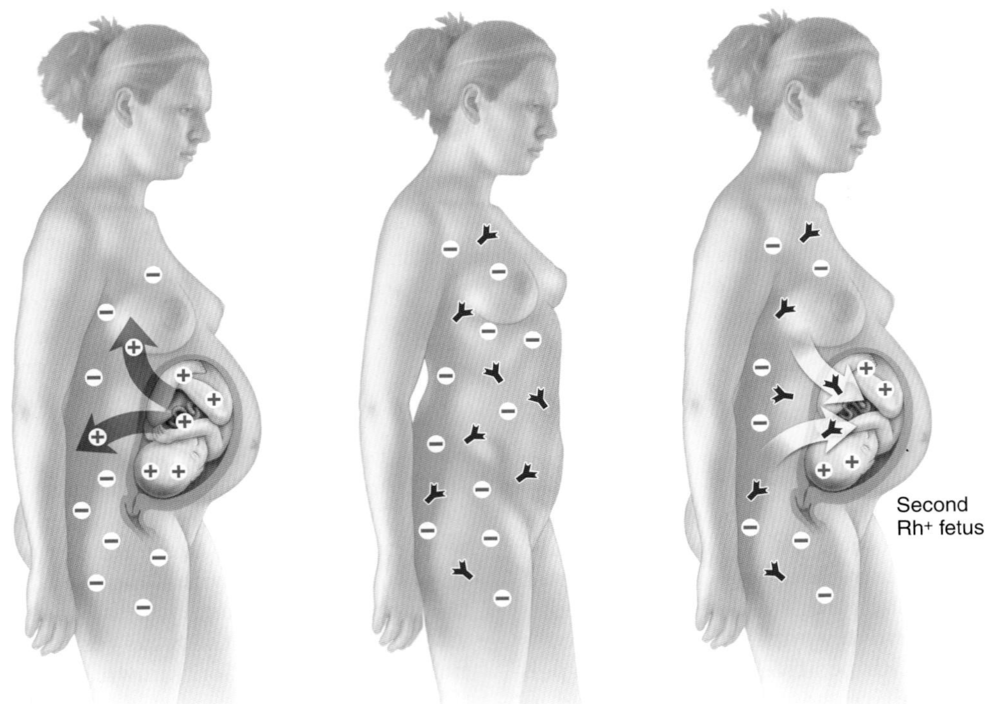

Figure 4.16. Maternal sensitization. (From Nath J. *Using Medical Terminology: A Practical Approach*. Baltimore, MD: Lippincott Williams & Wilkins; 2006.)

an invasive procedure with more risk than benefit. In a sensitized mother, the high-risk nature of the pregnancy requires careful screening of fetal status during growth in the uterus. Detection of the fetal RBCs antigen can be determined by performing an **amniocentesis** (insertion of a needle into the uterine cavity to obtain a sample of amniotic fluid) and by using the technique of genotyping. If the fetus is also Rh-negative, no further testing needs to be done because the fetus does not carry D antigen and therefore is unable to stimulate the maternal memory cells to initiate an immune response. A noninvasive method of determining fetal Rh status is to measure circulating fetal DNA in the maternal plasma.

In an Rh-positive fetus, measurements of amniotic components, including bilirubin, provide an indirect measure of hemolysis and anemia. Amniocentesis may be required several times during the pregnancy, or serially, to determine disease severity and progression. A noninvasive procedure may be used to reliably quantify fetal anemia and guide treatment decisions. Measurements of fetal middle cerebral artery peak systolic velocity (MCA PSV) using ultrasound can also provide information about fetal heart rate, tissue oxygenation, or blood **viscosity** (concentration) to detect fetal anemia.

TREATMENT

When hemolysis of fetal RBCs occurs, fetal oxygenation is decreased because of the decreased hemoglobin available to transport oxygen to cells and tissues. One of the primary treatments of a fetus with severe anemia is to provide healthy RBCs in exchange for hemolyzed RBCs, using an in-utero exchange transfusion. The need for transfusion is based on the determinations by amniocentesis or MCA PSV, as described previously. The transfusion procedure, completed under ultrasound guidance, uses the fetal umbilical cord arteries and vein to add healthy cells and remove damaged cells. The risks associated with this potentially dangerous procedure include infection, pregnancy loss, premature labor, rupture of membranes, worsening isoimmunization, and decreased fetal heart rate. The transfusion procedure may also need to be completed in a serial manner, depending on the progress of fetal disease. Once a mother is sensitized against the fetal D antigen, there are no procedures to desensitize her. The focus of managing disease in the fetus is the primary intervention.

The development of prevention strategies has reduced the rate of sensitization in at-risk mothers. This is accomplished by providing the Rh-negative mother with Rh immunoglobin (RhIg) when there is a risk of maternal exposure to fetal RBCs. Initiated in 1968, RhIg was administered to Rh-negative mothers by injection within 72 hours of delivering an Rh-positive fetus, when the risk of maternal and fetal circulations mixing is high. The RhIg binds to D antigen on fetal cells circulating in the maternal circulation, providing a protective coating around the cells and preventing detection by the maternal immune system and subsequent anti-D antibody production.

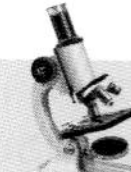

FROM THE LAB

Maternal antibodies to the fetal D antigen can be detected in the serum using an indirect Coombs test to determine whether the mother is sensitized. For sensitization to be prevented after maternal exposure to fetal D antigen, an adequate dosage of RhIg must be given. The standard prenatal dose is 500 IU and 1,500 IU at the time of delivery. If there is an increased risk of an excessive maternal exposure to fetal cells (i.e., after blunt trauma), testing to quantify the number of fetal cells present in the maternal circulation, the Kleihauer–Betke test, can be completed to assure adequate dosing of RhIg.

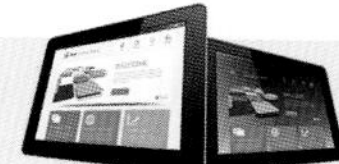

RESEARCH NOTES

RhIg has drastically reduced the number of women who become sensitized to the D fetal antigen. As a result, sensitization to other antigens in the Rh system (anti-FYa, anti-c, anti-E, and anti-K) is now getting more attention. No specialized treatments exist to prevent other forms of Rh sensitization. RhIg is often the treatment of choice in the protection against sensitization and has proven to be an effective strategy.[12]

Current prevention strategies include provision of RhIg administration to Rh-negative nonsensitized mothers during pregnancy at times when the likelihood of combined circulations is greatest and the fetal Rh factor is unknown. RhIg can be administered during invasive procedures, such as amniocentesis, upon early termination of pregnancy (as in the cases of abortion and ectopic pregnancy), following physical trauma and at 28 weeks' gestation to provide protection from inadvertent antigen exposure. RhIG continues to be administered to Rh-negative mothers within 72 hours of delivery if the newborn is Rh-positive. The optimal dosage and administration regimen of RhIg continues to be reevaluated to maximize effectiveness and safety.[11]

Stop and Consider

Is an Rh-positive mother at risk of becoming sensitized to her Rh-negative fetus? Why or why not?

SUMMARY

- The cellular components of the immune response work together to mount the third line of defense against invasion of pathogens.
- Innate and adaptive (cell-mediated and humoral) immune responses combine to provide protection against infection and illness.
- T lymphocytes proliferate and differentiate into cytotoxic or helper T cells when presented with an antigen, leading to cell-mediated immunity.
- B lymphocytes produce and secrete antibodies, each capable of detecting specific antigens, leading to humoral immunity.
- Granulocytes respond quickly and broadly to infectious agents.
- The lymphatic system traps antigens captured by cells of the immune system, allowing the antigen to be presented to antibody.
- Molecules known as major histocompatibility complex (MHC) or human leukocyte antigen (HLA) display antigens to T cells, stimulating the immune response.
- Receptors on T and B lymphocytes recognize unique antigen and antigen–MHC complexes in a specific manner resulting in targeted destruction of antigen-bearing cells.
- Altered immune function may be caused by inability to mount an immune defense, exaggerated immune responses, inappropriate immune responses to "self," and immune response directed toward transplanted tissues.
- Maladaptations in immune response, either exaggerated or impaired, contribute to acute and chronic disease.
- Immunosuppression is the result of a primary or secondary immunodeficiency.
- Hypersensitivity responses are mediated by IgE, antigen–antibody, immune complex, or cytotoxic reactions.
- Autoimmunity is the failure to distinguish "self" from "nonself," leading to an immune response against an individual's own tissues.

- Alloimmunity results from an immune response directed against the tissues of another individual of the same species, often seen in transplantation.
- Protection of immune function and the manipulation of the immune system to prevent disease are exciting prospects that will significantly decrease morbidity and mortality resulting from many chronic diseases in the United States and throughout the world.

CASE STUDY 4.1

C.J., a 19-year-old White female, has a history of hay fever, which seems to get worse during the summer months. After a weekend camping trip, she developed difficulty breathing and needed to seek care for these symptoms, which were diagnosed as an exacerbation of asthma. Think about which clinical model is most related to this process. From your reading related to inflammation and immune function, answer the following questions:

1. What anatomic problem would most likely lead to difficulty breathing as a consequence of allergy and asthma?
2. What is the injury in asthma?
3. How would the immune system respond?
4. Why is this a chronic problem?
5. What pathophysiologic changes would most likely occur with chronic asthma and allergy?
6. What would you expect to find as clinical manifestations?
7. What diagnostic tests might be used?
8. What treatment measures would you anticipate?

Log onto the Internet. Search for a relevant journal article or Web site that details asthma with an allergic component to confirm your predictions.

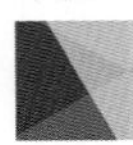

CASE STUDY 4.2

A.L., a 25-year-old Native American female, is pregnant with her second child. She was exposed to a child with chicken pox at a recent family event. A.L. has not had chicken pox, and she has not been immunized. Her 4-year-old son was immunized (initial and booster) against the varicella virus that causes chicken pox. From your reading related to immunity, answer the following questions:

1. What is A.L.'s risk for infection with the varicella virus?
2. Explain A.L.'s son's risk for infection with the varicella virus.
3. Discuss the risk for A.L.'s unborn child for infection with varicella.
4. Discuss prevention and treatment strategies that can be used to prevent varicella infection in each of these individuals.
5. What strategies should be used to protect other household family members?
6. Identify whether prevention strategies for A.L., her son and fetus stimulate passive or active immune responses.
7. How can it be determined if an individual has immunity to varicella?

Log onto the Internet. Search for a relevant journal article or Web site that details varicella infection prevention during pregnancy and childhood and special considerations in immune responses in these groups to confirm your predictions.

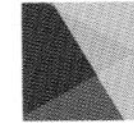

PRACTICE EXAM QUESTIONS

1. During flu season, you get exposed to the influenza virus. Which component of your immune system will be the first to respond to this foreign pathogen?
   a. Innate
   b. Adaptive
   c. Humoral
   d. T-cell mediated

2. The following season, you are concerned about getting the flu again. Which of the following statements is true?
   a. You continue to be at risk because nothing can protect you from reinfection.
   b. Vaccination for prevalent strains of influenza virus can provide improved protection against the disease.
   c. Premedication with immunosuppressants will provide protection against infection.
   d. Because you have had the flu once, you will be protected from getting it again.

3. Immune suppression in AIDS is related to:
   a. Decreased platelet count
   b. Decreased red blood cell count
   c. Decreased lymphocyte count
   d. Elevated lymphocyte count

4. Which of the following conditions represents pathologic responses caused by immunologic memory?
   a. Common cold
   b. Anaphylaxis
   c. Shingles
   d. Strep throat

5. The pathology related to systemic lupus erythematosus is due to:
   a. Neutrophil activation
   b. Delayed immunity
   c. Immunosuppression
   d. Immune complex deposition

6. Immunodeficiency is the result of:
   a. Failure of host defense mechanisms
   b. Hypersensitive immune responses
   c. Inappropriate immune response to self
   d. Immune response stimulated by antigens from other individuals

7. A hypersensitivity reaction resulting from a yellow jacket sting is an example of:
   a. Type I, immediate hypersensitivity reaction
   b. Type II, antibody-mediated reaction
   c. Type III, immune complex reaction
   d. Type IV, cell-mediated reaction

8. A hypersensitivity reaction resulting from complement activation due to insoluble antigen–antibody deposition is an example of:
   a. Type I, immediate hypersensitivity reaction
   b. Type II, antibody-mediated reaction
   c. Type III, immune complex reaction
   d. Type IV, cell-mediated reaction

9. Autoimmunity may be triggered by which one of the following?
   a. Elimination of self-reactive lymphocytes in central lymphoid tissues
   b. Persistent lymphocyte ignorance
   c. Impaired T-cell activation
   d. Close resemblance between foreign and self-antigen

10. Treatment of an altered immune response with corticosteroids is associated with which one of the following adverse effects?
    a. Decreased blood sugar
    b. Loss of bone mineral
    c. Thickening of skin
    d. Weight loss

11. The transfer of secretory IgA from mother to infant during breastfeeding is an example of
    a. Hypersensitivity reaction
    b. Active immunity
    c. Passive immunity
    d. Alloimmunity

12. Which of the following is true regarding cytotoxic T lymphocytes?
    a. Recognize the MHC class I–antigen complex
    b. Recognize the MHC class II–antigen complex
    c. Carry the CD4 marker
    d. Present antigen to B lymphocytes for antibody production

13. Which of the following are considered antigen-presenting cells?
    a. Dendritic cells
    b. Eosinophils
    c. B lymphocytes
    d. T lymphocytes

14. Which of the following markers identifies a nucleated body cell?
    a. CD4
    b. BCR
    c. MHC I
    d. MHC II

15. Which of the following is true regarding pharmacologic treatment for AIDS?
    a. Drugs are used to target increased red blood cell number
    b. Drugs are used to target increased white blood cell number
    c. Drugs are used to increase host DNA replication
    d. Drugs are used to inhibit HIV replication

DISCUSSION AND APPLICATION

1. What did I know about basic alterations in immunity before today?
2. What body processes are affected by altered immune function? How does immunity impact those processes?
3. What are the potential etiologies for altered immune function? How do alterations in immune function develop?
4. Who is most at risk for developing altered immunity? How can these alterations be prevented?
5. What are the human differences that affect the etiology, risk, or course of altered immunity?
6. What clinical manifestations are expected in the course of altered immunity?
7. What special diagnostic tests are useful in determining the diagnosis and course of illness due to altered immune function?
8. What are the goals of care for individuals with altered immunity?
9. How does the concept of altered immunity build on what I have learned in the previous chapter and in the previous courses?
10. How can I use what I have learned?

RESOURCES

AIDSinfo (a service of the US Department of Health and Human Services):
http://aidsinfo.nih.gov

The American College of Rheumatology:
http://www.rheumatology.org/
This site is a resource for information about autoimmune disorders.

Immune Deficiency Foundation:
http://www.primaryimmune.org/
Learn more about primary immune deficiency.

National Institute of Allergy and Infectious Disease (NIAID):
http://www3.niaid.nih.gov/
Find out more about general immune function.

References

1. Jackson KD, Howie LD, Akinbami LJ. *Trends in Allergic Conditions Among Children in the United States, 1997–2011.* NCHS Data Brief. No. 121. Hyattsville, MD: National Center for Health Statistics; 2013.
2. Bilò MB, Severino M, Cilia M, et al. The VISYT trial: venom immunotherapy safety and tolerability with purified vs nonpurified extracts. *Ann Allergy Asthma)Immunol*. 2009;103(1):57–61.
3. UNAIDS, World Health Organization. Fact sheets. 2015. http://www.who.int/mediacentre/factsheets/fs360/en/. Accessed November 11, 2015.
4. Centers for Disease Control and Prevention. HIV in the United States: at a glance. http://www.cdc.gov/hiv/statistics/overview/ataglance.html. Accessed November 11, 2015.
5. Gavin L, MacKay AP, Harrier S, et al. Sexual and reproductive health of persons aged 10–24 years—United States, 2002–2007. *MMWR Surveill Summ.* 2009;58(SS06):1–58.
6. Branson BN, Hansfield HH, Lampe MA. Revised recommendations for HIV testing of adults, adolescents, and pregnant women in health care settings. *MMWR Recomm Rep.* 2006;55(RR14):1–17.
7. Selik RM, Mokotoff ED, Branson B, et al. Revised surveillance case definition for HIV infection—United States, 2014. *MMWR Recomm Rep.* 2014;63(RR03):1–10.
8. Soriano V. Update of the DHHS antiretroviral treatment guidelines. *AIDS Rev*. 2014;16(2):117–118.
9. American College of Rheumatology Ad Hoc Committee on Systemic Lupus Erythematosus Guidelines. Guidelines for referral and management for systemic lupus erythematosus in adults. *Arthritis Rheum*. 1999;42(9):1788–1796.
10. Molino C, Fabbian F, Longhini C. Clinical approach to lupus nephritis: recent advances. *Eur J Intern Med*. 2009;20(5):447–453.
11. Pilgrim H, Lloyd-Jones M, Rees A. Routine antenatal anti-D prophylaxis for Rh-D negative women: a systematic review and economic evaluation. *Health Technol Assess.* 2009;13(10):1–126.
12. Gottvall T, Filbey D. Alloimmunization in pregnancy during the years 1992–2005 in the central west region of Sweden. *Acta Obstet Gynecol Scand*. 2008;87(8):843–848.

Find additional resources for this chapter at http:thePoint.lww.com thePoint®

Chapter 5

Infection

LEARNING OUTCOMES

1. Define and use the key terms listed in this chapter.
2. Relate the development of infection to breaks in the three lines of defense.
3. Identify the ways in which microbes can become pathogens to human host cells.
4. Differentiate the basic types of microbes.
5. Determine measures to break the chain of infection at each link.
6. Identify the phases of acute infection.
7. Discuss the potential complications of acute infection.
8. Distinguish common clinical manifestations related to infection.
9. Identify laboratory and diagnostic tests relevant to infection.
10. Discuss treatment modalities effective against various types of infection.
11. Apply concepts of infection to the clinical models in this chapter.

INTRODUCTION

How many infections have you had in your lifetime? You have probably had too many to count! **Infection** is a state of cellular, tissue, and sometimes even organ destruction resulting from invasion by microorganisms. Multiple sites throughout the body contain specialized defense mechanisms to protect against microbe invasion (Fig. 5.1). Unfortunately, with infection, harmful microorganisms have penetrated the three lines of defense and have caused disease.

Even with the advent of new antibiotics and vaccinations, infectious disease remains a health care challenge. The overuse or incomplete use of antimicrobial drugs has led to multiple drug-resistant microbes. Globalization has promoted the rapid spread of harmful microbes around the world. Importation and mass distribution of perishable food items has also contributed to infectious disease spread. A thorough understanding of infection is therefore critical to your work in the health professions.

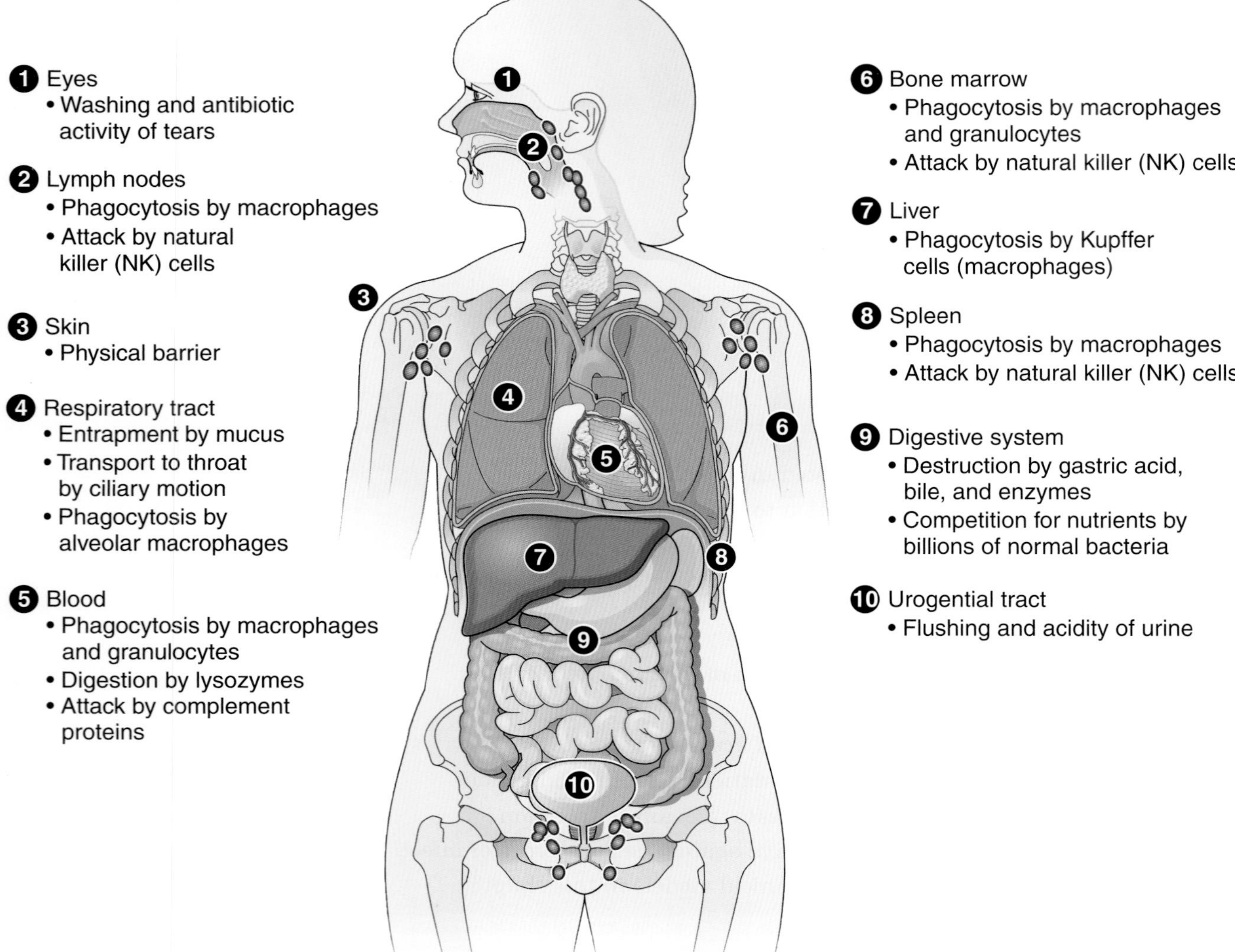

Figure 5.1. Nonimmune antimicrobial protective mechanisms. The numbered areas show the functions of various organs and systems that defend against bacteria and other microbes.

Module 1 Microbes

Microbes, including bacteria, viruses, fungi, and protozoa, are everywhere in the human environment. **Resident flora** are microorganisms that live on or within the body in nonsterile areas, such as the skin, mucous membranes, bowel, rectum, or vagina, without causing harm. Inflammatory and immune attacks are generally not waged against these inhabitants as long as the skin and mucosa remain intact. Resident flora compete with disease-producing microorganisms to protect the body against certain infections and to provide a type of natural immunity.

A delicate balance of homeostasis is needed because often more than one type of resident flora can be found in nonsterile areas. Destroying one type of resident flora can allow overproliferation of another competing type. For example, if a person experiences a bacterial infection and is prescribed an antibiotic, the antibiotic may also destroy the helpful resident bacteria living in nonsterile areas of the body. The resident fungi no longer have to compete with the destroyed resident bacteria. The fungi overproliferate, resulting in a fungal infection. This example helps to explain why vaginal yeast (fungal) infections are common in women who are on antibiotics.

Pathogens

A **pathogen** is a disease-producing microbe. To cause disease in humans, a pathogen must be capable of binding to specific receptors on the human host cell. This is a very important concept to understand. If the microorganism is not able to bind to the receptors, the host cell remains unaffected. This explains why some microorganisms found in the environment are not harmful to humans. Receptors also provide clues to the types of cells to which the pathogen will attach. For example, influenza virus attaches to receptors only in respiratory tract epithelial cells. The basic local clinical manifestations (i.e., cough, nasal congestion, and sore throat) reflect respiratory epithelial cell necrosis elicited by the pathogen. Receptor binding offers some clues to the racial and geographic differences in human infection. For example, some African American individuals lack receptors for the microorganism that causes malaria and are therefore not susceptible to this infection.

Once receptor attachment has been established, the mechanism by which the pathogen causes disease in the human host cell includes one or more of the following:

1. Direct destruction of the host cell by the pathogen
2. Interference with the host cell's metabolic function
3. Exposing the host cell to toxins produced by the pathogen

The **pathogenicity**, or qualities that promote the production of disease, involves multiple factors, including the pathogen's potency, invasiveness, ability to evade the immune system, speed of replication, production of toxins, adherence to the human host cell, and degree of tissue damage that is elicited. The following factors affect the variability with which the pathogen is able to elicit disease.

- **Virulence** is the potency of the pathogen indicated by the ratio of the number of cases of disease in a population compared with the number of people exposed to the microorganism. A more virulent microorganism is one that causes severe disease in a large proportion of those exposed to the microorganism.
- **Infectivity** is the proportion of exposures needed to cause infection in an individual based on the pathogen's ability to enter, survive in, and multiply in the host. Virulence and infectivity are related. A more infective organism is one that takes one exposure, takes hold, multiplies, and causes disease in the host.
- **Toxigenicity** is the ability of the pathogen to produce harmful toxins that increase host cell and tissue damage.
- **Antigenicity** is the level to which a pathogen is viewed by the host immune system as foreign. A more antigenic pathogen elicits a more prominent immune response. Those with low antigenicity can readily elude immune mechanisms and continue to survive in the host.
- **Antigenic variability** is a process of eluding the human host defenses and is often a result of altering the antigens present within or on the surface of the microorganism. This means that many infectious microorganisms can escape human host defenses through slight genetic variations unrecognized by the host. These mutations are responsible for much of the infectious disease burden throughout the world.
- **Pathogenic defense mechanisms** are the ways in which many pathogens have developed ways to avoid destruction by the host, such as through thick protective capsules, which prevent phagocytosis.
- **Coinfection** is a phenomenon of hosting two or more pathogens simultaneously. Certain pathogens, such as those that cause chlamydia and gonorrhea, are more likely to be transmitted and to coexist in the host. Coinfection presents a greater challenge to the immune system.
- **Superinfection** is when an infection arises in addition to one that is already present. Superinfection often results from compromised host defenses and overproliferation of resident flora.

TYPES OF PATHOGENS

Basic types of microorganisms that can cause disease include bacteria, viruses, fungi, and protozoa. Understanding the distinctive quality of each microorganism can provide clues to the transmission and spread of infectious disease.

Some microorganisms live and reproduce independently of the host. Other microorganisms are considered parasites. **Obligate parasites** require the host for metabolism and reproduction. **Facultative parasites** may live on the host but can also survive independently. Helminths (worms) are also capable of eliciting disease in humans. They are not considered microorganisms but rather are a highly diverse group of multicellular parasites. Helminth eggs can be found in contaminated food, water, or soil, as well as within infected insects. Once infected, the helminth matures within the host and can grow to be quite large.

Bacteria

Bacteria are single-celled microorganisms (Fig. 5.2). Most can reproduce outside of host cells. Bacteria that require oxygen for growth are called **aerobic**;

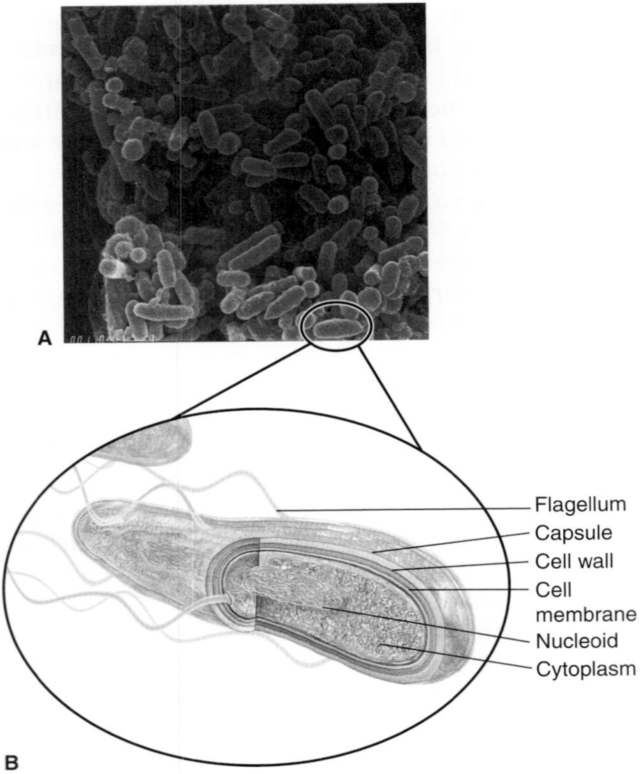

Figure 5.2. Bacterial cell **(A)** scanning electron microscopy; basic structure of bacteria **(B)**.

those that do not are called **anaerobic**. Oxygen requirements dictate where the bacteria can best survive. Anaerobic bacteria survive best in deep tissues of the body where oxygen supply is limited. This type is difficult to treat because antimicrobial drugs often travel within the vascular system to affect local tissues. Deeper tissues are much more difficult to penetrate. Some bacteria can survive in both aerobic and anaerobic environments.

Bacteria are often referred to by their shape: cocci (spheres), bacilli (rods), vibrio (comma-shaped), and spirochetes (spirals). They contain an indiscrete nucleus, a cytoplasm, and an outer cell membrane. The "indiscrete" nucleus does not have a nuclear membrane and is therefore not separate from the cytoplasm. Like the nucleus, the cytoplasm is also different from human cells. The cytoplasm of bacteria is referred to as **cytosol**. Cytosol contains extensive ribosomes, proteins, and carbohydrates but does not contain mitochondria, endoplasmic reticulum, or other membranous components.

The innermost cell membrane, also called the cell envelope, has multiple functions:

- Formation of a barrier surrounding the bacterial cell
- Protein and DNA synthesis
- Cell division

Most bacteria also include a rigid cell wall that surrounds this inner membrane. The cell wall provides shape and structure. Because human cells do not have a cell wall, antibiotic treatment is commonly aimed at inhibiting synthesis of the bacterial cell wall during bacterial replication. Therefore, the bacteria are destroyed and the human host cell is unharmed. Some bacteria can also have a capsule covering this cell wall. Bacteria with a capsule more easily adhere to host cells. The capsule is also highly resistant to phagocytosis. The variability of each type of cell envelope, cell wall, and capsule is important in the pathogenicity of the bacteria, and will often direct treatment decisions.

Stop and Consider
What aspects of bacteria would be effective targets for pharmacologic treatment?

The damage caused by bacteria can result from bacterial structural properties and exotoxin release. Structural properties critical to the pathogenicity of bacteria include:

- **Independent survival:** Bacteria can survive outside the human host and can infect and reinfect if not destroyed.
- **Stimulation of an inflammatory response:** Bacteria stimulate an inflammatory and immune response that will destroy surrounding host tissues in an effort to rid the body of the invader.
- **Bacterial capsule:** Encapsulated bacteria are adherent and highly resistant to phagocytosis.
- **Endotoxin:** The presence of endotoxin in the gram-negative bacterial cell envelope activates the plasma protein systems (Chapter 3). **Endotoxin** is a complex of phospholipid–polysaccharide molecules that form the structural component of the gram-negative cell wall. Endotoxin causes inflammatory mediators to be released, leading to a massive inflammatory response (Fig. 5.3). This in turn can result in a state of septic shock accompanied by severe diarrhea, fever, and leukocytosis. When inducing fever, these endotoxin-containing bacteria are referred to as **pyogenic** bacteria.
- **Endospores:** Some bacteria can produce spores that survive in a latent state that is resistant to environmental extremes and lack of nutrients. When the environment is more conducive to replication, the bacteria will emerge from the spore state, multiply, and may cause infection in a susceptible host.

Many bacteria are also capable of producing toxins, called **exotoxins**, and enzymes, which result in host cell dysfunction or lysis. Exotoxins are potent substances, often bacterial-derived proteins, released

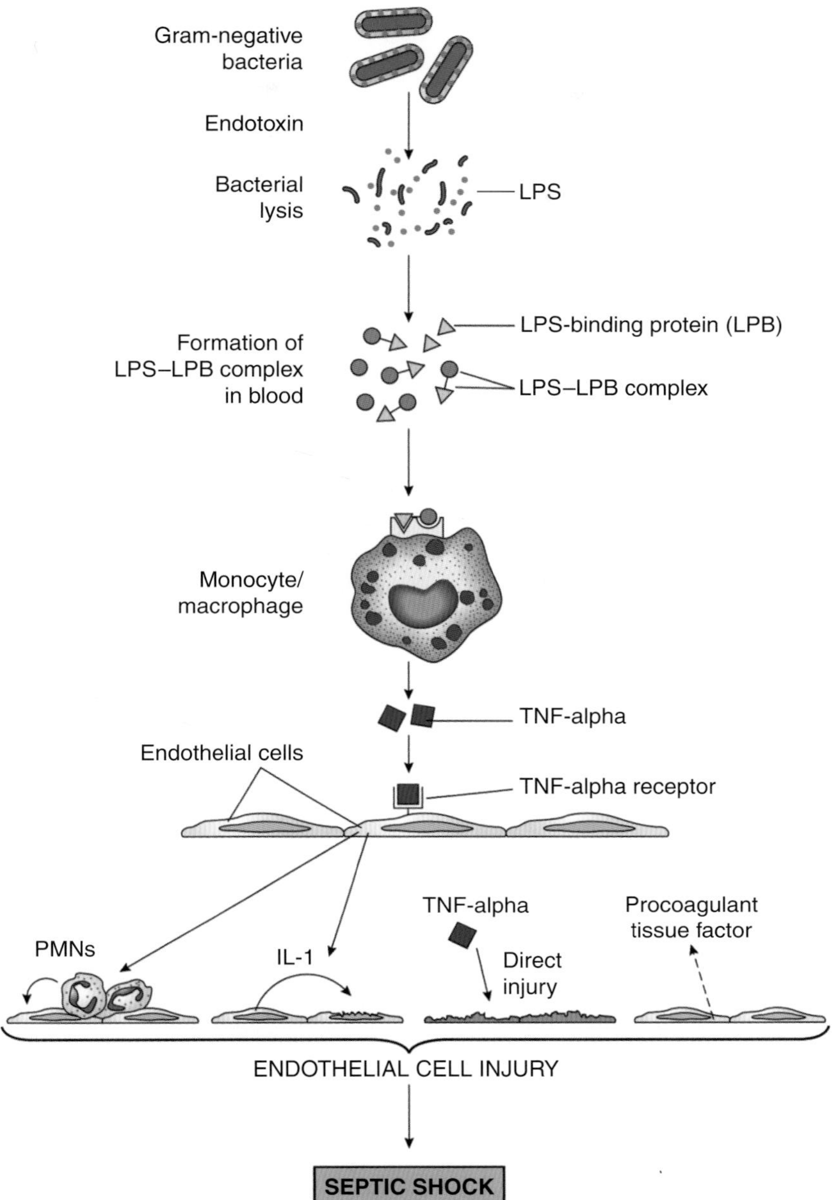

Figure 5.3. Pathogenesis of endothelial cell injury in endotoxic shock. In sepsis caused by gram-negative bacteria, the lysis of the organisms releases endotoxin into the circulation in the form of lipopolysaccharide (LPS), where it binds to the LPS-binding protein (LBP). The LPS–LPB complex binds to monocytes/macrophages, which are stimulated to secrete substantial quantities of tumor necrosis factor-alpha (TNF-alpha), a potent inflammatory mediator. TNF-alpha mediates septic shock by causing endothelial cell injury by a number of mechanisms: (1) direct cytotoxicity; (2) enhancing the adherence of polymorphonuclear leukocytes; (3) stimulating the release of interleukin-1 (IL-1), a cytokine that injures endothelial cells; and (4) promoting the expression of procoagulant tissue factor, thereby leading to thrombosis and local ischemia.

into the surrounding tissues that cause local or systemic injury to the host. The target tissue can be in the brain and spinal cord (neurotoxic), the gastrointestinal tract (enterotoxic), the liver (hepatotoxic), the blood (hemotoxic), and so forth. Figure 5.4 depicts examples of pathogenic bacteria and the sites of infection for each type.

Viruses

Viruses are considered obligate intracellular parasites. This means that viruses cannot replicate outside of the host cell. The virus binds to specific receptors on the host cell and then moves into the host cell. Once inside the host cell, the virus converts

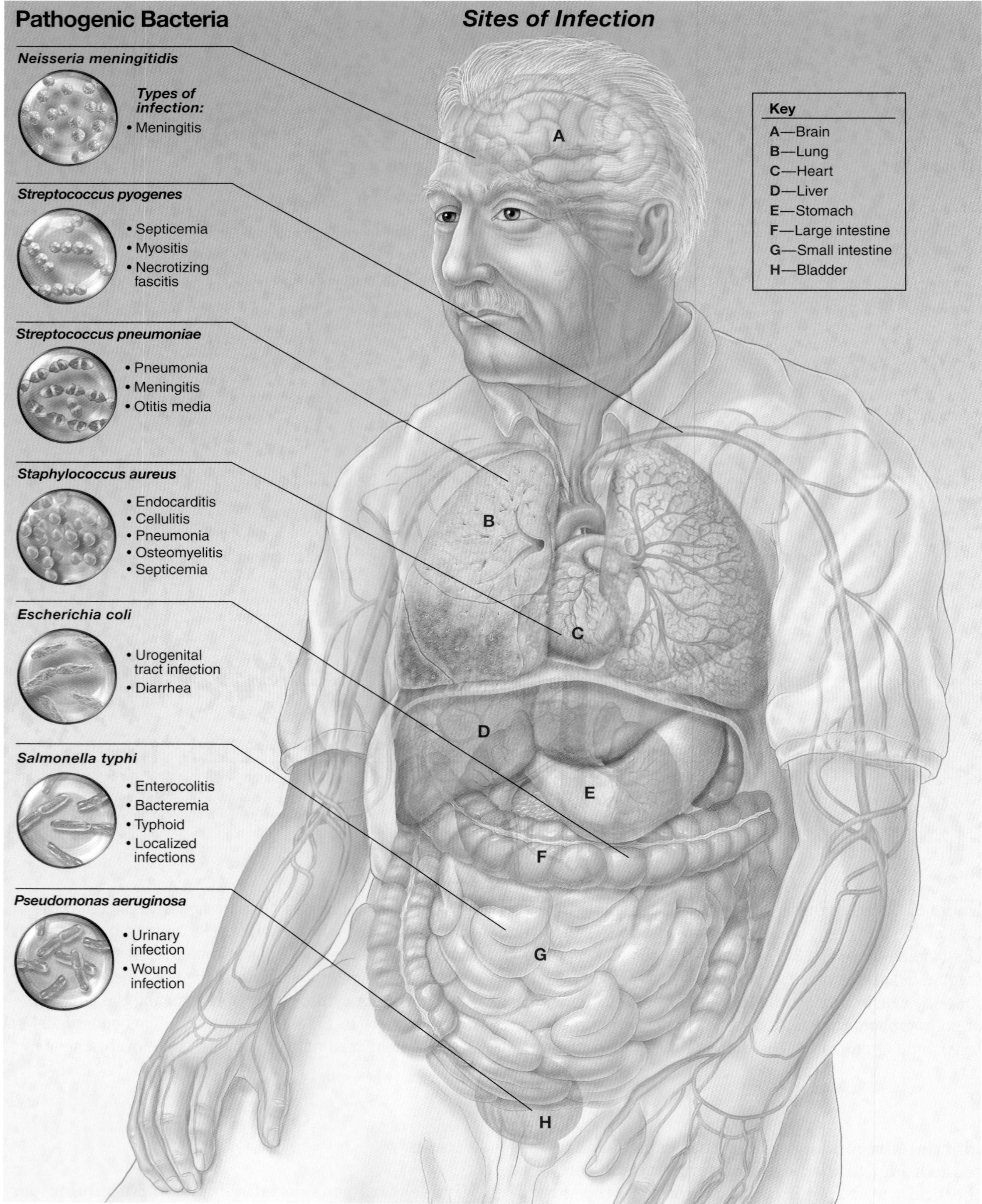

Figure 5.4. Sites of bacterial infection for each type of pathogenic bacteria. (Courtesy Anatomical Chart Company.)

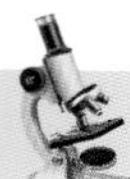

FROM THE LAB

Laboratory tests are important in differentiating the specific types of bacteria that are causing the infection. The goal is to "match the bug to the drug," that is, aiming treatment at the specific bacteria without harming the host cells or resident flora. Cultures can be obtained and the bacteria grown and identified. This usually takes 3 days or more. Two other important clues that allow more rapid identification of bacterial characteristics are the Gram stain and tests for coagulation. Bacterial cell walls, when exposed to a Gram stain in the lab, become either dark blue or red (when counterstained). Bacterial cell walls that preserve the stain and turn dark blue are considered gram-positive. Examples of gram-positive bacteria include *Staphylococcus aureus*, *Streptococcus pneumoniae*, and *Clostridium difficile*. Those that do not retain the dark blue color and instead turn red when another stain is applied are considered gram-negative. Examples of gram-negative bacteria include *Neisseria gonorrhoeae*, *Helicobacter pylori*, and *Escherichia coli*. Coagulase tests differentiate potentially pathogenic *Staphylococcus* species from other gram-positive cocci. Staphylococcal bacteria that cause coagulation (clotting) in the blood are more resistant to phagocytosis or antibody destruction. A coagulase-positive test indicates a pathogenic strain of staphylococcal bacteria that should be treated aggressively.

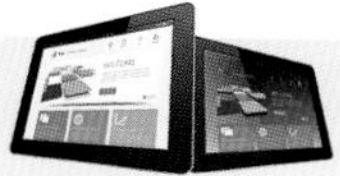

RESEARCH NOTES

Prions, transmissible protein particles that lack DNA or RNA, have been found to cause infectious disease in humans. Prion diseases, also known as spongiform encephalopathies, are implicated in rare, progressive neurodegenerative conditions such as Creutzfeldt–Jakob disease and bovine spongiform encephalopathy, also known as mad-cow disease. Interestingly, prion diseases are not known to elicit a notable immune response by the host, and the mechanism by which they destroy brain tissue is poorly understood. Prion diseases progress rapidly and are always fatal. Animal prion diseases pose a significant public health risk, with recent reports of secondary person-to-person spread.[1]

the host cellular metabolism to nucleic acids and proteins that are encoded and controlled by the virus. Viruses have the ability to either directly kill the cell or modify certain cellular functions, such as protein synthesis. Viruses can cause cells to proliferate rapidly and randomly, causing tumors to form in the body. The cell ultimately loses its ability to function. The virus next releases particles outside of the cell, called **virions**, which can enter and infect other nearby cells (Fig. 5.5).

Initially, viruses evade many defense mechanisms by hiding within host cells. As the virus moves from cell to cell, the immune response is activated. Viral infections are often severe enough to spark a strong, eradicating immune response. This exaggerated immune response allows neutralization of the virus and resolution of the infection. The infected host cells are eliminated, and the virus can no longer replicate. In this regard, many viruses, such as those associated with the common cold, are considered self-limiting; that is, the infection ceases after a certain period of time.

Some viruses are sustained for longer periods in the host. If the initial, acute infection does not provoke a strong viral-eradicating immune response, the individual is more likely to host a chronic viral infection. Chronic viral infections are promoted by various viral and host factors:

1. The size of the virus that is inoculated into the body
2. The process of viral replication
3. The viral genotype
4. Host susceptibility

For example, in an immunocompetent healthy adult, hepatitis B becomes a chronic infection in 10% of cases. This same virus, when spread to a fetus from an infected mother, becomes chronic in 90% of newborns. The major difference between the two scenarios is the immaturity of the newborn's immune system, allowing the virus to continue to replicate.

Also characteristic of chronic viral infections is a period of **latency**, or dormancy. During this period, the virus is integrating itself into the host cell's genetic material. The virus will reside in a host cell and cause minimal or no loss of functional capabilities for that cell. The virus demonstrates low antigenicity, although cellular mitosis continues and new cells that contain viral material are generated. Immunocompromise, including that induced by physical and emotional stress, provides a medium for active viral replication. Active viral replication can be triggered weeks to years after the initial inoculation with the virus. This process results in host cell death. Cell death leads to recognizable signs and symptoms of disease. A common example of a latent virus is herpes simplex virus, which causes cold sores. The virus remains dormant. Replication is triggered by immunocompromise (often stress related). The local clinical manifestations characteristic of herpes simplex infection (e.g., itching, blistering, and erythema) then become apparent. These local necrotic cells are removed from the body by inflammatory/immune

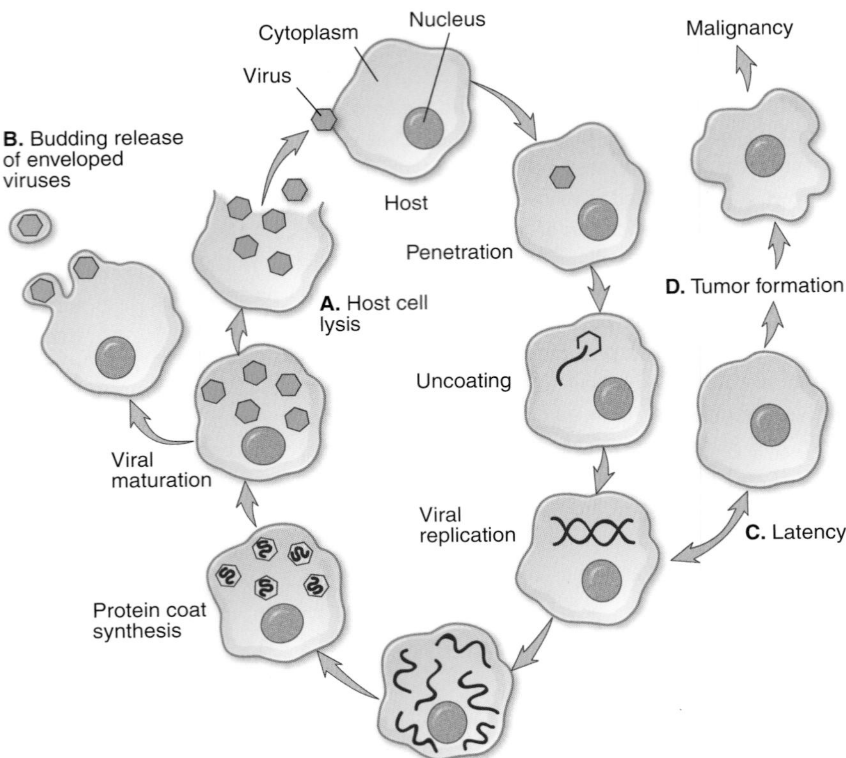

Figure 5.5. Consequences of viral infection in host cells. **A:** Cell lysis. **B:** Continuous release of budding viral particles. **C:** Latency. **D:** Tumor formation. (Modified from Porth CM. *Pathophysiology: Concepts of Altered Health States*. 7th ed. Philadelphia, PA: Lippincott Williams & Wilkins; 2004, with permission.)

mechanisms; however, other cells containing viral material remain and can cause active disease again at another time.

Another example of latency is a disease condition caused by herpes zoster virus. The original infection with herpes zoster virus causes varicella, or chicken pox. During the initial battle against the virus, some of the viral particles leave the skin blisters from the chicken pox and move into the nervous system. When the varicella virus reactivates, often years later, the virus moves back down the long nerve fibers from the sensory cell bodies to the skin, causing severe pain along these nerves. Blisters are often present as well. This disease recurrence is known as shingles. Examples of other select viral diseases are listed in Table 5.1.

Stop and Consider
Why are antiviral drugs difficult to develop and use effectively?

Rickettsiae, Mycoplasmas, and Chlamydiae

Rickettsiae, mycoplasmas, and chlamydiae are unique pathogens that have characteristics of both bacteria and viruses. Rickettsiae, like viruses, are obligate intracellular parasites that cannot replicate outside the host. However, rickettsiae are also gram-negative bacteria that are capable of producing energy. Rickettsiae target human endothelial cells of the blood vessels and capillaries. Mycoplasmas lack a cell wall and survive on the surface of host cells, but they do not enter the host cell for replication. Chlamydiae reproduce through binary fission yet are obligate intracellular parasites (Fig. 5.6). These pathogens use the host metabolism to reproduce. The life cycle of chlamydiae has the following distinct phases:

1. The metabolically inactive elemental body enters the body, attaches to, and internalizes the host cell.
2. The elemental body becomes metabolically active and transforms into a reticulate body, which takes over the host cell.
3. The chlamydiae are then capable of replication.
4. Each replicated pathogen goes through the life cycle, causing epithelial cell necrosis.

Fungi

Fungi are relatively large organisms compared to bacteria and viruses. They have a nuclear membrane, cytoplasm, and organelles. Unicellular forms

Table 5.1 Select Viruses and Related Disease Conditions

Virus	Transmission	Disease Condition	Clinical Manifestations
Respiratory syncytial virus (RSV)	Respiratory droplets	Lower respiratory tract infection in young children	Fever, runny nose, cough, wheezing
Paramyxovirus	Respiratory droplets	Measles	Fever, runny nose, cough, rash
Rotavirus	Primarily fecal–oral	Gastroenteritis	Severe, watery diarrhea; vomiting
Coxsackievirus	Direct contact with or stool infected secretions	Hand-foot-mouth disease	Fever, sores in the mouth, rash with blisters, especially on hands and feet
Human parvovirus B19	Respiratory droplets	Fifth disease	Mild rash with "slapped cheek" appearance on face, fever, malaise
Adenovirus	Respiratory droplets or fecal-oral	Common cold with respiratory droplets, gastroenteritis with fecal–oral transmission	Common cold: runny nose, sore throat, fever, malaise; gastroenteritis: diarrhea, vomiting
Rhinovirus	Respiratory droplets	Common cold	Fever, runny nose, sore throat, body aches, malaise
Coronavirus	Respiratory droplets	Severe acute respiratory syndrome (SARS)	High fever, headache, body aches, cough, pneumonia, diarrhea

are called **yeasts**; multicellular forms are called **molds** (Fig. 5.7). Yeasts reproduce by budding and form an elongated chain, called **pseudohyphae**. Mold colonies have tubules that branch to form **hyphae**; clusters of hyphae form **mycelium**. Some fungi can grow as either yeasts or molds. Superficial or deep-tissue invasion occurs when pseudohyphae or hyphae multiply. This invasion results in inflammatory and immune responses. Infections with fungi are referred to as **mycoses** or mycotic infections.

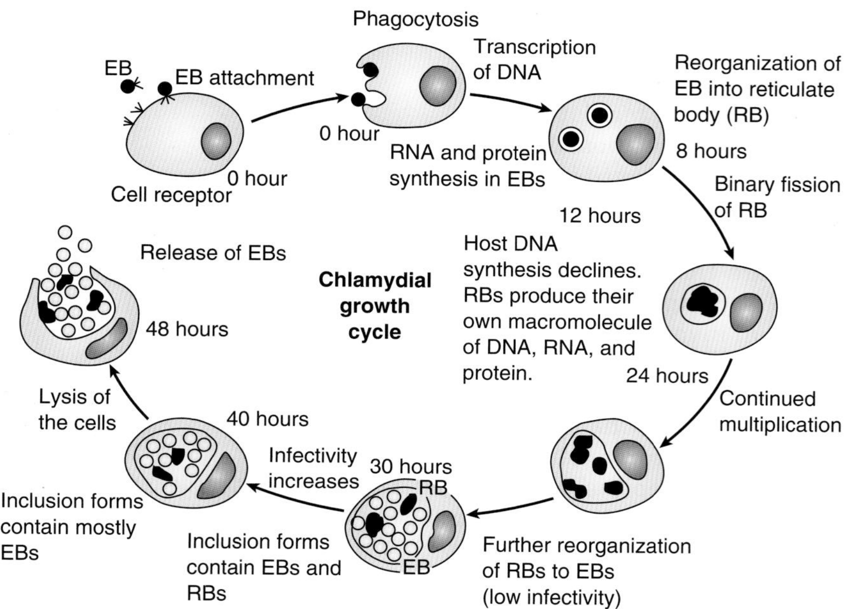

Figure 5.6. Chlamydial growth cycle. EB, elementary body; RB, reticulate body. (From Thompson SE, Washington AE. Epidemiology of sexually transmitted *Chlamydia trachomatis* infections. *Epidemiol Rev*. 1983;5:96–123, with permission.)

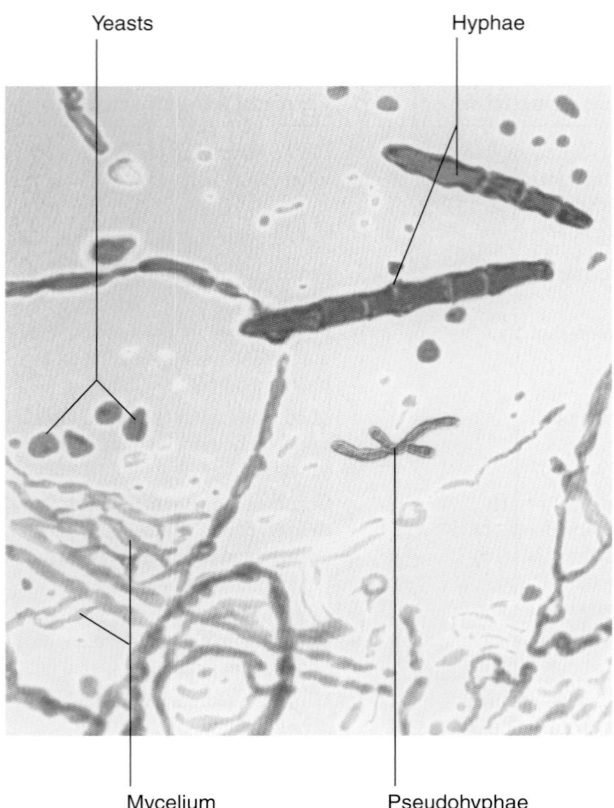

Figure 5.7. Basic structure of fungi. Molds grow as branching hyphae, forming a mycelium. Yeasts multiply by budding and form elongated pseudohyphae. (Courtesy Anatomical Chart Company.)

Fungi are common resident microbes. These organisms frequently inhabit the skin surface or mucous membranes and are kept at bay by intact integument, inflammatory, and immune cells. Resident bacteria also compete with and regulate growth of resident fungi. As previously mentioned, reduction of resident bacteria, often via antibiotics, disturbs this balance and allows fungal overgrowth.

Fungal infections can also be opportunistic. **Opportunistic pathogens** are those that cause disease only in a host with a compromised immune system. Patients with fungal invasion of tissues are frequently immunocompromised, such as persons with AIDS (Chapter 4). One of the most common opportunistic yeast infections involves *Candida*. Yeast grows well in warm, moist, dark environments; common sites for superficial candidal epithelial cell infection include those with skin–skin contact, such as beneath the breasts in women, the diaper area in infants, and the perineum, between toes, nail beds, and oral mucosa in susceptible individuals. **Maceration**, a softening and breaking down of these tissues, is often related to excessive moisture and is required for candidal infections to gain a foothold. Deep-tissue infections, such as those found in the lungs, kidney, and heart, are life-threatening and are found almost exclusively in immunocompromised patients.

Clinical manifestations of superficial *Candida* cutaneous invasion include skin redness, itching, and burning at the site. In oral candidiasis, lesions are white and resemble cottage cheese attached to an erythematous oral cavity; these lesions bleed easily and can be painful if scraped (Fig. 5.8). Vulvovaginal candidiasis also produces redness, itching, and burning at the site along with a thick, white, vaginal discharge.

Protozoa

Protozoa are unicellular, complex microorganisms. They are characterized by an irregular or fluctuant shape without a cell wall, and many are motile. Transmission can occur through sexual contact, contaminated food or water, or by an insect or other arthropod, which carries the protozoa. Some protozoa are parasites and some are capable of living independently of the host. Those that are parasites compete for and deprive host cells of nutrition, causing tissue destruction.

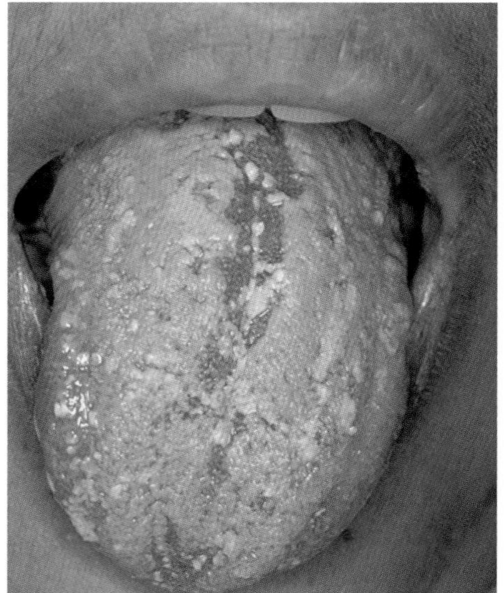

Figure 5.8. Oral candidiasis. These curd-like lesions can be easily removed with gauze. (From Goodheart HP. *Goodheart's Photoguide of Common Skin Disorders*. 2nd ed. Philadelphia, PA: Lippincott Williams & Wilkins; 2003, with permission.)

Module 2 Communicable Disease

Communicable diseases are those that are spread from person to person, often through contact with infected blood and body fluids. Although all communicable diseases are infectious, not all infectious diseases are communicable. Communicable diseases are infections caused by microorganisms that live and reproduce in a human host.

Stop and Consider
What sources of infection would not be considered communicable?

The chain of infection is a useful organization for recognizing the factors inherent in the transmission and spread of communicable diseases (Fig. 5.9). The infectious agent link refers to the pathogens described above. Infection control measures seek to break one or more of these links. For example, breaking the chain of infection at the level of the pathogen requires sterilization of the environment to remove all pathogens from contact with the human cell. Sterilization is performed using physical or chemical agents, heat being the most important.

Sterilization
INFECTIOUS AGENT
• Bacteria
• Fungi
• Viruses
• Rickettsiae
• Protozoa
Sanitizing environment
RESERVOIRS
• People
• Equipment
• Water
Antimicrobial drugs
Treatment of underlying diseases
SUSCEPTIBLE HOST
• Immunosuppression
• Diabetes
• Surgery
• Burns
• Elderly
Recognition of high-risk patients
PORTAL OF ENTRY
• Mucous membrane
• GI tract
• GU tract
• Respiratory tract
• Broken skin
Covering potential entry points
PORTAL OF EXIT
• Excretions
• Secretions
• Skin
• Droplets
Hand washing
Covering secretions
MEANS OF TRANSMISSION
• Direct contact
• Ingestion
• Fomites
• Airborne
Trash disposal
Hand washing
Isolation
Sterilization
Universal precautions
Airflow control
Food handling

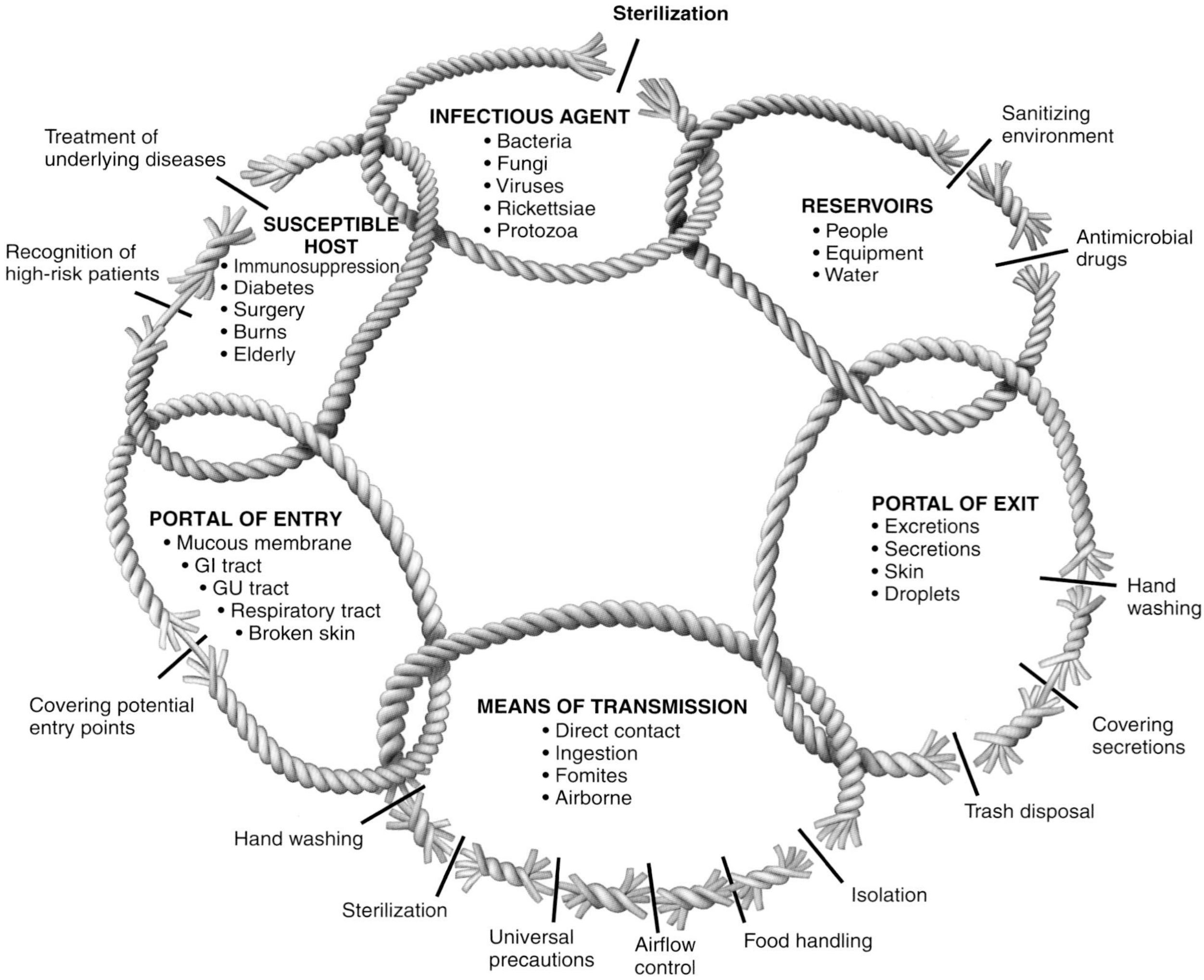

Figure 5.9. Chain of infection. Sources of infection are depicted along with interventions used to break the chain of infection at each link. GI, gastrointestinal; GU, genitourinary. (Modified from Smeltzer SC, Bare BG. *Textbook of Medical–Surgical Nursing*. 10th ed. Philadelphia, PA: Lippincott Williams & Wilkins; 2003, with permission.) To see a video on the chain of infection, visit http://thePoint.lww.com, using the scratch-off code on the inside front cover. thePoint®

An **autoclave** is a device that uses steam heat at high pressures to sterilize objects.

Reservoir

The reservoir is the "holding tank" for the microorganism. The reservoir could include an infected person, an animal, or the environment, such as pond water. Breaking the chain at the level of the reservoir includes providing antimicrobial drugs to the carrier or taking action to destroy the presence of the microorganism in the environment.

Portal of Exit

The portal of exit represents the passage by which the microorganism leaves the reservoir. In human hosts, common portals of exit include the respiratory tract, gastrointestinal tract, skin, mucous membranes, placenta, and blood. If you have a respiratory infection, wearing a mask or otherwise covering your mouth and nose during sneezing will help to block the portal of exit.

Mode of Transmission

All infections will occur through some form of contact with a pathogen. This contact can be direct or indirect. The mode of transmission refers to the mechanism of transference from the reservoir to the portal of entry. The modes of transmission include:

- **Direct contact:** As a mode of transmission, direct contact implies physically touching or otherwise coming in contact with the reservoir. Examples of direct contact transmission include touching the blood or body fluids of an infected person, kissing, or sexual intercourse. This mode can also involve close contact by touching another person or a surface in the environment that is holding the pathogen.
- **Droplet transmission:** Larger respiratory particles, produced by sneezing, coughing, or talking, can pass through the air from the reservoir to the host. For droplet transmission to occur, the host must be within 3 feet of the reservoir. The heavy droplet particles drop to the ground beyond this distance. Most respiratory illnesses are spread through droplet transmission.
- **Airborne transmission:** Smaller respiratory particles can remain suspended in the air and are subject to airborne transmission. The particles can remain in the area of the reservoir for an extended period. Infection can be transmitted to a person who enters this area and breathes the air. Tuberculosis and varicella (chicken pox) are examples of respiratory diseases spread through airborne transmission.
- **Vector transmission:** A **vector** is a vehicle that harbors the pathogen and carries it to the host. Biologic vectors are those that support the life cycle of the pathogen. Arthropods, such as mites, ticks, and spiders, and insects, are examples of biologic vectors. Mechanical vectors are not essential to the life cycle of the pathogen and can include dogs, mosquitoes, and even food.

Universal precautions are a standard of health care that recognizes all blood and body fluids as potentially infected. Universal precautions dictate that health care providers wear gloves when having *any* contact with blood and body fluids. Masks and protective eyewear are also recommended if splattering of blood or body fluids is anticipated. Additional precautions are implemented depending on the mode of transmission.

Stop and Consider
How can you break the chain of infection at each of the different modes of transmission?

Portal of Entry

The portal of entry refers to the access point for the microorganism into the **host**, or the individual who is exposed to, and contracts the infection. The most common locations for microorganisms to enter the body include through the mucous membranes, eyes, respiratory tract, genitourinary tract, gastrointestinal tract, or placenta.

Loss of physical (skin) and chemical barriers can also provide access to the portal of entry. Breaking the chain of infection at the level of the portal of entry involves covering and protecting potential entry points. Examples include wearing gloves, mask, protective eyewear, and condoms. Each of these measures prevents entry of the microorganism into host tissues.

Host Factors

When host lines of defense are compromised and microbes gain access to vulnerable areas, infection can result. Factors that increase host susceptibility to experiencing infection are primarily related to impaired host defense mechanisms (problems with skin/mucous membranes, impaired inflammation, and/or decreased immunity). Immunosuppression is often related to poor nutrition, the extremes of age, concurrent chronic illness, and severe stress. Coinfection and superinfection impact the load placed on the host immune defenses and can further complicate infectious processes.

Module 3 Acute Infection and Complications

Acute infection in both communicable and noncommunicable infectious disease progresses along five distinct phases (Fig. 5.10):

1. **Exposure:** Exposure is contact with the pathogen through any of the modes of transmission described above.

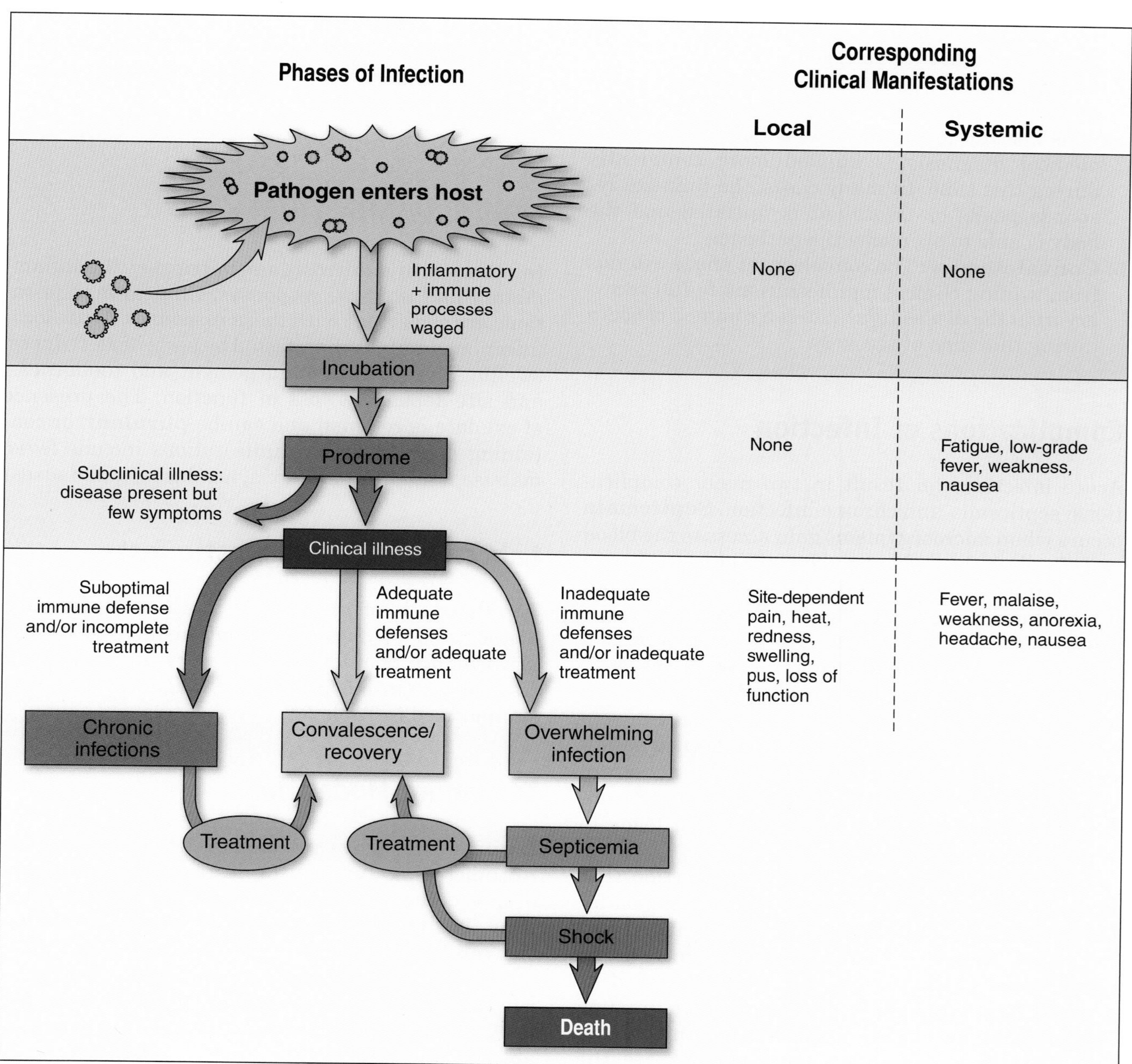

Figure 5.10. Concept map. Phases of infection and corresponding clinical manifestations.

2. **Incubation:** The incubation phase extends from exposure to the onset of any signs or symptoms. During the incubation period, the individual often has no idea that he or she has been exposed to, or will develop, the illness. With communicable disease, it is often during this incubation period that transmission of microorganisms to others is greatest. For example, chickenpox has an incubation period of 7 to 21 days from exposure to recognizable signs and symptoms.
3. **Prodrome:** The prodromal phase involves the onset of vague, nonspecific signs and symptoms, including fatigue, low-grade fever, nausea, weakness, and generalized muscle aches. This phase is often described as feeling "under the weather." The specific signs and symptoms related to the disease have not yet emerged.
4. **Acute clinical illness:** The clinical illness phase represents the manifestation of signs and symptoms specific to the disease. Often, the accurate medical diagnosis is applied more confidently during this time. In many cases, the immune response peaks or treatment is initiated and the body is able to overcome the pathogen.
5. **Convalescence:** The convalescent phase extends from waning clinical manifestations to full recovery from the disease. Fatigue is a common concern during this time of recovery.

Complications of Infection

Acute infection can result in two major complications: septicemia and chronic infection. **Septicemia** occurs when microorganisms gain access to the blood and circulate throughout the body. When septicemia is caused by bacteria, the term **bacteremia** is often used. The development of overwhelming systemic infection is based on the degree of microorganism pathogenicity and immunocompromise in the host. Once pathogens enter the blood and gain access to all perfused tissues, the infection can result in septic shock and become life-threatening. **Septic shock** is a process of systemic vasodilation due to severe infection, often with gram-negative bacteria (the endotoxin component). Massive vasodilation leads to poor perfusion of vital organs.

Chronic infection is defined as an infection that lasts for several weeks to years. The mechanism for eliciting a chronic viral infection was discussed earlier in the chapter. Chronic bacterial infection can result when pathogens are not fully destroyed as a result of a suboptimal inflammatory or immune responses or incomplete antibiotic treatment. The pathophysiologic processes and outcomes are the same as with chronic inflammation (Chapter 3).

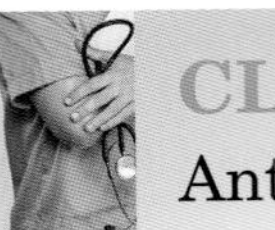

CLINICAL PRACTICE
Antibiotic Teaching Essentials

Antibiotic resistance is one of the most serious public health problems facing health care today. Overexposure to antibiotics or incomplete treatment can result in bacteria changing and becoming resistant to the prescribed antibiotic. Patients need to be clearly informed of the importance of taking an entire course of an antibiotic (even if feeling better) to prevent this complication. Health care providers can assist by teaching proper handwashing techniques and not prescribing antibiotics to treat viral infections. To maintain the benefit of antibiotic therapy, antibiotics should only be used when absolutely necessary.

Clinical Manifestations

Infection with a microorganism triggers the inflammatory and immune responses. Clinical manifestations are consistent with these responses. Acute local infection is usually manifested by pain, heat, redness, swelling, lymph node enlargement and tenderness, and site-dependent loss of function. The presence of exudate is common and can be **purulent**, or containing pus. Systemic manifestations include fever, malaise, weakness, anorexia, headache, and nausea.

Laboratory and Diagnostic Tests

The diagnosis of infection is based on a thorough history and physical examination along with the performance of relevant laboratory and diagnostic tests. Common laboratory and diagnostic tests are summarized in Table 5.2.

Treatment Modalities

Antimicrobial drugs are often used to treat infection. Antimicrobials function to destroy pathogens or to decrease the growth of the offending microorganisms. The major mechanisms of action are to alter the cellular structure of the microorganism or to disable enzymes produced by pathogens. Antibacterial drugs can inhibit synthesis of the bacteria cell wall, damage the cytoplasmic membrane, and disable nucleic acid metabolism or protein synthesis. Antifungals function by binding to the fungal cell

Table 5.2 Common Laboratory and Diagnostic Tests to Detect Infection

Test	Purpose	Interpretation
White blood cell count	A nonspecific test that examines an increase or decrease in white blood cells to assist in determining the presence of inflammatory or infectious process	**Leukocytosis:** elevation in white blood cells, which may indicate an infectious process, often bacterial in origin **Leukopenia:** decrease in white blood cells, which may indicate a viral infection or a problem with suppression of white blood cell production
Serum antibody levels	A specific blood test that detects the presence of certain antibodies against pathogens (see hepatitis)	Presence of specific antibodies indicates an exposure to the antigen at some point
Cultures	Identifies presence and density of microorganisms that grow in a specific medium over a period of time (usually 3 days or so); sample extracted from body tissues (including blood) or exudates	Positive test indicates the microorganism is present
Sensitivities	Identifies which antimicrobial drugs would be most effective for a specific pathogen	If the microorganism is sensitive to a certain antibiotic, that is the recommended treatment

membrane, increasing permeability, and reducing viability of the fungal cells. Because bacteria do not contain the same components as fungal cells, antifungal medications are not active against bacteria. Antiviral treatment has been met with limited success because viral growth employs the host cell. Therefore, destruction of the virus can significantly damage host cells as well. Symptomatic treatment, such as fluids, rest, and analgesics, are often recommended with all infections.

Module 4 Clinical Models

The following clinical models have been selected to aid in the application of knowledge related to infection. When reading through the clinical models, differentiate the type of pathogen, acute or chronic features of the disease, and the role of inflammatory and immune responses.

Influenza

Influenza is a viral infection of the epithelial cells of the airway. The virus is transmitted via respiratory droplets from another infected person or contaminated surface. Three different types of influenza viruses (A, B, or C) can cause influenza disease; each of these types also has several strains, or subtypes.

PATHOPHYSIOLOGY

The respiratory epithelial cells are armed with cilia, mucus, and antibodies. The influenza virus enters the respiratory tract, attaches to the surface epithelial cells, impairs cilia, mucus, and antibodies, moves into the cells, and replicates (Fig. 5.11). The virus causes these epithelial cells to die, resulting in necrosis and sloughing of the dead cells. In many cases, influenza results in an uncomplicated upper respiratory infection or can progress to viral pneumonia. In more severe cases, viral infection in the lung tissue can lead to bacterial pneumonia, impaired air exchange, and even death. Young children (under 2 years of age), adults 65 years of age and older, pregnant women, and individuals with chronic cardiopulmonary, renal, metabolic, or immunodeficient conditions are predisposed to greater morbidity and mortality when infected with influenza.

Influenza viruses are well adapted to escape host defenses and gradually change genetic composition during replication in the human host cell in a process called **reassortment**. This process results in viral offspring with altered antigenic properties. These minor genetic modifications result in ongoing host susceptibility to the influenza virus. The development of vaccines is adjusted yearly to take into account these shifts.

CLINICAL MANIFESTATIONS

The clinical manifestations of influenza are based on the inflammatory response and cell necrosis in

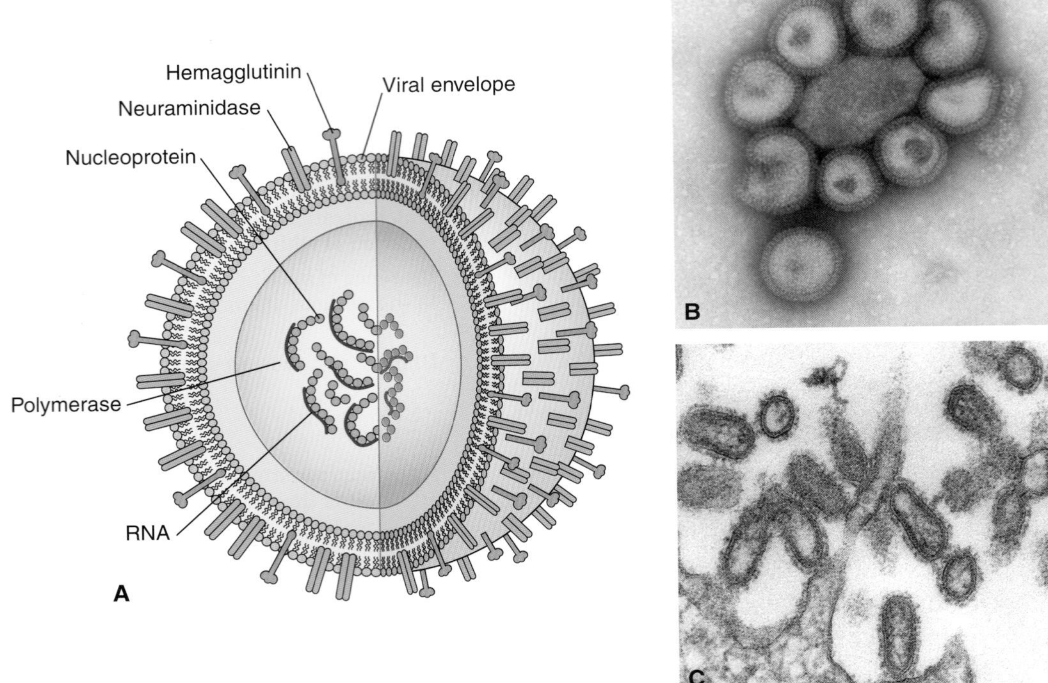

Figure 5.11. Influenza type A virus. **A:** Model of the RNA influenza A virus, showing the hemagglutinin and neuraminidase envelope glycoproteins that provide access to host cells. **B:** Negative-stained transmission electron micrograph (TEM) depicting the ultrastructural details of a number of influenza viral particles, or "virions." **C:** TEM revealing ultrastructural features of the 1918 influenza pandemic virus virions. (**B and C:** From the Centers for Disease Control and Prevention Public Health Image Library. Nos. 8432, 8996. **B:** Courtesy of F. A. Murphy; **C:** Courtesy of Cynthia Goldsmith.)

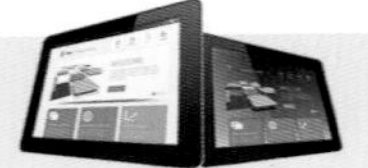

RESEARCH NOTES

Epidemiologists are concerned with tracking the movement of influenza viruses worldwide to predict the most effective vaccine strategy. Selection of the most appropriate vaccine combination is based on antigenic analyses of recently isolated influenza viruses, epidemiologic data, and postvaccination serologic studies in humans. The Food and Drug Administration's Vaccines and Related Biological Products Advisory Committee (VRBPAC) makes a final vaccine recommendation for the United States based on these data.[2]

the respiratory tract and include cough, sore throat, nasal congestion and drainage, and shortness of breath. Systemic signs of inflammation are also common and include chills, fever, body aches, weakness, and malaise.

DIAGNOSTIC CRITERIA

Diagnosis is based on a health history significant for the clinical manifestations described previously. Influenza is a clinical diagnostic challenge because many symptoms resemble that of the common cold. However, influenza is more likely to have an abrupt onset, severe body aches, fever, anorexia, headache, malaise, and a dry cough. During influenza outbreaks, rapid viral assays are available to identify type A and B viruses. These tests using nasopharyngeal secretions are quick (10 to 20 minutes) but can have a false-positive or false-negative error rate around 20% to 30%.

TREATMENT

Influenza is highly contagious and epidemics are common worldwide. Because this infection is viral, treatment is usually symptomatic and focuses on hydration, adequate nutrition, and control of body aches with analgesics. Aspirin use should be avoided in children to prevent the development of Reye syndrome. Antiviral drugs may help reduce the duration of disease if they are started early in the course of infection. Preventing the infection is an important strategy, such as through effective handwashing and annual vaccination.

Hepatitis

Hepatitis is inflammation of the liver. There are numerous causes, the most notable being viral infection. Hepatitis can also result from alcohol abuse or ingestion of other toxic substances that damage the liver.

The Function of the Liver

The major roles of the liver include:

- Secretion of bile
- Metabolism of bilirubin
- Blood storage
- Synthesis of clotting factors
- Metabolism of nutrients
- Metabolic detoxification
- Storage of minerals and vitamins

The liver has a major impact on health status and multiple important functions, but it also has excellent regenerative and restorative capabilities. Injury to the liver often affects the blood vessels, lymphatics, and nerves, which are concentrated in the outer coating of the liver, called the Glisson capsule. When inflamed or enlarged, the Glisson capsule causes right upper-quadrant abdominal pain.

The liver has an active role in venous blood return for the circulatory system. Deoxygenated blood from the gastrointestinal (GI) tract, spleen, and pancreas travels to the liver by way of the portal vein before moving on to the vena cava and heart. This blood bypass is called **portal circulation** (Fig. 5.12). Obstruction of portal circulation from liver damage causes backup of blood flow to the GI tract, spleen, and pancreas.

Within the capsule are hepatocytes, the functional cells of the liver that are capable of regeneration. Hepatocytes are responsible for secretion of bile. Bile contains bile salts, cholesterol, bilirubin, electrolytes, and water. Bile is needed for fat emulsification and absorption. Damage to hepatocytes therefore inhibits bile production and can affect fat absorption. The liver converts fats (primarily triglycerides) to glycerol and free fatty acids to provide energy to the cells. Glucose is another source of energy affected by liver disease, which causes blood glucose fluctuations. The liver is capable of releasing glucose during hypoglycemia, converting amino acids and glycerol to glucose if needed, and taking up glucose from the blood during hyperglycemia. Blood volume and pressure regulation is also aided by the work of the liver in producing plasma proteins.

The liver plays a critical role in detoxification. The liver alters substances, such as alcohol, medications,

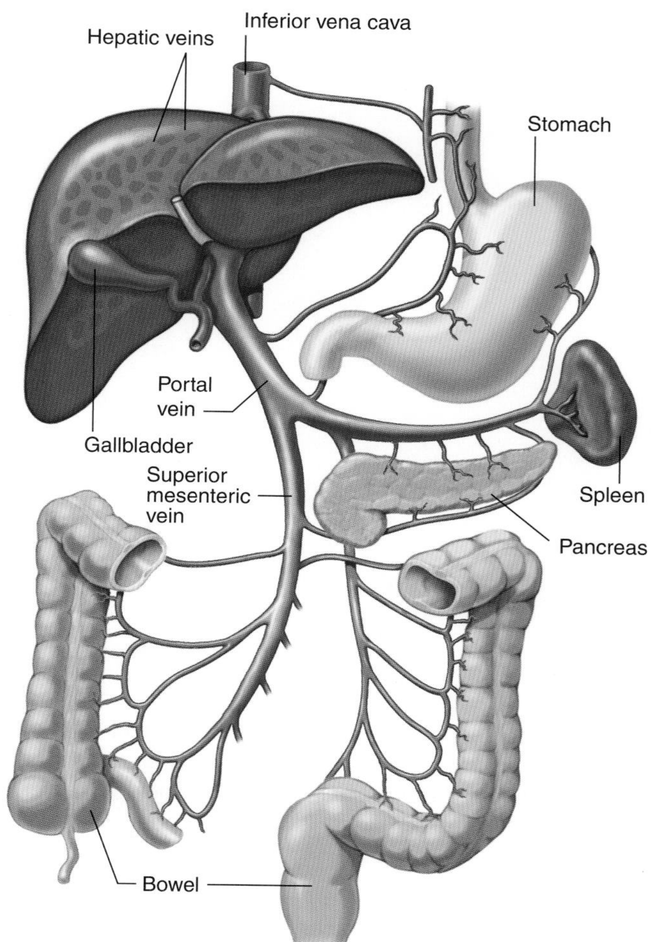

Figure 5.12. The portal circulation. Blood from the gastrointestinal tract, spleen, and pancreas travels to the liver via the portal vein before moving into the vena cava for return to the heart.

and hormones, and helps remove these from the body. Damage to the liver will affect the levels of toxic substances circulating in the body. Always use caution when administering medications to patients with liver disease, such as hepatitis. Most medications are metabolized in the liver and, with poor liver function, may continue to circulate at high levels without being inactivated and removed.

Not to be confused with bile production, bilirubin metabolism is another major role of the liver. Recall that bile contains bilirubin. Bilirubin results from the destruction of aged red blood cells. The liver is responsible for breaking down and removing these dying red blood cells. The aged red blood cells are engulfed and destroyed by phagocytes housed in the liver called **Kupffer cells**. Small capillaries perfuse the liver and are lined with Kupffer cells. Kupffer cells are phagocytes that readily engulf harmful substances. This helps to explain why bacterial and

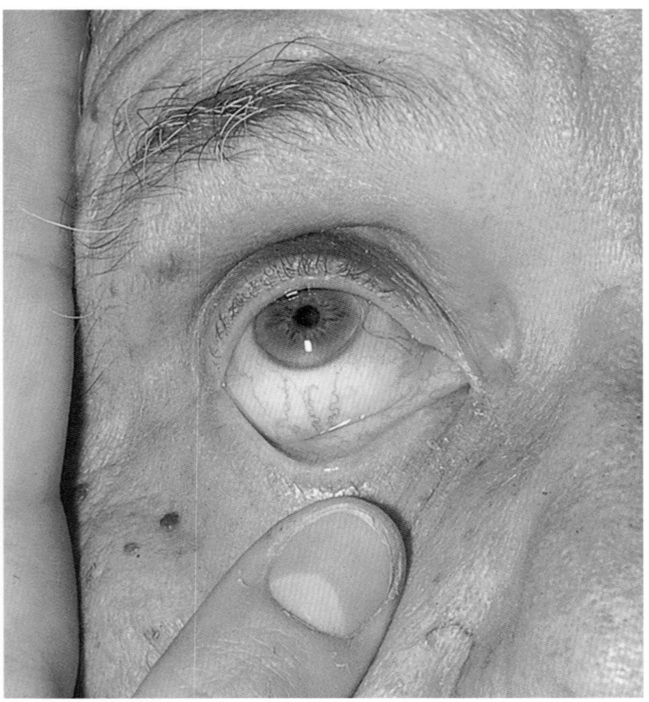

Figure 5.13. Jaundice marked by the presence of a yellow sclera. (From Bickley LS, Szilagyi P. *Bates' Guide to Physical Examination and History Taking*. 8th ed. Philadelphia, PA: Lippincott Williams & Wilkins; 2003, with permission.)

other foreign invaders in the liver are less likely to cause disease than viral microorganisms. When damage to the liver occurs, bilirubin is allowed to circulate freely. Bilirubin is responsible for the yellow-tinged skin color and sclera of the eyes (**jaundice**) in individuals with liver disease (Fig. 5.13). Similarly, the obstruction of bile flow can result in jaundice. The presence of liver disease marked by jaundice is often referred to as the **icteric phase**. Newborns often experience some degree of physiologic (expected) jaundice because of liver immaturity. In newborns, this physiologic jaundice typically resolves spontaneously within a week.

Kupffer cells separate hemoglobin into heme and globin. The globin is degraded into amino acids. The amino acids are then used again to form new protein. The iron cleaved from the heme component can be stored in the liver or used by the bone marrow for **erythropoiesis**, which is the formation of new red blood cells. In patients with protein and iron malnourishment, deficiencies are even more striking when liver disease is present. The liver also produces clotting factors, making those with liver disease more prone to bleeding and bruising.

Viral Hepatitis

Viral hepatitis refers to inflammation of the liver caused by viral infection. The hepatitis viruses (A, B, C, D, and E) are often implicated in this disease. These are referred to as HAV, HBV, and so forth. Table 5.3 details the route of transmission, incubation, and other characteristics of the major hepatitis viruses. Other viruses, including herpes simplex virus, Epstein–Barr virus, and even Ebola virus, can also cause liver inflammation.

PATHOPHYSIOLOGY

The major routes of transmission for the hepatitis viruses include fecal–oral contact or contact with

Table 5.3 Characteristics of Hepatitis Viruses

	Transmission	Incubation	Carrier State	Chronic	Vaccine	Diagnosis
Hepatitis A	Fecal–oral from another infected person; contaminated food and water supplies	1–2 months	No	No	Yes	Blood detection of anti-HAV
Hepatitis B	Contact with infected blood and body fluids; infected mother to fetus	2–3 months	Yes	Yes	Yes	Blood detection of HBsAg
Hepatitis C	Contact with infected blood	2–3 months	Yes	Yes	No	Blood detection of anti-HCV
Hepatitis D	Contact with infected blood and body fluids; infected mother to fetus; MUST have HBsAg to be infected with hepatitis D (coinfection or superinfection)	2–3 months	Yes	Yes	No	Blood detection of anti-HDV
Hepatitis E	Fecal–oral from another infected person	1–2 months	No	No	No	Blood detection of anti-HEV

infected blood and body fluids. Fecal–oral transmission is a problem of hand contact with infected feces in which the virus is transmitted to another when encountering the oral mucosa. For example, if a food preparation worker does not thoroughly wash his or her hands after toileting, he or she can transmit the virus to restaurant patrons who consume the handled food. Contact with blood and body fluids, as with hepatitis B, C, and D, is of particular concern for health care workers who are at high risk of contracting these infections because of frequent contact with blood and body fluids.

Once infected, hepatitis can lead to acute or chronic disease. Hepatitis B can also exist in an asymptomatic carrier state. In general, fecal–oral transmission leads to acute hepatitis, whereas transmission by blood and body fluids results in chronic disease. The level of damage in acute viral hepatitis can vary from death of a few hepatocytes to massive hepatic necrosis. An inflammatory response is waged and the local Kupffer cells help remove necrotic cells. Affected hepatocytes regenerate. Regeneration generally begins within 48 hours of hepatocyte necrosis. With severe infection, **fulminant hepatitis**, which is hepatic failure from severe acute hepatitis, can occur. Obstruction can occur in the blood vessels that perfuse the liver, resulting in tissue hypoxia. Bile flow can also become obstructed.

Stop and Consider
What is the role of bile and why is obstruction of bile flow problematic?

Likewise, chronic hepatitis can range from minimal damage to widespread hepatocyte necrosis, fibrosis, diffuse scarring, and cirrhosis. Chronic hepatitis is represented by impaired liver function for more than 6 months. The liver is infiltrated with macrophages and lymphocytes. Patients with chronic hepatitis also carry an increased risk of developing hepatocellular carcinoma related to persistent cell injury.

Cirrhosis is an end-stage liver disease marked by interference of blood flow to the liver and widespread hepatocyte damage. Interference of blood flow to the liver (1) exacerbates hypoxia of the hepatocytes and results in further cell death; (2) causes blood and bile to back up into the liver resulting in further injury and inflammation; and (3) obstructs blood flow from portal circulation. Liver failure and death may result.

Stop and Consider
Compare fulminant hepatitis and cirrhosis to general infection complications (septicemia and chronic infection).

CLINICAL MANIFESTATIONS

All types of viral hepatitis can cause acute, icteric illness. Three phases, similar to the general phases of infection, characterize acute hepatitis infection:

1. **Prodrome:** a period of fatigue, anorexia, malaise, headache, and low-grade fever. The prodrome usually lasts about 2 weeks.
2. **Icterus:** marked by the onset of jaundice, dark urine, and clay-colored stools 2 weeks after exposure to the virus. This phase corresponds to the clinical illness phase discussed previously and lasts approximately 2 to 6 weeks. The liver is enlarged and tender.
3. **Recovery:** marked by the resolution of jaundice around 8 weeks after the initial exposure to the virus. Signs and symptoms improve with the exception of the liver, which remains enlarged and tender for an additional 1 to 4 weeks.

A careful study of Figure 5.14 will reveal the connection between pathophysiologic processes and clinical manifestations of liver failure.

DIAGNOSTIC CRITERIA

Diagnosis is often based on detection of viral antibodies, such as anti-HAV, anti-HCV, anti-HDV, and anti-HEV, in the blood of the infected person. The core of the hepatitis B virus contains two antigens: the core antigen (HBcAg) and the e antigen (HBeAg). Since there are three possible clinical courses for hepatitis B: complete recovery, asymptomatic carrier state, or chronic infection, the health professional must look at the corresponding antigen and antibody levels. Antibodies to the hepatitis B core antigen (IgM anti-HBc) are required for the diagnosis of acute hepatitis B infection. Cells infected with hepatitis B virus also present surface antigens on the outer coating. The hepatitis B surface antigen (HBsAg) may be present in acute infection or in those who are chronic asymptomatic carriers. Other findings that may aid in diagnosis and prognosis include the detection of bilirubin in the urine, elevated serum bilirubin levels (more than 30 mg/dL indicates more severe disease), and prolonged clotting time (a grave finding that indicates impaired liver function).

TREATMENT

Hepatitis A and hepatitis B can be prevented through vaccination. Treatment of acute viral hepatitis, as with other viral infections, is symptomatic. Fluids, rest, and analgesics are recommended, particularly during the icteric phase of illness. Avoidance of strenuous physical activity or contact sports is often

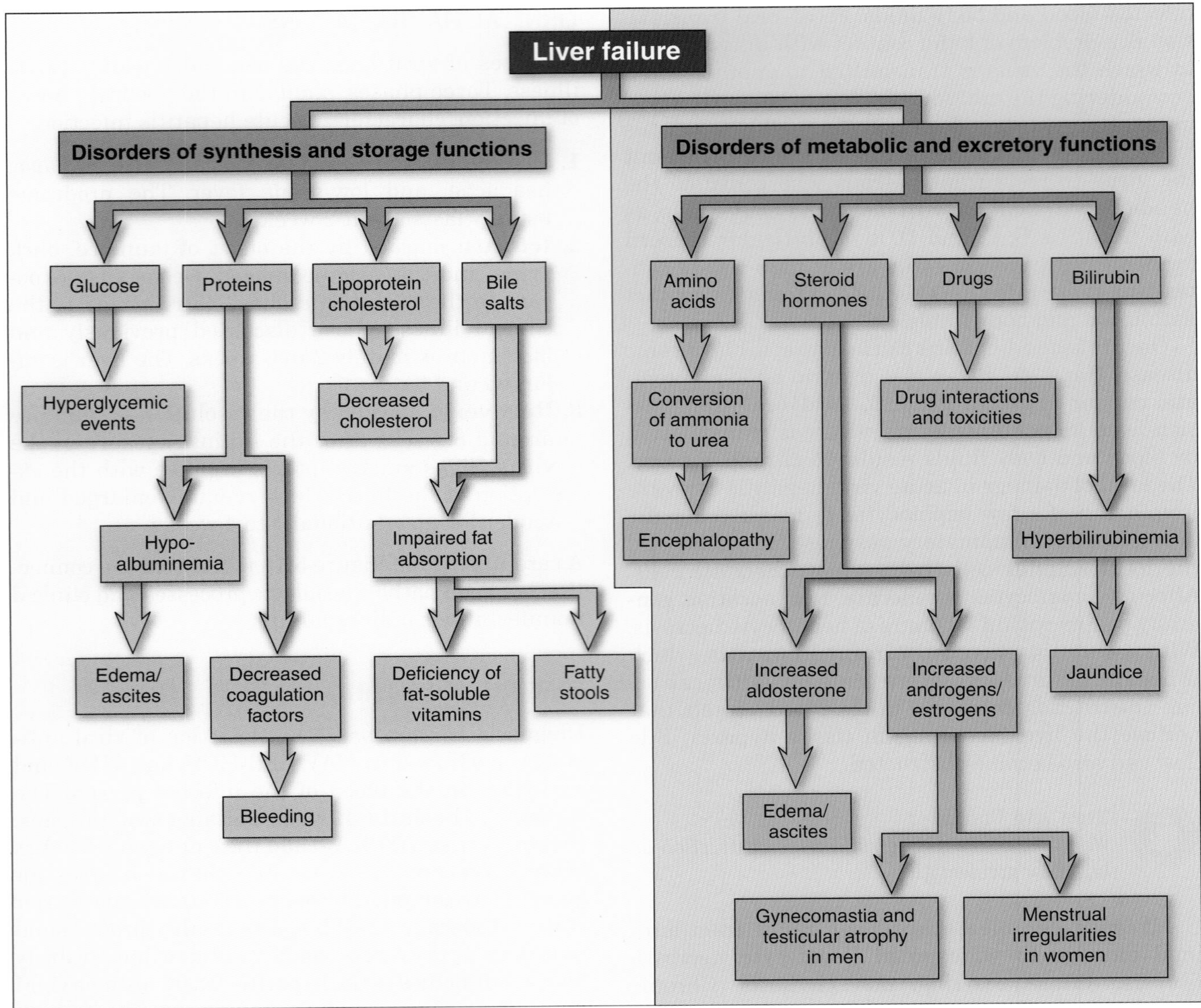

Figure 5.14. Concept map. Alterations in liver function and manifestations of liver failure. (Modified from Porth CM. *Pathophysiology: Concepts of Altered Health States*. 7th ed. Philadelphia, PA: Lippincott Williams & Wilkins; 2004, with permission.)

recommended to avoid liver injury. A low-fat diet is recommended because bile helps with fat emulsification and absorption and bile production may be impaired during liver disease. Antiviral medications may be used in chronic viral hepatitis to decrease viral replication. Avoidance of transmission to others is critical through careful hand washing, avoidance of contact with infected fecal material, and avoidance of contact with blood and body fluids where appropriate.

Tuberculosis

Tuberculosis (TB) is the most prevalent and deadly infectious disease worldwide. The Centers for Disease Control and Prevention (CDC) estimates that one-third of the world's population is infected with TB, and in 2013, 9 million new cases were reported. Another 3 million people worldwide die every year because of active TB infection and the accompanying complications.[3]

PATHOPHYSIOLOGY

Tuberculosis is an infectious disease caused by an aerobic, rod-shaped bacterium (bacillus) called *M. tuberculosis*. Humans are the only known reservoir. The primary site of infection is in the lungs, although TB can infect any organ in the body. TB differs from other respiratory infections in many ways, including the pathogen, mode of transmission, location of infection, clinical presentation, and chronicity.

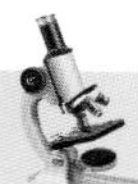

FROM THE LAB

The cell-mediated hypersensitivity reaction that occurs with TB is a key diagnostic feature of this condition. Exposure to *Mycobacterium tuberculosis* is determined via a tuberculin skin test using a purified protein derivative (PPD), formerly known as a Mantoux test. The health provider injects 5 tuberculin units of PPD intradermally. Exposure to TB is measured as the amount of induration (swelling at the local site) at 48 to 72 hours as a result of exposure to the PPD antigen. The size of induration, rather than erythema (redness), is critical for the diagnosis.

With TB, the route of transmission is through inhaling airborne droplet nuclei from an infected person. Airborne droplet nuclei, released within respiratory secretions through coughing, talking, or sneezing, are extremely small and remain suspended in the air longer than most other microorganisms. TB is therefore likely to infect a greater number of people within a common air space compared with illnesses spread by larger, heavier respiratory droplets that fall quickly to the floor.

When inhaled, droplet nuclei move past the bronchi directly to the terminal bronchioles and alveoli of the lung. Quick movement of the tiny microbes beyond the upper respiratory tract often prevents activation of the appropriate defense mechanisms in the upper airway, including the cough and sneeze reflexes. Upon encountering the bacilli, alveolar macrophages ingest but are unable to destroy the bacteria. As the bacilli proliferate within the macrophages, the macrophages present the bacilli as antigens to T lymphocytes (cell-mediated immunity). In an attempt to destroy the bacilli, the inflammatory and cellular immune responses are elicited, leading to one of the following:

1. Containment through an effective cellular immune response (asymptomatic primary TB)
2. Multiplication and the development of aggressive, symptomatic disease (progressive primary TB)
3. Dormancy with future multiplication or reinfection leading to aggressive, symptomatic disease (secondary TB)

Destruction or containment of TB largely depends on an effective cell-mediated immune response of the host, comprised of the production of lytic (killing) enzymes by sensitized macrophages and the development of activated T lymphocytes. Several characteristics of *M. tuberculosis* are important in the pathogenesis of TB. The bacilli are slow growing and resistant to destruction. The bacilli do not produce toxins; damage to the lung and other body tissues is through the hypersensitivity reaction elicited by the bacilli. When the number of inhaled pathogens is small and the host has a competent immune system, the bacilli can be successfully ingested, contained, and killed. If the immune system is compromised, the containment and destruction of the bacilli is less likely, and larger areas of necrosis can develop. The infection can then more easily spread through the lymph nodes to other organs in the body.

The initial containment and destruction of the bacilli occurs through a granulomatous inflammatory response. The formation of a granuloma, or walled-off area of bacteria, is referred to as a **Ghon focus**. The Ghon focus is considered the primary lung lesion. Often, particularly when the number of infecting bacilli is large, the center of the granuloma develops a distinct type of necrosis, termed **caseous necrosis**, which is pasty, yellow, and cheeselike. The *M. tuberculosis* within the Ghon focus drain along lymph channels to lymph nodes in the lungs and form further granulomas. The Ghon focus and the additional granulomas that develop through the lymph channels are referred to as the **Ghon complex** (Fig. 5.15). An intact inflammatory and immune response eventually results in the formation of scar tissue and calcification of these Ghon complex lesions. However, small numbers of dormant bacteria can survive within these calcifications for years.

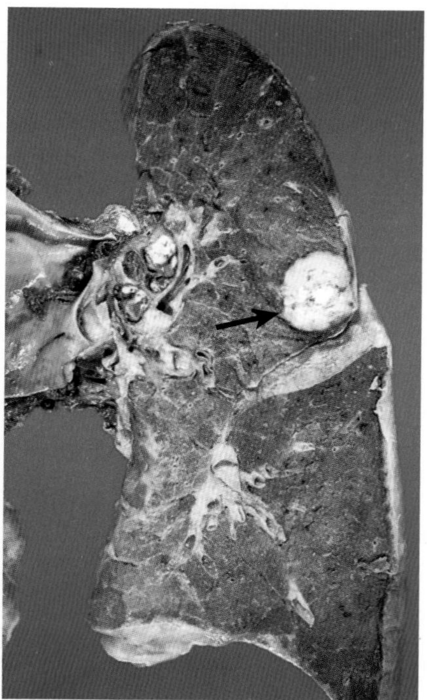

Figure 5.15. Tuberculosis showing a healed Ghon complex. (From Rubin E, Farber JL. *Pathology*. 4th ed. Philadelphia, PA: Lippincott Williams & Wilkins; 2005, with permission.)

Tuberculosis is often distinguished as either primary or secondary TB. Primary infection is the initial exposure and growth of the bacilli in an individual with or without symptoms. Individuals *with* symptoms are believed to have an aggressive and destructive disease, termed active infection. Individuals *without* symptoms exhibit an effective inflammatory and immune response, and a healed Ghon complex eventually forms, surrounding dormant bacilli. If the immune system becomes compromised and the bacteria are allowed to again proliferate, the infection becomes active and progresses to secondary TB. Secondary TB is characterized by reactivation of the primary infection after a long period of dormancy or by reinfection with the pathogens known to cause TB. Secondary TB, which can spread to other organs, is marked by aggressive, destructive cavitations of the lung tissue. **Cavitations** are areas of necrosis that erode surrounding structures of the lungs, including the bronchioles, bronchi, and surrounding blood vessels. If untreated, secondary TB can continue to spread, destroying tissues throughout the body. The pathogenesis of TB is depicted in Figure 5.16.

Stop and Consider
How does the development of granulomas, fibrosis, and calcification in TB compare with other chronic inflammatory conditions, such as rheumatoid arthritis?

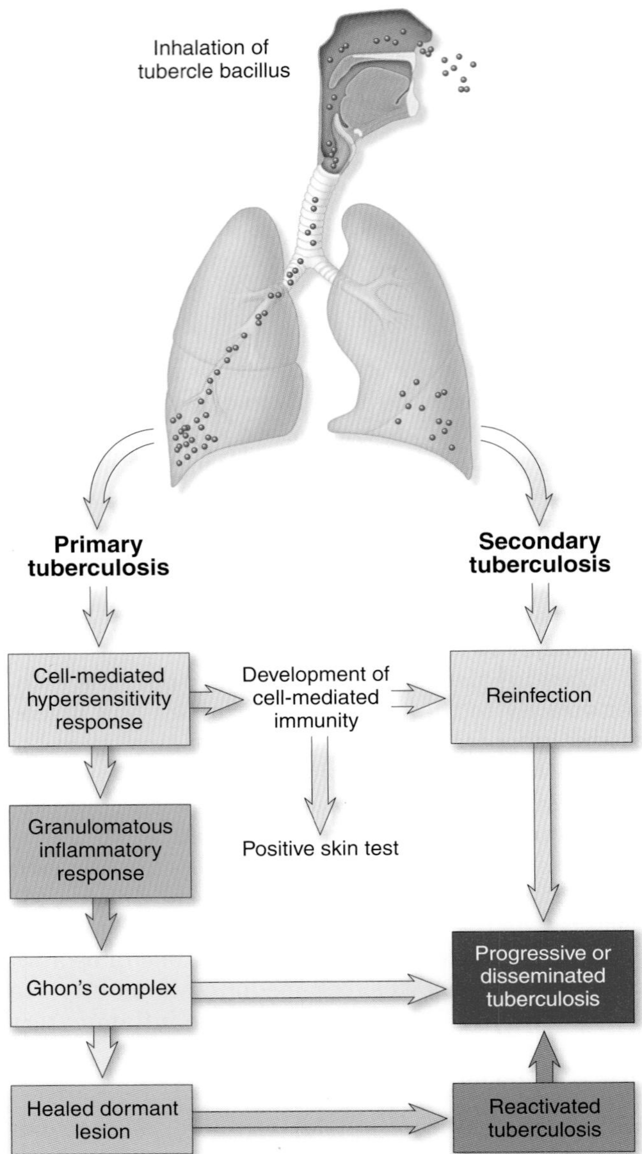

Figure 5.16. Pathogenesis of tuberculosis. (Modified from Porth CM. *Pathophysiology: Concepts of Altered Health States*. 7th ed. Philadelphia, PA: Lippincott Williams & Wilkins; 2004, with permission.)

CLINICAL MANIFESTATIONS

Most (90%) of individuals infected with primary TB are asymptomatic. In those individuals with progressive primary TB (10%), clinical manifestations may resemble those of chronic inflammation, such as malaise, weight loss, fatigue, anorexia, low-grade fever, and possibly night sweats. Ongoing destruction of lung tissue results in a severe chronic productive cough with **hemoptysis** (bloody sputum). The bacteria readily reside in sputum and can be transmitted to others. Because secondary TB infection can reside in other organs of the body, clinical manifestations may extend outside of the lungs. For example, TB found in the meninges of the brain will present with headache and mental status changes that may progress to coma over a period of days to weeks after infection.

DIAGNOSTIC CRITERIA

Active infection with TB is diagnosed through tuberculin skin tests (see From the Lab), chest radiograph, sputum culture, and sputum nucleic acid amplification. A chest radiograph in primary TB often shows patchy or nodular infiltrates or pleural effusion. The upper lobe of the lung is most commonly affected. Advanced infection is noted by the presence of cavitation. Inactive "old" disease is noted by the presence of calcification. A CT scan may be needed if the results of the chest radiograph are unclear or inconclusive.

Sputum specimens should be collected in the early morning of three consecutive days. Fiberoptic bronchoscopy with transbronchial biopsy and bronchial washings may be needed to obtain sputum and tissue specimens for further analysis, particularly in those patients who are unable to expectorate sufficient sputum. The advantage to using nucleic acid amplification over sputum culture is that these newer technologies identify TB within 24 hours compared to a week or more with sputum cultures.

TREATMENT

Treatment is achieved through the use of multiple antimicrobial drugs over several months. The treatment protocol should include directly observed therapy (DOT). This means that the patient must be observed taking the medications at each administration by the health professional or designated personnel. DOT is required to promote complete eradication of the bacteria through improved patient compliance with the prolonged treatment regimen. Typically, treatment involves the use of four antimicrobial drugs: isoniazid, rifampin, pyrazinamide, and either ethambutol or streptomycin. Multiple drug resistance is a major treatment issue related to TB. Resistance to the prescribed antimicrobials is suspected if the patient shows no improvement within 1 to 2 weeks after starting the four first-line drugs. Those individuals with multiple drug-resistant TB are prescribed medications for which the bacteria are susceptible. To prevent transmission to others, hospitalized patients with suspected or diagnosed TB must be placed in isolation. This includes a private room with negative pressure and adequate air exchange mechanisms. Persons entering the room must wear masks or respirators capable of filtering droplet nuclei.

Bacilli Calmette-Guérin (BCG) is a vaccine for TB that is used in many countries with a high prevalence of TB to prevent childhood tuberculous meningitis or miliary (disseminated in the blood) tuberculosis. It is not widely recommended in North America because of the relatively low risk of infection and variable effectiveness against adult pulmonary TB. Individuals who have been vaccinated with BCG will have a positive tuberculin reaction when the PPD is administered; therefore, the tuberculin skin test is not an effective screening tool to detect TB exposure in those individuals vaccinated with BCG.

Urinary Tract Infection

Urinary tract infections (UTIs) can occur anywhere along the urinary tract, from the urethral meatus (urethritis) to the bladder (cystitis). These infections are **ascending**; that is, microorganisms enter at the distal urethra and move up toward the bladder. The bacteria attach to the urinary tract epithelium, resulting in an acute inflammatory response.

PATHOPHYSIOLOGY

Escherichia coli is the most common microorganism implicated in urinary tract infection. *E. coli* is an aerobic, gram-negative bacterium and is resident flora in the gastrointestinal tract. When gaining access into the urinary tract (which is a sterile area of the body), *E. coli* causes infection. Women are particularly vulnerable because of a short urethra and close proximity between the urethra and anus. Mechanical obstruction of the urinary tract, such as with renal calculi (kidney stones) or an enlarged prostate, and introduction of urinary catheters into the urethra and bladder can also increase the likelihood of developing a urinary tract infection.

CLINICAL MANIFESTATIONS

The tissues in the urinary tract become edematous and hyperemic, which results in **dysuria** (pain with urination), urinary **urgency** (the need to immediately urinate), and urinary frequency. Tissue destruction in the urinary tract may result in **hematuria**, or blood in the urine. The inflammatory response to these bacteria produces a purulent exudate, which can be detected as cloudy urine from the increase in leukocytes.

DIAGNOSTIC CRITERIA

Diagnosis is based on the history of presenting symptoms along with physical examination and diagnostic tests. Physical examination may demonstrate suprapubic tenderness with palpation. Urinalysis and urine culture are required and must be obtained using a midstream or catheterized sample using the appropriate technique. **Pyuria**, or purulent exudate (pus) in the urine, found by performing the leukocyte esterase dip test, increases the likelihood of bacterial infection. The definition of UTI is based on a urine culture noting greater than 1,000 colonies of a single organism per mL. Imaging studies may be needed if urinary obstruction is suspected.

TREATMENT

The process of urination assists in "flushing" out much of the bacteria that attempt to ascend the urethra. For this reason, increasing fluid intake is important for patients with UTI. Drug therapy with an antibiotic effective against gram-negative aerobic bacteria is the primary treatment intervention. Patients with diabetes mellitus, immunosuppression, or urinary tract obstruction, or patients who are pregnant, are more likely to develop complications with a UTI and must be aggressively treated with a prolonged course of antibiotics. If UTI is untreated, the bacteria can continue to ascend into the kidneys and result in pyelonephritis.

Pyelonephritis

Pyelonephritis refers to infection and resulting inflammation of the renal parenchyma resulting in scarring. Pyelonephritis can be both acute and chronic. Acute pyelonephritis is discussed here. Chronic pyelonephritis occurs almost exclusively in patients with renal anatomic abnormalities, such as in children with vesicoureteral reflux, a condition characterized by an incompetent ureterovesical valve allowing retrograde urine flow. Repair of the anatomical abnormality is indicated for those with chronic pyelonephritis.

Function of the Kidneys

Each kidney is comprised of about a million filtering units called nephrons. Each nephron is responsible for filtering a small amount of blood. Within the nephron are a glomerulus and a tubule. The glomerulus lets fluid and waste products pass through but prevents the passage of red blood cells and large molecules, such as proteins. The filtered fluid then passes through the tubule, which sends needed minerals back to the bloodstream and removes wastes.

The kidneys serve a number of critical functions essential for homeostasis. Every day, the two kidneys filter about 120 to 150 quarts of blood to produce about 1 to 2 quarts of urine. Urine is composed of wastes and excess fluid. Other important kidney functions include:

- Keeping levels of electrolytes stable, such as sodium, potassium, and phosphate
- Producing hormones that regulate blood pressure, promote red blood cells, and strengthen bones

Acute Pyelonephritis

PATHOPHYSIOLOGY

Acute pyelonephritis results from bacterial infection of the renal parenchyma. The most commonly implicated bacteria is *E. coli*. Bacteria reach the kidney by ascending from the lower urinary tract through the ureters and to the nephrons (Fig. 5.17). Upon ascension, bacteria attach to the epithelium of the urinary tract and trigger the acute inflammatory response. Chemical mediators are released promoting the further movement of bacteria into the urine. Risk factors, which promote the development of pyelonephritis include:

- Urinary obstruction, such as with renal calculi
- Incomplete bladder emptying causing urine stagnation
- Frequent intercourse, which can irritate the urethra
- Exposure to sexually transmitted infection
- Pregnancy/hormonal changes decrease ureteral peristalsis

CLINICAL MANIFESTATIONS

Acute pyelonephritis often presents clinically as a triad of signs/symptoms: fever, costovertebral angle pain, and nausea and/or vomiting. Symptoms may be mild to severe and usually develop over the course of a day to several days. Patients may also report dysuria, urinary frequency, hesitancy, lower abdominal pain, urinary urgency, and even blood in the urine.

DIAGNOSTIC CRITERIA

The diagnosis of pyelonephritis is suggested by the clinical manifestation triad above and is supported by urine studies. Urinalysis screens for bacteriuria, microscopic evaluation reveals hematuria, and urine culture identifies the pathogen. Imaging studies may be used to visualize renal abnormalities.

TREATMENT

Uncomplicated pyelonephritis can be treated in the emergency department with IV fluids, IV antibiotics, and pain medications. Oral antibiotics are continued once the patient returns home. Hospitalization is appropriate for those with severe disease, or those who are pregnant, elderly, or have another chronic disease that may impact resolution. Surgery may be required to remove any abscesses or obstructions that may have occurred or to correct congenital anomalies that have contributed to the pyelonephritis.

Meningitis

Meningitis is inflammation of the membranes (meninges) of the brain and spinal cord. Meningitis commonly results from infection with bacteria or viruses. This section will focus on bacterial meningitis. Worldwide, the rates of meningococcal disease are highest in infants. Adolescents, young adults, and the elderly are also at increased risk.

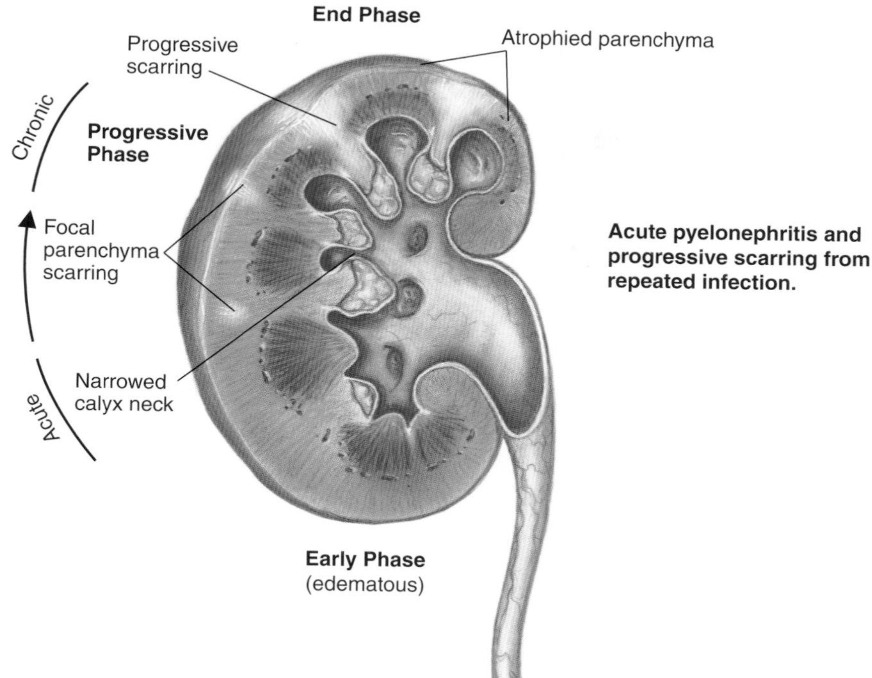

Figure 5.17. Acute pyelonephritis and progressive scarring from repeated infection.

Function of the Meninges

The meninges are comprised of the dura mater, arachnoid, and pia mater (Fig. 5.18). The dura mater is the durable layer; it is the toughest and outermost layer of the meninges. This layer has its own blood supply and is pain sensitive. The arachnoid layer is a web of collagen that provides a cushion. The pia mater forms the delicate inner lining of the brain.

The main functions of the meninges are to:

1. Protect the brain and spinal cord from injury
2. Provide blood supply to the skull and brain tissue
3. Allow for the flow of cerebral spinal fluid

Bacterial Meningitis

PATHOPHYSIOLOGY

The most common bacterial cause of meningitis is *N. meningitides*, an aerobic, gram-negative bacterium. There are at least 13 different *N. meningitidis* subtypes. Viral meningitis is often referred to as aseptic meningitis. It is generally less severe than bacterial meningitis and often resolves without specific treatment. Fungi can result in meningitis in individuals who are immunocompromised. Table 5.4 compares the different types of meningitis.

The mode of transmission for meningitis is respiratory droplets passed from an infected person to the host. The microorganism enters the respiratory tract and attaches to epithelial cells. Inflammatory and immune responses are waged. Immunoglobulins in the respiratory mucosa can provide protective immunity against the microorganisms. However, in some cases, the bacteria move through the mucosa and get into the central nervous system or the blood. The mechanism for entry into the blood and central nervous system is often unknown.

In the central nervous system, the bacteria multiply along the meninges and in the cerebral spinal fluid (CSF). The rapid proliferation of bacteria is related to few antibodies, complement components, and white blood cells in the CSF. The inflammatory response causes the brain tissues to become edematous (swollen) and **hyperemic** (filled with blood). The infectious process is perpetuated by the replication of bacteria (along with the influx of inflammatory cells) and increased capillary permeability. Exudate accumulates throughout the CSF, causing damage to cranial nerves, obstruction of CSF pathways, obstruction of blood flow to brain tissue, and reduced oxygen to the brain. Meningitis can result in septicemia. Septicemia damages endothelial cells of the vessels. Massive, systemic inflammation can then lead to septic shock.

CLINICAL MANIFESTATIONS

Acute bacterial meningitis is noted for a rapid and severe onset of symptoms (often within less than 24 hours). Irritation of the meninges results in the characteristic clinical manifestations: severe

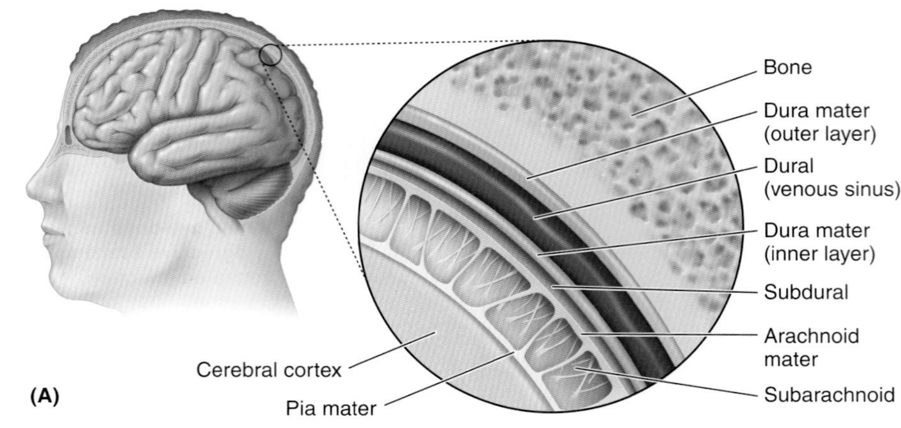

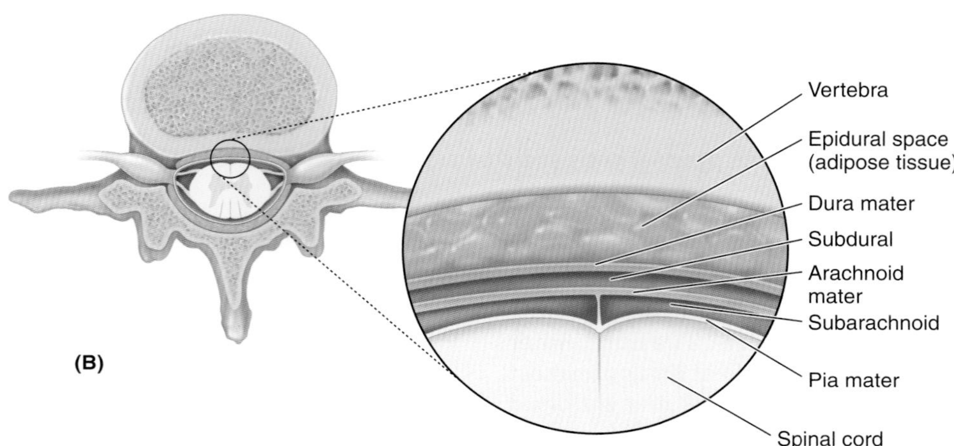

Figure 5.18. Meninges of the brain **(A)** and spinal cord **(B)**. (From Nath J. *Using Medical Terminology: A Practical Approach*. Baltimore, MD: Lippincott Williams & Wilkins; 2006, with permission.)

Table 5.4 Comparison of the Types of Meningitis

	Bacterial	Viral	Fungal
Common pathogens	*S. pneumoniae, N. meningitidis,* and *Haemophilus influenzae* (in those unimmunized)	Aseptic; variety of viral agents including enteroviruses, herpesviruses, HIV	Opportunistic fungi
Onset	Rapid (less than 24 hours)	1–7 days	>7 days
Severity of symptoms	Severe	Mild to moderate	Often mild
Predominant cells	Neutrophils	Lymphocytes	Lymphocytes
Changes in intracranial pressure	Increased	Normal or slightly increased	May be increased
CSF Gram stain	Positive bacteria	Negative	Negative
Glucose in CSF	Decreased	Normal	Decreased
Treatment	Antibiotics	Symptomatic, supportive	Antifungals

CSF, cerebral spinal fluid.

headache, light sensitivity (**photophobia**), and a hyperextended stiff neck (**nuchal rigidity**). The increase in intracranial pressure (ICP) from brain edema and resultant hypoxia (low oxygen) in the brain leads to decreased alertness, loss of consciousness, changes in mental status, vomiting, and seizures. Systemic manifestations include fever, leukocytosis, and anorexia.

DIAGNOSTIC CRITERIA

The diagnosis of meningitis is often made through history and physical examination, blood cultures, and CSF analysis and cultures. Meningeal irritation is related to the influx of chemical mediators, inflammatory cells, and exudate into the CSF and meningeal tissues. Kernig and Brudzinski signs are two common physical examination tests performed to determine the presence of meningeal irritation (Fig. 5.19). To elicit meningeal pain using the **Kernig sign**, the patient is placed supine with the knees bent and hips flexed. The practitioner lifts and extends one knee upward. The Kernig sign is considered positive if moving the leg upward stretches the irritated meninges and elicits pain. Similarly, with the **Brudzinski sign**, the patient is supine. The practitioner quickly flexes the neck to the chest. Again, this activity stretches the irritated meninges at the neck. A positive Brudzinski sign occurs when the patient protects the irritated meninges by involuntarily flexing the hips and knees.

TREATMENT

Treatment involves intravenous antibiotics, corticosteroids, fluids, and other methods to decrease inflammation, maintain adequate blood pressure, and maintain vital organ perfusion. Treatment should be started early in the disease to avoid septicemia and septic shock. The mortality rate is 50% to 90% for patients who are not diagnosed until after the onset of severe neurologic impairment. Appropriate antibiotic treatment of most common types of bacterial meningitis should reduce the risk of dying from meningitis to below 15%. However, even with early recognition and treatment, the mortality risk is higher among the elderly. Treatment is also indicated for close household contacts who may have been exposed to *N. meningitidis*. Hospitalization may require respiratory isolation until the patient has been on antibiotics for at least 24 hours to prevent bacterial spread to other patients.

Immunization is an important step in preventing bacterial meningitis in all populations. Vaccination for *H. influenzae* and meningococcal disease is part of the recommended vaccine schedule for children and adolescents. College students are at particular risk because of close living quarters, and should be appropriately vaccinated.

Tinea

Tinea is a group of fungal skin diseases that occur in various locations, including the feet (tinea pedis), nails (tinea unguium), scalp (tinea capitis), groin (tinea cruris), and skin (tinea corporis and tinea versicolor). Fungal infections of the skin, hair, and nails are also called **dermatophyte** infections and are considered minor but extremely common.

PATHOPHYSIOLOGY

The major mode of transmission is direct contact with another person or surface reservoir. Risk factors for the development of dermatophyte infections

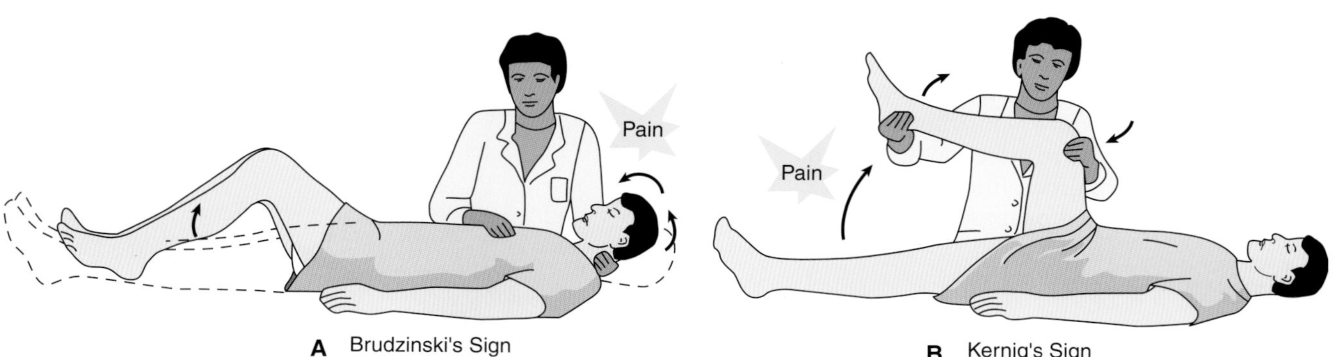

Figure 5.19. Signs of meningeal irritation include nuchal rigidity and positive Brudzinski and Kernig signs. **A:** Flexion of hips, knees, and ankles with neck flexion indicates meningeal irritation. **B:** Extension of the upper leg places a stretch on the meninges and causes pain. (From Nettina SM. *Lippincott Manual of Nursing Practice*. 9th edition. Philadelphia, PA: Wolters Kluwer Health; 2010.)

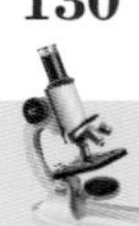

FROM THE LAB

The CSF in bacterial meningitis has a high concentration of neutrophils and protein related to the inflammatory response. The CSF has a low concentration of glucose related to energy needs and utilization by leukocytes and the bacterial cells.

include exposure to moist conditions, genetic predisposition, immunocompromise, and sharing of hygiene facilities (such as public showers) with infected persons. The dermatophyte attaches to and produces thickening of keratinized cells. The infection often remains localized. Complications include bacterial superinfection or generalized invasive dermatophyte infection.

CLINICAL MANIFESTATIONS

Clinical manifestations vary depending on the location of infection. All forms result in changes in the skin, hair, or nails. Tinea corporis is known as "ringworm" because the infection spreads circumferentially like an erythematous bull's eye (Fig. 5.20A). Tinea versicolor presents as patches of hypopigmentation on the skin of the trunk and extremities. Tinea capitis results in hair loss or breakage at the site of infection. Tinea pedis is notable for scaling, fissuring, and maceration, most often between or around the toes. Tinea cruris ("jock itch") is characterized by erythematous lesions that have central clearing and raised borders. Tinea unguium affects the nails and leads to thickened, discolored (white, yellow, brown, or black), dystrophic changes and nail plate separation from the nail bed (Fig. 5.20B). Most forms of tinea can also cause pruritus (itching).

DIAGNOSTIC CRITERIA

The diagnosis of tinea is based on physical examination and laboratory studies, including direct microscopic examination of infected skin, nail, or hair, fungal cultures, and wood light examination. Hyphae on skin or nails and spores within or around the hair shaft can be detected with microscopic examination. Wood light is a procedure of moving a portable ultraviolet light over the site of infection and noting a bright yellow-green or dull green fluorescence (i.e., glowing). This procedure is used primarily for tinea capitis.

TREATMENT

Fungal infections are treated with topical or oral antifungal agents. Treatment with topical therapy for dermatophyte infections of the skin commonly extends from 2 to 8 weeks. Topical therapy is ineffective for treating tinea in the hair and nails. These types require prolonged oral antifungal therapy. Prevention measures are also critical to avoid recurrence of infections. Practicing proper hygiene and avoiding contact with others who have suspicious lesions can deter infection.

Malaria

Malaria is a potentially life-threatening disease caused by infection with *Plasmodium* protozoa transmitted by mosquito. Malaria is currently eradicated in the United States and almost all cases in the US occur in patients who have recently traveled to the

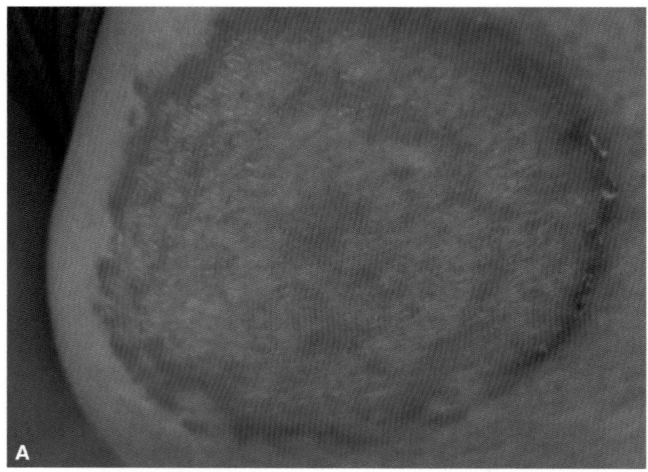

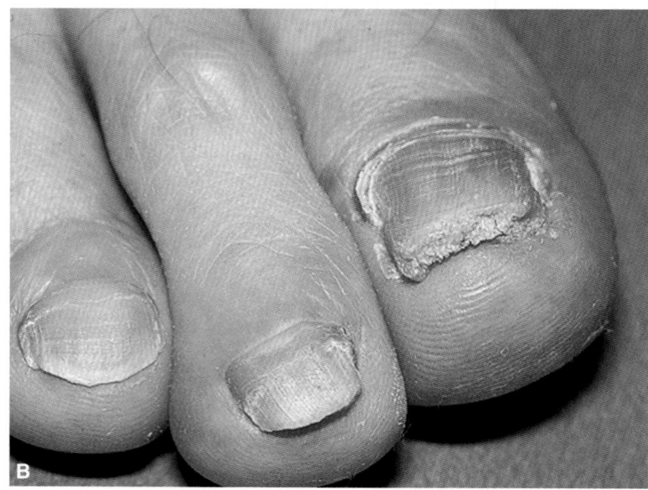

Figure 5.20. Tinea. **A:** Tinea corporis (ringworm). (Image provided by Stedman's.) **B:** Tinea unguium. (From Goodheart HP. *Goodheart's Photoguide of Common Skin Disorders*. 2nd ed. Philadelphia, PA: Lippincott Williams & Wilkins; 2003, with permission.)

US from malaria-endemic areas. Worldwide, however, malaria causes over a million deaths per year, often affecting children from sub-Saharan Africa. *Plasmodium falciparum* is the most lethal species and is responsible for 95% of these deaths.[4]

PATHOPHYSIOLOGY

Malarial infection is typically acquired in an endemic area following a mosquito bite. The *Anopheles* species of mosquito transmits plasmodia, contained in its saliva, into the host. Plasmodia enter circulating red blood cells and feed on hemoglobin and other proteins within the cells. The incubation period varies depending on the *Plasmodium* species, but infection typically develops within a month of exposure. Individuals with sufficient immunity can spontaneously clear the parasites and require no treatment. In many cases, however, the parasites evade the immune response and cause infection.

CLINICAL MANIFESTATIONS

A high index of suspicion is warranted if a patient has recently traveled to a tropical area and presents with the typical malaria symptoms a few weeks after the infection. Clinical manifestations include:

- Headache
- Shivering and chills
- High fever
- Excessive sweating
- Cough
- Fatigue
- Malaise
- Joint/muscle aching

DIAGNOSTIC CRITERIA

The diagnosis of malaria is made through history of travel to an endemic area, physical examination, and laboratory testing. Given the pathophysiology of malaria, which attacks proteins in red blood cells, hemoglobin levels are often low, as are platelet counts, and liver function tests are abnormal. A classical triad of thrombocytopenia, elevated lactate dehydrogenase (LDH), a liver enzyme, and atypical lymphocytes is a common presentation. Peripheral blood smears will show red blood cells infected with the malaria parasite (Fig. 5.21).

TREATMENT

The best treatment is prevention. This occurs by limiting exposure to infective mosquitoes, particularly at dawn and dusk, when feeding is highest, using a bed net during sleep, wearing long-sleeve clothing, and using insect repellants with 35% or greater DEET concentration (for adults); children should use concentrations of DEET at less than 35%. Use this product sparingly on exposed skin and remove when out of range of infective mosquitoes. Antimalarial drugs can be prescribed to those traveling to areas endemic to malaria.

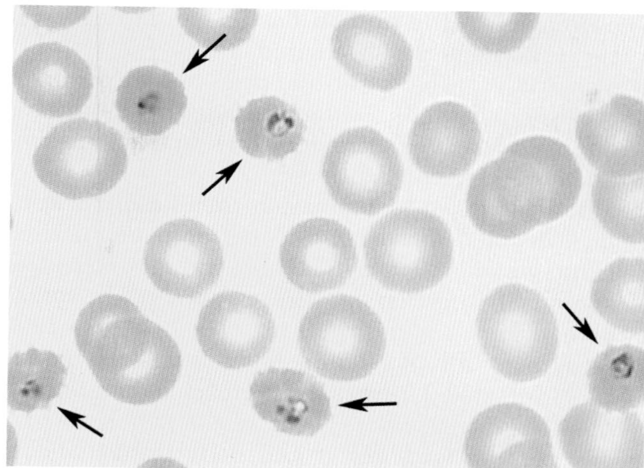

Figure 5.21. Peripheral blood smear shows several erythrocytes parasitized by malaria *(arrows)*.

Antimalarial drugs fall into four major drug classes: quinolines, antifolates, artemisinins, and antimicrobials. Multiple drugs must be used as no single drug has been shown to eradicate all forms of the parasite at all stages of its life cycle. A typical drug combination used is chloroquine (quinoline) and sulfadoxine-pyrimethamine (antifolate). Antipyretics can be used to reduce fever and promote comfort.

SUMMARY

- Exposure to a microorganism elicits the inflammatory and immune responses. Infection results from inadequacies of the three lines of defense and represents a state of tissue destruction resulting from invasion by microorganisms.
- The chain of infection is a useful organization for recognizing the factors inherent in the transmission and spread of communicable disease. The links in the chain include the pathogen, portal of entry, reservoir, portal of exit, mode of transmission, and host. Infection control measures seek to break one or more of these links.
- Microorganisms that cause infection are called pathogens. The pathogenicity, or qualities that promote the production of disease, involves multiple factors, including the pathogen's potency, invasiveness, ability to evade the immune system, speed of replication, production of toxins,

adherence to the human host cell, and degree of tissue damage that is elicited.

- Bacteria, viruses, fungi, and protozoa are common types of pathogens. Understanding the distinctive quality of each can provide clues to transmission and spread of each pathogen.
- Major modes of transmission include direct contact, droplet, airborne, and vector transmission. Hand washing is a critical step in preventing the spread of infection by direct contact. Universal precautions are a standard of health care that recognizes all blood and body fluids as potentially infected. Universal precautions dictate that health care providers wear gloves when having *any* contact with blood and body fluids. Masks and protective eyewear are also recommended if splattering of blood or body fluids is anticipated.
- Phases of an acute infection include exposure, incubation, prodrome, clinical illness, and convalescence. Clinical symptoms are dictated by the cells that are damaged by the invading microorganism.
- Complications of acute infection include septicemia and chronic infection with loss of function in the affected tissues.

CASE STUDY 5.1

You are the parent of a 6-month-old child who is fussy and is tugging on her ears. You take her to the clinic and are told that she has otitis media, a middle ear infection. From your reading and experience regarding infectious processes, answer the following questions:

1. Outline the process that is most likely occurring in this child's body.
2. What anatomic differences in a child would predispose to this type of infection?
3. What are the probable sources of this infection?
4. What would you expect for local and systemic clinical manifestations?
5. What diagnostic tests could be used? How could you differentiate between viral or bacterial pathogens?
6. What treatment measures would you anticipate?
7. What would be the potential complications?

Log on to the Internet. Search for a relevant journal article or Web site that details otitis media and confirm your predictions.

CASE STUDY 5.2

Jamie is a 48-year-old black woman who comes into the emergency department complaining of painful swelling, drainage, and redness over the past 5 days in the left hand. She spends a lot of time outdoors working in her garden and said she had a "pretty nasty" mosquito bite on the top of that hand before the swelling started. After 3 days of increased swelling and redness, she went to her doctor and received an oral antibiotic and was told it was probably a mild infection from the insect bite. Now, she presents because her hand is increasingly painful, tight, and the drainage has worsened. She noticed that she had a fever this morning of 102.9°F. Laboratory test results today show a WBC count of 18,500. After intravenous antibiotic treatment and hospitalization, the wound culture is found to be positive for methicillin-resistant *S. aureus* (MRSA). From your reading and experience regarding infectious processes, answer the following questions:

1. Outline the process that is most likely occurring in Jamie's body.
2. What is the probable source of this infection?
3. What would you expect for local and systemic clinical manifestations?
4. What diagnostic tests were used or could be used? How could you differentiate between viral or bacterial pathogens?
5. What additional treatment measures would you anticipate? How is MRSA treated differently than nonresistant pathogens?
6. What would be the potential complications?

Log on to the Internet. Search for a relevant journal article or Web site that details MRSA and confirm your predictions.

CASE STUDY 5.3

Kathy is a 55-year-old Caucasian woman who lives in northern Minnesota. Kathy was out walking her dog in the woods and upon returning home found a deer tick crawling on the back of her hand. Later that week she noticed a rash on her leg, forming the shape of a bull's eye around her knee. She experienced a fever, headache, and generalized body aches. She was tested and found positive for Lyme disease. Lyme disease is infection with the spirochete *Borrelia burgdorferi* transmitted through a tick bite. From your reading and experience regarding infectious processes, answer the following questions:

1. Outline the process that is most likely occurring in Kathy's body.
2. What is the source of this infection?
3. What would you expect for local and systemic clinical manifestations?
4. What diagnostic tests were used or could be used?
5. What additional treatment measures would you anticipate?
6. What would be the potential complications?

Log on to the Internet. Search for a relevant journal article or Web site that details Lyme disease and confirm your predictions.

PRACTICE EXAM QUESTIONS

1. You are looking to break the chain of infection by washing your hands frequently as you provide care for patients. Which of the following links in the chain will be broken by this activity?
a. Reservoir
b. Host
c. Portal of entry
d. Mode of transmission

2. Which of the following may make a person more susceptible to getting an infection?
a. Age between 6 and 46 years
b. Experiencing a surgery that is healing by primary intention
c. Final exams week
d. A functioning immune system

3. The feeling that "something is not quite right" is considered which stage in infection?
a. Point of infection with pathogen
b. Incubation
c. Prodrome
d. Acute symptoms

4. Which of the following clinical manifestations is not typically found with inflammation but is more characteristic of a bacterial infection?
a. Purulent exudate
b. Redness and swelling at the site
c. Lymphadenopathy
d. Fever

5. A white blood cell differential shows an increase in the number of monocytes and macrophages in the blood. This typically means that:
a. This is a new infection
b. This is a chronic infection
c. This is a viral infection
d. The differential provides no useful information

6. Given the mode of transmission for influenza, how would you break the chain of infection and prevent spread?
a. Administer antibiotics as directed
b. Wash hands after toileting
c. Disinfect table surfaces in the room
d. Wear a mask

7. Which of the following diagnostic tests would give information to the presence of a carrier-state asymptomatic hepatitis B infection?
a. Hepatitis B surface antigen (HBsAg)
b. Hepatitis B core antigen (HBcAg)
c. Prothrombin time (PTT)
d. There is no way to distinguish the different forms of hepatitis B

8. What is the most likely complication of an untreated UTI?
a. Glomerulonephritis
b. Pyelonephritis
c. Fulminant UTI
d. Urethritis

9. Treatment for tinea unguium must include:
a. Oral antifungals
b. Topical antifungals
c. Both topical and oral antifungals
d. Nail removal and topical antifungals

10. Which of the following scenarios is most likely in the CSF of a patient with bacterial meningitis?
a. CSF has high neutrophil count and high protein count.
b. CSF has high neutrophil count and low protein count.
c. CSF has high glucose level and high red blood cell count.
d. CSF has high lymphocyte count and low red blood cell count.

11. Which of the following is an important characteristic of *M. tuberculosis* (the microbe that causes TB) and helps to explain its pathogenesis?
a. It is a large and fast-growing microbe.
b. It produces toxins and these toxins destroy lung tissue.
c. It is resistant to destruction and can sit dormant for years.
d. It cannot be detected or diagnosed until the disease is well advanced.

12. An important aspect of infection is prevention. Which of the following would be an effective prevention measure for malaria?
a. Antibiotics
b. Avoiding international travel
c. Handwashing
d. Wearing long sleeves and pants

13. Infections cause a local inflammatory response at the site of infection, which leads to specific clinical manifestations. In the case of pyelonephritis, what would be a likely clinical manifestation?
    a. Dysuria
    b. Hyperglycemia
    c. Tachycardia
    d. Pruritis

14. The patient is diagnosed with influenza. Which of the following best describes the route of transmission for this disease?
    a. Airborne
    b. Respiratory droplets
    c. Direct contact
    d. Fecal–oral

DISCUSSION AND APPLICATION

1. What did I know about infection prior to today?
2. What body processes are affected by infection? What are the expected functions of those processes? How does infection affect those processes?
3. What are the potential etiologies for infection? How does infection develop?
4. Who is most at risk for developing an infection? How can infection be prevented?
5. What are the human differences that affect the etiology, risk, or course of infection?
6. What clinical manifestations are expected in the course of infection?
7. What special diagnostic tests are useful in determining the diagnosis and course of infection?
8. What are the goals of care for individuals with infection?
9. How does the concept of infection build on what I have learned in the previous chapters and in previous courses?
10. How can I use what I have learned?

RESOURCES

The World Health Organization (WHO) provides valuable information about the global infectious disease threat. The organization Web site can be accessed at: http://www.who.int/

An excellent review of the WHO Strategy for Containment of Antimicrobial Resistance can be found at:
www.who.int/drugresistance/en/

The Centers for Disease Control and Prevention (CDC) provides a wealth of information on infectious disease prevention and spread. The Web site can be accessed at:
http://www.cdc.gov/

The National Institute of Health provides research-based information related to allergy and infectious disease at:
http://www.niaid.nih.gov

References

1. Centers for Disease Control and Prevention. Prion diseases. 2015. http://www.cdc.gov/prions/
2. Centers for Disease Control and Prevention. Vaccines and preventable diseases. 2015. http://www.cdc.gov/vaccines/vpd-vac/default.htm
3. Centers for Disease Control and Prevention. Global tuberculosis (TB). 2014. http://www.cdc.gov/tb/topic/globaltb/default.htm
4. Perez-Jorge E. Malaria. 2014. http://emedicine.medscape.com/article/221134-overview

Find additional resources for this chapter at http:thePoint.lww.com thePoint®

Genetic and Developmental Disorders

Chapter

6

LEARNING OUTCOMES

1. Define and use the key terms listed in this chapter.
2. Identify the implications of alteration in the structure and function of genes and chromosomes.
3. Describe inheritance patterns in single gene disorders and chromosomal disorders.
4. Compare and contrast the inheritance patterns of multifactorial and altered chromosomal disorders.
5. Discuss the influence of gene–environment interactions on developmental disorders and future development of disease.
6. Analyze the biologic, social, and ethical implications of genetic screening.
7. Apply concepts of alterations in genetics and development to clinical models.

INTRODUCTION

How do you feel today? How will you feel a week from now? How about a month or year from today? Although you probably do not think that far ahead, the story of your future health and risk of disease can be told by your genetic makeup. The study of genetics is the study of **heredity**, the passage of characteristics from parent to offspring. Your story is but one chapter in your family's book of heredity. Your health has been influenced by the genetic contributions of your parents and the contributions from all of the generations before them. Your genes will contribute to future chapters when passed on to your children. The roadmap of your life's journey toward health is designed by the genes that make you who you are. Your genetic makeup can sometimes lead directly to disease or can just point you in that direction, which can be changed by other things that you encounter along the way. An understanding of the genetic influences of health and disease provides the basis for the application of these concepts to the promotion of health and the prevention of disease.

The advancement of knowledge in the genetic basis for disease is rapid, revealing new approaches to disease treatment and prevention. The Precision Medicine Initiative is a new approach, which takes into account each individual's genetics, environment, and lifestyle in determination of disease risk and personalized treatment (Fig. 6.1). The Precision Medicine Initiative includes voluntary contribution of health information by individuals, including health history and genomic data, forming a large repository of health data that will lead to new ways to prevent and treat disease. The health and genomic data will be made available to the individuals providing the data, providing control

THE PRECISION MEDICINE INITIATIVE®
WHAT IS IT?
Precision medicine is an emerging approach for disease prevention and treatment that takes into account people's individual variations in genes, environment, and lifestyle.
The Precision Medicine Initiative® will generate the scientific evidence needed to move the concept of precision medicine into clinical practice.
WHY NOW?
The time is right because of:
Sequencing of the human genome
Improved technologies for biomedical analysis
New tools for using large datasets

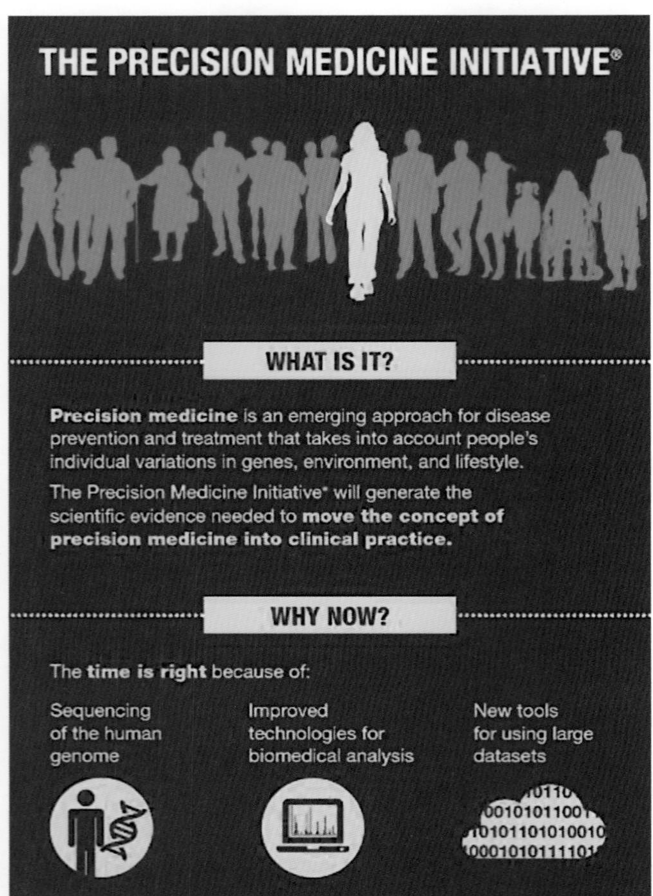

Figure 6.1. Precision Medicine Initiative. The Precision Medicine Initiative is a National Institutes of Health-supported approach to advancing novel methods to prevent and treat genomic-based disease in individuals.

over their own information. Data will also be available to researchers in deidentified aggregate form. This complex initiative leverages health information technology and the rapidly evolving methods needed to analyze large amounts of health data that can be used to forge new approaches to precise care, from populations to individuals.

Stop and Consider
What are the potential risks to security and privacy posed by provision of health and genomic data?

Module 1 Review of Genetic Processes

Chapter 2 introduced the basic components of the genetic system in the discussion of cellular structure. This chapter expands on the genetic components of the cell and introduces other influences that are important in genetic regulation of health and disease. The nucleus houses the genetic components essential to life processes. The organization of these components will be presented in an ordered fashion to provide an overview of both structure and function. The processes of transcription and translation of genes and the replication of chromosomes will be highlighted as the basis for improved application to genetic and developmental alterations discussed in the modules that follow this review.

Deoxyribonucleic Acid

Deoxyribonucleic acid (DNA) is a type of nucleic acid that contains a sugar (deoxyribose), and it is usually found in the cell nucleus and mitochondria. DNA is responsible for the storage of genetic information. It is made up of four nitrogenous bases, including the **purines**, adenine (A) and guanine (G), and the **pyrimidines**, cytosine (C) and thymine (T). DNA is usually double-stranded, with two single strands linked by the purine/pyrimidine combinations of A–T and C–G, also known as **base pairs**. These linked combinations bring the two single strands together in a double helix structure, connected by hydrogen bonds. These products combine in specific ways, forming genes and chromosomes.

Genes

Genes are small functional hereditary units located on a specific site of a chromosome. Made up of pieces of DNA, most genes contain the information, or **genetic code**, for making a specific protein. Genes vary in size, and associated DNA nitrogenous base pairs total anywhere between several hundreds and one million. Genes occur in pairs in somatic (body) cells and singly in gametes such as ova and sperm,

Table 6.1 Amino Acids and Their Genetic Codes

Amino Acid	Symbol	Codons
Alanine	Ala	GCA, GCC, GCG, GCU
Cysteine	Cys	UGC, UGU
Aspartic acid	Asp	GAC, GAU
Glutamic acid	Glu	GAA, GAG
Phenylalanine	Phe	UUC, UUU
Glycine	Gly	GGA, GGC, GGG, GGU
Histidine	His	CAC, CAU
Isoleucine	Ile	AUA, AUC, AUU
Lysine	Lys	AAA, AAG
Leucine	Leu	UUA, UUG, CUA, CUC, CUG, CUU
Methionine	Met	AUG
Asparagine	Asn	AAC, AAU
Proline	Pro	CCA, CCC, CCG, CCU
Glutamine	Gln	CAA, CAG
Arginine	Arg	AGA, AGG, CGA, CGC, CGG, CGU
Serine	Ser	AGC, AGU, UCA, UCC, UCG, UCU
Threonine	Thr	ACA, ACC, ACG, ACU
Valine	Val	GUA, GUC, GUG, GUU
Tryptophan	Trp	UGG
Tyrosine	Tyr	UAC, UAU

consistent with the chromosome makeup of those same cell types.

The four nitrogenous bases (adenine, guanine, cytosine, and thymine) that are the foundations for DNA base pairs are also important in the formation of the genetic code. The sequence of three of these bases forms a **codon** (nucleotide triplet), a fundamental triplet code necessary for protein synthesis. The basic compounds produced by these codons are **amino acids**. Twenty different types of amino acids combine to form the basis of human proteins, produced by **ribonucleic acid (RNA)** as a result of reading the genetic code. Redundancy is built into this process, allowing production of a single amino acid from more than one combination of triplet nitrogenous bases in most cases (Table 6.1). The base pairs in RNA are similar to those described for DNA, with the exception that T is substituted by uracil (U) in the genetic code, resulting in purine/pyrimidine combinations of A–U and C–G (Fig. 6.2). RNA delivers DNA's genetic message to the cytoplasm of a cell where proteins are made. The process of protein production by genes is complex. A brief overview is presented in Figure 6.3 to help apply this information to health and disease.

Three types of RNA are involved in the process of protein production. **Messenger RNA (mRNA)** provides a template for protein synthesis dependent on a codon sequence that is based on that of the complementary strand of DNA (cDNA). Through the process of **alternative splicing**, certain pieces of the RNA called **exons** are retained, and other segments, **introns**, are excised. The genetic code directs the specific splice location, allowing for a large variety of mRNA molecules to be transcribed from a single gene. **Transfer RNA (tRNA)** delivers these products for protein production (Fig. 6.3). Each tRNA recognizes and binds a specific amino acid, which it then transfers to organelles called ribosomes. Ribosomes are formed by a combination of **ribosomal RNA (rRNA)** produced in the nucleolus and nuclear ribosomal proteins. These ribosomes are transported from the nucleus to the cytoplasm where many attach to the endoplasmic reticulum, associate with mRNA, and begin protein synthesis, also known as **translation** of the genetic code.

The process of making a protein from a gene is highly complex and sometimes difficult to understand. One way to think of this process in a more simplified way is to consider the basic steps of transcribing and translating a gene with something more familiar, like reading. The nucleus is like the library. It contains the complete complement of genetic materials as the library has a full range of books needed to satisfy any reader. Within the nucleus are the chromosomes that contain genes. The genes are located along specific areas of each numbered chromosome. This is like the books arranged in the library by the Dewey Decimal or Library of Congress Classification Systems so that what is sought can be easily found. Within each section of books are those that are arranged by topic or subject matter. This is similar to the arrangement of the organization of exons and introns along genes that serve to provide the code and regulation for the transcription of the DNA nucleotide bases. The mRNA reads the series of DNA nucleotide bases and *transcribes* them into complementary RNA nucleotide bases, a process similar to identifying the letters in a word. Each letter is taken so that pieces of words or syllables are formed, like the process of sounding out each part of a word in the process of reading. This process is similar to taking the transcribed mRNA nucleotide bases and *translating* them into the nucleotide triplet, or codon. The nucleotide bases that make up each codon

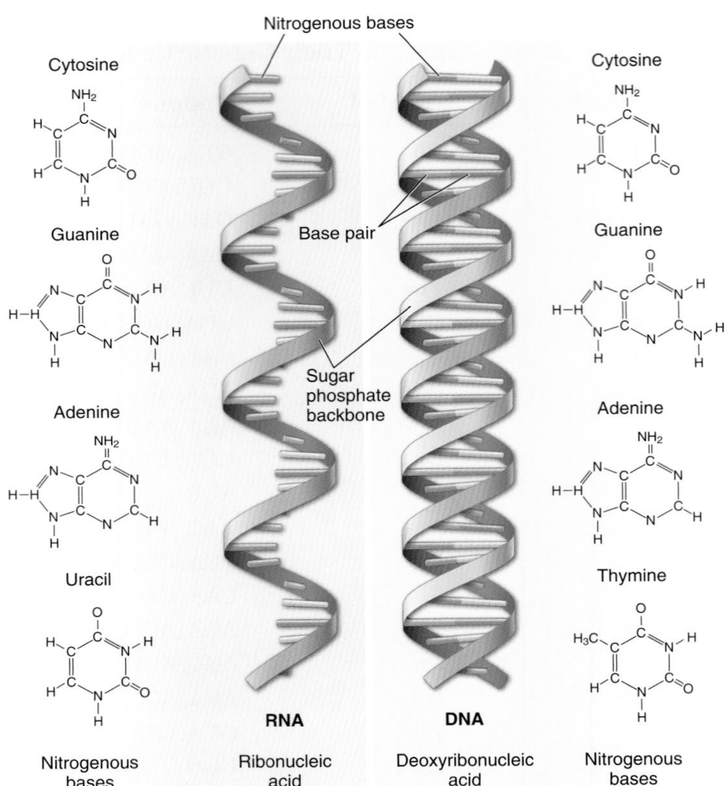

Figure 6.2. Base pairs in RNA and DNA. Uracil is the nitrogenous base in RNA, corresponding with the thymine base in DNA. Note the single helix structure of RNA in contrast to the double helix structure of DNA.

are translated by the tRNA, complementing those transcribed by the mRNA. Here, each syllable comes together to make a word. Specific tRNAs recognize each codon, binding to the codon in the ribosome and transferring it to the growing chain of amino acids, the process continuing until the production of the individual protein is complete. The amino acids combine in particular ways to form polypeptide chains, similar to how words form sentences. Finally, polypeptide chains combine to form large proteins of various sizes in a way that sentences come together to form paragraphs, chapters, and whole books.

Chromosomes

Chromosomes are composed of double-stranded DNA containing threadlike sections of genes, most commonly found in the cell nucleus (Fig. 6.4). During cell division, chromosomes reproduce their physical and chemical structures, passing on genetic information. The process of cell division and creation of new cells are a result of the processes of mitosis and meiosis. In mitosis, the chromosomes in the nuclei of somatic cells go through a series of phases (prophase, prometaphase, metaphase, anaphase, and telophase), resulting in the creation of daughter cells with the same chromosome number and genetic makeup as the original somatic cell. Chromatids, one of two strands newly formed during the early process of chromosome duplication, is joined together by a centromere. The somatic cells of the body each contain chromosome pairs. The end of each chromosome is composed of DNA segments known as telomeres. DNA is wound around spool-like protein cores known as histones. Each human somatic body cell contains 23 pairs of chromosomes, or a total of 46, also known as the **diploid** number of chromosomes. Of the total number of chromosomes, 44 are **autosomes** (chromosomes other than a sex chromosome) and 2 are **sex chromosomes**. The two sex chromosomes, known as X and Y, are the genetic determinants of the sex of an individual. Females possess two X chromosomes and males one X and one Y.

Gametes (ova and sperm) contain only one of the chromosome pairs, known as the **haploid** number of chromosomes. Germ cells (ova and sperm) are produced through a process known as meiosis. In meiosis, one cell produces four cells, each with half the number of chromosomes, known as gametocytes. When sperm divide, four spermatids result. When ova divide, three polar bodies and only one ovum are produced. These cell numbers reflect their roles in reproduction. The combination of ova and sperm genetic material at the time of conception results in a cell with the diploid number of chromosomes. In this way, each parent contributes one chromosome; therefore, children get half of their chromosomes from their mothers and half from their fathers.

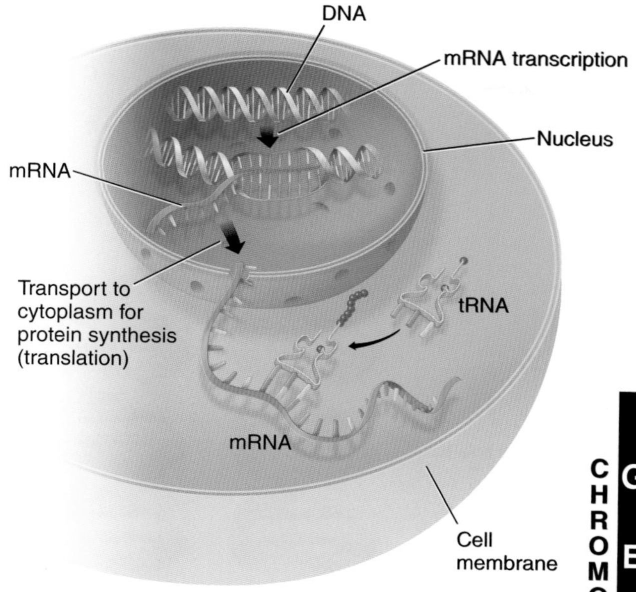

Figure 6.3. RNA in protein production. In the cell nucleus, the gene exon sequence is copied by mRNA, forming a template of the DNA nucleotide bases for transcription of the genetic code. The mRNA sequence of the 3 bases comprising a codon is translated to a specific amino acid. The codon is read in the ribosome, with the specific amino acid transferred by tRNA to the growing chain of amino acids leading to peptide and protein production.

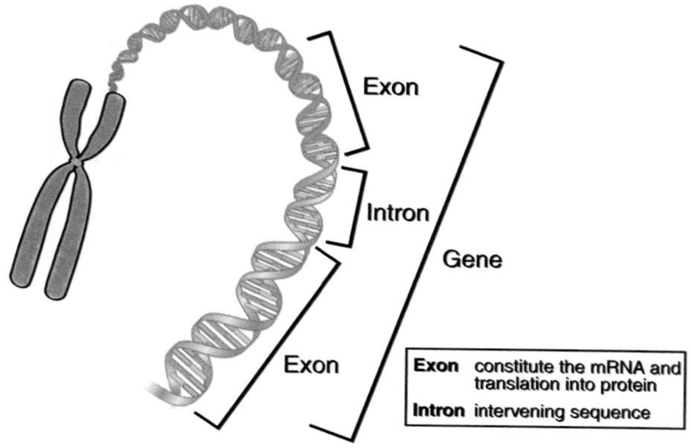

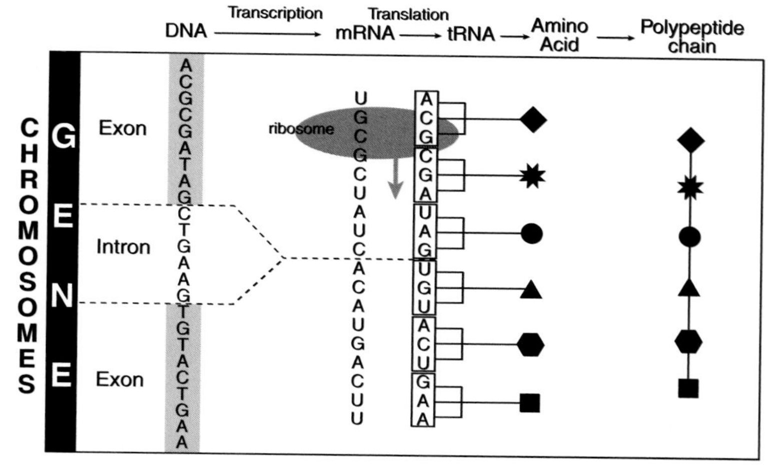

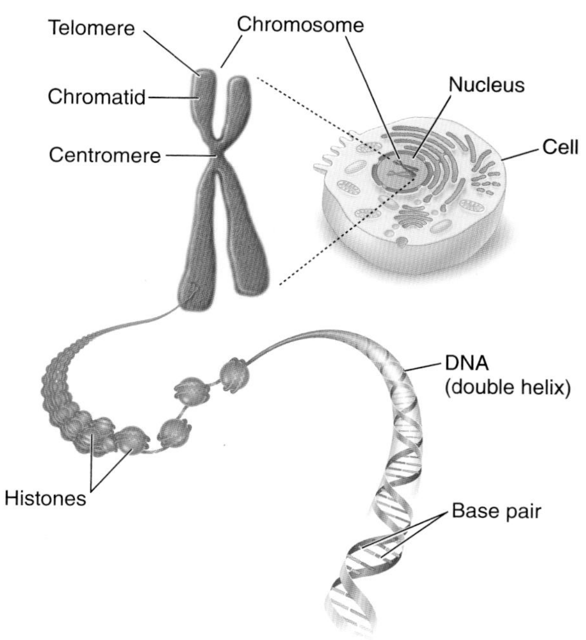

Figure 6.4. Nuclear chromosomes. Chromosomes are comprised of two chromatids joined by a centromere. Chromosomes contain compacted DNA with an individual's unique genetic information.

Chromosomal Replication

Each of the DNA strands of the double helix is important in replication of genetic information, but only one forms the template for **transcription**, or the transfer of the genetic code from one type of nucleic acid to another. The other strand serves as a complement to the strand used in transcription. Before cellular reproduction, the two DNA strands unwind from the helix, and each forms new strands made up of matching base pairs next to each original strand. The result is four strands, doubles of each of the two original strands (Fig. 6.5). When the cell divides by the process of mitosis, these duplicated molecules are separated and placed in a daughter cell, each with a double strand formed by the transcription strand and its complement.

Stop and Consider

What would happen to protein synthesis if the gene didn't turn on? If one of the nucleotide bases was substituted for another? If one extra nucleotide base was added to an exon?

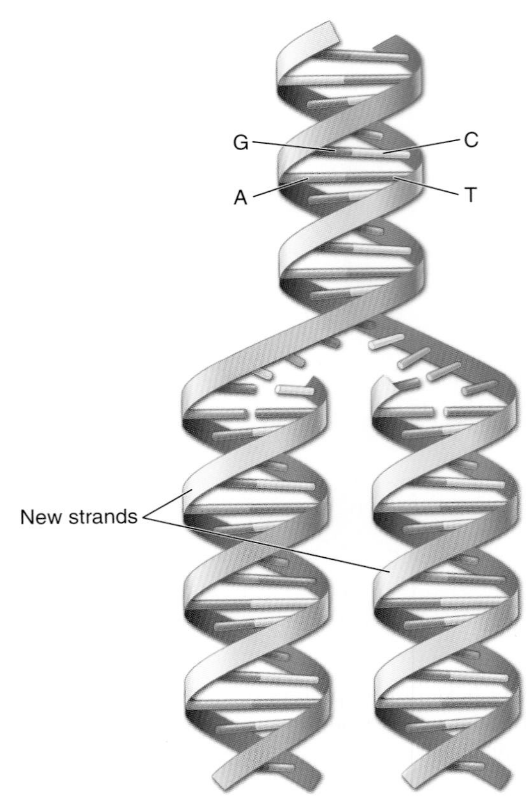

Figure 6.5. Genetic replication. The DNA strands in the double helix replicate to form two identical double helices to be placed in the daughter cells when the cell divides.

Module 2 Inheritance of Genetic Disorders

Since the 1850s, when Gregor Mendel began the first work on the study of genetics in his experiments with garden peas, much has been learned about human genetics and the way traits are passed on from one generation to the next. Although none of the genetic concepts was known at the time, Mendel recognized the presence of factors that controlled the physical features of plants. He also realized that some of these "factors" had more influence, or were more dominant, than others. Mendel determined laws of genetic traits, described by the following categories:

- Autosomal dominant
- Autosomal recessive
- Sex-linked dominant
- Sex-linked recessive

The discovery of the double helix structure of DNA by Watson and Crick in 1953 was followed by other discoveries that greatly improved our understanding of genetics.

Study of the human genome, or the full DNA sequence, is known as **genomics**. Genomics reflects not just the study of single genes but the functions and interactions of all the genes in the genome, including interactions between genes and with genes and the environment. An international research project, the Human Genome Project, was started in 1990 with goals to map each human gene and to completely sequence human DNA. After completion of the project in 2003, work continues to analyze the tremendous amount of data generated by this project. The identification of the location of specific genes on chromosomes provides an opportunity for scientists to pinpoint the cause of genetic disease, and is the basis for current and future strategies to prevent or treat genetic defects. The interactions between genes and the environment provide the basis for application in other areas of study including nutrigenomics (the effect of nutrients on health through nutrient–genome interactions) and pharmacogenomics (interactions between drugs and the genome that affect the efficacy or toxicity in the human response).

It may be possible to improve health by understanding the mechanisms of disease contributing to complex conditions such as hypertension, diabetes, and asthma through the study of the human genome.[1] Instead of targeting specific individuals for screening of genetic information to predict disease, genetic screening in the future will be done on entire populations, allowing the identification of risk groups to determine susceptibility to disease.[2]

Identification of individuals with risks for specific conditions provides an opportunity to intervene and initiate strategies to prevent the development of disease

Table 6.2 Common Newborn Screening Tests

Disease	Pathology	Newborns Affected	Consequences if Left Untreated	Treatment
Phenylketonuria (PKU)	Inability to break down amino acid phenylalanine	1 in 14,000	Brain damage, mental retardation	Avoid foods with phenylalanine
Hypothyroidism	Thyroid hormone deficiency	1 in 3,000	Retards growth and brain development	Replacement of thyroid hormone
Galactosemia	Inability to convert the sugar galactose into glucose for energy	1 in 50,000	Death, blindness, mental retardation	Avoid foods with galactose
Sickle cell anemia	Inherited blood disease causing abnormal shape and function in red blood cells	1 in 400 African Americans	Infection, pain, organ damage, and death	Early identification and treatment of symptoms and prevention of infection and triggers
Congenital adrenal hyperplasia (CAH)	Group of disorders from deficiencies in hormones	1 in 19,000	Altered genital development, kidney function, and death	Replacement of missing hormones
Biotinidase	Deficiency of biotinidase, an enzyme that recycles biotin, a B vitamin	1 in 60,000	Frequent infections, hearing loss, mental retardation, death	Replacement with additional biotin
Maple syrup urine disease	Inability to break down the essential amino acids leucine, valine, and isoleucine	1 in 230,000	Mental retardation, seizure, and death	Diet low in leucine, valine, and isoleucine
Homocystinuria	Inability to break down the amino acid methionine	1 in 340,000	Growth problems, developmental delay, mental retardation	Vitamin B_6 therapy
Medium-chain acyl-CoA dehydrogenase deficiency	Inability to use fat for energy	1 in 20,000	Sudden infant death and mental retardation	Steady food intake and avoidance of fasting

before it begins. Newborn screening is an example of this type of screening and has been in place since the 1960s. All states require newborns to be screened for certain genetic disorders, although not all states have the same requirements. Recommendations include testing for more than 30 specific conditions though states retain the legal authority to determine screening requirements based on criteria that include cost, frequency of the disorder, and treatment availability (genes-r-us.uthscsa.edu). Some of the most commonly tested newborn diseases are included in Table 6.2.

Transmission and Expression of Genetic Traits

Traits are transmitted to each generation by the gametes; the ova, and the sperm. Each parent contributes one set of chromosomes, ensuring that each offspring has two genes at each locus, or location on the chromosome, when these chromosomes combine. The combination of the ova and sperm at the time of conception determines the genetic makeup of an individual, or the **genotype**. The genotype of a person is not always apparent or visible. A person's **phenotype** refers to the traits that are apparent or observable. Examples of these kinds of traits include gender, blood type, and eye or hair color. Genes may have many forms, such as those determining hair or eye color, that determine offspring traits, due to **alleles** (a series of two or more different genes occupying the same location on a specific chromosome). Other traits, known as **polygenic**, result from the interaction of several genes and are influenced by environmental factors. The transmission of genetic traits is specific for the trait and can be a complex process.

Many diseases result from damage to genes or chromosomes. These defects can be the result of spontaneous damage (de novo), environmental insult or they can be an inheritable defect. Errors in DNA duplication can occur and result in genetic **mutations**. These mutations become permanent structural alterations in DNA. They are often resolved by DNA repair mechanisms, which prevent serious harm. However, when these repair mechanisms fail, the damaged genetic material can be passed on. The effects of mutations can be variable, ranging from no effect at all, to change in the expression of a trait or the function of a cell. Occasionally, a **somatic mutation** (not inheritable) can result in a **polymorphism** (gene occurring in more than one form). This common DNA variation can occur among individuals and have no impact on health (e.g., having one brown eye and one blue eye). Other mutations result in permanent change in genetic material, forming the basis of disease. In some cases, mutations affecting the control of cellular proliferation can result in cancer, which is discussed in Chapter 7. The transmission of genetic mutation is affected by the **expressivity** of the mutation, or the way the gene is expressed in the phenotype, which can range from mild to severe. **Penetrance**, the ability of a gene to express a mutation, can also influence the effects of genetic mutations. Obviously, many variables influence the complexity of the transmission of genetic traits.

Inheritance of Single Gene Disorders

Some traits are passed on by the transmission of a single gene and are known as **single gene traits**. When people have identical alleles on each chromosome, they are **homozygous** for that gene. If they have two different alleles on each chromosome, they are **heterozygous** (only one copy) for that gene. Inheritance of single gene traits follows a **Mendelian pattern** of predictable trait transmission based on autosomal dominant or recessive genotypes. On autosomal chromosomes, some alleles have more influence than others. **Dominant** forms of a gene are more likely to be expressed in a person. **Recessive** genes are less influential, requiring homozygous alleles to be expressed. A dominant allele, when combined with a recessive allele, may prevent the phenotypic expression of the recessive gene, although both alleles comprise the genotype. An example of the application of this concept is a person who is heterozygous for the alleles that contribute to eye color. That person may have a dominant allele for brown eyes and a recessive allele for blue eyes in his or her genotype but express the trait of brown eyes in his or her phenotype because of the imbalance in the influence of the two alleles. A person must be homozygous for a recessive gene in order for it to be expressed in the phenotype. Therefore, for a person to express the recessive trait of blue eyes, he or she must be homozygous for the allele for blue eyes (Fig. 6.6).

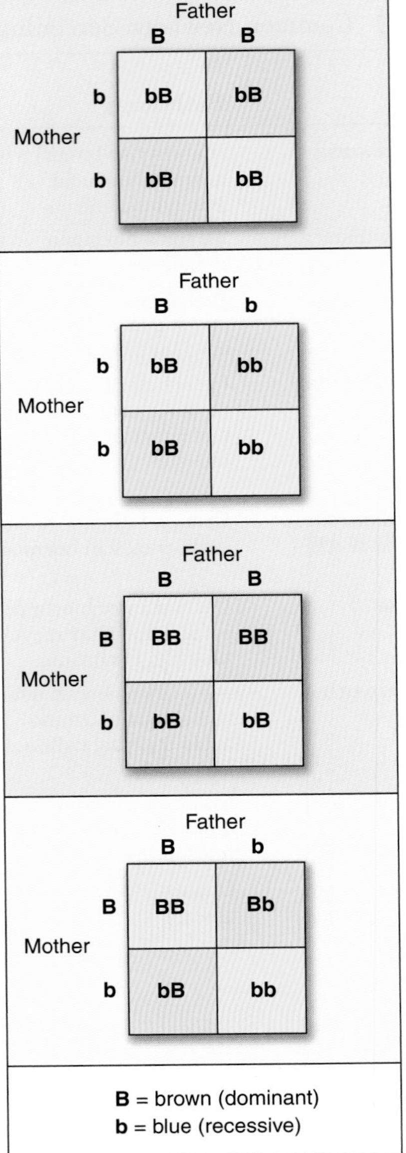

Figure 6.6. Eye color inheritance. Brown eye color will result if any of the combinations contain the dominant allele (BB, bB, Bb). Blue eyes will result from a combination of the recessive alleles (bb).

The sex chromosomes, X and Y, determine gender at conception. X chromosomes are much larger than Y and carry much more genetic material. Females have two copies of the X chromosome

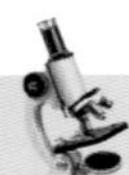

FROM THE LAB

Newborn screening is done using a variety of different types of tests. One of the oldest tests is the Guthrie bacterial inhibition assay, initially developed to identify infants with the metabolic disorder phenylketonuria (PKU). The use of tandem mass spectrometry allows for the identification of a wide array of amino acid, fatty acid, and organic acid metabolic disorders from a sample of dried blood on filter paper.[3] DNA testing of newborns for such diseases as cystic fibrosis can be done to get an early diagnosis and to initiate treatment for optimal wellness.

(XX), whereas males have one copy of X and one of Y (XY). The X chromosome is inherited from both parents in the female but only from the mother in the male. Traits passed on by sex chromosomes are known as **sex-linked**. These traits are most often recessive and are linked to the X chromosome. While females possess two copies of the X chromosome, one becomes inactivated, leading to variable expression patterns of X-linked genes. In males, the genes are inherited on the single copy of the X chromosome. Males are usually affected by this recessive disorder because they have only one X chromosome. Females are usually carriers because they have two copies of the X chromosome.

GENETIC MUTATIONS

Inheritable single gene mutations follow the Mendelian pattern of inheritance in a clearly identifiable and predictable manner. Single gene disorders occur at a specific, single site on the strand of DNA as a result of:

- Deletion
- Duplication
- Inversion
- Insertion
- Translocation

These mutations are caused by the substitution of a base pair that leads to an error in the transcription of a single codon, which in turn leads to the abnormal formation of proteins (Fig. 6.7). The resulting alteration in cellular function leads to the manifestation of disease. Specific mechanisms of genetic alterations can now be considered as causative factors of damage in autosomal and sex-linked gene errors. Table 6.3 describes the patterns of inheritance in single gene disorders.

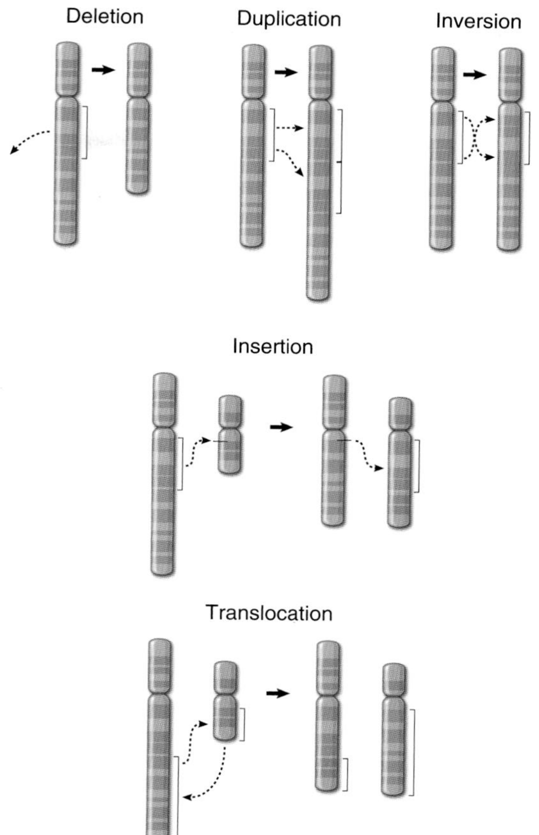

Figure 6.7. Common forms of genetic mutations. The alterations in cellular function caused by genetic mutation lead to the manifestation of disease.

AUTOSOMAL DOMINANT DISORDERS

Most hereditary disorders involve the genes on autosomes because there are more of these types of chromosomes (22 pairs) than sex chromosomes (1 pair). Because the genetic mutations occur on autosomes, the resulting disorders affect males and females equally (Fig. 6.8). If one parent is heterozygous for the autosomal dominant disorder, each child has a 50% chance of inheriting the damaged gene. In offspring who inherit the damaged allele, the dominant nature of the gene is likely to lead to disease, even

Table 6.3 Patterns of Inheritance in Single Gene Disorders

Inheritance Pattern	Allele Configuration	Transmission	Expression	Carrier	Non-Carrier
Autosomal dominant disorders	Heterozygous	One heterozygous parent	50%	0%	50%
Autosomal recessive disorders	Homozygous	One homozygous and one noncarrier parent	None	100%	0%
		Two heterozygous parents	25%	50%	25%
Sex-linked disorders	Paternal X link	Transmitted to daughters only	0%	100%	0%
	Maternal X link	Transmitted to daughters and sons	50% sons	50% daughters	50% sons 50% daughters
Mitochondrial gene disorders	Maternal link	Transmitted to daughters and sons	Variable	Variable	Variable

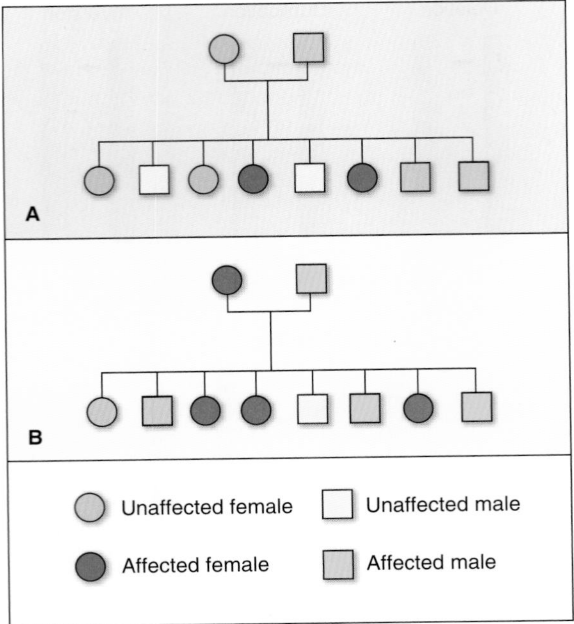

Figure 6.8. Autosomal dominant inheritance patterns. **A:** When only one parent is heterozygous for the dominant diseased gene, the child has a 50% chance of having the disease and a 50% chance of being unaffected. **B:** When both parents are heterozygous for the diseased gene, the child has only a 25% chance of being unaffected and a 75% chance of having the disease.

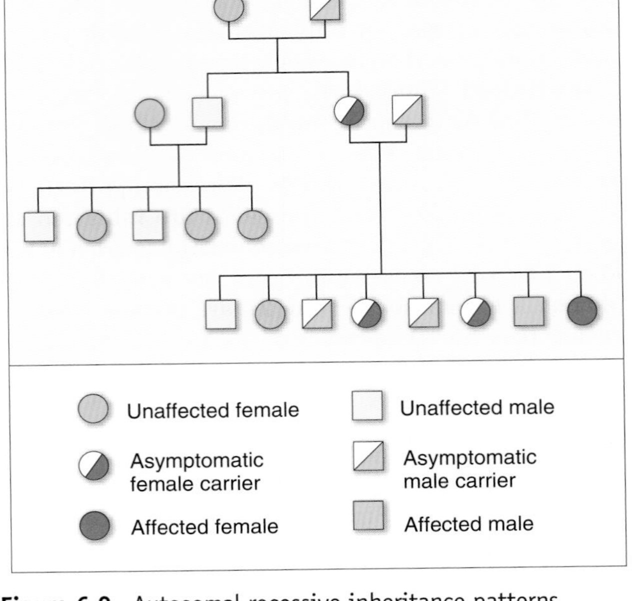

Figure 6.9. Autosomal recessive inheritance patterns. Recessive genes are expressed in the phenotype when the child is homozygous for the disease gene. If the inherited genotype is heterozygous, the child is a carrier of the disease gene and has the ability to continue this inheritance pattern. When one parent is a carrier, the children have a 50% chance of being a carrier themselves. If both parents are carriers, 25% of the children will be unaffected, 25% will be affected, and 50% will become carriers of the disease gene.

when the offspring is heterozygous for the allele. Examples of diseases having this type of autosomal dominant inheritance pattern include Huntington disease (HD) (described in detail in Clinical Models), Marfan syndrome, and osteogenesis imperfecta.

AUTOSOMAL RECESSIVE DISORDERS

Autosomal recessive inheritance patterns result in a different pattern of disease expression than the autosomal dominant disorders (Fig. 6.9). Because of the recessive nature of the genes involved, a child must be homozygous for the mutated gene to express the disease. This means that both parents must have at least one copy of the damaged gene for the disease to be passed on to their children. The mutated recessive gene may be present in their genotype but not in their phenotype. In other words, they may be unaware that they have the mutated gene because they do not have the disease. Individuals who are heterozygous for a recessive gene mutation are known as **carriers**.

If both parents are carriers, their child has a 25% chance of expressing the disorder. If only one parent is a carrier, the child has an equal chance of being a carrier (50%) or be completely unaffected (50%). If both parents are homozygous for the gene and have the disease, all of their children will also have the disease by inheriting both damaged alleles from their parents. When one parent is homozygous for the gene mutation and has the disease and the other does not carry the recessive gene mutation, all of their children will be carriers with the ability to pass on the mutated gene. Autosomal recessive disorders appear more frequently within specific populations, where the likelihood of carriers is greater. Examples of

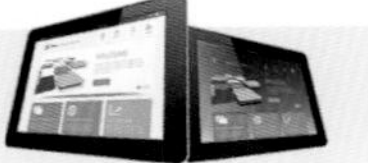

RESEARCH NOTES

Prostate cancer is the most common cancer among American men (usually over 65 years old), causing more than 40,000 deaths. It is estimated that approximately 181 of 100,000 African American men will be diagnosed with prostate cancer this year, with 54 of those dying from the disease. This disease appears to run in families, leading to investigation into the genetic link to the disease by scientists at the National Human Genome Research Institute (NHGRI). These scientists have identified the location of a gene, called *HPC-1*, that is associated with increased risk of prostate cancer.[4]

autosomal recessive disorders are cystic fibrosis, Tay-Sachs disease, thalassemia, and sickle cell disease (described further under Clinical Models).

SEX-LINKED DISORDERS

Mutations of genes located on the sex chromosomes, X or Y, are called sex-linked disorders. Many of these disorders are linked to genes on the X chromosome, or X-linked, and are usually recessive. For this reason, there is a gender difference in expression of X-linked disorders. Because females have two copies of the X chromosome, they are usually carriers of disease. Males have only one copy of the X chromosome and therefore are more likely to express the genetic disorder. Y-linked diseases result from the inheritance of a gene mutation on the Y chromosome from the father and are less common than X-linked disorders.

Sex-linked disorders are inherited based on which parent has the gene mutation. When the father carries the defective gene on the X chromosome, all daughters will be carriers and sons will be unaffected (Fig. 6.10A). When the mother is a carrier and passes the defective gene to her child, her daughters will have a 50% chance of being a carrier, and her sons will have a 50% chance of being affected (Fig. 6.10B). Hemophilia and X-linked severe combined immunodeficiency (XSCID), often referred to as "bubble boy disease," are examples of X-linked disorders, with females carrying the defect and only males expressing the disease.

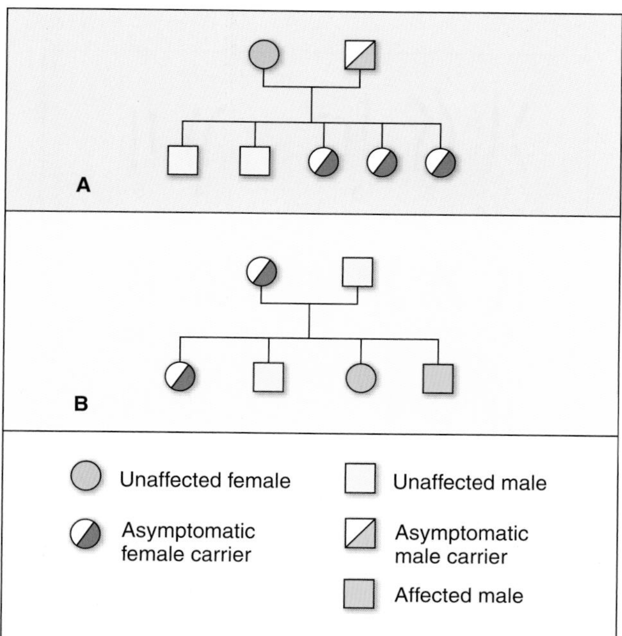

Figure 6.10. Sex-linked inheritance patterns. **A:** Expression of recessive X-linked traits occurs only in males when the defective gene is inherited from the mother. **B:** Carrier status is limited to female children and males are unaffected when the damaged gene is inherited from the father.

MITOCHONDRIAL GENE DISORDERS

The pattern of mitochondrial gene transmission is different from the transmission of nuclear genes.

Although most genes can be found in the cell nucleus, several dozen genes can be found in the mitochondria. The functions of these genes are associated with the overall function of mitochondria and are often related to energy production. Sperm do not carry a significant number of mitochondrial genes; therefore, men do not pass mitochondrial gene disorders on to their offspring. Most mitochondrial genes are passed on through the maternal gametes (ova), which are dense with these genes. For this reason, mitochondrial genes are transmitted only through female or maternal lines, in a **matrilineal** inheritance pattern.

Leigh syndrome is a condition involving mitochondrial DNA (mtDNA). Manifestations usually occur in the first year of life and include hypotonia, spasticity, peripheral neuropathy, encephalopathy, ataxia, and vision and hearing loss. Manifestations of mitochondrial gene disorders are variable because of the heteroplasmic features of these disorders. **Heteroplasmy** refers to the random distribution of mitochondria to daughter cells during embryonic cell division, leading to a variable distribution of mutant mitochondrial genes in tissues of an individual and between related individuals. Manifestations are revealed when the mutant mitochondria reach a critical level, or threshold.

Inheritance of Polygenic Disorders

Polygenic inheritance involves multiple alleles at different loci affecting phenotype. The expression of disease often involves a complex interaction of multiple factors that impact the interaction between genes and environment. Environmental influences modulate the phenotypic expression of a trait in multifactorial inheritance. An example of this type of inheritance is the height of an individual. Height is influenced by the combination of genes inherited from both parents, but it can also be influenced by environmental factors, including nutrition and hormones.

Certain environmental conditions must be present for expression of a genetic trait that leads to disease. Factors that can increase expression of disease include chemicals (alcohol, tobacco, drugs, and hormones), nutrition, and altitude. Clinical manifestations of multifactorial disorders may be seen at birth and include such disorders as cleft lip/palate, clubfoot, and neural tube defects, including anencephaly and spina bifida (discussed in more detail in Clinical Models). Other multifactorial disorders are not expressed until the person ages, including hypertension, coronary artery disease, diabetes, and many cancers.

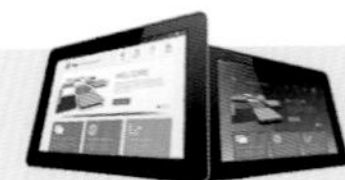

RESEARCH NOTES

Human genome mapping and improved technology identifying DNA patterns have stimulated applications of the gleaned information in areas beyond human health. These include the use of DNA as evidence in identifying criminals. First used in 1983, DNA evidence has been used to convict individuals of crimes and to exonerate innocent individuals.[6,7] This practice is commonly referred to as "DNA fingerprinting." Current DNA technology uses short tandem repeats (STRs), lengths of DNA stretches that are unique to an individual. STRs from suspect individuals are compared with national databases for rapid and accurate identification. In addition, mtDNA provides information about maternal lineage, and Y-specific STRs provide evidence for paternal lineage. These techniques are most often used in historical identification, such as the determination of lineage of the Russian royal family, the Romanovs. These techniques were especially useful in identifying the remains of victims of the World Trade Center disaster, leading to positive identification of more than 1,500 individuals.

Stop and Consider

The process of genetic selection is based on reproductive practices that result in offspring with desired traits. These practices are in use today in the animal industry, where animals are bred for desired qualities such as increased milk production in dairy cows or desired characteristics in show dogs. Food products are genetically manipulated to have traits of disease resistance. What are the health implications of genetic selection in humans? What are the social and ethical implications?

Inheritance of Chromosomal Alterations

Chromosomal alterations may result from the loss, addition, or rearrangement of genetic material. Chromosomal alterations can be detected by assessing an individual's karyotype, or chromosomal complement. A **karyotype** is a picture of arranged, paired, like chromosomes in order of largest to smallest (Fig. 6.11). Chromosomes are matched by centromere location and banding pattern (see From the Lab).

ALTERATIONS IN CHROMOSOMAL NUMBER

Chromosomes separate during mitosis and meiosis in a process known as disjunction. When chromosomes fail to separate, the result is **nondisjunction** (Fig. 6.12). Nondisjunction results in an unequal number of chromosomes between cells. The timing of nondisjunction determines the number of cells involved. If it occurs soon after conception, it may affect all of the resulting cells. If it happens later, some cells will be affected and others will be normal. The term **mosaicism** refers to the combination of cells with the regular chromosome number and those with an altered number of chromosomes; the effects are determined by the ratio. The risk of nondisjuncture increases with parental age.

Monosomy occurs when nondisjunction results in cells with one copy of a chromosome instead of two. If this occurs in autosomes, this defect is not compatible with life. Although monosomy in the sex chromosome is compatible with life, significant physical and mental defects result. An example of a condition that results from monosomy of the sex chromosome includes Turner syndrome (TS), described in more detail under clinical models.

Trisomy refers to the presence of three copies of a chromosome in a cell. The viability of the individual is determined based on which specific chromosome is affected. If a large chromosome is affected, trisomy is incompatible with life because large chromosomes contain a great deal of genetic material. When trisomy occurs in chromosome 21, the condition known as Down syndrome results. Children born with Down syndrome have characteristic facial features,

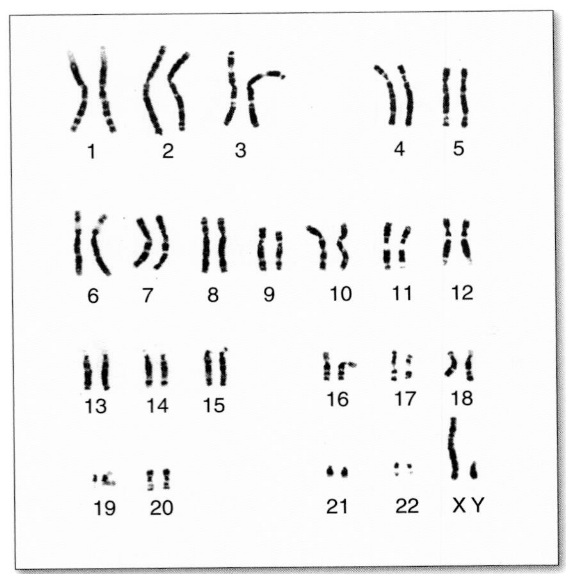

Figure 6.11. Karyotype. The karyotype shows the 23 pairs of chromosomes from a man. Notice the size of the Y chromosome compared with the X chromosome. (From Bear MF, Connors B, Paradiso M. *Neuroscience: Exploring the Brain*. Baltimore, MD: Lippincott Williams & Wilkins; 2006.)

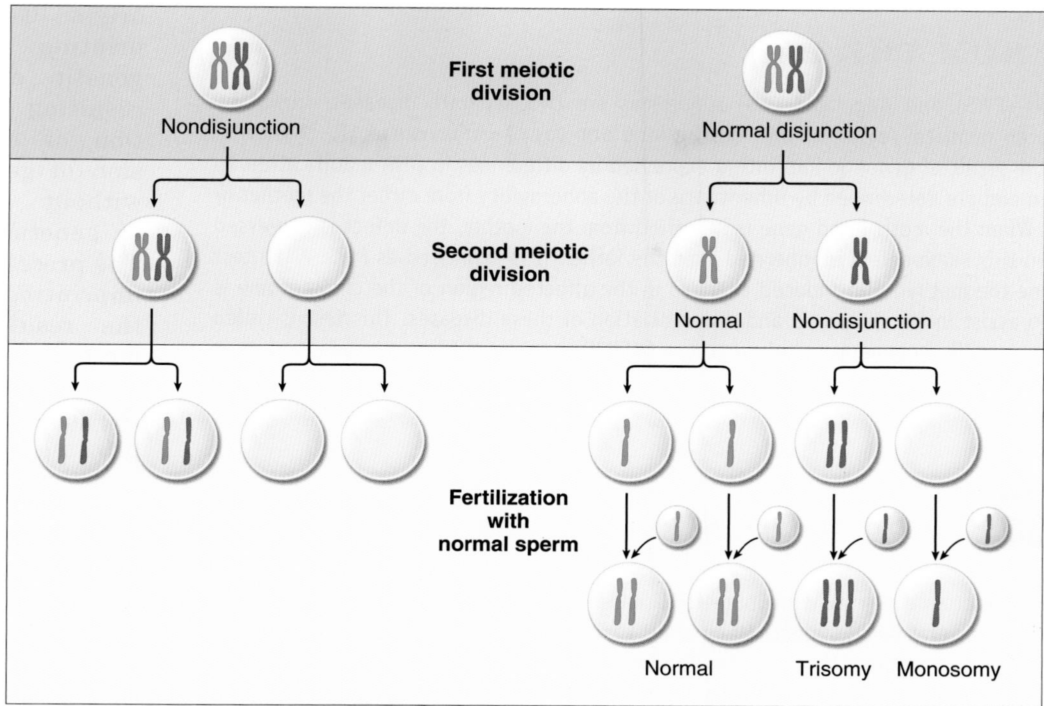

Figure 6.12. Chromosomal nondisjunction. Process of nondisjunction at the first and second meiotic divisions of the ovum and fertilization with normal sperm. (Modified from Pillitteri A. *Maternal and Child Nursing*. 4th ed. Philadelphia, PA: Lippincott Williams & Wilkins; 2003.)

small stature, physical defects, and neurologic involvement. The clinical manifestations for a person with Down syndrome can be modified by the degree of mosaicism (see Clinical Model: Down Syndrome).

ALTERATIONS IN CHROMOSOMAL STRUCTURE

Translocation occurs when a large segment of DNA breaks from one chromosome and reattaches to a different chromosome, often occurring during meiosis. If the translocation is balanced, this abnormal arrangement does not affect the individual because he or she still retains the same amount of genetic material. It can seriously affect any offspring who inherits the defective chromosome, as the genetic complement inherited on the altered chromosome will result in either missing or excessive genes in the offspring.

Epigenetic Inheritance

Epigenetic is defined as "above the genome." Epigenetic modifications are caused by environmental and metabolic agents that stimulate chemical modifications of genes. The chemical modifications typically include chemical modifications to histones (e.g., acetylation) and DNA (e.g., methylation). The epigenetic modifications change the expression of the gene without causing genetic mutation. The change in gene expression induced by epigenetic modification may persist even after removal of the initiating agent and has the potential to be passed to offspring. Epigenetic modifications of gene expression are heritable, with the potential to influence the health of future generations.

When genes are inappropriately silenced or activated through epigentics, disease may result. Examples include Wilms tumor, osteosarcoma,

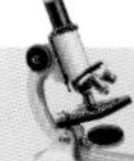

FROM THE LAB

Chromosomal abnormalities can be determined by examining the number and structure of chromosomes through evaluation of the karyotype. The first step in evaluating a person's karyotype is obtaining a cell sample. Cells are prepared and chromosomes removed during mitosis, at which time they can best be seen under a microscope. The chromosomes are attached to a slide and stained with a special dye called Giemsa. A striped, or banded, appearance results from the dye staining of regions rich in adenine and thymine base pairs. A picture of the chromosomes is then taken and the single chromosomes are matched with their pairs and arranged from largest to smallest. There are three criteria for matching chromosomes: size, Giemsa banding pattern, and centromere position.

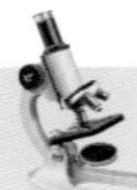

FROM THE LAB

Prader–Willi (PWS) and Angelman (AS) syndromes are two separate diseases caused by changes in an identical region of DNA on the long arm (q) of chromosome 15. These diseases are the result of genomic imprinting expressed by differences in DNA modification by methylation and are determined by inheritance of the abnormality from either the mother or the father. When the methylated gene is inherited from the mother, the defect is expressed as AS. When this same defect is inherited from the father, it is expressed as PWS. A lab test to determine the methylation-induced changes in the affected region of the chromosome is available to assist in the diagnosis and differentiation of these diseases. This test is called methylation-specific polymerase chain reaction (MSPCR).[5]

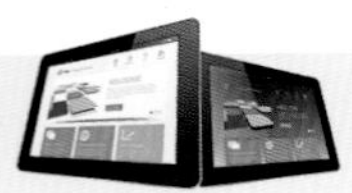

RESEARCH NOTES

Environmental factors that may contribute to disease in adulthood can be linked to events that occur during fetal development. Many adult diseases have been linked to a fetal environment that impairs growth of the developing fetus. The study of the fetal origins of disease suggests that the fetus whose intrauterine growth is restricted may be programmed to develop diseases, including hypertension, diabetes, and breast cancer. It may be that all of these individuals are born susceptible to these diseases, and therefore the expression of disease is determined by environmental influences.[8,9]

bilateral retinoblastoma, and embryonal rhabdomyosarcoma, forms of cancer resulting from gene silencing through DNA methylation. Some diseases are associated with repeated expansions of cytosine bases, targets for methylation, that may change gene expression. Examples of diseases involving repeat cytosine-linked expansions include myotonic muscular dystrophy (MMD) and fragile X syndrome (FXS) (see description in clinical model).

Genomic imprinting is the mechanism that controls expression of genes based on parental origin. Genomic imprinting is an epigenetic phenomenon resulting in regulation of the expression of gene activity without alteration of genetic structure. The process of genetic imprinting is usually the result of DNA methylation, preventing transcription of the gene. Genomic imprinting occurs when both maternal and paternal alleles are present, with only one allele expressed and the other imprinted allele inactive due to epigenetic silencing through DNA methylation. Approximately 20 known genes are affected by imprinting, causing different diseases based on whether they were inherited from the mother or the father. Two classic conditions that illustrate the influence of an imprinting defect on chromosome 15 include Prader–Willi (paternal-related) and Angelman (maternal-related) syndromes (see From the Lab).

Stop and Consider

Why does it take four generations for evidence of epigenetic inheritance?

Module 3 Developmental Disorders

Developmental disorders are usually the result of environmental influences that alter gene function, contributing to the expression of altered structure or function of the affected tissue or organ system. Developmental disorders occur after conception and therefore are not inherited and are hence disorders of development.

Congenital Disorders

Developmental disorders can be the result of chemicals, hormones, drugs, pathogens, or other environmental factors that cause congenital disorders in the developing child. The result of gene–environment interactions that occur during fetal development, congenital disorders are linked to events that occur at critical points in development. Factors may include the intrauterine and nutritional environments that impair appropriate anatomic and physiologic development of the embryo and fetus. Environmental influences may also be the result of a pathogen challenge prior to the fetus' ability to mount an adequate immune response. Exposure to drugs and toxins in the maternal system may also result in errors in morphogenesis, or the appropriate structure of organs and tissues. The period of intrauterine embryonic and fetal development is characterized by the dynamic processes of cellular proliferation and differentiation, increasing vulnerability to environmental insults that lead to altered function across the lifespan.

The risk of damage to a developing child is greatest during the embryologic period (weeks 3 through 8 of gestation). During this time, **organogenesis** (development of organ systems) is occurring. If damage occurs during this period, the organ systems most susceptible at the time of exposure are specifically affected. Damage prior to this time, the preembryologic period, may interfere with implantation or may be so significant that the pregnancy ends in spontaneous abortion. The fetal period begins during gestational week 9 and continues through the end of pregnancy (Fig. 6.13). Environmental insult during the fetal period has the potential to alter developing organ systems based on the timing of the challenge.

Substances that cause damage to developing embryos or fetuses are known as **teratogens**. Many substances that enter the mother's system are able to cross the placenta and enter the fetal circulation. If teratogen exposure is serious and occurs very early in the pregnancy, it can cause damage incompatible with life, resulting in spontaneous abortion or miscarriage. Damage later in fetal life is usually seen in specific organs, which were actively developing at the time of exposure. Teratogens can take many forms, including pathogens, drugs, alcohol, and environmental chemicals.

It is difficult to predict the effects of teratogen exposure because the effects are influenced by many variables. For example, it is known that maternal alcohol consumption during pregnancy is the sole causative factor identified for the development of **fetal alcohol syndrome (FAS)**. FAS is a condition characterized by significant mental handicap, growth deficit, and physical disability. The damage in FAS is linked to the amount and timing of alcohol exposure to the developing fetus. Not all babies exposed to alcohol develop FAS, suggesting the influence of environmental factors and varying susceptibility. Maternal abstinence from alcohol during pregnancy would result in the elimination of FAS, the leading cause of mental retardation in the United States.

Maternal infection during pregnancy can also result in congenital disorders in the fetus. The group of diseases described by the acronym known as TORCH is known to cause damage to the fetus if exposure occurs. These diseases are:

- *T*oxoplasmosis
- *O*ther (hepatitis)
- *R*ubella
- *C*ytomegalovirus
- *H*erpes

Many pathogens in addition to those described in the TORCH group have teratogenic effects and are often manifested by fetal loss, multiple fetal

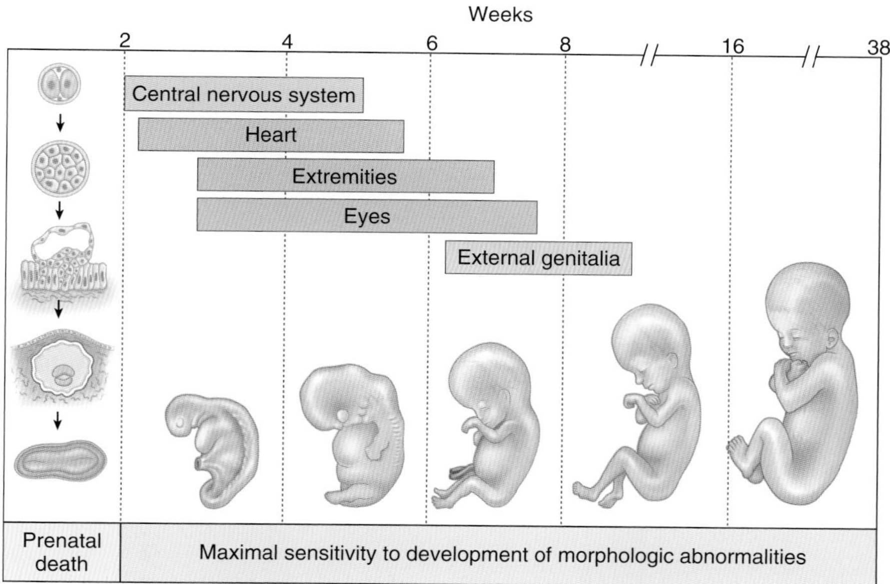

Figure 6.13. Critical periods of vulnerability. Preembryologic (weeks 0 to 2) exposure to teratogenic insult is often incompatible with life. The embryologic period (3 to 8 weeks) represents the most vulnerable period of teratogenic damage. During the fetal period (9 weeks to delivery), risk for teratogenic insult remains, especially for tissues of the neurologic system. (Modified from Rubin E, Farber JL. *Pathology*. 4th ed. Philadelphia, PA: Lippincott Williams & Wilkins; 2005.)

malformations, and neurologic involvement. Examples of common conditions include varicella (chicken pox) and parvovirus (fifth disease).

The presence or absence of agents in the environment can pose a risk for the development of genetic defects. An example of an environmental insult that can cause genetic damage is ionizing radiation. Radiation exposure to the fetus can cause genetic mutations. DNA repair mechanisms exist for this specific type of damage. If these repair mechanisms fail or if the damage is too great for adequate repair, permanent damage to DNA may result, leading to defects. There is no evidence that the radiation exposure delivered during diagnostic procedures causes damage, but women who are pregnant are cautioned to avoid radiographs unless absolutely necessary.

Maternal nutrient deficiency is linked to the development of congenital defects. Maternal folic acid deficiency is known to be a risk factor for the development of neural tube defects (NTDs), including anencephaly and spina bifida. Adequate maternal intake of folic acid prior to pregnancy is associated with a reduction in the occurrence of NTDs. Since 1998, foods have been fortified with folic acid, resulting in the prevention of NTDs by 50% in the United States.[10] There has been a call for a similar strategy internationally, where dietary recommendations alone are not adequate to reduce the incidence of NTDs.[11]

Developmental Origins of Adult Disease

Observations from the "Barker Hypothesis" during the 1980s demonstrated the link between low infant birth weight and future development of heart disease, suggesting that undernutrition during pregnancy permanently changed fetal structure, function, and metabolism, programming the fetus for future development of disease.[12] Current evidence implicates epigenetic modifications triggered by the adverse intrauterine environment during fetal development as the likely etiology of genetic predisposition to disease. As in other conditions with complex etiologies involving gene–environment interactions, the predisposition to adult disease due to fetal intrauterine adaptations requires an environmental trigger for expression of disease.[13]

The developing fetus is dependent on the maternal system for the delivery of oxygen and nutrients and the removal of wastes. The placenta is the interface between the maternal and fetal systems, playing an important role in support of fetal growth and development. The placenta has a significant endocrine function, providing hormones that support fetal and maternal adaptations needed for an optimal pregnancy outcome. Reduced maternal blood flow and variations in constituents in the maternal blood create an adverse intrauterine environment contributing to fetal adaptations that promote survival in utero, but may be mismatched with the environmental conditions of postnatal life.

Maternal nutritional status is central to the promotion of fetal development. Variations in maternal nutritional status including obesity, macronutrient and micronutrient excesses, and deficiencies are associated with future development of obesity, diabetes, and heart disease.[14] Alterations in maternal hormonal status may stimulate fetal adaptations that may predispose to future development of disease. Examples of maternal hormonal conditions that have been linked to future disease include stress due to alteration in stress hormone delivery to the fetus and deficiency in maternal prohormone vitamin D levels. Impaired nutrition and stress are some of the challenges in the extrauterine environment that may provide the trigger for expression of disease, including hypertension, obesity, and diabetes.

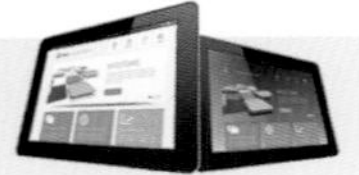

RESEARCH NOTES

Many adult-onset disorders can be predicted by genetic testing. Individuals should be counseled on the issues related to the knowledge that they have a predisposition to develop a disease. Identification of gene mutations that lead to disease may prevent a person from obtaining adequate insurance coverage for medical care. In addition, it is important to share this information with other family members who may also be at risk. Ethically, individuals should be encouraged to share their diagnosis of a genetic disorder, which the medical providers cannot themselves disclose to others because of patient confidentiality.[15] It is important to share knowledge of hereditary genetic disease with family members for them to make informed decisions about their future reproduction and health.

Module 4 Management of Genetic and Developmental Disorders

Unlike other pathologic alterations that present with symptoms restricted to one particular organ system, the clinical manifestations of developmental and genetic disorders are specific to the affected tissues and organ systems at the time of insult. Even among individuals with similar genetic alterations, manifestations are influenced by penetrance and expressivity. Clinical manifestations of specific syndromes are presented in the clinical models in this chapter that represent a variety of developmental, genetic, chromosomal, and epigenetic pathologies. General methods of identification and management of alterations in genetics and development are discussed in the next section.

Screening and Diagnosis

Screening and diagnosis can be completed in an individual across the lifespan. Individuals may request genetic screening when family history indicates a heritable genetic risk. Genetic screening may be done in order to determine treatment decisions when faced with a diagnosis associated with known genetic risk. Individuals during the childbearing years may consider genetic screening to determine the probability of genetic risk in offspring based on cues in maternal and paternal history or factors such as parental age. In all cases, the decision to pursue genetic screening has emotional, ethical, and economic implications.

PRENATAL SCREENING AND DIAGNOSIS

Ideally, counseling on the inheritance of genetic risk is completed prior to conception. Genetic risk can be determined when a complete family and pregnancy history is obtained. Maternal age (older than 35 years) or the family history of genetic disorders represents some of the most common reasons for seeking prenatal diagnosis. The decision to undergo screening may be made when a woman has had repetitive (three or more) spontaneous abortions, which suggests the potential for a chromosomal abnormality. Individuals who present with manifestations classically linked to single gene alterations or clinical subjective and objective findings that form a syndrome may undergo genetic screening to identify a defect and determine whether the defect can be passed on to offspring.

The goal of prenatal diagnosis is to determine recognizable chromosomal or genetic defects in the growing fetus. Initially, screening techniques can be used to determine genetic risk. Screening of maternal serum may be completed to identify NTDs or Down syndrome risk. Ultrasound is used to screen for abnormalities in the physical structure of the fetus. Although these techniques suggest risk, they are not diagnostic. Screening tests that suggest genetic abnormalities are usually followed by diagnostic testing. Cell samples of fetal origin must be used to diagnose fetal abnormalities. Fetal cells can be obtained from the chorionic villi, which contain cells of trophoblastic origin and therefore are fetal. The amniotic fluid that surrounds the fetus is another source of fetal genetic material and can also be used to identify genetic disorders. Finally, percutaneous blood sampling can be used to examine fetal cells obtained from a sample of fetal blood from the umbilical cord.

When the risk of transmission of a genetic defect is identified, prenatal counseling should include the option of preimplantation genetic diagnosis. **Preimplantation genetic diagnosis** is an alternative to prenatal diagnosis, and it allows for identification of abnormalities before implantation. Preimplantation genetic diagnosis requires the use of in vitro fertilization, embryo culture, and biopsy of the **blastomere** (early embryo). This procedure is costly and invasive, and its use is restricted to those individuals with identified risks, including single gene defects, X-linked disorders, **aneuploidy** (abnormal chromosome number), and those with balanced translocation.[16] Balanced translocation refers to the exchange of entire chromosome segments between two different chromosomes. Individuals with balanced translocations have the appropriate amount of genetic material, so appear phenotypically normal. However, these individuals are carriers of this chromosomal anomaly and are able to pass one of the altered chromosomes, producing an unbalanced chromosomal complement in the offspring.

A thorough family history is often the first step toward a genetic diagnosis. Review of generational information is important in the determination of trends. This information is often depicted graphically as a pedigree, tracing genetic disorders through generations. Pedigrees are helpful in the tracking of inheritable single gene, chromosomal, and multifactorial disorders. A karyotype helps determine the presence of chromosomal abnormalities. When using a karyotype to identify chromosomal abnormalities as a cause for repeated abortion, cell samples from both parents are needed. Prenatal counseling of families with genetic disorders involves providing information to support decisions about pregnancy outcome and determining support services needed for the best possible outcome.

POSTNATAL SCREENING AND DIAGNOSIS

In the newborn period, screening for the most common genetic conditions results in earlier identification and treatment of many disorders. Learning more about genetics increases the ability to identify genetic causes of many diseases, including cancer, Parkinson disease, and Alzheimer disease. Although not all individuals with these diseases have a readily identifiable genetic mutation, many who have a family history of the disease have a genetic link. Once the gene responsible for the disease is identified, individuals at risk can be screened for the particular mutation. Disorders are discovered by determining the sequencing of DNA and identifying variations consistent with mutations that result in disease.

Genetic screening of carriers and affected individuals may provide predictive, preventive, and personalized medical care. The trend of the future is to use population-based screening to predict risk for adult-onset disorders in different ethnic and cultural groups. Knowledge of the molecular basis of disease is progressing faster than our grasp on the ethical and social implications of that knowledge. Complex implications related to the nature of patient relationships, antidiscrimination laws, and legal rules related to medical care and public health are challenges that need to be determined.[17]

Stop and Consider
What are some instances in which identifying genetic information can be harmful?

Treatment Strategies

Treatment of genetic disorders is disease specific. When anatomic anomalies exist, surgical correction is often implemented. If the disease results in deficiency of a particular enzyme, replacement of the missing protein is instituted, if possible. Treatment of disorders is unique to the genetic deficit and is primarily geared toward alleviation of the associated clinical manifestations.

Counseling individuals and families with genetic alterations must include communication of implications of the defect and the risk of reoccurrence. Counseling can occur in families when a risk of having children with genetic defects exists or when an affected child is born. It is important to understand the effects of the genetic condition on the individual as well as the family. A complete explanation of diagnostic strategies necessary to help the family identify risk is important. Discussion of genetic risk with families must be presented in a manner that is understood by the patients and that meets individual patient and family needs. The following are some of the strategies used:

1. Assess literacy level of the individual and family
2. Ask for interpretation of information about testing procedures and possible outcomes
3. Provide information about rates of risk in both positive and negative terms
4. Promote ability to make informed decisions

Module 5 Clinical Models

The following clinical models have been selected to illustrate the concepts of alterations in genetics and development. As you read the descriptions that follow, think about the processes of altering genetic traits as they apply to the specific conditions to help in the understanding and application of these concepts. Figure 6.14 provides a summary of genetic alterations in human disease.

Autosomal Dominant Genetic Disorder: Huntington Disease

HD is a neurologic disorder caused by degeneration of the basal ganglia and cortical regions of the brain. HD affects approximately 5 of 100,000 predominantly White males and females of northern European ancestry.[18] A parent with HD has a 50% chance of passing the condition on to each child because of the autosomal dominant transmission of this condition. All individuals who inherit the significantly mutated gene will eventually develop the clinical manifestations of this fatal condition (full penetrance). Manifestations usually appear by the mid-40s and include impaired function of movement, emotion, and cognition. There is no known cure for this condition.

PATHOPHYSIOLOGY

HD is a progressive, autosomal dominant disorder caused by a defect in the huntingtin gene on

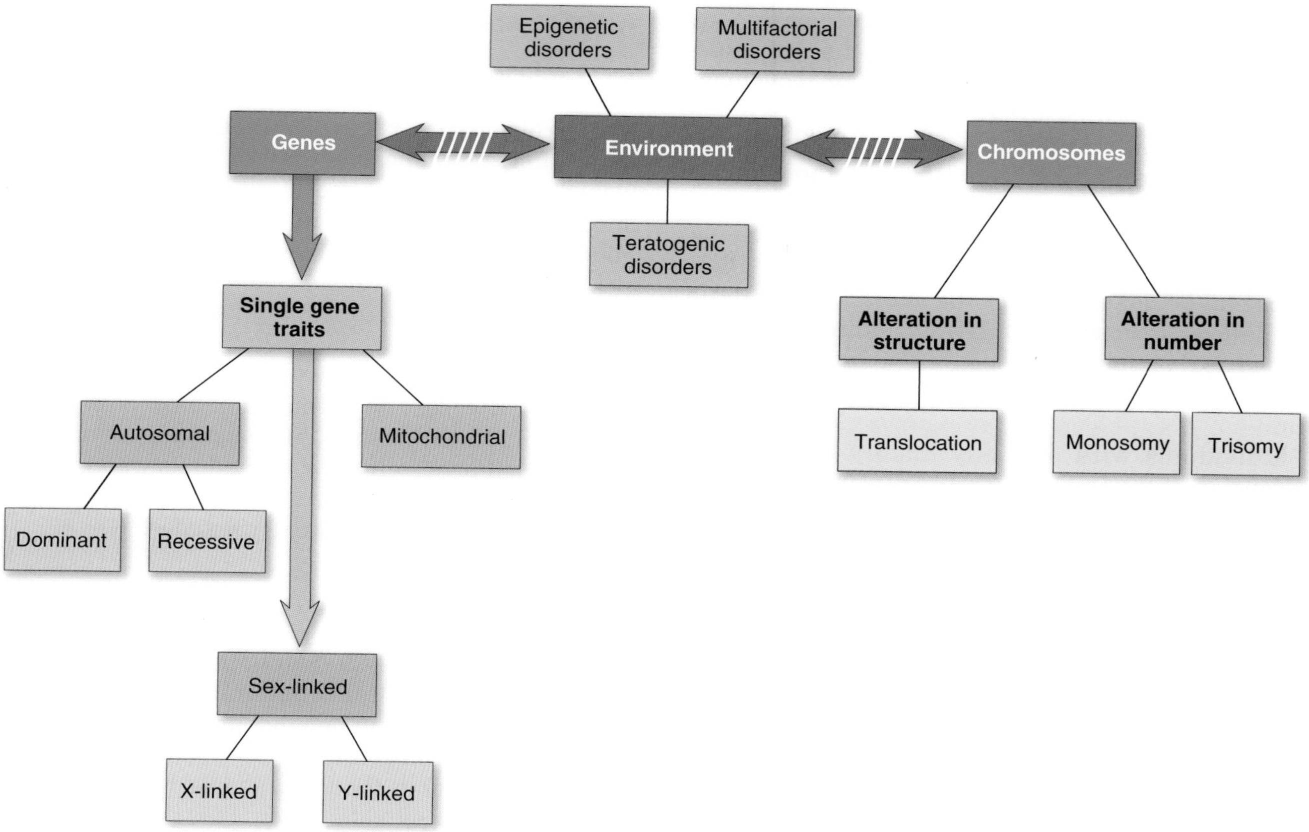

Epigenetic disorders
Multifactorial disorders
Genes
Environment
Chromosomes
Teratogenic disorders
Single gene traits
Alteration in structure
Alteration in number
Autosomal
Mitochondrial
Translocation
Monosomy
Trisomy
Dominant
Recessive
Sex-linked
X-linked
Y-linked

Figure 6.14. Concept map. Genetic alterations in human disease.

chromosome 4. The gene defect results in a triplet cytosine–adenine–guanine (CAG) expansion mutation in the huntingtin (*HTT*) gene, with an increased number of mutations associated with earlier onset of the clinical manifestations of the disease. Full penetrance is observed when there is an expansion of >38 CAG repeats. The genetic mutation generates a code for the abnormal huntingtin protein, which then accumulates to toxic levels and destroys nerve cells, resulting in atrophy in the brain. A protein fragment of the huntingtin protein produced by caspase (an enzyme that breaks down protein) may also be involved in the pathology associated with HD. As the CAG expansion is a target for methylation, epigenetic mechanisms underlying the damage of HD are under investigation.

CLINICAL MANIFESTATIONS

Individuals with HD suffer from involuntary movements, cognitive impairment, and emotional disturbance. Early psychologic manifestations include personality changes, loss of memory, antisocial and impulsive behaviors, and emotional lability. Altered motor function in the early stage of disease manifestation includes restlessness, fidget-like activity and abnormal eye movements, representing early signs of **dyskinesia** (difficulty in performing voluntary movements). Chorea (rapid, involuntary, nonrepetitive movement of the face, trunk, and limbs) is a key feature of HD. The progressive nature of the condition leads to immobility, severe loss of cognitive function, intellectual deterioration, delusions, and paranoia.

DIAGNOSTIC CRITERIA

Diagnosis of HD is based on a complete family and personal medical history and physical examination.

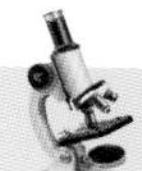

FROM THE LAB

Screening for HD can be accomplished by analyzing DNA from a blood sample to determine if the genetic mutation is present. CAG repeats are counted, with the number of repeats considered in diagnosis. CAG repeats of 28 or fewer do not indicate HD. Individuals with CAG repeats greater than 40 are diagnosed with HD. Because of the serious nature of the diagnosis and lack of an available cure, the decision to test for the defect is a difficult one.

Mental, cognitive, and emotional evaluation may provide indications of early signs of disease, especially when coupled with early signs of movement disorders. Genetic testing can definitively diagnose HD, revealing the associated mutation on the huntingtin gene. Blood samples from the affected individual, as well as a close family member, can precisely diagnose HD. In symptomatic individuals, CT, MRI, or positron emission tomography (PET) scans can be done to detect the characteristic brain anomalies associated with HD, including shrinkage of the basal ganglia components, caudate nuclei and putamen, and enlargement of the ventricles of the brain.

Individuals with a family history of HD have the option of genetic testing prior to onset of symptoms; this is known as presymptomatic testing. Counseling should be provided before presymptomatic testing considering the profound impact a diagnosis of HD can have on an individual and the family.

TREATMENT

There is currently no cure for this condition. Supportive care including occupational, physical, and speech therapies, and nutrition management may optimize quality of life. Underlying movement and psychiatric disorders may be treated with pharmacologic therapy. Research into potential treatment options has identified new pathways to preserving brain function and preventing disease. Epigenetic targets are being studied as the basis for treatment, targeting regulation of gene expression.[19] The use of stem cells to foster protection of the neurologic system is also a potential future treatment.[20] Investigation into pharmacotherapy to treat or cure HD has shown promise for the use of caspase inhibitors[21] and cannabinoids,[22] though efficacy is uncertain. Clinical trials will provide data on patients that will ultimately determine the effectiveness of these treatments.

Stop and Consider
What are the risks and benefits of testing for HD? Are there reasons why a person would not want testing?

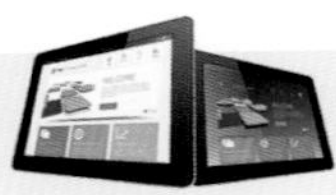

RESEARCH NOTES

A group of researchers studied residents from an endemic population of people afflicted with HD in Venezuela. A model was developed that determined the variables contributing to age of onset of symptoms. Variables accounting for age of onset included number of repetitive triplets in the Huntington gene as the primary determinant (72%), although other genes and environmental factors, including poverty and nutrition, explained the remaining variation.[23]

Autosomal Recessive Disorder: Sickle Cell Disease

Sickle cell disease is an inherited homozygous disorder affecting hemoglobin in red blood cells. Hemoglobin A (adult) in the red blood cells is replaced by another form of hemoglobin, hemoglobin S (sickled). Following an autosomal recessive inheritance pattern, sickle cell disease is transmitted from parent to child. Sickle cell disease is commonly found in individuals of African ancestry. In the United States, 9% of African Americans have sickle cell trait and 1 in 600 have sickle cell disease.[24] As a result of improved screening, treatment, and education, life expectancy is increasing.[25,26] Median survival for individuals was 14 years in 1973. Recently, median survival has increased to 42 years for males and 48 years for females.[27]

PATHOPHYSIOLOGY

Sickle cell disease is the result of a single gene mutation that follows Mendelian inheritance patterns. Red blood cells contain hemoglobin A (HbA), or adult hemoglobin. Hemoglobin S (HbS) is an abnormal type of hemoglobin found in people with sickle cell anemia. Red blood cells with HbA are soft, round, and pliable enough to circulate through the small blood vessels in the microcirculation. HbS changes the phenotype of red blood cells, making them stiff and distorted. Red blood cell life span is reduced from approximately 120 days to 16 days when red blood cells carry HbS, further contributing to symptoms of anemia and increased demand to produce additional red blood cells. The form of hemoglobin produced is determined by the two beta globin genes located on chromosome 11. The defect in sickle cell anemia is a point mutation, in which the amino acid valine is substituted for glutamine on the beta chain of hemoglobin of red blood cells. The phenotypic expression of this genetic mutation in an individual who is homozygous for the sickle beta globin gene (bS) is sickle cell anemia.

When exposed to conditions of low oxygen tension, the hemoglobin's shape is distorted into a sickled shape, known as **hemoglobin S** (Fig. 6.15). The irregularly shaped hemoglobin causes damage to the endothelial cells that line blood vessels and to the red blood cells themselves. Trapping of the red blood cells in the spleen causes **hemolysis**, or breakdown of red blood cells, resulting in anemia. The altered shapes of the red blood cells cause difficulty in

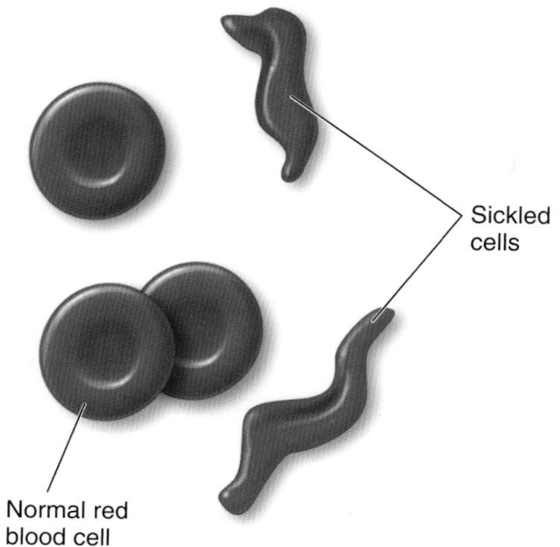

Figure 6.15. Red blood cells in sickle cell anemia. When red blood cells are exposed to conditions of low oxygen tension, it results in the sickle shape of the cells. (Courtesy Anatomical Chart Company.)

their passage through small blood vessels, resulting in decreased oxygenation. Pain related to ischemia results and can develop into necrosis and organ failure if left untreated.

As expected in autosomal recessive disorders, the genetic mutation associated with sickle cell anemia is recessive. For individuals to have the disease phenotype, their genotype must be homozygous for the defective allele. An individual who is heterozygous for the genetic mutation is a carrier and is considered to have **sickle cell trait**.

CLINICAL MANIFESTATIONS

Clinical manifestations including hallmarks of vaso-occlusion and hemolysis are related to the proportion of HbS in the circulation. Pain is also characteristic of sickle cell disease, often stimulated by events including infection, dehydration, and stress, though a precipitating event is not always identifiable.

Hemolysis, shortened red blood cell life, and splenic trapping result in breakdown of red blood cells, releasing contents into the circulation. The two clinical manifestations, jaundice and anemia, result. Jaundice results from the release of **bilirubin**, a yellow, lipid-soluble byproduct of hemoglobin, as a result of RBC damage. The loss of RBCs results in anemia, making it difficult to oxygenate tissues adequately. This, combined with the blockade of small vessels by the sickled RBCs, further adds to the problems of tissue oxygenation. Tissue ischemia often results, promoting the development of recurrent, painful episodes. Because of the resultant systemic tissue ischemia, the location of pain can occur in the chest, extremities, or abdomen. Stroke and priapism (painful, prolonged erection) can also result. Organ damage to the spleen, kidneys, and liver can result from sickle cell crisis, contributing to significant morbidity and mortality. Splenic damage can contribute to decreased immune defense, increasing the risk of overwhelming infection. In children, infection and stroke are common manifestations of sickle cell anemia.[26] Microvascular occlusion may lead to necrosis and cell death. Neurologic complications include risk for stroke, neurocognitive decline, and intracranial hemorrhage.

DIAGNOSTIC CRITERIA

Early identification of individuals with sickle cell disease is vital to decreased morbidity and mortality. Prenatal and newborn screening for sickle cell disease has improved treatment of complications, particularly for infection in the newborn period when the risk is highest. Laboratory testing for sickle cell disease includes:

- Hemoglobin electrophoresis (see From the Lab below)
  - Identifies hemoglobin types (HbA, HbS)
  - Differentiates homozygosity from heterozygosity by proportion of hemoglobin types
  - Homozygous: 80% to 90% HbS of total hemoglobin
  - Heterozygous: 35% to 40% HbS of total hemoglobin
- Isoelectric focusing
  - Method used to separate proteins based on their isoelectric point, based on the pH when the protein net charge is zero
  - Adjunct in determination of hemoglobin type
- High-performance liquid chromatography (HPLC)
  - Method used in the identification of hemoglobin variants
- DNA analysis

Prenatal diagnosis can be done by analysis of fetal DNA obtained from chorionic villus sampling or amniotic fluid. Newborn screening should be initiated

FROM THE LAB

Hemoglobin electrophoresis is used to identify specific forms of hemoglobin. This test is completed on a blood sample drawn from a person suspected or known to have sickle cell anemia. An electric charge is passed through a solution of hemoglobin. Hemoglobin varieties move to specific distances through the solution, based on composition. A person with sickle cell disease will have a predominance of HbS.

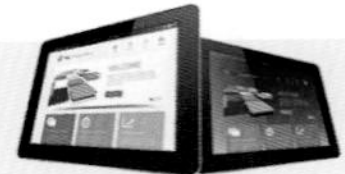

RESEARCH NOTES

Gene therapy in the treatment of sickle cell anemia represents an effective strategy in the prevention of disease-associated complications. Research is currently in the early stages, but recent studies show promise for this potential therapy. One approach reported in a recent study of gene therapy involved the manipulation of the differential expression of the globin genes, inducing preferential expression of HbF.[28] Therapy involving substitution of HbS with HbF through the transcriptional control of globin genes was studied as a potential therapy for sickle cell anemia. The focus of this study was to find the right DNA sequence to target and to test its effectiveness in promoting expression of HbF. Using an in vitro method involving cells, the researchers were able to selectively express HbF, reinforcing the importance of the continued development of this strategy as an effective treatment for sickle cell anemia.

in the first 6 months of life, with hemoglobin F (HbF) included in the distribution of hemoglobin types expected. Laboratory follow-up of individuals diagnosed with sickle cell anemia who are not experiencing complications includes evaluation of hemolysis and anemia with yearly complete blood counts (CBC) and urinalysis. Tests of liver (liver function tests: AST, ALT) and kidney (serum creatinine and blood urea nitrogen [BUN]) function should be completed every 2 to 3 years. Retinal examinations should also be completed to determine evidence of damage or disease.

TREATMENT

Prevention of complications related to infection is important in the management of sickle cell anemia. Immunization against childhood and community illnesses, such as pneumococcal pneumonia, influenza, and meningococcal meningitis, are important to protect from infection. Penicillin prophylaxis is an important intervention designed to support immune defense.

Treatment for patients with sickle cell anemia is usually symptom specific. Pain management is critical to the management of sickle cell anemia. Identification and avoidance of precipitating factors, including infection, extremes of temperature, and emotional/physical stress, is important for pain prevention. Lab evaluation of a complete blood count (hemoglobin, reticulocytes, white blood cells, granulocytes, and bands) can help determine anemia and infection. Severe episodes of pain often require the use of opiates. Blood transfusion addresses the anemia associated with sickle cell disease and decreases the proportion of circulating HbS by adding healthy donor RBCs with HbA. Transfusion has also been shown to decrease the risk of stroke in children. Folic acid supplementation is frequently used to prevent megaloblastic erythropoiesis.

Pharmacologic measures for the prevention of complications include the use of hydroxyurea. Hydroxyurea increases the production of HbF, preventing the formation of HbS. Hydroxyurea kills bone marrow cells, inducing an increased production of cells with higher hemoglobin F content, promoting life span of cells and depressing production of HbS. Increases in HbF have been associated with improvement of the clinical manifestations related to sickle cell anemia. The use of nitric oxide during acute chest crisis may promote relaxation of the resistance arteries to promote perfusion to ischemic tissues. Future treatments in clinical development include the use of gene therapy and stem cell allogenic approaches that would not only treat the symptoms, but would provide the potential for a cure.[29]

Stop and Consider

What are the risks to the fetus when the father has sickle cell anemia? What are the risks to the fetus when the mother has sickle cell anemia?

Mitochondrial Gene Disorder: Mitochondrial Encephalomyopathy, Lactic Acidosis, and Stroke

Mitochondrial encephalomyopathy, lactic acidosis, and stroke (MELAS) is mitochondrial gene disorder. Although uncommon, MELAS is considered a significant cause of stroke-like manifestations in individuals less than 45 years of age.[30] Mean life span of those with the full clinical syndrome ranges from 20 to 40 years, with cardiopulmonary failure, pulmonary disease, and status epilepticus the most commonly reported causes of death. There is no gender or ethnic predilection for MELAS.[31]

PATHOPHYSIOLOGY

MELAS is a maternally inherited condition, characterized by mtDNA point mutations. The ovum is the source of mtDNA; therefore, this condition is maternally inherited. To date, eight mtDNA point mutations and one deletion mutation have been identified as genetic causes of MELAS. Most of the mutations are in genes that encode tRNA for the amino acids leucine and valine. A substitution of adenine to guanine in the gene-encoding tRNA accounts for approximately 80% of MELAS cases. Mutations may also affect **cytochrome oxidase (COX)**, an enzyme important in catalyzing oxidation–reduction mitochondrial reactions in cellular respiration. The prevailing theory on the underlying mechanism involved in MELAS is that a decrease in oxidative phosphorylation creates an imbalance between ATP production and usage, contributing to neuronal dysfunction.[30]

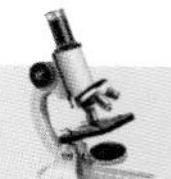

FROM THE LAB

Diagnosis of mitochondrial abnormalities is often determined by biochemical assays that detect specific disease markers. The most common of these markers are COX and succinate dehydrogenase (SDH), both of which play a significant role in mitochondrial cellular respiration.[32] An increase in SDH leads to altered structure of muscle fibers, impairing muscle function. On microscopic evaluation, muscle fibers exposed to trichrome stain turn a bright red color, leading to the common term "ragged red fibers," characteristic of many mitochondrial gene disorders. Ragged red fibers may also be stained with other dyes to characterize presence of COX and SDH.

CLINICAL MANIFESTATIONS

The manifestations of MELAS are variable because of the heteroplasmic nature of this condition. Clinical manifestations of MELAS develop when mutant mtDNA reaches a threshold of 56% to 95%. The age of onset of clinical manifestations averages 10 years. Classic symptoms of MELAS include:

- Stroke-like episodes in individuals younger than 40 years of age
- Encephalopathy, including seizures and dementia
- Lactic acidosis

Other associated manifestations include hearing loss, blindness, migraine headaches, vomiting, short stature, hemiparesis, hemiplegia, cardiomyopathy, diabetes, and myopathy.

DIAGNOSIS

Diagnosis of MELAS is based on family history and documentation of clinical manifestations, and it is confirmed with laboratory studies. Biochemical analyses can determine respiratory chain dysfunction and lactic acidosis. Muscle biopsy demonstrates the characteristic findings of myopathy in MELAS: the presence of ragged red fibers (see From the Lab, below). Common lab studies used in the diagnosis of MELAS include:

- Serum and cerebrospinal fluid levels of lactic acid and pyruvic acid
- Serum creatine kinase
- Skeletal muscle biopsy to determine activity of substances involved in cellular respiration
- Blood, skeletal muscle, or hair follicle samples for determination of mtDNA mutations

Imaging studies can be added to laboratory studies to confirm a diagnosis of MELAS. CT or MRI brain scans can detect neurologic damage related to seizure activity and stroke. PET scans can determine the cerebral metabolic rate for oxygen. Electroencephalogram (EEG) is useful in identifying neural activity indicating a seizure disorder. Cardiomyopathy can be detected with echocardiography (ultrasound determination of heart structure and function) or electrocardiography (ECG), a test that indicates the neural conduction in the heart.

TREATMENT

Currently, treatment strategies are focused on management of manifestations. Examples include the use of anticonvulsant medications directed at controlling seizure activity and cochlear implants to improve hearing. Treatment strategies in development include the use of agents that affect oxidative phosphorylation. Agents of this type include coenzyme Q, riboflavin, and creatine. Clinical trials are investigating the use of dichloroacetate, a compound that promotes the conversion of pyruvate (a byproduct of carbohydrate metabolism) to acetyl-CoA instead of the usual product lactate, reducing the risk for development of lactic acidosis (further discussed in Chapter 8).

Alteration in Chromosome Number (Autosome): Down Syndrome

Trisomy that results in excess genetic material is often incompatible with life, especially when the defect involves larger chromosomes. When trisomy occurs on chromosome 18, the clinical manifestations are severe. Congenital heart defects, multiple joint contractures, spina bifida, hearing loss, underdevelopment or missing radial bone of forearm, cleft lip, birth defects of the eye, and small size at birth are the most common developmental complications of this syndrome. Among infants born with trisomy 18, median survival is estimated at 6 days.[33]

Down syndrome is named for Dr. John Langdon Down, who identified the syndrome in the 1860s based on the pattern of manifestations he recognized in the residents of an asylum for children with mental illness in England. The genetic basis of chromosome 21 trisomy was not identified until 1959. Down syndrome is one of the most common genetic birth defects, affecting approximately 1 in 800 to 1,000 babies of both genders. According to the National Down Syndrome Society, there are approximately 350,000 people living with Down syndrome in the United States. Life expectancy among adults with Down syndrome is about 55 years, although life span varies depending on the individual and his or her medical condition. An increase in the incidence of Down syndrome was expected because of delayed childbearing and an increased birth rate in women over 35 years.

PATHOPHYSIOLOGY

Down syndrome is a condition characterized by alteration in chromosome number. Also known as trisomy 21, children born with Down syndrome have three copies of chromosome 21. The additional chromosome can be caused by fertilization of a gamete with two copies of chromosome 21, by nondisjuncture during cell division, or by translocation. When an error in cell division occurs after fertilization, the child may develop two cell lines: one with the usual chromosome complement and one with trisomy 21, known as mosaic Down syndrome.

CLINICAL MANIFESTATIONS

Children born with Down syndrome have a combination of birth defects, including mental retardation, characteristic facial features, and health problems including cardiac defects, intestinal malformations, and visual and hearing impairment. The severity of expression of these problems varies greatly among affected individuals. Increased risk of infection, thyroid problems, and leukemia are also possible sequelae of Down syndrome. Facial features characteristic of Down syndrome include eyes that slant upward, small, low-set ears that fold at the top, small mouth, flattened nose bridge, and short neck (Fig. 6.16). Short stature, short fingers, and decreased muscle tone are also characteristic outward manifestations of Down syndrome.

When parents have a balanced translocation, they may be free of the disease phenotype but can pass on the defect, resulting in trisomy of their child. Balanced translocation in a parent is the only inheritable form of trisomy. Other mechanisms leading to trisomy 21 represent spontaneous events. The risk of trisomy as a result of nondisjuncture increases with age. Maternal age over 35 years is associated with a greater risk of Down syndrome. The risk of Down syndrome increases with age, from about 1 in 1,250 for a woman at age 25, to 1 in 1,000 at age 30, 1 in 400 at age 35, and 1 in 100 at age 40. Strikingly, the risk is increased to 1:60 by age 42, further rising to

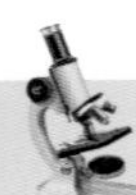

FROM THE LAB

Screening for Down syndrome can be done during the prenatal period. Noninvasive methods of screening may include biochemical analysis of substances in maternal blood, using the quadruple test, which includes measurement of serum alpha-fetoprotein, unconjugated estradiol, human chorionic gonadotropin (hCG) hormone, and inhibin A during the second trimester, after 14 weeks' gestation. When the quadruple test was combined with an ultrasound evaluation of nuchal translucency and pregnancy-associated plasma protein-A (PAPP-A) at 10 weeks (integrated test), this two-step evaluation was very accurate in detecting Down syndrome (see Research Notes, below).[34]

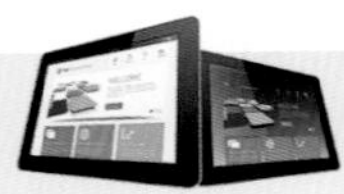

RESEARCH NOTES

Traditionally, determination of effective antenatal screening for Down syndrome was hindered by variations in study design, preventing generalizability of study findings to the population. In a recent large prospective study of 47,053 singleton pregnancies, testing of maternal serum and urine samples, as well as nuchal translucency, was conducted to determine reliable biomarkers of Down syndrome.[35] The false-positive rates for specific prenatal tests were as follows:

- Integrated test (nuchal translucency and PAPP-A at 11 weeks of pregnancy; alpha-fetoprotein, unconjugated estriol, free beta or total hCG, and inhibin A in the early second trimester): 0.9%
- Serum integrated test (nuchal translucency, free beta hCG and PAPP-A at 11 weeks of pregnancy): 4.3%
- Quadruple test (alpha-fetoprotein, free beta, or total hCG and inhibin A): 6.2%
- Nuchal translucency at 11 weeks: 15.2%

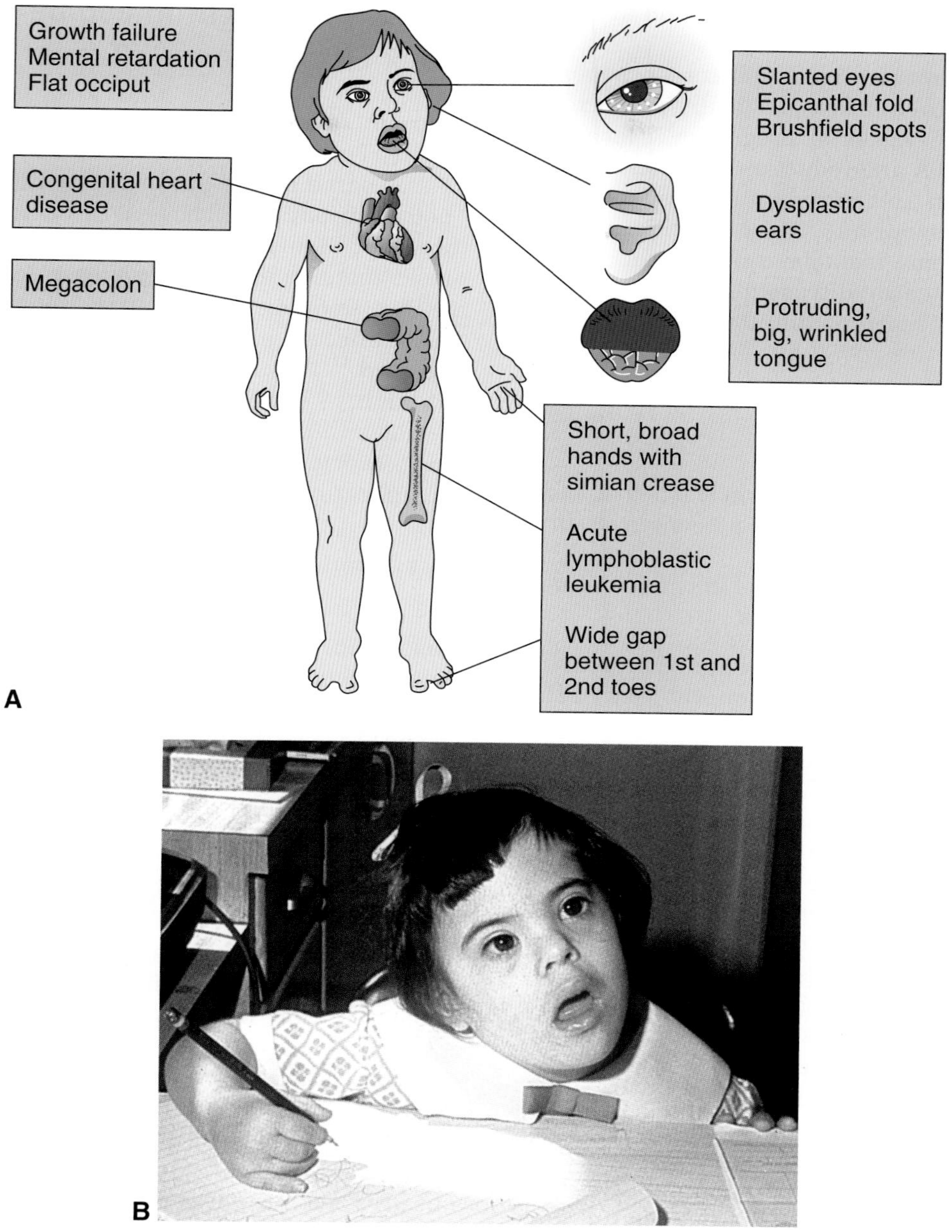

Figure 6.16. Typical clinical manifestations of a child with Down syndrome. The clinical manifestations of Down syndrome include organ system anomalies with long-term health implications **(A)** in addition to characteristic physical features **(B)**. (Modified from Rubin E, Farber JL. *Pathology*. 4th ed. Philadelphia, PA: Lippincott Williams & Wilkins; 2005.)

1:12 by age 49. However, it is important to note that about 75% of babies with Down syndrome are born to women who are under age 35, as younger women have far more babies.

DIAGNOSTIC CRITERIA

Screening for Down syndrome in the first trimester can be accomplished by looking for increased **nuchal translucency (NT)** or thickness of the nape of the neck, a common finding in fetuses with chromosomal abnormalities. Evaluation of NT uses ultrasound to measure a fluid-filled sac at the back of the fetus' neck during early pregnancy. The best time for NT testing is between 10 and 14 weeks. After that time, the fluid collected is able to drain via a more developed lymph system. When NT is combined with maternal serum PAPP-A and free or total hCG hormone, screening reliability is increased. Diagnostic genetic testing requires the more invasive procedures of chorionic villus sampling (completed between 11 and 13 weeks of pregnancy). These invasive procedures carry more risk and are associated with a 1% risk of pregnancy loss.

The second trimester quadruple screen, a measure of four biochemical markers, is ideally conducted between 15 and 18 weeks of pregnancy. Elevation of hGG and inhibin A and reduction in maternal serum alpha-fetoprotein and unconjugated estriol suggest risk for Down syndrome. More specific screening for Down syndrome includes a pattern of anatomic anomalies detected by ultrasound. Some of the distinctive physical features detectable by ultrasound include:

- Short humerus
- Short femur
- Hydronephrosis
- Echogenic cardiac foci (areas in the heart, usually the left ventricle, identified as echoes or bright areas)
- Echogenic bowel (bright areas in the intestine)
- Other major anatomic defects

These findings individually may not be unusual, but when they appear in combination, the risk of Down syndrome must be addressed.

A limitation of some screening tests includes a high rate of "false-positive" results, meaning that the positive screening result is present in the absence of disease. Further, there is a risk of "false-negative" results, meaning the actual disease condition was not detected by the screening test, leaving families with a false assurance. Tests with high rates of "false-positive" and "false-negative" results have limited use in the identification and management of disease. When the findings from any screening tests suggest Down syndrome, further testing is offered to provide an accurate diagnosis.

Second trimester amniocentesis (completed between 15 and 19 weeks of pregnancy) provides an opportunity to collect samples of amniotic fluid, grow fetal cells in culture, and evaluate the fetal karyotype to determine the presence of chromosomal abnormalities. Future diagnostic tests cell free DNA collected from maternal blood as a reliable method for rapid prenatal diagnosis of Down syndrome.[36]

TREATMENT

Treatment in Down syndrome is focused on promotion of maximal independence and quality of life. Early intervention programs, including speech, language, and physical therapy, promote optimal function. Congenital heart disease remains the most frequent cause for early death. Treatment of cardiac or gastrointestinal complications may require surgical repair. Overall life expectancy is shorter than the general population.

Alteration in Chromosome Number (Sex Chromosome): Turner Syndrome

Turner syndrome is a condition named after Dr. Henry Turner, who first identified the condition in the 1930s based on the pattern of manifestations identified in his patients. The genetic basis of the syndrome was not identified for another 30 years. TS is the most common fetal monosomy in females, occurring with a frequency of approximately 3%. Of those fetuses affected, approximately 99% are spontaneously aborted.[37] TS occurs in 1 in 2,500 to 1 in 3,000 girls at birth, or in 25 to 55/100,000 predominantly white females. Individuals with TS have a decreased life expectancy, usually related to the associated medical complications of diabetes and heart disease.

PATHOPHYSIOLOGY

TS occurs in females when the chromosome number is altered, resulting from the loss of all or part of the sex chromosome X. Of those affected by TS, about 50% have true monosomy with only one X chromosome (45, X), 10% have structural abnormality of the X chromosome, and remaining cases exhibit one or more additional cell lines or a mosaic karyotype (45, X/46, XY).[38]

CLINICAL MANIFESTATIONS

Clinical manifestations vary based on the type of abnormality, the point in time when nondisjuncture occurred, and the proportion of damaged cells in each tissue type (true monosomy versus mosaicism). Manifestations common across TS include short stature and ovarian failure. Intelligence is usually normal, but girls with TS often have some learning and social problems. Other associated symptoms can be grouped into three categories:

- Skeletal abnormalities
  - Short fingers
  - Short neck
  - Cleft palate
  - Osteoporosis
- Soft tissue abnormalities
  - Lymphatic obstruction
  - Webbed neck
  - Low hairline
- Organ abnormalities
  - Cardiac abnormalities
  - Kidney abnormalities
  - Liver abnormalities
  - Hearing loss

In addition to reproductive effects, adult women with TS may also suffer from hypothyroidism, deafness, osteoporosis, and problems related to estrogen deficiency.[39] Altered morphology of structures in the inner ear results in conductive hearing loss and otitis media.[40] Growth hormone administration promotes optimal height development. Life span in these women is decreased secondary to cardiovascular problems, including atherosclerosis.[41] Congenital malformations of the left heart, aortic rupture and dissection, hypertension, and ischemic heart disease are all risks for women with TS.

Klinefelter syndrome (KS) is another condition characterized by abnormal number of sex chromosomes, and it is considered a counterpart to TS. In KS, an abnormal ovum carrying an additional X chromosome (XX) is fertilized by a normal male sperm (Y). The child, with a karyotype of 46XXY, is phenotypically male. The male phenotype after puberty includes scant pubic hair, atrophic testes, and a small penis. Functionally, men with KS are infertile. They may also have feminine features, including lack of facial hair, female hip shape, and breast development. Figure 6.17 illustrates some of the physical characteristics of TS and KS.

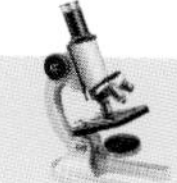

FROM THE LAB

Karyotyping is used to identify partially or completely missing X chromosomes, diagnostic of TS. Efforts to find a more affordable and quicker method are ongoing. Molecular detection of nonmethylated segments of the X chromosome, characteristic in TS, may be useful in screening high-risk groups.[42] MSPCR may also prove effective in diagnosing TS.[43]

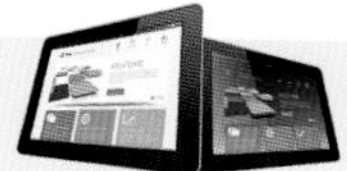

RESEARCH NOTES

Individuals with TS are at increased risk of type 2 diabetes because of decreased insulin secretion.[49] Prolonged treatment with growth hormone, commonly used in TS, can also contribute to an increased risk of insulin resistance.

DIAGNOSTIC CRITERIA

Early ultrasound (14 to 16 weeks) can identify characteristics that increase suspicion of TS. These findings include a large, septated, cystic **hygroma** (cyst with a diameter larger than the biparietal diameter of the head) on the back of the neck, edema, short femur, and narrow aortic arch. Live born females are not routinely screened unless they present with behavioral or physical characteristics consistent with the diagnosis of TS.[44] Parents report behaviors of delayed development, feeding problems, and crying during infancy in their daughters diagnosed with TS.[45] Physical findings in the newborn period include puffy hands and feet from lymphedema, extra nuchal skin from the remaining cystic hygroma, and heart defects, including hypoplastic heart and coarctation of the aorta.[38] Short stature may be the only physical characteristic in girls diagnosed in mid-childhood.

Many mosaic individuals affected with TS are not diagnosed until later in life, when gonadal failure alters reproductive development. Delayed puberty and infertility related to premature ovarian failure are common problems that lead to the identification of TS in women without other classic characteristics. Puberty and the development of adult female physical characteristics must often be induced by estrogen hormone administration.[45,46] Although ovarian follicle development in fetal life is significantly reduced, individuals who have a mosaic karyotype may have spontaneous pregnancies.[48] Repeated spontaneous miscarriage may be the characteristic leading to screening and diagnosis in these women. Women with TS often experience premature menopause.

TREATMENT

There is no specific management plan for treatment of TS. The phenotypes are varied and determine screening for related health concerns and treatment of altered function. In addition to management of medical complications, assistance in socialization facilitates independent living and function. Some women require assisted reproduction techniques to achieve pregnancy, supported by hormone administration. In vitro fertilization via an oocyte donation may be needed to promote pregnancy, although these women may face increased risk of aortic rupture related to the physical stressors of pregnancy.[50]

Sex-Linked Genetic Disorder: Fragile X Syndrome

FXS is an example of a sex-linked genetic disorder that follows Mendelian inheritance patterns. As its name implies, the defect that causes the disorder is located on the X chromosome. Fragile X is the leading cause of inherited intellectual disability in the

Small Stature
Webbed neck
Coarctation of the aorta
Poor breast development
Widely spaced nipples
Wide carrying angle of arms
Rudimentary ovaries-gonadal streak
Primary amenorrhea
Multiple pigmented nevi
A
↑FSH, LH
Tall, slim eunuchoid stature
Gynecomastia
Feminized habitus (↑estradiol)
Testicular atrophy
Barr body
XXY
B

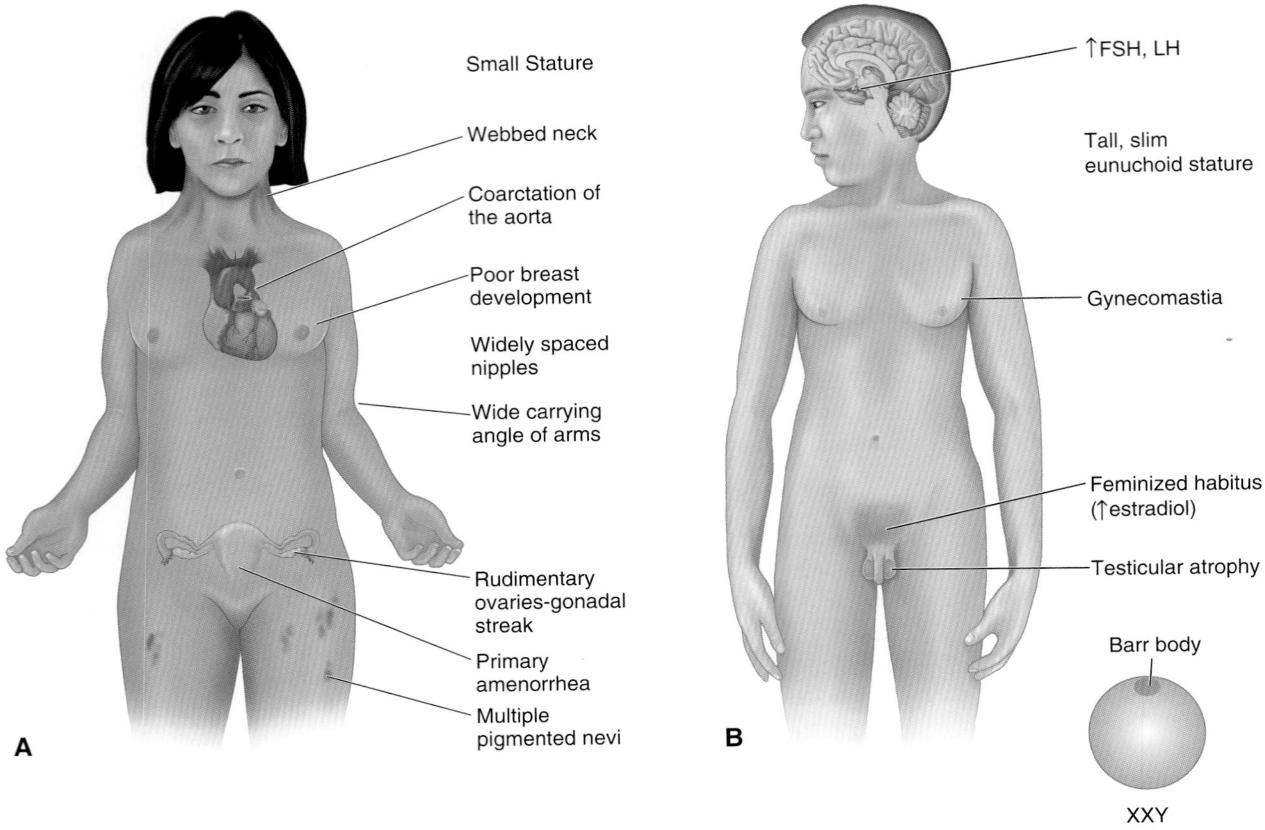

Figure 6.17. Clinical manifestations of Turner syndrome **(A)** and Klinefelter syndrome **(B)**. Turner syndrome is characterized by physical manifestations of altered female reproductive development resulting from complete or partial monosomy of the X chromosome. (Modified from Rubin E, Farber JL. *Pathology*. 4th ed. Philadelphia, PA: Lippincott Williams & Wilkins; 2005.)

United States. The prevalence of FXS with the full mutation affects an estimated 1:4,000 males and 1:5,000–8,000 females, though it is felt that this syndrome is underdiagnosed.[51] Approximately 1:250 women are carriers of the defective gene.

PATHOPHYSIOLOGY

Located on the long arm of the X chromosome, a nucleotide mutation in the fragile X mental retardation 1 (*FMR1*) gene has been identified as the molecular basis of the syndrome. The unusual mutation is characterized by a variable trinucleotide repeat of the nitrogen base combination of cytosine–guanine–guanine (CGG). The number of CGG repeats within a gene determines if a person has a typical allele (less than 55 repeats), premutation (55 to 200 repeats), or a full mutation (more than 200 repeats).[52] This defect results in the impaired ability to produce the fragile X mental retardation protein (FMRP). Under normal circumstances, DNA methylation of *FMR1* reduces gene activity, decreasing FMRP production. As the CGG triplet repeats increase, the targets for DNA methylation increase resulting in further reduction of FMRP protein production and risk for impaired postnatal brain development and worsening severity of phenotype. As is typical in sex-linked disorders, males are affected by the disorder and females are carriers.

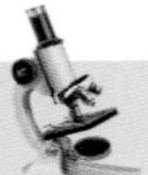

FROM THE LAB

The *FMR1* gene test is specific for diagnosing FXS. Laboratory testing for FXS is done by detection of the triplet expansion region of the *FMR1* gene. The laboratory test polymerase chain reaction (PCR) amplifies the specific alleles. After amplification, Southern blot analysis is performed to detect the expanded alleles.[53] This test has been shown to detect and measure the CGG repeat effectively, with more than 99% sensitivity and 100% specificity.

CLINICAL MANIFESTATIONS

The hallmarks of FXS include behavioral and cognitive manifestations. Unlike other sex-linked disorders, the variations in the gene mutation can lead to clinical signs in female carriers.

Behavioral manifestations in males include attention deficit/hyperactivity, expressive delay, negative response to touch, repetitive speech, and social anxiety, the common manifestations of autism spectrum disorder. Cognitive manifestations include mental impairment, with some affected males affected by seizures. Typical physical features include distinctive facial features (protruding lower jaw, large head with broad forehead), connective tissue problems (hyperflexible joints), below-average height, and macroorchidism (enlarged testicles); however, they are not specific enough to diagnose the condition.

Female carriers have fewer and less severe clinical manifestations including mild cognitive or behavioral defects, possible autistic behaviors, premature ovarian failure, and fragile-X-associated tremor/ataxia syndrome (FXTAS) in more severe degrees of mutation.[52]

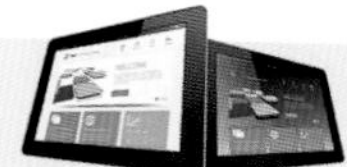

RESEARCH NOTES

The use of gene therapy in the treatment of FXS holds promise for a potential treatment or cure. With current technology, significant challenges exist in determining the delivery of gene therapy and an effective method to target the damaged cells.[54]

DIAGNOSTIC CRITERIA

Screening for the disorder includes family history or manifestations of fragile X. The risk of recurrence is high in carrier relatives, presenting an important consideration for prenatal testing. Prenatal screening is completed using the techniques of chorionic villus sampling or amniocentesis to collect samples for definitive genetic diagnosis based on the length of CGG repeats in the *FMR1* gene. Because the clinical manifestations are vague and can be associated with many other disorders, individuals with a family history of FXS should be screened for the disorder. Currently, FXS is not among the usual disorders detected by routine newborn screening.

TREATMENT

No cure currently exists for FXS. Behavioral and educational management and treatment of physical symptoms are recommended. Treatment of the behavioral problems associated with FXS is important to individual and family functioning and include developmental, educational, and behavioral interventions. The use of pharmacotherapy to manage distractibility, hyperactivity, and impulsivity has been shown to be helpful. Antidepressants can help manage anxiety, obsessive-compulsive behaviors, and mood changes. Aggression may be treated with the use of antipsychotic medications. The combination of these psychopharmacologic agents for specific manifestations of fragile X can contribute to enhanced individual functioning.[55]

Stop and Consider

What are the benefits of early prenatal diagnosis in a child with FXS?

Epigenetic Inheritance: Beckwith–Wiedemann Syndrome

Beckwith–Wiedemann Syndrome (BWS) is associated with pediatric overgrowth and predisposition to tumor growth, linked to genetic and epigenetic alterations. The phenotype ranges in severity and has equal prevalence among males and females, occurring spontaneously in the majority of individuals affected.

PATHOPHYSIOLOGY

BWS results from disordered epigenetic regulation of imprinted genes. Regulation of the imprinted genes insulin-like growth factor 2 (*IGF2*) and *H19*, located in the same region of chromosome 11 (11p15.5, band 15.5 on the short arm of chromosome 11), is altered because of changes in DNA methylation in the imprinting center in the *KCNQ1* gene. Nearby *KCNQ10T1* and *CDKN1C* genes may have a change in expression because of DNA methylation changes or genetic mutation. Like other imprinted genes, both *IGF2* and *H19* are monoallelic, transmitted by a single parent. *IGF2* is paternally inherited and expressed, functioning as a growth factor. Altered *IGF2* imprinting and loss of DNA methylation increase gene expression and associated growth function. *H19* is maternally inherited and expressed, functioning as a tumor suppressor. Altered *H19* imprinting and gain of DNA methylation decrease gene expression and associated tumor suppressor function. Changes in gene expression contribute to overgrowth and tumor development.

CLINICAL MANIFESTATIONS

Characteristic manifestations of BWS are associated with overgrowth, including macrosomia (increased birth weight), macroglossia (large tongue), cardiomegaly, and enlarged abdominal organs. Abdominal wall defects (omphalocele) may also be part of the BWS phenotype. Metabolic disorders including hypoglycemia appear soon after birth. Tumors of embryonic origin including Wilms tumor, neuroblastoma, hepatoblastoma, and rhabdomyosarcoma may occur in children during the first 8 years of life. Clinical manifestations of overgrowth and metabolic disorders can range from mild to severe and do not reflect tumor risk.[56]

DIAGNOSTIC CRITERIA

BWS is suspected based on clinical manifestations and family history, though few cases of BWS are familial. Genetic testing is indicated in the complex diagnosis of BWS and includes analysis of epigenetic and genetic alterations. As DNA methylation can vary by tissue type, often two tissues/cell populations are required for definitive testing. Karyotype determination can identify translocations, inversions, and duplications. DNA sequencing to detect genetic mutations may also be conducted.

TREATMENT

Management of BWS during infancy includes assuring airway sufficiency and feeding ability, both potentially limited by macroglossia. Tumor surveillance includes abdominal ultrasound, MRI, CT examination, and chest X-ray conducted at regular intervals through the first 8 years of life. Alpha-fetoprotein may also be measured for detection of hepatoblastoma. Cardiac evaluation including electrocardiogram and echocardiogram may be conducted because of cardiomyopathy. Treatment of metabolic disorders, including hypoglycemia, is critically important in the newborn period to reduce the risk of central nervous system complications. Genetic testing is indicated in the affected individual and family if the genetic etiology is found to be a mutation or translocation.

Developmental Maladaptation: Neural Tube Defects

NTDs are a group of serious birth defects involving the tissues of the nervous system (the brain and spine). The fortification of foods with folic acid is recognized as an important public health strategy in the prevention of NTDs. Pregnancies affected by spina bifida decreased from 2,490 to 1,640 annually since fortification of food with folic acid began in 1998. The number of infants born with anencephaly decreased from 1,640 to 1,380 annually during the same period. The overall risk for development of NTDs decreased by 26%.[57]

To see a video on lumbar myelomeningocele, visit http://thePoint.lww.com, using the scratch-off code on the inside front cover.

PATHOPHYSIOLOGY

NTDs are examples of developmental disorders during embryologic development. NTDs result from incomplete closure of the neural tube during embryonic life, typically during the first 3 to 4 weeks after conception. The degree of neural tube closure distinguishes between the different types of defects. The most common conditions resulting from neural tube anomalies include spina bifida and anencephaly. Each of these conditions has clinical manifestations specific to the condition. Causes that may contribute to these disorders include teratogenic or genetic insult. This defect may occur alone or in combination with other anomalies as part of a syndrome or result from a genetic or chromosomal abnormality. One of the major risks identified with the increased incidence of NTDs is maternal folic acid deficiency. There is still much to understand about the underlying biochemical and genetic mechanisms that lead to folic acid-associated NTDs.[58] Despite the currently unexplained mechanism of disease development, the recognition of folic acid as a cause of NTDs has resulted in successful efforts in prevention. In 1992, the US Department of Health and Human Services, Public Health Service, and the Centers for Disease Control and Prevention issued recommendations for the use of folic acid supplementation to reduce the number of NTDs in childbearing women. Recommendations included the dietary consumption of folic acid 0.4 mg/day, or as a supplement. Because folic acid deficiency interfered with NTD development early in pregnancy, the recommendations included all childbearing-age women, including those not currently pregnant. Not all women who are folate deficient have babies with NTDs, suggesting the influence of genetic mechanisms in the development of the disease phenotype.

CLINICAL MANIFESTATIONS

The stimulus that results in incomplete neural tube closure is initiated early, often before many women even realize they are pregnant. Neural tube closure occurs between embryologic days 24 and 28, beginning cranially at the head and moving distally toward the spine. In anencephaly, the closure defect is located in the skull area, with all or part of the top of the skull and portions of the brain absent. Spina bifida is the result of a closure defect in the spine. There are three main variations of spina bifida:

1. **Spina bifida occulta:** incomplete closure of vertebrae without protrusion of the meninges or spinal cord
2. **Meningocele:** incomplete closure with protrusion of meninges and cerebrospinal fluid

3. **Myelomeningocele:** incomplete closure with protrusion of meninges, cerebrospinal fluid, and spinal cord/nerve roots

In most cases, anencephaly involves a significant portion of the brain, resulting in fatality. The severity of spinal bifida is determined by the involvement of the spinal nerves. Clinical manifestations can range from a dimple at the base of the spine in occulta to lower body paralysis in myelomeningocele. Variations in types of NTDs are depicted in Figure 6.18.

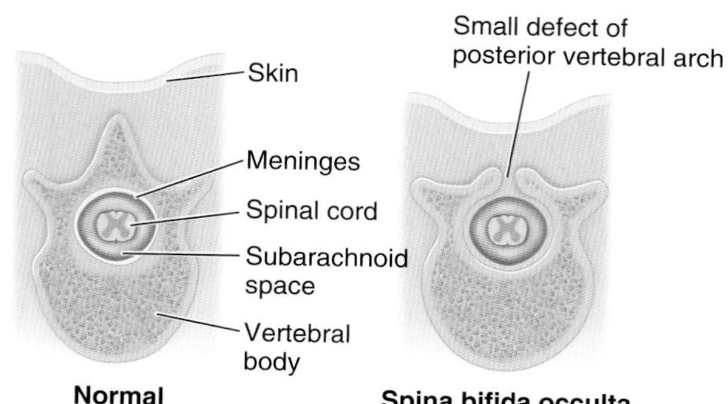

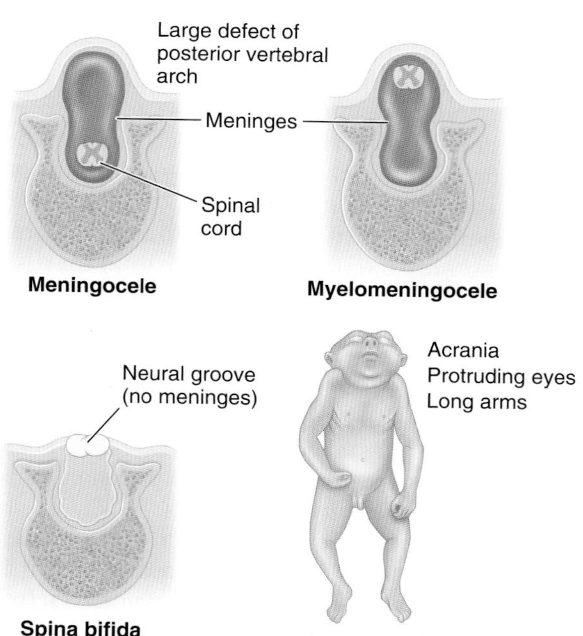

Figure 6.18. Neural tube defects. Variations in neural tube defects result from incomplete fusion of the neural tube with bone, soft tissues, or skin. (Modified from Rubin E, Farber JL. *Pathology*. 4th ed. Philadelphia, PA: Lippincott Williams & Wilkins; 2005.)

DIAGNOSTIC TESTING

Prenatally, when meninges are in communication with amniotic fluid, alpha-fetoprotein leaks from the cerebrospinal fluid into the amniotic fluid. This can be measured indirectly through determination of alpha-fetoprotein from a maternal blood sample (maternal serum alpha-fetoprotein [MSAFP]). A more direct measurement of alpha-fetoprotein can be obtained using amniotic fluid via amniocentesis. Anatomic anomalies may also be detected by ultrasound, detection influenced by the location, and size of defect.

TREATMENT

Treatment in anencephaly is usually limited to supportive care and comfort. Treatment for meningocele and myelomeningocele requires surgical correction to prevent complications, but it does not alter neurologic damage.

Stop and Consider

Are there any risks related to fortifying foods with folic acid? Are there risks in other non–childbearing populations (elderly, children, men) to folic acid food fortification? Is the economic cost associated with food fortification justified?

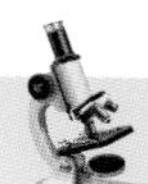

FROM THE LAB

Maternal serum alpha-fetoprotein levels were measured in a large study that compared measurements before and after mandatory supplementation in the United States.[57] Consistent with the decreased incidence of NTDs, the incidence of high MSAFP values was similarly decreased by 32%, supporting the effectiveness of folic acid fortification efforts.

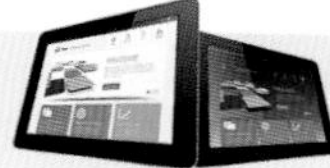

RESEARCH NOTES

Technologic advances in fetal surgery have contributed to the possibility of intrauterine closure of myelomeningocele as a preferred therapy for the future.[59] Current studies are underway to determine whether the benefits of intrauterine surgical closure are great enough to overcome the risks associated with this type of surgery.

SUMMARY

- Alterations in genetic structure and function form the basis of many diseases.
- Components of the genetic system include genes and chromosomes.
- The double helix structure, DNA, is composed of specific combinations of four nitrogenous bases, forming genes and chromosomes.
- The sequence of nitrogenous bases in genes produces amino acids, which combine to form proteins.
- Three types of RNA are involved in protein production and include messenger RNA, transfer RNA, and ribosomal RNA.
- The somatic cells of the body each contain 46 chromosomes: 44 autosomes and 2 sex chromosomes.
- The influence of genetics can be exerted by expression of a trait, the inheritance of a trait, or the establishment of a predisposition for disease.
- Single gene traits are inherited in an autosomal dominant, autosomal recessive, or sex-linked pattern or via a mitochondrial gene disorder.
- Syndromes caused by alterations in chromosome number or structure are associated with multiple clinical manifestations.
- Epigenetics regulate gene expression through chemical modifications of genes.
- Epigenetic modifications direct gene expression during development and disease and are influenced by endogenous and exogenous factors including environment and lifestyle.
- Multifactorial disorders involve both genetic and environmental factors.
- Identification of risk for genetic disorders is based on family history and genetic screening.
- The combination of environment and genetics may underlie diseases that affect morbidity and mortality in the United States and throughout the world.
- As continued investigation reveals information that unlocks many genetic mysteries, the social and ethical implications of such findings must keep pace with the science.

CASE STUDY 6.1

J.S., a 13-year-old male, has hemophilia A. He is entering middle school and wants to play intramural football. Think about a clinical model most related to this diagnosis. From your reading related to genetic disorders, answer the following questions:

1. What is the pathology associated with hemophilia?
2. What are the clinical manifestations?
3. What are the risks of his passing hemophilia on to his future daughters? Sons?
4. What are the treatment options for hemophilia?
5. What are the risks related to treatment of hemophilia?
6. What recommendations should be made in light of his request to play football?

Log onto the Internet. Search for a relevant journal article or Web site that details hemophilia to confirm your predictions.

CASE STUDY 6.2

William, a 2-year-old male, has a history of delayed motor milestones. He was delayed in rolling over, sitting, and standing. He began to walk at 18 months. He has a waddling gait and difficulty climbing stairs. After genetic testing, William was diagnosed with Duchenne muscular dystrophy (DMD).

1. What is the genetic defect associated with DMD?
2. What are the clinical manifestations of DMD?
3. What are the risks of his passing DMD on to his future daughters? Sons?
4. What are the treatment options for DMD?
5. What is the life expectancy for William?

Log onto the Internet. Search for a relevant journal article or Web site that details DMD to confirm your predictions.

CASE STUDY 6.3

Susie is a 30-year-old female diagnosed with leukemia. Leukemia is a cancer that targets blood forming tissue and is associated with silencing of tumor suppressor genes.

1. What effect does silencing of tumor suppressor genes have in leukemia?
2. Identify how DNA methylation contributes to tumor suppressor gene silencing?
3. Substances called DNA methyltransferases (DNMT) inhibitors are used to reverse epigenetic silencing. How might this have potential for treatment of leukemia?

Log onto the Internet. Search for a relevant journal article or Web site that details epigenetic etiology in cancer and epigenetic modifiers in the treatment of cancer to confirm your predictions.

PRACTICE EXAM QUESTIONS

1. A person's phenotype can be best described as:
   a. The genetic makeup of an individual
   b. Traits that are observable or apparent
   c. Traits that are inherited in a recessive pattern
   d. Traits that are inherited in a dominant pattern

2. A person's genotype can be best described as:
   a. The genetic makeup of an individual
   b. Traits that are observable or apparent
   c. Traits that are inherited in a recessive pattern
   d. Traits that are inherited in a dominant pattern

3. Which of these conditions follows a Mendelian pattern of recessive inheritance?
   a. Coronary artery disease
   b. Down syndrome
   c. Marfan syndrome
   d. Tay-Sachs disease

4. Which of these conditions follows a multifactorial pattern of inheritance?
   a. Coronary artery disease
   b. Down syndrome
   c. Marfan syndrome
   d. Tay-Sachs disease

5. Fortification of foods with folic acid has resulted in a significant reduction in the incidence of:
   a. Huntington disease
   b. Turner syndrome
   c. Neural tube defects
   d. Cleft lip and palate

6. Which of the following chromosomal abnormalities can result in an inheritable form of trisomy?
   a. Nondisjunction during meiosis
   b. Balanced translocation
   c. Insertion
   d. Deletion

DISCUSSION AND APPLICATION

1. What did I know about genetic and developmental disorders before today?
2. What body processes are affected by genetic and developmental disorders? How do genetic and developmental disorders affect those processes?
3. What are the potential etiologies for genetic and developmental disorders? How do genetic and developmental disorders develop?
4. Who is most at risk for developing genetic and developmental disorders? How can these alterations be prevented?
5. What are the human differences that affect the etiology, risk, or course of genetic and developmental disorders?
6. What clinical manifestations are expected in the course of genetic and developmental disorders?
7. What special diagnostic tests are useful in determining the diagnosis and course of genetic and developmental disorders?
8. What are the goals of care for individuals with genetic and developmental disorders?
9. How does the concept of alteration in genetics build on what I have learned in the previous chapter and in the previous courses?
10. How can I use what I have learned?

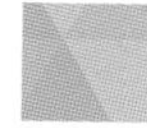

RESOURCES

Fragile X Syndrome: NIH Genetics Home Reference
https://ghr.nlm.nih.gov/condition/fragile-x-syndrome

National Institute of Neurological Disorders and Stroke Huntington's Disease Information Page:
http://ninds.nih.gov/health_and_medical/disorders/huntington.htm

March of Dimes:
http://modimes.org
Find out more about newborn screening, including state-specific requirements.

National Down Syndrome Society:
http://www.ndss.org/

National Human Genome Research Institute, National Institutes of Health:
http://www.genome.gov/
Find out about genetic disorders, definitions of common genetic terms, and current genetic research.

Sickle Cell Disease Association of America:
http://www.sicklecelldisease.org/

American Heart Association. Heart Disease and Stroke Statistics—2009 Update. Dallas, TX: American Heart Association; 2009.
http://www.americanheart.org/presenter.jhtml?identifier=3000090

References

1. Guttmacher AE, Collins FS. Genomic medicine—a primer. *N Engl J Med.* 2002;347(19):1512–1520.
2. Khoury MJ, McCabe LL, McCabe ER. Population screening in the age of genomic medicine. *N Engl J Med.* 2003;348(1):50–58.

3. Banta-Wright SA, Steiner RD. Tandem mass spectrometry in newborn screening: a primer for neonatal and perinatal nurses. *J Perinat Neonatal Nurs*. 2004;18(1):41–58; quiz 59–60.
4. Powell IJ, Carpten J, Dunston G, et al. African-American heredity prostate cancer study: a model for genetic research. *J Natl Med Assoc*. 2001;93(12, suppl):25S–28S.
5. Buller A, Pandya A, Jackson-Cook C, et al. Validation of a multiplex methylation-sensitive PCR assay for the diagnosis of Prader-Willi and Angelman's syndromes. *Mol Diagn*. 2000;5(3):239–243.
6. Gill P. DNA as evidence—the technology of identification. *N Engl J Med*. 2005;352(26):2669–2671.
7. Rothstein MA. Genetic justice. *N Engl J Med*. 2005;352(26):2667–2678.
8. Ahlgren M, Melbye M, Wohlfahrt J, et al. Growth patterns and the risk of breast cancer in women. *N Engl J Med*. 2004;351(16):1619–1626.
9. Barker DJ, Eriksson JG, Forsen T, et al. Fetal origins of adult disease: strength of effects and biological basis. *Int J Epidemiol*. 2002;31(6):1235–1239.
10. Mills JL, Signore C. Neural tube defect rates before and after food fortification with folic acid. *Birth Defects Res A Clin Mol Teratol*. 2004;70(11):844–845.
11. Botto LD, Lisi A, Robert-Gnansia E, et al. International retrospective cohort study of neural tube defects in relation to folic acid recommendations: are the recommendations working? *BMJ*. 2005;330(7491):571.
12. Wadhwa PD, Buss C, Entringer S, et al. Developmental origins of health and disease: brief history of the approach and current focus on epigenetic mechanisms. *Semin Reprod Med*. 2009;27(5):358–368.
13. Swanson JM, Entringer S, Buss C, et al. Developmental origins of health and disease: environmental exposures. *Semin Reprod Med*. 2009;27(5):391–402.
14. Symonds ME, Sebert SP, Hyatt MA, et al. Nutritional programming of the metabolic syndrome. *Nat Rev Endocrinol*. 2009;5(11):604–610.
15. Clayton EW. Ethical, legal, and social implications of genomic medicine. *N Engl J Med*. 2003;349(6):562–569.
16. Sampson JE, Ouhibi N, Lawce H, et al. The role for preimplantation genetic diagnosis in balanced translocation carriers. *Am J Obstet Gynecol*. 2004;190(6):1707–1711; discussion 1711–1713.
17. Offit K, Groeger E, Turner S, et al. The "duty to warn" a patient's family members about hereditary disease risks. *JAMA*. 2004;292(12):1469–1473.
18. Anderson KE. Huntington's disease and related disorders. *Psychiatr Clin N Am*. 2005;28:275–290.
19. Glajch KE, Sadri-Vakili G. Epigenetic mechanisms involved in Huntington's disease pathogenesis. *J Huntingtons Dis*. 2015;4(1):1–15. doi:10.3233/JHD-159001.
20. Fink KD, Deng P, Torrest A, et al. Developing stem cell therapies for juvenile and adult-onset Huntington's disease. *Regen Med*. 2015;10(5):623–646. doi:10.2217/rme.15.25.
21. Wong BK, Ehmhoefer DE, Graham RK, et al. Partial rescue of some features of Huntington disease in the genetic absence of caspase-6 in YAC128 mice. *Neurobiol Dis*. 2015;76:24–36. doi:10.1016/j.nbd.2014.12.030.
22. Koppel BS, Brust JC, Fife T, et al. Systematic review: efficacy and safety of medical marijuana in selected neurologic disorders: report of the Guideline Development Subcommittee of the American Academy of Neurology. *Neurology*. 2014;82(17):1556–1563. doi:10.1212/WNL.0000000000000363.
23. Wexler NS, Lorimer J, Porter J, et al. Venezuelan kindreds reveal that genetic and environmental factors modulate Huntington's disease age of onset. *Proc Natl Acad Sci U S A*. 2004;101(10):3498–3503.
24. Steinberg MH. Management of sickle cell disease. *N Engl J Med*. 1999;340(13):1021–1030.
25. McKerrell TD, Cohen HW, Billett HH. The older sickle cell patient. *Am J Hematol*. 2004;76(2):101–106.
26. Quinn CT, Rogers ZR, Buchanan GR. Survival of children with sickle cell disease. *Blood*. 2004;103(11):4023–4027.
27. Platt OS, Brambilla DJ, Rosse WF, et al. Mortality in sickle cell disease: life expectancy and risk factors for early death. *N Engl J Med*. 1994;330(23):1639–1644.
28. Talano JA, Cairo MS. Smoothing the crescent curve: sickle cell disease. *Hematology Am Soc Hematol Educ Program*. 2014;2014(1):468–474. doi:10.1182/asheducation-2014.1.468.
29. Graslund T, Li X, Magnenat L, et al. Exploring strategies for the design of artificial transcription factors: targeting sites proximal to known regulatory regions for the induction of gamma-globin expression and the treatment of sickle cell disease. *J Biol Chem*. 2005;280(5):3707–3714.
30. Matsumoto J, Saver JL, Brennan KC, et al. Mitochondrial encephalomyopathy with lactic acidosis and stroke (MELAS). *Rev Neurol Dis*. 2005;2(1):30–34.
31. Majamaa K, Moilanen JS, Uimonen S, et al. Epidemiology of A3243G, the mutation for mitochondrial encephalomyopathy, lactic acidosis, and strokelike episodes: prevalence of the mutation in an adult population. *Am J Hum Genet*. 1998;63(2):447–454.
32. Cao Z, Wanagat J, McKiernan SH, et al. Mitochondrial DNA deletion mutations are concomitant with ragged red regions of individual, aged muscle fibers: analysis by laser-capture microdissection. *Nucleic Acids Res*. 2001;29(21):4502–4508.
33. Benachi A, Letourneau A, Kleinfinger P, et al. Cell-free DNA analysis in maternal plasma in cases of fetal abnormalities detected on ultrasound examination. *Obstet Gynecol*. 2015;125(6):1330–1337. doi:10.1097/AOG.0000000000000874.
34. Alfirevic Z, Neilson JP. Antenatal screening for Down's syndrome. *BMJ*. 2004;329(7470):811–812.
35. Wald NJ, Rodeck C, Hackshaw AK, et al. SURUSS in perspective. *BJOG*. 2004;111(6):521–531.
36. Taylor-Phillips S, Freeman K, Geppert J, et al. Accuracy of non-invasive prenatal testing using cell-free DNA for detection of Down, Edwards and Patau syndromes: a systematic review and meta-analysis. *BMJ Open*. 2016;6(1):e010002. doi:10.1136/bmjopen-2015-010002.
37. Bronshtein M, Zimmer EZ, Blazer S. A characteristic cluster of fetal sonographic markers that are predictive of fetal Turner syndrome in early pregnancy. *Am J Obstet Gynecol*. 2003;188(4):1016–1020.
38. Sybert VP, McCauley E. Turner's syndrome. *N Engl J Med*. 2004;351(12):1227–1238.
39. Ostberg JE, Conway GS. Adulthood in women with Turner syndrome. *Horm Res*. 2003;59(5):211–221.
40. Serra A, Cocuzza S, Caruso E, et al. Audiological range in Turner's syndrome. *Int J Pediatr Otorhinolaryngol*. 2003;67(8):841–845.

41. Cooley M, Bakalov V, Bondy CA. Lipid profiles in women with 45,X vs 46,XX primary ovarian failure. *JAMA*. 2003;290(16):2127–2128.
42. Longui CA, Rocha MN, Martinho LC, et al. Molecular detection of XO—Turner syndrome. *Genet Mol Res*. 2002;1(3):266–270.
43. Pena SD, Sturzeneker R. Fetal diagnosis of monosomy X (Turner syndrome) with methylation-specific PCR. *Prenat Diagn*. 2003;23(9):769–770.
44. Gunther DF, Eugster E, Zagar AJ, et al. Ascertainment bias in Turner syndrome: new insights from girls who were diagnosed incidentally in prenatal life. *Pediatrics*. 2004;114(3):640–644.
45. Starke MK, Albertsson W, Moller A. Parents' descriptions of development and problems associated with infants with Turner syndrome: a retrospective study. *J Paediatr Child Health*. 2003;39(4):293–298.
46. Piippo S, Lenko H, Kainulainen P, et al. Use of percutaneous estrogen gel for induction of puberty in girls with Turner syndrome. *J Clin Endocrinol Metab*. 2004;89(7):3241–3247.
47. Hanton L, Axelrod L, Bakalov V, et al. The importance of estrogen replacement in young women with Turner syndrome. *J Womens Health (Larchmt)*. 2003;12(10):971–977.
48. Reynaud K, Cortvrindt R, Verlinde F, et al. Number of ovarian follicles in human fetuses with the 45,X karyotype. *Fertil Steril*. 2004;81(4):1112–1119.
49. Bakalov VK, Cooley MM, Quon MJ, et al. Impaired insulin secretion in the Turner metabolic syndrome. *J Clin Endocrinol Metab*. 2004;89(7):3516–3520.
50. Karnis MF, Zimon AE, Lalwani SI. Risk of death in pregnancy achieved through oocyte donation in patients with Turner syndrome: a national survey. *Fertil Steril*. 2003;80(3):498–501.
51. Lyons JI, Kerr GR, Mueller PW. Fragile X Syndrome: Scientific Background and Screening Technologies. *J Mol Diagn*. 2015;17(5):463-471. doi:10.1016/j.jmoldx.2015.04.00.
52. Song FJ, Barton P, Sleightholme V, et al. Screening for fragile X syndrome: a literature review and modelling study. *Health Technol Assess*. 2003;7(16):1–106.
53. Gold B, Radu D, Balanko A, et al. Diagnosis of fragile X syndrome by Southern blot hybridization using a chemiluminescent probe: a laboratory protocol. *Mol Diagn*. 2000;5(3):169–178.
54. Rattazzi MC, LaFauci G, Brown WT. Prospects for gene therapy in the fragile X syndrome. *Ment Retard Dev Disabil Res Rev*. 2004;10(1):75–81.
55. Berry-Kravis E, Potanos K. Psychopharmacology in fragile X syndrome—present and future. *Ment Retard Dev Disabil Res Rev*. 2004;10(1):42–48.
56. Mussa A, Russo S, Larizza L, et al. (Epi)genotype-phenotype correlations in Beckwith-Wiedemann syndrome: a paradigm for genomic medicine [published online ahead of print July 3, 2015]. *Clin Genet*. doi:10.1111/cge.12635.
57. Centers for Disease Control. Spina bifida and anencephaly before and after folic acid mandate—United States, 1995–1996 and 1999–2000. *MMWR Morb Mortal Wkly Rep*. 2004;53(17):362–365.
58. Stover PJ. Physiology of folate and vitamin B_{12} in health and disease. *Nutr Rev*. 2004;62(6, pt 2):S3–S12; discussion S13.
59. Bruner JP, Tulipan N, Reed G, et al. Intrauterine repair of spina bifida: preoperative predictors of shunt-dependent hydrocephalus. *Am J Obstet Gynecol*. 2004;190(5):1305–1312.

Find additional resources for this chapter at http:thePoint.lww.com thePoint®

Chapter 7

Altered Cellular Proliferation and Differentiation

LEARNING OUTCOMES

1. Define and use the key terms listed in this chapter.
2. Recognize the role of genetic mutations in the development of neoplasms.
3. Discuss major carcinogens and their role in carcinogenesis.
4. Outline the characteristics of tumor cells.
5. Differentiate benign and malignant tumors.
6. Explain the mechanisms of cancer spread.
7. Classify tumors based on staging and grading criteria.
8. Identify local and systemic clinical manifestations of neoplasia.
9. Describe cancer treatment strategies.
10. Apply the principles of carcinogenesis to select clinical models.

INTRODUCTION

"You have cancer." Very little strikes more fear than those three words. Although many cancers are curable and current research continues to support prevention, early detection, and effective treatment options, cancer continues to affect millions of lives each year and is one of the leading causes of death in the United States.

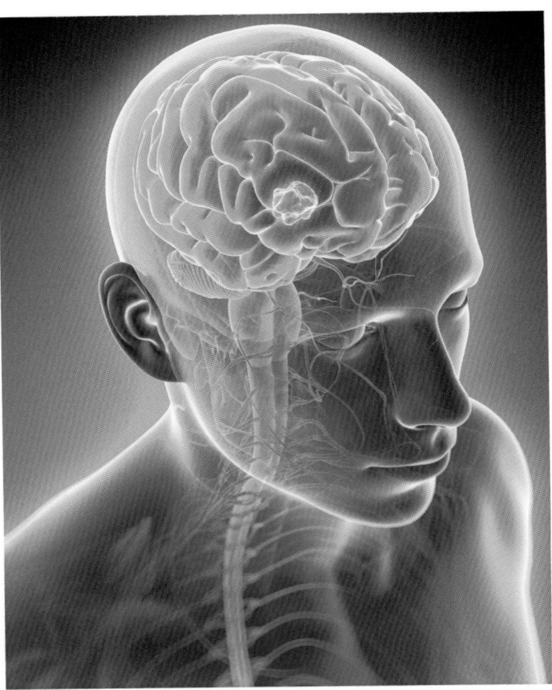

Brain tumor, 3D-rendered illustration. © Sebastian Kaulitzki.

Module 1 The Impact of Cancer on the Cell

Cellular **proliferation** is the generation of new, daughter cells divided from progenitor (parent) cells. Meiosis is a process of dividing germ cells, resulting in ovum and sperm. Mitosis is the division and proliferation of all other nongerm cells. Cellular proliferation through mitosis occurs continuously and/or in response to needs. For example, epithelial cells of the skin constantly reproduce to replace those damaged by the external environment. These cells can increase the rate of division in times of need, such as occurs with a wound injury. Similarly, red blood cell (RBC) proliferation replaces RBCs at the end of the cell's 120-day lifespan and also increases exponentially in the case of excessive blood loss to maintain blood volume and oxygenate tissues. A regulated balance of cell growth and cell death is needed to maintain homeostasis in the body. We are concerned here with the loss of regulated balance of cell division resulting in the *overproliferation* and crowding of cells.

Differentiation refers to the orderly process of cellular maturation to achieve a specific function. Regulation of proliferation and differentiation are under the control of genes, growth factors, nutrients, and stimulation from the external environment. As with proliferation, a balance of differentiated (cells with a specific function, such as RBCs) and undifferentiated cells (stem cells and progenitor cells) is necessary to respond to the needs of the body (Fig. 7.1).

Stem cells are highly undifferentiated units that have the potential to divide into progenitor cells, then daughter cells, which can then mature into more differentiated units with a specific function. Undifferentiated cells are valued for their flexibility and adaptability. With each step toward differentiation, the cell loses its ability to flexibly respond and adapt but gains the ability to carry out an important physiologic function. For example, with extensive blood loss, daughter cells are directed to differentiate into RBCs to replace the lost blood. Again, a balance of undifferentiated and differentiated cells is needed to maintain homeostasis. We are concerned in this chapter with the loss of differentiation, rendering the cell incapable of carrying out a designated function.

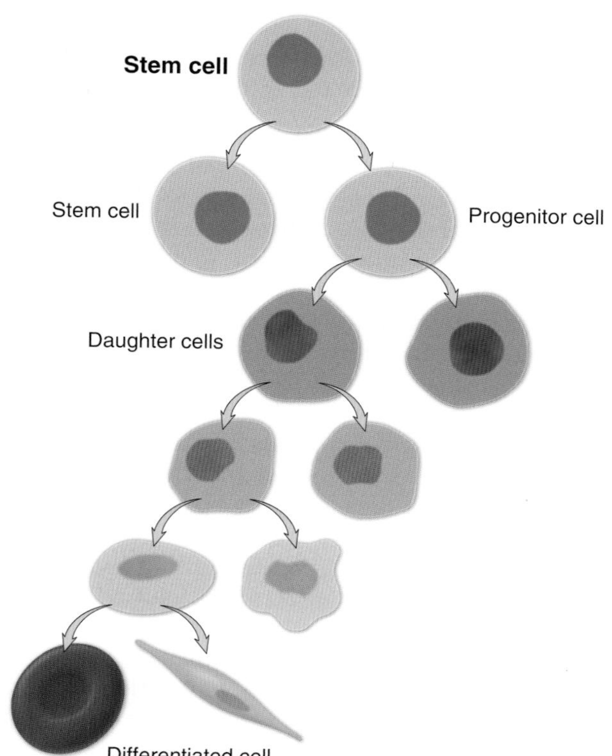

Figure 7.1. Cellular differentiation is the process by which cells become more specialized. Undifferentiated stem cells divide into like stem cells and parent (progenitor) cells, which continue to divide and further differentiate into highly specialized and functional cells. (Modified from Porth CM. *Essentials of Pathophysiology: Concepts of Altered Health States*. Philadelphia, PA: Lippincott Williams & Wilkins; 2003, with permission.)

Altered Cellular Proliferation and Differentiation

At the cellular level, cancer occurs because of gene malfunction that goes unrepaired. More specifically, cancer is caused by altering those genes that control cell reproduction, growth, differentiation, and/or death. The cell is therefore allowed to grow uncontrollably (altered proliferation). The cell also loses its ability to carry out its specified function (altered differentiation) and does not die when expected. **Cancer** is a term used to describe highly invasive and destructive **neoplasms**, which are irreversible deviant cell clusters. These neoplastic cells ignore the genetic controls placed on cellular proliferation and differentiation; they are uncontrolled and unregulated.

Neoplasms can emerge from proliferating parenchymal (functional tissue and organ) or stromal (supportive structure) cells. Rapidly dividing labile cells, such as epithelial cells and blood cells, are highly prone to the development of neoplasms. Permanent (undividing) cells, such as cardiac myocytes, mature neurons, and the lens of the eye, are not.

CARCINOGENESIS

Mutations, gene variants, and epigenetics are heavily implicated in **carcinogenesis**, which is the origin and development of cancerous neoplasms. Mutations are abnormal changes in the DNA of a gene (Chapter 6). There are two major types of gene mutations which can affect cell growth and division:

- *Inherited* gene mutations (about 5% of cancers) are present in the egg or sperm as they combine to become the zygote. These are called germline or hereditary mutations. In general, inherited mutations leading to cancer have incomplete penetrance, meaning not everyone with the mutation will get cancer. Since it takes more than one mutation in a cell for cancer to occur, those who have inherited an abnormal copy of a gene already have one strike against them. Additional mutations lead to a greater likelihood of developing cancer and developing it earlier in life. Also, all cells in the person with the inherited gene mutation hold this mutation (including some of the person's germ cells) and can be passed onto the next generation.
- *Acquired* gene mutations (about 95% of cancers) are those that occur after conception (are not present in the parent egg or sperm). Some acquired mutations are caused by environmental exposures, such as smoke or radiation, and others have no clear cause. Since we have two copies of most genes (one from each chromosome pair), both copies must mutate for the gene to lead to unregulated cell growth and division. Acquired gene mutations leading to cancer often occur much later in life because the number of gene mutations required to cause cancer build up over time. Mutations, upon cell division, are passed onto new cells. These mutations are called somatic or spontaneous mutations and are not passed onto subsequent generations.

GENETIC MUTATIONS

DNA is constantly being damaged by the environment. Mutator genes repair DNA and protect the genome. By disabling the protective, DNA-repairing mutator genes, the environment is conducive to neoplastic development as mutations go unrepaired and the cell becomes unstable. Two major categories of genes exist that, when altered, can lead to cancerous transformations. Typically, a combination of mutations involving more than one gene category is needed for neoplasms to develop. This mutation–transformation–neoplasia evolution is unique to each cancer type, and the process often takes several years (Fig. 7.2). These categories include:

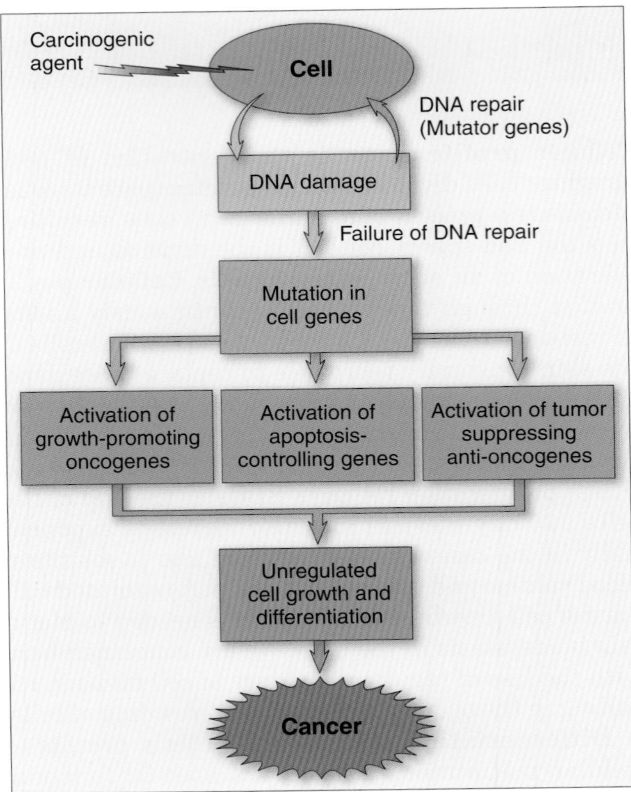

Figure 7.2. Concept map. The genomic mechanisms of cancer. (Modified from Porth CM. *Essentials of Pathophysiology: Concepts of Altered Health States*. Philadelphia, PA: Lippincott Williams & Wilkins; 2003, with permission.)

- **Oncogenes:** genes that code for proteins involved in cell growth or regulation
- **Tumor suppressor genes:** genes that prohibit overproliferation of cells and regulate apoptosis

Oncogenes

Oncogene literally means "cancer gene." Oncogenes promote unregulated cell growth and development and can also inhibit cell death. The activation of oncogenes in germline cells is often incompatible with life and results in spontaneous abortion. Those germline mutations that are not lethal can develop into inheritable neoplasms. More commonly, however, activation of oncogenes is seen in the spontaneous mutation of somatic cells.

The conversion from a "normal" gene to one that induces neoplasia depends on the mutation of protooncogenes. **Protooncogenes** are important "normal" genes in the body with a vital role in regulating cell function. Protooncogenes are also considered precursor genes that, when activated, become oncogenes through one of three ways:

1. Point mutation
2. Translocation
3. Gene amplification

A point mutation damages a single nucleotide base pair in the DNA that leads to the development of altered, unregulated proteins in somatic cells. Point mutations can arise spontaneously or from exposure to environmental influences, such as cancer-inducing chemicals or ultraviolet radiation.

Chromosomal translocations have also been implicated in the activation of oncogenes. The chromosome breaks, relocates, and unites with another chromosome. Encoded proteins become excessive, and the cell deviates from expected growth, differentiation, and death cycles. Common types of cancers that result from chromosomal translocations include leukemias, lymphomas, and many solid tumors.

Gene amplification is a process of altering the chromosome by accelerating the replication of genes. Similar to translocations, this is a problem of overproducing gene products. Gene amplification is implicated in many solid tumors, including breast cancer and neuroblastoma. In many cases, the greater the gene amplification, the poorer the prognosis.

With each type of oncogene transformation, the basic mechanisms of action include:

- Encoding growth factors to stimulate cell overproliferation
- Disturbing cell surface receptors and restricting cell-to-cell communication
- Encoding proteins in the cell nucleus to alter the cell cycle, restrict apoptosis, and impact differentiation of the cell

Although oncogenes are often categorized as either viral or cellular/chromosomal, both types result in similar alterations to the cell phenotype. With viral oncogenes, the virus inserts itself into the genetic material of the host cell, replicates, and then moves on to infect other cells. During this process, the virus may capture a portion of the host cell's genetic material along with its own. The proper regulation of genes may not be possible if this occurs because the genetic repertoire of the retrovirus is limited.

The notations for oncogenes are three-letter abbreviations, such as *ras, neu,* or *myc.* The origin or location of the gene is indicated by the prefix of "v-" for virus or "c-" for cell or chromosome; additional prefixes, suffixes, and superscripts provide further delineation. For example, breast cancer has been linked to the c-*neu* oncogene and lung cancer to the c-L-*myc* gene. More than 40 human oncogenes have been identified.

Tumor Suppressor Genes

Tumor suppressor genes are the genes that regulate the rate at which cells divide and die. A major mechanism for regulating proliferation is to control apoptosis (programmed cell death) so that the optimal number of cells is maintained for homeostasis. When mutated, tumor suppressor genes are inactivated and the cell becomes "immortal," most likely through alteration of the cell mitochondria. This can occur in germline or somatic cells as inherited or spontaneous mutations. The cell undergoes unrestricted proliferation, and neoplastic transformations are supported. Tumor suppressor genes can be likened to a wall or gate. When intact, growth is restricted. A mutation is like a large hole in the gate, allowing unrestricted growth of the cell.

Several tumor suppressor genes exist. Three common tumor suppressor genes that can allow neoplasias to form when mutated are the *TP53* gene, retinoblastoma (*Rb*) gene, and *BCL-2* gene. The *TP53* gene has been implicated as the most common mutation that leads to the development of cancer. Located on chromosome 17, this gene is deleted or mutated in three of four types of colorectal cancer and is found in many other malignancies. The *TP53* gene is responsible for opposing cell division in response to cell DNA damage by delaying cell development. This delay allows time for DNA to be repaired. If the cell cannot be repaired, the *TP53* gene can also force the damaged cell to undergo apoptosis. Without *TP53*, cells are unresponsive to the need for repair. Cells with damaged DNA are able to reproduce and can become neoplastic.

The *Rb* gene is a tumor suppressor gene that, when mutated, can result in a rare childhood cancer of the retina of the eye (retinoblastoma). Just

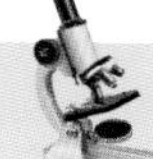

FROM THE LAB

Genetic testing may be sought by individuals newly diagnosed with cancer or those who have family members with cancer. Gene testing involves examining a person's DNA, typically taken from cells in a sample of blood, for mutations linked to that type of cancer. Specific genetic mutations have been linked to certain types of cancer, and for some cancer types, this information has been converted into a clinical test. An accurate gene test can determine whether a mutation is present but does not guarantee that the disease will develop. For example, a woman with the *BRCA1* breast cancer susceptibility gene has an 80% chance of developing breast cancer by age 65. A woman in that same family could test negative for *BRCA1* and still acquire the disease over time at the same rate as the general population. Although gene testing poses little physical discomfort or risk, the emotional and psychological consequences may be severe, particularly if there are limited prevention, early detection, or treatment interventions.

less than half of the cases are germline cell mutations; the remaining are spontaneous mutations in somatic cells. Inheritance of retinoblastoma follows a dominant pattern. The *Rb* gene has a major role in suppressing tumor proliferation. Development of other types of cancer, including osteosarcoma, breast cancer, pancreatic cancer, and lung cancer, has also been connected to inactivation of the *Rb* gene.

The *BCL-2* gene has been discovered to inhibit apoptosis. If gene *BCL-2* becomes mutated and permanently activated, the cell with the altered gene ignores all of the normal triggers to die and thereby becomes immortal. This altered cell continues to divide by mitosis, passing along the altered gene to progeny cells. These cells accumulate and form neoplasms. *BCL-2* mutations were first found in leukocytes and are known to lead to one form of leukemia.

ROLE OF GENE VARIANTS AND EPIGENETICS

Gene variants are inherited differences in genes that are not mutations but can still have an impact on cell growth and division. Gene variants are referred to as polymorphisms. Commonly, individuals have an inherited difference in one nucleotide of a gene (a single nucleotide polymorphism). Some of these variants have no obvious effect on the gene; some can have minor effects, such as impacting estrogen levels and contributing to hormone-dependent cancers. Gene variants do not cause cancer directly but can set the stage for the development of neoplasms.

Epigenetic changes (turning genes on and off but not as a result of polymorphisms or mutations) can also influence carcinogenesis. These epigenetic changes are primarily through one of the following:

- DNA methylation
- Histone modification
- RNA interference

Each of these processes interrupt the gene expression by adding or subtracting substances that activate or deactivate DNA, chromosomes, or RNA. In effect, epigenetic changes can alter the parts of the genes that control cell growth and division.

Stop and Consider

Why would someone with Down syndrome (trisomy 21) have an increased risk of developing leukemia?

In summary, genetic mutations, gene variants, and/or epigenetic changes are necessary but not sufficient factors in developing cancerous neoplasms. Additional alterations in the host cell genetic material, influenced by carcinogens, is required to develop into invasive cancerous transformations.

CARCINOGENS

The identification of cancer-causing agents is based on epidemiological studies, experimental research, and knowledge of cellular and molecular pathology. A **carcinogen** is a known cancer-causing agent. Carcinogens are agents that interfere with molecular pathways and can initiate or promote tumors to form in the body. Some carcinogens are considered direct because they cause modification of cell DNA and interfere with cell function. Others are considered indirect because they induce immunosuppression or chronic inflammation or act in conjunction with other carcinogens to induce DNA damage.

Certain substances or exposures are known to cause or promote cellular mutations, such as radiation, exposure to reactive oxygen species (free radicals), hormones, tobacco, infectious microorganisms, and chemicals (Fig. 7.3). Because cancer exhibits a prolonged latent period between the initiation and onset of clinical manifestations, identification of a precise carcinogen can be difficult.

Radiation

Ionizing radiation is both a potential cause of, and treatment for, cancer. Although radiation has many diagnostic and therapeutic applications, high-energy ionizing radiation (gamma rays, X-rays, and ultraviolet) is capable of causing genetic damage in a cell and can also kill cells directly. Radiation induces injury by producing reactive oxygen species. These unstable molecules damage the cell membrane, allowing the radiation energy to interrupt cell DNA and invoke mutations.

Labile cells are most affected by radiation exposure. Radiation treatment takes advantage of this feature with the treatment aimed at directly killing cells that are highly proliferative—most notably, cancer cells. The accumulative effect of low-dose radiation exposure is an area of extensive debate. Because all individuals are exposed to low-dose radiation over time, it is difficult to discern whether the radiation is to blame for carcinogenesis.

Ultraviolet radiation is short wavelength electromagnetic energy that, within a certain range, is also capable of inducing carcinogenesis. Sun exposure is the primary source. The risk for developing neoplasms, such as with skin cancer, from radiation exposure depends on the length of exposure, frequency of burn injuries from sun exposure, and skin tone. Similar to other types of radiation injury, the ultraviolet exposure (290 to 320 nm wavelengths) directly kills cells and can induce cellular mutation.

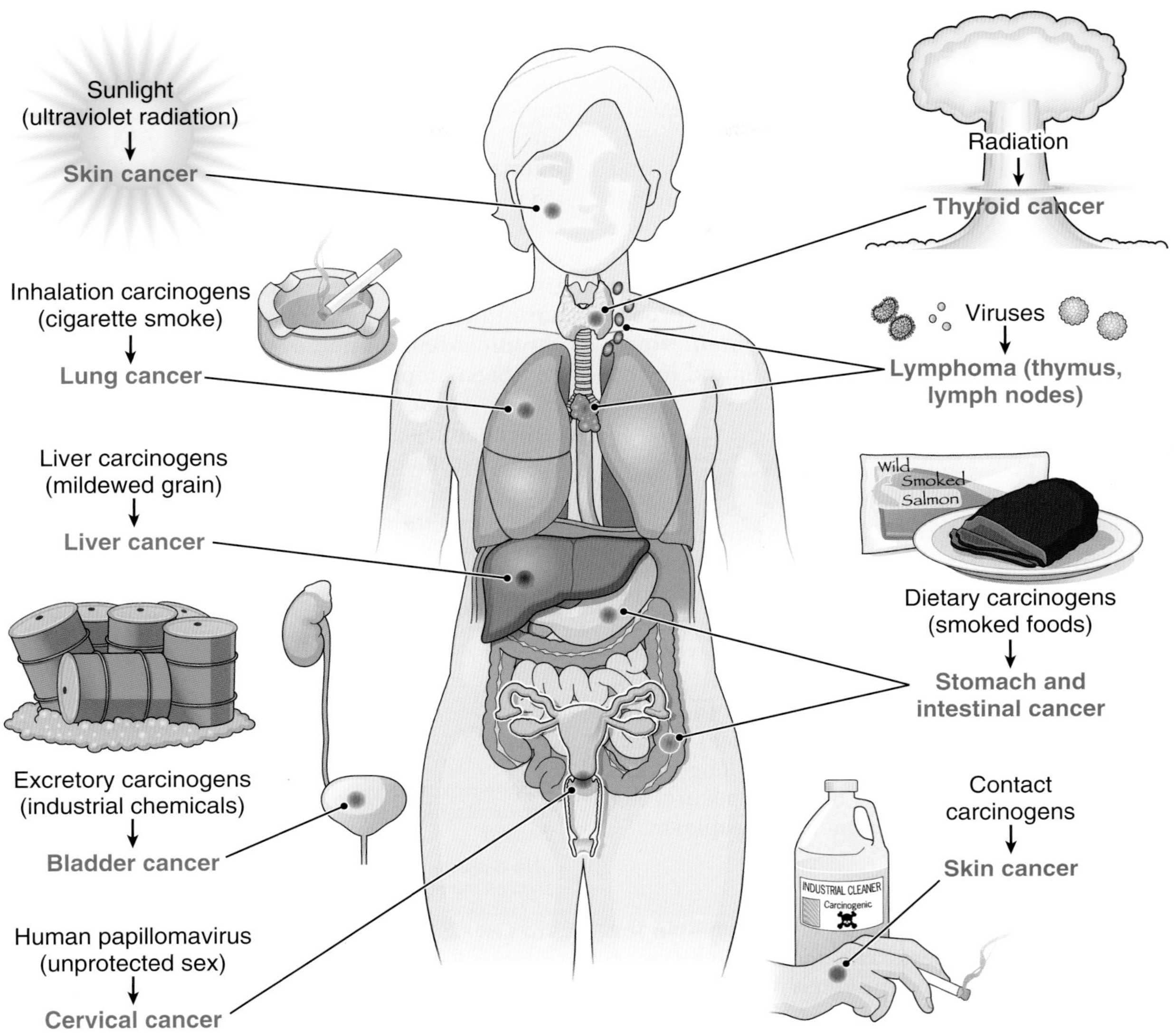

Figure 7.3. Potential carcinogens and corresponding cancers.

Stop and Consider
Do you think microwave ovens, electromagnetic fields, and ultrasound, as energy transmitters, would induce cellular injury?

Hormones

Hormones, like radiation, are also a cancer promoter and treatment. Some tumor cells are responsive to, or dependent on, hormones for growth. Tumors of the breast, uterus, prostate, and adrenal glands often contain receptors that are responsive to hormone levels in these tissues.

Hormones can also be considered a cancer treatment. They can be therapeutically administered to block the effects of tumor growth. For example, the adrenal corticosteroid hormones (i.e., prednisone) can directly kill tumor cells, especially lymph cells, and can inhibit mitosis. These drugs also have potent anti-inflammatory effects. Removal of organs or tissues that secrete specific hormones in the body will also affect tumor growth. Hormones such as estrogen and testosterone can be manipulated to "starve" the tumor and prohibit further growth. Tamoxifen is a drug commonly used in breast cancer treatment. Tamoxifen blocks the action of estrogen and inhibits tumor growth in the estrogen-sensitive breast tissues.

Chemicals

Many chemicals have been implicated in carcinogenesis, such as tobacco, asbestos, benzene, insecticides, and formaldehyde. The basic mechanism for direct or indirect chemical carcinogenesis include the development of highly reactive species, such as free radicals, that induce cell mutation or alter cell proteins or enzymes to interfere with cell regulation. Enzymes in the body are responsible for metabolizing and inactivating potentially carcinogenic chemicals. Genetic factors, environmental factors, and lifestyle (especially diet) influence these enzyme levels and therefore influence the development of chemical carcinogenesis. Predicting who will develop cancer from exposure to specific chemicals is very difficult given our frequent contact with numerous sources of varying potencies. A complete list of known, probable, and possible chemical carcinogens is maintained by the American Cancer Society and is found in the reference section of this chapter.

Tobacco

Cigarette tar contains thousands of substances, many of which are carcinogenic. Approximately one in three cancer deaths in the United States can be linked to tobacco.[1] Inhaling cigarette and cigar smoke is toxic to respiratory mucosa and is known to cause lung cancer. Use of tobacco is also responsible for initiating or promoting many other types of cancer, such as laryngeal, lip, esophageal, and bladder cancer. Smoking, as with other chemical carcinogens, exhibits a dose effect; that is, the longer and heavier the smoking or tobacco use or exposure, the greater the risk for the development of neoplasms.

Microbes

Viral infections are estimated to be responsible for 15% of all human cancers. The most prevalent of these is caused by human papillomavirus (HPV) and the hepatitis viruses. HPV is transmitted during sexual intercourse to the female cervix where certain strains of the virus can lead to cervical cancer. The hepatitis B or C viruses can lead to hepatocellular cancer.

Viruses vary by the mechanisms leading to neoplasia. For example, retroviruses, such as HIV, can alter genes or proteins that regulate these genes directly and also render the immune system defenseless. In the process of carcinogenesis, viral proteins are necessary to initiate, maintain, or enhance the malignant phenotype. A few bacteria, such as *Helicobacter pylori*, are also considered carcinogenic. Chronic inflammation, a common complication of chronic infection, is known to support tumor growth.

Initiation–Promotion–Progression Theory

Carcinogenesis is a highly complex process. Multiple steps are involved in the development of neoplasms, and several theories have been suggested. One such theory proposes that an initiating event must be combined with a promoting event for cancer to develop and then progress (Fig. 7.4). This initiation–promotion–progression theory underscores the idea of cofactors in cancer etiology. The **initiating event** causes a mutation in a cell. The initiating event may eventually be identified, but many times it is not. The **promoting event** is an expansion of the mutated cell's growth and reproduction. The continued growth of the cell depends on continued exposure to the promoter. A common cancer promoter is chronic inflammation. For example, chronic gastritis has been implicated in the development of gastric cancer. Other cancer promoters include hormones and chemicals in the environment. **Progression** is an extension of the promotion phase with one exception: now the cancerous growth is no longer dependent on continued exposure to the promoter. The growth now becomes autonomous. The cell is capable of functioning outside of the rules that regulate cell growth, division, and death. If either the

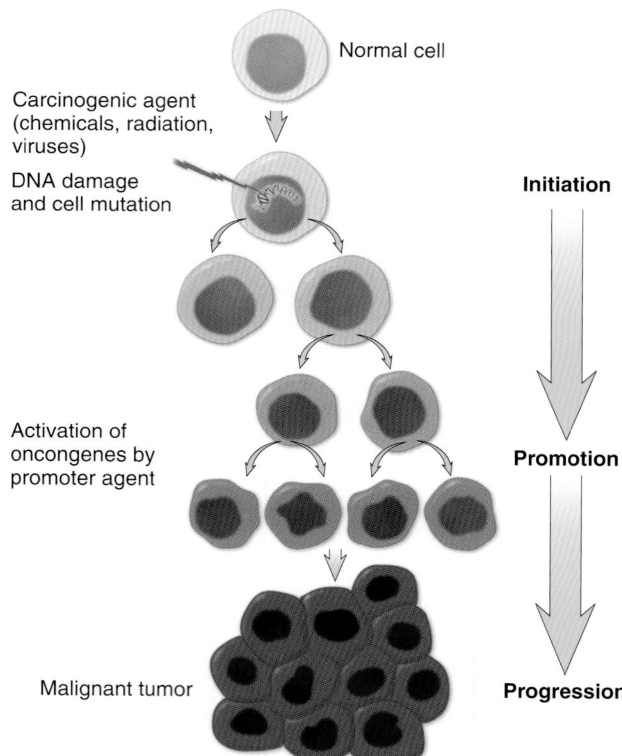

Figure 7.4. Initiation–promotion–progression theory. Initiation involves the exposure of cells to a carcinogenic agent. A promoter agent activates promotion and unregulated cell growth begins. Progression is the acquisition of independent growth of tumor cells. (Modified from Porth CM. *Essentials of Pathophysiology: Concepts of Altered Health States*. Philadelphia, PA: Lippincott Williams & Wilkins; 2003, with permission.)

initiating or promoting event occurs in isolation, or if the promoter occurs before the initiator, cancer does not develop.

Often, the exact initiator-promoter event is not clearly identified. Also, and perhaps most importantly, not all individuals who are exposed to a cancer-causing agent develop cancerous neoplasms. This fact highlights the complex interaction of heredity and the environment in the etiology and promotion of cancer.

Module 2 The Impact of Cancer on Tissues, Organs, and Organ Systems

Neoplasms exhibit autonomy and anaplasia. **Autonomy** refers to the unregulated proliferation of the neoplasm. **Anaplasia** refers to the loss of cell differentiation and therefore the loss of cell function. The greater the degree of anaplasia the more aggressive, or malignant, the tumor will be. When analyzing cells under a microscope, those with greater anaplasia show wide variation in size and shape with enlarged nuclei and rapid, atypical mitosis (Fig. 7.5).

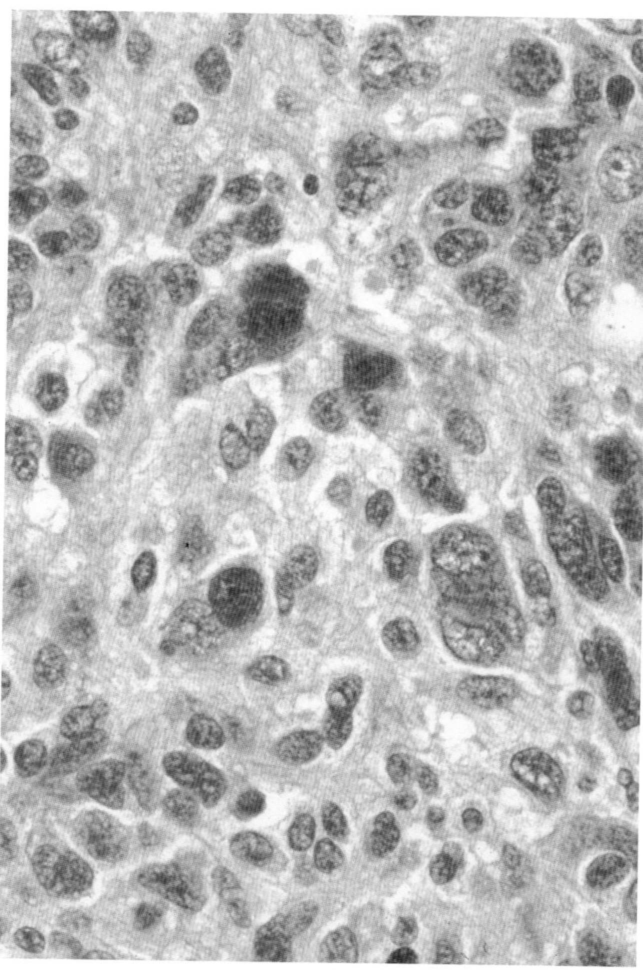

Figure 7.5. Cells with greater anaplasia show wide variation in size and shape with enlarged nuclei.

Neoplasms exhibit several other distinct characteristics:

- Loss of cell-to-cell communication, which allows further unrestricted growth of tumor cells
- Increased energy expenditure, which deprives unaffected cells of nutrients
- Increased motility and loss of cohesion/adhesion, which promotes movement to other locations
- Rapid angiogenesis, which provides extensive blood flow to the tumor cells
- Substance secretion, which alters the metabolism and degrades neighboring unaffected cells
- Presence of foreign antigens on the cancer cell surface, which can trigger the immune response

Proliferating cells are typically sensitive to the presence of neighboring cells. During wound healing, when cell-to-cell contact is established, the cells no longer reproduce. When this contact is lost, DNA, RNA, and proteins are triggered to synthesize new cells. Neoplastic cells are not sensitive to cell-to-cell messages. The neoplastic cells do not recognize that other cells are nearby and do not respond accordingly by decreasing the rate of reproduction. Neoplasms exhibit deviant and excessive growth factors that allow rapid reproduction and angiogenesis (development of new blood vessels) to meet the extreme nutrient demands of the tumor cells. The blood flow demands of neoplastic cells deprive neighboring tissues of adequate oxygen and other nutrients, which result in tissue ischemia and necrosis. The tumor cells can also secrete enzymes that degrade the extracellular matrix and allow the tumor to move into neighboring tissues.

Cellular mutations and aberrations are seen as a type of cellular injury that is subject to destruction by the inflammatory and immune responses. The tumor cells express antigens seen as foreign to the host. Many cellular transformations are removed from the body by these active defense mechanisms and never progress to form tumors in the body. Immunodeficiency, therefore, results in a much higher risk for the development of cancer.

Benign Versus Malignant

Tumors are classified as benign or malignant (Fig. 7.6). The terms benign and malignant refer to the tumor location and appearance related to the tissue of origin (the unaffected tissue surrounding the neoplasm). Typically, tumors that remain localized and closely resemble the tissue of origin are considered **benign**. In other words, benign tumors overproliferate but do not demonstrate a significant loss of differentiation. Benign tumors are often met with a sigh of relief; however, benign is not always equivalent to harmless. Large benign tumors can impinge on nearby structures, obstruct vital functions, and can even result in death. In some cases, benign growths, such as polyps or skin tags, are recognized as tumors but are not actually neoplastic.

Tumors that are invasive, destructive, proliferate rapidly, spread to other sites (metastasize), and do not resemble the tissue of origin are considered **malignant**. Malignant tumors can promote ischemia and necrosis of tissue because the tumor uses energy and nutrients needed by unaffected tissues. As stated previously, the term cancer is usually equated with malignant neoplasms.

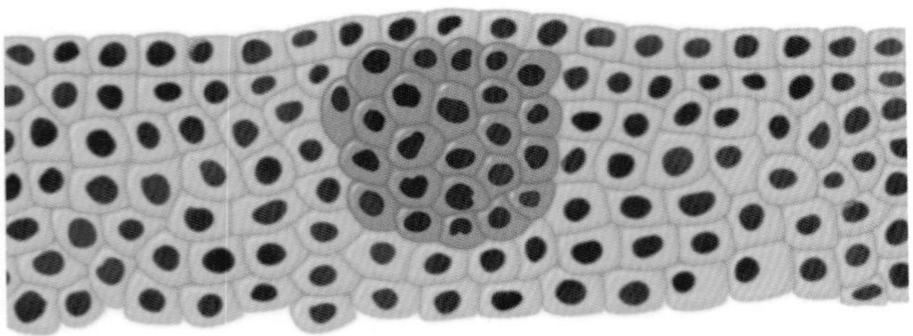

A

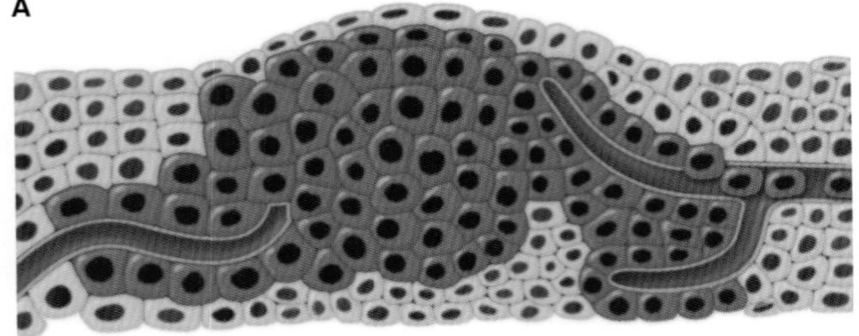

B

Figure 7.6. Benign versus malignant tumors. **A:** Benign tumor shows a slow-growing mass that has not yet invaded nearby tissues. **B:** Malignant tumor shows aggressive cell growth and invasion into nearby tissues and blood vessels.

Cancer Spread

Neoplasms invade locally by impinging on and moving into nearby tissues. **Local spread** is the proliferation of the neoplasm within the tissue of origin. Enlargement of tumors within the tissue or organ promotes loss of function and can result in obstruction, hemorrhage, and necrosis. Although the tumor is getting larger, it remains localized at this early stage. Obviously, confined neoplastic growths equate to a more favorable prognosis.

Direct extension is a process of tumor cells moving into adjacent tissues and organs. This aspect of invasion beyond the local tissues is a defining characteristic of malignancy. Penetration of the basement membrane is the first step for epithelial tumors. Those tumors located in areas without a basement membrane incur less resistance to invade distally. The neoplastic cells adhere to the extracellular matrix by expressing surface adhesion molecules. The tumor proceeds by releasing enzymes that dissolve the extracellular matrix. Once free of the confines of the local tissue or organ, the tumor travels to nearby structures, adheres to adjacent extracellular matrices, and again releases enzymes that degrade the neighboring matrix and allow the tumor to move into the nearby tissues and organs. **Seeding** is a form of direct extension in which neoplastic proliferation occurs within peritoneal and pleural cavities surrounding the affected tissue or organ. The malignant tumors move along these membranes and can gain easy access to other organs supported within these cavities.

Metastases occur when neoplasms are spread to distant sites often by way of the lymphatics or blood vessels (Fig. 7.7). The lethal aspect of cancer is metastatic growth. Once the neoplasm has moved to a distant site, detection and treatment become much more complex.

The mechanism for movement of neoplasms to distant sites is a process of adherence and degradation with the addition of access to the blood and lymphatics. The tumor cells accomplish this by:

1. Breaking through the basement membrane (if present) and extracellular matrix
2. Gaining access to and circulating within the blood vessels or lymph system
3. Leaving the blood vessels or lymph system and adhering to distant tissues
4. Establishing a new nutrient network at the distant tissues through a process of angiogenesis

Tumors can access distant sites most readily through the lymphatic system. Lymphatic capillaries and venules are thinner than other blood and lymphatic vessels and are therefore less resistant to

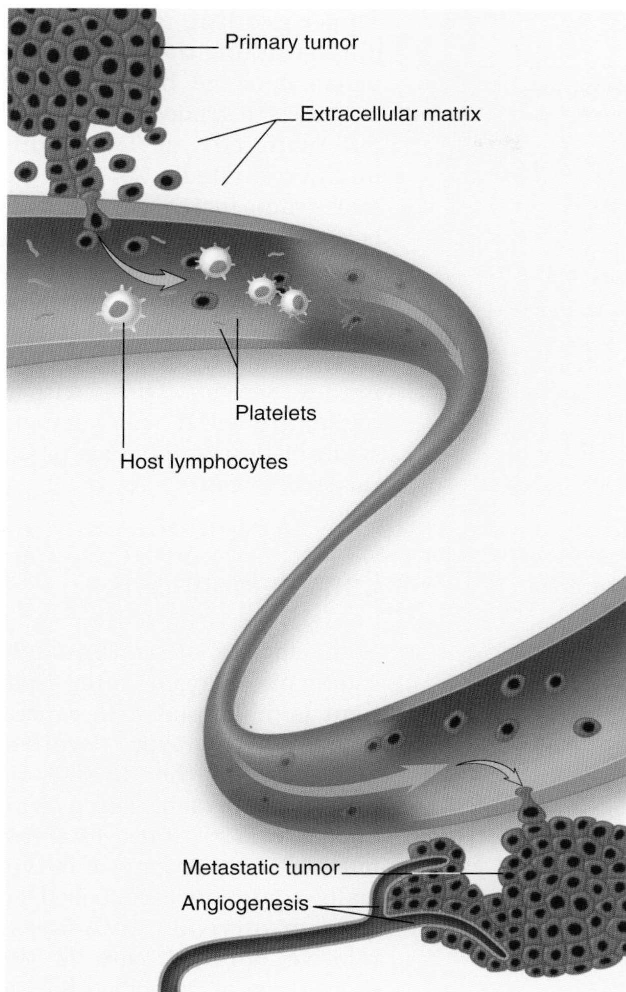

Figure 7.7. Metastatic spread of tumors through the vascular system. A primary benign tumor shows a slow-growing mass that has not invaded nearby tissues. A malignant tumor shows aggressive cell growth and invasion into nearby tissues and blood vessel.

invasion by neoplasms. The neoplasm binds to endothelial cells in the vessels, releases enzymes that degrade the vessel wall, and moves into the blood or lymph circulation. If the immune defense is unsuccessful, the tumor cells then travel through the circulation to distant sites, attach and move through vessel walls, exit the circulation, and move into the distant site. Once inside the new location, the neoplasm must reestablish a nutrient network through a process of angiogenesis. The tumor secretes growth factors that allow the development of vascular flow to the proliferating neoplasm at the distant site. Vessels are generated, and the tumor continues to proliferate.

The preferred location of the newly settled neoplasm is somewhat predictable. Organ **tropism** is a term used to describe the affinity of a primary tumor to a specific distant site. Factors that promote preferential relocation include:

1. A favorable environment offered by the new tissue or organ
2. Adherence molecule compatibility between the neoplasm and the new tissue or organ
3. The location of the organ in relation to the path of blood flow

For example, tumors that originate in the colon are prone to metastasizing in the liver. This is related to easy access of colon tumor cells through the veins of the portal circulation, which travels directly to the liver, allowing adherence of tumor cells to this organ. Another common site for metastatic growth is the lung, where tumor cells adhere after being transported through the vena cava. Organ tropism is also demonstrated in tumors that move from the lung to the brain and from the breast or prostate to the bone.

Cancer Nomenclature

Identification of the tumor type based on the tissue of origin is a common method of naming neoplasms. Although not used consistently, the suffix "oma" is often employed to designate tumors based on cell or tissue of origin. The cell or tissue of origin is placed directly before this suffix in *benign* tumors. For example, a benign tumor of the squamous epithelium is referred to as an **epithelioma**. When the same cell origin presents as fingerlike projections, it is referred to as a **papilloma**. Benign tumors of glandular epithelial origin are termed **adenomas**; those that arise from germ cells are called **teratomas**; those that arise from bone cells are known as **osteomas**; and those stemming from chondrocytes are called **chondromas**.

When the tumor is *malignant*, the cell or tissue prefix and the suffix "oma" remain with one addition: "carcin" is placed in the middle to designate malignant epithelial cells, and "sarc" is placed in the middle to designate malignant connective tissue cells. For example, a malignant tumor of epithelial cells is called an **adenocarcinoma**. A malignant tumor of chondrocytes is a **chondrosarcoma**. As indicated, this nomenclature does not always follow a consistent pattern. Lymphoma, melanoma, leukemia, and hepatoma are all malignant neoplasms. Table 7.1 further distinguishes benign and malignant tumor nomenclature.

Carcinoma in situ is a unique term used to describe carcinomas confined to the epithelium that have not yet penetrated the basement membrane. These neoplasms remain "in situ" for an indefinite

Table 7.1 Tumor Nomenclature

Tissue Type	Benign Tumors	Malignant Tumors
Epithelial		
Surface	Papilloma	Squamous cell carcinoma
Glandular	Adenoma	Adenocarcinoma
Endothelial		
Blood vessels	Hemangioma	Hemangiosarcoma
Lymph vessels	Lymphangioma	Lymphangiosarcoma
Connective		
Fibrous	Fibroma	Fibrosarcoma
Adipose	Lipoma	Liposarcoma
Cartilage	Chondroma	Chondrosarcoma
Bone	Osteoma	Osteosarcoma
Muscle		
Smooth muscle	Leiomyoma	Leiomyosarcoma
Striated muscle	Rhabdomyoma	Rhabdomyosarcoma
Neural		
Glial tissue	Glioma	Glioblastoma, astrocytoma, medulloblastoma, or oligodendroglioma
Meninges	Meningioma	Meningeal sarcoma
Blood		
Granulocyte		Myelocytic leukemia
Erythrocyte		Polycythemia vera
Plasma cells		Multiple myeloma
Lymphocyte		Lymphocytic leukemia or lymphoma

period. During this time, the tumor is often asymptomatic. Detection of tumors in situ represents a favorable prognosis. However, many carcinomas are not detected until the tumor cells penetrate the basement membrane and metastasize to distant organs.

Cancer Classifications

Staging is a process of classifying the extent or spread of neoplasms and refers to the tumor size, location, lymph node involvement, and spread (Fig. 7.8). The higher the number, the more extensive the tumor size and spread. Treatment decisions are often based on staging criteria. The TNM classification system is frequently used to stage tumors (Table 7.2). TNM stands for:

- T = tumor size. Indicates the presence and size of the primary tumor.
- N = node (lymph) involvement. Indicates involvement of regional lymph nodes.
- M = metastases. Indicates the extent of metastases.

Tumor **grading** is a process of differentiating the level of anaplasia depicted by the tumor. Tumors are graded from I (well differentiated) to IV (highly undifferentiated). As the tumor grade increases, the cells become more deviant from the tissue of origin. Those that are graded lower (I or II) resemble the tissue of origin in terms of size, shape, structure, and mitotic activity. Those with a higher grade (III or IV) demonstrate little resemblance to the tissue of origin.

Cancer Prognosis

Many factors affect the likely course and outcome after a patient is diagnosed with cancer, including the type, location, and stage of the disease, as well as the person's age, overall health, and response to treatment. Cancer prognosis is typically communicated based on a 5-year survival rate. A 5-year relative survival rate is the percentage of persons who are living 5 years after diagnosis. The 5-year survival rate includes those who are cancer free, in remission, or living with cancer.

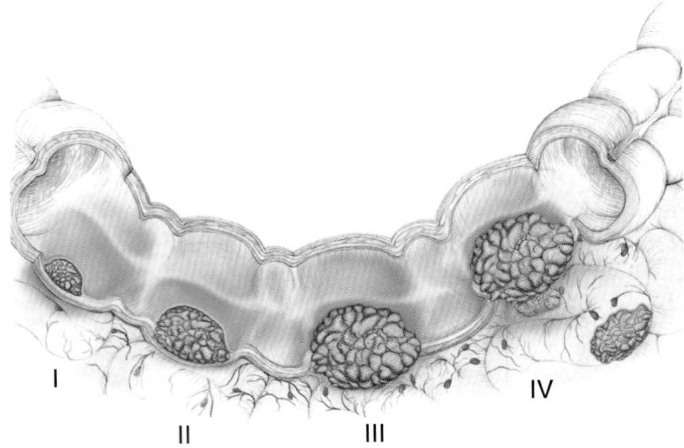

Figure 7.8. Tumor staging, I through IV. The size of the tumor and local to distant invasion increases with higher numeric staging. (Asset provided by Anatomical Chart Company.)

Table 7.2 TNM Classification System

Classification	Description
Primary Tumor (T)	
TX	Primary tumor cannot be evaluated
T0	No evidence of primary tumor
Tis	Carcinoma in situ (early cancer that has not spread to neighboring tissue)
T1, T2, T3, T4	Size or extent of the primary tumor
Regional Lymph Nodes (N)	
NX	Regional lymph nodes cannot be evaluated
N0	No regional lymph node involvement (no cancer found in the lymph nodes)
N1, N2, N3	Involvement of regional lymph nodes (number and/or extent of spread)
Distant Metastasis (M)	
MX	Distant metastasis cannot be evaluated
M0	No distant metastasis (cancer has not spread to other parts of the body)
M1	Distant metastasis (cancer has spread to distant parts of the body)

TNM, tumor size, node, metastases.
Reprinted with permission from Greene F, Page D, Morrow M, et al. *AJCC Cancer Staging Manual*. 6th ed. New York, NY: Springer; 2002.

General Manifestations

Early manifestations of neoplasms are often vague and ignored and are a result of:

1. Inflammatory and immune responses to the neoplasm
2. Increased metabolic rate induced by the neoplasm
3. Local effects of neoplastic cell encroachment or obstruction on neighboring tissues
4. Systemic effects of the neoplasm seemingly unrelated to cancer (paraneoplastic syndromes)

General manifestations indicating inflammatory and immune responses include lymphadenopathy, fever, and anorexia. Lymphadenopathy, a condition of enlarged lymph nodes throughout the body, is a condition of hyperplasia of the lymph nodes from lymphocyte activity, specifically against the developing neoplasm. The immunoreactivity that accompanies neoplasias is often a low-grade, chronic hyperplasia that is nontender. The supraclavicular nodes are often described as sentinel lymph nodes—these are often the first lymph nodes to receive lymphatic drainage from a malignant tumor.

Unexplained fever is also a common manifestation of cancer. Fever results from the release of pyrogens directly from cancer cells and other cells active in the inflammatory response (Chapter 3). Similarly, anorexia (loss of appetite) is a manifestation present within the inflammatory response caused by the presence of circulating chemical mediators. Anorexia can also result from changes in taste receptors (the mechanism is unclear) that can accompany tumor cell growth.

Neoplastic cells require a lot of energy for rapid, uncontrolled proliferation. Inflammatory mediators, along with excess energy use by the proliferating neoplastic cells, can result in unexplained weight loss and tissue wasting. When severe, neoplasias can lead to a syndrome called **cachexia** (Fig. 7.9). Cachexia is believed to be a result of early feelings of fullness with eating coupled with the release of chemical mediators, such as tumor necrosis factor, that induce a lack

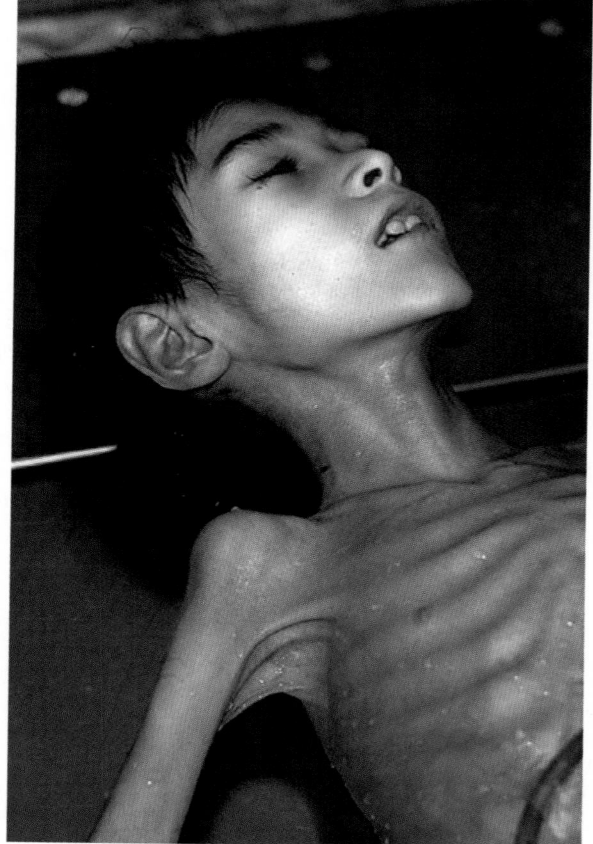

Figure 7.9. Cachexia of malignancy. This photo is of a patient with pancreatic carcinoma. The wasting away of body tissue is not entirely a matter of lost appetite.

of appetite. Tumor necrosis factor also suppresses the enzymes that are needed to release fatty acids from lipoproteins for use by tissues. The presence of high levels of tumor necrosis factor makes lipid energy unavailable to the tissues and promotes tissue wasting.

Local manifestations are site dependent and are related to (1) the space occupied by the tumor that impinges on the local structures; and (2) the loss of function in the tissue or organ that is being "taken over" by the tumor. Tumor cells are destructive to neighboring tissues and cause bleeding, bruising, and poor wound healing. Crowding of blood cells in the bone marrow can result in suppression of RBC and platelet production. Hemorrhage, also a common manifestation of tissue destruction caused by tumor-secreted enzymes, contributes to loss of blood cells. Anemia, bruising, and poor clotting are common effects of these alterations in the blood.

A palpable mass is often the first clinical manifestation that may present in tumors such as those found in the breast, testicle, and lymph nodes. In later stages, compression on nearby structures can elicit a pain response, such as a chronic headache with brain tumors, bone pain with proliferating cells crowding in the bone marrow, and abdominal pain that can occur in pancreatic cancer. Loss of function may also provide clues to the presence of neoplasms. Constipation, diarrhea, and blood in the stool may be evident in colon cancer. Cough, hemoptysis (blood in sputum), and shortness of breath are often present in lung cancer (Box 7.1).

Stop and Consider

How is delayed wound healing, as a clinical manifestation of cancer, explained by the deregulation of the destruction and regeneration/repair balance of the extracellular matrix during tumor invasion?

Paraneoplastic syndromes are hormonal, neurologic, hematologic, and chemical disturbances in the body, which are not directly related to invasion by the primary tumor or metastasis. Along with the local effects exerted by a growing tumor, paraneoplastic syndromes are often responsible for the range of clinical manifestations that can occur. For example, a significant characteristic of many neoplasms is the ability to produce and secrete ectopic hormones. **Ectopic** refers to hormone secretion from a site outside of an endocrine gland. The ectopic hormones are not under the regulatory control of the endocrine system and do not respond to the feedback mechanisms typical of that system. In some cases, substances are secreted by the tumor that mimic the hormone function and result in clinical manifestations characteristic of an oversecretion of that hormone. For example, some tumors secrete excess antidiuretic hormone. This hormone signals the body to retain water and sodium. The individual will present with widespread edema; this condition, when severe, can lead to coma and death.

Paraneoplastic syndromes can also present as a disturbance in neurologic function. As presented in the previous example, tumors can secrete hormones that disturb fluid and electrolyte balance, and this directly affects neurologic functioning. Tumors can also cause generalized numbness, weakness, and loss of neurologic function through several mechanisms, including promoting brain hemorrhage, promoting infection in the central nervous system, or denying the vascular supply and oxygen to neuronal tissues.

Box 7.1 ABCDE: The Warning Signs of Skin Cancer

The following characteristics warrant further examination by a health care practitioner:

Asymmetry: A mole that is irregularly shaped
Border: A mole with jagged edges without clear definition
Color: A growth that is multicolored or that changes color
Diameter: A sudden increase in a mole size, especially one that is greater than 6 mm across (the size of a pencil eraser)
Elevation: A flat mole that becomes elevated

Diagnostic Tests

Coupled with a complete history and physical examination, the following diagnostic tests can be used to determine the presence and extent of neoplasms:

- Imaging studies
- Biopsy and cytology studies
- Tumor markers and other blood, urine, or tissue tests

Imaging studies allow direct visualization of tumor masses via radiographs (X-rays), endoscopic examination, ultrasound, computed tomography (CT), or magnetic resonance imaging (MRI) scans. These tests are useful in determining the presence, size, and location of tumors. Once the tumor has been located, tissue samples can be removed (biopsy) and these cells examined (cytology) to determine the presence and stage of neoplasms. In most cases, a definitive diagnosis of cancer can be made only with a microscopic examination of tumor cells.

Tumor markers are substances that may be detected in cells or body fluids and can provide clues to the presence, extent, and treatment response of certain neoplasms. Tumor markers may be produced by the tumor itself or by unaffected cells in the body in response to the presence of a malignant or benign tumor. Hundreds of tumor markers are used to identify various types of tumors.

Tumor markers can be comprised of hormones, enzymes, and immunoglobulins. Many tumor markers are expressed as protein antigens. For example, prostate-specific antigen (PSA), produced by cells in the prostate, is present in low concentrations in adult males. Elevations of PSA may be found in the blood of men with inflammation (prostatitis), benign enlargement (benign prostatic hypertrophy), and malignant neoplasms of the prostate. Similarly, CA 125 is an antigen-expressed tumor marker for ovarian cancer, but it may also be increased in uterine, cervical, pancreatic, lung, colon, breast, and gastrointestinal cancers. This tumor marker can also be increased in noncancerous conditions, such as pregnancy, pelvic inflammatory disease, pancreatitis, liver disease, and inflammatory conditions of the lung. Measurement of carcinoembryonic antigen (CEA) is primarily used to monitor colorectal cancer disease and treatment; however, a wide variety of other cancers can also produce elevations in CEA, including cancer of the lung, breast, pancreas, stomach, cervix, bladder, kidney, thyroid, liver, and ovary. Inflammatory conditions, such as inflammatory bowel disease, pancreatitis, and hepatitis, can also cause elevations in CEA levels.

As indicated previously, tumor markers can also be expressed in some noncancerous conditions and are not elevated in every person with cancer, especially in the early stages. In addition, many tumor markers are not specific to one type of cancer; that is, a tumor marker level can be elevated by more than one type of cancer. Therefore, tumor marker results are interpreted with caution. The measurement of tumor marker levels alone is *not* sufficient to diagnose cancer. Rather, these tests are most informative after diagnosis when results are compared over time. Monitoring tumor marker trends allows the ability to determine treatment effectiveness and to determine recurrence of the tumor after treatment.

Cancer Treatment

Treatment of cancer has three possible goals:

1. Completely eradicate the neoplasms
2. Control continued growth and spread
3. Reduce symptoms without curing the cancer

Major treatment strategies to achieve these goals include surgery, chemotherapy, radiation, hormones, and immunotherapy. Each of these therapeutic strategies can be used alone or in combination. Surgery, chemotherapy, and radiation are compared in Table 7.3. Bone marrow transplantation may also be used to replace or supplement blood cells in the bone marrow. Stem cell transplantation in the bone marrow has also shown promise as a therapeutic strategy for some types of cancer.

Table 7.3 Cancer Treatment Strategies

Treatment Strategy	Mechanism of Action	Adverse Effects/ Complications
Surgery	Directly removing the tumor, organ, or affected lymph nodes through a variety of surgical techniques; pathologic specimens are examined for clear margins denoting complete tumor removal	Inability to remove all of the tumor cells; bleeding; infection.
Chemotherapy	Administering medications systemically to interrupt tumor growth or kill tumor cells; combination therapy with two or more agents is common	Nausea, vomiting, hair loss, poor wound healing, immunosuppression, infections, bleeding.
Radiation	Using focal ionizing radiation to damage cell DNA and prevent further replication of the proliferating cells; external radiation (most common) is aimed at the tumor from outside of the body; internal radiation is implanted into or near the tumor in small capsules or other container; systemic radiation is a process of administering (oral or injected) unsealed radioactive materials that travel throughout the body	Skin penetration causes skin redness, irritation, itching, poor wound healing, skin ulceration, and, over time, hyperpigmentation and atrophy. Bleeding, infection, and anemia can result from loss of blood cells. Fibrosis of tissues and organs can occur, leading to diarrhea, esophageal or intestinal strictures, and fibrosis of the heart and lungs.
Biologic response modifiers (BMRs)	Altering the biologic response of the host most often achieved through stimulating the host immune response	Few, if any, adverse effects; BMRs selectively aid in destroying tumor cells without affecting the host cells.
Hormones	Manipulating tumors that depend on hormones by inhibiting RNA and protein synthesis and binding to receptor sites	Dependent on the expected response of the hormone used; the actions of the hormone are exaggerated.

Although treatment of the tumor is important, care of the *patient* with cancer and his or her family involves the provision of psychosocial support needed to address the anxiety and depression that may accompany such a diagnosis. This support may include addressing sexuality, spirituality, and other personal issues related to the diagnosis, treatment, and coping with cancer. The health professional must also be aware of and open to discussing alternative, complementary, or experimental therapies.

Palliative care is another important aspect of cancer treatment. **Palliative** care is the term frequently used to describe treating symptoms, such as pain, without curing the cancer. Common side effects of treatment include fatigue, nausea, vomiting, pruritus, and diarrhea. Care of the patient includes addressing complications of treatment and providing nutritional support for optimal health.

Cancer Prevention

Prevention of cancer involves avoiding known carcinogens, participating in health promotion activities, such as exercising moderately and consuming a balanced healthy diet, accepting vaccinations when indicated, and taking measures to protect against chronic injury, including exposure to reactive oxygen species. Individuals with light skin are most at risk for basal cell carcinoma and melanoma. Those with darker skin are protected by melanin pigment. The melanin absorbs ultraviolet radiation. Although those with darker skin are more protected, the skin is still vulnerable to burn injuries, and cancer can develop. Using sunscreen and keeping exposed skin areas covered help protect against and prevent skin cancers.

Many other types of cancer are also considered preventable, including those caused by tobacco use, heavy alcohol consumption, infection with carcinogenic microorganisms, and obesity. The American Cancer Society estimates that one in three cancer deaths are caused by tobacco use.[1] In addition, preventable cancer deaths can be linked to nutritional factors, physical inactivity, or obesity.[1] Vaccination against certain viral infections may also reduce the cancer incidence. For example, vaccination against hepatitis B virus should decrease the incidence of hepatocellular cancer.

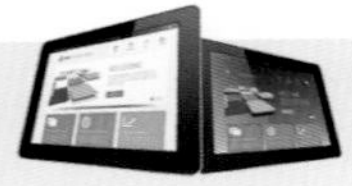

RESEARCH NOTES

Cancer drugs are broadly classified into two categories: cytotoxic chemotherapies (those that directly kill cancer cells) and targeted therapies (those that modulate the activity of one or more proteins involved in cancer). Research has focused more recently on developing targeted therapies, specifically to interfere with oncogenes. The researchers report, "... novel approaches, including synthetic lethality and collateral vulnerability screens, are now being developed to target gene defects in p53, PTEN, and BRCA1/2." These show promise in targeting tumor suppressors in cancer therapeutics.[2]

Children and Cancer

Although rare, cancer is the leading cause of death by disease in children ages 1 through 14 years. Whereas most adult cancers involve tissues and solid organs with an epithelial origin (carcinomas), such as colon cancer, lung cancer, and breast cancer, most childhood cancers originate in the mesodermal germ layer, which develops into bone, blood, blood vessels, muscle, lymphatics, connective tissue, and kidneys. Therefore, the types of cancer most prevalent in childhood are leukemia (31%), brain/spinal cord tumors (21%), neuroblastoma (7%), Wilms tumor (6%), Hodgkin lymphoma (4%), non-Hodgkin lymphoma (4%), rhabdomyosarcoma (3%), retinoblastoma (3%), osteosarcoma (3%), and Ewing sarcoma (2%). Neoplasms that resemble embryonic tissue can originate during embryonic and fetal development and persist to form tumors in the body. These embryonic tumors are most often manifested prior to age 5 years.

The cause of childhood cancer more often has an inherited, gene variant, or epigenetic basis because children have had limited exposure to environmental exposures, such as chemicals, and limited time to participate in harmful health behaviors, such as smoking. Those with inherited mutations include retinoblastoma (retina), Wilms tumor (kidney), and osteosarcoma (bone).

Detection of cancer in children is often difficult. Unexplained clinical manifestations that should alert parents and health professionals to a potential problem include: unusual mass or swelling, pallor, persistent malaise, bruising, sudden and persistent pain, limping gait, fever, prolonged illness, headaches, vision changes, and excessive, rapid weight loss. Dramatic improvements in survival of children have occurred over the past 20 years because of advances in treatment. The average 5-year survival rate for all cancer types is greater than 75%.

Module 3 Clinical Models

The following clinical models were selected to help apply knowledge related to altered cellular proliferation and differentiation. Note the commonalities of cellular autonomy and anaplasia. Recognize the differences in clinical manifestations and diagnosis based on the tumor types and locations.

Lung Cancer

Carcinoma of the lung is the leading cause of cancer deaths in the world. Smoking and other environmental toxin exposures are unequivocally implicated in the carcinogenesis.

PATHOPHYSIOLOGY

The onset of lung cancer is most often the result of environmental exposures to particular toxins combined with a genetic susceptibility to these toxins. Active smoking is responsible for approximately 90% of lung cancer cases. The majority of remaining cases are attributed to occupational exposures, such as with asbestos and radon. In a very small percentage, there are no known environmental triggers. For the vast majority, repeated exposure to smoking and environmental toxins cause DNA damage and induce mutations in the *ras* family of oncogenes, *Rb*, *p53* and other tumor suppressor genes. Specific to adenocarcinoma, which is the most common type of lung cancer, *ras* gene activation contributes to tumor progression. There are two major categories of lung cancer:

- Non-small cell lung cancer (85%)
  - Adenocarcinomas are the most common form of lung cancer in the United States. Neoplasms develop in the peripheral bronchiolar and alveolar lung tissue leading to pleural fibrosis and adhesions (Fig. 7.10).
  - Squamous cell carcinoma begins with injury to the bronchial columnar epithelium (i.e., from smoking) and leads to squamous metaplasia, dysplasia, carcinoma in situ, and an invasive tumor.
  - Large cell carcinomas are those that are neither adenocarcinomas nor squamous cell. The tumor cells are large and show a high level of anaplasia.
- Small cell lung cancer (15%) is a highly malignant epithelial tumor that grows and metastasizes rapidly. This form of cancer is highly linked to smoking.

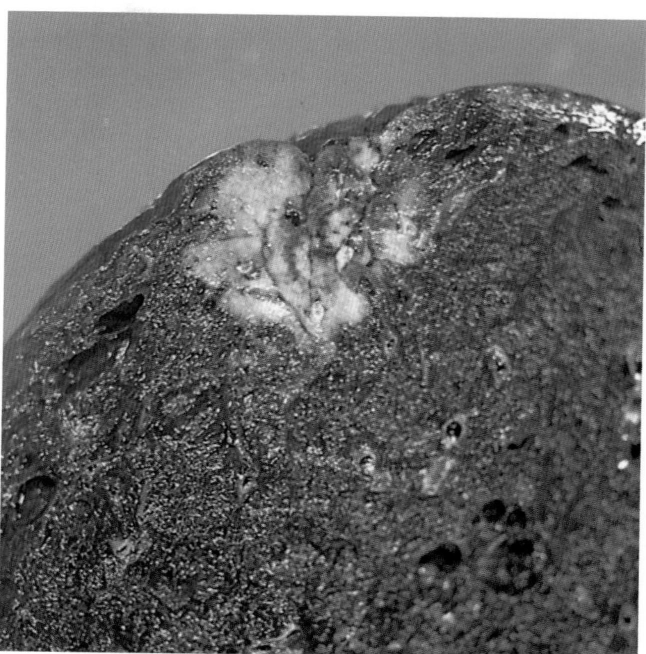

Figure 7.10. Adenocarcinoma of the lung. Adenocarcinoma is the most common type of lung cancer and often begins in the peripheral bronchiolar and alveolar lung tissue. This tumor is found in the upper right lobe of the lung. (Modified from Rubin E, Farber JL. *Pathology*. 4th ed. Philadelphia, PA: Lippincott Williams & Wilkins; 2005.)

In all forms of lung cancer, the neoplasms can penetrate epithelial layers and move into the lung tissue, pleural cavity, chest wall, and beyond. The location of large lung tumors allows compression on lower cervical and upper thoracic nerves. Metastatic spread occurs via lymph channels and the vascular system. Lung carcinoma is organ tropic to the bone, liver, and the brain.

CLINICAL MANIFESTATIONS

The most common clinical manifestations for all lung cancer subtypes are persistent cough, hemoptysis (bloody sputum), chest pain, and shortness of breath. These clinical manifestations are often ignored and explained away as "smoker's cough" or bronchitis. General systemic manifestations and paraneoplastic syndromes discussed earlier also apply to lung carcinoma.

DIAGNOSTIC CRITERIA

A physical examination, complete blood count, and chest X-ray are completed when the patient presents with cough, hemoptysis, chest pain, and or shortness of breath. The diagnosis is confirmed and the type of cell identified through bronchoscopy, sputum cytology, and tissue biopsy.

Staging lung cancer is based on whether or not the cancer has spread from the lungs to the lymph nodes or other organs. Because signs and symptoms are often ignored, early-stage lung cancer (stages I and II) is difficult to detect. Most people with lung cancer are diagnosed at stages III and IV.

- **Stage I:** The cancer is located only in the lungs and has not spread to any lymph nodes.
- **Stage II:** The cancer is in the lung and nearby lymph nodes.
- **Stage III:** Cancer is found in the lung and in the lymph nodes in the middle of the chest, also described as locally advanced disease.
- **Stage IV:** This is the most advanced stage of lung cancer, and is also described as advanced disease. This is when the cancer has spread to both lungs, to fluid in the area around the lungs, or to another part of the body, such as the liver or other organs.[3]

TREATMENT

Lung cancer has a high mortality rate. Treatment selection is based on identification of the tumor type as either small cell or non–small cell (adenocarcinoma, squamous cell, and large cell) lung carcinoma. Small cell carcinoma is more likely to respond to chemotherapy, yet is also more likely to be widely disseminated at diagnosis. Because patients with small cell carcinoma tend to develop distant metastases, surgical resection and radiation rarely contribute to long-term survival.

Treatment of non–small cell carcinomas is often based on the ability or inability to resect (surgically remove) all or part of the tumor. If non–small cell carcinomas (adenocarcinoma, squamous carcinoma, and large cell carcinoma) can be surgically removed, the cancer may be cured by surgery alone or by surgery and chemotherapy. If the tumor cannot be surgically removed, local control of the tumor may be achieved with radiation therapy, but cure is unlikely. The 5-year survival rate is dependent upon the stage at diagnosis. For those with early recognition and a local tumor, the 5-year survival rate is 49%; however, this drops to 16% for those with regional involvement, and to 2% for those with distant metastases.[3]

Colon Cancer

Colon cancer is the most frequently occurring type of gastrointestinal (GI) tract cancer. As with other forms of cancer, it is multifactorial in origin and occurs as a result of genetic changes, environmental exposures, dietary influences, and is increased with those who have chronic inflammatory conditions of the GI tract.

PATHOPHYSIOLOGY

Although the exact cause is often not clearly established, the primary risk factor is age. More than 90% of cases are diagnosed in adults over the age of 50 years. Other risk factors include family history of colorectal cancer, smoking, alcohol consumption, chronic inflammatory bowel disease, obesity, and physical inactivity, and a diet high in fat and low in fruits and vegetables. Although this finding is controversial, higher amounts of fiber in the diet have been shown to bind to potential mutagens and move contents more quickly through the colon and therefore may prevent neoplasms. A reduced fat diet may decrease the secretion of bile into the intestine and limit the exposure of the bowel to the tumor-promoting effects of bile acids. Nutrients with a protective effect against colorectal cancer include selenium and vitamins E, C, and A, as well as vegetables such as broccoli, cauliflower, cabbage, and brussels sprout.

Tumors in the colon or rectum can range from benign polyps to invasive tumors and are most often of epithelial origin, termed adenomas or adenocarcinomas. These are classified according to three groups:

1. Nonneoplastic polyps (not generally considered a cancer precursor)
2. Neoplastic polyps (adenomatous polyps, adenomas; increased risk of developing carcinoma of the colon/rectum)
3. Cancers (most often adenocarcinomas)

An average of nine major deleterious mutations are harbored within cancerous tumors of the colon/rectum and five to seven mutations are needed to promote the development of malignant tumors. At least two pathways have been identified that can lead from healthy epithelium to carcinoma:

1. A series of events triggering chromosomal instability (85%)
2. Replication errors (15%)

Chromosomal instability is based on alterations in chromosome number (aneuploidy) and chromosomal deletions, particularly of chromosomes 5q, 18q, 17p, and the mutation of the *KRAS* oncogene.[4] Chromosomal instability leads to a loss of tumor suppressor function, and impaired DNA repair is heavily implicated in the transformation to adenocarcinomas. Early activation of neoplasia is often related to a mutated loss of a tumor suppressor gene called *APC* (adenomatous polyposis coli) gene. Mutations in the *APC* gene lead to adenomatous polyps, which are considered a major precursor to malignant tumor development. Replication errors differ in that the chromosomes remain intact, but the patient has still acquired defects in DNA repair, allowing mutated neoplasia-promoting genes to promote cancerous transformations.

In both scenarios (chromosomal instability and replication errors), the cellular transformation that forms in the mucosal epithelium of the bowel begins at the base of the **crypts**, or mucosal epithelial depressions (Fig. 7.11). This is the area where mitosis occurs. As the cell matures, it moves up the crypt and eventually reaches the surface of the bowel where the cell then dies and is sloughed off and removed through the colon. With *APC* gene mutation, tumor cells in the bowel resist apoptosis and accumulate on the bowel surface. The cells continue to proliferate to form benign adenomatous polyps. Removal of benign adenomatous polyps can reduce the risk of the development of adenocarcinomas. Other mutations further promote the transformation to a malignant tumor, such as the deletion of other tumor suppressor genes: the *DCC* ("deleted in colon cancer") gene and the *p53* gene.

CLINICAL MANIFESTATIONS

Because of the widespread public health campaign promoting screening, colon cancer is now often detected before it starts to cause symptoms. When present, clinical manifestations of colorectal cancer depend on the location and characteristics of the tumor. Early stages of tumor development are often asymptomatic. As the tumor enlarges, ulceration and hemorrhage can result in **occult**, or hidden, blood in the stool if the tumor is along the ascending colon. **Frank**, or visible, blood in the stool, abdominal pain, and bowel obstruction are more likely if the tumor is located along the descending colon or in the rectum. Anemia, caused by blood loss in the stool, or a change in bowel habits may be the first diagnostic clue. General systemic manifestations and paraneoplastic syndromes also apply for colorectal cancer.

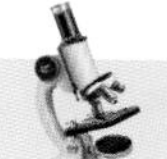

FROM THE LAB

Testing for occult blood in the stool involves taking a small sample of the stool and combining this with a chemically impregnated test strip. Guaiac or orthotolidine is an often-used chemical. These tests are often referred to as guaiac or Hemoccult tests. A positive test indicates the presence of occult blood in the stool and warrants further evaluation.

DIAGNOSTIC CRITERIA

Guidelines from the American College of Gastroenterology recommend colonoscopy every 10 years, beginning at age 50, as the preferred screening

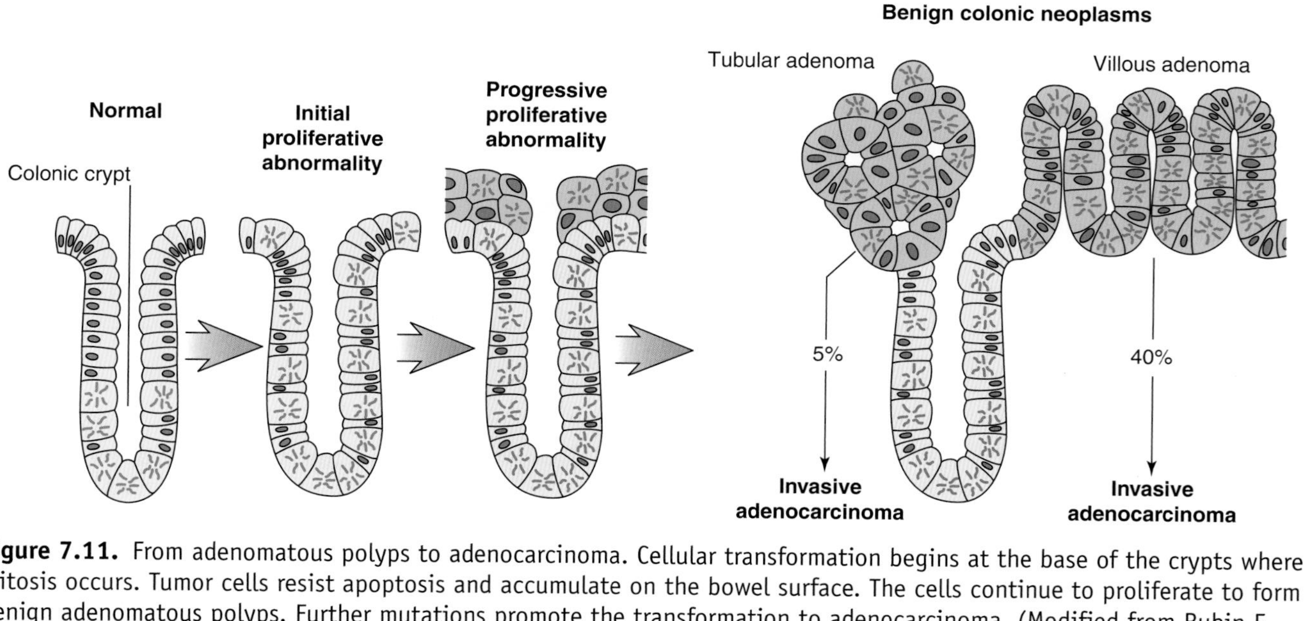

Figure 7.11. From adenomatous polyps to adenocarcinoma. Cellular transformation begins at the base of the crypts where mitosis occurs. Tumor cells resist apoptosis and accumulate on the bowel surface. The cells continue to proliferate to form benign adenomatous polyps. Further mutations promote the transformation to adenocarcinoma. (Modified from Rubin E, Farber JL. *Pathology*. 4th ed. Philadelphia, PA: Lippincott Williams & Wilkins; 2005.)

strategy.[4] Laboratory studies and diagnostic tests that may be helpful include:

- Complete blood count
- Liver function tests (colon cancer is organ tropic to the liver)
- Serum carcinoembryonic antigen (CEA)
- Colonoscopy
- Sigmoidoscopy
- Biopsy of suspicious lesions

The American Joint Committee on Cancer (AJCC) has designated staging of colorectal cancer using a modified TNM classification. Nodal and metastatic designations are identical to the classic TNM system. The tumor aspect of the classification depends on the extent of tumor progression through the bowel wall versus the size of the tumor. The modifications and staging for colorectal cancer are found in Table 7.4. Distant metastases, when present, are most often found in the liver.

TREATMENT

Colorectal cancer is highly treatable and often curable when localized in the bowel. Surgical treatment is required and results in cure (with localized tumors) in about 50% of patients. Those with unresectable, locally advanced, or metastatic disease are treated with combination drug chemotherapy, biological agents, and radiation as indicated. The prognosis of colorectal cancer is directly related to the location and degree of penetration of the tumor through the bowel, the presence of bowel obstruction or perforation, lymph node involvement, and the presence of distant metastases. The 5-year survival rate ranges from 95% for those with stage I disease to 10% for those diagnosed at stage IV.[4]

Table 7.4 TNM Classification and Staging for Colorectal Cancer

Classification or Stage	Description
Primary Tumor (T)	
TX	Primary tumor cannot be assessed
T0	No evidence of primary tumor
Tis	Carcinoma in situ
T1	Tumor invades submucosa
T2	Tumor invades muscularis propria
T3	Tumor invades through and into subserosa, or into perirectal tissues
T4	Tumor directly invades other organs or structure, and/or perforates visceral peritoneum
Regional Lymph Nodes (N)	
NX	Regional lymph nodes cannot be assessed
N0	No regional lymph node metastasis
N1	Metastasis in 1–3 regional lymph nodes
N2	Metastasis in 4 or more regional lymph nodes
Distant Metastasis (M)	
MX	Distant metastasis cannot be assessed
M0	No distant metastasis
M1	Distant metastasis
Staging Based on TNM	
Stage 0	Tis, N0, M0
Stage I	T1 or T2, N0, M0
Stage IIA	T3, N0, M0
Stage IIB	T4, N0, M0
Stage IIIA	T1 or T2, N0, M0
Stage IIIB	T3 or T4, N1, M0
Stage IIIC	Any T, N2, M0
Stage IV	Any T, Any N, M1

TNM, tumor size, node, metastases.
Reprinted with permission from Greene F, Page D, Morrow M, et al. *AJCC Cancer Staging Manual*. 6th ed. New York, NY: Springer; 2002.

Brain Cancer

Brain cancer is highly feared because of the possibility of developing severe disability, seizures, paralysis, and cognitive impairment. Brain tumors are one of the most common cancers in children, second to leukemia. Brain cancer, as a result of metastatic spread from another site such as the lungs, is much more common that primary brain tumors (those originating from the neural tissue). For example, it is estimated that upon autopsy, around 20% of patients with systemic cancer have brain metastases.[5] This may be due in part to exposure to cancer treatment with ionizing radiation, which increases the risk of developing tumors in the nervous system.

PATHOPHYSIOLOGY

Brain metastasis (spread from other tumor sites) along with gliomas, meningiomas, pituitary adenomas, and acoustic neuromas accounts for 95% of all brain tumors. Adults are more likely to develop primary supratentorial brain tumors.

Children are more likely to develop primary infratentorial brain tumors. Figure 7.12 depicts the distribution of these and other common intracranial tumors.

Gliomas, more specifically astrocytomas, are the most common tumor type originating in the brain. The specific genetic mutation or chromosomal aberration is variable depending on the subtype. For example, grade II diffuse astrocytomas most often occur in patients with inherited *p53* germline mutations or with a deletion of chromosome band 17p13.1.[5] Astrocytomas most often present in the brainstem or cerebellum of the child, spinal cord of young adults, and cerebral hemispheres of the adult. Astrocytomas vary in the level of differentiation at diagnosis. Approximately 20% are well differentiated, 40% are highly undifferentiated, and the remaining are somewhere in between. Gliomas can be benign or malignant. As gliomas enlarge, tumors impinge on vital brain structures and become fatal. Unlike other tumors, gliomas rarely metastasize outside of the CNS. Prognosis is based on the level of anaplasia; that is, the more undifferentiated the tumor, the poorer the prognosis.

The TNM classification is not used for brain tumors the following reasons:

- Tumor size is less relevant than the location and histology
- The brain and spinal cord have no lymphatics
- Most patients with CNS tumors do not live long enough to develop metastatic disease

Rather, the World Health Organization classification of CNS tumors is often used as it incorporates morphology, genetics, and immunologic markers (Table 7.5).

CLINICAL MANIFESTATIONS

Clinical manifestations of intracranial tumors depend on the size and location of the tumor. Neurologic deficits are created when the tumor erodes functional neurons. This results in specific motor or sensory losses, such as vision changes, numbness, weakness, or paralysis. Cognitive, behavioral, and personality changes are also common and may manifest as irritability, forgetfulness, and depression. Pressure increases in the cranium from the growing tumor, along with inflammation and fluid accumulation, lead to headaches (often a later sign) and vomiting. Seizures can also result from irritation and the subsequent disorderly discharge of neurons. Tumor compression on the respiratory and cardiac centers can result in death.

DIAGNOSTIC CRITERIA

Diagnosis of brain tumors is based on history and physical examination, including a complete neurologic examination. This neurologic examination involves testing cranial nerves, reflexes, sensory function, and motor function. Direct visualization of tumor growth via brain scans, radiographs, CT, MRI, and cerebral angiography will also aid in the diagnosis and prepare for removal of the tumor. Positron emission tomography (PET) scanning and spectroscopic evaluations are current strategies for diagnosing metastasis in the cerebrum. These tests are

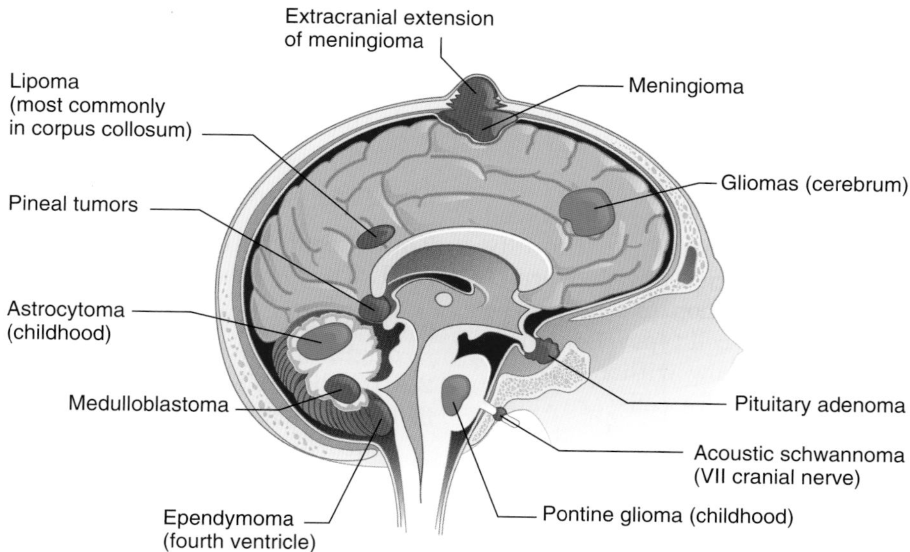

Figure 7.12. The most common locations for select intracranial tumors. Note that most tumors arise in the cerebral hemispheres. (Modified from Rubin E, Farber JL. *Pathology*. 4th ed. Philadelphia, PA: Lippincott Williams & Wilkins; 2005, with permission.)

Table 7.5 World Health Organization Grading of Central Nervous System Tumors

Grade	Description
Grade I	Lesions with low proliferative potential, discrete borders, and likely to be cured with surgical resection
Grade II	Lesions that are generally infiltrating and low in mitotic activity but recur; may progress to higher grades of malignancy
Grade III	Lesions with histologic evidence of malignancy associated with elevated mitotic activity, are infiltrative, and anaplastic
Grade IV	Lesions that are mitotically active, necrosis-prone, and generally associated with rapid proliferation

Reprinted with permission from Kleihues P, Burger P, Scheithauer B. The new WHO classification of brain tumours. *Brain Pathol.* 1993;3:255–268.

also useful for differentiating the metastases from other lesions in the brain.

TREATMENT

The treatment of brain cancer varies depending on the location, extent, and nature of the neoplasms. Primary tumors are treated with surgical resection whenever feasible. The goal of surgery is to remove the tumor as completely as possible while still preserving neurologic function. Radiation therapy also has a major role in treatment and is almost universally indicated. Chemotherapy, often administered into the spinal canal, may also be used to treat certain chemosensitive tumor types, such as gliomas, medulloblastomas, and some germ cell tumors. Chemotherapy may also be placed directly in the brain during surgery as a local treatment. For patients with metastases to the brain, whole brain radiation therapy (WBRT) may be needed because of widespread tumors. Palliative care is essential and may include the use of anticonvulsants to treat seizures.

Leukemia

Leukemias are malignant neoplasms of the blood and blood-forming organs. Leukemia (literally, "white blood") is most often associated with overproliferation and lack of differentiation in white blood cells, but it can also affect other cell types. Leukemia replaces cells in the bone marrow with immature, proliferating neoplasms. Immature cells are called **blast cells**. Nonfunctioning leukemic blast cells then circulate in the vascular system.

DNA changes in the blood cells can result from environmental exposures to ionizing radiation, alkylating drugs, chemicals, or internal factors, such as chromosomal abnormalities. Chromosomal abnormalities can activate cellular oncogenes that promote proliferation of blast cells.

The leukemias are classified as acute or chronic and are also classified according to cell type. Acute leukemias, as is the case with other acute conditions, are sudden and result in a rapid and noticeable loss of function. Chronic leukemias are more gradual in onset, and early symptoms, if any, are vague. The different cells affected by leukemia are either lymphoid or myeloid types. Lymphocytic leukemias involve immature lymphocytes that originate in the bone marrow. Myelogenous leukemias involve myeloid stem cells in the marrow. Leukemias can interfere with the maturation of all blood cells, including erythrocytes and platelets.

Acute Leukemias

Acute lymphocytic leukemia (ALL) is the most common cancer in children whereas acute myeloid leukemia (AML) more commonly occurs in adults. In ALL, lymphoid progenitor cells (lymphoblasts) are arrested in their early stage of development because of faulty expression of genes. In AML, it is the hematopoietic precursor cells of the bone marrow which are affected (Fig. 7.13).

PATHOPHYSIOLOGY

Once established, the deviant blast cells replace the normal marrow elements, resulting in a marked decrease in the production of functional white blood cells, RBCs, and platelets. The deviant cells can then move into organs other than the marrow, particularly the liver, spleen, and lymph nodes.

CLINICAL MANIFESTATIONS

The clinical manifestations are similar in ALL and AML. They are sudden in onset and are related to:

1. Immaturity of white blood cells and other cells originating in the bone marrow
2. Crowding of leukemic cells in the bone marrow
3. Infiltration of leukemic cells in the CNS, lymph nodes, liver, and spleen

Immaturity of white blood cells leads to increased infections. Crowding of leukemic cells in the bone marrow can suppress erythrocyte and platelet production, leading to anemia, bruising, and bleeding problems, such as frequent **epistaxis**, or nose bleeds. Anemia leads to fatigue. Cell crowding also increases

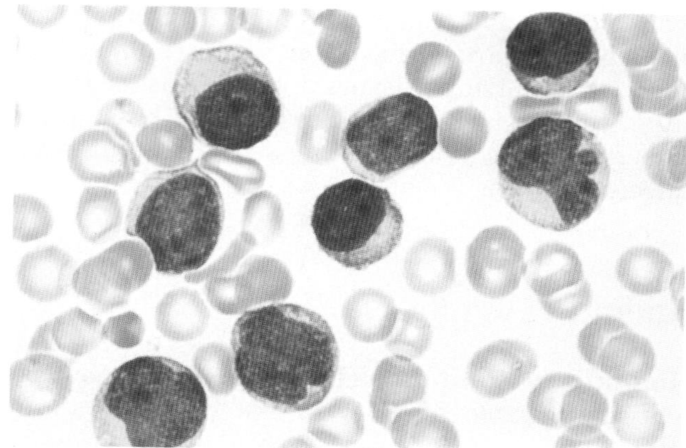

Figure 7.13. Acute lymphoblastic leukemia. The lymphoblasts contain irregular, prominent, and indented nuclei. (From Rubin E, Farber JL. *Pathology*. 4th ed. Philadelphia, PA: Lippincott Williams & Wilkins; 2005, with permission.)

pressure and resorption within the bone and can result in bone pain. Infiltration into the CNS causes headaches, visual disturbances, nausea, vomiting, seizures, and coma. Infiltration in the lymph nodes, spleen, and liver causes enlargement and tenderness of these organs. Unexplained weight loss and fever are also common clinical manifestations.

DIAGNOSTIC CRITERIA

Diagnosis is based on patient history and physical examination. The blood cell count demonstrating blast (immature white blood cells) cells greater than 20% and microscopic examination of blood cells is diagnostic. Further cytologic analysis differentiates the specific leukemia subtype.

TREATMENT

The most common treatment protocol for ALL includes a systemic combination of chemotherapy and specific prophylactic central nervous system intrathecal chemotherapy with or without cranial radiation. The treatment protocol is divided into stages that include induction, intensification, and maintenance. Close monitoring is required during treatment because of the myelosuppression and immunosuppression that is expected with intense chemotherapy. The goal is to achieve remission (blast cells less than 5%). Among children with ALL, more than 95% attain remission and the 5-year survival rate is over 80%.

Treatment for AML also includes systemic combination chemotherapy in two phases: induction (to achieve remission) and postremission. Because only 5% of those with AML develop CNS disease, prophylactic CNS intrathecal chemotherapy is rarely indicated. Approximately 70% of adults with AML can expect to attain complete remission after induction therapy. Success with therapy is related to younger age, lack of CNS involvement, lack of systemic infection at diagnosis, and lower immature WBC counts.

Chronic Lymphocytic and Myelogenous Leukemias

Chronic leukemias have a more gradual onset and are found most commonly in middle and older adults. Chronic lymphocytic leukemia (CLL) results in hypoproliferative, immunologically dysfunctional small B lymphocytes (Fig. 7.14). The cells do not readily form antibodies in the presence of antigens, and infection is common. Chronic myelogenous leukemia (CML) is similarly insidious in onset and characterized by uncontrolled proliferation of granulocytes, erythroid cells, and megakaryocytes (myelogenous cells types); again, these cells are relatively mature but not fully functional.

PATHOPHYSIOLOGY

The chronic leukemias are acquired mutations resulting in clonal B cells or hematopoietic stem cells disrupted along the differentiation pathway. In 50% of those with CLL, an abnormal deletion of 13q is noted. Other chromosome abnormalities associated with CLL include the deletion of the short arm of chromosome 17 (associated with loss of function of tumor suppressor gene *p53*) and the presence of trisomy 12. Similarly, in CML, a 9 and 22 chromosome

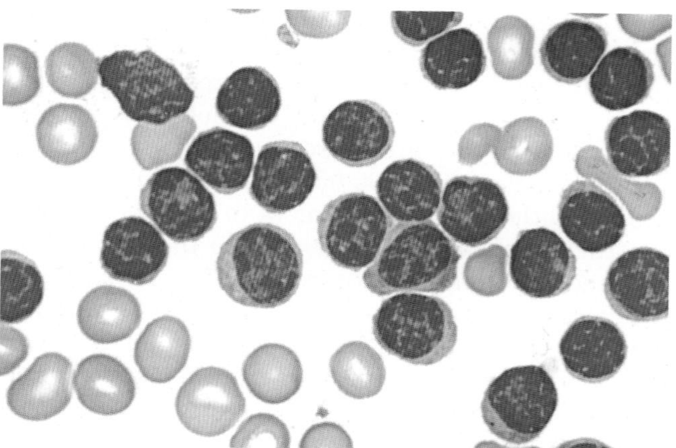

Figure 7.14. Chronic lymphocytic leukemia. A peripheral blood smear shows numerous small-to-medium sized lymphocytes. (From Rubin E, Farber JL. *Pathology*. 4th ed. Philadelphia, PA: Lippincott Williams & Wilkins; 2005, with permission.)

translocation is present in 95%. The resultant shortening of chromosome 22, referred to as the **Philadelphia chromosome**, activates oncogenes. The *BCR* and *ABL* genes become rearranged, allowing production of abnormal tyrosine kinase protein, leading to disordered myelopoiesis (formation of bone marrow).

CLINICAL MANIFESTATIONS

Clinical manifestations for chronic leukemias are often subtle or not present until the disease is well advanced. When present, the clinical manifestations are similar to acute leukemias: fatigue, lymph node enlargement (particularly with CLL), hepatomegaly, splenomegaly, recurrent or persistent infections, low-grade fever, anemia, weight loss, bleeding, bruising, and bone pain.

DIAGNOSTIC CRITERIA

Diagnosis prior to the onset of recognizable symptoms is often made incidentally; the individual is seeking care for another purpose, a blood cell count is performed, an elevation in the WBC count is noted, and the patient undergoes further investigation. The patient may have detectable spleen enlargement on physical examination. A bone marrow biopsy is often performed and detects a greater proportion of immature myeloid cells. Cytologic analysis is used to determine specific chromosomal aberrations or genetic mutations. For example, CML is further distinguished by the presence of the Philadelphia chromosome.

TREATMENT

The optimal treatment for CML and CLL at diagnosis has not yet been established. Patients with early-stage CLL are often not treated until becoming symptomatic. More than half of patients may be cured with bone marrow or stem cell transplantation. However, eligibility is restricted by age, overall health status, and inability to locate a suitable donor. Patients with extremely high circulating WBCs (greater than 100,000/mm^3) require immediate chemotherapeutic treatment to avoid death from obstruction of blood vessels leading to vital organs. Splenectomy may be required in those with physical discomfort and hematologic disorders related to massive splenic enlargement. The median survival rate is around 5 to 10 years, with a 5-year survival rate of 50% to 60%.

Lymphomas

Lymphomas, malignant lymphocytes or lymphoblasts, are commonly classified as either Hodgkin lymphoma or non-Hodgkin lymphoma. Lymphomas, like leukemia, are derived from WBCs (namely lymphocytes) and lymph tissues. Lymphomas form solid organ tumors in the lymph tissue and later in the bone marrow. Lymphomas can also be present in the spleen and liver.

Hodgkin Lymphoma

Hodgkin lymphoma (HL) is a malignant but potentially curable disorder of the lymphoid tissue often characterized by the painless, progressive enlargement of cervical (neck) lymph nodes. Risk factors include exposure to viruses such as Epstein–Barr virus (EBV), genetic factors, and immunosuppression. Incidence is highest in those between the ages of 10 and 30 years and in those older than 50 years. Interestingly, the childhood form of HL is similar in biology and pathogenesis to the adult-onset form. The mortality rate has declined dramatically for adults with HL at a greater pace than any other malignancy, also largely because of the effectiveness of contemporary radiation and chemotherapeutic treatments.

PATHOPHYSIOLOGY

Classic HL is characterized by the presence of multinucleated giant cells (macrophages), called Reed–Sternberg cells, or mononuclear giant cells, called Hodgkin cells, surrounded by multiple other inflammatory cells, such as neutrophils, eosinophils, plasma cells, small lymphocytes, and fibroblasts. HL can be classified into five types. The first four types encompass "classic HL," and the fifth type is a distinct entity with its own clinical presentation and treatment plan.

1. Nodular sclerosing
2. Mixed cellularity
3. Lymphocyte depletion
4. Lymphocyte rich
5. Nodular lymphocyte-predominant

The pathogenesis of HL is still under investigation. The Reed–Sternberg or Hodgkin cell has been identified as the neoplastic origin, capable of clonal expansion. In classic HL, the **Reed–Sternberg cell** (Fig. 7.15) originates in the cell components of lymph nodes following a B-lymphocyte lineage; it is the neoplastic cell diagnostic for HL. Susceptibility to specific viral oncogenes or certain HLA subtypes suggests a multifactorial etiology with a genetic influence. HL typically arises in B cells that cannot synthesize immunoglobulin and are resistant to apoptosis. Speculation about a viral etiology is

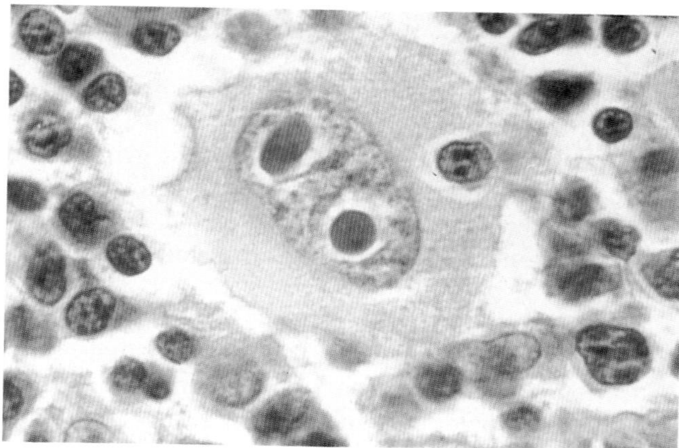

Figure 7.15. Classic Reed–Sternberg cell. The Reed–Sternberg cell is derived from B lymphocytes and suggests the presence of Hodgkin lymphoma. The cell is large and binucleated or multinucleated with eosinophilic nucleoli. (From Rubin E, Farber JL. *Pathology*. 4th ed. Philadelphia, PA: Lippincott Williams & Wilkins; 2005, with permission.)

evidenced by EBV genetic material, which can often be detected in these affected cells. The risk of developing EBV-positive HL is increased significantly in those infected with this virus. Other increased incidence is found in children who have parents with a history of HL. Once the primary tumor is established, the neoplasm may spread to connecting lymph channels and can also infiltrate the vascular system. HL is organ tropic to the lung, liver, bones, and bone marrow.

CLINICAL MANIFESTATIONS

The vast majority of individuals with HL present with a nontender enlarged lymph node or group of nodes in the neck. The enlarged nodes are generally firm and rubbery in texture. Other manifestations, such as low-grade fever, fatigue, weight loss, pruritus, and drenching night sweats, are associated with the release of lymphokines and cytokines (inflammatory mediators) by Reed–Sternberg or Hodgkin cells. Approximately 20% of patients will have a mass at the mediastinum that is greater than one-third of the chest diameter. Splenomegaly and hepatomegaly may also be detected.

DIAGNOSTIC CRITERIA

The diagnosis and staging of HL is based on the patient history, physical examination, laboratory studies, and thoracic and abdominal CT scans. The most significant diagnostic feature of Hodgkin lymphoma is the presence of Reed–Sternberg cells. The Ann Arbor classification is used to stage HL:

- Stage I: A single lymph node area or single extranodal site
- Stage II: Two or more lymph node areas on the same side of the diaphragm
- Stage III: Lymph node areas on both sides of the diaphragm
- Stage IV: Disseminated or multiple involvement of the extranodal organs

TREATMENT

Treatment is based on clinical staging of HL. Chemotherapy, radiation, and hematopoeitic stem cell transplantation are the primary treatment modalities. Patients with stage I or II disease are considered to have clinical early-stage disease and are treated with chemotherapy, combined chemotherapy–radiation therapy, or radiation therapy alone. Patients with stage III or IV disease or those with the presence of systemic symptoms at any stage require combination chemotherapy with or without adjunct radiation therapy. Reduced dosages, particularly lower-dose radiation, are used when treating children. Poor prognosis is based on the presence of systemic symptoms, the stage of the disease, the presence of large masses, treatment effectiveness, the extremes of age, expansive disease spread, and the presence of immunodeficiency. The overall 5-year survival rate for patients with HL is around 85%.

Stop and Consider
How are leukemias and lymphomas similar?

Non-Hodgkin Lymphoma

Non-Hodgkin lymphoma (NHL) is a generic classification made up of a broad range of B-cell and T-cell malignancies within the lymph nodes. NHL occurs much more frequently than HL, does not exhibit the malignant Reed–Sternberg cell, and is more likely to affect noncontiguous (unconnected) lymph nodes. Similar to HL, the etiology of NHL is often unknown; however, chromosomal translocations, infections, chronic inflammation, viruses, immunodeficiency, environmental factors, and genetic factors are implicated.

PATHOPHYSIOLOGY

The precise genetic mutation for NHL is highly variable, depending on the specific cell affected by neoplasia. Mutations can affect protooncogenes or tumor suppressor genes resulting in a deviant clonal expansion of B cells (85%) or T cells (15%). There are at least 10 NHL subtypes. As with HL, spread can occur via the lymphatic and vascular systems. NHL is organ tropic to the liver, spleen, and bone marrow.

CLINICAL MANIFESTATIONS

Clinical manifestations can vary somewhat depending on the tumor type and extent of disease. The most common occurrence, as with HL, is painless and slowly progressive enlargement of lymph nodes. Those with NHL can experience systemic manifestations, such as fever, night sweats, weight loss, an increased risk of infection, and paraneoplastic syndromes as with other malignant neoplasms.

DIAGNOSTIC CRITERIA

Diagnosis is based on patient history and physical examination, along with confirmation via lymph node biopsy. Chest and abdominal CT scans can also be used to visualize the tumor size and location. Examination of the cells in the cerebrospinal fluid may be positive for metastases in patients with aggressive NHL.

The staging system (I through IV) is similar to that of HL. Histologic classification is based on three major categories of lymphoid malignancies based on morphology and cell lineage: B-cell neoplasms, T-cell/natural killer (NK)-cell neoplasms, and HL. Both the lymphomas (solid tumors in lymph) and leukemias (circulating neoplasms with immune cell lineage) are included in this classification and there can be crossover between leukemias and lymphomas given the impact on lymphocytes. For example, B-cell CLL and B-cell small lymphocytic lymphoma are, in essence, the same neoplasm.

TREATMENT

Currently, treatment is based on categorizing the NHLs into two prognostic groups: the indolent (painless, passive) lymphomas and the aggressive lymphomas. Early-stage (stage I and stage II) indolent NHL can be treated effectively with radiation therapy. Later-stage indolent and aggressive NHLs require intensive combination chemotherapy regimens with or without radiation therapy and stem cell transplantation. Prognosis for NHL is based on the stage, cell characteristics, age, treatment response, tumor size, lactate dehydrogenase (LDH) values, and the number of affected lymph node sites outside of those surrounding the primary tumor. In general, the 5-year survival rate for all types of NHL is around 60%.

SUMMARY

- Neoplasia is a disorder of cellular proliferation and differentiation.
- Mutations of genes that regulate cell growth, reproduction, and death are responsible for neoplastic transformations.
- Carcinogenesis is complex and involves multiple stages.
- Certain substances or exposures are known to cause or promote cellular mutations, such as radiation, exposure to reactive oxygen species (free radicals), hormones, tobacco, infectious microorganisms, and chemicals.
- Cancer often exhibits a prolonged latent period between the initiation and onset of clinical manifestations, making identification of a precise carcinogen difficult.
- Neoplastic cells are autonomous, anaplastic, and energy-dependent. They undergo extensive angiogenesis, deprive unaffected tissues of oxygen and other nutrients, and secrete substances that can alter metabolic processes.
- General manifestations related to systemic inflammatory and immune systems include lymphadenopathy, fever, and anorexia.
- Local clinical manifestations are site dependent and are related to (1) the space occupied by the tumor that impinges on the local structures; and (2) the loss of function in the tissue or organ that is being "taken over" by the tumor.
- Tumors spread locally and to distant sites through the vascular and lymphatic systems.
- Metastases are distant relocations of the tumor that contribute to the lethal aspect of cancer.
- Major treatment strategies for neoplasia include surgery, chemotherapy, radiation, hormones, and immunotherapy.

CASE STUDY 7.1

A 65-year-old Hispanic woman recently underwent a mammogram offered by a community "health on wheels" clinic. The radiologist detected a breast mass on the right side. She has a younger sister who had breast cancer as well. Her sister died 2 years ago at the age of 62. Her menses began at age 11 and cessation of menstruation occurred around age 58. She is overweight and is on estrogen replacement therapy. She does not have any children.

1. Outline the process that has occurred in her body.
2. What were the risk factors that she demonstrated?
3. What would you expect for clinical manifestations?
4. What additional diagnostic tests could be used?
5. What treatment measures would you anticipate?

Log on to the Internet. Search for a relevant journal article or Web site (such as www.cancer.gov/cancertopics/pdq/genetics/breast-and-ovarian/healthprofessional) that details breast cancer and confirm your predictions.

CASE STUDY 7.2

A 51-year-old Caucasian man is being evaluated for headaches, hypertension, severe skin itching, and liver and spleen enlargement. He has a ruddy complexion. Laboratory and diagnostic tests reveal that he has an elevated hematocrit and RBC count. He is diagnosed with polycythemia vera, on overproliferation of RBCs. Although not described in your reading, use what you know about overproliferation/differentiation and apply this to what might happen if RBCs were involved.

1. Outline the process that has mostly likely occurred in his body.
2. What would you expect for clinical manifestations?
3. What diagnostic tests were used and what do these tell you?
4. What treatment measures would you anticipate?

Log on to the Internet. Search for a relevant journal article or Web site (such as http://www.cancer.gov/cancertopics/pdq/treatment/myeloproliferative/HealthProfessional/page4) that details polycythemia vera and confirm your predictions.

CASE STUDY 7.3

An 11-year-old boy presents to the emergency department with low back pain and a palpable mass on his right side near his hip. His parent also reports intermittent, low-grade fever and weight loss over the past 3 months. After careful physical examination, laboratory studies, and imaging studies, a diagnosis of Ewing sarcoma is determined.

1. Outline the process that has mostly likely occurred in his body.
2. What would you expect for clinical manifestations?
3. What diagnostic tests were used and what do these tell you?
4. What treatment measures would you anticipate?

Log on to the Internet. Search for a relevant journal article or Web site (such as http://www.cancer.gov/types/bone/hp/ewing-treatment-pdq) that details Ewing sarcoma and confirm your predictions.

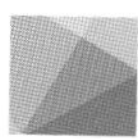

PRACTICE EXAM QUESTIONS

1. A patient comes to the clinic concerned about a painless lymph node in the neck. A diagnosis of lymphoma is made. Which of the following would indicate that the lymphoma was Hodgkin lymphoma versus non-Hodgkin lymphoma?
   a. The location of the enlarged lymph nodes
   b. The presence of Reed–Sternberg cells
   c. Spread to the spleen, liver, and bone marrow
   d. The age of the patient

2. Which of the following genes, when mutated, is NOT implicated in the development of neoplasms?
   a. Cancinogenes
   b. Tumor suppressor genes
   c. Oncogenes
   d. Mutator genes

3. Which of the following cells is least likely to develop into a neoplasia?
   a. Epithelial cell
   b. Cardiac myocyte
   c. Lymphocyte
   d. Hepatocyte

4. Which gene has been implicated most frequently in the development of cancer?
   a. *p53* gene
   b. *Rb* gene
   c. *T21* gene
   d. None of these is implicated in the development of cancer.

5. Which of the following is characteristic of benign neoplasms?
   a. Highly undifferentiated
   b. Invasive
   c. Destructive
   d. Cell overproliferation

6. Which is the most significant difference between acute lymphocytic and acute myelogenous leukemia?
   a. ALL affects adults and AML affects children most often
   b. Cell type affected
   c. Diagnostic tests used
   d. Clinical manifestations

7. Your grandfather has colon cancer but then it migrates to the liver. The affinity for movement to another specific organ is called:
   a. Tropism
   b. Migratism
   c. Magnetism
   d. Malignancy

8. You are a public health official and want to make the greatest difference in reducing cancer deaths across the globe. Which intervention would have the greatest impact?
   a. Smoking cessation programs
   b. Routine genetic testing
   c. Distribute sunscreen to all adults and children
   d. Eliminate unnecessary uses of radiation

9. What sign/symptom might indicate that you are experiencing a paraneoplastic syndrome?
   a. Bone pain
   b. Edema
   c. Cough
   d. Hematuria

10. Which type of cancer would most likely spread through the process called seeding?
   a. Lung
   b. Colon
   c. Ovarian
   d. Bone

DISCUSSION AND APPLICATION

1. What did I know about altered cellular proliferation and differentiation prior to today?
2. What body processes are affected by altered proliferation and differentiation? What are the expected functions of those processes? How does altered proliferation and differentiation affect those processes?
3. What are the potential etiologies for altered cellular proliferation and differentiation? How does altered proliferation and differentiation develop?
4. Who is most at risk for developing altered cellular proliferation and differentiation? How can altered proliferation and differentiation be prevented?
5. What are the human differences that affect the etiology, risk, or course of altered cellular proliferation and differentiation?
6. What clinical manifestations are expected in the course of altered cellular proliferation and differentiation?
7. What special diagnostic tests are useful in determining the diagnosis and course of altered proliferation and differentiation?
8. What are the goals of care for individuals with altered cellular proliferation and differentiation?
9. How does the concept of altered cellular proliferation and differentiation build on what I have learned in the previous chapters and in previous courses?
10. How can I use what I have learned?

RESOURCES

American Cancer Society:
http://www.cancer.org/docroot/home/index.asp

National Cancer Institute:
http://www.nci.nih.gov/

American Association for Cancer Research:
http://cancerres.aacrjournals.org/

Intercultural Cancer Council:
http://www.iccnetwork.org

References

1. American Cancer Society. *Cancer Facts and Figures, 2014*. Atlanta, GA: American Cancer Society; 2014. http://www.cancer.org
2. Yunhua L, Xiaoxiao H, Cecil H, et al. Targeting tumor suppressor genes for cancer therapy. *Bioessays*. 2015;37(12):1277–1286. doi:10.1002/bies.201500093.
3. Tan WW. Non-small cell lung cancer. 2015. http://emedicine.medscape.com/article/279960-overview
4. Dragovich T. Colon cancer. 2015. http://emedicine.medscape.com/article/277496-overview
5. SEER cancer statistics factsheets: brain and other nervous system cancer. Bethesda, MD: National Cancer Institute; 2015. http://seer.cancer.gov/statfacts/html/brain.html

Find additional resources for this chapter at http:thePoint.lww.com thePoint®

Altered Fluid and Electrolyte Balance

Chapter

8

LEARNING OUTCOMES

1. Define and use the key terms listed in this chapter.
2. Compare and contrast the distribution of fluid in body compartments.
3. Differentiate between cations and anions, including expected concentrations within specific body compartments.
4. Identify the influences that promote fluid movement between and within compartments.
5. List four potential sources of body fluid loss.
6. Describe the clinical implications of alterations in fluid and electrolyte balance.
7. Apply concepts of altered fluid and electrolyte balance to selected clinical models.

INTRODUCTION

Have you ever been thirsty on a hot, sunny day? What about after a long workout or after eating a bag of pretzels? Thirst is the way the body communicates the need to increase fluid intake. Fluid intake must make up for fluid lost through sweating, breathing, and urinating. In addition to fluids, electrolytes and specialized compounds that control acid–base balance are necessary for cell and organ functioning. This chapter reviews the mechanisms involved in the dysregulation of fluid, electrolyte, presented in individual modules. It also covers interactions between these concepts and the clinical consequences that may result. Selected clinical models that highlight specific alterations are presented in module 3 to allow the student to apply the learned concepts.

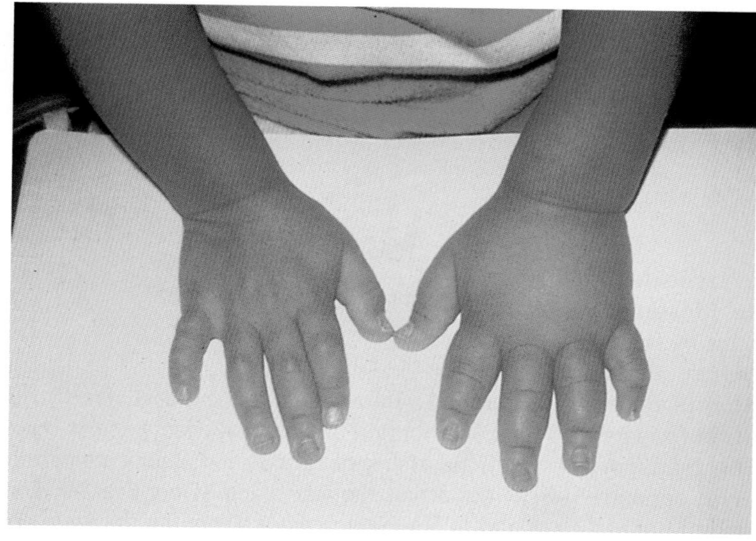

Lymphedema

Module 1 Electrolyte Imbalance

Body fluid contains dissolved particles known as electrolytes. **Electrolytes** are electrically charged particles, or **ions**. Ions with a positive charge are called **cations** and include sodium (Na^+), calcium (Ca^{2+}), hydrogen (H^+), and potassium (K^+). Negatively charged ions are called **anions** and include chloride (Cl^-), bicarbonate (HCO_3^-), sulfate (SO_4^{2-}), and phosphate (PO_4^{3-}). Ions with opposite charges are attracted to each other and form molecules. An example of this is the bonding of the cation Na^+ to the anion Cl^- to form the molecule NaCl, or sodium chloride.

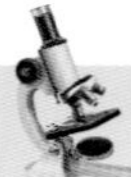

FROM THE LAB

The amount of electrolytes in body fluids is described by the concentration of solute in a particular volume of fluid. Measurements are often described as milligrams per deciliter (mg/dL), the solute weight in one-tenth of a liter (dL), also equivalent to 100 microliters (μL) of solution. Electrolytes can also be expressed in measurements of milliequivalents per liter (mEq/L), which considers the charge equivalency for a specific weight of electrolyte. Based on electroneutrality, cations and anions must be balanced in the body. The combination of anions and cations results from the attraction based on ionic charge rather than molecular weight. Therefore, 1 mEq of sodium has the same number of charges as 1 mEq of chloride. Clinical measurements of electrolytes are determined by their concentration in the plasma.

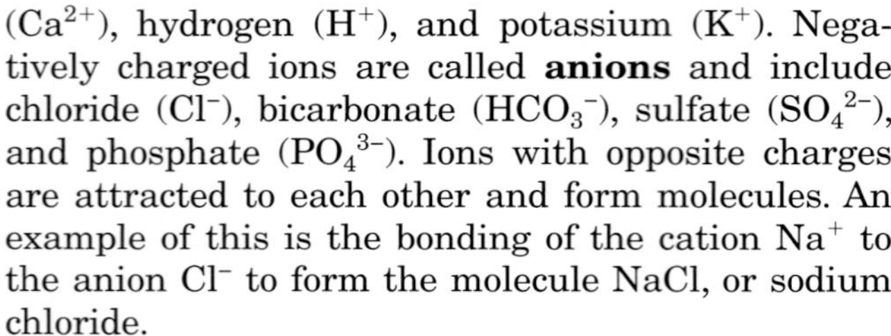

The plasma within the vascular space and the interstitial fluid of the extracellular compartment are high in sodium, chloride, and calcium; low in potassium, magnesium, and phosphate; and contain moderate levels of bicarbonate. The intracellular fluid contains extremely low levels of calcium; small amounts of sodium, bicarbonate, and chloride; and moderate amounts of phosphate and magnesium. Potassium is found in greatest concentrations in the intracellular fluid. Figure 8.1 illustrates the concentrations of electrolytes inside and outside of a cell.

Electrolyte Transport

The cell membrane forms a barrier between the intracellular and extracellular compartments. Movement of electrolytes across the cell barrier occurs by transport mechanisms, some that require energy (active transport) and others that follow gradients determined by charge/electrical or concentration (passive transport), as detailed in Chapter 2. The transport of one positively charged ion for another in opposite directions across the cell membrane is called **cation exchange**. Similarly, when reciprocal transport of negatively charged ion occurs, it is called **anion exchange**. The exchange of like-charged ions between cellular compartments provides a homeostatic mechanism to maintain electrolyte and acid–base balance.

Stop and Consider
Calcium is one of the electrolytes important in muscle contraction. Large amounts of calcium must be available inside the cell to promote the development of tension in muscle cells. What must happen to intracellular calcium levels for this to occur?

Altered Electrolyte Balance

Regulation of electrolyte balance is critical to metabolic function of cells. Alterations in electrolytes can disrupt many processes, including generation of action potentials and maintenance of fluid and acid–base balance.

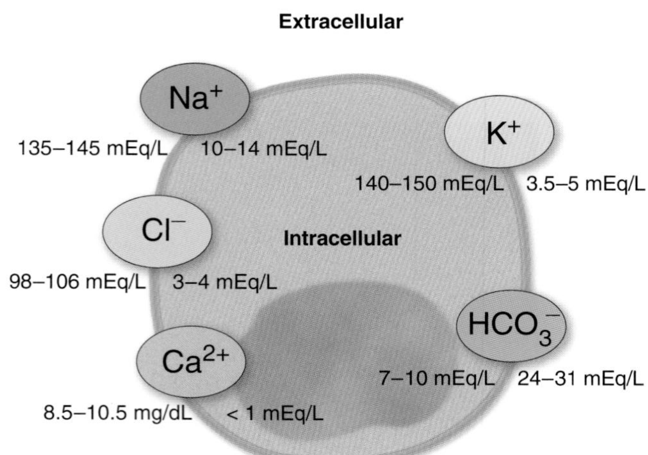

Figure 8.1. Intracellular and extracellular distribution of ions. Distribution of electrical charge across the membrane. Electroneutrality of cations and anions promote balanced charges across the membrane. (From Bear MF, Connors BW, Paradiso MA. *Neuroscience: Exploring the Brain*. 3rd ed. Baltimore, MD: Lippincott Williams & Wilkins; 2006.)

ALTERED SODIUM BALANCE

Sodium is the most abundant cation in the extracellular compartment and serves as the primary determinant of blood osmolality. Transport of sodium out of the cell occurs against its concentration gradient, requiring active transport through the energy-dependent Na^+/K^+-2ATPase membrane pump (Fig. 8.2). Alterations in sodium balance can alter acid–base balance, fluid balance, and neural conduction. Dietary sources provide sodium, which is excreted mainly by the kidneys, along with water.

Hyponatremia

Hyponatremia is characterized by decreased levels of sodium in the blood. Sodium loss most often occurs through vomiting, diarrhea, and sweating. Blood sodium levels of less than 135 mEq/L are diagnostic of hyponatremia. Osmotic swelling of cells contributes to muscle twitching and weakness. Reduced extracellular circulating volume may lead to hypotension, tachycardia, and reduced or absent urine output (**oliguria** and **anuria**, respectively). Altered neuronal function may lead to nausea and vomiting, lethargy, confusion, seizures, or coma.

Stop and Consider
Why is sodium balance especially critical to fluid balance?

Hypernatremia

Excessive dietary intake of sodium and loss of body water are the primary causes of hypernatremia. **Hypernatremia** is characterized by blood sodium levels of greater than 145 mEq/L. Cell metabolism is altered, as evidenced by agitation, restlessness, and decreased levels of consciousness. Fluid shifts caused by hypernatremia may result in thirst, hypertension, tachycardia, edema, and weight gain.

ALTERED POTASSIUM BALANCE

Potassium is the most abundant intracellular cation. Because most potassium is found in muscle, total body potassium is determined in large part by body size and muscle mass.

Hypokalemia

Loss of potassium may result from excessive loss due to diuretic use, severe vomiting, or diarrhea. Potassium levels of less than 3.5 mEq/L in the blood indicate **hypokalemia**. These levels of potassium alter membrane potential, which may result in dizziness, hypotension, cardiac arrhythmias, muscle weakness, and leg cramps. Decreased smooth muscle motility contributes to nausea, anorexia (loss of appetite), and abdominal distention.

Hyperkalemia

Potassium levels of more than 5 mEq/L in the blood are diagnostic of **hyperkalemia**. Causes of hyperkalemia are often iatrogenic, that is, caused by inappropriate use of drugs or their management, leading to increased potassium levels. Movement of potassium from the intracellular to the extracellular space may also lead to hyperkalemia. Inadequate excretion of potassium, as in renal failure (see Chapter 18), can also lead to hyperkalemia. These levels can alter membrane potential and are associated with the

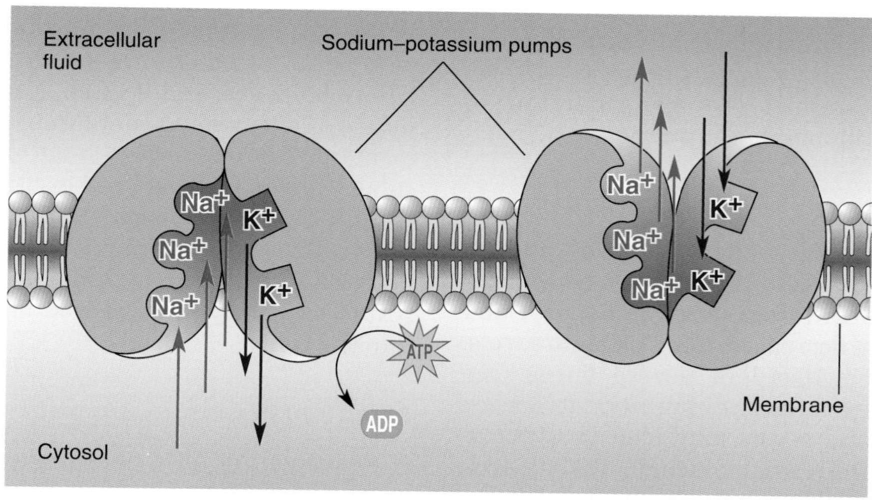

Figure 8.2. The sodium-potassium pump. This membrane-associated ion pump uses energy in the form of ATP to transport sodium and potassium across the membrane against their concentration gradient. (From Bear MF, Connors BW, Paradiso MA. *Neuroscience: Exploring the Brain*. 3rd ed. Baltimore, MD: Lippincott Williams & Wilkins; 2006.)

development of cardiac arrest, abdominal cramping, and flaccid paralysis because of their effects on sodium channels.

ALTERED CHLORIDE BALANCE

Chloride is a major extracellular anion. Chloride movement is often associated with sodium and plays a role in regulation of acid–base balance.

Hypochloremia

Hypochloremia is determined when blood chloride levels are less than 98 mEq/L. Common reasons for chloride loss include vomiting, diarrhea, and the use of diuretics. Hypochloremia is often associated with hyponatremia, hypokalemia, and metabolic alkalosis. Muscle effects include excessive tone and tetany (sustained contraction), weakness, and twitching. Shallow, depressed breathing, paralysis, or mental confusion may result.

Hyperchloremia

Hyperchloremia can result from severe dehydration, kidney failure, hemodialysis, and traumatic brain injury. Diagnosed by blood chloride levels of more than 108 mEq/L, hyperchloremia may result in hyperchloremic metabolic acidosis. Deep rapid breathing, weakness, headache, diminished cognitive ability, and cardiac arrest may result from hyperchloremia.

ALTERED CALCIUM BALANCE

Most calcium is contained within bones and teeth; only a small fraction is located in the extracellular fluid. Although the concentration of calcium in the extracellular fluid is relatively small, calcium plays an essential role in many metabolic processes, including activity of enzyme systems, generation of action potentials, and muscle contraction.

Hypocalcemia

Calcium blood levels of less than 8.5 mg/dL, indicative of **hypocalcemia**, lead to enhanced neuromuscular irritability. Medications, such as heparin and glucagon, can cause decreased blood calcium levels. In addition, thyroid disorders, severe burns (see Chapter 16), kidney failure, vitamin D deficiency (see Chapter 17), and sepsis may lead to hypocalcemia. Clinical manifestations include anxiety, irritability, muscle twitching, cramps, spasms, tetany, laryngospasm, and seizure. Hypotension and cardiac arrhythmia may occur because of decreased calcium entry into the cell.

Hypercalcemia

Blood calcium levels greater than 10.5 mg/dL indicate **hypercalcemia**. Increased blood calcium levels may result from excessive bone breakdown, thyroid disease, and excessive intake of calcium supplements, including calcium-containing antacids. Decreased neuromuscular irritability caused by increased threshold accounts for the main manifestations of hypercalcemia. These manifestations include confusion, fatigue, constipation, nausea and vomiting, muscle weakness, cardiac arrhythmia, headaches, and irritability.

ALTERED MAGNESIUM BALANCE

Magnesium has functions similar to the cations calcium and potassium. Much of the body's magnesium is contained in bone, similar to calcium. Soft tissues and muscle cells also contain significant concentrations of magnesium.

Hypomagnesemia

Hypomagnesemia, characterized by blood levels less than 1.5 mEq/L, usually occurs in association with hypokalemia and hypocalcemia. Inadequate intake of magnesium because of malnutrition, malabsorption syndromes, severe burns, or alcoholism is the most common cause of hypomagnesemia. Diuretic use is also associated with a risk of hypomagnesemia. Tetany, muscle cramping, and seizures are possible manifestations resulting from altered neuromuscular transmission. Cardiac arrhythmia and hypotension occur from the alteration of electrical currents because of the concurrent effects of sodium, potassium, and calcium imbalances.

Hypermagnesemia

Magnesium levels greater than 2.5 mEq/L measured in the blood define **hypermagnesemia**. This imbalance occurs with less frequency than other electrolyte imbalances, and it often results from excessive intake of magnesium-containing products or supplements or from end-stage renal disease. Neuromuscular transmission and cell excitability are reduced, resulting in hypotension, diminished reflexes, muscle weakness, flaccid paralysis, and respiratory depression. Cardiac arrhythmia and bradycardia may result secondary to decreased movement of sodium into the cell.

ALTERED PHOSPHATE BALANCE

A component of ATP, phosphate, is essential to cellular metabolism. Cellular functions of glycolysis and many enzyme reactions depend on phosphate. The major intracellular anion phosphate is stored in bones and teeth, in conjunction with calcium.

Hypophosphatemia

Blood phosphate levels less than 2.5 mg/dL are associated with **hypophosphatemia**. Often associated with hypomagnesemia and hypokalemia, hypophosphatemia may result from severe burns, malnutrition, malabsorption, alcoholism, kidney disease, vitamin D deficiency, or prolonged diuretic use. Manifestations of hypophosphatemia include muscle weakness, tremor, **paresthesia** (abnormal sensation such as tingling or burning), weight loss, and bone deformities.

Hyperphosphatemia

Hyperphosphatemia occurs when blood phosphate levels rise above 4.5 mg/dL, and it often occurs in tandem with hypocalcemia. Conditions resulting in hyperphosphatemia include fractures, bone disease, hypoparathyroidism, acromegaly (see Chapter 2), systemic infection (see Chapter 5), and intestinal obstruction (see Chapter 18). There are no associated symptoms of hyperphosphatemia, unless it is accompanied by other electrolyte imbalances.

Manifestations of electrolyte imbalances are summarized in Table 8.1.

Table 8.1 Manifestations of Electrolyte Imbalances

Electrolyte	Blood Level	Imbalance	Manifestations
Sodium	<135 mEq/L	Hyponatremia	Muscle cramps, twitching, weakness Volume deficit, hypotension, oliguria Headache, anxiety, altered consciousness
	>145 mEq/L	Hypernatremia	Thirst, dry skin and mucous membranes Decreased excretions Headache, restlessness, altered consciousness
Potassium	<3.5 mEq/L	Hypokalemia	Dizziness, muscle weakness, leg cramps Cardiac arrhythmia, hypotension Thirst, nausea, anorexia Poorly concentrated urine, polyuria
	>5 mEq/L	Hyperkalemia	Cardiac arrest Abdominal cramping, flaccid paralysis
Chloride	<98 mEq/L	Hypochloremia	Increased muscle tone, twitching, weakness, tetany Shallow, depressed breathing, respiratory arrest Mental confusion
	>108 mEq/L	Hyperchloremia	Hyperchloremic metabolic acidosis Deep, rapid breathing Weakness, headache, diminished cognitive ability Cardiac arrest
Calcium	<8.5 mg/dL	Hypocalcemia	Enhanced neuromuscular irritability Anxiety, irritability, seizure Muscle twitching, cramps, spasm, tetany, laryngospasm Hypotension, cardiac arrhythmia
	>10.5 mg/dL	Hypercalcemia	Decreased neuromuscular irritability Confusion, fatigue, headache, irritability Constipation, nausea, vomiting Cardiac arrhythmia
Magnesium	<1.5 mEq/L	Hypomagnesemia	Tetany, muscle cramping Seizures Cardiac arrhythmia, hypotension
	>2.5 mEq/L	Hypermagnesemia	Reduced neuromuscular transmission and cell excitability Flaccid paralysis, diminished reflexes, muscle weakness Hypotension, respiratory depression
Phosphate	<2.5 mg/dL	Hypophosphatemia	Muscle weakness, tremor, paresthesia Weight loss, bone deformity
	>4.5 mg/dL	Hyperphosphatemia	No associated manifestations

Module 2 Fluid Imbalance

The body is mostly fluid, accounting for a significant percentage of body weight. Total body water can vary by gender, age, and amount of body fat. Sixty percent of the body is comprised of fluids distributed between two compartments: 40% is located in the intracellular compartment and 20% is located in the extracellular compartment (Fig. 8.3). The **intracellular compartment** consists of the fluid inside the cells, containing approximately two-thirds of the body water and accounting for 40% of body weight.

The smaller **extracellular compartment** contains the remaining one-third, or 20%, of body fluid in the interstitial tissue and plasma outside the cells. Fluid in the plasma compartment accounts for 5% of body weight, and the interstitial fluid accounts for 14% of body weight. A third, minor extracellular compartment is the transcellular compartment, separated by a layer of endothelium. The fluid in this compartment is contained in body spaces such as the spinal cord, peritoneal, pleural, pericardial, and joint spaces. This relatively small compartment of fluid is often referred to as a "third space" because it is unavailable for exchange between the other extracellular compartments.

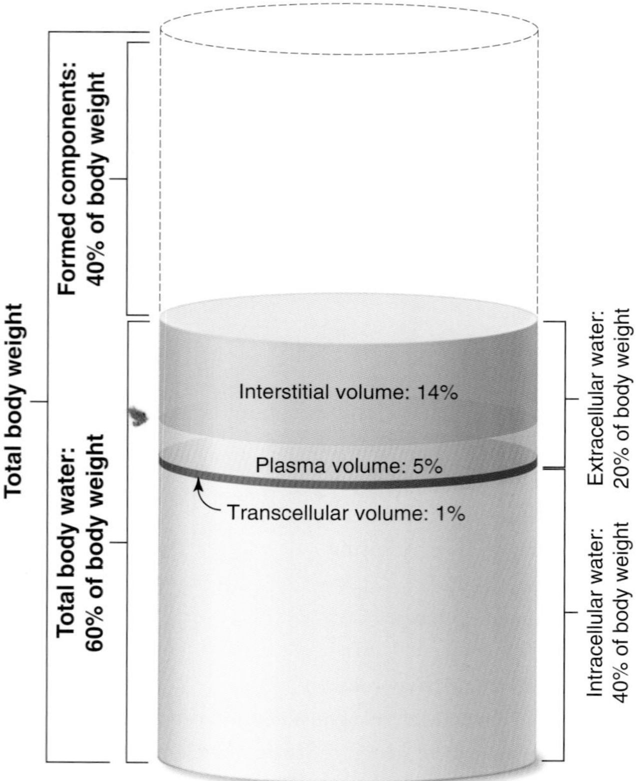

Figure 8.3. Body fluid compartments. Extracellular water makes up 20% of body weight, and intracellular water makes up 40% of body weight.

Fluid Balance

Body fluid volume is regulated directly in the extracellular compartment and indirectly in the intracellular compartment by the kidneys. This process involves water and ion movement across the cell membranes of the renal tubules and close association with the vasculature of the kidneys (Fig. 8.4).

FLUID TRANSPORT

Water is able to move between compartments through special channels in the cell membrane, called **aquaporins**. Movement of water is stimulated by a concentration gradient, moving to an area of higher concentration of particles (less water content) from an area of lower concentration of particles (more water content). This process, **osmosis**, is regulated by the concentration of particles that do not diffuse across the semipermeable membrane. Some characteristics that make particles nondiffusible include large size or lipid solubility. **Osmotic pressure** is generated as water moves through the membrane. An osmole is the unit of measure reflecting the osmotic activity that nondiffusible particles exert in pulling water from one side of the semipermeable membrane to the other. Osmolarity is the osmolar concentration in 1 L of solution (mOsm/L) and is used when referring to fluids outside the body. Osmolality is the osmolar concentration in 1 kg of water (mOsm/kg of H_2O), and is used to describe fluids within the body. Table 8.2 summarizes active and passive transport mechanisms.

Fluid also moves between extracellular compartments, with forces promoting fluid movement balance. **Hydrostatic forces** (pressure of fluid) can promote movement of fluid based on the pressure gradient, also known as **filtration pressure**. The pressure of the blood on the capillary walls (semipermeable membranes) can force fluid movement from within the vessel to the interstitial space; this movement is called filtration. Capillary filtration pressure is countered by interstitial fluid pressure, which opposes fluid movement out of the capillary. Conversely, capillary osmotic pressure caused by proteins or other molecules can pull fluid from the interstitial space into the intravascular space;

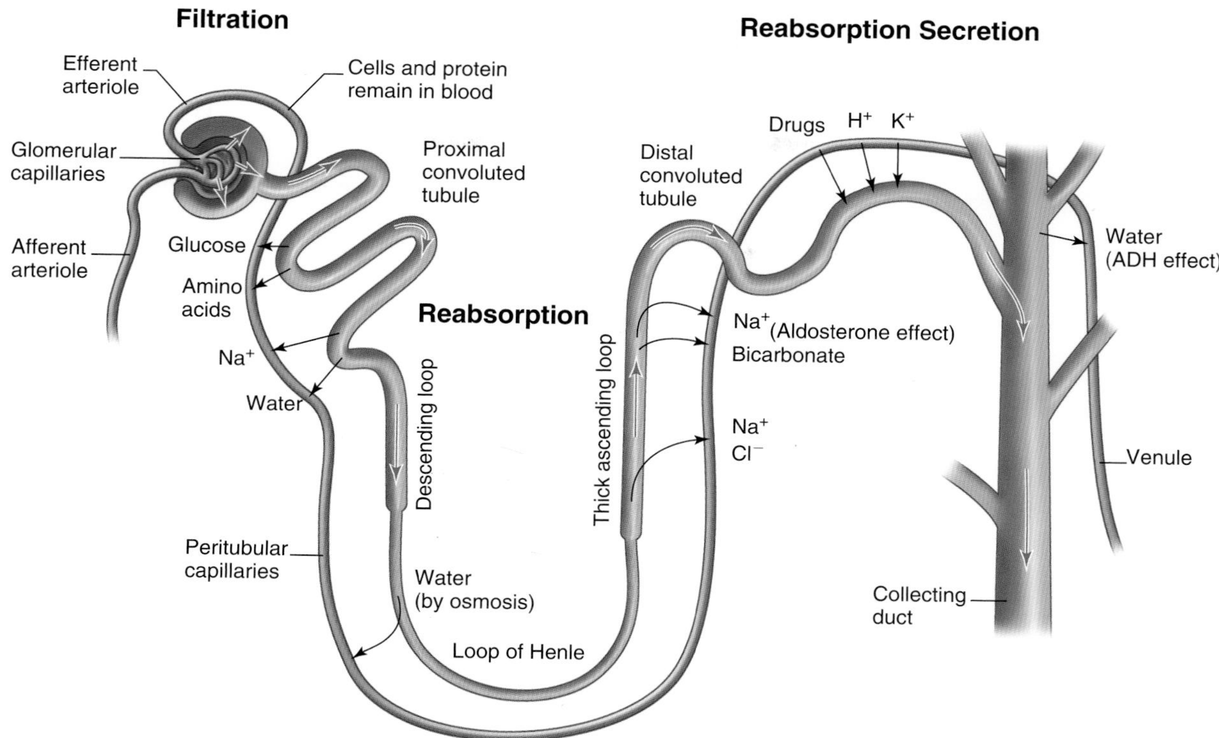

Figure 8.4. Renal regulation of fluid and electrolytes. Filtration, reabsorption, and secretion processes are illustrated between the renal structures and associated vasculature. Note the movement of ions and water along the tubules. ADH, antidiuretic hormone. (Modified from Premkumar K. *The Massage Connection: Anatomy and Physiology*. Baltimore, MD: Lippincott Williams & Wilkins; 2004.)

this movement is called reabsorption. This force is countered by tissue osmotic pressure, which opposes such movement (Fig. 8.5). In vessels with intact endothelial cells, fluid moves out of the capillary at the arteriolar end of the capillary bed where the hydrostatic pressure is greater, and it moves back in at the venous end where oncotic pressure is greater. The small amount of fluid that remains in the interstitium is removed by the lymphatic system and returned to the circulation.

FLUID REGULATION

Mechanisms regulating total body water include those that promote thirst and water excretion. Neural and hormonal mechanisms work in concert to attain or maintain fluid balance.

Mechanisms to Promote Fluid Intake

Thirst is an important mechanism contributing to increased fluid intake. Thirst is characterized by a desire to drink fluids high in water content, which is prompted by uncomfortable sensations in the mouth and pharynx.[1] The sensory neurons known as **osmoreceptors** in the hypothalamic thirst center that promote thirst are activated by:

- Cellular dehydration resulting from increased extracellular osmolality
- Decrease in blood volume

Stop and Consider
Are there any risks to drinking too much water?

Stretch receptors in the carotid and aorta (high-pressure baroreceptors) and the left atrium (low-pressure baroreceptors) sense change in arterial blood pressure and contribute to the development of thirst. The hormone, angiotensin II, also indirectly contributes to thirst in response to low blood volume and low blood pressure. The renal hormone, renin, is released from the kidneys and serves as an enzyme, converting angiotensinogen to angiotensin I. Angiotensin I is converted to angiotensin II by angiotensin-converting enzyme, primarily in the lungs. Angiotensin II also regulates aldosterone, a hormone produced in the adrenal cortex. The increase in sodium retention that results from the effects of aldosterone may have the indirect effect of increasing thirst.

Table 8.2 Mechanisms of Membrane Transport

Transport Mechanism	Type of Transport	Stimulus for Transport	Outcome of Transport
Diffusion 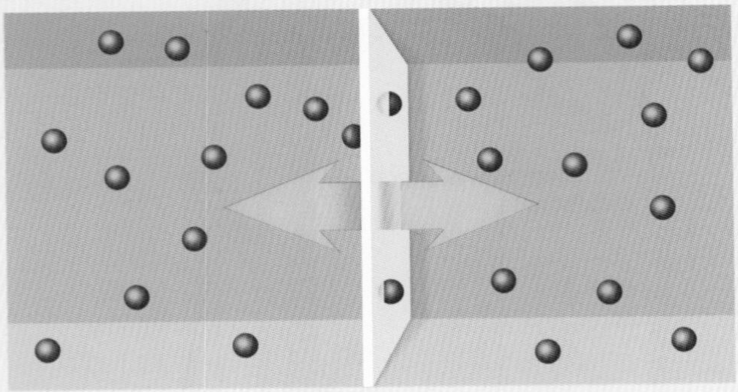	Passive	Chemical or electrical gradient	Particles are evenly distributed across the membrane
Osmosis 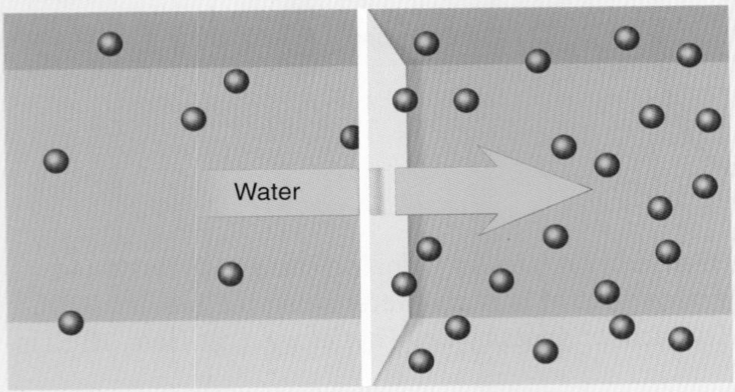 (Water)	Passive	Concentration gradient	Flow of water is directed by osmotically active particles
Facilitated diffusion 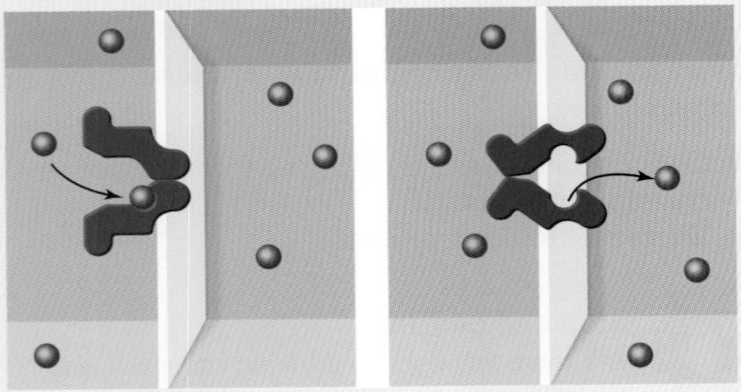	Passive	Binding of substance to transporter	A carrier system moves particles across the membrane
Active transport 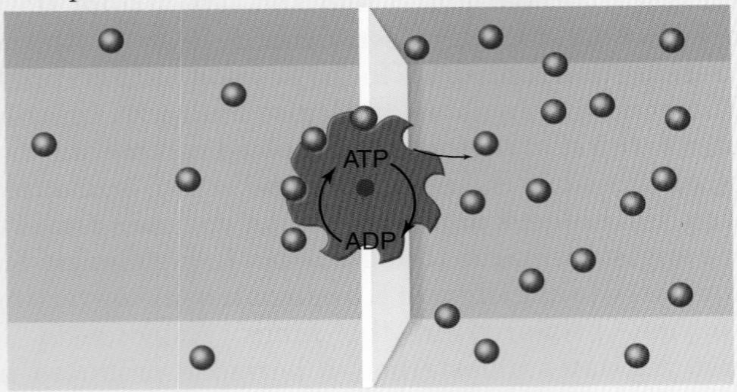 (ATP, ADP)	Active	Proteins using energy pump ions across the membrane	Energy (ATP) moves to particles against a gradient across the membrane

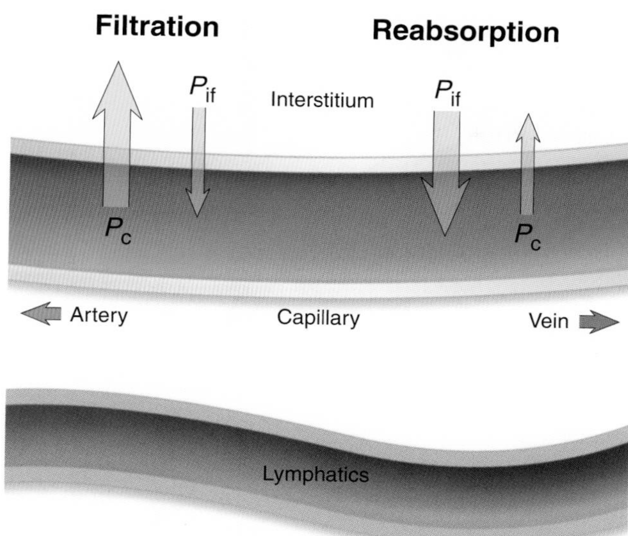

Figure 8.5. Forces for fluid movement across the capillary. P_c is the capillary lumen hydrostatic pressure, and P_{if} is the interstitial hydrostatic pressure. When P_c is greater than P_{if}, filtration processes are dominant. When P_{if} is greater than P_c, reabsorption processes are "favored" or dominant.

Antidiuretic hormone (ADH) regulates fluid volume by controlling excretion of total body water. Produced in the hypothalamus, ADH is transported to the posterior pituitary where it is stored until needed. Production and release of ADH is stimulated by hypothalamic osmoreceptor detection of increased blood osmolality. Also known as vasopressin, ADH works at the level of the kidney to promote the reabsorption of water via aquaporins from the renal-collecting ducts into the vasculature, reducing fluid loss through decrease in urine output. The mechanisms that promote fluid intake are illustrated in Figure 8.6.

Mechanisms to Promote Fluid Excretion

The most common method for increasing fluid excretion is the use of diuretics. **Diuretics** are drugs that increase urine production. The kidneys are the target of the effects of diuretics, which are designed to decrease reabsorption of sodium in the kidney. This mechanism is effective because water moves together with sodium.

Different types of diuretics work on different structures of the kidney. The **loop diuretics** reduce reabsorption of sodium in the thick ascending loop of Henle, causing a decreased osmolality in the interstitial fluid of the collecting ducts and impair the ability to concentrate urine at the loop. **Thiazide diuretics** prevent NaCl reabsorption in the distal convoluted tubule. This action is coupled with increased potassium loss in the urine and uric acid retention. Potassium-sparing diuretics, also known as aldosterone antagonists, reduce sodium reabsorption in the late distal tubule and collecting tubule, functions regulated by aldosterone. The effects of aldosterone at this site are inhibited, promoting excretion of sodium and water. The simultaneous effect of increased potassium reabsorption prevents the potential for excessive loss associated with other types of diuretics. The secretion of hydrogen ions may be altered, increasing the risk for metabolic acidosis, discussed later in this chapter.

Tonicity

The osmotic pressure or tension of a solution is known as tonicity.[1] Tonicity is determined by solutes that cannot cross the semipermeable cell membrane, producing an osmotic force that transports water. Cell size can be affected by tonicity, promoting fluid movement in or out of cells. **Hypertonic** solutions have a greater osmolality than the intracellular fluid (ICF). When cells are in a hypertonic solution in which the extracellular osmotic force is greater, water moves out of the cell causing cells to shrink. **Hypotonic** solutions have a lower osmolality than the ICF. The osmotic forces outside the cells are less than that of the intracellular environment, promoting water movement into the cell and causing cells to swell. An example of cellular changes in response to sodium concentration is shown in Figure 8.7, with hypernatremia serving as an example of a hypertonic solution, and hyponatremia representing a hypotonic solution. Cells in an **isotonic** solution, which has the same osmolality as the ICF,

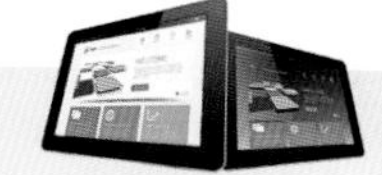

RESEARCH NOTES

In addition to chemical diuretics, certain foods can have diuretic effects. The American Heart Association has long advocated the Dietary Approaches to Stop Hypertension (DASH) diet for blood pressure-lowering effects. The DASH diet is rich in fruits and vegetables. Although it was recognized that the DASH diet lowered blood pressure, the explanation for these effects was unknown until a group of researchers determined that the DASH diet promoted salt excretion and increased urine production, similar to the mechanism of action of diuretic drugs.[2]

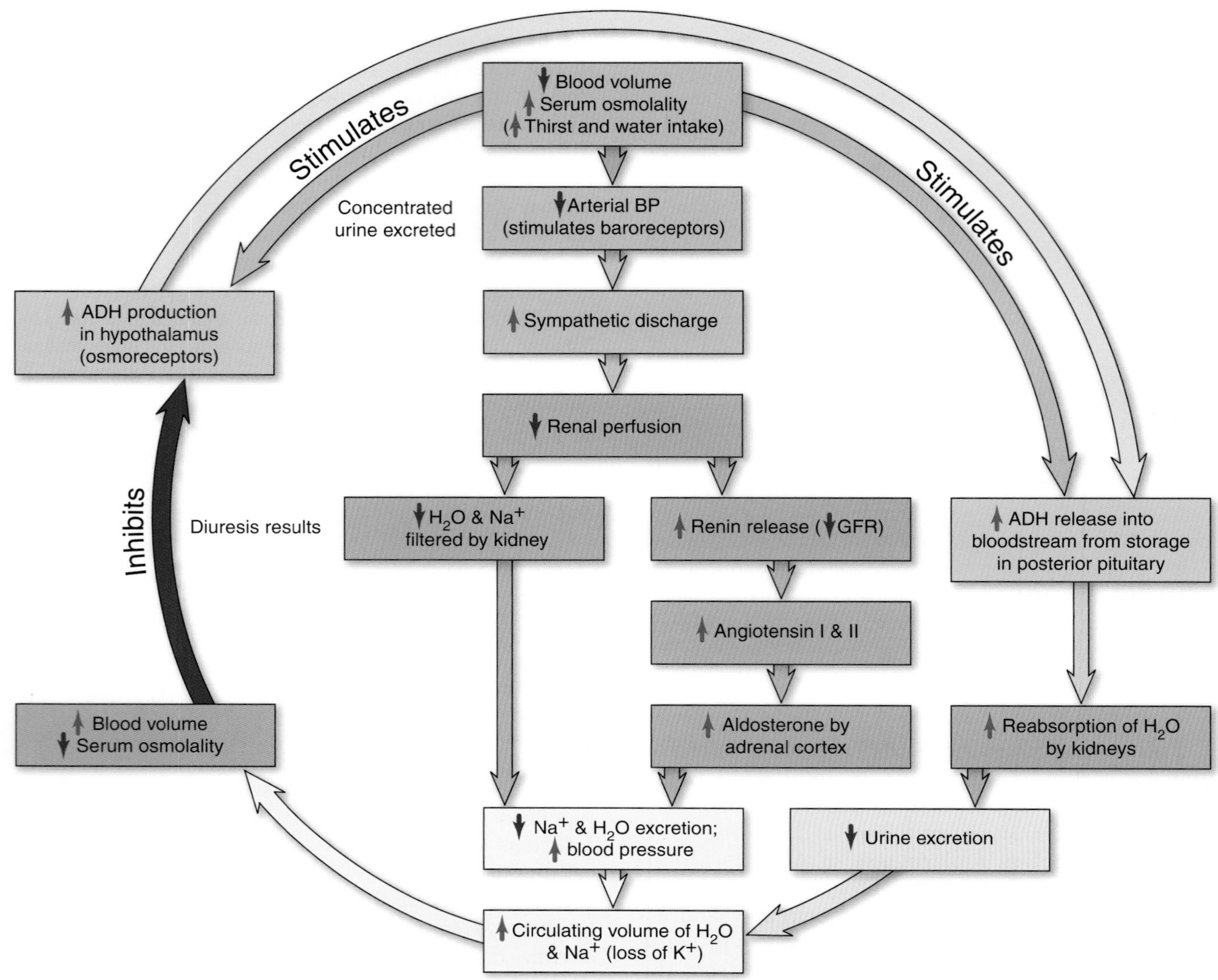

Figure 8.6. Fluid regulation cycle. Negative feedback mechanisms promote regulation of body fluid. Decreased blood volume and increased serum osmolality promote water intake via thirst. Decreased blood pressure (BP) increases sympathetic nervous stimulation, triggering reduced renal perfusion and the renin–angiotensin–aldosterone system. Reabsorption of water through the actions of antidiuretic hormone (ADH) combined with reduced sodium and water secretion through the effects of aldosterone leads to increased circulating volume of water and sodium. Increased blood volume and low serum osmolality inhibit ADH production, promoting diuresis. GFR, glomerular filtration rate. (From Smeltzer SC, Bare BG. *Textbook of Medical-Surgical Nursing*. 10th ed. Philadelphia, PA: Lippincott Williams & Wilkins; 2003.)

are unchanged with osmotic forces balanced within and outside of the cell.

Altered Fluid Balance

The imbalance of hydrostatic and osmotic forces can result in alterations in fluid balance. Total body fluid can also be altered by increases or decreases in fluid ingestion and excretion. Excretion of bodily fluids, such as urine, emesis, sweat, or blood, as well as insensible fluid loss during respiration, can significantly alter fluid balance. Fluid gain or loss can be measured by serial (repeated) measures of body weight, as 1 L of water weighs 1 kg or 2.2 lb.

WATER CONTENT

Alterations in water and sodium can affect total body fluid balance. Decreased vascular volume is known as **hypovolemia**, often the result of inadequate fluid intake or excessive excretion. **Hypervolemia** is an excessive increase of fluid in the extracellular compartment.

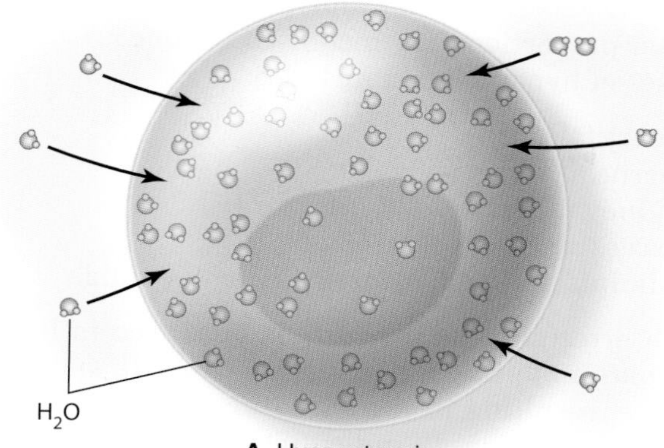

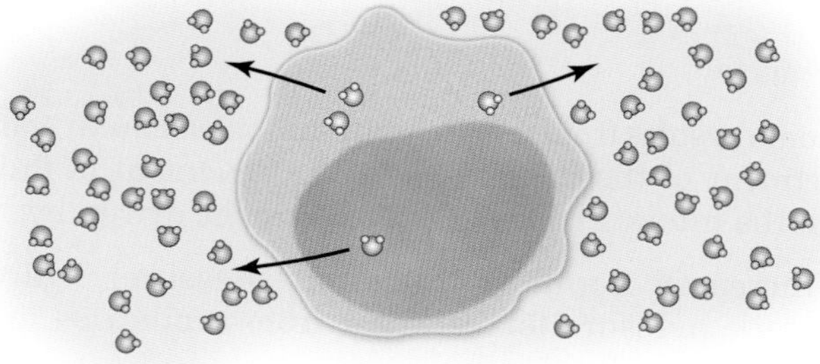

Figure 8.7. Effect of tonicity on cell size. **A:** The cell swells as water is pulled in from extracellular fluid. **B:** The cell shrinks as water is pulled out into extracellular fluid.

Hypovolemia

Hypovolemia is a deficit of body fluid volume. Causes of hypovolemia can be attributed to excessive body fluid loss, reduction of fluid intake, or loss of fluid to a third space resulting in decreased extracellular fluid volume. Decreased intravascular volume results in decreased capillary hydrostatic pressure. Blood circulation and transport of oxygen and nutrients to tissues may be impaired.

Clinical manifestations of hypovolemia, from least to most severe, include:

- Thirst
- Dry mucous membranes
- Weight loss
- Flattened neck veins
- Diminished skin **turgor** (fullness) (Fig. 8.8)
- Prolonged time for capillaries to refill after blanching (more than 3 seconds)
- Decreased urine output
- Increased heart rate
- Decreased blood pressure
- Altered level of consciousness

The body attempts to compensate with physiologic responses to counter the manifestations of hypovolemia. Decreased blood flow to the kidneys triggers the activation of the renin–angiotensin–aldosterone system (RAAS), increasing sodium and water reabsorption.

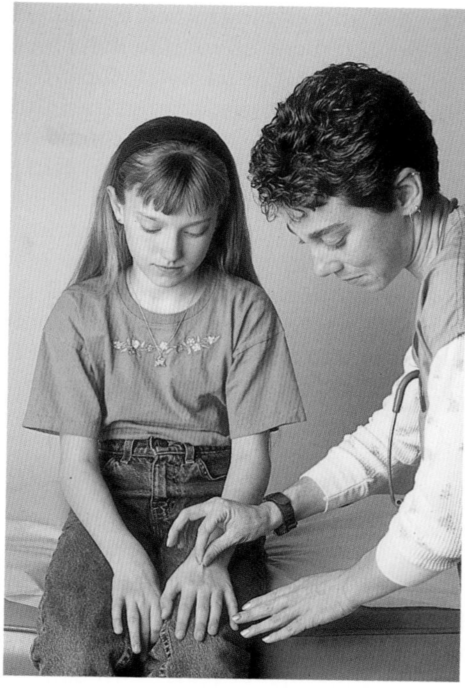

Figure 8.8. Skin turgor evaluation. After squeezing the skin together, release should result in the ridges immediately returning to a normal appearance. Dehydration should be suspected when evidence of ridges remain after release. (Courtesy Lesha Studios, with permission.)

Decreased blood pressure sensed by baroreceptors stimulates the sympathetic nervous system to increase heart rate, constrict arteries, and increase contractility of the heart. The expected response to compensate for decreased intravascular fluid volume is increased cardiac output and mean arterial pressure. ADH and aldosterone work together to decrease urine output and increase fluid intake by stimulating thirst. Failure to compensate adequately may impair cellular function significantly, resulting in multisystem failure.

The type of fluid loss that leads to hypovolemia may affect tonicity of the extracellular fluid. The diagnosis and management of alterations in fluid balance may depend on the circumstances contributing to hypovolemia. Laboratory testing of hemoglobin, hematocrit, blood urea nitrogen (BUN), serum creatinine, urine-specific gravity, blood glucose, electrolytes, and plasma proteins can provide dditional information to guide treatment strategies.

Hemorrhage

Hemorrhage, or excessive bleeding, may result in hypovolemia. Because water and sodium are lost at comparable rates, this condition is isotonic. Hemoglobin and hematocrit are decreased and BUN may be increased early in hemorrhage. Damage to other organ systems may be evident if hypovolemia is not corrected. Fluid replacement for volume expansion is often necessary and is determined by the amount of blood loss. Replacement of volume with blood products, either whole blood or packed (concentrated) red blood cells, provides the necessary extracellular fluid expansion as well as the cellular components lost with bleeding. The crystalloid solution **Ringer lactate** intravenous fluid contains sodium, chloride, potassium, calcium, and lactate in concentrations that mirror those found in plasma and may also be an appropriate treatment in large volume fluid resuscitation.[3] Fluid replacement with osmotically active fluids helps promote the movement of fluid from the interstitial space to the intravascular space.

Dehydration

Dehydration is the result of decreased extracellular fluid volume or increased sodium content in relation to water content, representing a hypertonic condition. Excessive watery diarrhea, sweating, and insensible respiratory water loss during hyperventilation or fever may lead to dehydration. Intravascular volume may become viscous, with evidence of an increase in hematocrit caused by hemoconcentration. Thirst may be stimulated, and urinary output decreased. Movement of fluid from the intracellular to the extracellular compartment promotes cell shrinkage. Dehydration of brain and nerve cells may result in headache, decreased reflexes, seizures, and coma. Expansion of extracellular volume with oral or intravenous rehydration, such as Ringer lactate, is indicated to prevent organ damage. When chloride loss complicates dehydration, intravenous replacement with an isotonic solution of normal saline may be indicated to address the underlying ionic alteration.

Water Intoxication

Hypotonic hypovolemia, also known as water intoxication, results from decreased sodium concentration, often the result of water replacement after strenuous activity or excessive loss of sodium from diuretic therapy inhibiting ADH. Cellular swelling occurs because of movement of water from the extracellular space to the intracellular space. Increases in cellular water trigger clinical manifestations, including muscle weakness, cramps, and fatigue, and central nervous system involvement such as headache, confusion, and depression of deep tendon reflexes (DTRs). Treatments including limiting water or increasing sodium intake target the underlying cause of the condition. Hypertonic saline solutions and loop diuretics to increase water elimination are also optional treatments.

Hypervolemia

Hypervolemia is an expansion of extracellular volume involving the interstitial or vascular space.

When excess sodium and water are retained in similar proportions, the increased volume is isotonic. Causes of hypervolemia include:

- Heart failure
- Cirrhosis of the liver
- Kidney failure
- Excessive fluid replacement
- Administration of osmotically active fluids

Mean arterial blood pressure is increased in hypervolemia, inhibiting the secretion of ADH and aldosterone, resulting in increased urinary sodium and water elimination. In individuals who are unable to mount these compensatory mechanisms, heart failure and pulmonary edema may result.

Edema

Edema results from increases in the extracellular compartment of the interstitial fluid. Movement of fluid into the interstitial compartment can be driven by:

- Increased capillary filtration pressure: hydrostatic pressure forces water from capillaries into interstitial fluid
- Decreased capillary osmotic pressure: fluid moves to the interstitium across the concentration gradient
- Increased capillary permeability: altered integrity of the capillary wall allows proteins to leak from the capillaries into the interstitial space, increasing interstitial osmotic pressure
- Obstructed lymph flow (**lymphedema**): fluid in the interstitium cannot be returned to the systemic circulation

The mechanisms for the development of edema are depicted in Figure 8.9. Edematous tissues may be at risk for damage because of the resulting increased distance for diffusion and the compression of the vasculature supplying oxygen and removing waste. The clinical manifestations of edema are determined by the sites of occurrence. When located in the joints, pain and impaired movement may result. When located in the brain or lungs, function may be so impaired that death may result. When fluid accumulation in the peripheral interstitium exceeds the tissues' ability for absorption, the fluid becomes mobile when pressure is exerted upon it. When pressure over an edematous area forces fluid movement and leaves an indentation, the edema is referred to as **pitting** (Fig. 8.10). Edema may be recognized as a local area of swelling, increased body weight, and pain.

Body weight measurements provide an effective evaluation of edema, with increased body weight reflecting an increase in total body fluid. Visual inspection of extremities helps to identify peripheral edema. Evaluation of edema within organ systems not readily visible depends on the involved tissues. Auscultation of heart and lungs may reveal excessive fluid.

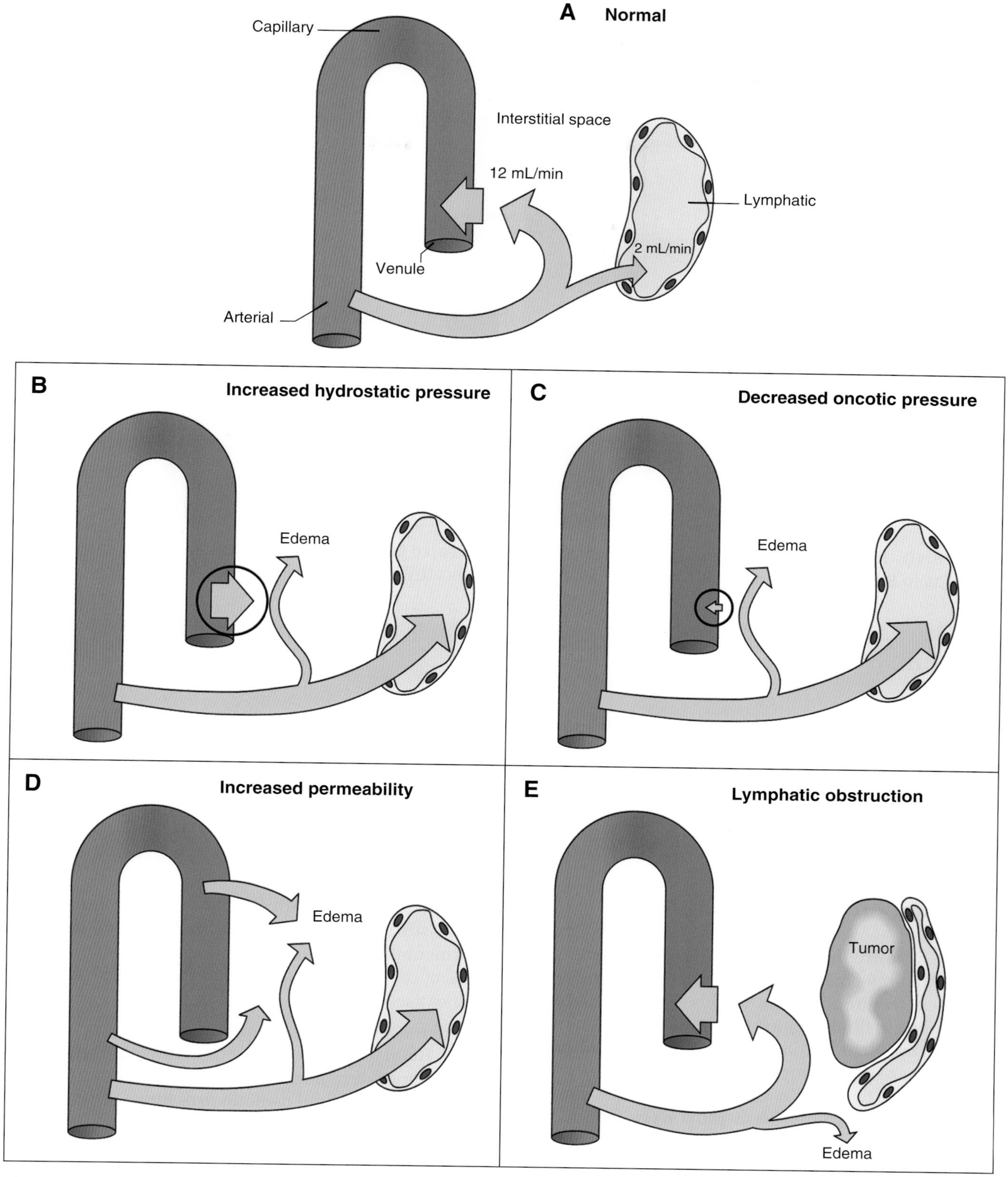

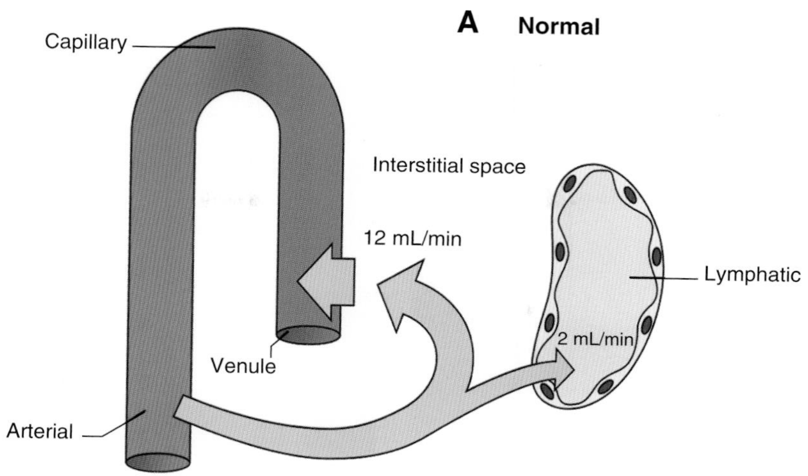

Figure 8.9. Mechanisms of edema in the capillary system. **A:** Normal. The differential between the hydrostatic and oncotic pressures at the arterial end of the capillary system is responsible for the filtration into the interstitial space of approximately 14 mL of fluid per minute. The fluid is reabsorbed at the venous end at the rate of 12 mL/min. Lymphatic capillaries drain fluid at a rate of 2 mL/min. **B:** Edema caused by increased hydrostatic pressure. Elevation at the venous end of the capillary decreases reabsorption. If the lymphatic capacity to drain fluid is exceeded, fluid accumulates. **C:** Edema caused by decreased oncotic pressure. Decreased oncotic pressure in the vascular space promotes reduced fluid reabsorption. **D:** Edema caused by increased permeability results from endothelial injury, allowing fluid to leak from the vascular space. **E:** Lymphedema results from accumulation of fluid caused by lymphatic obstruction. (From Rubin E, Farber JL. *Pathology*. 4th ed. Philadelphia, PA: Lippincott Williams & Wilkins; 2005.)

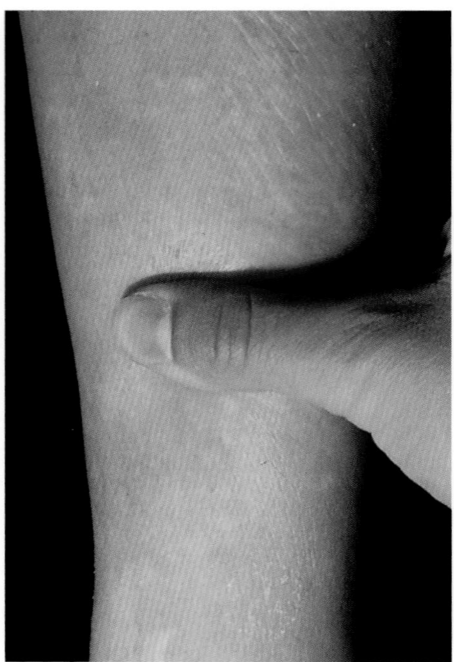
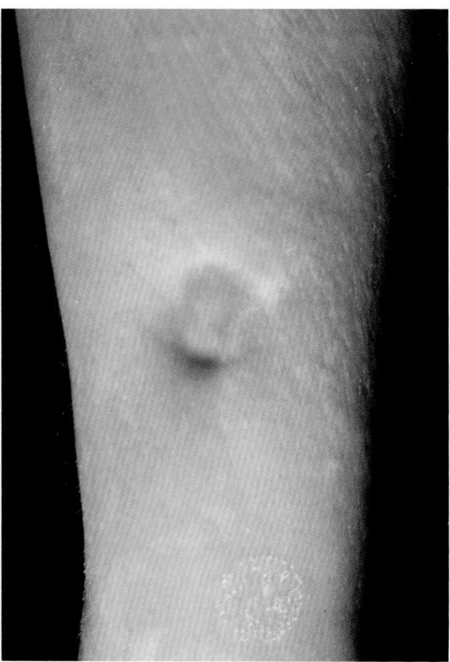

Figure 8.10. Pitting edema. Palpation causes a depression when released because of movement of fluid in the interstitium. (From Rubin E, Farber JL. *Pathology*. 4th ed. Philadelphia, PA: Lippincott Williams & Wilkins; 2005.)

Module 3 Clinical Models

The clinical models presented in this chapter incorporate the concepts of altered fluid and electrolyte balance. Each concept is individually highlighted, although clearly each is related to the other. When reviewing the clinical models, the student should apply the concepts he or she has learned about these alterations.

Altered Fluid Balance: Cirrhosis

Chapter 5 introduced the liver disease known as cirrhosis. In this chapter, the discussion of cirrhosis focuses on the implications of this disease related to alterations in fluid balance. Cirrhosis and chronic liver disease represent leading causes of mortality, although the rates are decreasing. From 1980 to 1989, hospitalization rates for women were less than that for men by one-third. Hospitalization rates were 20% to 30% lower in Whites as compared to Blacks. Increasing age was associated with increased death rates in men (15.2 to 49 in 100,000) and in women (4.8 to 26.7 in 100,000) when rates for age groups in the 35 to 44 and 65 to 74 (men) and 75 to 84 (women) range were compared.[4]

PATHOPHYSIOLOGY

As previously discussed, **cirrhosis** is a form of liver disease characterized by the interference of local blood flow and hepatocyte damage. Cirrhosis is often (but not always) the result of hepatitis and liver damage from alcohol exposure. The most common complication of cirrhosis is **ascites**, accumulation of fluid in the peritoneal cavity. This is an example of fluid loss to a "third space," making it unavailable for use in the remaining extracellular or intracellular compartments.

Ascites is the manifestation of the combination of hydrostatic pressure, oncotic pressure, and capillary permeability, similar to other forms of edema. Examples of conditions leading to ascites and the underlying causes include:

- Increased hydrostatic pressure
  - Budd–Chiari syndrome (hepatic vein obstruction)
  - Congestive heart failure
- Decreased colloid osmotic pressure
  - Malnutrition
  - Nephrotic syndrome
- Increased capillary permeability
  - Malignancy
  - Bacterial peritoneal infection

Increased vascular resistance to blood flow in the liver causes a condition known as **portal hypertension**, elevation in the portal (hepatic) pressure of the liver. Increased pressure promotes movement of fluid out of capillaries through hydrostatic mechanisms.

The movement of fluid into the interstitium exceeds the ability of the lymphatic system to recirculate fluid to the systemic circulation, leading to accumulation. Increased vascular resistance triggers the production of vasodilators to decrease vascular resistance and increase blood flow. The dilation of the portal arteries eventually results in a decrease in blood volume and a drop in arterial pressure. To compensate for the drop in blood pressure, arterial pressure is maintained by activating mechanisms, which results in sodium and water retention and expands plasma volume. Intestinal capillary pressure and permeability are altered by the combination of portal hypertension and arterial dilation, promoting the transport of fluid to the abdominal cavity. In the advanced state, cirrhosis is associated with protein wasting. This leads to loss of albumin in the circulation, further altering fluid balance through loss of fluid to the extravascular space.

Progressive pathology may lead to renal impairment, including impaired free water excretion that leads to dilutional hyponatremia and renal vasoconstriction, which increases the risk of **hepatorenal syndrome** (renal failure caused by severe renal vasoconstriction). Increased levels of renin and aldosterone further contribute to altered fluid balance.

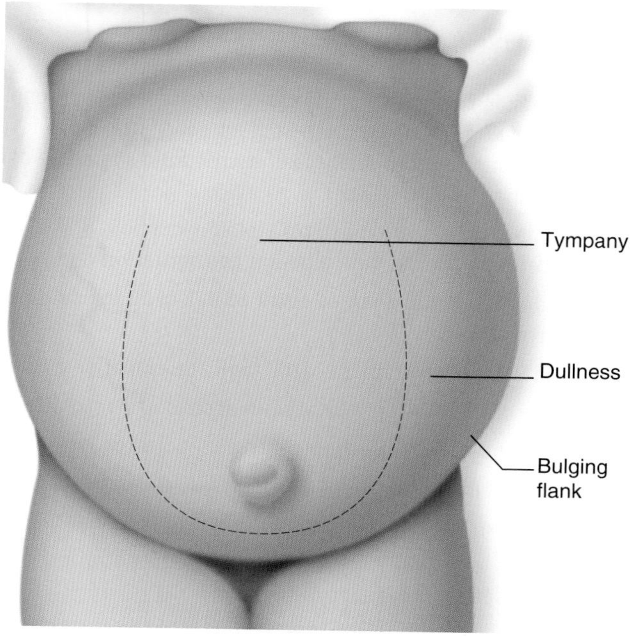

CLINICAL MANIFESTATIONS

The severity of ascites is related to the manifestation of clinical signs and symptoms (Fig. 8.11). Ascites can be described based on volume of fluid in the peritoneum (moderate to large volume) and is often associated with the following manifestations:

- Moderate to severe abdominal discomfort
- Increased abdominal girth
- Increased weight
- Severe sodium retention
- Dilutional hyponatremia
- Renal failure (oliguria and increase in serum creatinine)

Figure 8.11. Clinical evidence of ascites. Fluid accumulation in the abdominal cavity causes distention and bulging flanks and umbilicus. Tympany over the intestines and dullness over fluid in abdomen and flanks are also noted.

TREATMENT

The volume of ascites is a primary determinant of treatment. Diuretics are often used to promote ascitic fluid loss and normalize sodium balance. Caution must be used to avoid excessive diuresis, which results in hypovolemia and increases risk of renal failure. In severe cases, paracentesis may be necessary. **Paracentesis** is the insertion of a cannula into the peritoneal cavity to remove ascitic fluid (Fig. 8.12). Intravenous albumin may be administered to expand plasma volume in individuals who have had a large volume of fluid removed to reduce the risk of circulatory dysfunction and rapid recurrence of ascites.

DIAGNOSTIC CRITERIA

Physical examination and change in body weight are used to diagnose ascites. Measurement of abdominal girth or circumference may be useful. Evaluation of liver, renal, and cardiac function should be completed to determine systemic damage or dysfunction.

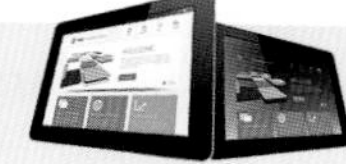

RESEARCH NOTES

Ascites can lead to the development of shock, renal failure, respiratory failure, and hypoperfusion as a result of abdominal pressure. In a recent case report, a 67-year-old woman came into the emergency room who reported mild difficulty breathing. Her abdomen was obese and tense on examination. While being evaluated in the emergency room, the patient developed severe hypotension, oliguria (decreased urine output), and an increased serum creatinine level consistent with acute onset renal failure. She required ventilatory support because of decreased oxygen saturation of her tissues. An ultrasound revealed severe ascites. Paracentesis was done with removal of 4,500 mL of fluid, reducing abdominal pressure.[5]

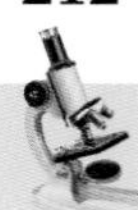

FROM THE LAB

Urinary sodium concentration provides a measurement of renal sodium retention. In patients with large volume ascites, urine sodium concentrations of 10 mmol/L are consistent with severe sodium retention. Analysis of ascitic fluid should be done to help determine etiology. Ascitic fluid analysis involves:

- Determination of serum-ascitic albumin gradient (SAAG): calculated from the difference between ascitic fluid albumin concentration and serum albumin concentration
  - Gradients greater than or equal to 1.1 g/dL indicate portal hypertension or transudative ascites
  - Gradients lesser than 1.1 g/dL indicate exudative ascites
- Amylase concentration: elevated in ascites of pancreatic origin
- White blood cell (WBC) count: increase indicates infection
  - Predominantly polymorphonuclear WBC indicates bacterial infection
  - Predominantly mononuclear WBC indicates fungal or tuberculin infection
- Red blood cell (RBC) count: increased concentration indicates hemorrhagic ascites, often caused by malignancy
- Gram stain and culture: determination of pathogen involved in infection
- Cytology: examination of cells for signs of malignancy

Stop and Consider
Why does ascites often return after fluid removal by paracentesis?

Altered Sodium Balance: Dehydration

Dehydration is characterized by negative fluid balance. Diarrhea is the most common cause of dehydration, although a variety of other conditions can lead to dehydration. According to the World Health Organization, dehydration secondary to diarrheal illness is the leading cause of infant and child mortality. It was estimated that between 2000 and 2003, diarrhea was the cause of death in 17% of children younger than 5 years and in 3% of babies younger than 28 days of age. A worldwide problem linked to 4% of all deaths, diarrhea kills approximately 2.2 million people in the world each year, mostly affecting children in developing countries.

PATHOPHYSIOLOGY

Fluid deficit associated with dehydration involves both intracellular and extracellular volume. Causes of dehydration resulting in fluid depletion include:

- Decreased fluid intake
- Increased fluid output
  - Renal
  - Gastrointestinal
  - Insensible
- Fluid shift between compartments
  - Ascites
  - Capillary leakage (burns and sepsis)

Dehydration is categorized based on blood sodium concentration, providing information about the type of fluid loss and the potential complications associated with coexisting electrolyte imbalance. Categories of dehydration are described in Table 8.3. Volume deficit coupled with altered sodium balance stimulates further fluid shifts, determined by the amount of circulating sodium in the blood. In hyponatremic dehydration, the fluid lost contains more sodium than the amount contained in the blood, leading to a hypotonic state. Seeking equilibrium, fluid shifts from the intravascular compartment to the extravascular compartment because of the low level of sodium in the blood. This step results in further volume depletion of the intravascular space, exaggerating the effect of actual volume loss. Conversely, hypernatremic dehydration is associated with hypotonic fluid loss. Because less sodium is lost relative to the fluid amount, loss of hypotonic fluid leads to a hypertonic state, promoting fluid movement from the extravascular space to the intravascular space. This type of fluid shift actually minimizes the effects of the fluid loss, maintaining vascular volume and potential for perfusion.[6]

CLINICAL MANIFESTATIONS

Identification of clinical manifestations of dehydration helps to determine dehydration severity. Estimates of fluid deficit are based on age and body size. In newborns, dehydration is classified by loss of body weight, with 5% considered mild, 10% considered moderate, and 15% considered severe. In children who weigh more than 10 kg, mild dehydration is associated with a 3% weight loss, moderate is associated with a 6% loss, and severe equates to a 9% loss. Mild dehydration is associated with mild manifestations, with signs and symptoms worsening as the severity of dehydration increases. Manifestations of dehydration include:

- Decreased level of consciousness
- Prolonged capillary refill time

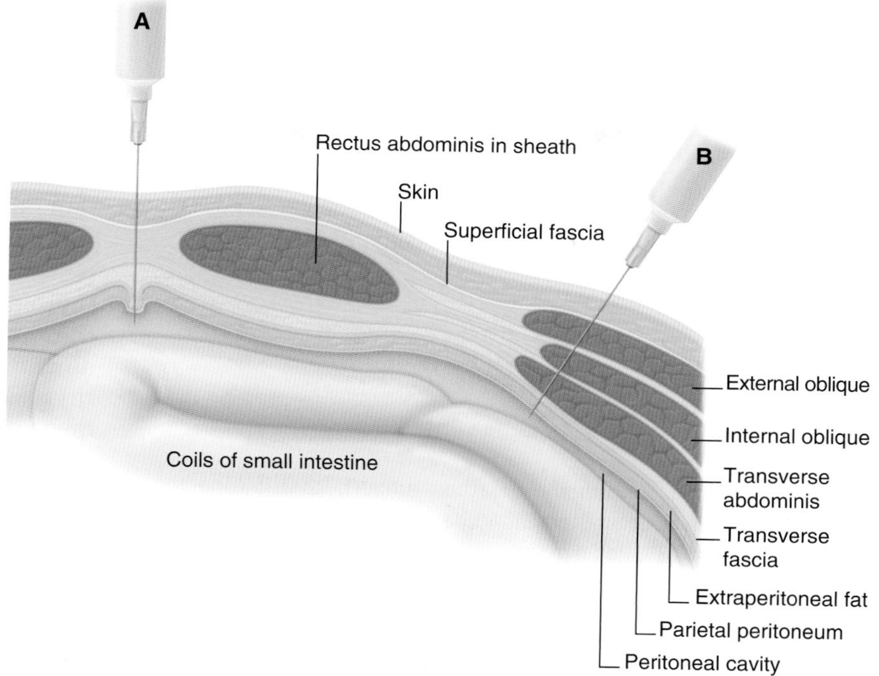

Figure 8.12. Paracentesis of the abdominal cavity. **A:** Midline approach. **B:** Lateral approach. (From Snell MD. *Clinical Anatomy*. 7th ed. Philadelphia, PA: Lippincott Williams & Wilkins; 2003.)

Table 8.3 Classifications of Dehydration: Sodium Considerations

Dehydration Category	Sodium Concentration	Frequency of Diagnosis	Type of Fluid Loss	Fluid Shifts
Hyponatremic	<130 mEq/L	5%–10%	Hypertonic	Intravascular to Extravascular
Isonatremic	130–150 mEq/L	80%	Isotonic	None
Hypernatremic	> 150 mEq/L	5%–10%	Hypotonic	Extravascular to Intravascular

- Dry mucous membranes
- Decreased or absent tears
- Change in vital signs
  - Increased respiratory rate
  - Decreased blood pressure
  - Weak pulse
- Depressed fontanel (areas not enclosed by cranium, or "soft spots" on infants heads)
- Sunken eye
- Decreased or absent urine output

DIAGNOSTIC CRITERIA

A recent history helps determine the cause and severity of dehydration. Fluid intake, including volume and type (hypertonic or hypotonic), as well as fluid output, quantity, and characteristics (urine, stools, emesis, and sweat), are important in determining fluid balance. Appetite patterns and recent weight loss may provide an indication of malnutrition. Underlying medical condition, recent exposure to illness, or recent travel may point to an infectious cause of fluid imbalance.

History and evaluation of clinical manifestations provide the basis of diagnosis. Laboratory analyses are generally reserved for severe cases of dehydration. Blood concentrations of sodium, potassium, and chloride may indicate associated electrolyte and acid–base imbalances. Poor perfusion may promote buildup of lactic acid, consuming bicarbonate. Measures of circulating bicarbonate may provide another indication of acid–base balance. Hypoperfusion may also lead to renal damage, which can be determined by evaluation of BUN and creatinine. Urine can be evaluated for concentration by measurement of specific gravity and for electrolyte content (see From the Lab, below). Results of the laboratory evaluation may assist in the treatment plan.

TREATMENT

Oral rehydration for mild to moderate dehydration helps restore fluid balance. Fluids intended for

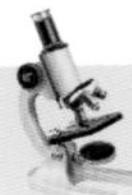

FROM THE LAB

Urine-specific gravity measures the concentration of particles in the urine, comparing the weight of urine to the weight of water. A value between 1.010 and 1.025 suggests fluid balance. Concentrated urine contains more particles and has a higher specific gravity (more than 1.025). Dilute urine has a lower concentration of particles and has a lower specific gravity (less than 1.010). Urine osmolality measures indicate the kidney's ability to excrete or conserve water, or the ability to concentrate urine, providing additional information on the renal contributions to fluid and electrolyte balance.

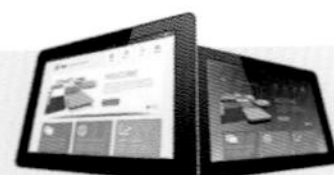

RESEARCH NOTES

Hyponatremia is becoming an increasing concern for marathon runners, contributing to race-related morbidity and mortality.[7] In a recent study of 488 athletes participating in the Boston Marathon, researchers found that 13% had hyponatremia and 0.6% had critical hyponatremia with extremely low serum sodium concentrations. Excessive fluid intake during the race was the strongest single predictor for the development of hyponatremia. The researchers found no association with the type of fluid intake among the runners (plain water or electrolyte solutions) and the risk for hypovolemia, emphasizing the greater role of volume in the development of fluid imbalance. The risk was significantly increased in women and in individuals with extremes of body mass index.

rehydration contain sodium, potassium, and glucose in the appropriate proportions, promoting ready absorption from the gastrointestinal system into the circulation. Rehydration fluids must be administered frequently and in small amounts. Severe dehydration with hypovolemia requires intravenous administration of Ringer lactate or isotonic saline solution to promote intravascular volume. Ideally, volume replacement should be determined based on calculation of fluid deficit. Care must be taken to avoid rapid correction of hyponatremia, which is associated with neurologic complications. Rapid rehydration in hypernatremia may cause cellular swelling to the point of cellular rupture.

Altered Calcium Balance: Hypoparathyroidism

Calcium homeostasis is tightly controlled through negative feedback regulation. Availability of calcium within a narrow range in the blood promotes optimal cellular and tissue function including generation of action potentials, muscle contraction and enzyme activity throughout the body. The parathyroid glands play an essential role in regulation of calcium, participating in negative feedback regulation to maintain calcium blood levels between 8.5 and 10.5 mg/dL. Alterations in parathyroid function contribute to loss of negative feedback regulation, leading to alterations in blood calcium levels.

Hypoparathyroidism is a condition characterized by a low level of parathyroid hormone secretion. One of the most common reasons for hypoparathyroidism is damage to the parathyroid glands during thyroid surgery or thyroid radiation treatment because of the close proximity of the parathyroid and thyroid glands. Hypoparathyroidism may also be congenital, identified in infants early in life. Autoimmune causes of hypoparathyroidism involving parathyroid injury due to autoantibodies can also lead to reduced parathyroid function. Reduction or loss of parathyroid function and resulting consequences in calcium homeostasis is the focus of this clinical model.

PATHOPHYSIOLOGY

There are four parathyroid glands located posterior to the thyroid gland. The parathyroid glands produce parathyroid hormone in response to the need to increase blood calcium. Parathyroid hormone targets sources of calcium, mobilizing calcium from intracellular calcium stores to the blood for participation in calcium-required functions. The bones represent a major target for parathyroid hormone as they serve as a large calcium storage site. The kidneys are also responsive to parathyroid hormone, increasing reabsorption of calcium from the urinary filtrate and moving the calcium back into the blood. Indirectly, parathyroid hormone assists in intestinal reabsorption of calcium via activated vitamin D. When calcium levels rise to target levels in the blood, the parathyroid glands receive signals to reduce production of parathyroid hormone. This negative feedback system is essential in maintaining calcium homeostasis.

When the parathyroid gland function is impaired and unable to respond to signals to increase production of parathyroid hormone in response to low calcium levels, the triggers for mobilizing calcium stores and enhancing renal reabsorption have reduced or no effectiveness. The inability to increase calcium levels due to lack of parathyroid hormone leads to hypocalcemia.

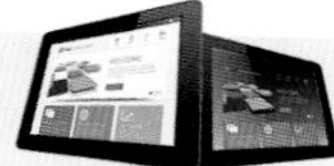

RESEARCH NOTES

Recombinant parathyroid hormone (rhPTH) was investigated in clinical trial designed to determine effectiveness in treatment of hypoparathyroidism. Research participants received injections of rhPTH in a variety of doses to determine effectiveness in regulating calcium levels while reducing supplemental calcium and vitamin D treatments. FDA approval of rhPTH was based on the clinical trials results, providing the foundation of current treatment recommentations.[8]

CLINICAL MANIFESTATIONS

The signs and symptoms of hypoparathyroidism are general and may make diagnosis challenging without laboratory confirmation. There is significant overlap between the clinical manifestations of hypoparathyroidism with hypocalcemia including enhanced neuromuscular irritability, seizure and muscle cramping. Clinical manifestations of hypothyroidism in adults include:

- Hair dryness and loss
- Nail ridges and breakage
- Skin dryness
- Bone loss
- Tingling in extremities (parathesia)
- Visual changes
- Muscle cramps
- Seizures
- Fatigue

Children with congenital hypoparathyroidism are particularly susceptible to the neurologic consequences of low calcium levels. Congenital hypoparathyroidism is associated with seizures, growth and neurological deficits along with unusual facial characteristics.

DIAGNOSTIC CRITERIA

Past medical and surgical history are important considerations in the determination of hypoparathyroidism. Physical examination that includes the objectives signs of hypoparathyroidism will provide evidence of clinical manifestations, prompting laboratory evaluation to confirm diagnosis. Laboratory measures of parathyroid hormone, blood calcium, phosphorus, and magnesium will be important to determine electrolyte imbalance and the underlying cause. Measurement of urinary calcium provides evidence for efficiency of renal calcium reabsorption.

TREATMENT

Hypoparathyroidism is a chronic condition requiring long-term treatment with supplemental calcium (carbonate or citrate) and vitamin D (calcitriol) with the objective of maintenance of blood calcium levels at the lower range of normal and optimal calcium reabsorption. Achievement of calcium homeostasis will reduce manifestations and long-term consequences of hypocalcemia. Recently, a new treatment for hypoparathyroidism was approved. Recombinant parathyroid hormone, given in conjunction with calcium and vitamin D supplementation, has been approved for treatment of hypoparathyroidism.[8]

Stop and Consider

What changes in other electrolytes would be expected in hypoparathyroidism-associated hypocalcemia, and what are the expected manifestations that are likely?

SUMMARY

- Fluid and electrolyte balance are important to homeostasis and cellular function.
- Fluid represents 60% of body weight, with two-thirds of body fluids contained in the intracellular compartment and the remaining one-third contained in the extracellular compartment.
- Fluid transport is accomplished based on concentration and chemical gradients. Osmotic pressure is generated by charged particles and pressure gradients are generated by hydrostatic forces.
- Thirst, stimulated by hormonal mechanisms, is important in the regulation of fluid intake. Diuretics stimulate excretion of fluid through actions within the kidneys.
- Alterations in fluid balance may result from imbalance between hydrostatic and osmotic forces and from altered capillary permeability. Hypervolemia and hypovolemia are examples of altered fluid balance.
- Alterations in fluid and electrolyte balance can occur because of other diseases or can cause illness.
- Electrolytes contain positive charges (cations) or negative charges (anions) that determine attractive forces and movement caused by differing concentrations between compartments.

- Low blood levels of electrolytes are indicated by the prefix "hypo"; increased blood levels of electrolytes are indicated by the prefix "hyper," followed by the term for the specific electrolyte involved (i.e., -natremia [sodium], -kalemia [potassium], and -phosphatemia [phosphate]).
- Correction of fluid and electrolyte imbalances is critical to the maintenance of bodily functions.
- To correct imbalances in fluid and electrolyte, careful consideration must be given to the potential impact across body systems and compartments.

CASE STUDY 8.1

Jenny, a 19-year-old college student, was injured in a fire resulting from a car accident. She experienced full-thickness burns over approximately 10% of her body. Consider the clinical model that is most related to this process. From your reading related to fluid, electrolyte, and acid–base balance, answer the following questions:

1. What anatomic problem would most likely lead to fluid shifts because of burn injury?
2. What is the cause of fluid shifts in burn injury?
3. How would you manage fluid shifts in burn injury?
4. What would you expect for clinical manifestations?
5. What diagnostic tests might be used?

Log onto the Internet. Search for a relevant journal article or Web site that details fluid resuscitation after burn injury, to confirm your predictions.

PRACTICE EXAM QUESTIONS

1. Fluid loss in response to hypervolemia is promoted by:
   a. Stimulating secretion of ADH, promoting urinary sodium and water elimination
   b. Inhibiting the secretion of aldosterone, promoting urinary sodium and water elimination
   c. Lowering mean arterial pressure
   d. Administering osmotically active fluids

2. Which of the following ions is most closely related to water movement?
   a. Potassium
   b. Sodium
   c. Chloride
   d. Calcium

3. Which compartment contains the greatest amount of body water?
   a. Transcellular
   b. Plasma
   c. Interstitial
   d. Intracellular

4. Which of the following transport mechanisms is associated with movement of water across a semipermeable membrane?
   a. Diffusion
   b. Osmosis
   c. Facilitated diffusion
   d. Active transport

5. Which one of the following conditions will most likely result in edema?
   a. Intravascular filtration pressure greater than interstitial filtration pressure
   b. Intravascular reabsorption greater than interstitial reabsorption
   c. Intravascular oncotic pressure greater than interstitial oncotic pressure
   d. Increased lymphatic reabsorption

6. Ascites is the primary mechanism of body fluid imbalance in which of the following conditions?
   a. Salt-losing tubulopathy
   b. Cirrhosis
   c. AIDS
   d. Isonatremic dehydration

7. Hypokalemia is a hallmark of the following conditions?
   a. Salt-losing tubulopathy
   b. Cirrhosis
   c. AIDS
   d. Isonatremic dehydration

8. Hypotonic fluid loss may result in
   a. Hyponatremic dehydration
   b. Isonatremic dehydration
   c. Hypernatremic dehydration
   d. None of the above

DISCUSSION AND APPLICATION

1. What did I know about alterations in fluid and electrolyte balance before today?
2. What body processes are affected by alterations in fluid and electrolyte balance? How do fluid and electrolyte imbalances affect those processes?

3. What are the potential etiologies for alterations in fluid and electrolyte balance? How do fluid and electrolyte imbalances develop?
4. Who is most at risk for developing fluid and electrolyte imbalances? How can these alterations be prevented?
5. What are the human differences that affect the etiology, risk, or course of alterations in fluid and electrolyte balance?
6. What clinical manifestations are expected during fluid and electrolyte imbalances?
7. What special diagnostic tests are useful in determining the diagnosis and course of alterations in fluid and electrolyte balance?
8. What are the goals of care for individuals who have alterations in fluid and electrolyte balance?
9. How does the concept of alterations in fluid and electrolyte balance build on what I have learned in the previous chapter and in the previous courses?
10. How can I use what I have learned?

RESOURCES

American Burn Association:
http://www.ameriburn.org/

US FDA Natpara (parathyroid hormone) for injection: US prescribing information. 2015:
http://www.fda.gov/

References

1. *Stedman's Electronic Dictionary*. Philadelphia, PA: | Lippincott Williams & Wilkins; 2004.
2. Akita S, Sacks FM, Svetkey LP, et al. Effects of the Dietary Approaches to Stop Hypertension (DASH) diet on the pressure-natriuresis relationship. *Hypertension.* 2003;42(1):8–13.
3. Liamis G, Filippatos TD, Elisaf MS. Correction of hypovolemia with crystalloid fluids: individualizing infusion therapy. *Postgrad Med.* 2015;127(4):405–412.
4. Centers for Disease Control and Prevention. Deaths and hospitalizations from chronic liver disease and cirrhosis—United States, 1980–1989. *MMWR Morb Mortal Wkly Rep.* 1993;41(52/53):969–973.
5. Etzion Y, Barski L, Almog Y. Malignant ascites presenting as abdominal compartment syndrome. *Am J Emerg Med.* 2004;22(5):430–431.
6. Reynolds RM, Padfield PL, Secki JR. Disorders of sodium balance. *BMJ.* 2006;332(7543):702--705.
7. Almond CS, Shin AY, Fortescue EB, et al. Hyponatremia among runners in the Boston marathon. *N Engl J Med.* 2005;352(15):1550–1556.
8. Kim ES, Keating GM. Recombinant parathyroid hormone (1–84): a review in hypoparathyroidism. *Drugs.* 2015;75(11):1293–1303.

Find additional resources for this chapter at http:thePoint.lww.com thePoint®

Chapter

9 Altered Acid–Base Balance

LEARNING OUTCOMES

1. Define and use the key terms listed in this chapter.
2. Differentiate between acids and bases, including expected concentrations to pH.
3. Compare and contrast buffer systems involved in acid–base balance.
4. Outline the critical components that determine pH.
5. Describe the clinical implications of alterations in acid–base balance.
6. Compare and contrast mechanisms leading to metabolic acidosis and metabolic alkalosis.
7. Apply concepts of altered fluid, electrolyte, and acid–base balance to selected clinical models.

INTRODUCTION

When was the last time you thought about the intricate balance of integrated body systems that are required to sustain a physiologic pH? Fortunately, the systems involved in regulation of acid–base balance to maintain a normal pH are active continually, responsive to even small changes that threaten the delicate balance. The redundancy in systems to achieve optimal pH is needed in order for cells to function optimally. This chapter builds on content related to fluid and electrolyte balance and includes a review of the mechanisms involved in acid–base balance, presented in individual modules. It also covers interactions between concepts and the clinical consequences that may result. Selected clinical models that highlight specific alterations are presented in Module 2 to allow the student to apply the learned concepts.

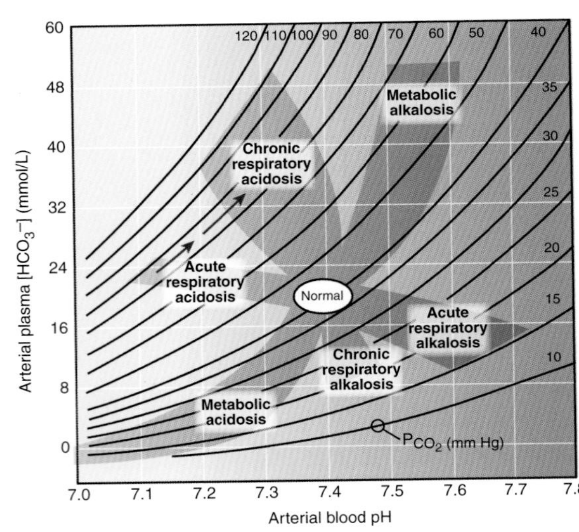

pH-bicarbonate diagram. The diagram shows the relationship between arterial pH, bicarbonate, and Pco2 and provides a useful way of determining a patient's acid–base disturbance. Normal values are shown in the elliptical area in the center. Values left of normal represent acidemia, which may be caused by respiratory acidosis or metabolic acidosis. Values to the right of normal represent alkalemia, which may be caused by respiratory alkalosis or metabolic alkalosis. Pco2, partial pressure of carbon dioxide (mm Hg). From Rhoades RA, Bell DR. Medical Physiology. Philadelphia: Wolters Kluwer Health, 2012.

Module 1 Acid–Base Imbalance

Regulation of acids and bases is critical to the metabolic activities of the body. A narrow physiologic pH range is required for the function of cells, tissues, and organs.

Regulation of Acid and Base

Acids are substances that donate hydrogen ions, and **bases** are substances that accept hydrogen ions. Weak acids in plasma include albumin and inorganic phosphorus. Strong ions almost completely dissociate, or separate, when in solution. In plasma, the strong cations include Na^+, K^+, Ca^{2+}, and Mg^{2+}. The strong anions are Cl^- and lactate.[1] The ratio between acids and bases in the extracellular fluid of the body is closely regulated to provide a favorable environment for metabolic cellular functions. The clinical measurement of this balance is known as **pH**. Hydrogen ion concentration represents the inverse of the pH so that when the pH is low, there is a high amount of H^+; when the pH is high, there is a low amount of H^+.

The ions involved in acid–base balance are reflected in the determination of the anion gap. The **anion gap** is a calculation of the major measured cations and anions in the plasma, providing an indication of acid–base balance. The clinical calculation of anion gap uses sodium (major measurable cation), chloride, and bicarbonate (major measurable anions), and it reflects the difference between the unmeasurable anions, including phosphates, sulfates, organic acids, and proteins. The difference in the concentrations of the cation sodium (140 mEq/L) and the anions chloride (102 mEq/L) and bicarbonate (26 mEq/L) in the blood is known as the anion gap. In other words, $Na^+ - (Cl^- + HCO_3^-) =$ 140 mEq/L − (102 mEq/L + 26 mEq/L) = anion gap (Fig. 9.1). Therefore, the anion gap is 12 mEq/L, with a variation of 2 mEq/L, which results in a normal range of 10 to 14 mEq/L. The anion gap serves as a measurement of acid–base balance. Occasionally, other electrolytes may be considered, resulting in a different reference range distinguishing a normal from an abnormal value. An example of this variation includes the addition of the cation potassium to sodium, which changes the anion gap to 16 mEq/L (range 14 to 18 mEq/L).

BUFFER SYSTEMS

The balance of pH involves **buffer systems** (mixing of acid and base to resist pH change), which are responsible for trading stronger acids and bases for weaker varieties. Acid–base balance is regulated by the actions of buffer systems, working together to respond to conditions threatening acid–base balance. The onset of action in each system varies, leading to rapid responses to correct acute insults, followed by more prolonged correction via a slower onset of action. These buffer systems include:

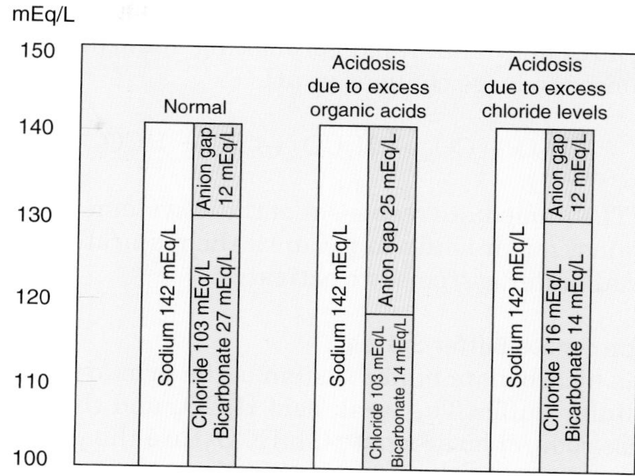

Figure 9.1. Anion gap. Excess organic acids replace bicarbonate in metabolic acidosis with increased anion gap. Rise in chloride is offset by decline in bicarbonate in hyperchloremic acidosis with normal anion gap.

1. **Plasma buffer system:** reacts within seconds in response to hydrogen ion concentration
2. **Respiratory buffer system:** reacts within minutes to excrete CO_2 through change in respiratory rate
3. **Renal buffer system:** reacts within hours to days through the production, absorption, and excretion of acids, bases, and ions

Plasma Buffer Systems

Plasma buffer systems depend on rapid responses of chemical systems in the extracellular and intracellular compartments. The primary plasma buffer systems include the bicarbonate and protein buffer systems and the H^+/K^+ cation exchange system. The buffering of free hydrogen ions is central to the effectiveness of each of the plasma buffer systems. Hydrogen ion can be incorporated into substances, which reduces the amount of freely circulating H^+. Conversely, hydrogen ion can be released from substances to increase the amount of free H^+ circulating in the blood. In this way, changes in pH can be addressed in a rapid way by simply regulating the amount of free H^+ in the blood. One of the primary chemical reactions that regulate these processes involves water, carbon dioxide, carbonic acid, and bicarbonate. The chemical alteration of water and carbon dioxide is catalyzed by the enzyme carbonic anhydrase, present in many body cells. The reaction is reversible and rapid, promoting immediate responses to large changes in pH.

$$H_2O + CO_2 \leftrightarrow H_2CO_3 \leftrightarrow H^+ + HCO_3^-$$

The immediate responses of these systems protect against major shifts in pH until the respiratory and renal buffer systems are activated.

Bicarbonate Buffer System

The bicarbonate buffer system is the primary extracellular buffer. The weak acid H_2CO_3 and the weak base sodium bicarbonate ($NaHCO_3$) are the primary substances involved in the bicarbonate buffer system (Fig. 9.2). The bicarbonate buffer system makes CO_2 available, which can replace HCO_3^- lost as a result of added base or eliminated with the addition of acid.

Protein Buffer System

The protein buffer system responds to the moment-to-moment changes to retain pH in the narrow range necessary for optimal cell function. Proteins serve as the largest buffering system. The protein buffer system involves intracellular proteins and the proteins albumin and plasma globulins in the vascular compartment. Able to function as either acid or base, proteins are referred to as **amphoteric**. The protein buffers can both accept or donate H^+ ions. The H^+ and CO_2 ions that are released because of these reactions can then freely diffuse across cell membranes.

Potassium–Hydrogen Exchange

Ionic exchange of the potassium (K^+) and hydrogen (H^+) cations contributes to regulation of acid–base balance. Excess H^+ in the extracellular compartment can diffuse across the cell membrane inside the cell for buffering. The entry of H^+ prompts the exit of K^+ from within the cell to the extracellular space, potentially resulting in hyperkalemia. Conversely, if the extracellular level of K^+ falls, as in the case of hypokalemia, K^+ then moves out of the cell in parallel with H^+ entry into the cell, decreasing extracellular concentrations of H^+, thereby increasing pH. The regulation of acid–base and electrolyte balance is closely tied in an effort to maintain homeostasis.

A. $HCL + NaHCO_3 \rightleftharpoons H_2CO_3 + NaCl$

B. $NaOH + H_2CO_3 \rightleftharpoons NaHCO_3 + H_2O$

Figure 9.2. Bicarbonate buffer systems. **A:** The strong acid HCl is substituted for the weaker acid H_2CO_3 through a reaction with the weak base $NaHCO_3$. **B:** The strong base sodium hydroxide (NaOH) is substituted for the weak base $NaHCO_3$ through a reaction with the weak acid H_2CO_3.

Respiratory Buffer System

The respiratory buffer system is the second system that responds to changes in pH, contributing to regulation of CO_2. H_2CO_3 is an acid that is estimated by blood levels of dissolved carbon dioxide (CO_2). CO_2 in gas form is considered **volatile** because it can be excreted by the lungs. Because CO_2 is excreted by the lungs, respiratory function contributes to H_2CO_3 levels. When pH levels fall (acidosis), increased respiratory rate increases excretion of CO_2 and lowers H_2CO_3 levels, promoting restoration of acid–base balance. In the case of an increase in pH (alkalosis), reduced respiratory rate promotes retention of CO_2, increasing H_2CO_3 levels. The respiratory buffer system is important in compensation for alterations in acid–base balance but is unable to completely restore homeostatic pH. Respiratory compensation is essential to provide the additional time needed for renal correction of acid–base imbalances.

Renal Buffer System

The kidneys are the primary regulators of the balance between acids and bases. Circulating fixed acids are considered **nonvolatile** because they are unable to be excreted by the lungs and require buffering and excretion by the kidneys. Renal regulation of pH is accomplished through generating, buffering, and eliminating acids and bases. The main mechanisms of renal regulation of pH include hydrogen ion elimination/bicarbonate conservation, tubular buffer systems (phosphate, ammonia), potassium–hydrogen exchange, and chloride–bicarbonate exchange.

Hydrogen Ion Elimination/Bicarbonate Conservation

Excretion of excess H^+ promotes regulation of pH. When pH is low, excess H^+ ions are secreted from the blood into the renal tubular filtrate where they can ultimately be excreted in the urine. The kidney can regulate HCO_3^-, conserving it when excess acid is added and excreting it in the presence of excess base. The kidneys contribute to plasma regulation of HCO_3^- by the reabsorption of HCO_3^- from the urine into the bloodstream, or by the elimination of buffered hydrogen ions. Reabsorption of basic bicarbonate ions is among the ways the kidneys work to obtain a pH between 7.35 and 7.45, thereby promoting optimal cellular functioning. A pH of

7.4 requires a 20:1 ratio of bicarbonate (HCO_3^-) base to carbonic acid (H_2CO_3). Rather than the absolute concentration of a substance, the ratio of substances provides the balance, which serves as the determinant of pH.

Tubular Buffer Systems

The tubule structures of the kidney are protected by the regulation of urine pH. Intratubular buffers bind unbuffered H^+ to maintain local pH for kidney cell function. The phosphate buffer system uses HPO_4^{2-} to bind H^+, resulting in $H_2PO_4^-$, allowing the kidney to secrete H^+ ions. The ammonia buffer system promotes excretion of H^+ and generates HCO_3^- in a series of ion exchanges between ammonium (NH_4^+) and HCO_3^-. The secreted H^+ ions combine with ammonia (NH_3) and are then eliminated in the urine as NH_4Cl.

Potassium–Hydrogen Exchange

Cation exchange of K^+ and H^+ occurs in the renal tubular cells in a similar manner described in the discussion of plasma buffering systems. Hypokalemia promotes movement of K^+ out of the tubular cells in exchange for H^+ movement into the cells, promoting loss of circulating H^+ and increase in pH. A lowering of pH occurs in hyperkalemia, when K^+ moves into the tubular cells in exchange for H^+, leading to an increase in circulating H^+. The cation exchange between H^+ and K^+ is tightly aligned with changes in pH, with acidosis promoting an increase in H^+ excretion and decrease in K^+ excretion while alkalosis promotes a decrease in elimination of H^+ and increase in elimination of K^+.

Chloride–Bicarbonate Exchange

Renal regulation of HCO_3^- can also be accomplished by anion exchange with Cl^- Chloride typically is absorbed along with sodium in the renal tubule cells. Under certain conditions including volume depletion due to vomiting and other causes of chloride loss, anion exchange between HCO_3^- and Cl^- occurs. Anion exchange between HCO_3^- and Cl^- can lead to alterations in acid–base balance because of manipulation of HCO_3^-. In hypochloremia alkalosis, an excess HCO_3^- results from increased reabsorption of HCO_3^- from the filtrate to the blood due to low circulating Cl^- levels, increasing pH. A decrease in pH is the result of reduced HCO_3^- reabsorption due to an increase in circulating Cl^- levels, known as hyperchloremic acidosis. Because the change in HCO_3^- is offset by the change in Cl^-, the anion gap is normal in hyperchloremic acidosis (Fig. 9.1).

Stop and Consider

What other organ systems are important in the regulation of fluid, electrolyte, and acid–base balance?

Altered Acid–Base Balance

Acid and base disorders can be respiratory or metabolic in origin. Respiratory acidosis is described in detail in Chapter 15. This chapter focuses on metabolic alterations in acid–base balance. Metabolic disorders result in an alteration in HCO_3^- caused by the addition or loss of nonvolatile acid or base in the extracellular fluid. Metabolic acidosis results in a reduction of HCO_3^-, prompting a decrease in ph. Increased levels of HCO_3^- result in an increase of pH, known as metabolic alkalosis. Initiating events that cause altered HCO_3^- levels trigger compensatory mechanisms to maintain acid–base balance. Kidneys compensate efficiently by conserving HCO_3^- or H^+ ions until the pH has returned to normal. These compensatory mechanisms adjust pH without altering underlying cause. Arterial blood gas (ABG) analysis is the lab test used to determine acid–base balance. Anion gap, base excess or deficit, CO_2 and HCO_3^- levels, and pH can be measured in an arterial blood sample. These variables not only determine balance but point to causes that might result in altered balance. Base excess or deficit represents the amount of fixed acid or base needed to achieve a pH of 7.4 in the blood sample.

METABOLIC ACIDOSIS

A base deficit of HCO_3^- characterizes metabolic acidosis. Metabolic acidosis may occur secondary to an increase in strong anions (Cl^-) or to an increase in weak acids. The levels of circulating albumin must also be considered when determining the presence of metabolic acidosis. Hypoalbuminemia may mask the presence of metabolic acidosis caused by an alkalizing effect.[2] Mechanisms contributing to the development of metabolic acidosis include:

- Increased production of nonvolatile acids; caused by fasting, ketoacidosis, and lactic acidosis
- Decreased secretion of acids by the kidneys; leads to renal failure
- Increased loss of bicarbonate; caused by diarrhea, gastrointestinal suction
- Increase in Cl^-; caused by excessive chloride reabsorption in the kidney, sodium chloride infusion

The clinical manifestations of metabolic acidosis include anorexia, nausea, vomiting, weakness, lethargy, confusion, coma, vasodilation, decreased heart rate, and flushed skin. Laboratory findings include decreased pH (less than 7.35) and HCO_3^- less than 24 mEq/L. The anion gap may increase when the cause of the metabolic acidosis is due to excess metabolic acids. When acidosis is caused by increased chloride, the anion gap remains normal. Compensatory mechanisms in metabolic acidosis include increased breathing rate and depth, hyperkalemia, and increased ammonia in urine. Treatment is aimed to correct the primary cause of metabolic acidosis, replace fluid and electrolytes, and correct the pH.

METABOLIC ALKALOSIS

Increased pH caused by plasma excess of HCO_3^- characterizes metabolic alkalosis. Mechanisms contributing to the development of metabolic alkalosis include:

- Decreased H^+ ions
- Increased HCO_3^- ions
- Loss of Cl^- ions

Impaired excretion of excess HCO_3^- may be promoted by contraction of extracellular fluid volume, hypokalemia, and hypochloremia. Clinical manifestations of metabolic alkalosis by be asymptomatic or have signs related to extracellular volume depletion, or hypokalemia. Laboratory findings include increased pH (greater than 7.45) and HCO_3^- greater than 31 mEq/L. Treatment of the underlying cause is a primary target of therapy, in addition to correction of chloride deficit (if present) and circulating potassium in addition to volume replacement.

Stop and Consider
Why can excessive, prolonged vomiting promote the development of metabolic alkalosis?

Module 2 Clinical Models

The clinical models presented in this chapter incorporate the concepts of altered acid–base balance. The clinical models will highlight concepts of fluid and electrolyte balance covered in Chapter 8 as they are intricately related to acid–base balance. When reviewing the clinical models, the student should apply the concepts he or she has learned about the alterations in fluid, electrolyte and acid–base balance in the application to clinical models that illustrate these concepts. An overview of the relationship between fluid, electrolyte, and acid–base balance is shown in Figure 9.3.

Altered Acid–Base Balance: Highly Active Antiretroviral Therapy (HAART)-Associated Acidosis

As discussed in Chapter 4, the treatment of HIV has been effective in prolonging life and decreasing the incidence and severity of many HIV-associated pathologies. Although HIV treatments have improved outcomes, there are known drug-related adverse effects. The use of nucleoside-analog reverse transcriptase inhibitors (NRTIs) for the treatment

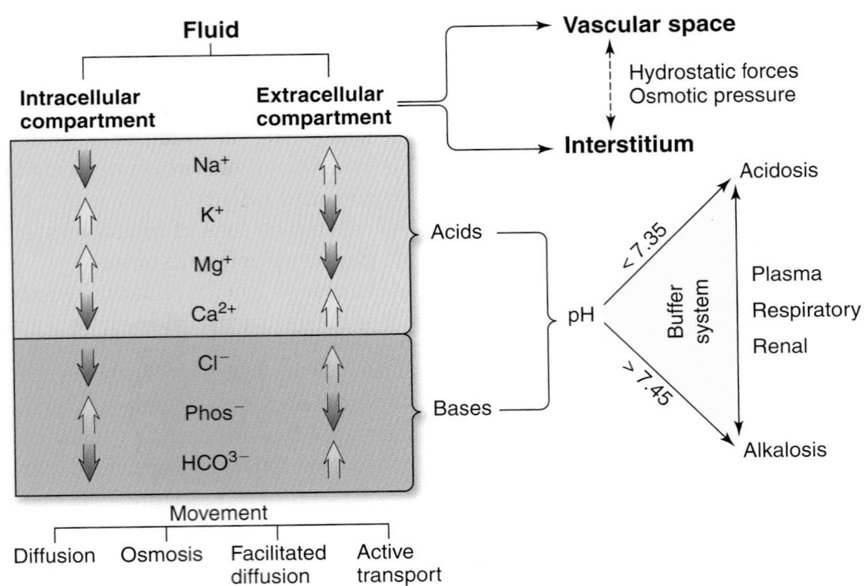

Figure 9.3. Concept map. Fluid, electrolyte, and acid–base balance.

of HIV has improved morbidity and mortality significantly. As more infected individuals take NRTIs and are on them for longer periods, some significant adverse drug effects are being uncovered. Among them is the development of **hyperlactatemia**, or an elevation of lactic acid in the blood. Many individuals who develop hyperlactatemia, also known as **lactic acidemia**, are not symptomatic, and they experience subclinical episodes that are self-limiting. Other individuals suffer from a life-threatening form of metabolic acidosis known as **lactic acidosis** that results from hyperlactatemia,[3] a rare, but serious, complication of NRTI use. Asymptomatic lactic acidemia associated with elevated lactate levels and normal pH affects approximately 8% to 21% of individuals taking at least one NRTI, with lactic acidosis occurring in about 1.5% to 2.5%.[4]

PATHOPHYSIOLOGY

Inhibition of the enzyme DNA polymerase by NRTIs may lead to mitochondrial dysfunction and is believed to be responsible for the development of hyperlactatemia. Loss of mitochondrial DNA prevents production of the necessary components of the electron transport chain in the mitochondria. Oxidative phosphorylation is impaired, promoting the formation of lactic acid for use by the cells for energy. The buildup of lactic acid in the blood reduces pH and predisposes affected individuals to developing lactic acidosis.

CLINICAL MANIFESTATIONS

Symptoms are related to the severity of the metabolic acidosis developing from hyperlactatemia. Most individuals with hyperlactatemia are asymptomatic and do not demonstrate any clinical manifestations.[4] Mild hyperlactatemia can induce symptoms such as nausea, vomiting, abdominal discomfort, and weight loss. **Hepatic steatosis** (fatty liver) is often associated with symptomatic hyperlactatemia, resulting from NRTI-stimulated fat deposition in the liver. Severe hyperlactatemia is the disease subtype associated with a form of metabolic acidosis known as lactic acidosis syndrome (LAS). Lactic acidosis is associated with pH levels of less than 7.3.[5] Liver involvement, including **hepatomegaly** (enlarged liver), elevated liver enzymes, and hepatic failure, is often associated with LAS. LAS may potentially result in coma and multiorgan failure.

DIAGNOSTIC CRITERIA

Early recognition and treatment of hyperlactatemia in HIV-infected individuals taking NRTIs are critical factors in decreasing morbidity and mortality because of this adverse drug effect. The clinical manifestations and laboratory determination of the amount of lactate in the blood assist in the diagnosis and form the basis of treatment strategies. Liver function tests may be completed to identify hepatic dysfunction. Electrolyte and blood pH levels may also be analyzed.

TREATMENT

Subclinical hyperlactatemia requires no treatment. This condition is usually transient and resolves without intervention. Drug selection may influence the development of hyperlactatemia; certain drugs deplete mitochondrial DNA more than others. NRTI treatment may be stopped or altered in individuals who develop symptoms of hyperlactatemia, but have not developed metabolic acidosis, in an attempt to prevent the development of LAS. NRTI treatment is stopped in individuals with LAS, although recovery cannot be assured. Intravenous administration of fluids can be used to expand intravascular volume, prevent cardiovascular collapse, and promote renal clearance of lactate. A period of weeks may be needed before lactate levels return to normal. Resolution of LAS is confirmed by:

- Normalization of sodium bicarbonate
- Normalization of pH
- Serum lactate of less than 3.0 mmol/L
- Normalization of liver function

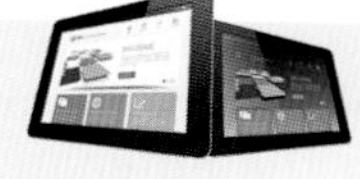

RESEARCH NOTES

The influence of mitochondrial DNA depletion and increases in serum lactate levels vary among different NRTIs. A study was done on patients taking NRTIs to determine the origin of hyperlactatemia. Blood samples were taken to determine serum lactate levels, and mitochondrial DNA concentrations were determined from liver biopsy samples. Depletion of mitochondrial DNA was increased by 47% in individuals taking the NRTIs zalcitabine, didanosine, and stavudine when compared to patients taking zidovudine, lamivudine, and abacavir. Increased lactate levels were also associated with the use of the drugs, which depleted mitochondrial DNA at a higher rate.[6]F

Stop and Consider
How is lactic acidosis different from other types of metabolic acidosis?

Altered Acid–Base Balance: Renal Tubulopathy

Hypokalemic salt-losing tubulopathies (SLTs) are a group of autosomal recessive disorders characterized by metabolic alkalosis. Many of the same physiologic abnormalities are common between the groups, although the age of onset varies between conditions. Four variants of this disorder are known:

1. Classic Bartter syndrome (cBS)
2. Gitelman syndrome (GS)
3. Hyperprostaglandin-E syndrome (HPS), also known as antenatal Bartter syndrome (aBS)
4. Hyperprostaglandin-E syndrome with sensorineural deafness (HPS + SND)

Bartter and Gitelman syndromes are characterized by hypokalemia and hypochloremic metabolic alkalosis.[7] The prevalence of Bartter syndrome worldwide is not currently known. Studies have been conducted in Australia, Europe, the Middle East, and the United States. A study of patients in Costa Rica revealed a high frequency of Bartter syndrome (1.2 cases per 100,000 live births). The incidence of Bartter syndrome is estimated to be 25.4 cases per 100,000 in preterm births.[8]

PATHOPHYSIOLOGY

In SLTs, electrolyte reabsorption in the renal tubules is impaired because of a gene defect altering five renal membrane proteins. The effects are related to specific protein alterations characteristic of each condition and have been likened to the effects of diuretics.[9] The cBS and HPS syndromes manifest alterations similar to those induced by the loop diuretics, inhibiting reabsorption of sodium and chloride in the loop of Henle. GS-associated electrolyte alterations mimic those induced by thiazide diuretics, blocking sodium reabsorption in the distal renal tubule. Inhibition of sodium reabsorption is desirable because excretion of sodium in the urine is accompanied by the excretion of water. Potassium may also be excreted, resulting in hypokalemia. Excessive loss of the strong cations sodium and potassium lead to the development of metabolic alkalosis.

CLINICAL MANIFESTATIONS

Manifestation of HPS occurs in utero; neonates present with severe effects. The initial manifestation is maternal hydramnios (excessive amniotic fluid) because of increased fetal urine output. Bartter syndrome and Gitelman syndrome often present in early infancy through childhood and adolescence. The neonatal (first 28 days of life) course is complicated by polyuria (excessive urine output), hypercalciuria (excessive calcium excreted in urine), and affects from increased levels of prostaglandin, including fever, vomiting, and diarrhea, further contributing to altered fluid and electrolyte balance.[10]

Metabolic alkalosis is associated with contracted extracellular fluid volume because of sodium chloride loss. This decreased intravascular volume limits the space for distribution of bicarbonate, amplifying the hyperbicarbonatemia. Sodium chloride loss also contributes potassium loss and increased renal reabsorption of bicarbonate, further increasing blood pH and worsening metabolic alkalosis.[11]

DIAGNOSTIC CRITERIA

Renal structures can be evaluated with ultrasound. Determination of electrolyte and fluid imbalances can be evaluated by measurements of electrolytes in serum and urine. ABGs, anion gap, and base excess measures can be used to determine the presence of metabolic alkalosis and to guide treatment strategies. Fluid balance may be determined by urine-specific gravity measurement. Laboratory evaluations to detect renal failure (discussed in more detail in Chapter 18) are done serially in these chronic conditions. In families with known risk for these disorders, DNA testing for the genetic defect located on chromosome number 1 can be accomplished on amniotic fluid in the antenatal period or from a cell sample taken directly from the neonate after birth.

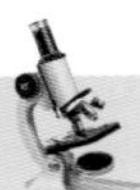

FROM THE LAB

As in evaluation of ascites, urinary sodium concentration can be used to provide a measurement of renal sodium retention. In patients with dehydration, urine sodium concentrations help determine etiology. Urinary sodium concentrations of less than 20 mEq/L indicate a nonrenal cause of fluid loss, such as ascites, vomiting, or diarrhea. Hypovolemia associated with urinary sodium concentration of more than 20 mEq/L indicates fluid loss of renal origin. Fluid loss of renal origin may be caused by drugs such as thiazide diuretics because they alter urine concentration. Renal causes of hypovolemia can also include excessive salt loss because of renal failure.

TREATMENT

Treatment strategies are focused on the correction of renal salt and fluid losses. Sodium and potassium supplements are used to correct hyponatremia and hypokalemia. Diuretics that spare potassium excretion, including spironolactone and amiloride, may also be used. Indomethacin, a prostaglandin inhibitor, may be used to reduce prostaglandin production. Calcium and magnesium supplements may also be used to correct hypocalcemia and hypomagnesemia.

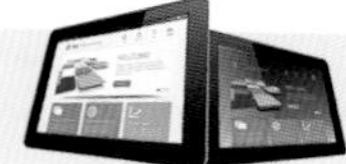

RESEARCH NOTES

Salt transport depends on the recycling of potassium in the thick ascending limb of the loop of Henle. The genetic alterations associated with Bartter syndrome contribute to the loss of potassium channel secretory activity, accounting for the alteration in electrolytes characteristic of the syndrome.[12]

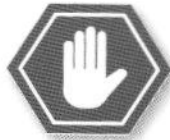

Stop and Consider

Why are potassium-sparing diuretics the preferred treatment of fluid and electrolyte imbalances associated with Bartter syndrome?

Altered Acid–Base Balance: Metabolic Acidosis in Parenteral Nutrition

Parenteral nutrition is an example of supplemental nutrition that bypasses typical processes of eating and digestion (Fig. 9.4). Alterations in the ability for individuals to obtain oral nutrition can result from a variety of conditions including altered function of the gastrointestinal track. In cases where individuals are unable to eat or drink, supplemental nutrition must be provided to delivery essential energy and nutrients necessary for survival. The duration of parenteral nutrition is typically short, though may be extended over a longer term in unique circumstances.

PATHOPHYSIOLOGY

Parenteral nutrition is designed to meet nutritional needs through the delivery of water, glucose or dextrose, amino acids, lipids, vitamins, minerals, electrolytes, acetate, and trace elements through the venous system. The formulation of parenteral nutrition is designed to meet the unique needs of the individual. Hydrochloric and organic acids are added to the formulation of parenteral nutrition as they are required for chemical interaction between solution components. The solution acidity is countered by the addition of base to reach a pH of 7.4 prior to infusion. Hydrochloric acid infused as a component of parenteral nutrition may contribute to increase blood chloride levels with a simultaneous reduction in base, promoting conditions that favor metabolic acidosis. Metabolic acidosis may also result from metabolism of amino acids, leading to increased H^+ production and need for buffering by HCO_3^-. Further complicating the development of metabolic acidosis are the disrupted carbohydrate and lipid metabolic pathways that produce acidic byproducts and impaired buffer systems among severely ill patients who are likely candidates for parenteral nutrition. When the individual's condition is complicated by thiamine deficiency, the risk for metabolic acidosis is even greater because of a buildup of lactic acid as thiamine is required for lactic acid metabolism.[13]

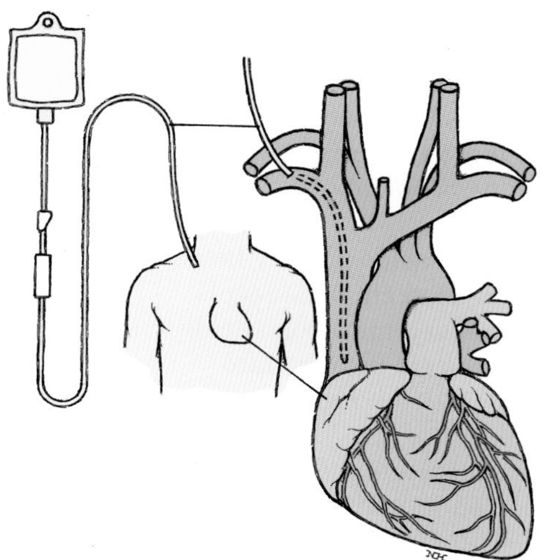

Figure 9.4. Parenteral nutrition. Delivery of intravenous nutrition, bypassing the gastrointestinal system.

CLINICAL MANIFESTATIONS

The symptoms of metabolic acidosis are variable, dependent in part on the severity of the condition. Typical manifestations of anorexia, nausea, vomiting, weakness, lethargy, confusion, coma, vasodilation, decreased heart rate, and flushed skin can be masked by the underlying condition, prompting the need for parenteral nutrition. Extreme symptoms may include neurologic manifestations including coma and seizures as well as alteration in cardiac rhythm.

DIAGNOSTIC CRITERIA

As with other causes, individuals with metabolic acidosis secondary to parenteral nutrition are diagnosed through ABG sampling to determine pH. Along with a pH of <7.35, decreased HCO_3^- levels and possible signs of respiratory compensation (decreased CO_2) may be associated with low pH. Electrolyte balance and calculation of anion gap will provide greater detail regarding the nature of the acidosis.

TREATMENT

The approach to treatment is dependent on the laboratory assessment and complicating factors associated with the acidosis. Adjustment of parenteral nutrition solution components and intake are important targets to consider. Treatment with HCO_3^- base may be needed to correct a base deficit. Hydration and oxygen may also improve response to definitive treatment of metabolic acidosis.

SUMMARY

- Acid–base balance is important to homeostasis and cellular function.
- Alterations in acid–base balance can occur because of other diseases or can cause illness.
- Alterations in acid–base balance are associated with altered regulation of fluid and electrolyte.
- Acid–base balance is regulated by buffer systems, working in concert to maintain pH balance.
- Correction in pH alterations resulting from acid base imbalance are redundant and include rapid acting and long acting buffer systems that respond to immediate and long term need to restore acid–base balance.
- Anion gap, based on calculation of measurable cations and anions, provides an indication of acid–base balance.
- Metabolic acidosis is characterized by a deficit in base. Metabolic alkalosis is characterized by an excess in base.
- Correction of acid–base imbalances is critical to the maintenance of bodily functions.
- To correct imbalances in acid–base, careful consideration must be given to the potential impact of interactions with all body systems.

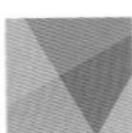

CASE STUDY 9.1

Scott, a 2-year-old male, was in the garage with his father while he was working on his car. When his father was distracted, Scott drank from a container of antifreeze containing methanol and ethylene glycol. Consider the impact of this event on Scott's acid–base balance and answer the following questions:

1. What are the pathologic consequences on organ systems resulting from ingestion of methanol and ethylene glycol?
2. What are the symptoms associated with methanol and ethylene glycol ingestion?
3. What are the acid–base alterations that are expected with ingestion of methanol and ethylene glycol?
4. What would you expect for clinical manifestations related to acid–base imbalance after methanol and ethylene glycol ingestion?
5. What diagnostic tests might be used?
6. What treatment is needed?

Log onto the Internet. Search for a relevant journal article or Web site that details methanol and ethylene glycol ingestion to confirm your predictions.

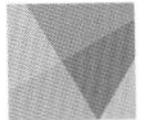

PRACTICE EXAM QUESTIONS

1. Which of the following is an example of a strong acid?
   a. Albumin
   b. Inorganic phosphorus
   c. Sodium
   d. Lactate

2. An anion gap of 16 can be calculated by which of the following scenarios?
   a. Sodium 146, chloride 102, bicarbonate 26 mEq/L
   b. Sodium 140, chloride 102, bicarbonate 26 mEq/L
   c. Sodium 136, chloride 122, bicarbonate 30 mEq/L
   d. Sodium 148, chloride 100, bicarbonate 28 mEq/L

3. A pH of 7.5 is defined as
   a. Alkalosis
   b. Acidosis
   c. Acidemia
   d. Alkalemia

4. An example of anion exchange includes:
   a. Sodium and hydrogen exchange
   b. Sodium and chloride exchange
   c. Bicarbonate and chloride exchange
   d. Hydrogen and bicarbonate exchange

5. Hypokalemia is often associated with which one of the following conditions?
   a. Metabolic alkalosis
   b. Metabolic acidosis
   c. Hyperchloremia
   d. None of the above

6. Metabolic acidosis may be associated with
   a. Increased chloride levels
   b. Increased metabolic acids
   c. Decreased bicarbonate
   d. All of the above

7. Hyperlactatemia due to drug treatment is a complication in which of the following conditions?
   a. Salt-losing tubulopathy
   b. Cirrhosis
   c. AIDS
   d. Isonatremic dehydration

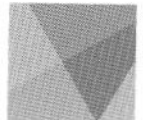

DISCUSSION AND APPLICATION

1. What did I know about alterations in acid–base balance before today?
2. What body processes are affected by alterations in acid–base balance? How do acid–base imbalances affect those processes?
3. What are the potential etiologies for alterations in acid–base balance? How do acid–base imbalances develop?
4. Who is most at risk for developing acid–base imbalances? How can these alterations be prevented?
5. What are the human differences that affect the etiology, risk, or course of alterations in acid–base balance?
6. What clinical manifestations are expected during acid–base imbalances?
7. What special diagnostic tests are useful in determining the diagnosis and course of alterations in acid–base balance?
8. What are the goals of care for individuals who have alterations in fluid, electrolyte, and acid–base balance?
9. How does the concept of alterations in fluid, electrolyte, and acid–base balance build on what I have learned in the previous chapter and in the previous courses?
10. How can I use what I have learned?

RESOURCES

Renal Tubular Acidosis—National Kidney and Urologic Diseases Information Clearing House: http://www.niddk.nih.gov/health-information/health-topics/kidney-disease/renal-tubular-acidosis-rta/Documents/renaltubularacidosis_508.pdf

Chronic Kidney Disease and Diet: Assessment, Management and Treatment: http://www.niddk.nih.gov/health-information/health-communication-programs/nkdep/a-z/Documents/ckd-diet-assess-manage-treat-508.pdf

References

1. Leblanc M. Acid-base balance in acute renal failure and renal replacement therapy. *Best Pract Res Clin Anaesthesiol.* 2004;18(1):113–127.
2. Levraut J, Grimaud D. Treatment of metabolic acidosis. *Curr Opin Crit Care.* 2003;9(4):260–265.
3. Izzedine H, Harris M, Perazella MA. The nephrotoxic effects of HAART. *Nat Rev Nephrol.* 2009;5(10):563–573.
4. McComsey GA, Yau L. Asymptomatic hyperlactataemia: predictive value, natural history and correlates. *Antivir Ther.* 2004;9(2):205–212.
5. Monier PL, Wilcox R. Metabolic complications associated with the use of highly active antiretroviral therapy in HIV-1-infected adults. *Am J Med Sci.* 2004;328(1):48–56.
6. Walker UA, Bauerle J, Laguno M, et al. Depletion of mitochondrial DNA in liver under antiretroviral therapy with didanosine, stavudine, or zalcitabine. *Hepatology.* 2004;39(2):311–317.
7. Seyberth HW. An improved terminology and classification of Bartter-like syndromes. *Nat Clin Pract Nephrol.* 2008;4(10):560–567.
8. Madrigal G, Saborio P, Mora F, et al. Bartter syndrome in Costa Rica: a description of 20 cases. *Pediatr Nephrol.* 1997;11(3):296–301.
9. Reinalter SC, Jeck N, Peters M, et al. Pharmacotyping of hypokalaemic salt-losing tubular disorders. *Acta Physiol Scand.* 2004;181(4):513–521.
10. Jeck N, Reinalter SC, Henne T, et al. Hypokalemic salt-losing tubulopathy with chronic renal failure and sensorineural deafness. *Pediatrics.* 2001;108(1):E5.
11. Adrogue HJ, Madias NE. Management of life-threatening acid-base disorders. Second of two parts. *N Engl J Med.* 1998;338(2):107–111.
12. Lu M, Wang T, Yan Q, et al. ROMK is required for expression of the 70-pS K channel in the thick ascending limb. *Am J Physiol Renal Physiol.* 2004;286(3):F490–F495.
13. Dounousi E, Zikou X, Koulouras V, et al. Metabolic acidosis during parenteral nutrition: pathophysiologic mechanisms. *Indian J Crit Care Med.* 2015;19:270–274.

Find additional resources for this chapter at http:thePoint.lww.com thePoint®

Chapter 10

Altered Neuronal Transmission

LEARNING OUTCOMES

1. Define and use the key terms listed in this chapter.
2. Describe outcomes related to altered voltage during the phases of action potential.
3. Differentiate between types of injury in the central and peripheral nervous systems.
4. Analyze potential targets of impaired function in altered reflex response.
5. Describe factors associated with altered synaptic transmission.
6. Compare and contrast neurologic transmission patterns and outcomes in the somatic, sympathetic, and parasympathetic nervous systems.
7. Identify common signs and symptoms of altered neuronal transmission.
8. Describe diagnostic tests and treatment strategies relevant to altered neuronal transmission.
9. Predict expected functional impairment from altered neurologic transmission based on type, severity, and site of neurologic injury.
10. Apply concepts of altered neuronal transmission to select clinical models.

INTRODUCTION

We often take for granted the simple things that are part of our daily life, such as walking, swallowing food, balancing a checkbook, or singing a favorite song. These activities are a reflection of the high-level functioning of nervous cells and tissues. This chapter highlights impaired neural function and the consequences of these alterations. A review of normal neural transmission is presented, followed by a discussion of the pathologic changes associated with impaired conduction of neural impulses in the various nervous system tissues and organs. Finally, these concepts are applied to selected models of clinical disease.

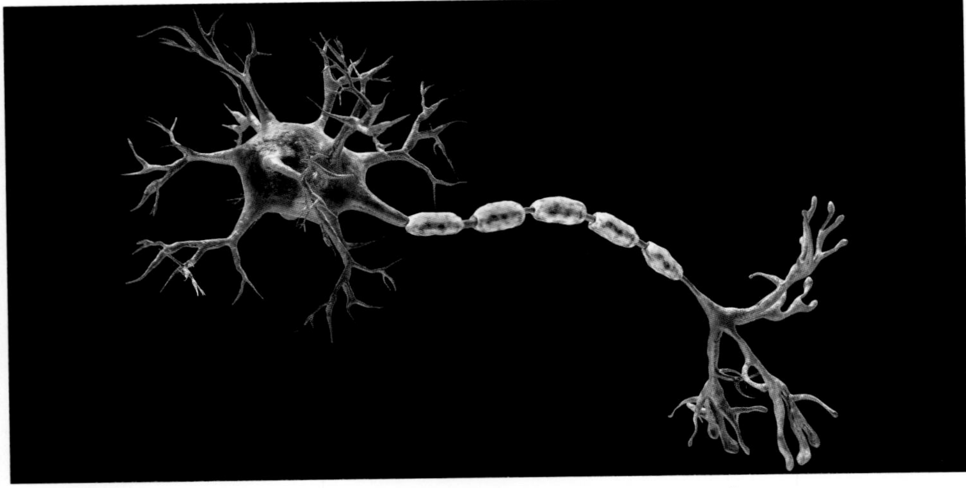

Digital illustration of a neuron. Image © vitstudio.

Module 1 Alterations in Neuronal Impulse Conduction

Neuronal transmission of impulses is critical to maintain vital functions. Disruption of any component required for conduction of nerve impulses may alter neural signaling. The basic structural components of the neuron must be intact to function properly. The organelles must support the function of neural cells through such things as the genetic regulation of essential functions and the production of proteins, neurotransmitters, and energy required for optimal cell functioning. The propagation of the neural impulses through development of synapses, availability of receptors, release and uptake of neurotransmitters, generation of action potentials, and target organ responsiveness is also required. The external environment, including ion concentrations and fluid balance, must be in harmony for optimal neural cell functioning. Neural impulse conduction requires a complex organization of neural structures for physiologic functioning.

Neurons

The **neuron** (nerve cell) is the fundamental functional unit of the nervous system. Composed of a central cell body, one axon, and a variable number of dendrites, neurons are excitable cells that contribute to the highly specialized cell function of the transmission of nerve impulses throughout the body. The **cell body**, or **soma**, is filled with cytoplasm and contains processes, including the nucleus, that support the metabolic demands of the cell. The cytoplasm of the cell body is also contained in the dendrites and axons. **Dendrites** are multiple, branched extensions of the cell body that transmit impulses to the cell body. The **axon** carries impulses away from the cell body. The transmission speed of nerve impulses from the dendrites to the synaptic terminals is enhanced by the myelin sheath, which is interrupted by the nodes of Ranvier. Figure 10.1 illustrates the structures of a neuron.

Neurons are categorized based on their highly specialized functions. **Sensory neurons**, also known as **afferent neurons,** carry impulses from receptors in the periphery to the brain and spinal cord in the central nervous system (CNS). **Motor neurons**, also known as **efferent neurons**, carry signals away from the spinal cord and brain to targets in the body that regulate activity. **Interneurons** are the most abundant neuron type. Interneurons provide connections between neurons, transmitting signals between afferent and efferent neurons.

Supporting Cells

The brain contains approximately 100 billion neurons and many trillions of glia, neural support cells. Glia, derived from the Greek meaning "glue," provide support and nutrition, maintain homeostasis, and form the myelin that covers the neurons of the brain. Support cells provide neurons with protection and metabolic support, and they help segregate neurons to promote optimal functioning. Support cell types vary depending on the component of the nervous system; that is, central nervous system or peripheral nervous system, which is discussed further in the next section. The specific cell types are outlined in Table 10.1.

Myelin, a protein high in lipid content, is important to neural cell functioning. The insulating properties of myelin increase the speed of nerve impulse by

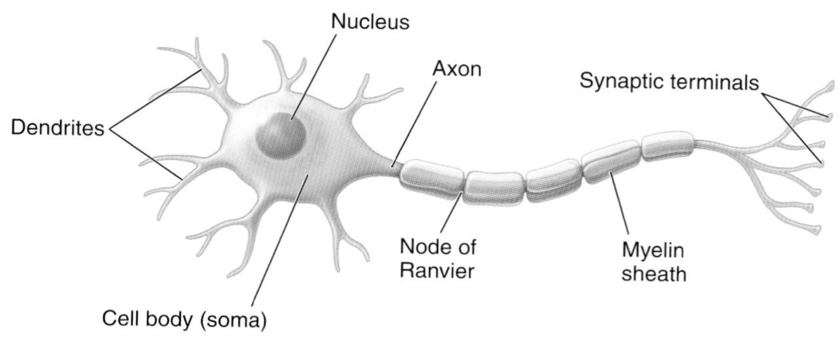

Figure 10.1. Components of the neuron.

Table 10.1 Supporting Cells of the Nervous System

Nervous System	Supporting Cell Type	Function
Central nervous system	Glial cells	
	Oligodendroglia (also known as oligodendrocytes)	Control myelin production and maintenance
	Astroglia (also known as astrocytes)	Provide transport mechanisms for the exchange of oxygen, carbon dioxide, and metabolites between blood vessels and neurons; stimulate phagocytosis; provide support to neural structures
	Microglia	Control phagocytosis of injured or damaged cells
	Ependymal cells	Line the ventricular system
Peripheral \nervous system	Schwann cells	Stimulate myelin production and maintenance
	Satellite cells	Provide physical support of neurons

containing the current in a small space surrounding the axon. The specific cell type supporting production and maintenance of myelin varies depending on the type of neuron involved. **Oligodendrocytes** are responsible for the formation of multilayered myelin segments around multiple axons in the brain, promoting the speed of nerve impulse conduction in the CNS. **Schwann cells** produce myelin on long, single axons of the peripheral nervous system. In myelinated axons, the myelin sheath is interrupted at intervals by the **nodes of Ranvier**. These nodes are rich in sodium channels and are necessary to promote the movement of the nerve impulse over long distances. Impulses traveling down the axon jump from node to node in a stepwise fashion in a process known as **saltatory conduction**.

Neuronal Transmission

Transmission of neuronal impulses requires complex coordination between neuronal structures and the surrounding environment. Alterations in any aspect of neuronal communication may result in manifestations of impaired function. Neurons communicate with other neurons and cells in the body through the generation of electrical signals called **action potentials**. Action potentials are electrical events that travel along the entire neuron by allowing charged ions to flood through channels in the semipermeable membrane around the nerve cell. Action potentials are regulated by changes in membrane potential. **Membrane potential** is the difference in electrical charge between the inside and outside of the cell. An excitable neuronal cell is **polarized** when at rest. The inside of the cell is more negative compared with the outside of the cell; the difference is measured at approximately −70 mV. Cell bodies and dendrites have few voltage-gated channels, which results in changes in membrane potential that do not reach the threshold (**subthreshold**), or the point at which the cell is committed to an action potential. Voltage-gated channels are found in the **axon hillock**, the point at which the axon is joined to the cell body. Subthreshold potentials converge from the cell body and dendrites at the axon hillock, where a full action potential is generated and conducted down the length of the axon.

At rest, the neuron and the surrounding space act as a **capacitor**, storing current, which is released during the action potential. Myelin insulation reduces loss of current, limiting drift of sodium ions away from the neuron. Action potential is determined at the point when sodium channels open, allowing the flow of sodium into the cell. There are three components of the action potential in the neuron:

1. Resting membrane potential
2. Depolarization phase
3. Repolarization phase

The membrane potential of a cell at rest is known as the **resting membrane potential (RMP)**. RMP refers to the membrane potential (or state of tension) inside a cell membrane, measured relative to the fluid just outside in the absence of significant electrical activity. **Depolarization** is the result of rapid movement of sodium into the cell through sodium channels in the cell membrane. This inflow generates an electrical impulse. This impulse is transmitted along the axon to trigger the release of neurotransmitters. The **repolarization** phase is initiated by the flow of potassium ions out of the cell. The efflux of potassium ions promotes return of the cell to RMP (Fig. 10.2).

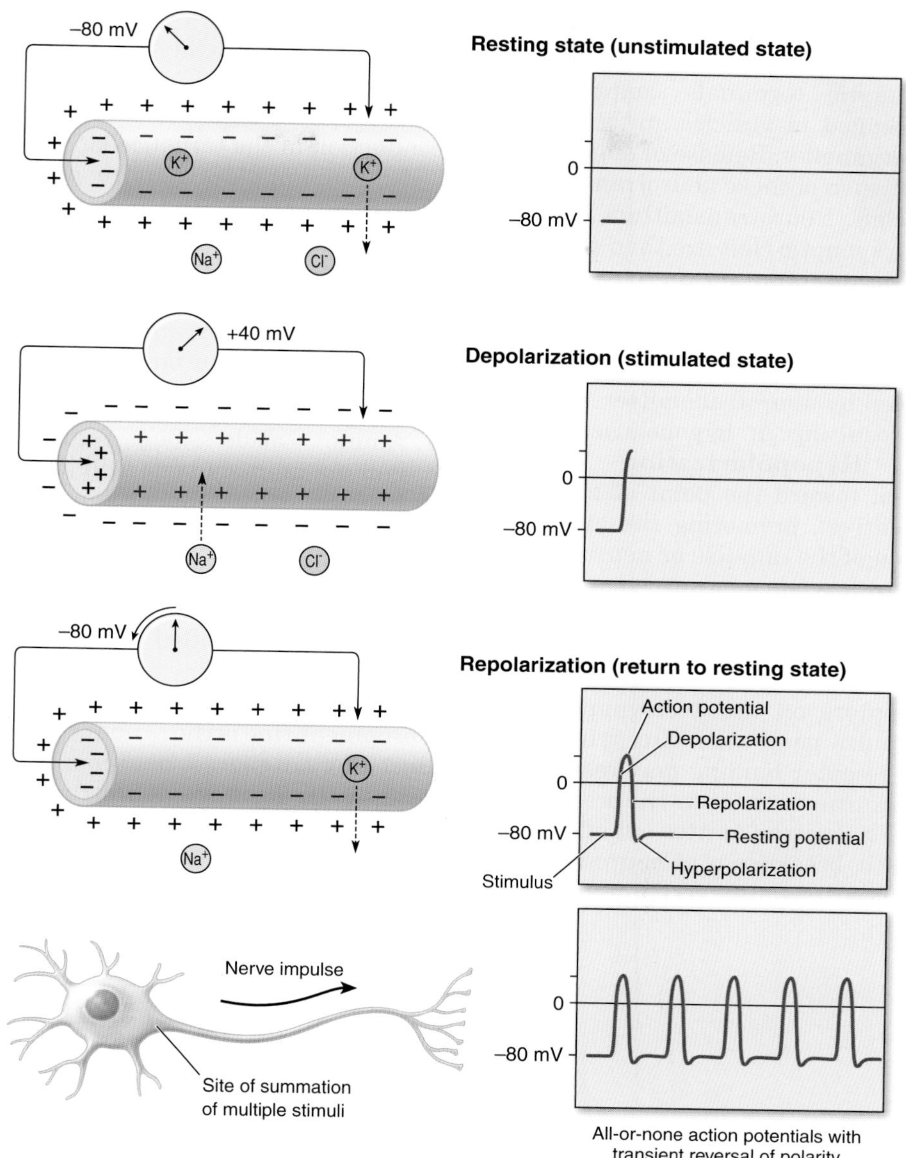

Figure 10.2. Electrical charges at rest and with stimulation. Influx of sodium ions into the cell promotes depolarization and the development of an action potential. Efflux of potassium ions causes repolarization and return to resting membrane potential. (Modified from Snell R. *Clinical Neuroanatomy*. Philadelphia, PA: Lippincott Williams & Wilkins; 2003.)

Communication Between Neurons

Information from one neuron flows to another neuron across a **synapse**. The synapse is a small gap or junction separating neurons. Electrical and chemical synapses are typically found in the nervous system.

Electrical synapses transmit impulses by passage of current-carrying ions through small openings known as **gap junctions**. The transmission of electrical impulses through gap junctions is fast and direct. This mode of neural transmission is multidirectional. Gap junctions are commonly involved in the transmission of electrical impulses that lead to cardiac contractions.

Chemical synapses involve specific structures important for impulses stimulated by **neurotransmitters**, chemical agents affecting the function of another nearby cell or cells. Neurotransmitters carry signals between nerve cells and other excitable cells, including other nerve cells and muscle cells, to trigger a response in another cell. The synaptic structures involved in this type of neural transmission include:

- Presynaptic terminals
- Synaptic cleft
- Postsynaptic membrane

Chemical synaptic transmission is unidirectional, limited to one-way communication between neurons.

Synaptic arrangements can include contacts between axon and dendrite, axon and soma, and axon and axon. Presynaptic terminals contain neurotransmitters packaged in vesicles, mitochondria, and other cellular organelles. Release of neurotransmitters permits diffusion of these neurotransmitters into the synaptic cleft. Neurotransmitters released from vesicles at the synaptic cleft are then available to bind with specific receptors on the postsynaptic membrane, promoting excitation or inhibition of the postsynaptic neuron. These effects are caused by changes in membrane potential of the postsynaptic neuron induced by neurotransmitter–receptor binding, thereby resulting in hypopolarization or hyperpolarization. **Hypopolarization** changes membrane potential toward the point of threshold potential (less negative), promoting the excitatory effect of propagation of the impulse or neuron firing. **Hyperpolarization** has the opposite effect of moving the membrane potential away from threshold (more negative), promoting an inhibitory effect.

Neurotransmitter released into the synaptic cleft must bind to receptors on the postsynaptic neuron to achieve impulse generation. Interruption in neurotransmitter–receptor binding may result from reuptake of the neurotransmitter into the presynaptic neuron, diffusion of neurotransmitter out of the synaptic cleft, enzymatic breakdown of neurotransmitter in the synapse or postsynaptic receptor alteration that impairs neurotransmitter binding (Fig. 10.3). Alteration in the control of neurotransmitter–receptor binding impairs postsynaptic impulse generation and the physiologic outcome associated with neural conduction in the target cells.

Neural impulses require precise control, determined in part by the neurotransmitter type, the postsynaptic receptor with affinity for binding a specific neurotransmitter and modulators of neural transmission. Neurotransmitters are produced in the neuron, determined by the enzyme systems present in the neuron. Neurotransmitters can be grouped into three major types:

1. Amino acids (e.g., glutamic acid and gamma-aminobutyric acid [GABA])
2. Peptides (e.g., endorphins, enkephalins, substance P)
3. Monoamines (e.g., serotonin, dopamine, norepinephrine)

Neurons are classified by the primary neurotransmitter produced. For example, dopaminergic neurons produce dopamine as the primary neurotransmitter; norepinephrine is the primary neurotransmitter produced by adrenergic neurons; gamma-aminobutyric acid is the primary neurotransmitter produced by GABA-ergic neurons.

Typically, there are multiple receptor types and subtypes that can bind a single neurotransmitter.

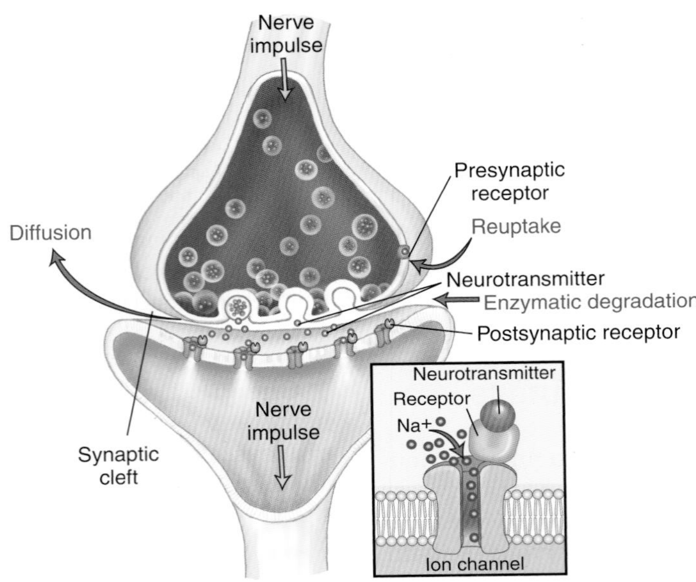

Figure 10.3. The action potential generated at the axon hillock of the presynaptic neuron leads to release of neurotransmitter from the synaptic vesicle. Neurotransmitter enters the synaptic cleft and either binds to a receptor on the postsynaptic neuron, is taken back up into the presynaptic receptor, is degraded by enzymes in the synaptic cleft or diffuses away from the synapse. When neurotransmitter binding to a postsynaptic receptor occurs, a change in potential occurs. An inhibitory impulse results in a more negative potential, moving further away from threshold. An excitatory impulse raises voltage to a less negative membrane potential. When threshold is reached, an action potential results. The impulse is transmitted on the length of the postsynaptic neuron to the target cells, resulting in a physiologic outcome.

The receptor determines the character of the neural impulse, either inhibitory or excitatory. The impulses generated by neurotransmitter-receptor binding are linked to a physiologic outcome in the target cells. For example, when norepinephrine binds to the alpha-adrenergic receptor, smooth muscle contraction results. Norepinephrine binding to the beta-adrenergic receptor results in smooth muscle relaxation. In this way, a small number of neurotransmitters can induce multiple effects due to the much larger number of receptors available for binding. The effects of neurotransmitters can be altered by **neuromodulators**, released from axon terminals. The effects of neuromodulators may inhibit, potentiate, or prolong the effects of neurotransmitters.

Processes of Neuronal Injury

Mature neurons do not divide, a fact that is an important consideration when neurons are injured. Unlike most other cells, new neurons are not generated to replace those that have lost function through damage or death. Myelin that has been damaged is not replaced, leading to permanent neurologic deficits. The loss of neurons through cell damage or as a process of aging contributes to disability and is the basis for a variety of neurologic disorders. Damage to neurons results from the following processes:

- **Chromatolysis:** The swelling of a neuron because of injury
- **Atrophy:** Decrease in the size of the cell (neuron)
- **Neuronophagia:** Phagocytosis and inflammatory responses caused by a dead neuron damaging neighboring cells
- **Intraneuronal inclusions:** Distinctive structures formed in the nucleus or cytoplasm

Developmental Considerations

The neural tube develops early in embryonic life. Alterations in cellular differentiation, proliferation, or migration can result in significant neurologic impairment. At birth, almost all of the neurons necessary for functioning during adult life are present. By the age of 2 years, the brain achieves 80% of its adult size. The brain continues to develop and mature for the first few years of life. Glial cells divide and multiply, myelin deposition on neural fibers increases, and new connections are forged.

As individuals age, altered nervous system function may result from a decreased number of neurons, altered structure, or responsiveness of neural tissues. The characteristic brain changes that may occur with aging include:

- Enlargement in the size of the ventricle system
- Widening of sulci
- Decreased brain volume and weight
- Increase in the appearance of neurologic disorders, such as stroke, Alzheimer disease, and Parkinson disease (PD)
- Sensory changes, including cataract development, loss of focus, hearing, smell, and taste

Module 2 Alterations in CNS Function

The nervous system is divided into systems which connect and function as a unit. Functional distinctions are sometimes made, though it is important to recognize the broad scope of impact of neuronal impairment across systems. This chapter discusses the nervous system by organizing the nervous system into the CNS and the peripheral nervous system, which is further divided into the autonomic and somatic nervous systems. Involuntary nervous control is regulated by the visceral and autonomic nervous systems. The **somatic nervous system** refers to voluntary nervous control in skeletal muscles.

CNS Organization

The CNS is composed of the brain and spinal cord. The brain weighs approximately 3 lb (1.36 kg) in an average adult and is composed of neurons and support cells. The brain receives and processes sensory information, initiating and coordinating motor responses. The spinal cord conducts sensory information from the peripheral nervous system and motor information from muscle to the brain for processing.

BRAIN

The brain is divided into lobes and hemispheres. Four separate lobes of the brain are divided by **sulci** (fissures) and **gyri** (irregular convolutions on the surface) and have specialized functions (Fig. 10.4). The lobes and their functions include:

- Frontal lobe: reasoning, planning, speech, and movement
- Parietal lobe: perception of touch, pressure, temperature, and pain

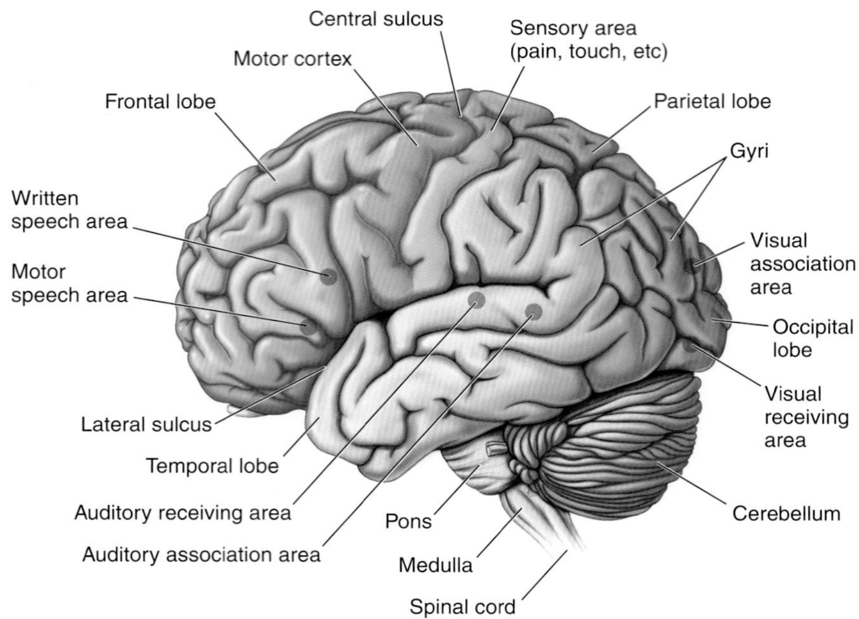

Figure 10.4. Lobes of the brain. External view with motor and sensory areas. (Modified from Bear MF, Connors BW, Parasido MA. *Neuroscience: Exploring the Brain*. 3rd ed. Philadelphia, PA: Lippincott Williams & Wilkins; 2006.)

- Temporal lobe: perception, memory, and recognition of auditory stimuli
- Occipital: vision

The brain is also divided into two halves, or hemispheres, each containing the four lobes of the brain. The right and left hemispheres communicate with each other through a bundle of nerve fibers known as the **corpus callosum**. Neural activity in the *right hemisphere* of the brain involves functional capacity of the left side of the body. The *left hemisphere* of the brain also demonstrates this contralateral pattern. Functions have been attributed to the control of specific brain hemispheres as follows:

- Left hemisphere
  - Speech and language
  - Calculations
  - Math
  - Logical abilities
- Right hemisphere
  - Visual imagery
  - Face recognition
  - Music
  - Spatial abilities

Brain structures can be characterized further by their location. These categories include:

- Forebrain
  - Telencephalon
    - Cerebral cortex
    - Basal ganglia
    - Hippocampus
    - Amygdala
  - Diencephalon
    - Hypothalamus
    - Thalamus
- Midbrain
  - Mesencephalon
    - Tectum
    - Tegmentum
- Hindbrain
  - Metencephalon
    - Cerebellum
    - Pons
  - Myelencephalon
    - Medulla oblongata

The structures of the brain and related functions are outlined in Table 10.2. The cerebrum includes the telencephalon structures cerebral cortex and basal ganglia. Figure 10.5 highlights the location of specific brain structures, which can be seen with a coronal view. The structure of the brain is also revealed by the composition of tissue in the lobes of each hemisphere. The tissue of the cerebral cortex, basal ganglia, hypothalamus, and thalamus is **gray matter**, primarily composed of cell bodies; whereas other brain structures are composed of **white matter**, tissue composed primarily of myelinated axons and dendrites.

SPINAL CORD

The spinal cord serves as the primary pathway for communication of messages or impulses from the

Table 10.2 Brain Structures and Functions

Brain Structure	Anatomic Significance	Function
Cerebral cortex	Located in the telencephalon of the forebrain; convoluted layer of cerebrum that contains gray matter (unmyelinated cell bodies)	Controls higher-order functions including language and information processing
Basal ganglia	Located in the telencephalon of the forebrain; includes structures of the globus pallidus, caudate nucleus, subthalamic nucleus, putamen and substantia nigra	Control voluntary movement; establish posture
Hippocampus	Component of the limbic system located in the telencephalon of the forebrain; convoluted structure located in the temporal lobe; forms the medial margin of the cerebral hemisphere	Controls impulses of emotion, hunger, sexual arousal, and aggression; involved in memory and learning
Amygdala	Component of the limbic system located in the telencephalon of the forebrain; almond-shaped structure of gray matter in the temporal lobe	Produces and responds to nonverbal signs of anger, avoidance, defensiveness, fear, and inspiring aversive cues
Hypothalamus	Located in the diencephalon of the forebrain; the hypothalamus is critical to the integration of homeostatic control of the internal environment; borders the posterior pituitary, the third ventricle, and the thalamus	Controls body temperature, appetite, water balance, secretion from the pituitary gland, emotions, and autonomic functions, including sleep and wakefulness
Thalamus	Located in the diencephalon of the forebrain; consists of two large egg-shaped masses of tissue, one on each side of the third ventricle	Relays sensory information (including pain) through an ascending pathway via the thalamus to the cerebral cortex, focusing of attention and organization of incoming stimuli
Tectum	Located in the dorsal region of the mesencephalon (midbrain); contains visual and auditory receptors	Controls auditory and visual responses
Tegmentum	Located in the ventral region of the mesencephalon (midbrain); consists of the cerebral aqueduct and reticular formation	Controls motor functions; regulates awareness, attention, and some autonomic functions
Cerebellum	Located in the metencephalon of the hindbrain; separated from the central hemispheres by a fold in the dura mater superior to the pons	Maintains muscle tone; coordinates muscle movement and balance
Pons	Located in the metencephalon of the hindbrain; serves as the connection between the cerebellum and the cerebrum and between the midbrain and the medulla oblongata	Assists in controlling autonomic functions, arousal, and sleep
Medulla oblongata	Located in the myencephalon of the hindbrain; a component of the brainstem, the medulla is the most caudal segment of the neural tube of the brain	Regulation of vasomotor, cardiac, and respiratory function
Reticular activating system (RAS)	A network of hyperexcitable neurons extending from the brainstem through the cerebral cortex	Routes incoming information to the appropriate location in the brain; RAS activity also involved in wakefulness

periphery and the brain. The spinal cord is also central to the control of reflex responses. The length of the spinal cord varies from an average of 43 cm in an adult female to 45 cm in an adult male. The vertebral column housing the spinal cord is approximately 70 cm long, far exceeding the length of the spinal cord. Because the spinal cord ends at the last of the thoracic vertebra, nerves branching from the spinal cord below the lumbar and sacral levels must extend for a distance before they exit the vertebral column. The extension of nerves in this portion of the vertebral canal is called the **cauda equina**.

The nervous tissue of the spinal cord is composed of both white and gray matter, based on the presence or absence of myelin. The proportion of gray matter to white matter in the spinal cord is determined by the amount of tissue innervated. Differences in proportion of gray and white matter are seen in the various segments of the cord. The lower lumbar and upper sacral segment innervate the lower

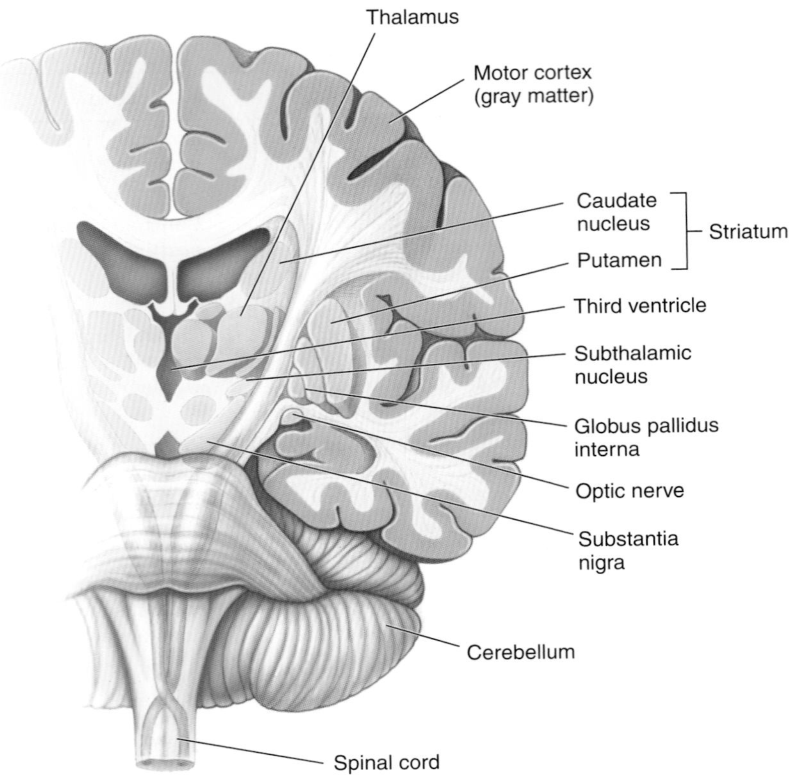

Figure 10.5. Coronal view of the brain. (Courtesy Anatomical Chart Company.)

extremities and contain larger amounts of gray matter. The white matter proportion increases as the cord approaches the brain due to the greater number of ascending fibers.

The gray matter contains synapses between sensory, motor, and interneurons. On cross-section of the spinal cord, the gray matter has a butterfly-like appearance and contains nerve cell bodies. The posterior extensions are the **dorsal horns**, which contain sensory neurons that receive afferent impulses via the dorsal roots. The anterior extensions are known as the **ventral horns**, which contain efferent motor neurons that leave the cord through the ventral roots. **Upper motor neurons** (UMN) include cell bodies in the motor cortex and the axons extending to the brain stem and spinal cord. **Lower motor neurons** (LMN) are located in the ventral horns of the spinal cord. Interneurons connect UMNs with LMNs in the spinal cord.

Surrounding this gray matter is the white matter, composed of the axons of the spinal cord. The white matter contains myelinated axons, giving the lighter-colored appearance reflected by its name (Fig. 10.6). Myelin produced by Schwann cells increases the velocity and survival of nerve impulses along longer neuronal processes.

The white matter contains ascending sensory and descending motor tracts with axons that communicate impulses within the CNS. The ascending tracts communicate sensory information from the periphery to the CNS and will be discussed in more detail in Chapter 12. The **pyramidal motor system**, composed of the axons in the descending corticospinal and corticobulbar tracts, provides

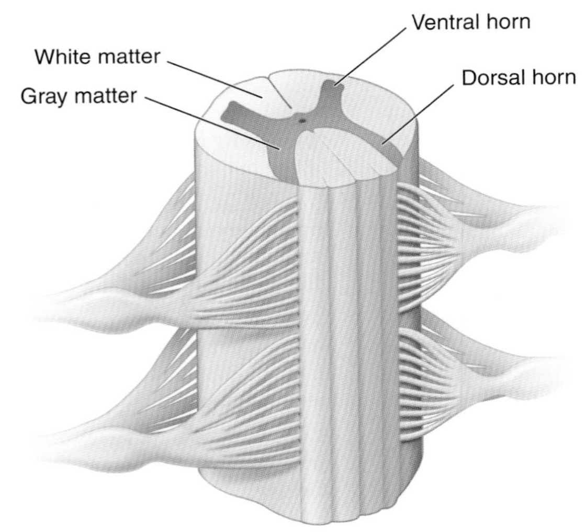

Figure 10.6. Spinal cord structures. The spinal cord runs inside the vertebral column. Axons enter the spinal cord through the dorsal roots and exit by the ventral roots.

control of voluntary movement. Motor nerves of the pyramidal tract originate in both hemispheres of the sensorimotor areas of the cerebral cortex and extend through the medullary brainstem, condensing to form pyramids. The majority of UMNs of the corticospinal tract cross over in the medulla, descending on the contralateral side. The UMNs synapse onto the LMNs, leaving the spinal cord via the ventral root. The UMNs that do not cross over in the medulla travel down the ipsilateral spinal cord, crossing over and synapsing on the LMN at the level of spinal cord exit. The LMNs synapse onto motor fibers in the peripheral nervous system, providing innervation and motor function to the legs. Injury to axons before they cross over results in spastic paralysis on the opposite side of the body, whereas injury to axons after they cross over exerts its effect on the same side of the body. Axons of the corticobulbar tract provide innervation to the muscles of the face, controlling motor neurons located in cranial nerve brain nuclei.

The **extrapyramidal system**, separate from the pyramidal motor system, modulates motor function, attenuating erratic motions and maintaining muscle tone and stability of the trunk. Functions associated with the extrapyramidal system are associated with the basal ganglia. The subcortical nuclei of the basal ganglia include the structures of the caudate nucleus, putamen, subthalamic nucleus, substantia nigra, and globus pallidus, which comprise the main structures of the extrapyramidal system.

Protective Structures of the CNS

The maintenance of a stable environment provides a source of protection for the neurologic system. The interconnected circulatory systems confer neurologic protection via the blood–brain barrier and cerebrospinal fluid (CSF).

NEUROCIRCULATORY SYSTEM

The nervous system is perfused by two parallel communicating systems. These systems include the cerebrovascular circulation and the CSF circulation.

Cerebrovascular Circulation

The vascular supply of the CNS provides oxygenation and nutrients for optimal metabolism and function. Maintenance of perfusion to the brain is essential for prevention of cellular injury and death. Neurons in the brain are sensitive to hypoxia, requiring adequate perfusion. Arterial supply to the brain includes the vertebral, basilar, and carotid arteries. The circle of Willis is a cerebral arterial structure that connects the vertebral and carotid circulations. This structure is important as a route of collateral circulation in case perfusion is impaired in another arterial system. The primary vascular drainage of the brain occurs via the jugular veins. Perfusion to the spinal cord is supplied by the spinal arteries and drained by the spinal veins. Removal of excess fluid in the CNS occurs between the pia matter of the meninges and the blood vessels because typical lymphatics are absent in the brain.

Stop and Consider

The preferred energy source for the brain is glucose. What manifestations can be expected when adequate levels of glucose are unavailable?

Blood–Brain Barrier

The brain is protected from exposure to potentially hazardous substances by reduced permeability in capillaries that supply the brain, known as the **blood–brain barrier (BBB)**. The BBB transports substances in a selective manner because of the tight junctions in the endothelial cells lining the capillaries of the brain. Transport across the BBB of large molecules, molecules with low lipid solubility, and molecules with high electrical charge are resisted. Substances that are small, highly lipid soluble, and have a low electrical charge are able to cross the BBB more readily. The BBB functions include:

- Protection of the brain from foreign substances
- Protection of the brain from hormones and neurotransmitters in the systemic circulation
- Protection against drastic environmental fluctuations

Cerebrospinal Fluid

The **meninges** of the CNS include three membranes that protect tissue surfaces, containing CSF. These membranes and their relative locations include:

1. Dura mater (outer layer)
2. Arachnoid mater (middle layer)
3. Pia mater (inner layer)

The surface of the CNS is bathed by the **cerebrospinal fluid**, which flows from four fluid-filled interconnecting cavities of the brain, known as the **ventricles**. CSF is produced by the **choroid plexus**, a structure located in the two lateral and single third and fourth ventricles of the brain. CSF flows from the lateral ventricle to the third ventricle through the **interventricular foramen** (also called the foramen of Monro). The third and fourth ventricles are connected by the **cerebral aqueduct** (also known as the aqueduct of Sylvius). CSF then

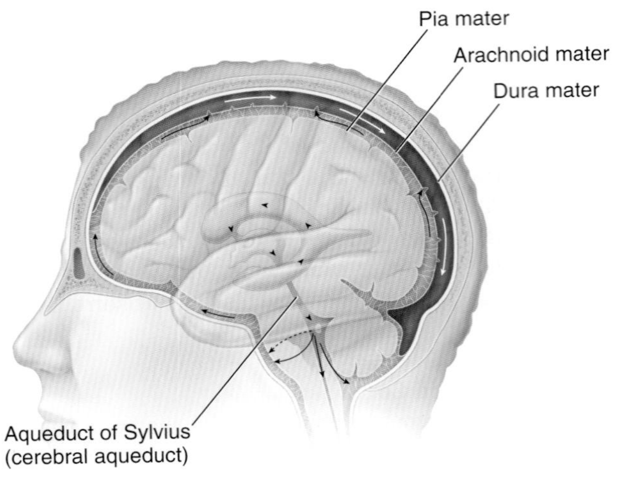

Figure 10.7. Cerebrospinal fluid flow in the ventricular system. Arrows indicate the direction of cerebrospinal fluid flow.

flows into the subarachnoid space (Fig. 10.7). CSF protects the CNS by:

- Providing a cushion for brain structures
- Reducing the pressure on brain structures
- Removing harmful substances
- Transporting hormones to remote sites in the brain

The total volume of CSF in the CNS at any one time is approximately 125 to 150 mL. The choroid plexus produces 400 to 500 mL CSF per day to maintain a resting pressure of 150 to 180 mm H_2O. When CSF pressure exceeds venous pressure, CSF can be absorbed into the blood via the arachnoid. This movement of fluid from the CSF to the circulation is unidirectional, preventing the absorption of fluid from the blood into the CSF.

Stop and Consider
How would CSF volume be altered if fluid could move directly from the blood into the CSF?

CNS Cellular Injury

Responses to injury vary based on the specific cell type involved. These responses mirror the major functional properties of the cells. In the CNS, astrocytes respond to local tissue injury through proliferation, forming a "glial scar." This process is known as **astrogliosis**. Common tissue injuries that are likely to cause this response include contusions, wounds, tumors, abscesses, and hemorrhages. Unchecked proliferation may result in neoplastic transformation responsible for the development of gliomas, as discussed in Chapter 7.

Microglia, like astrocytes, mount an immune response to areas of injury. Reactive changes seen in microglia include extension of the nucleus, leading to their description as "rod cells" when in this state. When joined together with astrocytes, microglia combine to form **microglial nodules.** Oligodendroglial damage leads to demyelination of axons. Ependymal cell damage is linked to alterations in CSF production and transfer, affecting intracranial pressure (ICP).

Neurologic transmission is impaired in the presence of significant neuronal damage or death. The manifestations of altered function reflect the site of injury and the functions that are controlled by those particular neurons. The nervous system responses to injury include degeneration of axons, demyelination, and neuropathy. Alteration in neuronal transmission underlies the manifestations that result from these types of injuries.

MECHANISMS OF INJURY TO THE CNS

Functions of the brain and spinal cord can be impaired because of injury. Mechanisms of injury may result from trauma, ischemia, excitatory response to neurotransmitters, or pressure.

Traumatic CNS Injury

Traumatic injury can impair neurologic functioning locally or systemically. When injury is restricted to a structure innervating a specific area, a local effect may be seen. Injury to neural tissue responsible for the integrated transmission of impulses to multiple, distant sites is likely to have a more systemic effect. Examples of these types of major injuries include trauma to the components of the CNS (the brain and spinal cord).

Traumatic Brain Injury

Automobile accidents, falls, sports-related accidents, and "shaken baby syndrome" are conditions that may result in traumatic brain injury (TBI), also known as concussion. Groups at highest risk for TBI include persons 65 years of age or older due to falls, children and young adults age 5 to 24 due to motor vehicle accidents and children age 0 to 4 due to assault.[1] Head trauma that results in TBI may lead to changes in physical, intellectual, emotional, or social abilities. Head trauma from a blunt force injury (e.g., when the head strikes a hard surface or is struck by a rapidly moving object [coup/countercoup]) is an example of a closed head injury. The force of the acceleration impact causes injury to the tissue in the local area (coup), and the deceleration impact leads to injury on the opposite side of the skull (countercoup). Lacerations and contusions of the brain tissue may result from contact with the rough surface of the skull. The cerebral cortex may suffer effects of movement within the skull, increasing the likelihood of damage to the frontal, temporal, and occipital lobes of the brain as well as the upper midbrain. Open traumatic injury involves exposure of brain structures (e.g., dura, meninges, and brain tissue) to the environment. The risk of infection and injury to brain tissue is significant with this type of injury.

TBI may lead to seizure activity, concussion, contusion, hematoma (epidural, subdural, or intracerebral), edema, or skull fracture. Increased ICP, respiratory depression/failure, and herniation of the brainstem may also occur. Manifestations are caused by axonal injury from the original trauma and by spread of damage that causes secondary injury. Diagnosis is often made using brain imaging techniques, including computerized tomography (CT) or magnetic resonance imaging (MRI). Brain activity can be determined with an electroencephalogram (EEG). Lumbar puncture (spinal tap) with removal and analysis of CSF may determine the presence of blood, indicating intracranial hemorrhage.

Treatment is directed toward the specific injury and diagnosis. Surgery may be necessary to evacuate a hematoma or to remove foreign fragments from brain tissue. Supportive care includes determination of the extent and progression of neurologic damage, reduction of increased ICP, pain control, provision of anticonvulsant medications to prevent seizures, respiratory support, and antibiotics to prevent or treat infection.

Traumatic Spinal Cord Injury

According to the National Spinal Cord Injury Statistical Center, spinal cord injury (SCI) primarily affects young adults. The average age at injury has increased from 28.7 years in the 1970s to an average age of 40.7 years since 2005. Most spinal cord injuries (approximately 81%) are among males. Although frequency among Caucasians has steadily decreased over the past two decades, the incidence of SCI has increased among African Americans, Asians, and Hispanics.[2] The leading causes of SCI include motor vehicle accidents and acts of violence (e.g., gunshot). Spinal cord injuries may be the result of fractures, contusions, or compression of the vertebral column. These injuries may also stem from trauma to the head or neck. Neurologic damage resulting from pulling, twisting, severing, or compressing the neural tissue of the spinal cord is a serious, potentially life-threatening condition. The level of injury within the spinal cord is the determining factor for the clinical consequences. The most common spinal cord injuries occur at C5-C7, T12, and L1.

Traumatic injury to the spinal cord is often secondary to motor vehicle accidents, falls, acts of violence and recreational injuries, similar to the events leading to brain injury. Injury often extends two segments above and below the site of damage. Diving into shallow water may also cause serious spinal cord damage. Damage results from hyperextension and hyperflexion due to rapid acceleration/deceleration, excessive pressure to the top of the head causing compression injury, and rotational forces causing trauma from twisting of the spinal cord. Hemorrhage in the gray matter and the pia mater/arachnoid may lead to necrosis. Extension of hemorrhage into the white matter and the development of local edema decreases perfusion to the cord, leading to ischemia. Phagocytic activity in the gray matter results in macrophage engulfment of axons, replacing neural tissue with nonfunctional connective tissue. Scarring and thickening of the meninges alters neural conduction and function.

A clinical manifestation of vertebrae fracture may be pain. When SCI results, responses can range from mild **paresthesia** (abnormal sensation, such as burning, pricking, tickling, or tingling) to **quadriplegia** (paralysis of all four extremities). The level of the SCI and the severity of injury (complete or incomplete transection) also contribute to the neurologic deficit. Table 10.3 presents the possible consequences of serious SCI.

Diagnosis of SCI can be made by radiograph (fracture), neurologic examination, lumbar puncture, CT scan, or MRI scan. Immediate treatment includes immobilization of the spine to prevent further injury. Once the spine is stabilized, corticosteroids are given to lessen inflammation. Traction, casting, and surgery may also be necessary.

Ischemic CNS Injury

Ischemic injury occurs when there is inadequate perfusion to neurologic tissue, resulting in impaired oxygenation. **Focal ischemia** in the brain is confined to a specific brain region while **global ischemia** includes larger areas of brain tissue. Reduction in the supply of oxygen leads to tissue necrosis. The cause of decreased perfusion and oxygenation may be local or may be a systemic condition. For example, occlusion of blood supply may result from a thrombosis in a local vessel, embolism from a thrombus originating in a distant site, or from local hemorrhage. A global ischemic event is associated with a wide area of hypoxia, as is seen in the case of cardiac arrest or profound hemorrhage (Fig. 10.8). Spinal cord ischemia is often due to occlusion of spinal blood vessels resulting from dissecting aortic aneurism or emboli. Malformations in the spinal vasculature may also impair perfusion leading to ischemia and neural injury.

The pathology underlying ischemic injury is related to oxygen and nutrient deprivation to neurologic tissue. Impaired blood flow for longer than a few minutes results in tissue infarction in brain tissue with high metabolic demands. Cellular function ceases because of the inability to use anaerobic metabolic processes or uptake glucose and glycogen. Infarction stimulates a response to tissue injury that results in an inflammatory response and the development of edema, leading to increased ICP. Cell injury leads to changes in the transport of ions leading to local water and electrolyte imbalances (Chapter 8) and acidosis (Chapter 9). Calcium, sodium, and water build up in the area of cellular damage. Free radical formation and increased release of excitatory neurotransmitters may potentiate the effects of the ischemic injury.

Clinical manifestations of ischemic injury are related to the functional areas involved. Sensory and motor functions are often affected. When the injury occurs in the brain, the manifestations reflect the specific associated functions with motor deficits evident on the **contralateral**, or opposite, side of the body. Loss of consciousness, weakness, difficulty speaking or swallowing, impaired vision, and paresthesias may result.

CT scan, MRI, and angiography can be used to diagnose ischemic blockages. Altered metabolism in surrounding regions may be identified by positron

Table 10.3 Potential Results of Serious Spinal Cord Injury

Condition	Pathophysiology	Clinical Manifestations
Spinal shock	Loss of autonomic, reflex, motor, and sensory activity below the injury	Flaccid (without tone) paralysis Loss of deep tendon reflexes (DTRs) Loss of perianal reflexes Loss of motor and sensory function
Autonomic dysreflexia	Occurs after resolution of spinal shock Associated with injuries at or above T6 Stimulated by noxious stimuli (distended bowel or bladder, skin lesion)	Alteration in heart rate Hypertension Cold/gooseflesh skin below the lesion
Neurogenic shock	Altered vasomotor response secondary to impaired sympathetic impulse transmission from the brain stem to the thoracolumbar region Most common with cervical spinal cord injury	Orthostatic hypotension Bradycardia Loss of ability to sweat below the level of injury

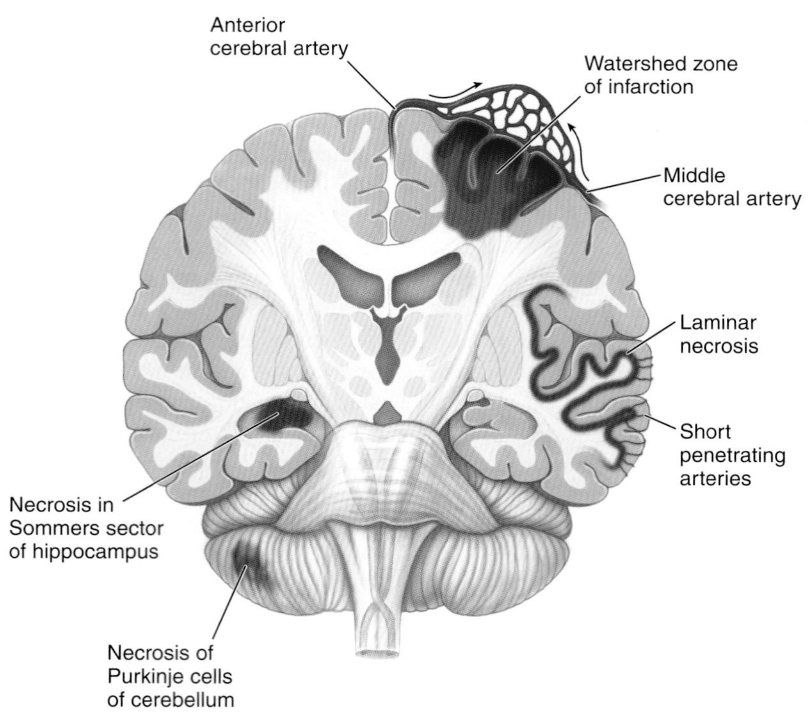

Figure 10.8. Global ischemia. Consequences of global ischemia include lesions related to cerebral vasculature and the sensitivity of individual neurons. (From Rubin E, Farber JL. *Pathology*. 4th ed. Philadelphia, PA: Lippincott Williams & Wilkins; 2005.)

emission tomography (PET) scanning. Treatment includes management of increased ICP, insertion of a stent to restore perfusion, thrombolytic therapy to dissolve the obstructive clot, and anticoagulation therapy to prevent future clot development.

EXCITATION INJURY

Neurons that are easily depolarized or hyperexcitable may cause altered transmission of signals. Increased neuron impulse frequency, intensity, or cascade of transmission can lead to pathologic consequences because of excitation injury. Injury to brain neurons may result from the effects of excitatory neurotransmitters, such as the amino acid glutamate. **Glutamate** is the main excitatory neurotransmitter in the body, active in the promotion of many higher-order functions. The effects of glutamate are exerted when it binds to its receptors, stimulating a cascade of signal transduction events. One receptor with affinity for glutamate is the ***N*-methyl-D-aspartate (NMDA) receptor**. When glutamate binds to the NMDA receptor, alterations in ion channel openings lead to prolonged action potentials. Damage to neurons from protein breakdown, free radical formation, DNA damage, and breakdown of the nucleus is stimulated by these prolonged action potentials.

Excitation injury may result from the inability to meet the metabolic demands of the cells. Oxygen needs dramatically increase with enhanced neurologic activity, increasing the risk of hypoxia development in affected tissues. Prolonged ischemia permits intracellular glutamate to move from the highly concentrated intracellular space to the extracellular environment, making more glutamate available for receptor binding, thereby intensifying the excitatory effects. In tissues sensitive to hypoxia, such as the brain, permanent brain injury may result.

The neurons of the hippocampus and cerebral cortex are particularly sensitive to the excitatory effects of glutamate and increases in calcium that result from changes in ion transport. The neurotoxic effects may be manifested by reductions in higher-order functions and cognitive and memory abilities. Neuronal cell death may result from prolonged exposure to the effects of glutamate.

Cell death may be prevented if the effects of glutamate can be blocked or the excessive level of glutamate removed from the neuronal synapses. Because glutamate is required by a wide variety of cells for normal functioning, the development of drugs to block or promote reuptake of glutamate has been hampered.

Excitatory responses may predominate during periods of deteriorating brain function. Loss of consciousness may promote the development of **decerebrate posturing**, the result of increased extensor muscle excitability, or **decorticate posturing**, the result of increased flexor muscle excitability (Fig. 10.9).

CNS PRESSURE INJURY

The skull and vertebral column provide the rigid structure surrounding the brain and spinal cord, restricting the potential area of expansion. Increases in pressure may result in neuronal injury and cell death. Increased pressure in the brain and spinal cord may result from excessive CSF volume, cerebral edema, or space-occupying lesions.

Increased CSF volume is the result of increased production or decreased absorption of CSF.

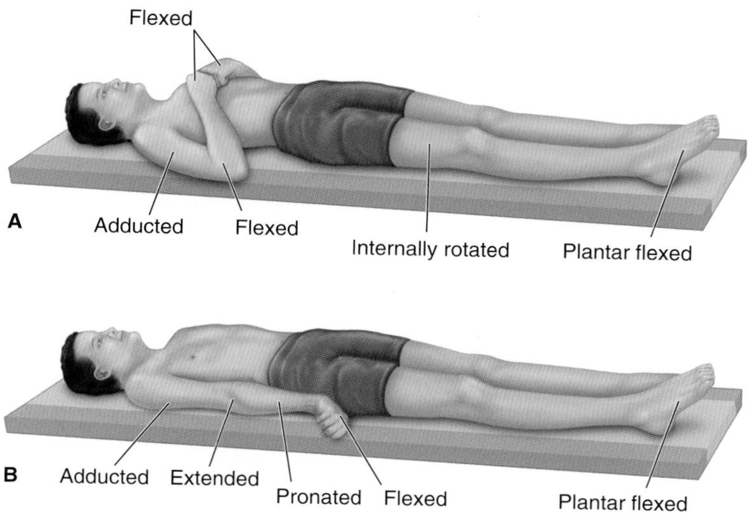

Figure 10.9. Posturing in brain injury. **A:** Flexor, or decorticate posturing response, is characterized by flexion of elbows, wrists, and fingers. **B:** Extensor, or decerebrate posturing response, is characterized by neck extension and clenching of the jaw. Arms are extended with flexion of wrists and fingers.

Obstruction of the ventricular system prevents CSF from reaching the arachnoid villi. Flow of the CSF may be obstructed by inflammation, tumor, hemorrhage, or congenital anomaly, promoting buildup in the ventricular system. Cerebral hemisphere enlargement and dilation of the ventricles result from pressure increases. Brain structures affected by the increased pressure respond with altered functional capacity. Responses may be altered by age and associated brain development.

Cerebral edema caused by abnormal water accumulation may also contribute to pressure injury. Edema may be a result of the transfer of water and protein from the vascular to the interstitial space, as discussed in Chapter 8. Edema may also be caused by an increase in intracellular fluid caused by a hypoosmotic state, such as occurs with water intoxication. Severe ischemia can also contribute to cerebral edema. Swelling of brain cells increases tissue volume, causing injury to cells. Manifestations of cerebral edema include disturbances in consciousness, intracranial hypertension, and neurologic deficit.

CNS tumors (discussed in Chapter 7) can also promote pressure injury. Brain and spinal cord compression, tumor infiltration, altered blood flow, and edema are often the sequelae of pressure injuries resulting from tumors. Tumors may obstruct CSF flow and promote brain displacement to an area of lower pressure, known as brain herniation. Stimulation of the vomiting center of the medulla may contribute to severe nausea. Personality and mental changes, including loss of memory and the development of depression, may result. The tumor location and site of pressure injury determine the specific signs and symptoms evidenced. Clinical manifestations of pressure injury are determined by the sites of injury and severity of damage, ranging from leg weakness to respiratory arrest.

A common response to pathologic events in the brain is ICP. Increased ICP can lead to blood flow reduction, death of brain cells, and damage to brain structures. Common symptoms of increased ICP include:

- Headache
- Vomiting
- **Papilledema** (edema of the optic disc)
- Mental deterioration

When increased ICP is caused by excessive CSF ventricular fluid volume, surgical shunting of CSF from the intraventricular spaces to the peritoneum may be required. A catheter is inserted into the left lateral ventricle and passed through the internal jugular vein into the right atrium (ventriculoatrial shunt) or the peritoneal cavity (ventriculoperitoneal shunt). For increased ICP caused by cerebral edema, osmotic diuretics such as mannitol are often used to promote fluid removal and excretion. Corticosteroids may also be used to stabilize cell membranes.

Module 3 Alterations in Peripheral Nervous System Function

The peripheral nervous system connects the CNS to limbs and organs, transmitting neural impulses via sensory pathways into the dorsal horn and extending motor pathways beyond the ventral horn. Located outside of the boundaries of the CNS, the peripheral nervous system is not protected by the blood–brain barrier or bony support of the CNS, increasing the potential for damage due to toxic and mechanical injury.

Peripheral Nervous System Organization

Functionally, the peripheral nervous system includes the somatic and the autonomic nervous systems. Motor and sensory nerves carrying nerve impulses to and from the periphery of the body are part of the peripheral nervous system, including the cranial and spinal nerves. Cranial nerves that mediate peripheral responses originate in the brain. There are twelve paired cranial nerves, each named, numbered, and specific in the sensory and motor functions they mediate (Table 10.4). There are 31 pairs of spinal nerves, each consisting of sensory/afferent and motor/efferent neurons. They are named for the vertebra immediately below their exit point from the spinal cord and include 8 cervical, 12 thoracic, 5 lumbar, 5 sacral, and 1 coccygeal nerve pairs. Table 10.5 provides further detail on the location and function of these nerves. Spinal nerves carry information to and from particular body regions, or **dermatomes** (Fig. 10.10). Manifestations of pain, numbness, or tingling can be linked to pressure or inflammation of the spinal nerves associated with specific dermatomes. Spinal nerves form together in an interconnection of fibers known as a **plexus**. Peripheral nerves arise in new combinations from each plexus. Common plexuses include the cervical, brachial, lumbar, and sacral.

Table 10.4 Cranial Nerves

Number	Name	Location	Type	Function
I	Olfactory	Cerebral cortex, amygdala, hippocampus, basal ganglia (caudate nucleus, putamen, globus pallidus)	Sensory	Smell reflexes
II	Optic	Hypothalamus, thalamus	Sensory	Vision
III	Oculomotor	Basal ganglia, substantia nigra, central gray matter	Motor	Extraocular eye movement (superior, medial and inferior lateral), pupil constriction, upper eyelid elevation
IV	Trochlear	Pons	Motor	Extraocular eye movement (inferior medial)
V	Trigeminal	Pons	Sensory	Corneal reflex, transmission of stimuli from face to head
			Motor	Lateral jaw movement, chewing, biting
VI	Abducens	Pons	Motor	Extraocular eye movement (lateral)
VII	Facial	Pons	Sensory	Taste (anterior two-thirds of tongue)
			Motor	Movement of facial muscles and muscles of expression in forehead, around eyes and mouth
VIII	Acoustic (vestibulocochlear)	Pons	Sensory	Hearing, balance
IX	Glossopharyngeal	Medulla	Sensory	Taste (posterior one-third of the tongue), sensations of the throat
			Motor	Swallow
X	Vagus	Medulla	Sensory	Sensations of larynx, throat, abdominal (gastrointestinal tract), and thoracic viscera (heart, lungs, bronchi)
			Motor	Palate movement, swallow, gag, activity of thoracic and abdominal viscera (including heart rate and peristalsis)
XI	Spinal accessory	Medulla	Motor	Movement of shoulders, head rotation
XII	Hypoglossal	Medulla	Motor	Tongue movement

Table 10.5 Spinal Nerves

Spinal Nerves	Location	Function
Lower cervical	C5-C8	Proprioception, deep tendon reflexes, movement, posture
Thoracic	T1-T12	Proprioception, movement, posture, respiration, sensation, sympathetic reflexes (vasomotor control, sweating, piloerection)
Lumbar	L1-L5	Proprioception, deep tendon reflexes, movement, posture, reflexes
Sacral	S1-S5	Proprioception, reflexes, defecation, urination, erection
Coccygeal	Co1-2	Proprioception, posture

Stop and Consider

When having a heart attack, a common manifestation is pain in the left arm or shoulder. How are dermatomes related to this phenomenon?

SOMATIC NERVOUS SYSTEM

Coordination of body movement, reception of external stimuli and regulation of activities under conscious control are the primary functions of the somatic nervous system. The somatic nervous system includes the peripheral fibers that transmit sensory impulses including body position, pain, temperature, and touch to the CNS and motor impulses to skeletal muscle from cell bodies located in the brain or spinal cord. Targets for innervation include skeletal muscle, skin and sensory organs. A review of somatic and special sensory function and dysfunction is included in Chapter 12.

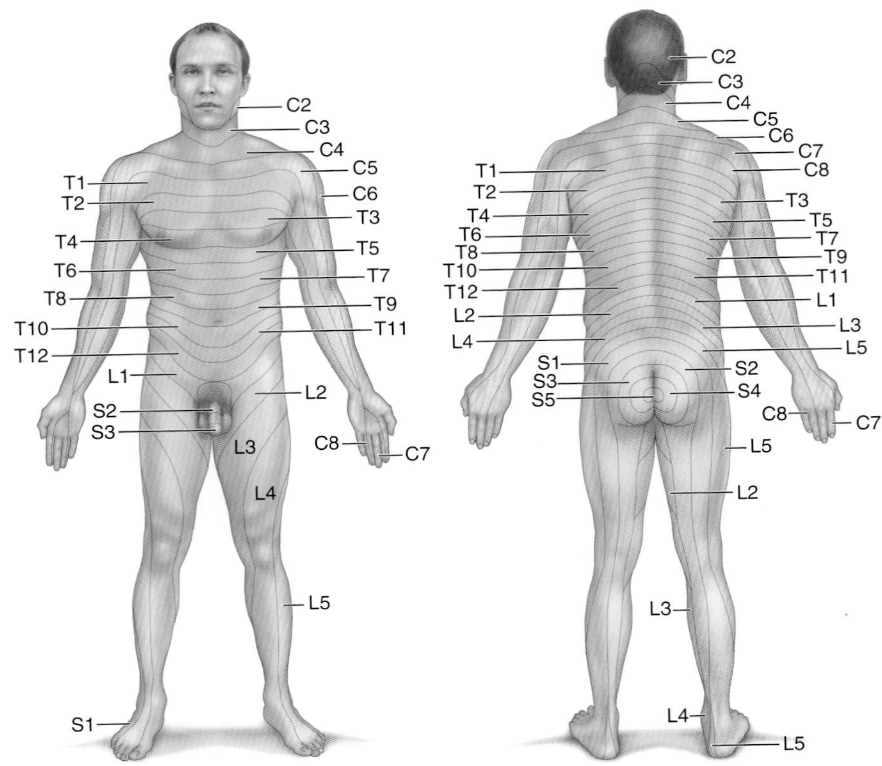

Figure 10.10. Distribution of dermatomes. Spinal nerves transmit impulses to specific areas known as dermatomes.

AUTONOMIC NERVOUS SYSTEM

The autonomic nervous system (ANS) controls involuntary functions of organs. All internal organs are innervated by the ANS, which transmits messages from the brain and neuroendocrine system. The two major divisions of the ANS are the sympathetic nervous system (SNS) and parasympathetic nervous system (PNS). These systems generally work in opposition to one another, working toward homeostatic balance.

Axon fibers extending from cell bodies in either the brain or spinal cord project to an autonomic **ganglion** (group of nerve cell bodies) known as **preganglionic neurons**. Fibers projecting from the autonomic ganglion to a target organ are known as **postganglionic neurons**. The SNS has short preganglionic fibers that synapse outside the spinal cord with secondary neurons. Long SNS postganglionic fibers synapse on target organs. The exception to this pattern is in the case of the adrenal medulla. Here, the unusually long preganglionic fibers of the SNS synapse directly onto the adrenal medulla, with the adrenal medulla itself serving as the secondary fiber.

The PNS organization differs from the SNS, with long preganglionic fibers extending to the walls of target organs. There, they synapse with secondary neurons, extending short postganglionic fibers into the organ walls. PNS is often linked with *vagal stimulation* because approximately 75% of all PNS impulses travel along the vagus nerve (cranial nerve X). One of the differences between the ANS and the somatic nervous system is that the latter involves only one neuron, whereas the ANS requires two.

Sympathetic Nervous System

The **sympathetic nervous system** is also known as the **thoracolumbar nervous system** because of the location of the nerve exit sites. Spinal cord exit sites of the SNS neurons are located between the first thoracic and second lumbar vertebrae. The nerves leave the spinal cord to merge with ganglia. The preganglionic neurons enter ganglia near the cord, where the impulse is then carried to the postganglionic neurons (Fig. 10.11). Sympathetic activity is responsible for:

- Increased heart rate and contractility
- Smooth muscle relaxation of the bronchioles
- Decreased peristalsis of the gastrointestinal (GI) tract and constriction of anal sphincter
- Decreased bladder tone and constriction of urinary sphincter

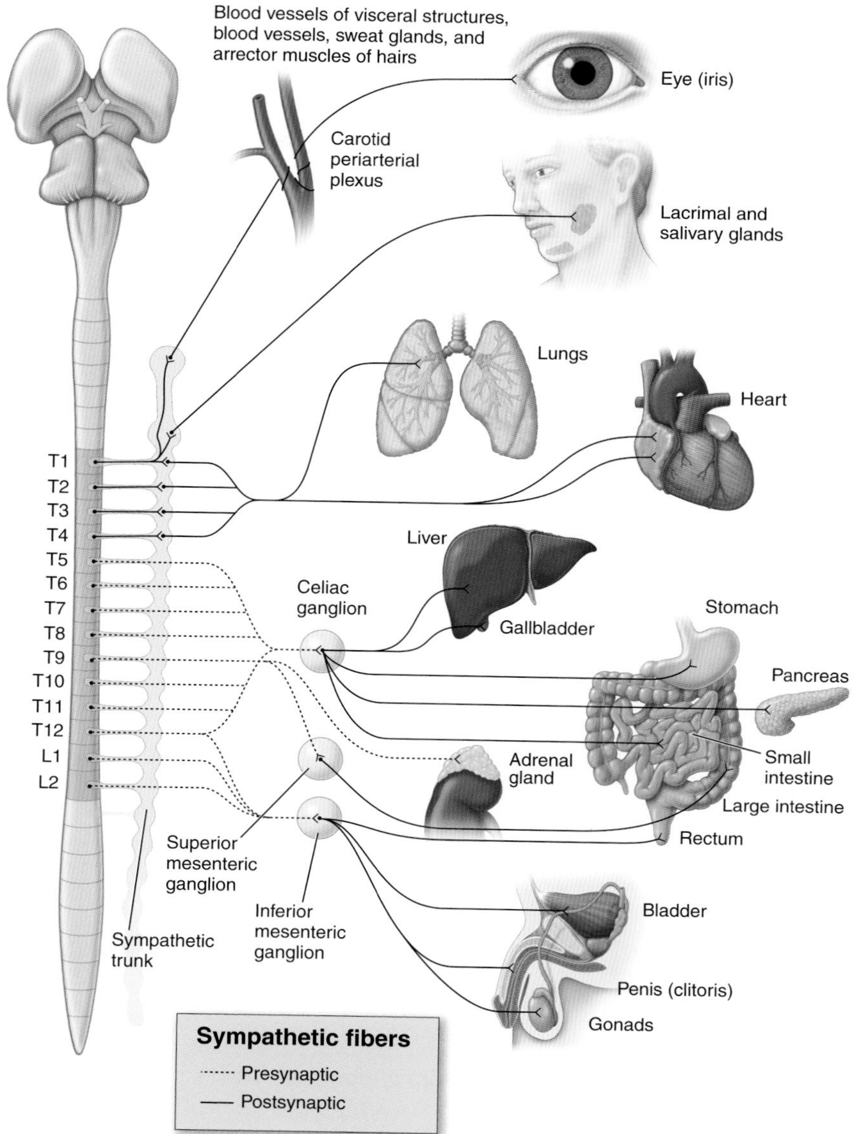

Figure 10.11. Distribution of sympathetic nerve fibers. (Modified from Moore KL, Agur A. *Essential Clinical Anatomy*. 2nd ed. Philadelphia, PA: Lippincott Williams & Wilkins; 2002.)

- Vasoconstriction and elevated blood pressure
- Increased respiratory rate
- Pupil dilation and ciliary muscle relaxation
- Reduced secretion of the pancreas
- Increased sweat gland secretion

Parasympathetic Nervous System

The neurons of the PNS leave the CNS via the cranial nerves from the midbrain and the medulla, and with the spinal nerves between S2 and S4 (craniosacral). The preganglionic neurons of the PNS are long, traveling close to organs or glands. The shorter postganglionic fibers innervate organs and glands, stimulating specific responses in the targets (Fig. 10.12). The typical effects of PNS innervation include:

- Decreased heart rate, contractility, and velocity of conduction
- Constriction of bronchial smooth muscle
- Increased peristalsis and GI tone with relaxation of anal sphincter
- Increased bladder tone and relaxation of urinary sphincter
- Vasodilation of arteries supplying external genitalia
- Constriction of pupils
- Increase in pancreatic, salivary, and eye secretions

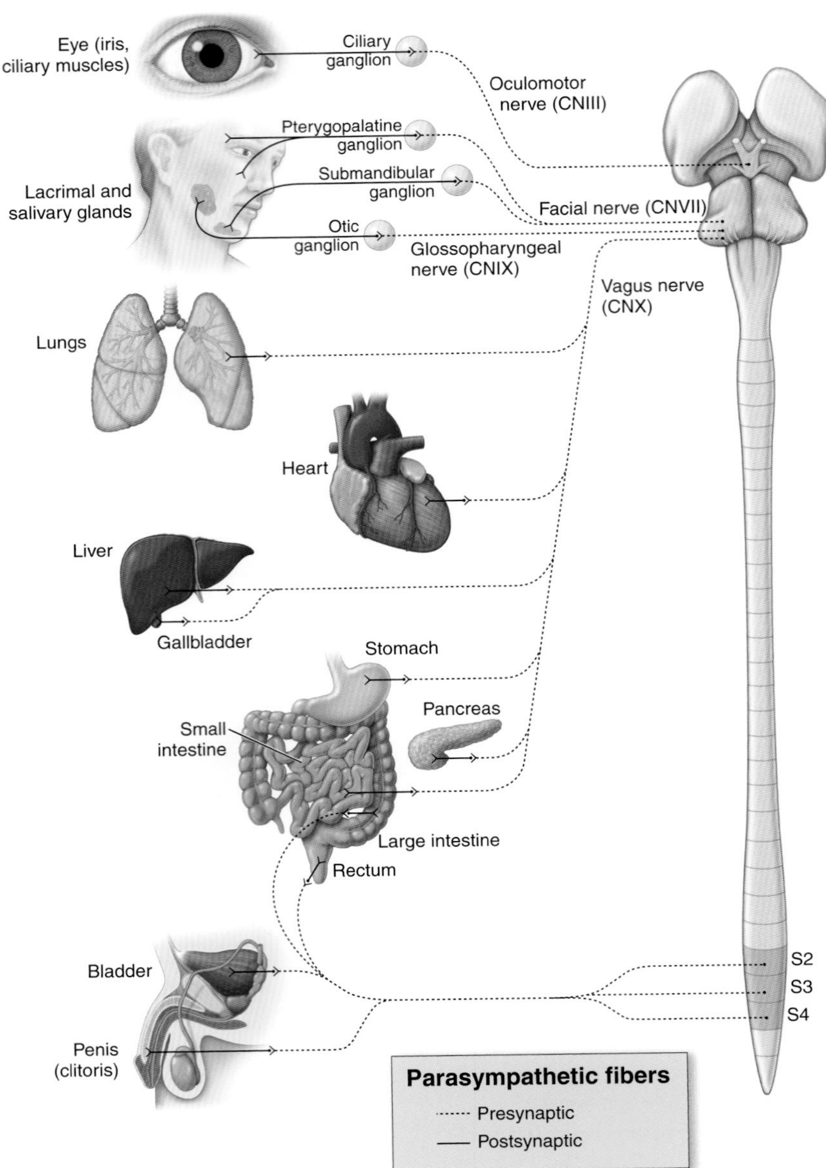

Figure 10.12. Distribution of parasympathetic nerve fibers. (Modified from Moore KL, Agur A. *Essential Clinical Anatomy*. 2nd ed. Philadelphia, PA: Lippincott Williams & Wilkins; 2002.)

Reflex Arcs

Communication between various segments of the nervous system can be illustrated by the reflex arc. A basic functional pathway of the nervous system, the **reflex arc** represents the process by which stimuli are received and interpreted, and in turn stimulate a response. For example, the knee-jerk response, also known as the patellar or deep tendon reflex (DTR), is a basic reflex requiring one sensory neuron and one motor neuron with a synapse in the CNS. A tap on the patellar tendon causes a sudden contraction of the anterior thigh muscles through conduction of the nerve impulse through the sensory afferent to the dorsal horn of the spinal cord. There, the impulse is conducted to an interneuron, then to the motor neuron, and away to the peripheral target, which is the skeletal muscle spindle of the anterior thigh (Fig. 10.13). Using this simple test, the function of the following components of the nervous system can be determined:

- Peripheral afferent neuron
- Peripheral muscle sensory response

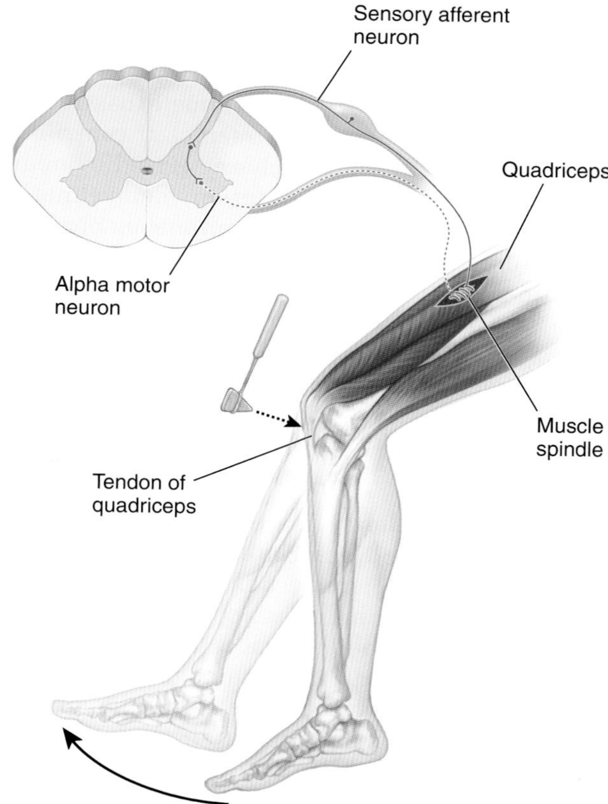

Figure 10.13. Reflex arc pathway. Reflex arc demonstrating the pathway of impulses between the receptor, spinal cord, and target organ. (From Bear MF, Connors BW, Parasido MA. *Neuroscience: Exploring the Brain*. 3rd ed. Philadelphia, PA: Lippincott Williams & Wilkins; 2006.)

- Dorsal root ganglia
- Dorsal and ventral horn
- Motor neuron
- Neuromuscular synapse
- Muscle fiber contractile response
- Selected spinal and cranial nerves
- Brainstem

Although this example represents the reflex arc in its simplest form, stimulation of DTRs and other more complex reflex arcs are significant clinical tools used to quickly evaluate neurologic status.

Peripheral Nervous System Cellular Injury

The peripheral nerves and their connective tissue support are vulnerable to injury due to the lack of protection afforded by the blood–brain barrier and bony limits of the CNS. Peripheral nerve injury is often the result of damage due to trauma or pressure. Injury to the cells of the peripheral nervous system shows a more limited scope of responses, including degeneration of the axons and segmental demyelination. Responses of peripheral nervous system cells to injury differ from CNS cell responses in that peripheral nervous system cells have some capacity for regeneration, repair, and reinnervation.

MECHANISMS OF INJURY TO THE PERIPHERAL NERVOUS SYSTEM

Axonal degeneration is caused by necrosis in response to significant injury to the cell body or axon of the neuron. In this process, an inflammatory response is stimulated, leading to phagocytosis of cellular debris by macrophages. **Distal axonopathy** occurs when the injury affects cells in distal areas of the body, such as the hands and feet. Regeneration of axons may be possible if the cell body and proximal axons are not damaged. When axonal degeneration occurs because of damage to the cell body (**neuronopathy**), the chance for regeneration is greatly reduced. When degeneration of the axon is caused by a crushing injury, it is known as a **Wallerian degeneration**. The clinical manifestations of damage to peripheral nerves are called **peripheral neuropathy**. Basic responses of peripheral nerves to injury are described in Figure 10.14.

Traumatic Peripheral Nerve Injury

Traumatic injury to peripheral nerves can occur because of the crushing or cutting of neurons. The area of nerve fiber that is severed from the cell body degenerates (Wallerian degeneration), stimulating the inflammatory processes induced by necrosis. Chromatolysis is induced in the injured neurons. Damage to peripheral nerves from traumatic injury manifests with sensory symptoms. These may include:

- Numbness
- Paresthesia
- Pain

The symptoms that result from peripheral nerve trauma are related to the number of axons involved and the ability of axons to regenerate. Regeneration of peripheral nerve fibers depends on the distance the regrowing fiber must go to restore communication. Because crushing injuries do not involve the complete separation of the axon and cell body from the target organ, regeneration success is much greater in these injuries than in fibers damaged by cutting injuries. When nerve trauma is limited to a single area (**mononeuropathy**), conditions such as

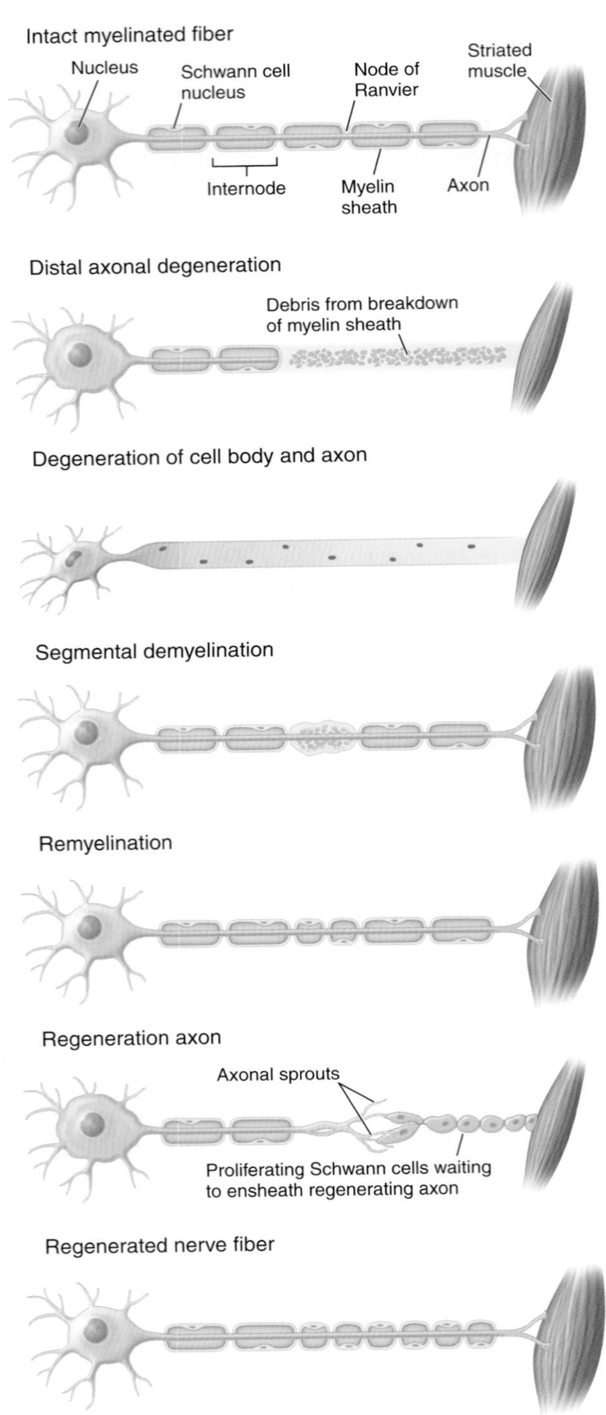

Figure 10.14. Basic responses of peripheral nerve fibers to injury. (From Rubin E, Farber JL. *Pathology*. 4th ed. Philadelphia, PA: Lippincott Williams & Wilkins; 2005.)

nerve entrapment and compression may contribute to impaired functional responses. Sensory responses to traumatic nerve injury can result from scar tissue formation entrapping a regenerating nerve.

Peripheral nerve damage involving multiple axons is known as **polyneuropathy**. Polyneuropathy can occur secondary to disease processes such as multiple sclerosis (MS), diabetes mellitus, nutrient deficiency, and toxic agents (arsenic). It contributes to multisystemic responses characterized by neural degeneration, neuroma formation, demyelination, and generation of abnormal, spontaneous nerve impulses from injured neurons. Responses may involve alterations in sensation, motor, or mixed responses. If the autonomic nervous system is involved, systemic alterations affecting blood pressure, evacuation of bowel or bladder, and erectile function may result.

Peripheral Nervous System Pressure Injury

Pressure on peripheral nerves may also contribute to nerve injury and associated symptoms. Edema in constricted spaces may cause this type of injury. Symptoms may be mild, as in the case of carpal tunnel syndrome when edema causes pain and paresthesia in the hands. This damage is usually reversible by correcting the edema. Trauma may lead to edema formation impinging on a nerve plexus, as in the case of birth trauma leading to **brachial plexus palsy**. The brachial plexus provides innervation to the shoulder, arm, forearm, wrist, and hand. Flaccid paralysis of the affected arm, which is usually temporary, occurs from altered neural transmission caused by edema-induced compression. Neuroma may develop during the process of injury repair, resulting in more significant impairment.

Peripheral Nervous System Motor Dysfunction

Disorders of motor function may be the result of peripheral nerve injury that alters reflex circuits. These disorders also can result from neuromuscular junction abnormalities, damage in skeletal muscle fibers, or SCI with damage to the corticospinal system or spinal nerve roots. Changes in skeletal muscle mass, such as occurs with atrophy or dystrophy, may contribute to impaired responses to adequate neural transmission. Movement disorders may be caused by excessive inhibitory or excitatory responses in nervous tissue that control functions such as coordination and proprioception. Movement disorders are characteristic of **extrapyramidal disorders**, which involve brain structures with the exclusion of the motor neurons, motor cortex, and pyramidal tract (corticobulbar and corticospinal). The extrapyramidal system (EPS) is often

Box 10.1 Movement Disorders

Ataxia—Inability to coordinate muscle activity
Athetosis—Involuntary movements of flexion and extension, pronation and supination of hands, toes, and feet; slow, writhing-type movements
Ballismus—Jerking, swinging, sweeping motions of the proximal limbs
Bradykinesia/hypokinesia—Decrease in spontaneity and movement
Chorea—Irregular, spasmodic, involuntary movements of the limbs or facial muscles, often accompanied by hypotonia
Cogwheel—Resistance to movement; rigidity decreasing to stiffness after movement begins
Dystonia—Abnormal tonicity; difficulty maintaining posture
Hyperkinesis—Excessive motor activity
Tic—Repeated, habitual muscle contractions; movements that can be voluntarily suppressed for short period only
Tremor—Oscillating, repetitive movements of whole muscles; irregular, involuntary contractions of the opposing muscle

specifically referring to the structures of the basal ganglia, substantia nigra, and subthalamic nucleus. Neurotransmitter excesses or deficiency may also contribute to movement disorders. Box 10.1 lists terms used to describe specific disorders of movement. Sensory deficits may also result from altered neuronal transmission. These alterations are explored in Chapter 12.

Stop and Consider
Why is it important to characterize specific types of altered movement?

Stop and Consider
What are the challenges of maintaining a treatment plan for a person with clinical signs and symptoms related to altered neuronal transmission?

Module 4 Clinical Models

Manifestations of neurologic alterations are often specific to the location of injury or damage. Alterations in mental status may include symptoms of altered consciousness, confusion, depression, anxiety, psychosis, inattentiveness, loss of rational thought, impaired memory, and poor judgment. Alterations in coordination lead to poor balance, injury from falls, difficulty in performing the **activities of daily living (ADL)**, and movement disorders. Sensory deficits include blindness, deafness, pain, loss of the ability to smell or taste, and lack of sensation. Manifestations of motor deficits may involve paralysis, impaired voluntary movements, or enhanced involuntary movement.

A complete neurologic examination may be necessary to identify and diagnose neurologic disorders. When specific symptoms point to a particular injury or type of disorder, a more focused examination may be performed. Table 10.6 outlines the components of a general neurologic examination. Treatment of neurologic disorders is focused on curing, treating, or alleviating symptoms. Psychiatric disorders of altered mental status are often managed with behavioral, cognitive, and pharmacologic methods and are detailed in Chapter 11. Synthetic drugs that alter neurotransmitter function may help manage psychiatric, motor, coordination, and sensory alterations. Symptom management can include treatments to reduce spasticity, increase muscle strength and tone, and improve memory. A review of underlying mechanisms leading to manifestations of neuronal disease is summarized in Figure 10.15.

The clinical models presented in this chapter incorporate the concepts of altered neuronal transmission. Individual concepts are highlighted, although, clearly, each is related to the other. When reviewing the clinical models, apply previously learned concepts to each alteration.

Cerebral Palsy

Cerebral palsy (CP) is a group of disorders resulting from damage to upper motor neurons. Symptoms appear during the first few years of life. The neuromuscular disorders that comprise CP stem from an event that occurs during the prenatal, perinatal (20 weeks' gestation through 28 newborn days), or postnatal (after birth) periods. According to the March of Dimes, CP affects approximately 1 in 300 children, diagnosed at the age of 2 years.[3]

PATHOPHYSIOLOGY

Central control of movement by the brain is altered in CP. Although the exact cause is not fully known, cerebral anoxia, hemorrhage, and other neurologic insults are likely involved. Classifications of CP can be based on the type of motor dysfunction or by the anatomy affected, as listed below:

- Motor dysfunction classifications
  - **Spastic:** inability of muscles to relax
    - Hemiplegia: involving one arm and one leg on the same side of the body
    - Diplegia: involving both legs
    - Quadriplegia: involving all four extremities, the trunk, and neck muscles
  - **Athetoid or dyskinetic:** inability to control muscle movement
  - **Ataxic:** inability to control balance and coordination

Table 10.6 Components of a General Neurologic Examination

Examination Component	Findings
Mental status	Orientation: time, place, and person; memory, attention, judgment, reasoning
Language	Expressive aphasia; problems with expression: receptive aphasia; problems with understanding: dysarthria; problems with word formation
Sensory function	Vision: pupil responsiveness, acuity, visual fields, extraocular eye movements
	Hearing, touch, pain, temperature, pressure, taste, position sense, gag reflex
Coordination	Tremor, rapid alternating foot and hand movements, finger to nose, toe to finger
	Gait
Motor function	Movement: voluntary, reflexive
Muscle tone	Cogwheeling, spasticity, rigidity
Muscle strength	Hand grasp, strength of flexors and extensors

CLINICAL MANIFESTATIONS

Symptoms of CP vary among individuals, involving altered body movement and muscle coordination. Early signs of motor involvement included delay in reaching milestones in infancy. Typical developmental milestones in infancy are based on motor function, including:

- Reaching for toy, 3 to 4 months
- Sitting, 6 to 7 months
- Walking, 10 to 14 months

Impairment may be manifested by mild motor dysfunction during physical activities, such as running, or by severe disability. Individuals with CP may have trouble with their fine motor skills or coordination for balance and walking. Cognitive function, speech, and seizure disorders are also common manifestations associated with CP. Seizures and mental disorders represent the more severe consequences of

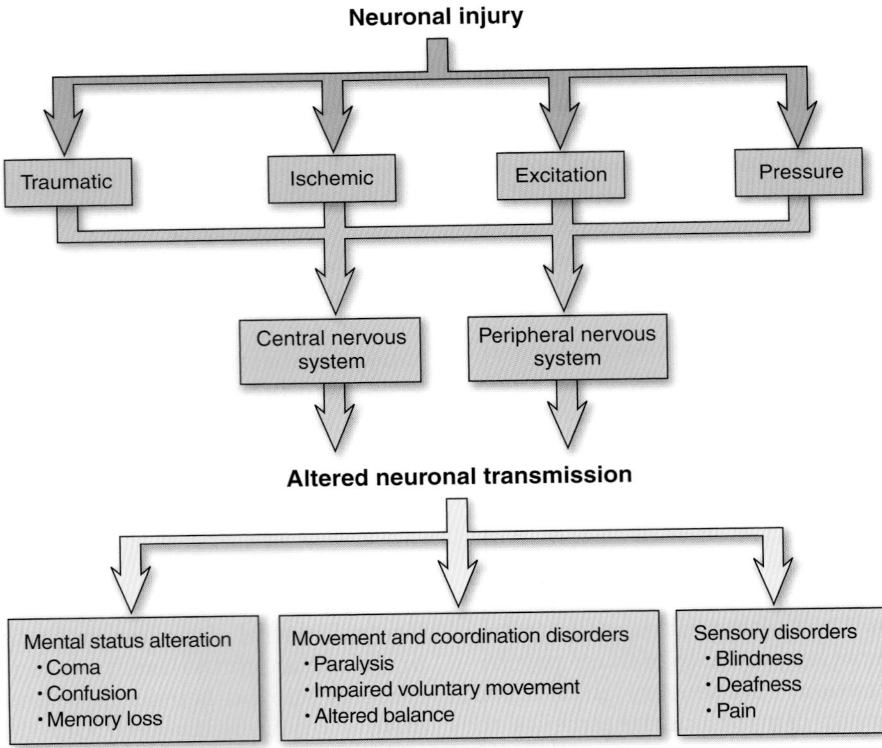

Figure 10.15. Concept map. Mechanisms of neuronal disorders.

CP. Signs of milder forms of CP may be seen during infancy, when developmental milestones are not achieved as expected. CP is not a progressive disease; therefore, worsening disabilities and deterioration of neural function are not expected with this diagnosis.

The development of seizures is often associated with CP, especially when the underlying event results in hypoxic insult.[4] Excitotoxic injury of the brain caused by excessive glutamate-mediated transmission may represent sequelae of neonatal brain injury. Glial uptake of glutamate may be impaired, resulting in overstimulation of glutamate receptors, NMDA, and alpha-amino-3-hydroxy-5-methyl-4-isoxazole propionic acid (AMPA).[5]

The neonatal brain, still undergoing maturation, is extremely vulnerable to cell death because of this excitotoxic injury. Neonatal seizures may reflect the consequences of brain injury. Seizure disorder, or *epilepsy*, is the result of impaired chemical and electrical neurotransmission. Impulses are spread in a disorderly way resulting from abnormal firing of neurons in the cerebral cortex. During the neonatal period, seizures may be subtle, limited to eye movements, sustained eye opening, tongue movement, or lip smacking. Over time, seizure activity may become more obvious.

Partial seizures begin locally in a small group of neurons in one hemisphere, spreading impulses throughout that hemisphere or to the other side of the brain. *Simple partial seizures* are limited to the originating hemisphere and can involve either motor or sensory brain components. Symptoms are sensory and autonomic without promoting an altered state of consciousness. *Complex partial seizures* involve both hemispheres and result in loss of consciousness and lack of memory about events during and after seizure. Partial seizures are short lived, lasting a few seconds in simple seizures and a few minutes in complex seizures.

Generalized seizures are caused by a more generalized electrical transmission. Absence seizures, characterized by a brief change in level of consciousness (LOC) and eye and mouth movements, can occur up to 100 times a day. *Myoclonic seizures* are characterized by involuntary muscle movements of the extremities or body, and are not associated with LOC. *Tonic–clonic seizures* are convulsive and are associated with **tonic** (a state of continuous muscle contraction) or **clonic** (rapid successions of alternating muscle contraction and relaxation) motions. Loss of consciousness and traumatic injury related to a fall may result. The seizures resolve in 2 to 5 minutes, depending on the duration of the altered electrical current. Recovery from the seizure is manifested by extreme fatigue, headache, muscle pain, and weakness, also referred to as the **post-ictal** state. *Status epilepticus* is a potentially life-threatening condition characterized by a continuous tonic–clonic seizure, which leads to hypoxia (Fig. 10.16).

DIAGNOSTIC CRITERIA

Pinpointing a specific time or event that resulted in the manifestations of CP is often difficult. The American College of Obstetricians and Gynecologists has attempted to define criteria to help determine the effects of a damaging neurologic event during labor or delivery.[6] These criteria include:

1. Apgar score (measures of heart rate, respiratory effort, color, reflexes, muscle tone) less than 7 at 5 minutes after birth.
2. Metabolic acidosis determined from analysis of the fetal umbilical artery cord blood at delivery that includes a base deficit of 12 mmol/L or more and pH less than 7.

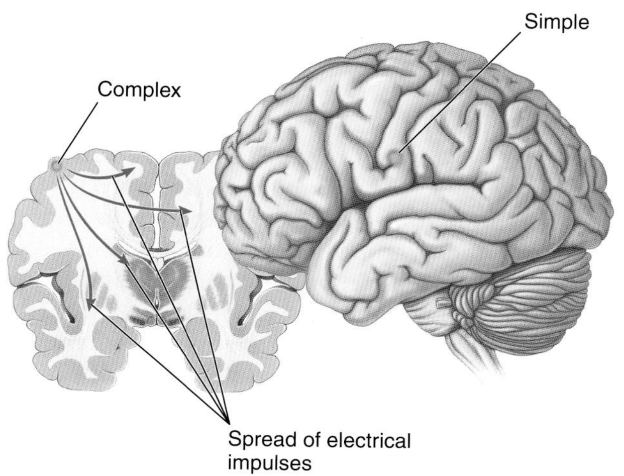

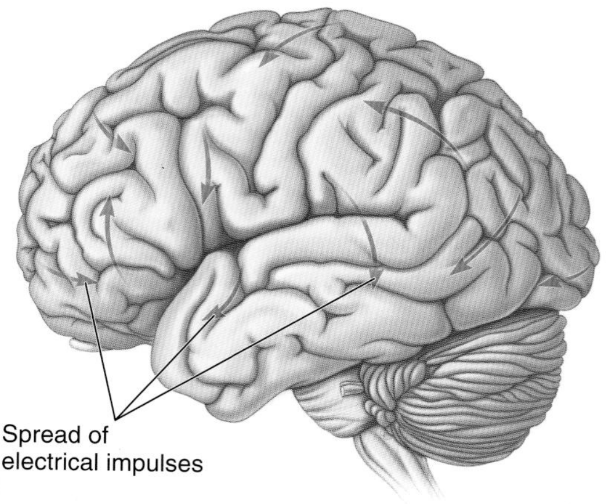

Figure 10.16. Seizure activity in the brain. **A:** Simple and complex partial seizures. **B:** Generalized seizures.

3. Evidence of cerebral hypoxic–ischemic injury based on MRI imaging.
4. Organ system failure (renal, liver, cardiac, gastrointestinal) due to hypoxic–ischemic encephalopathy.

The timing and character of events during pregnancy and in labor may provide further evidence of cause of hypoxic–ischemic injury consistent with CP. A combination of a thorough neurologic examination, including testing of motor skills and reflexes, along with a complete medical history provides evidence for a diagnosis consistent with spastic quadriplegia or dyskinetic CP. Consideration of developmental milestones, evaluation of muscle tone, and presence of abnormal movements and reflexes contribute to the diagnosis of CP. Children may be as old as 18 months before a diagnosis can be made.

TREATMENT

No cure exists for CP. Individuals are treated based on the signs and symptoms they manifest. Drugs to control seizures (e.g., lamotrigine, valproate) and muscle spasms (e.g., botulinum toxin type A, dantrolene, baclofen) may be necessary. Mobility may be improved with the use of special braces and mechanical aids. Physical, occupational, emotional, and speech therapy may support maximal functioning and independence.

Stop and Consider
Why is it important to determine the timing of neurologic injury related to CP?

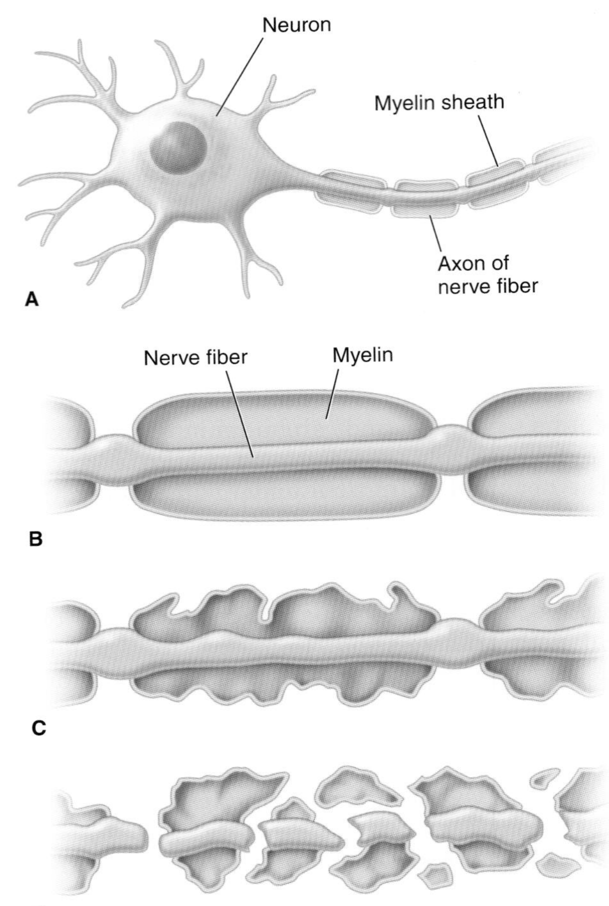

Figure 10.17. Process of demyelination. **A** and **B:** Show normal nerve cells with intact myelin sheaths. **C** and **D:** Show degenerating myelin, disrupting signal transduction in the axon.

Multiple Sclerosis

Multiple sclerosis is a disease of the CNS neurons and is characterized by the degeneration of myelin, a process known as **demyelination** (Fig. 10.17). MS is a progressive neurodegenerative disease affecting nerves in the CNS and peripheral nervous system. Although a great deal of research has been done to determine the exact cause of MS, currently none has been identified. Demographic characteristics of people most likely to develop MS include Caucasian women of northern European ancestry, ages 25 to 49 years. Environmental factors including viral infections, geographic location, place of birth, sunlight exposure, and vitamin D levels influence risk for MS. There are geographic differences that may be associated with the development of MS. Individuals who are born and continue to live in regions north of 40 degree latitude for the first 15 years of life have a higher risk (Fig. 10.18) though other factors may also contribute to observations of geographic risk. Prevalence is highest in northern and central Europe; northern regions of North America; Italy; and southern Australia. Family history also contributes to an individual's risk of developing MS.

PATHOPHYSIOLOGY

MS is a disease of multifactorial origin characterized by microglial activation and chronic neurodegeneration. Inflammatory T and B lymphocytes and macrophages and presence of IgG and IgM in the CSF provide evidence for immunopathology and predominance of the Th1 immune response. Axon injury and formation of demyelinated plaques predominantly in the optic nerves, spinal cord, brainstem, cerebellum, and the juxtacortical and periventricular white matter impair neural transmission and are associated with the clinical manifestations of the disease. Genetic and environmental factors play a role in an individual's risk for developing MS. Regional

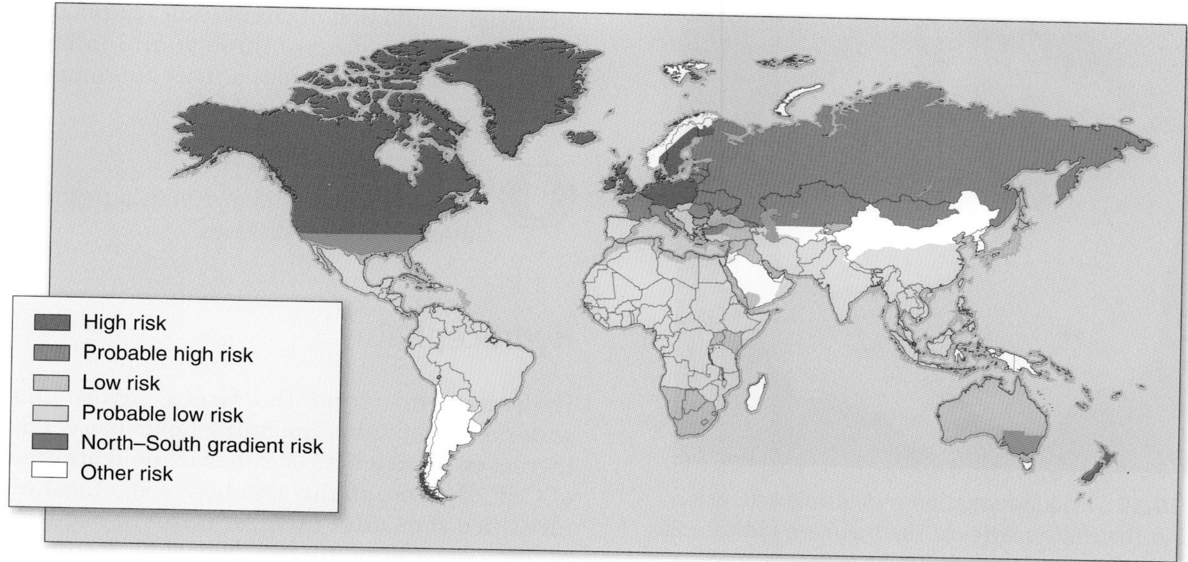

Figure 10.18. Worldwide distribution of multiple sclerosis.

variations may be caused by predominant pathogens of the regions, triggering MS through the process of molecular mimicry in genetically susceptible individuals, as discussed in Chapter 4. Factors including exposure to viral pathogens, vitamin D deficiency, exposure to sunlight and ultraviolet radiation, and genetic predisposition have been implicated in this complex disease of unknown origin.[7]

CLINICAL MANIFESTATIONS

The clinical manifestations of MS relate to the slowing of nerve conduction impulses down the nerve axon. Specific nerves are affected at different times, contributing to the variations seen in the time course and in the signs and symptoms of the disease. Clinical classification of relapsing and progressive disease can be further categorized into subtypes based upon the timing and character of clinical manifestations:

1. Clinically isolated syndrome (CIS): initial presentation of symptoms
2. Relapsing-remitting (RR): characterized by periods of acute neurologic symptoms (flare-ups, exacerbations, relapses) alternating with periods of symptom relief or return of neurologic function (remissions)
3. Primary progressive: slow, chronic deterioration of neurologic function with occasional plateaus, not associated with exacerbations or remissions
4. Secondary progressive: initially presenting with RR characteristics of exacerbations and remissions, followed by a pattern of slow, chronic deterioration as seen in primary progressive

MS **exacerbation**,[8] a demyelinating event of at least 24-hour duration in the absence of fever or infection, results in symptoms associated with impaired neurologic transduction. Common effects of MS are manifested by unilateral vision loss, cognitive loss, bowel and bladder dysfunction, altered gait and balance, spasticity, paresthesias, slurred speech, fatigue, and pain. More rarely, a condition known as **pseudobulbar affect** (uncontrollable laughing or crying) can result from cerebral involvement, leading to altered control of emotional responsiveness. Impaired vision, one of the most common symptoms of MS, may be caused by optic neuritis or impaired extraocular eye movements, contributing to loss of visual fields, unilateral vision loss, altered color perception, **nystagmus** (irregular eye movements), and pain.

DIAGNOSTIC CRITERIA

Diagnosis of MS is based on the presence of signs and symptoms consistent with the disease. A complete medical history and a thorough neurologic examination are the first steps toward diagnosis. An MRI may be completed to detect scarring or plaques in the CNS (Fig. 10.19). It is also important to determine the response of the CNS to peripheral sensory stimuli, inducing *evoked potentials* which may be indicative of abnormal nervous system function. Lumbar puncture to evaluate CSF may be done to determine the presence of IgG. The Revised McDonald Criteria is used in diagnosis of individuals presenting with MS symptoms consistent with CIS. MRI evidence of at least one lesion in two to four

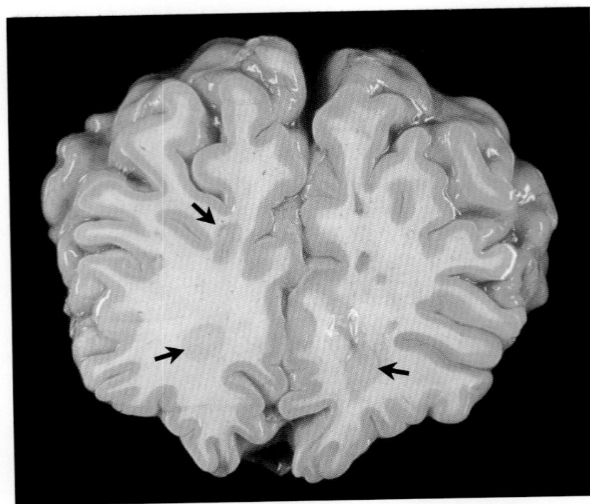

Figure 10.19. Plaque formation in multiple sclerosis. Plaques in the white matter of the brain are indicated by arrows. (From Rubin E, Farber JL. *Pathology*. 4th ed. Philadelphia, PA: Lippincott Williams & Wilkins; 2005.)

locations in areas of the juxtacortical, periventricular, infratentorial, and spinal cord and lesions in areas associated with symptoms including the optic nerve, brainstem/cerebellum, spinal cord, or cerebral hemispheres suggest a diagnosis of MS.[8]

TREATMENT

There is currently no cure for MS. A great deal of progress has been made in the use of drugs, known as disease-modifying drugs, to target symptoms and delay progression of the disease. In the most common form of MS (relapsing-remitting), early initiation of drugs is highly recommended. The immunomodulators Betaseron, Avonex, Extavia, and Rebif, all forms of beta interferon (IFN-β), are the mainstays of treatment. In addition, Copaxone, a drug that mimics the effects of myelin, is commonly used. Aubagio works through inhibition of mitochondrial enzymes needed for increased production of circulating lymphocytes. Tecfidera modulates disease through anti-inflammatory actions. Table 10.7 provides a more thorough description of treatment options in MS.[9]

Stop and Consider

How will regrowth of myelin help treat or cure other neurologic diseases?

Hydrocephalus

Hydrocephalus, from the Greek "hydro" meaning water and "cephalus" meaning head, is a condition of increased ventricular or subarachnoid accumulation of CSF. Hydrocephalus can be a congenital disorder identified soon after birth, or it can be acquired later in life. According to the National Hydrocephalus Foundation, approximately 1 in 500 births are affected by hydrocephalus in the United States. More than half of the cases of hydrocephalus are congenital. Long-term consequence of hydrocephalus may include motor disability, intellectual disability and problems with memory. The incidence of acquired hydrocephalus is unknown because of the relationship to the underlying causes.

PATHOPHYSIOLOGY

Because of an imbalance between the amount of fluid produced and the rate of fluid reabsorption, the accumulation of CSF leads to ventricular enlargement and increased ICP. Classifications of hydrocephalus reflect the underlying cause and include **noncommunicating hydrocephalus** because of CSF flow obstruction and **communicating hydrocephalus** because of impaired CSF absorption.

Hydrocephalus can be congenital, often identified during fetal life or at birth. Congenital hydrocephalus may be caused by neural tube defects, including spina bifida, or by an alteration in the structure of the cerebral aqueduct or choroid plexus. Acquired hydrocephalus is secondary to another disease process. Common conditions resulting in acquired hydrocephalus include:

- Brain tumor
- Intraventricular hemorrhage
- Meningitis
- Traumatic injury to the head

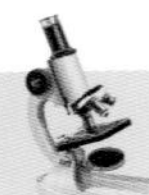

FROM THE LAB

Evoked potential testing provides information about the electrical activity in specific sensory nerve pathways. The altered transduction along these pathways may be too subtle to determine by routine neurologic examination. Stimulation of the pathways is measured by wires placed on the scalp over the areas of interest of the brain. There are three types of evoked potential tests:

1. Visual evoked potentials (VEP): stimulation induced by viewing an alternating checkerboard pattern
2. Brainstem auditory evoked potentials (BAEP): stimulation induced by clicking sounds in each ear
3. Sensory evoked potentials (SEP): stimulation induced by electrical impulses to the arm or leg

Table 10.7 Treatment Options in Multiple Sclerosis

Brand Name	Generic Name	FDA Approval Date	Administration Information	Common Side Effects
Avonex	Interferon beta-1a	1996	Weekly intramuscular injection	Flu-like symptoms
Betaseron	Interferon beta-1b	1993	Every other day subcutaneous injection	Flu-like symptoms
Extavia	Interferon beta-1b	2009	Every other day subcutaneous injection	Flu-like symptoms
Rebif	Interferon beta-1a	2002	Three times/week subcutaneous injection	Flu-like symptoms
Copaxone	Glatiramer acetate	1996	Daily subcutaneous injection	Injection site reaction
Aubagio	Teriflunomide	2012	Oral tablet daily	Diarrhea, abnormal liver tests, nausea, and hair loss
Tecfidera	Dimethyl fumarate	2013	Oral capsule, twice daily in first week, then daily	Flushing, nausea, vomiting, and diarrhea, decreased white blood cell count
Gilenva	Fingolimod	2010	Oral capsule twice daily	Headache, diarrhea, back pain, elevation of liver enzymes, cough, reduced heart rate
Lemtrada	Alemtuzumab	2014	Intravenous infusion	Rash, headache, fever, nausea, infection, fatigue, insomnia, thyroid gland disorders, pain in joints, extremities and back, diarrhea, sore mouth and throat, tingling, dizziness
Tysabri	Natalizumab	2004/2006	Intravenous infusion	Headache, fatigue, urinary tract infection

FDA, Food and Drug Administration.

Hydrocephalus often results from an episode of intraventricular hemorrhage in the newborn period, also a common consequence of prematurity.[10] Management strategies are directed toward controlling CSF volume and flow to maintain ventricle size and normal ICP (15 mm Hg or 150 to 200 mm of water). Increased ICP is a common consequence of hydrocephalus. The pathology associated with increased ICP includes:

1. Impaired perfusion leading to ischemia and cell death
2. Atrophy caused by impaired circulation

CLINICAL MANIFESTATIONS

Age of onset, underlying pathology, and severity of brain tissue compression contribute to the clinical manifestations of hydrocephalus. The skull of the newborn is less restrictive because of the presence of fontanels (often referred to as soft spots) and the unfused sutures of the skull bones. These conditions allow for the increase in head circumference, a cardinal sign in a newborn with hydrocephalus. Scalp vein distention, bulging fontanels, separation of bony sutures, and vomiting may also be seen. Infants with hydrocephalus may have difficulty feeding and may have a shrill, high-pitched cry. Symptoms in older children and adults include impaired motor and cognitive function and incontinence (Fig. 10.20). Unresolved hydrocephalus may lead to impaired neurologic function and death because of increased ICP.

Signs and symptoms resulting from increased ICP include:

- Increased blood pressure in an attempt to promote perfusion in cerebral vessels
- Altered heart rate
  - Initially increased (tachycardia) to increase cerebral blood flow; followed by a decreased heart rate (bradycardia) caused by stimulation of the baroreceptor reflex
- Headache resulting from stretching of the vessel walls or meninges
- Vomiting
- Decreased level of consciousness
- Papilledema

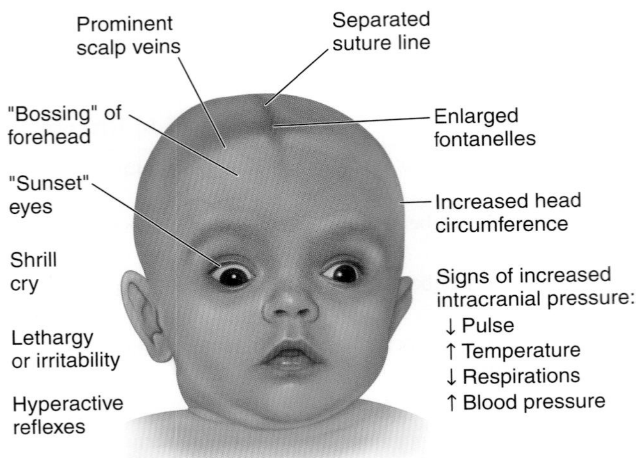

Figure 10.20. Clinical manifestations of hydrocephalus.

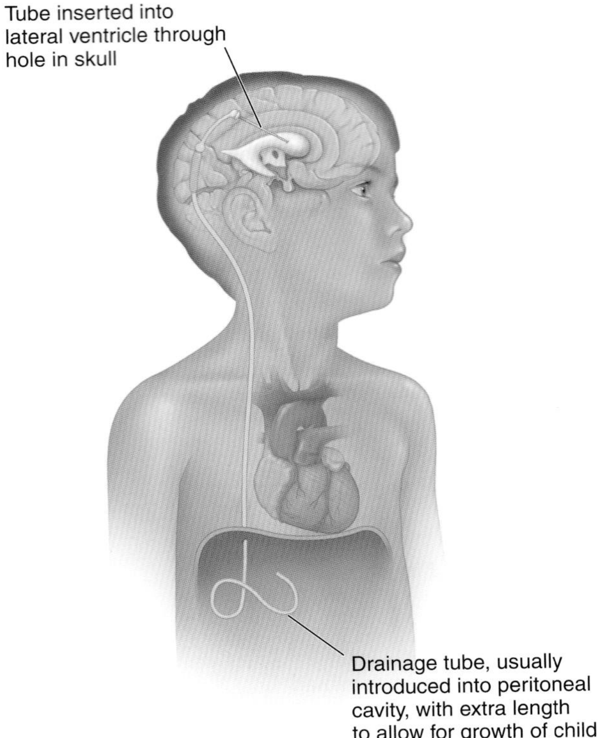

Figure 10.21. Ventriculoperitoneal shunt placement in hydrocephalus. (From Bear MF, Connors BW, Parasido MA. *Neuroscience: Exploring the Brain*. 3rd ed. Philadelphia, PA: Lippincott Williams & Wilkins; 2006.)

DIAGNOSTIC CRITERIA

Diagnosis of hydrocephalus may be made by the noninvasive techniques of measurement of head circumference and transillumination. **Transillumination** is accomplished by shining a light against the head to see accumulations of fluid in the tissue. Ultrasound examination is limited to infants with open anterior fontanelle and provides evidence of lateral ventricle size. In children and adults, diagnostic techniques include CT or MRI scan of the head for examination of ventricle size and CSF flow. Skull radiograph may be used to determine separation of skull bones.

TREATMENT

The treatment of hydrocephalus includes establishing and maintaining normal CSF volumes and ICP. One of the most common treatments for communicating or noncommunicating hydrocephalus is the surgical placement a ventriculoperitoneal shunt, a flexible tube placed into the ventricle to shunt excess CSF into the peritoneal cavity (Fig. 10.21). Another potential treatment option includes placement of a shunt that drains CSF fluid into the right atrium of the heart, called a ventriculoatrial shunt. The flow of CSF out of the ventricular system is controlled by a one-way valve, which helps control appropriate regulation. Observation of shunt-related complications, including infection, blockage, and malfunction, must be carried out to promote maintenance of normal CSF volume and ICP.

A possible alternative treatment for obstructive noncommunicating hydrocephalus is a procedure known as endoscopic third ventriculostomy (ETV). This procedure involves surgically placing an opening in the floor of the third ventricle to allow free-flowing release of CSF into the basal cisterna for absorption.

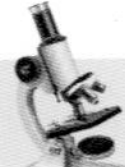

FROM THE LAB

The circulatory dynamics of both cerebral blood flow and cerebral spinal fluid contribute to ICP. Direct determinations of ICP measurements require invasive monitoring. This monitoring is achieved via an intraventricular drain connected externally to a transducer. Measurements are averaged over a minimum 30-minute period to take into account the dynamic fluctuations characteristic of CSF pressure.[11] ICP should be monitored for a period of 24 to 48 hours to determine trends or effectiveness of treatments to reduce pressure.

Incomplete Spinal Cord Transection

Many variables are associated with the degree of dysfunction experienced because of SCI. Spinal segmental level, type of injury, and degree of cord transection contribute to the manifestations and complications associated with SCI. An estimated 250,000 to 400,000 individuals live with SCI or spinal dysfunction. The condition of many individuals with SCI improves from the time of diagnosis, but few fully recover.

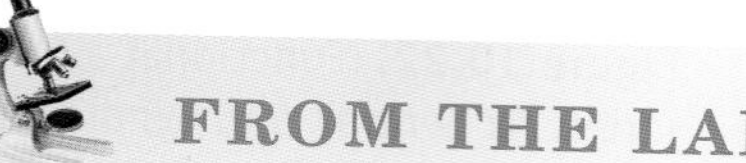

FROM THE LAB

Bowel and bladder storage require autonomic reflexes to coordinate involuntary smooth muscle activity of the urinary tract and voluntary contraction of the sphincter. Complex mechanisms involving the spinal and supraspinal nerve pathways may be impaired because of SCI. A process known as functional electrical stimulation (FES) may serve to generate artificial autonomic reflexes to promote mechanisms regulating bowel and bladder function. Electrical stimulation of efferent nerves to promote muscle contraction is accomplished through a process known as neurostimulation. Microstimulation provides electrical stimuli to preganglionic neurons and interneurons controlling bladder function via a microelectrode implanted within the spinal cord. Afferent fibers may be activated to adjust stimuli, a function known as neuromodulation.[12]

PATHOPHYSIOLOGY

SCI is due to nerve root or myelinated tract damage, impairing the transduction of afferent or efferent neural impulses. Damage to the gray matter of the central cord may result in loss of motoneurons and interneurons. The pathogenesis is related to the location, classification, type, and severity of the injury. SCI may result from complete or partial transection (Fig. 10.22). In complete injury, sensation and motor function below the level of injury are lost. Partial cord transections can be categorized into three types of syndromes (central cord, anterior cord, and Brown–Séquard syndrome), described in Table 10.8.

CLINICAL MANIFESTATIONS

SCI may be complicated by ischemia, hemorrhage, or necrosis. Injury to the neuronal fibers that carry impulses may be worsened by pressure from the edema related to the primary injury. The level of injury determines the nerves involved and helps anticipate the degree of functional loss. Loss of function in incomplete transection can be variable, based on the area and level of cord involved. In general, injuries to the cervical spine often result in quadriplegia. High injuries at the level of C1-C2 may result in loss of involuntary function, including sweating, blood pressure regulation, and body temperature regulation. Respiratory support with artificial ventilation may be required for injuries above C4. Injury to lower cervical segments is associated with preservation of upper body function. C7 through T1 injuries allow individuals to straighten their arms, but they may result in impaired fine motor skills. Paraplegia usually results from injuries at the thoracic level. Trunk and lower body control are lost at T1, with return of sitting balance and abdominal muscle control from T9 through T12. Injuries in the lumbar and sacral segments result in loss of control of the lower extremities. Bowel, bladder, and sexual function may be affected with SCI.

DIAGNOSTIC CRITERIA

When SCI is suspected, it is important to diagnose, begin immediate treatment, and prevent further damage. SCI can be diagnosed in a conscious person based on findings from testing of cognitive, motor, and sensory function. If the injured individual has manifestations of neck pain or weakness or is unable to respond because of loss of consciousness, diagnostic testing may be done. Commonly used tests to diagnose SCI include radiograph, CT scan, MRI, and myelography (imaging after injection of dye into the spinal canal).

TREATMENT

Traction may be used to immobilize the spine in the acute phase of SCI in an attempt to prevent further damage. Surgical treatment to correct fractures and decompress the spinal cord may be indicated. Lack of evidence to support the use of pharmacologic agents limits use in acute SCI.[12] Promotion of functional abilities is a priority of treatment after the acute phase of injury. The work of many researchers is targeted toward a cure for SCI.

To achieve a return of motor, sensory, and autonomic function, the regeneration of axons and reestablishment of neuronal transmission must occur. Regeneration of the pyramidal, extrapyramidal, autonomic, sensory, and cerebellar pathways, integrated reflex responses, and the required neurotransmitters are necessary for return of function.

Parkinson Disease

Parkinson disease is a chronic, progressive neurologic condition that affects the pigmented dopaminergic neurons of the substantia nigra and locus ceruleus of the basal ganglia. Degeneration of neurons is associated with impaired motor function, and onset occurs predominantly in individuals of middle to old age. First described in the early 1800s as "shaking palsy" by Dr. James Parkinson, the disease did not bear his name until half a century later, when Jean-Martin Charcot honored the early pioneer.[13] Although much has been learned, the condition still has no cure.

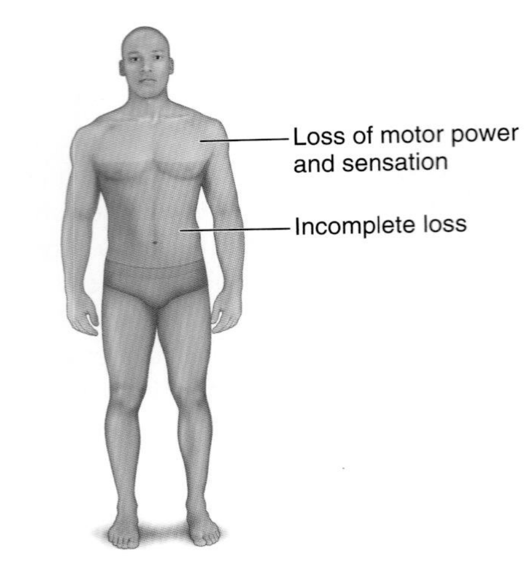

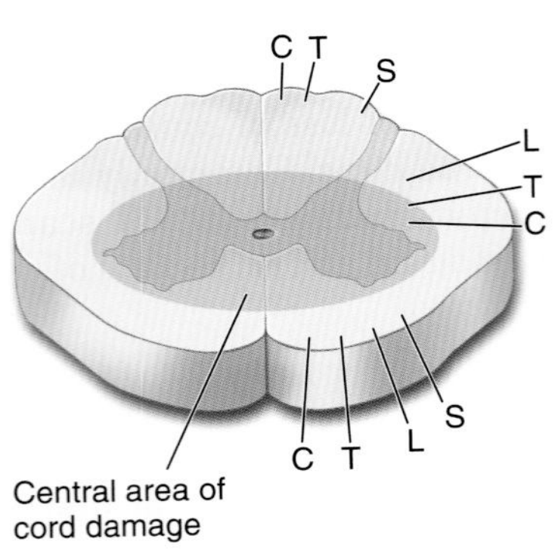

A

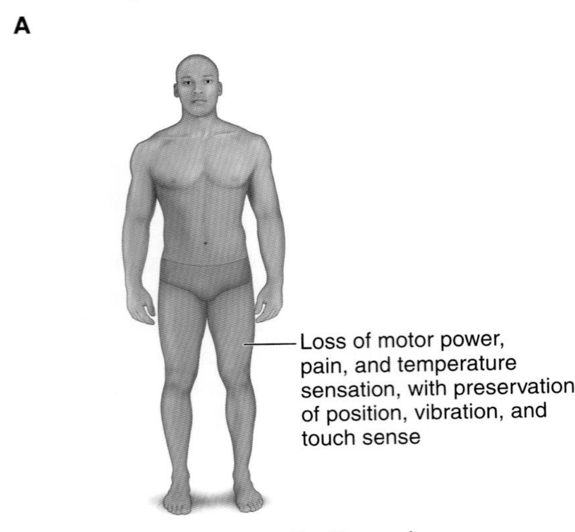

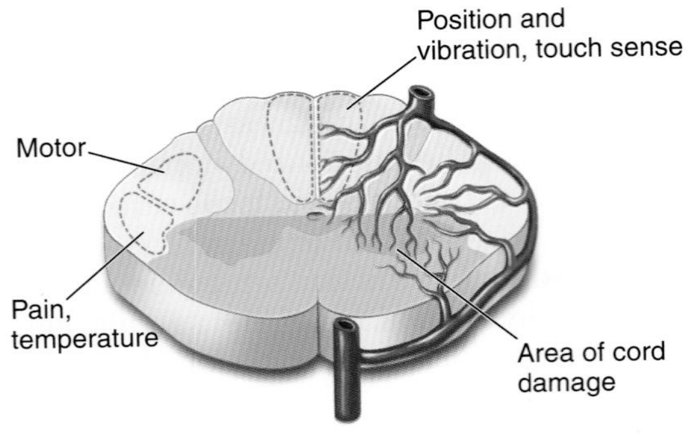

B

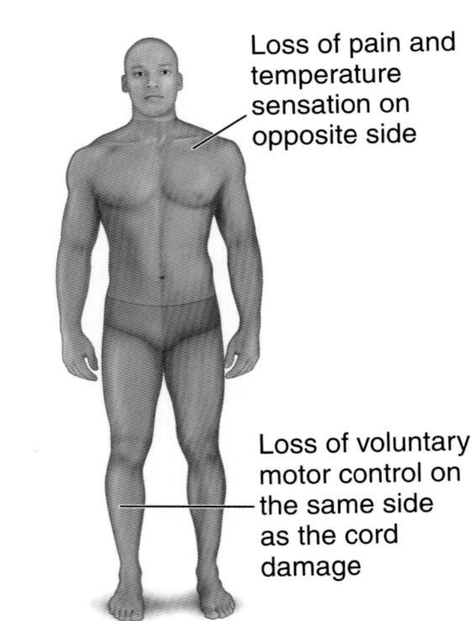

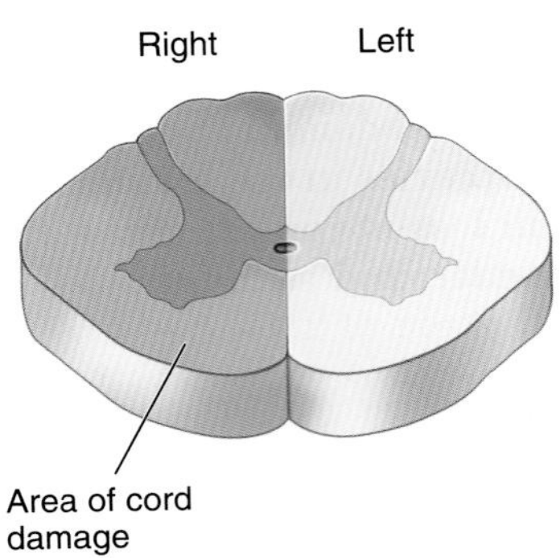

C

Figure 10.22. Functional alterations in incomplete spinal cord injuries. **A:** Central cord syndrome. **B:** Anterior cord syndrome. **C:** Brown–Séquard syndrome. (From Hickey JV. *The Clinical Practice of Neurological and Neurosurgical Nursing*. 5th ed. Philadelphia, PA: Lippincott Williams & Wilkins; 2003:420–421.)

Table 10.8 Categories of Partial Spinal Cord Transections

Syndrome	Area of Cord Affected	Common Cause	Manifestations
Central cord syndrome	Center cord affected	Usually caused by hyperextension injury	Motor deficits prominent in upper extremities Bladder dysfunction of variable severity
Anterior cord syndrome	Anterior cord affected	Occlusion of the anterior spinal artery Bone fragments	Loss of motor function, temperature, and pain below the level of injury Sensations of touch, pressure, vibration, and position intact
Brown–Séquard syndrome	Hemisection of the anterior and posterior cord	Usually the result of stabbing or gunshot injury with damage localized to only one side of the cord	Ipsilateral (same side) complete or partial paralysis, loss of touch, pressure, vibration, and positions sense below the level of injury Loss of temperature sensations contralaterally

According to the National Institute on Neurologic Disorders and Stroke, approximately 500,000 people in the United States are diagnosed with PD.[14] Annually, approximately 50,000 new cases are reported. More common in men than in women, the average age of onset is 60 years, with prevalence and incidence increasing with age.

PATHOPHYSIOLOGY

The basal ganglia are important in the control of movement through regulation of inhibitory and excitatory stimuli. The basal ganglia are composed of the forebrain structures of the striatum (caudate nucleus and putamen) and globus pallidus interna, the subthalamic nucleus (diencephalon), and the substantia nigra (midbrain) (Fig. 10.23). The substantia nigra is named for the black appearance of cells caused by the pigment melanin. Secreted by the cells of the substantia nigra, the neurotransmitter dopamine is transported to the striatum via the nigrostriatal pathway. PD is characterized by degeneration of the nigrostriatal pathway, which leads to a reduction in the neurotransmitter dopamine. Dopamine modulates balance between the excitatory and inhibitory neural motor pathways.

Impaired transport of dopamine alters excitability of the striatum and the release of other neurotransmitters. Neurons in the substantia nigra lose their pigment and their characteristic black color. In addition to pigment loss in the cells of the substantia nigra, neurons are atrophied, with some containing Lewy bodies. Lewy bodies are protein aggregations composed of the protein alpha-synuclein located primarily in the cells of the substantia nigra.

No specific mechanism explaining PD has been found. Neuronal injury from oxidative damage is suspected to play a role in the pathology associated with PD, potentially causing impaired mitochondrial function and antioxidant protection of neurons. The onset of the disease may also be related to a decline in the endogenous defense mechanisms associated with aging. Depigmentation of neurons may contribute to an inflammatory response to extracellular melanin in surrounding brain tissue.

PD can be an inherited disease, or it may occur sporadically. Although the genetic predisposition to PD in families is well known, recent developments in molecular biology have led to the identification of several genetic loci and alteration in mitochondrial function associated with familial PD.[15] Recent insights may lead to more effective treatments and markers of disease before the onset of symptoms.

CLINICAL MANIFESTATIONS

Most neural degeneration in PD occurs before the onset of the manifestations of this disease, also known as the preclinical period. The four primary manifestations of overt PD include (Fig. 10.24):

1. Tremor
2. Rigidity
3. Bradykinesia
4. Postural instability

Tremors usually involve the hands, arms, legs, and face, and they occur when the body is at rest. Tremors are progressive, initially manifesting in an isolated area and often beginning in one hand. Bradykinesia (slowed movement) is associated with initiation of movement and may progress to akinesia, or the inability to move (Fig. 10.25). Sudden halting of movement is also a cardinal sign of bradykinesia. Individuals with PD often walk with a

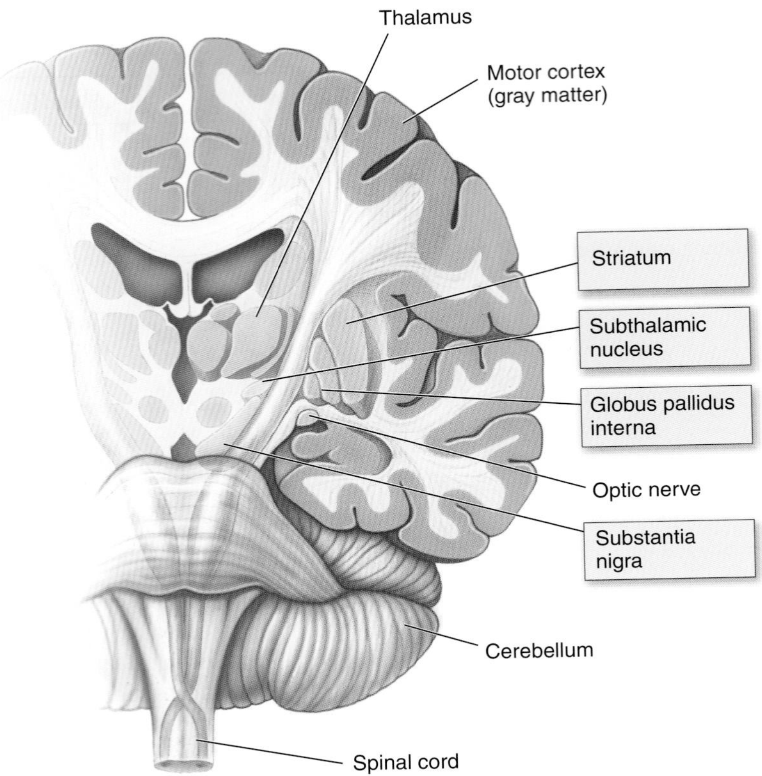

Figure 10.23. Pigmented neurons of the substantia nigra. Neurons of the substantia nigra and the locus ceruleus are heavily pigmented with neuromelanin.

shuffling gait and stooped posture. Rigidity caused by resistance to movement by both flexors and extensors manifest as jerky movements, also known as cogwheel rigidity. Involvement of the tongue, throat, and palate may increase the likelihood of feeding difficulties and aspiration caused by muscle rigidity. Speech may also be affected by oral manifestations, resulting in monotone, expressionless inflections in voice. Stiffness of the limbs and trunk, bradykinesia, and postural instability contribute to decreased coordination and impaired balance. A flat, or expressionless, affect may be the result of facial stiffness (Fig. 10.26).

Indirect manifestations of PD involve the influence of basal ganglia in autonomic nervous system responses. Increased sebaceous, sweat, and saliva secretions are common. Other autonomic dysfunctions, including altered blood pressure and thermal regulation, constipation, incontinence, and impotence, may occur. Cognitive and personality changes may be associated with PD. Dementia is also a common manifestation of PD.[16]

Stop and Consider
Why are individuals on antipsychotic medications at risk for development of Parkinsonian-like symptoms?

DIAGNOSIS

No single, definitive test exists to diagnose PD. Clinical findings based on the history and manifestations of the disease are used to obtain diagnosis. The Movement Disorder Society Task Force for Rating Scales for PD confirms the reliability of the Hoehn and Yahr (HY) scale as an indicator of stage progression and severity.[17] The Hoehn and Yahr scale includes the following criteria[18]:

- Stage one
  - Signs and symptoms on one side only
  - Symptoms mild
  - Symptoms inconvenient but not disabling
  - Usually presents with tremor of one limb
  - Friends have noticed changes in posture, locomotion, and facial expression
- Stage two
  - Symptoms are bilateral
  - Minimal disability
  - Posture and gait affected
- Stage three
  - Significant slowing of body movements
  - Early impairment of balance upon walking or standing
  - Generalized dysfunction that is moderately severe

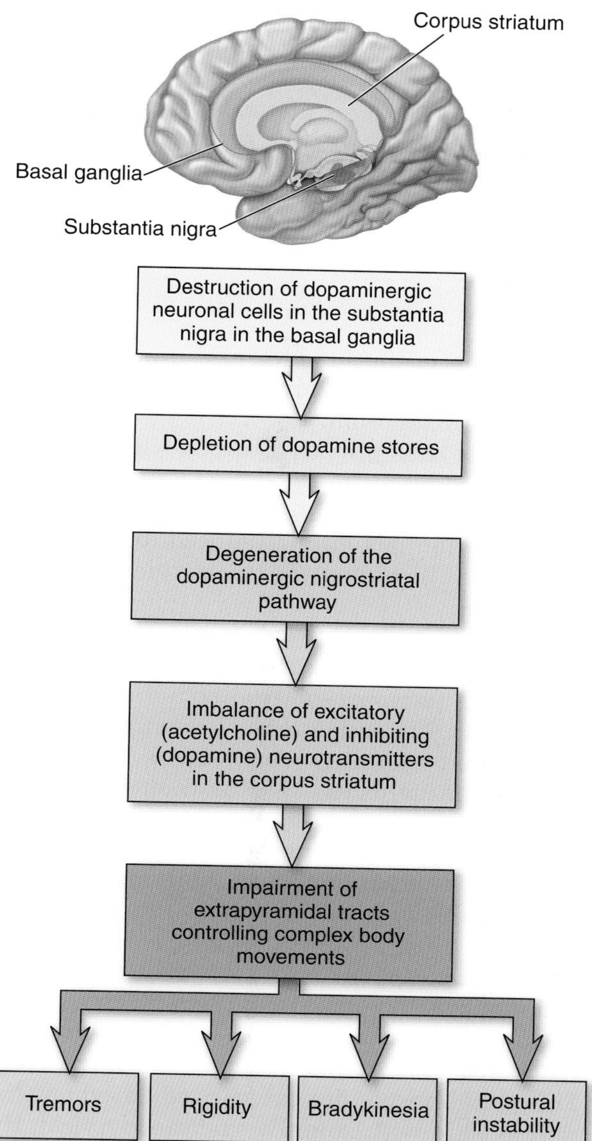

Figure 10.24. Pathophysiology and clinical manifestations of Parkinson disease. The nuclei in the substantia nigra project fibers to the corpus striatum, the pathway of dopamine transport. Loss of dopaminergic neurons in the substantia nigra is associated with manifestations of Parkinson disease. (Modified from Smeltzer SC, Bare BG. *Textbook of Medical-Surgical Nursing*. 10th ed. Philadelphia, PA: Lippincott Williams & Wilkins; 2003, with permission.)

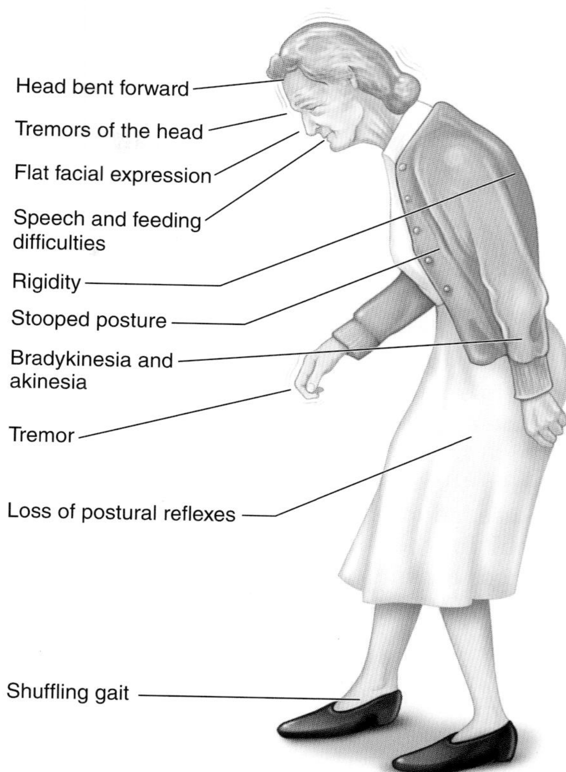

Figure 10.25. Mobility deficits in Parkinson disease. Musculoskeletal manifestations of Parkinson disease include tremors, rigidity, bradykinesia, and postural instability affecting the entire body. (Modified from Rosdahl CB. *Book of Basic Nursing*. 7th ed. Philadelphia, PA: Lippincott-Raven; 1999, with permission.)

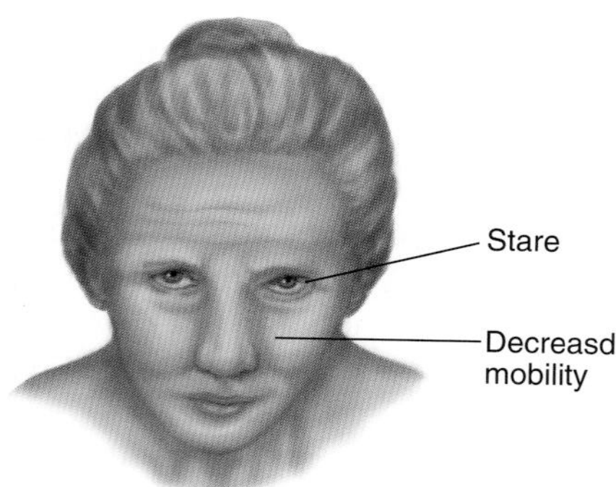

Figure 10.26. Facial features of Parkinson disease. Blunted expression, decreased blinking, and stare are characteristic manifestations. (Bickley LS, Szilagyl P. *Bates' Guide to Physical Examination and History Taking*. 8th ed. Philadelphia, PA: Lippincott Williams & Wilkins; 2003, with permission.)

- Stage four
  - Severe symptoms
  - Can still walk to a limited extent
  - Rigidity and bradykinesia
  - No longer able to live alone
  - Tremor may be less than earlier stages
- Stage five
  - Cachectic stage
  - Complete invalidism (i.e., disability)
  - Cannot stand or walk
  - Requires constant nursing care

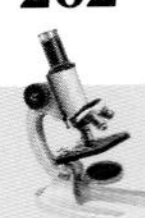

FROM THE LAB

Development of an early marker of disease before the onset of symptoms has been a focus of investigation in PD. No tests have demonstrated adequate sensitivity or specificity of practical use for the early diagnosis of PD.

TREATMENT

Pharmacologic management is a first-line treatment for PD. Levodopa is a dopamine precursor used as therapy to replace dopamine. Effective at ameliorating the symptoms associated with PD, there are many side effects, including nausea and vomiting, that make the drug difficult to tolerate. After prolonged use, additional dosing is often required and may result in other side effects, including dyskinesias and periods of time when the medication seems ineffective. Levodopa is often combined with carbidopa (Sinemet) which delays the conversion of levodopa to dopamine until it reaches the brain. When combined with the drug carbidopa, lower doses of levodopa and a decline in the incidence of side effects are possible while retaining effectiveness. A combination drug that adds entacapone to carbidopa and levodopa in the same formulation (Stalevo) extends the duration of action of levodopa. Amantadine (Symmetrel), alone or combined with an anticholinergic drug, may reduce the symptoms of PD along with the dyskinesia that results from use of levodopa. Anticholinergic agents often increase the effectiveness of levodopa, although the undesirable side effects of dry mouth, blurred vision, and urinary retention may occur and should be reserved for use in younger individuals. Dopamine agonists activate receptors and are a useful strategy for the treatment of PD. Drugs in this class include bromocriptine (Parlodel), pramipexole (Mirapex), rotigotine (Neupro) and ropinirole (Requip). The drug Apokyn (apomorphine) is used for the treatment of hypomobility or "off periods" when immobility prevents completion of activities of daily living.

Surgical options for the treatment of PD include pallidotomy and deep brain stimulation. These strategies are reserved for more advanced disease because of the risk involved with the treatments. Pallidotomy, an irreversible procedure involving destruction of the globus pallidus, is designed to decrease nerve firing in the damaged tissue. Deep brain stimulation (DBS) is a reversible procedure designed to alter abnormal function of the brain tissue through insertion of a neurostimulator designed to deliver electrical signals to a targeted area of the brain. Stimulation is intended to block abnormal nerve signals, resulting in tremor and other PD symptoms. The exact location of the brain tissue responsible for generation of nerve signals causing PD symptoms is identified before the procedure via an MRI or a CT scan.

SUMMARY

- The neuron is the fundamental unit of the nervous system; it has highly specialized functions in impulse transmission.
- Supporting cells provide neurons with metabolic support and protection.
- Impulse transmission is regulated by changes in membrane potential, induced by a variety of stimuli, including chemical, electrical, and mechanical.
- The nervous system is composed of the central nervous system (brain and spinal cord) and the peripheral nervous system (spinal and cranial nerves; somatic and autonomic [sympathetic and parasympathetic] nervous systems).
- Nervous tissue of the CNS is composed of both white and gray matter, based on the primary types of component neurons.
- Meninges (dura, arachnoid, pia) and the CSF provide protective and metabolic functions in the CNS.
- The brain is divided both by lobes (frontal, parietal, temporal, occipital) and hemispheres (right, left), each associated with highly specialized functions.
- The spinal nerves are categorized based on their relationship with spinal vertebrae (cervical, thoracic, lumbar, sacral).
- Autonomic functions are carried out by the sympathetic and parasympathetic nervous system.
- Neuronal injury contributes to disability and is the basis for a variety of neurologic disorders. Peripheral nerves have limited capacity for regeneration and reinnervation.
- Trauma represents the most common cause of injury to the nervous system, leading to neurologic impairment because of brain, spinal cord, or peripheral nerve injury. Ischemic, excitation, and pressure injury may represent primary or secondary causes of neurologic impairment.
- Disorders of neurologic function may be characterized by specific manifestations, pointing to the origin of pathology.
- Altered neuronal transmission and conduction has implications for all body systems and whole body function.

- A thorough understanding of the concepts that govern neuronal transmission will promote your ability to apply your knowledge in a variety of conditions and pathologies.

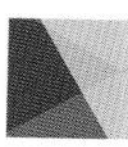

CASE STUDY 10.1

Carolyn, a 17-year-old soccer player, had a collision with another player and lost consciousness for a few minutes. When she regained consciousness, she had complaints of a headache and dizziness. She was confused and began to vomit, prompting her to go to the emergency room for evaluation. She was diagnosed with concussion, a form of mild traumatic brain injury.

1. In addition to those that Carolyn presented, what are the clinical manifestations associated with mild traumatic brain injury?
2. What is the etiology of Carolyn's injury?
3. How is concussion diagnosed?
4. What is the standard management for TBI?
5. Postconcussion syndrome may result from mild TBI. Describe the symptoms and treatment of this syndrome.

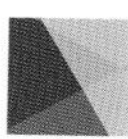

PRACTICE EXAM QUESTIONS

1. Neurons that carry sensory information to distant parts of the brain and spinal cord are called:
   a. Efferent neurons
   b. Afferent neurons
   c. Interneurons
   d. Extraneurons

2. Depolarization involves:
   a. The rapid movement of sodium into the cell
   b. The movement of potassium ions out of the cell
   c. Movement of potassium ions into the cell
   d. The absence of electrical activity

3. The lobe of the brain primarily involved in functions related to vision is the:
   a. Frontal lobe
   b. Parietal lobe
   c. Temporal lobe
   d. Occipital lobe

4. Which of the following areas of the spinal cord contains 12 segments?
   a. Cervical
   b. Thoracic
   c. Sacral
   d. Lumbar

5. Which cell type has the most potential for regeneration after injury?
   a. Astrocyte
   b. Peripheral axon
   c. Glial cell
   d. Oligodendrocytes

6. Coup/countercoup occurs due to which type of injury mechanism?
   a. Traumatic injury
   b. Pressure injury
   c. Excitation injury
   d. Ischemic injury

7. Neurogenic shock is due to altered transmission in which conduction system?
   a. Sympathetic
   b. Parasympathetic
   c. Somatic
   d. Peripheral

8. Seizure disorders are associated with which type of injury mechanism?
   a. Traumatic injury
   b. Pressure injury
   c. Excitation injury
   d. Ischemic injury

9. Which type of spinal cord injury is associated with the clinical manifestation of ipsilateral loss of motor and sensory function?
   a. Anterior cord syndrome
   b. Central cord syndrome
   c. Brown–Séquard syndrome
   d. Complete cord transection

10. Which type of neuron synthesizes and secretes norepinephrine as the primary neurotransmitter?
    a. Serotonergic
    b. Cholinergic
    c. Nicotinic
    d. Adrenergic

11. Parkinson disease is characterized by
    a. Neurofibrillary tangles
    b. Amyloid plaque
    c. Lewy bodies
    d. Tau

12. Which one of the following neurotransmitters is deficient in Parkinson disease?
    a. Dopamine
    b. Serotonin
    c. Norepinephrine
    d. Acetylcholine

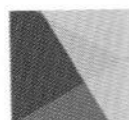

DISCUSSION AND APPLICATION

1. What did I know about altered neuronal transmission before today?
2. What body processes are affected by altered neuronal transmission? How do neuronal transmission patterns affect those processes?
3. What are the potential etiologies for altered neuronal transmissions? How do conduction defects develop?
4. Who is most at risk for developing altered neuronal transmission? How can these alterations be prevented?
5. What are the human differences that affect the etiology, risk, or course of altered neuronal transmission?
6. What clinical manifestations are expected in the course of altered neuronal transmission?
7. What special diagnostic tests are useful in determining the diagnosis and course of altered neuronal transmission?
8. What are the goals of care for individuals with altered neuronal transmission?
9. How does the concept of altered neuronal transmission build on what I have learned in the previous chapter and in previous courses?
10. How can I use what I have learned?

RESOURCES

March of Dimes:
http://www.modimes.org

National Hydrocephalus Foundation:
http://nhfonline.org/

National Institute of Neurological Disorders and Stroke:
http://www.ninds.nih.gov/

National Parkinson Foundation:
http://www.parkinson.org/

References

1. Centers for Disease Control and Prevention, National Center for Health Injury Prevention and Control. *Traumatic Brain Injury*. Bethesda, MD: US Department of Health and Human Services. http://www.cdc.gov/traumaticbraininjury/get_the_facts.html. Accessed November 24, 2015.
2. National Spinal Cord Injury Statistical Center. Spinal cord injury: facts and figures at a glance. *J Spinal Cord Med.* 2012;35(1):68–69. doi:10.1179/2045772 12X13237783484262.
3. March of Dimes. Cerebral palsy. http://www.marchofdimes.com/professionals/14332_1208.asp#howcommon. Accessed November 25, 2015.
4. Pisani F, Spagnoli C. Neonatal seizures: a review of outcomes and outcome predictors. *Neuropediatrics.* 2016;47(1):12–19. doi:10.1055/s-0035-1567873.
5. Ferriero DM. Neonatal brain injury. *N Engl J Med.* 2004;351(19):1985–1995.
6. American College of Obstetricians and Gynecologists. Task force on neonatal encephalopathy neonatal encephalopathy and neurologic outcome. *Obstet Gynecol.* 2014;123(4):896–901. doi:10.1097/01.AOG.0000445580.65983.d2.
7. Milo R, Kahana E. Multiple sclerosis: geoepidemiology, genetics and the environment. *Autoimmun Rev.* 2010;9(5):A387–A394.
8. Polman CH, Reingold SC, Banwell B, et al. Diagnostic criteria for multiple sclerosis: 2010 revisions to the McDonald Criteria. *Ann Neurol.* 2011;69(2):292–302. doi:10.1002/ana.22366.
9. Torkildsen Ø, Myhr KM, Bø L. Disease-modifying treatments for multiple sclerosis—a review of approved medications. *Eur J Neurol.* 2016;23(suppl 1):18–27. doi:10.1111/ene.12883.
10. Christian EA, Melamed EF, Peck E, et al. Surgical management of hydrocephalus secondary to intraventricular hemorrhage in the preterm infant [published online ahead of print November 13, 2015]. *J Neurosurg Pediatr.* 1–7. PMID: 26565942.
11. Czosnyka M, Pickard JD. Monitoring and interpretation of intracranial pressure. *J Neurol Neurosurg Psychiatry.* 2004;75(6):813–821.
12. Hurlbert JR, Hadley MN, Walters BC, et al. Pharmacologic therapy for acute spinal cord injury. *Neurosurgery.* 2013;72:93–105. doi:10.1227/NEU.0b013e31827765c6.
13. Burch D, Sheerin F. Parkinson's disease. *Lancet.* 2005;365(9459):622–627.
14. National Institute of Neurologic Diseases and Stroke. Parkinson's disease backgrounder. Washington, DC: National Institute of Health; 2004. http://www.ninds.nih.gov/disorders/parkinsons_disease/parkinsons_disease_backgrounder.htm
15. Hang L, Thundyil J, Lim KL. Mitochondrial dysfunction and Parkinson disease: a Parkin-AMPK alliance in neuroprotection. *Ann N Y Acad Sci.* 2015;1350(1):37–47. doi:10.1111/nyas.12820.
16. Zweig RM, Disbrow EA, Javalkar V. Cognitive and psychiatric disturbances in Parkinsonian syndromes. *Neurol Clin.* 2016;34(1):235–246. doi:10.1016/j.ncl.2015.08.010.
17. Goetz CG, Poewe W, Rascol O, et al. Movement disorder society task force report on the Hoehn and Yahr staging scale: status and recommendations. *Mov Disord.* 2004;19(9):1020–1028.
18. Hoehn MM, Yahr MD. Parkinsonism: onset, progression and mortality. *Neurology.* 1967;17:427–442.

Find additional resources for this chapter at http:thePoint.lww.com thePoint®

Altered Mood, Attention, and Behavior

Chapter 11

LEARNING OUTCOMES

1. Define and use the key terms listed in this chapter.
2. Differentiate mood, attention, and behavior.
3. Recognize neuronal pathways that regulate mood, attention, and behavior.
4. Identify common signs and symptoms of altered mood, attention, and behavior.
5. Describe diagnostic tests and treatment strategies relevant to altered mood, attention, and behavior.
6. Apply concepts of altered mood, attention, and behavior to select clinical models.

INTRODUCTION

How does being a student of pathophysiology affect your mood, attention, and behavior? Hopefully it triggers a good mood and positive regard as you accomplish your learning goals. Or maybe it causes you anxiety and challenges your focus. No matter how you would answer that opening question, this chapter's focus on mood, attention, and behavior is an important link in the study of pathophysiology. Patients are biopsychosocial beings. The previous chapters have focused on the "bio" part of this equation. Now it is time to turn our attention to the "psychosocial" aspects and the corresponding alterations.

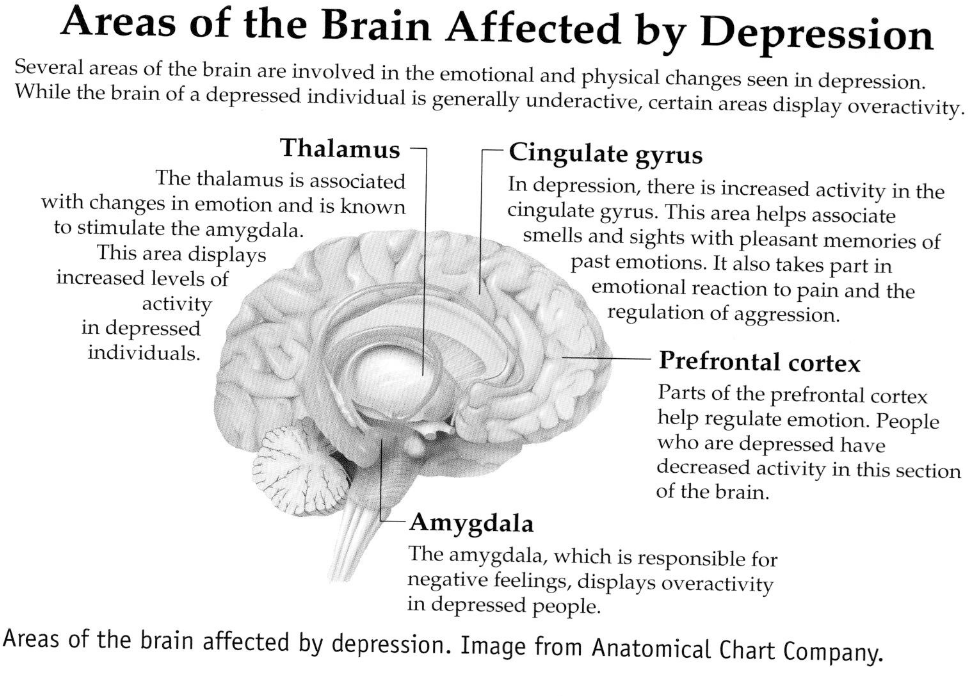

Areas of the brain affected by depression. Image from Anatomical Chart Company.

Module 1 Regulation of Mood, Attention, and Behavior

Regulation of Mood

Mood is an internal, subjective psychological state, which directs how a person feels and perceives the world. It is usually referred to as a good mood or bad mood. A positive (good) mood has been shown in numerous studies to enhance creative thinking, imagination, and problem solving. Mood changes gradually over time and is influenced by internal and external stimuli, such as sleep or stress. Similar terms used to describe mood are feelings, emotions, and temperament, but there are differences. Based on timing fluctuations, **emotions** (feelings) would be the most fluid, quickly moving minute-by-minute from happy to sad to disappointed. **Temperament** (personality), a stable representation of outlook, is less likely to change over time. Mood falls somewhere in between these two extremes.

The major brain structures that regulate mood are found in Figure 11.1. Each structure has a specific function:

- **Hypothalamus:** Regulates the autonomic nervous system during expression of emotions.
- **Prefrontal cortex:** Controls judgment, decision-making, and problem solving; involved in emotional responses; controls amygdala during stress; involved in short-term memory and in retrieving long-term memories. The left half appears to establish positive feelings and the right half establishes negative feelings. Sections of the prefrontal cortex also have significant functions:
  - **Lateral:** Controls consideration of alternatives and choosing a course of behavior.
  - **Orbitofrontal:** Controls delayed gratification; suppresses impulses.
  - **Ventromedial:** Connects emotions with meaning.
- **Amygdala:** The centers of emotionally charged memories, senses danger, and controls persistent negative thoughts, especially fear and aggression, are active during stress, anxiety, and depression. Connects with hippocampus, septal nuclei, thalamus, and prefrontal cortex.
- **Hippocampus:** Helps to create and file long-term memory.
- **Anterior cingulate cortex:** Has a wide variety of autonomic functions; regulates blood pressure

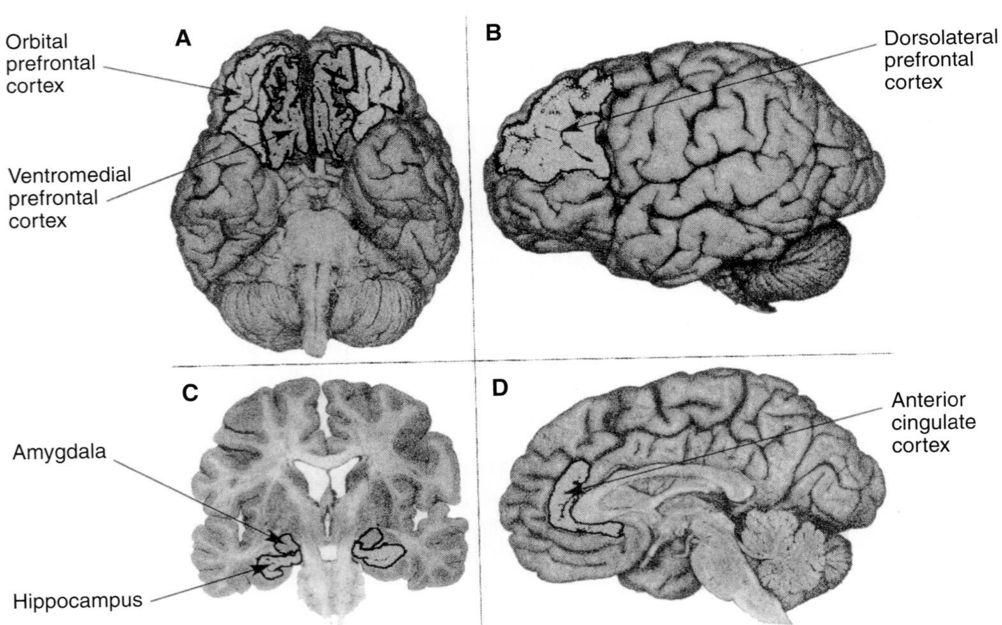

Figure 11.1. Key brain regions involved in mood regulation. **A:** Orbital prefrontal cortex and the ventromedial prefrontal cortex. **B:** Dorsolateral prefrontal cortex. **C:** Hippocampus and amygdala. **D:** Anterior cingulate cortex. (From Sadock BJ, Sadock VA, Ruiz P. *Kaplan & Sadock's Comprehensive Textbook of Psychiatry*. 9th ed. Philadelphia, PA: Lippincott Williams & Wilkins; 2009.)

and heart rate; involved in cognitive functions and emotion, such as empathy, impulse control, and decision-making.

- **Cingulate gyrus:** Located between the cingulate sulcus and corpus callosum; coordinates sights and smells with previous emotionally charged memories, involved in the emotional reaction to pain and impacts aggressive behavior.

More important, however, are the circuits which connect one's cognitive activity, expression of emotions, and behavior. This idea was first suggested in 1930 by James Papez (called the circuit of Papez) and later expanded by Paul MacLean, where it was referred to as the **limbic system**. These complex mood–attention–behavior connections of the limbic system can be traced through the hypothalamus, thalamus, hippocampus, anterior cingulate cortex, cingulate gyrus, amygdala, and prefrontal cortex (Fig. 11.2).

Neurotransmitters also play a critical role in mood regulation. Pharmacologic intervention in mood disorders most often targets one or more neurotransmitters. The various neurotransmitters and their actions on mood, attention, and behavior are summarized in Table 11.1.

Regulation of Attention

Attention is a culturally influenced process of selectively concentrating on information. It is both a cognitive process and a behavior as it involves the interaction of sensory cues and the corresponding actions. Attention processing and action occurs throughout the brain in both a reflexive, reactive manner and a thoughtful, intentional manner. For example, people automatically attend to a loud unexpected noise. This reflexive attention occurs "bottom up" and is largely regulated by the reticular activating system (RAS). The RAS is comprised of several neuronal pathways beginning with startling sensory input moving through reticular formation to the nuclei of the thalamus and outward to the parietal and temporal cortices and limbic system. In this way, the RAS facilitates neuronal activity during tasks requiring alertness and attention (Fig. 11.3). On

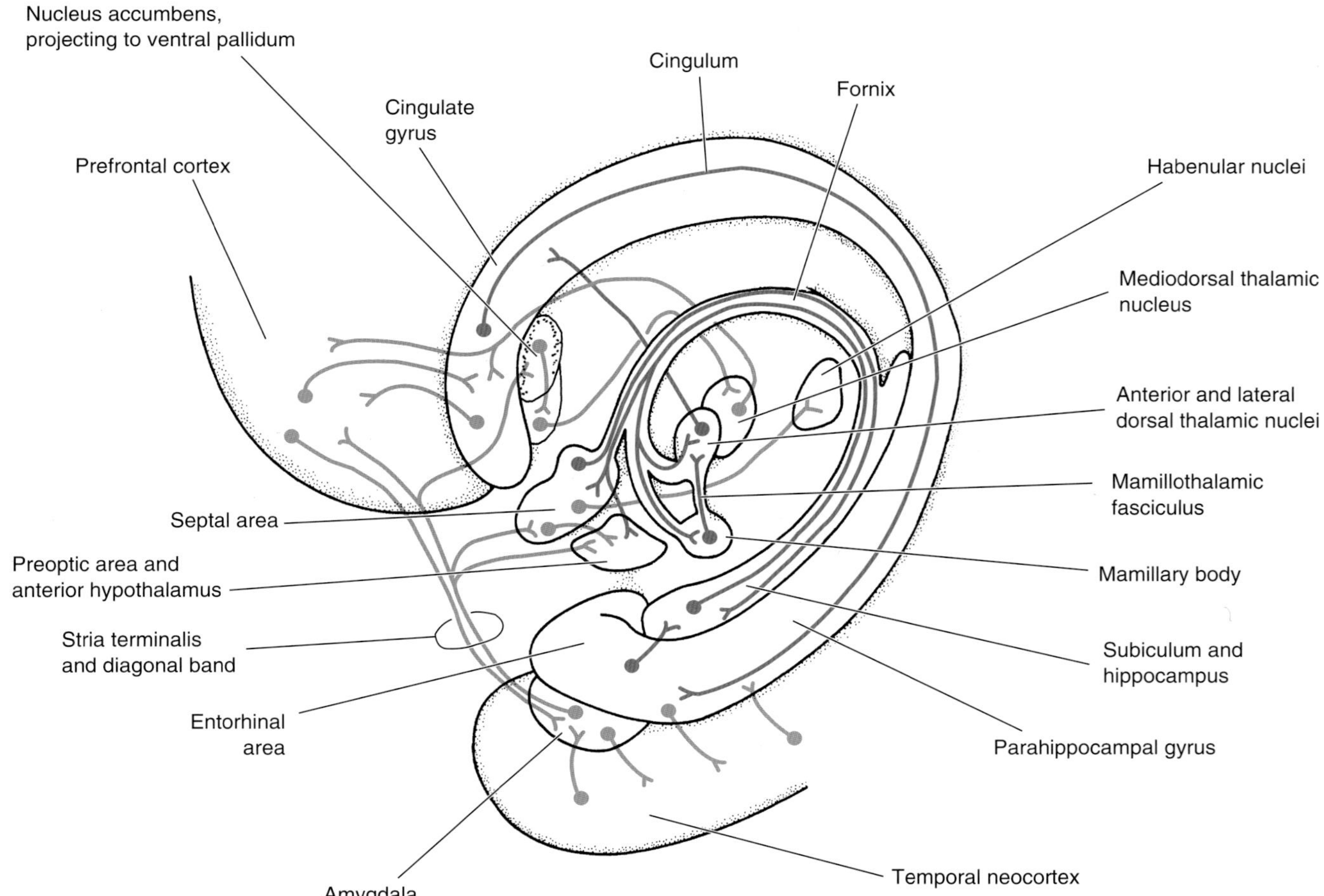

Figure 11.2. Complex connections of the hippocampal formation and amygdala in the forebrain and diencephalon, including the circuit of Papez *(red)* and other limbic system connections *(blue)*.

Table 11.1 Neurotransmitters Regulating Mood, Attention, and Behavior

Neurotransmitter	Function	Controls
Dopamine	Inhibitory	Voluntary movements of the body
		Mood
		Pleasurable emotions
Norepinephrine	Excitatory	Physical and mental arousal (fight or flight)
		Mood
		Heart rate and blood pressure
Serotonin	Inhibitory	Mood
		Perception
		Appetite
		Sleep
		Body temperature
Glutamate	Excitatory	Attention
		Learning
		Memory
Gamma-aminobutyric acid (GABA)	Inhibitory	Mood
		Muscle activity
		Visual sensory input
Acetylcholine	Excitatory	Attention
		Arousal
		Learning
		Memory
		Muscle activity

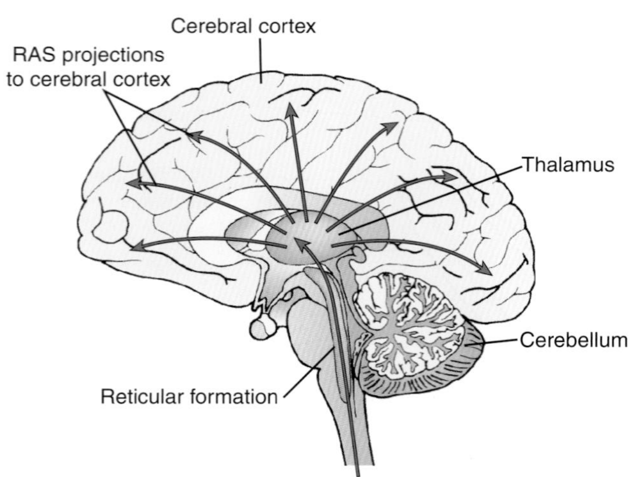

Figure 11.3. The reticular activating system (RAS). Ascending sensory tracts send axon collateral fibers to the reticular formation. These give rise to fibers synapsing in the nonspecific nuclei of the thalamus. From there, the nonspecific thalamic projections influence widespread areas of the cerebral cortex and limbic system.

the other hand, people can filter distractions and attend only to things that are important to him or her. This is referred to as "top down," or executive processing, and is mediated by the frontal lobe and basal ganglia. Executive processing allows attention to become connected with working memory, problem solving, and other higher-order functions. Neurotransmitters are also active in attention processes as illustrated in Table 11.1.

Visual attention, such as you are experiencing as you read this text, is an important form of sensory input requiring executive processing. With visual input, attention is distributed over the whole scene (or chapter colors, headings, pictures, as in this case). Second, attention is concentrated and focused on a specific area (such as this sentence). This results in high attention and visual resolution toward the focus, less attention and "blurriness" at the fringe, and virtually no attention beyond the margin. Try this while you are reading. See where your attention lies as your eyes move across the page.

Simultaneously, higher-level cognitive processes are placing the attended items into memory and giving the information meaning. There are several theories related to attention and various classifications. One way to organize attention is in five types, moving from simple to complex:

- **Focused:** Noticing and responding to one specific stimulus.
- **Sustained:** Sustaining concentration with vigilance over time.
- **Selective:** Noticing and responding to a stimulus while filtering distractions.
- **Alternating:** Moving between tasks having different cognitive requirements.
- **Divided:** Responding simultaneously to multiple tasks or demands.

The attention system has limits on what and how much can be processed. For example, driving while talking or texting on a cell phone leads to poor driving performance, more accidents, and veering toward the median or shoulder of the road. In addition, attention is divided and it is much more difficult to concentrate on both when studying while listening to the radio.

Stop and Consider
What are some examples of situations where you have experienced the types of attention above? What are other activities in which you participate where your attention is divided and attention resources are taxed?

Regulation of Behavior

Behavior is how people respond and act in a given situation. As with mood, the frontal lobe of the brain is the primary region responsible for regulating behavior. This lobe integrates all aspects of behavior including personality, perception, planning, self-awareness, judgment, mood, attention, memory, motivation, sexuality, expressive language, and social and emotional intelligence.

Generating appropriate behaviors for a given situation requires a complex interplay of cognitive and behavioral processes. For example, consider receiving bad news. Behavior will be based on noticing, perceiving, short-term and long-term memory (past experiences), current social expectations, mood, personality, motivation/inhibition, culture, consideration of all possible actions, planning, and deciding. All these occur within a matter of seconds and with little conscious effort.

Module 2 Alterations in Mood, Attention, and Behavior

Alterations in Brain Structure and Function

Alterations in the brain, limbic system connections, or neurotransmission can result in impairments of mood, attention, and behavior. A major cause of mood, attention, and behavior disorders is traumatic brain injury. The frontal lobe and corresponding limbic system structures are particularly vulnerable. When the prefrontal cortex suffers an injury, the patient loses the sense of social responsibility, concentration, abstract thinking, and problem solving. The patient displays a flat affect, an observed emotional response, with no signs of joy, sadness, hope, or affection. Destruction of the amygdala also has a significant impact. There is a reduction of fear and aggression and a loss of social intelligence. When both amygdalas are impaired, the connection between social intelligence and memory is also impaired. Patients lose facial expression recognition and cannot interpret what the other person is thinking or feeling. Similarly, emotional reactivity is impaired with damage to limbic system structures including the thalamus, prefrontal cortex, and hypothalamus. Lesions of the hypothalamus interfere with appropriate responses to thermal regulation, hunger, thirst, sexuality, and aggression toward others.

Neurotransmission impairments, such as levels of neurotransmitters or receptor issues, can lead to apathy, inattentiveness, and motor deficits as with low levels of dopamine, or agitation, restlessness, and psychosis as with high levels of dopamine. Deficits in serotonin have been associated with anxiety, obsessions, and compulsions. These various alterations are discussed in greater detail in Module 3.

Recognizing Alterations in Mood, Attention, and Behavior

Rarely are there laboratory tests or imaging studies that can confirm a psychiatric diagnosis. Diagnosis most often relies on patient history and reported observations of others. A number of valid and reliable screening tools are currently being used to attempt to identify patients with mood, attention, and behavioral disorders, such as the Mood Disorder Questionnaire. Sometimes the diagnosis is achieved only after other alternatives have been ruled out.

The most widely used categorical criteria for diagnosing alterations in mood, attention, and behavior are found in the American Psychiatric Association's fifth edition of the *Diagnostic and Statistical Manual of Mental Disorders* (DSM-5), and the World Health Organization's *International Statistical Classification of Diseases and Related Health Problems* (ICD-10). The DSM-5 is commonly used in the

Categorical Traits

Bipolar Disorder
Elevated Mood
Flight of Ideas
Pressured Speech

Schizophrenia
Disorganized Speech
Disorganized Behavior

Hallucinations
Suicidality
Delusions

Insomnia
Irritability
Impaired Concentration

Flat Affect
Avolition

Major Depression
Depressed Mood
Appetite Disturbance
Anergy
Guilt/Worthlessness

Figure 11.4. Categorical traits as conceptualized by the *Diagnostic and Statistical Manual* (DSM-5) represent a "menu-based" approach to psychiatric disorders. Individuals are assessed for a checklist of signs and symptoms that are then used to categorize the individual as "affected" according to a specific diagnosis. Not all symptoms are present in samples of individuals who carry a particular DSM diagnosis, and many of these symptoms occur across diagnostic boundaries, as illustrated in this Venn diagram. (From Sadock BJ, Sadock VA, Ruiz P. *Kaplan & Sadock's Comprehensive Textbook of Psychiatry*. 9th ed. Philadelphia, PA: Lippincott Williams & Wilkins; 2009:325.)

United States and the ICD-10 is used internationally. Figure 11.4 illustrates the categorical approach to diagnosing alterations in mood, attention, and behavior.

Treating Alterations in Mood, Attention, and Behavior

Treatment for alterations in mood, attention, and behavior must be individualized and can include (alone or in combination) in hospital or community settings the following:

- Psychotherapy—Conducted with a qualified mental health professional; explores thoughts, feelings, and behaviors, and seeks to improve well-being, such as through cognitive-behavioral therapy, exposure therapy, etc.
- Pharmacotherapy—Prescribed by a qualified mental health professional; drug therapy can help with management of symptoms related to alterations in mood, attention, and behavior, such as with antidepressant drugs.
- Counseling—Can help facilitate a number of strategies to promote wellness, including stress reduction, lifestyle changes, and community resource utilization.
- Alternative/complementary therapies—A number of alternative and complementary therapies can be used to alleviate symptoms, such as herbal remedies, acupuncture, homeopathy, and many others.
- Individual or family support group—Offers support and advice from others who have had similar needs and experiences, where the group is working toward a shared goal.

Stop and Consider
There is an inordinate amount of stigma involved in mental illness. What do you see in your community as barriers to patients seeking appropriate mental health treatment?

Module 3 Clinical Models

The following clinical models were selected to help apply knowledge related to altered mood, attention, and behavior. What you will notice is that these clinical models rely heavily on patient history and observations using screening tools for diagnosis. Treatments most often involve a combination of psychotherapy and pharmacotherapy and an emphasis on family support.

Generalized Anxiety Disorder

Anxiety disorders are a group of chronic psychiatric conditions characterized by overwhelming and irrational feelings of fear or worry. These feelings may cause physical symptoms, such as a stomachache, headache, racing heart, and shakiness. It is often the physical symptoms that cause the patient to seek medical care. There are several types of anxiety disorders, often organized into three distinct groups:

1. Anxiety disorders
2. Obsessive-compulsive disorders
3. Trauma/stress-related disorders

Figure 11.5 illustrates a decision-tree, which can be used to differentiate the various types of anxiety. The anxiety disorders are the most common category and

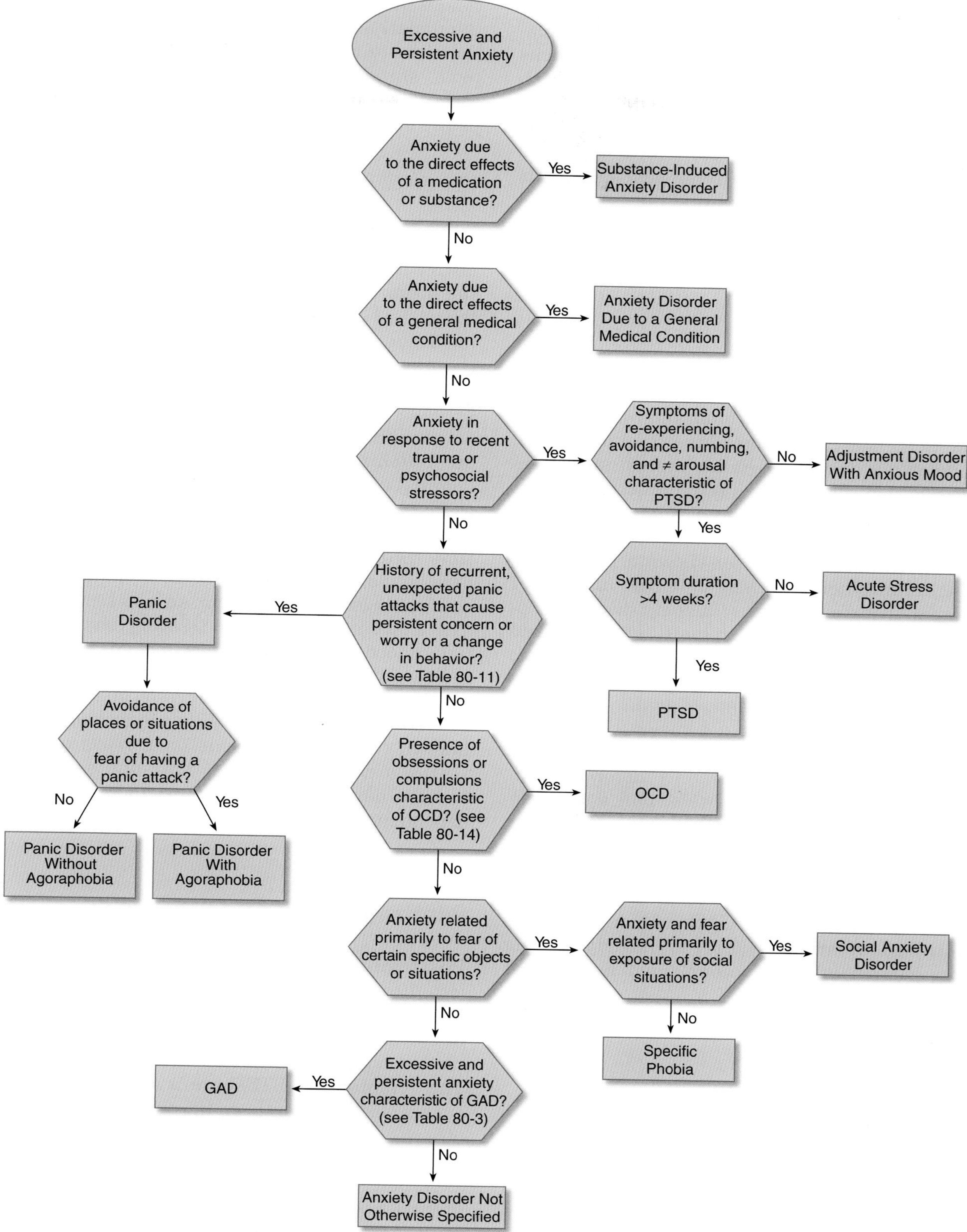

Figure 11.5. Diagnostic decision-tree for anxiety disorders. GAD, generalized anxiety disorder; OCD, obsessive-compulsive disorder; PTSD, posttraumatic stress disorder. (From Alldredge BK, Corelli RL, Ernst ME, et al. *Koda-Kimble and Young's Applied Therapeutics*. 10th ed. Philadelphia, PA: Lippincott Williams & Wilkins; 2012.)

include panic disorder, generalized anxiety, social anxiety, phobias, separation anxiety, and medication/illness-induced anxiety. This section will focus on **generalized anxiety disorder (GAD)**, which is characterized by excessive, uncontrollable, and irrational worry lasting greater than 6 months. The anxiety interferes with daily life due to irrational thinking about everyday matters, such as health, money, death, family, friends, work, etc. Around 6% of the US population is affected by GAD.[1] Posttraumatic stress disorder is also discussed in greater detail as a select clinical model in this module.

PATHOPHYSIOLOGY

Brain structure and function studies indicate that the amygdala is key in modulating fear and anxiety. Patients with anxiety disorders often show a greater response in the amygdala to anxiety-provoking events. The amygdala and other limbic system structures are closely connected to the prefrontal cortex. When treated with psychologic therapies or medications, amygdala abnormalities exerted on the limbic system and prefrontal cortex have been shown to be relieved. In the central nervous system (CNS), the major mediators of the symptoms of anxiety disorders appear to be norepinephrine, serotonin, dopamine, and gamma-aminobutyric acid (GABA). The autonomic nervous system, especially the sympathetic nervous system, mediates the symptoms of anxiety.

The cause of GAD is often not known. Genetic factors can influence risk; anxiety disorders are more likely to occur in those with a family history of anxiety. Environmental factors may also play a role, particularly exposure to traumatic events.

CLINICAL MANIFESTATIONS

Clinical manifestations of GAD include excessive, uncontrolled, irrational worry or anxiety lasting greater than 6 months, accompanied by at least three of the following:

- Restlessness
- Fatigue
- Difficulty concentrating
- Irritability
- Tension
- Sleep disturbance

Patients with GAD are also at risk for suicidal ideation and should be evaluated and treated accordingly.

DIAGNOSTIC CRITERIA

Diagnosis of GAD requires a thorough medical history and physical examination to rule out a medical condition or substance-abuse problem that may be the underlying cause for the generalized anxiety. In the absence of an underlying cause for GAD symptoms, standardized rating scales can be used to assess severity and to monitor progress with therapeutic interventions.

TREATMENT

Cognitive-behavioral therapy (CBT), alone or in addition to pharmacotherapy, is currently the most effective treatment for GAD. Cognitive therapy opens the doors to knowledge and understanding so that the patient can more clearly understand how irrational thoughts and beliefs lead to anxiety. Behavioral therapy involves gradual exposure of the patient to anxiety-provoking stimuli. Over time, the patient becomes desensitized and realizes that the feared, catastrophic, irrationally anticipated event does not occur. Relaxation techniques, including effective abdominal breathing, can also help control anxiety.

Pharmacologic treatment for GAD most commonly involves selective serotonin reuptake inhibitors (SSRIs). These drugs work by providing more serotonin at the synapse to allow for amplified nerve cell conduction resulting in an elevation of mood. The exact mechanism for treating anxiety is less understood. Benzodiazepines are also sometimes indicated for short term or as needed to reduce immediate overwhelming feelings of anxiety. The exact mechanism of action of benzodiazepines is not known; these drugs appear to increase activity of GABA, a neurotransmitter that suppresses the activity of nerves. Benzodiazepines do carry a risk for dependence and should be used cautiously.

Posttraumatic Stress Disorder

Posttraumatic stress disorder (PTSD) is an anxiety disorder caused by extreme traumatic events, commonly affecting those who have experienced military combat, victims of natural disasters, concentration camp survivors, and victims of violent crime. The symptoms of PTSD are a result of witnessing events such as death or life-threatening injury of others and/or serious personal harm where feelings of intense horror, fear, powerlessness, and guilt were experienced. It is estimated that more than 60% of men and 50% of women experience at least one traumatic event in their life. The most frequently reported traumatic events by men are rape, combat, and childhood neglect or physical abuse. Women most frequently report instances of rape, sexual molestation, physical attack, being threatened with a weapon, and childhood physical abuse. However, not all people who experience trauma develop PTSD. In the United States, it is estimated that 10% of women and 4% of men will develop PTSD at some point in their lives. Rates among veterans vary by service area but is estimated at 11% to 20% per year with a rate of 30% over a veteran's lifetime.[2]

PATHOPHYSIOLOGY

PTSD is caused by a combination of experiencing one or more traumatic events coupled with biologic susceptibility. The more severe the trauma and the more susceptible the individual, the more likely that person is to develop PTSD. Risk factors include prior exposure to trauma, particularly in childhood, where the child dissociated from the trauma. Others include close proximity, long duration, and high severity of the trauma, anxiety, depression, a heightened startle response, smaller hippocampal volume, alcohol and drug abuse, a family history of mental health issues, impaired social support, and the absence of early interventions.

Similar to other mental health disorders, there is a hereditary component to PTSD with about 30% of the risk explained by genetics. Experiencing traumatic events can result in fear reactions, which activate the prefrontal cortex and amygdala, and release stress hormones, which suppress the hypothalamus (Fig. 11.6). The adrenal response results in the creation of neuroendocrine patterns that persist beyond the traumatic event(s). Most notably, impairment in hypothalamic–pituitary axis, and subsequently the fight or flight response occurs, where cortisol levels become suppressed and catecholamine levels (such as epinephrine, also known as adrenaline, norepinephrine, and dopamine) are elevated. High norepinephrine levels in the prefrontal cortex promote flashbacks and nightmares. High dopamine levels induce anxiety and psychosis. Suppression of cortisol levels prohibits the restoration of homeostasis after the traumatic event. Future fearful events are marked by an overexaggerated fight or flight response (high catecholamines) with a restricted ability toward homeostasis (low cortisol).

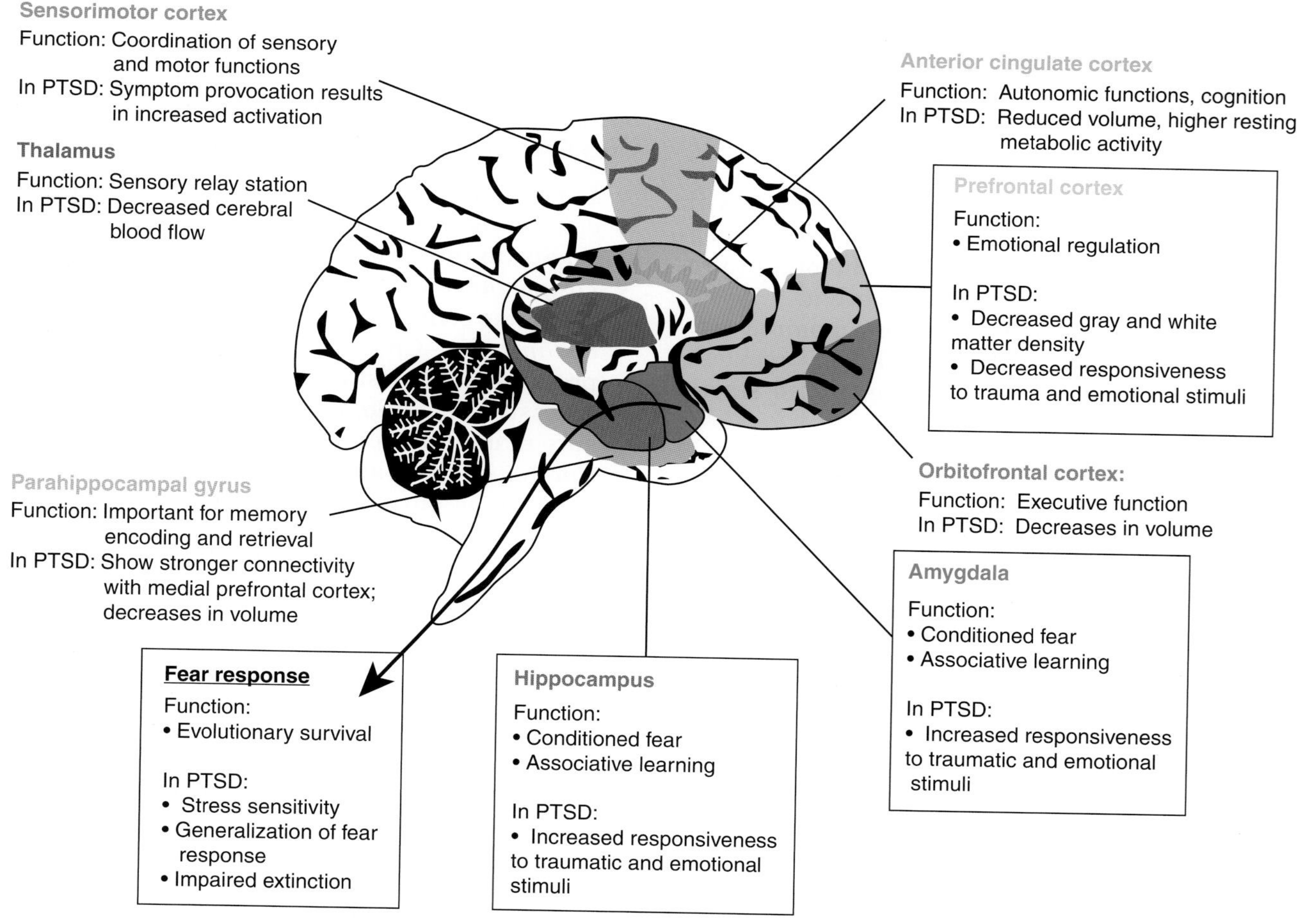

Figure 11.6. Brain regions associated with PTSD. (From Mahan AL, Ressler KJ. Fear conditioning, synaptic plasticity and the amygdala: implications for posttraumatic stress disorder. *Trends Neurosci*. 2012;35(1):24–35.)

CLINICAL MANIFESTATIONS

Clinical manifestations in PTSD appear after the traumatic event, often within 3 months, but emergence can occur beyond this time. Initial clinical manifestations can include avoidance and suppression of thoughts and emotions about the trauma. However, PTSD is characterized by reliving the traumatic event through intrusive nightmares and flashbacks.

For children, clinical manifestations generally differ from adults and can include excessive reactions to caregiver separation, crying, screaming, trembling, regression, withdrawal, disruptive behavior, inattentiveness, anger outbursts, sleep problems, irrational fears, and somatic complaints.

DIAGNOSTIC CRITERIA

The DSM-5 outlines the diagnostic criteria for PTSD (see Resources). Clinical manifestations must be present for at least 1 month, must cause impaired functioning, and cannot be attributed to any other medical condition. Other components must also be met to be diagnostic:

1. Experiencing/witnessing the traumatic event(s).
2. Persistently reexperiencing the traumatic event(s) through thoughts, dreams, hallucinations, dissociative flashbacks, etc.
3. Avoiding stimuli associated with the traumatic event(s) and numbing of responsiveness.
4. Distorting cognitions and mood associated with the traumatic event(s) such as a persistent negative emotional state or complete inability to remember important aspects of the event.
5. Reacting in an exaggerated or impaired way such as through irritability, anger, recklessness, hypervigilance, or an exaggerated startle response.

TREATMENT

Early intervention for those experiencing traumatic events, even prior to diagnosis with PTSD, can help to effectively ameliorate the symptoms. For those diagnosed with PTSD, psychotherapy often with medications for symptom management is the current treatment. Psychotherapy approaches, particularly through the use of trauma-focused cognitive-behavioral therapy (TFCBT) and eye movement desensitization and reprocessing (EMDR), have been shown to be effective. Both seek to change the trauma victim's thinking and behaviors surrounding the traumatic experience. In EMDR, eye movements are added to aid in the information-processing mechanisms of the brain. Play therapy is commonly employed for children with PTSD.

Medications are important for relieving symptoms, such as anxiety, depression, nightmares, and impulsivity. Commonly prescribed are antidepressant drugs, benzodiazepines for short-term anxiety relief, glucocorticoids (short term) to assist with neurocellular homeostasis, anticonvulsants for impulsivity, and clonidine (a centrally acting alpha-agonist hypotensive agent) for nightmares.

Major Depressive Disorder

Depression is a condition of altered mood, which can be short term and situationally dependent, such as with normal bereavement, or chronic and severe, as can occur with a major depressive disorder. **Major depressive disorder (MDD)** is a condition characterized by a pervasive and persistent low mood that is accompanied by low self-esteem and **anhedonia**, or loss of interest or pleasure in normally enjoyable activities. It is a disabling condition that adversely affects the patient's family, work or school life, sleep, eating habits, and overall health.

MDD is diagnosed upon the patient experiencing major depressive episodes, which are characterized by the presence of a severely depressed mood that persists for at least 2 weeks. Episodes may be acute or chronic/recurrent and are categorized as mild, moderate, or severe. The DSM-5 further differentiates five subtypes of MDD:

- *Seasonal affective*—Characterized by depressive episodes occurring in the late fall and winter, resolving in the spring/summer.
- *Postpartum*—Characterized by disabling depression after giving birth lasting up to 3 months.
- *Melancholic*—Characterized by pronounced depression often most notable in the early morning, excessive weight loss, excessive guilt, loss of pleasure in most/all activities.
- *Catatonic*—Rare and severe, characterized by immobility or purposeless movements, inability to speak, stupor.
- *Atypical*—Characterized by mood reactivity, weight gain, excessive sleep, social impairment.

During 2009 to 2012, 7.6% of Americans aged 12 and over had depression (moderate or severe depressive symptoms in the past 2 weeks). Depression was more prevalent among females and persons aged 40 to 59 and persons living below the poverty level were nearly 2½ times more likely to have depression than those at or above the poverty level.[3]

PATHOPHYSIOLOGY

Although the exact cause of depression has not been identified, a biopsychosocial model illustrates biologic, psychologic, and social factors all play a role. The heritability of depression, that is, the degree to which genetics plays a role, has been estimated at 40% for women and 30% for men.[4] Significant research on biologic factors has pointed to several potential influences:

- Damage to the cerebellum can directly cause depression;
- Those with one or two short alleles of the *5-HTT* gene (the serotonin transporter gene) are more likely to develop depression given very stressful life events;
- Excessive use and/or withdrawal from alcohol, illicit drugs, and certain sedative/hypnotic drugs are associated with the development of major depression;
- The levels of brain-derived neurotropic factor, responsible for neuron generation, are reduced in those with depression;
- Brain structural differences in neuroimaging studies have noted:
  - Increased adrenal gland and lateral ventricle volumes
  - Reduced volumes of the basal ganglia, thalamus, hippocampus, and frontal lobe
  - Loss of neurons in the hippocampus
- A hyperactive pituitary–adrenal axis and subsequent increased levels of cortisol have been associated with depression;
- Estrogen levels may play a role given the higher incidence in women, particularly after puberty, before menopause, and during pregnancy;
- Higher levels of circulating inflammatory cytokines, particularly IL-6 and TNF-alpha, are associated with depression.

Most notably, depression is believed to be a condition resulting from a deficiency in neurotransmitters or alterations in the synapses that use these neurotransmitters in critical areas of the brain. Although, as you will soon see, the phrase "chemical imbalance" is an oversimplification.

The specific neurotransmitter systems involved include norepinephrine (NE), dopamine (DA), and serotonin (5-HT). These neurotransmitters are also referred to as monoamines. For perfect neurotransmission, the following must take place:

- Presynaptic neurons are functional and release neurotransmitters at a normal rate;
- Enzymes are effectively active and break down neurotransmitters;
- Membrane transporters from the synaptic cleft are functional, allowing uptake, reuptake, and recycling of the active neurotransmitters;
- Receptors that detect neurotransmitters and control the release and flow of impulse through the neuron are functional;
- Postsynaptic neurons contain needed regulatory mechanisms to promote signal transduction.

The monoamine hypothesis of depression emphasizes the interplay of the NE, DA, and 5-HT neurotransmitters in regulating mood. In this theory, serotonin (5-HT) regulates the other neurotransmitter systems. Therefore, low levels of serotonin would result in low levels of norepinephrine and dopamine and lead to depression. This theory is supported by current pharmacologic treatment of depression, which targets the neurotransmitters and receptors, to improve mood (Fig. 11.7). The counterargument is that antidepressant drugs take weeks for their full effect, even though the boost of monoamines occurs within hours of taking the drugs. Also, not all patients with low monoamines exhibit symptoms of depression. These theories and counterarguments illustrate the complexity of pinpointing the biologic basis of depression.

Social and psychological influences on depression cannot be ignored. Isolation, social rejection, loss or lack of significant relationships, issues with family functioning, unemployment, poverty, abuse,

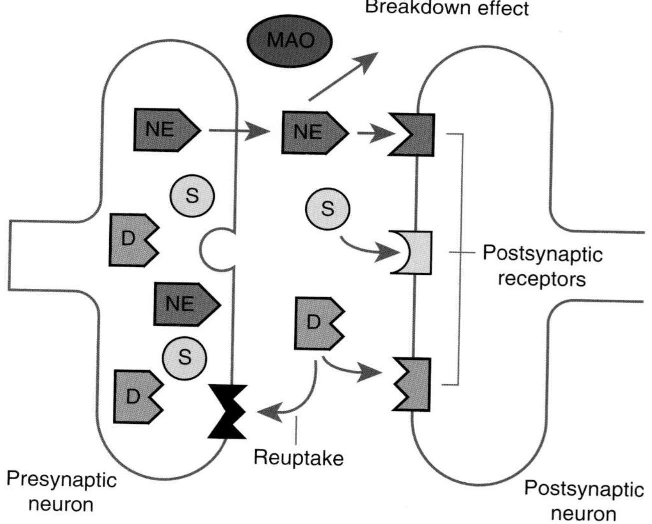

Figure 11.7. Schematic representation of the mechanism of action of antidepressant agents. Neurotransmitters (NE, S, D) are released from the presynaptic neuron into the synaptic space. They interact with the postsynaptic receptors and continue the neuronal transmission. After release from the postsynaptic neuron, these agents can be broken down by the enzyme monoamine oxidase (MAO) and the components recycled into the presynaptic neuron or they can be taken up again through the reuptake mechanism. Antidepressant agents can (1) block the MAO enzymes—MAO inhibitors; or (2) block the reuptake of the neurotransmitter. In effect, each mechanism increases the intrasynaptic concentration of the particular neurotransmitter.

alcohol/drug abuse, and other severe life stressors are important social influences. Psychologically, negative approaches to coping with adversity, low self-esteem, self-concept, and/or self-efficacy, distorted thinking, and low resilience are significant risk factors.

CLINICAL MANIFESTATIONS

Sadness is an expected part of being human. MDD, however, is characterized by a persistent very low mood and anhedonia, which pervades all aspects of life. Feelings of worthlessness, guilt, helplessness, hopelessness, and self-hatred are also often reported. Patients have interruptions in sleep patterns, unrelenting fatigue, and changes in appetite, weight, and sex drive. Cognitive features include changes in attention span and memory, frustration, intolerance, and negative cognitive distortions. Psychosomatic complaints include muscle tension, chronic pain, stomach aches, digestive problems, and headaches. Changes in impulse control may lead to suicidal or homicidal ideations and actions.

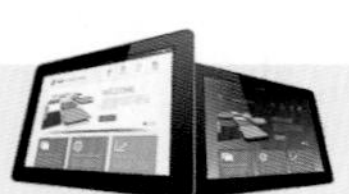

RESEARCH NOTES

Research on which therapies are most effective for depression in children and adolescents has shown mixed results. For example, a 2014 Cochrane review suggested that an overall prevalence of depressive disorders in children under 13 years is 2.8% compared to adolescents at 5.7%. In this review, 11 randomized-controlled studies compared psychotherapy, medications, and the combination of these with over 1,300 pediatric patients. Results of the trials showed differing conclusions, some of which were directly contradictory. At the conclusion of the review, the researchers noted: we do not know whether psychological therapy, antidepressant medication, or a combination of the two is most effective to treat depressive disorders in children and adolescents.[5]

DIAGNOSTIC CRITERIA

The diagnosis of MDD is based on the patient history, reported behaviors observed by relatives or friends, and a mental status examination. There is no laboratory test for major depression, although it is important to rule out any physical conditions that may cause similar symptoms. Diagnostic criteria, using the DSM-5, indicate that a major depressive episode must include the onset of five or more symptoms persisting over a 2-week period. One of these symptoms must reflect depressed mood or loss of interest or pleasure. There are many reliable and valid rating scales that may assist the practitioner in determining the severity of MDD. One example is the Beck Depression Inventory.

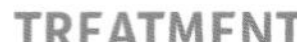

TREATMENT

The three most common treatments for depression are psychotherapy/counseling, antidepressant medications, and electroconvulsive therapy (ECT). The classes of drugs used to treat depression include selective serotonin reuptake inhibitors (SSRI), selective norepinephrine reuptake inhibitors (SNRI), norepinephrine and dopamine reuptake inhibitors (NDRI), tricyclic antidepressants (TCA), and monoamine oxidase inhibitors (MAOIs). ECT is used as a last line of therapy for MDD. Other potential therapies include transcranial magnetic stimulation (TMS), herbal or other alternative therapies, and light therapy. Treatment should be tailored based on severity of symptoms, effectiveness of prior treatments, presence of comorbid conditions, and patient preference.

Bipolar Affective Disorder

Bipolar affective disorder, also known as manic-depression, is a condition characterized by periods of **mania** (elevated mood and erratic behavior) and depression. Mania is the defining feature of bipolar affective disorder. In **hypomania** (a mild form of mania), patients are energetic, excitable, hyperactive, and may be highly productive. As mania worsens, patients become erratic and display impulsive behavior, resulting in poor decisions, and require very little, if any, sleep. At the most severe level, manic patients can experience **psychosis**, a complete mental and emotional loss of touch with reality. A depressive episode commonly follows an episode of mania. The biologic mechanisms responsible for switching between mania and depression are poorly understood. About 3% of people in the United States have bipolar disorder at some point in their life; lower rates are found in other countries. The most common age at which symptoms begin is from late adolescence to early adulthood.

PATHOPHYSIOLOGY

The exact cause of bipolar affective disorder has not been identified; however, a strong hereditary component (estimated to explain 60% to 80% of the risk) points to complex genetic and epigenetic influences. Researchers have identified multiple different disease alleles (heterogeneity). In isolation, one of these alleles, when affected, does not increase disease risk. However, when certain clusters of these disease alleles (referred to as loci) are affected, the patient is much more likely to develop bipolar affective disorder. These different disease allele clusters associated with bipolar affective disorder are referred to as the major affective disorder (MAFD) loci. At this time, there are around nine MAFD loci centralized on different chromosomes, but refinement of discovery is likely as research continues. The expressions of two particular genes (*ANK3* and *CACNA1C*) and their gene variants have been associated with the various bipolar phenotypes. In addition, genetic similarities between bipolar affective disorder, schizophrenia, and other psychiatric disorders indicate common expression of genetic variants and biologic origins.

Postmortem and neuroimaging studies have uncovered a number of brain findings associated with bipolar affective disorder, which further the understanding of its pathophysiology:

- Alterations in hippocampal neurons (atrophy and cell loss);
- Increased brain volume in the lateral ventricles and dorsal pallidum;
- Poor modulation between prefrontal and limbic regions of the brain, particularly the amygdala;
- High dopamine levels during the manic phase and low levels in the depressive phase;
- High glutamate (excitatory neurotransmitter) levels in the prefrontal cortex during the manic phase.

Individual psychological, environmental, and social factors, which interact with the genetic risk factors, play a significant role in the development of bipolar affective disorder. Examples include traumatic life events, such as childhood abuse, a harsh home environment, and disruptions in interpersonal relationships.

CLINICAL MANIFESTATIONS

Bipolar affective disorder is marked by clinical manifestations indicative of mania, which interrupt work and/or relationships, and last at least 1 week. These include a significant elevation in mood or irritability, rapid and excessive speech, distractibility, racing thoughts, impaired judgment, impulsivity, especially with spending money, hypersexuality, extreme focus or goal-orientation, or frustration. Patients also exhibit a decreased need for sleep and can have issues with substance abuse. The most extreme clinical manifestations are delusions, hallucinations, and psychosis. Hypomania is a milder form of mania and does not typically interrupt work and/or relationships. Signs and symptoms of the depressive phase include those described with MDD above.

DIAGNOSTIC CRITERIA

The diagnosis of bipolar affective disorder is based on the patient history, reported behaviors observed by relatives or friends, and a mental status examination. The diagnosis is often delayed because it can be difficult to distinguish bipolar from depressive (unipolar) disorders. There is no laboratory test, although it is important to rule out any physical conditions that may cause similar symptoms.

Diagnostic criteria, using the DSM-5, distinguish seven different subtypes of bipolar affective disorder: bipolar I disorder, bipolar II disorder, cyclothymic disorder, substance/medication-induced bipolar, bipolar and related disorder due to another medical condition, other specified bipolar, and unspecified bipolar. Each subtype has a variation in its diagnostic criteria. For example, the bipolar I disorder criteria represent classical manic-depressive disorder but without the experience of an MDD. Bipolar II requires at least one lifetime experience of major depression and at least one hypomanic episode. The cyclothymic disorder diagnosis is given to adults who experience at least 2 years (for children, a full year) of both hypomanic and depressive periods without ever fulfilling the criteria for an episode of mania, hypomania, or major depression and so forth. Diagnosis is confirmed with the specified clinical presentation over the requisite amount of time and without another underlying cause.

TREATMENT

Bipolar affective disorder is treated with psychotherapy and medications. Psychotherapy goals are to alleviate symptoms, recognize and reduce triggers, and build resilience. Medications generally fall into the categories of mood stabilizers or atypical antipsychotic drugs. Lithium carbonate and sodium valproate, both mood stabilizers, are commonly prescribed and have strong evidence supporting efficacy. A challenge of pharmacologic treatment is adherence to the medication regimen. Those in a manic phase often feel great, energetic, and focused, are impulsive, and make poor decisions. This, along with potential medication side effects of hand tremors, nausea, polyuria, and thirst among others can result in refusal to take medications.

Attention-Deficit Hyperactivity Disorder

Attention-deficit hyperactivity disorder (ADHD), as its name suggests, is a neurodevelopmental disorder of cognitive functions, causing attention deficit, hyperactivity, and impulsiveness. The DSM-5 further distinguishes three subtypes: (1) ADHD inattentive type; (2) ADHD hyperactive-impulsive type; and (3) ADHD combined type (inattentive and hyperactive-impulsive). Affected cognitive (executive) functions include those needed to manage daily life tasks such as attending to, organizing, and processing information, regulating emotions, motivation, and creating a working memory. ADHD affects around 5% of those under age 18, mostly boys, and persists to adulthood in about 30% to 50% of cases.[6]

PATHOPHYSIOLOGY

The exact cause of ADHD is often unknown and, similar to other alterations in mood, attention, and behavior, appears to be triggered by a combination of genetic and environmental factors. Previous infection or trauma of the brain has been implicated in some cases. Heritability has been estimated at 75%; siblings with ADHD are three to four times more likely to develop ADHD than those without affected siblings.[6] Specifically, gene variants associated with impairment of dopamine transmission are the likely genetic contributor. In about 9% of cases, the gene variant *LPHN3* is implicated. Potential environmental risk factors, in children who are genetically susceptible, include alcohol use or smoking during pregnancy, exposure to lead, insecticides, or food preservatives and dyes, very low birth weight, experiencing violence or abuse, and traumatic brain injury.

Changes in the brain structure and function associated with ADHD include the following:

- Impairment of dopamine and norepinephrine and lack of modulation of executive functions in the prefrontal cortex
- Reduced volume of the left-sided prefrontal cortex
- Thinning of the posterior parietal cortex

Clinical Manifestations

Clinical manifestations are related to reduced executive functioning and present as inattention, hyperactivity, restlessness, impulsivity, disruptive behavior, difficulties in school or work, and difficulties in social situations. Table 11.2 differentiates predominantly inattentive type from predominantly hyperactive-impulsive type.

DIAGNOSTIC CRITERIA

The diagnosis of ADHD is based on the patient history, reported behaviors observed by parents or teachers, and a mental status examination. There is no laboratory test for ADHD, although it is important to rule out any physical or other mental health conditions that may cause similar symptoms. The DSM-5 criteria are three to four times more likely to reach the conclusion of ADHD than the ICD-10. As mentioned, there are three subtypes. Diagnosis is based on the presence of clinical manifestations onset prior to age 12, across multiple settings (home, school, etc.), for at least 6 months, and ultimately causing interruptions in school or work, home, and social situations.

Table 11.2 Manifestations of ADHD Based on DSM-5 Subtype

Predominantly Inattentive	Predominantly Hyperactive-Impulsive
• Easily distracted • Missing details • Forgetful • Difficulty focusing attention on a task or when learning something new • Losing pencils, books, or other things needed to complete assignments or tasks • Daydreaming • Easily confused • Difficulty processing information as quickly and accurately as others • Struggles to follow instructions • Miss social cues	• Unable to sit still at school, during dinner, doing homework, or while doing any activities requiring stillness • Continuous talking • Touch and play with everything, moving quickly from one item to the next • Constantly in motion • Difficulty doing quiet tasks or activities • Impatient • Emotionally demonstrative • Act without regard for consequences • Difficulty waiting • Interruptive • Difficulty managing anger

ADHD, attention-deficit hyperactivity disorder.

TREATMENT

Treatment involves psychotherapy and medications alone or in combination. Physical exercise has been shown in multiple studies to improve behavior and motor skills in those with ADHD. Cognitive-behavioral therapy or just behavioral therapy are mainstays of treatment and have shown to be highly effective and often used as first-line treatment. Paradoxically, stimulant drugs are the most often used medications to treat ADHD. Although usually safe, their use is controversial and highly debated due to the potential for adverse effects, addiction, and dependence if misused or if use is prolonged. In short-term use, however, the vast majority of patients experience at least some improvements in attention, hyperactivity, and impulsivity.

Autism Spectrum Disorders

Autism is a neurodevelopmental disorder with its onset in early childhood. It is characterized by the classical triad of: impaired social interaction, impaired verbal and nonverbal communication, and a repetitive pattern of movement, interests, or behaviors. Autism is considered one of the autism spectrum disorders (ASDs). The other two ASDs are Asperger syndrome, similar to autism but with higher cognitive functioning and language development, and pervasive development disorder, which is diagnosed when the complete criteria for autism or Asperger syndrome are not met. Autism affects over 20 million people worldwide. In the United States, about 1 in 68 children were identified with an ASD; boys are diagnosed five times more often than girls.[7]

PATHOPHYSIOLOGY

Autism affects the information-processing centers of the brain, altering nerve cell-to-synapse connections. Although the exact etiology has not been determined, a complex interplay of environmental and genetic factors is suspected. The risk for autism is known to be increased with maternal exposure to teratogens, such as pollution, infections, heavy metals, and toxins, most notably within the first 8 weeks after conception. There is also a high risk with maternal valproate (a seizure drug) use during pregnancy. For these reasons, it is believed that autism is triggered very early in fetal development. The genetic basis is still under investigation. Autism cannot be traced to a single-gene mutation or to a single chromosomal abnormality. The genetic defect is not inherited, that is, it is not found in the (parent) germ cells. There is evidence, however, that autism is heritable and involves multiple genes, the environment, and epigenetic factors. For example, in identical twins, the rate of autism in one sibling is significantly increased if the other twin is diagnosed with autism.

The pathophysiologic changes and clinical manifestations that occur as a result of autism are evident among several regions of the brain, including the cerebellum, and frontal and temporal lobes. Deficits are universally found in social and emotional functioning. Patients with autism show a strong preference for nonsocial situations and stimuli, difficulties with language and face processing, difficulties empathizing, and delays in processing or rejection of certain visual and auditory stimuli (Fig. 11.8). One theory posits that autism results from low connectivity and thereby underfunctioning of neurons in high-level processes, such as those between the cortex and frontal lobe. This is coupled with high connectivity in lower-order brain areas, such as within the hemispheres of the cortex. Specific findings include:

- Reduced neuroanatomical connections to the frontal lobe
- Disrupted synaptic formation
- Thinning of the corpus collosum
- Greater myelination in the frontal cortex and less myelination in the temporal/parietal junction
- Reduced GABA-β receptors in the limbic cortex
- Disorganization of the architecture of the prefrontal cortex and temporal cortex

Endocrine and immune systems also appear to play an important role. A number of studies have uncovered biochemical changes that may occur with autism. For example, elevated serotonin levels, lactic acid, and cytokines are noted in some patients with autism pointing toward neuroendocrine and inflammatory influences.

CLINICAL MANIFESTATIONS

Clinical manifestations in ASD tend to become noticeable after 6 months of age and are well-established by 3 years of age. Manifestations are highly variable and represent the spectrum of autism from very mild displays of odd social, communication, and behavior (Asperger's) to completely silent, severe repetitive behaviors as with pervasive developmental disorder. The following are potential manifestations that can occur in each characteristic of the ASD triad:

- Impaired social interaction
  - Lack intuition and inattentive to social cues

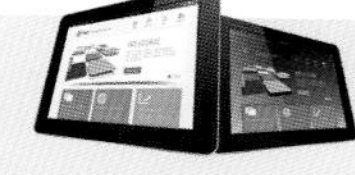

RESEARCH NOTES

The media is saturated with reports of children getting autism from the measles, mumps, and rubella (MMR) vaccine. The concern is most notably the time of diagnosis, which often occurs just weeks to months after routine scheduled childhood vaccinations. These anecdotes that autism may be linked with vaccinations have not been supported by research. A large study of 1,000 children over 5 years, conducted by the Centers for Disease Control and Prevention, found that vaccinations have no effect on the risk of developing an ASD. More specifically, exposure to antibody-stimulating proteins or polysaccharides from vaccines administered between the ages of 3 months and 2 years did not increase a child's risk of developing an ASD.[8]

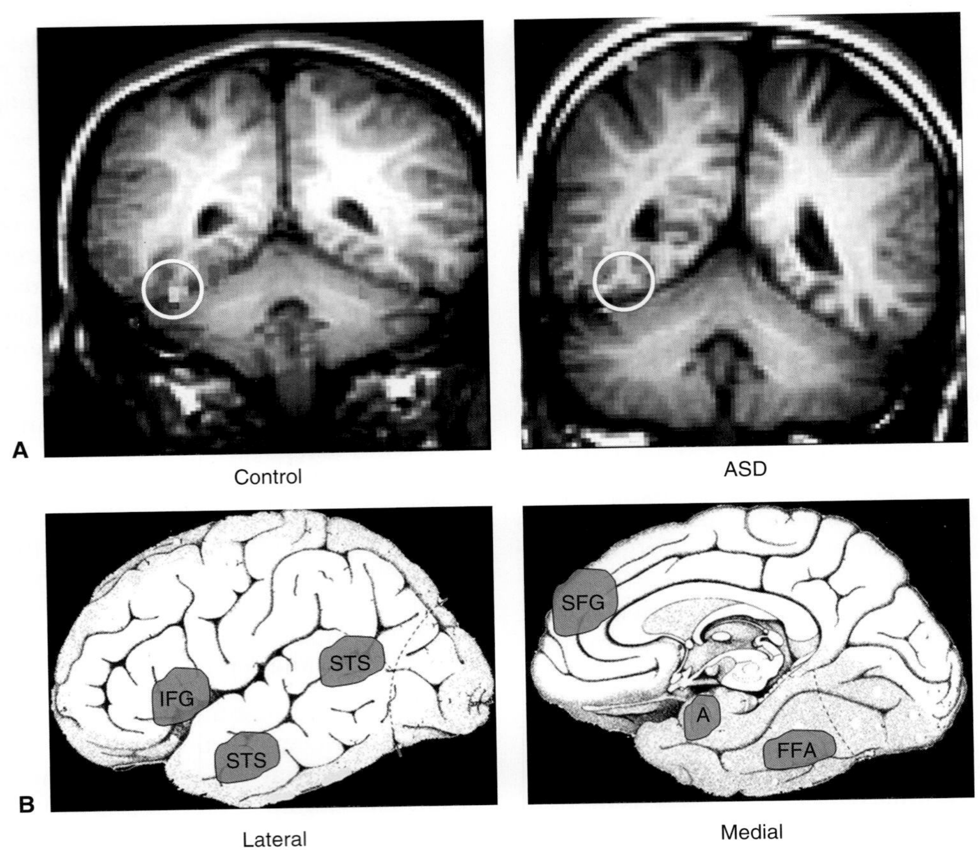

Figure 11.8. Functional magnetic resonance imaging (MRI) abnormalities observed in autism spectrum disorder (ASD). **A:** These coronal MRI images show the cerebral hemispheres above, the cerebellum below, and a circle over the fusiform gyrus of the temporal lobe. The examples illustrate the frequent finding of hypoactivation of the fusiform gyrus to faces in an adolescent boy with ASD **(right)** compared with an age- and IQ-matched unaffected control subject **(left)**. Note the lack of face activation in the boy with ASD but average levels of nonface object activation. **B:** Schematic diagrams of the brain from lateral and medial orientations illustrating the broader array of brain areas found to be hypoactive in ASD during a variety of cognitive and perceptual tasks that are explicitly social in nature. Some evidence suggests that these areas are linked to form a "social brain" network. A, amygdale (hypoactive during a variety of social tasks); FG, fusiform gyrus, also known as the fusiform face area (hypoactive during perception of personal identity); IFG, inferior frontal gyrus (hypoactive during facial expression imitation); pSTS, posterior superior temporal sulcus (hypoactive during perception of facial expressions and eye gaze tasks); SFG, superior frontal gyrus (hypoactive during theory of mind tasks, i.e., when taking another person's perspective). (Reprinted from Volkmar F, Lord C, Klin A, et al. Autism and the pervasive developmental disorders. In: Martin A, Volkmar F, eds. *Lewis' Child and Adolescent Psychiatry*. Philadelphia, PA: Lippincott Williams & Wilkins; 2007:387.)

    - Less eye contact, smiling, responsiveness to own name
    - Unable to recognize emotions or empathize with others
    - Difficulty with imaginative play
    - Exaggerated negative response to social stimuli, such as being touched
- Impaired verbal and nonverbal communication
    - Delayed speech development
    - Lack of integration between gestures, words, and intent (i.e., do not point at objects to show want or interest)
    - Display **echolalia** (repeating another's words)
- Repetitive pattern of movement, interests, or behaviors
    - Hand flapping, head rolling, body rocking, picking at skin, head banging
    - Compulsive or ritualistic behaviors, such as repeatedly arranging objects in a line or sorting
    - Resistance to change in the environment and routine
    - Narrow or restricted focus, interests, or activities

In addition, many of those with autism have poor muscle tone, incoordination, or toe walking. There can be developmental **regression**, that is, loss of previously achieved developmental milestones, such as loss of verbal skills. A high pain tolerance and lack of response to injury can occur.

DIAGNOSTIC CRITERIA

The DSM-5 outlines diagnostic criteria for ASD using the classical triad of symptoms above. Reliable and valid screening tools have been developed to aid in determining the presence of symptoms, severity, and impact. The classical triad of symptoms above must be present starting in early childhood and impair or limit daily functioning. Both components are required for diagnosis of ASD.

TREATMENT

Treatment for autism includes intensive, individualized, socially and behaviorally oriented therapeutic and educational programs guided by a qualified therapist and special education teacher. Therapy may include speech, occupational, and physical therapies. Commonly employed therapies include cognitive-behavioral interventions and language training. Pharmacologic approaches are not indicated for autism but may help with comorbid conditions, such as anxiety or ADHD.

Schizophrenia

Schizophrenia is a psychotic mental health disorder that affects how patients perceive the world. Patients with schizophrenia experience hallucinations, seeing or hearing things that are not actually there, delusions, fixed false beliefs, and disorganized speech and behavior. The onset is most commonly in late adolescence and early adulthood. Worldwide prevalence is estimated at 4 per 1,000 population.[9]

PATHOPHYSIOLOGY

The exact cause of schizophrenia is not known. The complex interactions of genetics, perinatal risks, and socioenvironmental triggers are implicated. The greatest risk factor is having a family history of schizophrenia (Fig. 11.9). Patients who have a first-degree relative with schizophrenia have a 10% higher risk. This percent jumps to 40% for the child when both parents have been diagnosed with schizophrenia. Similarly, concordance among monozygotic twins is 40% to 50%. Gene studies have identified over 100 potential gene loci and potential structural variants, some of which overlap with bipolar disorder and alcohol dependence. In patients who have no family history of schizophrenia, this may be the result of a spontaneous mutation.

Prenatal/perinatal infection (particularly certain viral infections such as influenza), fetal hypoxia, and malnourishment have been found to act in a synergistic way to promote the onset of schizophrenia in offspring who are genetically susceptible. Heavy marijuana and other drug use may hasten the onset of schizophrenia as well in susceptible individuals.

The development of schizophrenia leads to changes in the immune system, specifically overactive inflammatory cytokines, and subtle structural and functional brain changes in the frontal lobes, hippocampus, and temporal lobes. Specific changes include (Fig. 11.10) the following:

- Enlarged ventricles
- Decreased brain volume in temporal and prefrontal areas
- Loss of gray and white matter
- Dopamine cortical hyperactivity and limbic hypoactivity
- Reduced glutamate (neurotransmitter) receptor function and low glutamate levels

CLINICAL MANIFESTATIONS

The onset of clinical manifestations often occurs in adolescence and young adulthood and can range from mild to severe psychosis. Signs and symptoms include hallucinations (such as hearing voices), delusions, and disorganized thoughts and speech. Patients with schizophrenia can also present with social withdrawal, poor hygiene, poor judgment, and loss of motivation. There can be paranoia and

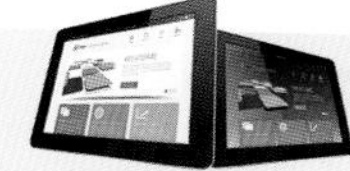

RESEARCH NOTES

The National Autism Center has completed the second phase of the National Standards Project, which has the goal of establishing a set of evidence-based standards for educational and behavioral interventions for children and young adults with ASDs. From this 2014 report, 14 interventions were identified as established and known to be effective. These include cognitive-behavioral interventions, language training, modeling, parent training, scripting, and peer training. Examples of therapies with a lack of evidence supporting effective use include auditory integration training, facilitated communication, gluten-free diets, and others. A full copy of this report can be requested at: http://www.nationalautismcenter.org/resources/.

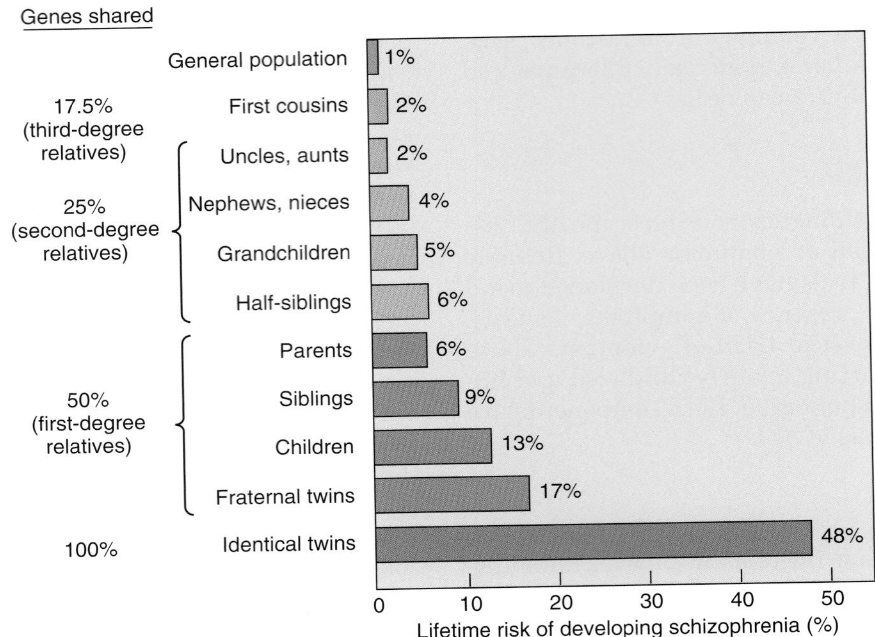

Figure 11.9. The familial nature of schizophrenia. The risk of developing schizophrenia increases with the number of shared genes, suggesting a genetic basis for the disease. (Adapted from Gottesman II. *Schizophrenia Genesis.* New York: WH Freeman, 1991, p. 96.)

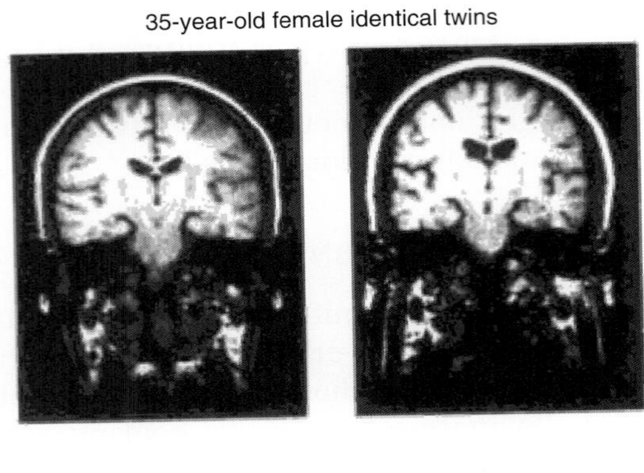

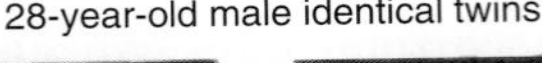

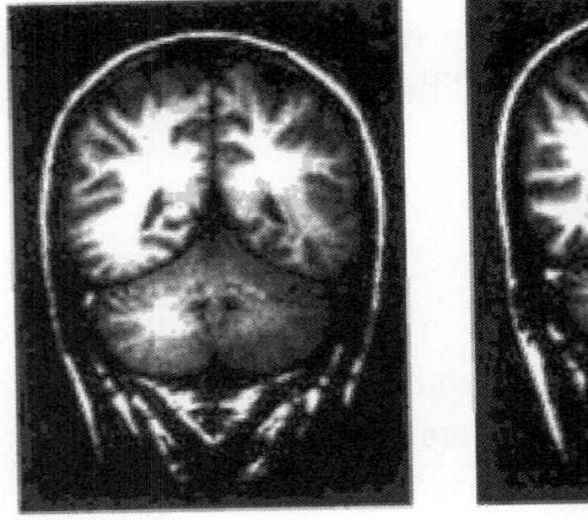

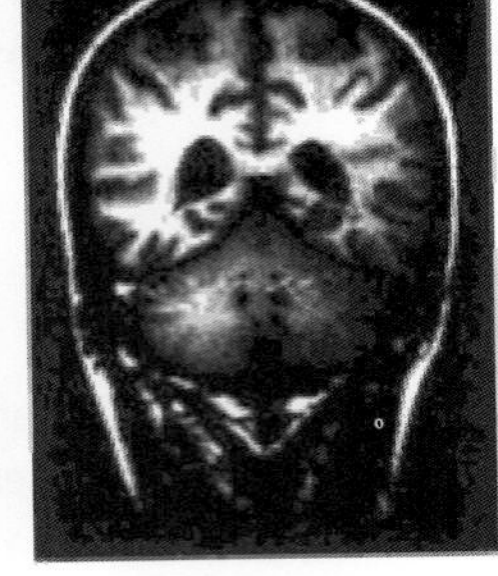

Figure 11.10. Coronal magnetic resonance imaging of two sets of twins discordant for schizophrenia. The enlarged lateral ventricles are readily apparent in the subjects on the right. (Courtesy of Drs. E. Fuller Torrey and Daniel Weinberger.)

impairments of memory, attention, and cognitive processing speed.

DIAGNOSTIC CRITERIA

The diagnosis of schizophrenia is based on the patient history, reported behaviors observed by others, and a comprehensive clinical assessment. There is no laboratory test for schizophrenia, although it is important to rule out any physical or other mental health conditions that may cause similar symptoms. To be diagnosed with schizophrenia, at least two indicators (delusions, hallucinations, or disorganized speech) have to be met for at least 1 month, with a significant impact on school or work, home, and social functioning for at least 6 months.

TREATMENT

Schizophrenia is treated with antipsychotic medications, and psychological and social support. Treatment can be a challenge since many patients with schizophrenia have irrational or even paranoid thinking and do not believe they have a disease. Medication side effects are also a major issue and often impact adherence. Hospitalization may be necessary if the behavior is threatening to the patient or society.

SUMMARY

- Mood is an internal, subjective psychological state, which directs how a person feels and perceives the world. Regulation of mood can be traced through the limbic system.
- Neurotransmitters also play a critical role in mood regulation. Pharmacologic intervention in mood disorders most often targets one or more neurotransmitters.
- Attention is a culturally influenced process of selectively concentrating on information. It is both a cognitive process and a behavior as it involves the interaction of sensory cues and the corresponding actions. Attention processing and action are largely regulated by the reticular activating system (RAS). The RAS is comprised of several neuronal pathways beginning with startling sensory input moving through reticular formation to the nuclei of the thalamus and outward to the parietal and temporal cortices and limbic system. Executive processing (frontal lobe and basal ganglia) allows attention to become connected with working memory, problem solving, and other higher-order functions.
- Behavior is how people respond and act in a given situation. As with mood, the frontal lobe of the brain is the primary region responsible for regulating behavior. This lobe integrates all aspects of behavior including personality, perception, planning, self-awareness, judgment, mood, attention, memory, motivation, sexuality, expressive language, and social and emotional intelligence.
- Generating appropriate behaviors for a given situation requires a complex interplay of cognitive and behavioral processes. Behavior will be based on noticing, perceiving, short-term and long-term memory (past experiences), current social expectations, mood, personality, motivation/inhibition, culture, consideration of all possible actions, planning, and deciding. All these occur within a matter of seconds and with little conscious effort.
- Alterations in the brain, limbic system connections, or neurotransmission can result in impairments of mood, attention, and behavior. The frontal lobe and corresponding limbic system structures are particularly vulnerable.
- When the prefrontal cortex suffers an injury, the patient loses the sense of social responsibility, concentration, abstract thinking, and problem solving. Impaired amygdalas sever the connection between social intelligence and memory. Lesions of the hypothalamus interfere with appropriate responses to thermal regulation, hunger, thirst, sexuality, and aggression toward others.
- Neurotransmission impairments can lead to apathy, inattentiveness, and motor deficits as with low levels of dopamine, or agitation, restlessness, and psychosis as with high levels of dopamine. Deficits in serotonin have been associated with anxiety, obsessions, and compulsions.
- Rarely are there laboratory tests or imaging studies that can confirm a psychiatric diagnosis. Diagnosis most often relies on patient history and reported observations of others.
- The most widely used categorical criteria for diagnosing alterations in mood, attention, and behavior are found in the American Psychiatric Association's fifth edition of the *Diagnostic and Statistical Manual of Mental Disorders* (DSM-5) and the World Health Organization's *International Statistical Classification of Diseases and Related Health Problems* (ICD-10).
- Treatments for alterations in mood, attention, and behavior include psychotherapy, pharmacotherapy, counseling, alternative/complementary therapies, and social support.

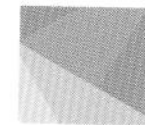

CASE STUDY 11.1

KT, age 42, presents to the emergency department with a complaint of having a "heart attack." She reports chest pain, apprehension, trembling, shaking, confusion, dizziness, nausea, and difficulty breathing. Her EKG is normal and she is found not to be experiencing a myocardial infarction. After further exploration, it is discovered that KT has a significant number of life stressors and a family history of anxiety. She is diagnosed with panic disorder.

1. Outline the process that is most likely occurring in this woman's body.
2. What is the etiology of panic disorder?
3. How do the expected clinical manifestations match what she is presenting?
4. What diagnostic tests could be used?
5. What treatment measures would you anticipate?

Log on to the Internet. Search for a relevant journal article or Web site (such as http://emedicine.medscape.com/article/287913-overview) that details panic disorder, and confirm your predictions.

CASE STUDY 11.2

PJ, 21 years old, is a nursing student at a small liberal arts college. He has always been told that he is "quirky" by others but has recently begun repetitively counting the stairs to his apartment and, if he misses one or it is not timed perfectly, he must go to the bottom and begin again. He is not sure why he participates in this ritual, but he explains that he is terrified of personal harm if he does not. He is diagnosed with obsessive-compulsive disorder.

1. Outline the process that is most likely occurring in this man's body. What specific brain changes are seen in OCD?
2. What is the etiology of OCD?
3. How do the expected clinical manifestations match what he is presenting?
4. What diagnostic tests could be used?
5. What treatment measures would you anticipate?

Log on to the Internet. Search for a relevant journal article or Web site (such as http://emedicine.medscape.com/article/1934139-overview) that details OCD, and confirm your predictions.

PRACTICE EXAM QUESTIONS

1. A patient is considering various treatment alternatives and choosing a course of action. Which prefrontal region is active during this process?
   a. Lateral
   b. Orbitofrontal
   c. Ventromedial
   d. Retroparietal

2. Given the action of each, which neurotransmitter is responsible for your heightened alertness during your tour through a haunted house?
   a. Epinephrine
   b. Norepinephrine
   c. Serotonin
   d. Dopamine

3. Executive processing refers to the ability to:
   a. Move quickly to get out of harm's way
   b. Apply for a job
   c. Solve problems
   d. See an oncoming car

4. Psychosis, or the loss of touch with reality, is characterized by:
   a. Aggressive anger
   b. Excess neurotransmitters
   c. Anhedonia
   d. Delusions

5. Which of the following is not a general treatment measure for altered mood, attention, or behavior?
   a. Electoconvulsant therapy
   b. Pharmacotherapy
   c. Psychotherapy
   d. Social support

6. Those with generalized anxiety disorder are likely to have overactivation of ______ with anxiety-provoking events:
   a. Serotonin
   b. The amygdala
   c. Norepinephrine
   d. The hypothalamus

7. Which of the following clinical manifestations is typical of PTSD?
   a. Hyperthyroidism
   b. Exaggerated startle response
   c. Repeated traumatic events
   d. Apathy

8. Which of the following best describes melancholic depression, one of the subtypes of major depressive disorder?
   a. Depressive episodes in the late fall and winter with excessive anhedonia
   b. Depressive episodes most notable in the early morning with excessive weight loss and guilt
   c. Disabling depression after giving birth and lasting up to 3 months
   d. Depression characterized by immobility or purposeless movements, the inability to speak, and stupor

9. Which of the following is not a brain change noted in those with ADHD?
   a. Impairment of dopamine and norepinephrine
   b. Reduced volume of the left-sided prefrontal cortex
   c. Thinning of the posterior parietal cortex
   d. Enlarged bilateral ventricles

10. A child with autism repeats everything you say. You recognize this behavior as:
    a. Echolalia
    b. Intentional antisocial behavior
    c. Lack of integration between gestures, words, and intent
    d. Delayed speech development

DISCUSSION AND APPLICATION

1. What did I know about altered mood and behavior before today?
2. What body processes are affected by altered mood and behavior?
3. What are the potential etiologies for altered mood and behavior?
4. Who is most at risk for developing altered mood and behavior? How can these alterations be prevented?

5. What are the human differences that affect the etiology, risk, or course of altered mood and behavior?
6. What clinical manifestations are expected in the course of altered mood and behavior?
7. What special diagnostic tests are useful in determining the diagnosis and course of altered mood and behavior?
8. What are the goals of care for individuals with altered mood and behavior?
9. How does the concept of altered mood and behavior build on what I have learned in the previous chapter and in previous courses?
10. How can I use what I have learned?

RESOURCES

Attention Deficit Disorder Association:
http://www.add.org

Autism Society:
http://www.autism-society.org/

Diagnostic and Statistical Manual of Mental Disorders (DSM-5):
http://www.psychiatry.org/psychiatrists/practice/dsm/dsm-5

International Classification of Diseases (ICD-10):
http://www.icd10data.com/

National Institute of Mental Health:
http://www.nimh.nih.gov

References

1. Kessler RC, McGonagle KA, Zhao S, et al. Lifetime and 12-month prevalence of DSM-III-R psychiatric disorders in the United States: results from the National Comorbidity Survey. *Arch Gen Psychiatry*. 1994;51(1):8–19.
2. U.S. Department of Veterans Affairs. PTSD: National Center for PTSD. http://www.ptsd.va.gov/public/PTSD-overview/basics/how-common-is-ptsd.asp. Accessed November 13, 2015.
3. Pratt LA, Brody DJ. Depression in the United States household population, 2009–2012. http://www.cdc.gov/nchs/data/databriefs/db172.pdf. Accessed November 13, 2015. National Center for Health Statistics Data Brief, December 2014, No. 172.
4. Kendler KS, Gatz M, Gardner CO, et al. A Swedish national twin study of lifetime major depression. *Am J Psychiatr*. 2006;163(1):109–114. doi:10.1176/appi.ajp.163.1.109. PMID: 16390897.
5. Cox GR, Callahan P, Churchill R, et al. Psychological therapies versus antidepressant medication, alone and in combination for depression in children and adolescents. *Cochrane Database of Syst Rev.* 2014;11:CD008324. doi:10.1002/14651858.CD008324.pub3. PMID: 25433518.
6. Centers for Disease Control and Prevention. Attention-deficit/hyperactivity disorder (ADHD). http://www.cdc.gov/ncbddd/adhd/data.html. Accessed November 13, 2015.
7. Centers for Disease Control and Prevention. Prevalence of autism spectrum disorder—autism and developmental disabilities monitoring network, 11 sites, United States, 2010. *MMWR* 2014;63(No. SS 2):1–21.
8. Hammer LD, Curry ES, Harlor AD, et al. Increasing immunization coverage. *Pediatrics*. 2010;125(6):1295–1304.
9. Saha S, Chant D, Welham J, et al. A systematic review of the prevalence of schizophrenia. *PLoS Med*. 2005;2(5):e141. doi:10.1371/journal.pmed.0020141.

Find additional resources for this chapter at http:thePoint.lww.com thePoint®

Chapter

12 Altered Somatic and Special Sensory Function

LEARNING OUTCOMES

1. Define and use the key terms listed in this chapter.
2. Describe the mode of transmission of neural impulses involved with the sensations of pain, vision, and hearing.
3. Identify pathways for the integration of neural and sensory experiences.
4. Indicate common mechanisms of alterations in vision and hearing.
5. Determine processes that contribute to the perception of pain.
6. Describe alterations in sensory experiences and the associated pathophysiologic manifestations.
7. Identify common signs and symptoms of alterations in sensation.
8. Describe diagnostic tests and treatment strategies relevant to alterations in hearing, vision, and pain management.
9. Predict functional impairments resulting from alterations in sensation.
10. Apply concepts of sensory alterations to select clinical models.

INTRODUCTION

How do you feel when you see a beautiful sunset? Hear the voice of someone special? Smell your favorite meal cooking on the stove? Close your fingers in the car door? Many sensations cause responses such as wonder, happiness, contentment, and pain. Your perceptions of the world around you are shaped by the many sensory cues you take in, which stimulate predictable reactions. Alterations in these sensations can cause significant impairment in physical, psychologic, and social functioning. A basic understanding of the function of sensory systems promotes the ability to anticipate deficits that may occur when these systems are altered. The focus of this chapter is alteration in somatosensory and special sensory function. Table 12.1 provides a description of sensations resulting from stimulation of specific somatosensory and special sensory receptors. The modules target pain and alterations in the special senses of vision and hearing. The clinical models in this chapter are selected to help apply concepts of altered somatosensory and sensory function.

Table 12.1 Neurons of the Somatosensory System

Neuron Type	Receptor Location	Sensation
General somatic afferent neurons	Wide distribution with branches throughout the body	Pain, touch, temperature
Special somatic afferent neurons	Muscle, tendons, and joints	Position and body movement
General visceral afferent neurons	Visceral structures	Fullness and discomfort

Module 1 Pain

Pain is a common, yet complex sensation. The typically unpleasant sensation is often associated with an emotional response and evidence of tissue damage. Protective reflex responses often limit the damage caused by an injury-provoking stimulus. Continued pain sensation reminds us of the damage and us helps to protect the injury during the healing process. Pain is transmitted by the somatosensory system, along with the sensations of touch, temperature, and body position.

Somatosensory System

Sensory systems relay information throughout the body from the periphery to the central nervous system (CNS) using sensory receptors, ascending pathways, and processing centers. Stimuli are received, which allow people to respond to the world around them. Afferent pathways, introduced in Chapter 10, promote communication from structures in the periphery to processing centers in the brain.

The diversity of the somatosensory system is the result of the receptors and pathways that are associated with the sensations of pain (nociception), touch, temperature, and proprioception (body position). A variety of receptor types result in specific somatosensory responses. These types include:

1. Mechanoreceptors: mechanical forces—receptor stretching alters membrane permeability
   a. Stretch receptors of muscles
   b. Skin receptors: touch, pain, cold, heat
2. Thermoreceptors: radiant heat energy
3. Nociceptors: pain

Table 12.2 describes the neurons responsible for some of these specific functions.

Stop and Consider
Based on the sensations involved, what other nerves do you think are involved in the somatosensory system?

SOMATOSENSORY NEURONAL ORGANIZATION

Neurons are organized in an ordered series, and information is directed toward the processing centers in the thalamus and cerebral cortex (Fig. 12.1). These neurons are categorized as follows:

- First-order neurons: communicate sensory information from the periphery to the CNS
- Second-order neurons: relay sensory input from reflex networks and sensory pathways directly to the thalamus
- Third-order neurons: communicate sensory information from the thalamus to the cerebral cortex

Interneurons are active throughout this network and modify the sensory information before it arrives at the processing centers. The numbers of neurons increase consistent with their order; third-order neurons are present in the greatest quantity.

SOMATOSENSORY NEURONAL TRANSMISSION

Somatosensory impulses are transmitted by a unique system of receptors and pathways. The sensory unit comprising the dorsal root ganglia (cell body, peripheral branch, and central axon) responds in distinct ways to different stimuli because of the specific nature of their associated receptors and nerve fibers.

Dorsal Root Ganglia Fibers

Transmission of nerve impulses along the fibers of the dorsal root ganglia depends on the diameter

Table 12.2 Sensory Receptor Forms and Functions

Receptor Type	Function	Example
Mechanoreceptor	Tactile skin sensation	Merkel cells
	Deep-tissue sensation	Ruffini endings
		Meissner corpuscles
		Pacinian corpuscle
		Hair follicle end organ
		Free nerve endings
	Hearing	Cochlear sound receptors
	Proprioception	Merkel cells
		Ruffini endings
		Pacinian corpuscles
Photoreceptor	Vision	Rods and cones
Chemoreceptor	Taste	Taste bud receptors
	Smell	Olfactory epithelium receptors
Nociceptor	Pain	Free nerve endings

of the nerve fiber and nerve fiber myelination. The three types of nerve fibers that are involved in the conduction of somatosensory impulses are type A, B, and C. Type A fibers have the largest diameter and are myelinated, accounting for their rapid rate of impulse conduction. The sensations transmitted by type A delta fibers include pressure, touch, cold sensation, and heat pain. Type A alpha and beta fibers may promote inhibitory effects, diminishing the sensation of pain. Type B fibers are also myelinated but have a smaller diameter than type A fibers, accounting for their slower rate of conduction. Mechanoreceptors in the cutaneous and subcutaneous areas of the skin stimulate nerve impulses along type B fibers. Type C fibers are unmyelinated and have the smallest diameter, leading to the slowest conduction rate of these three fiber types. Warm-hot sensation, as well as mechanical, chemical, heat-induced, and cold-induced pain sensations, is transmitted along type C fibers.

Dermatome Innervation

Dermatomes are innervated by a single pair of dorsal root ganglia and reflect the segmental organization of the spinal cord, as described in Chapter 10. Overlap of dermatome processes occurs in peripheral

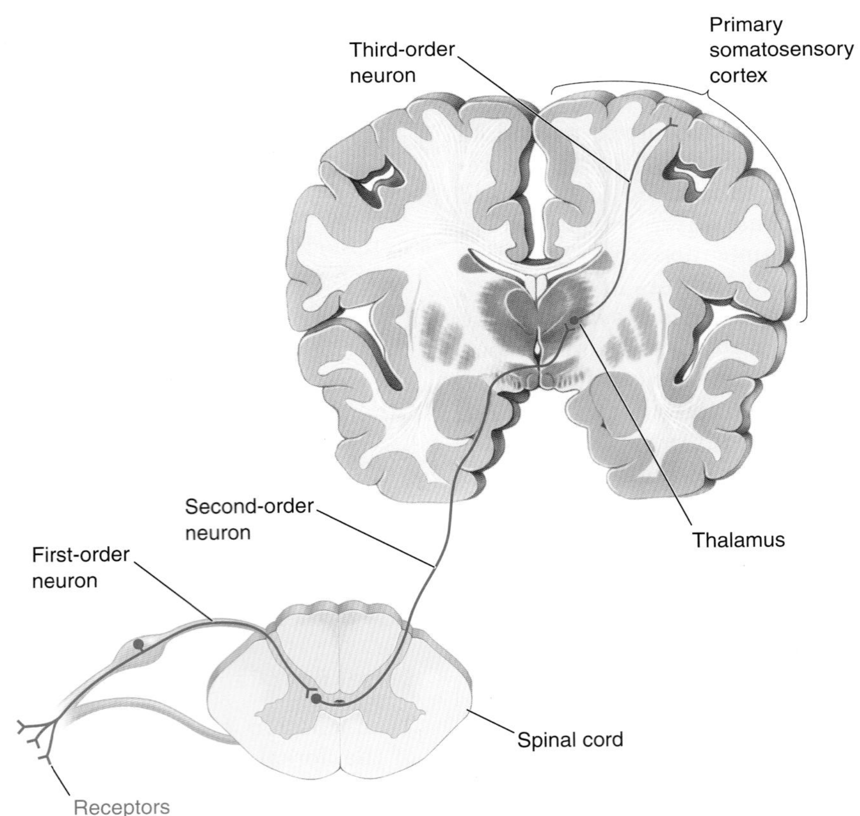

Figure 12.1. Arrangement of first-, second-, and third-order neurons of the somatosensory system.

processes on the body surface and central processes in the spinal cord, providing some redundancy of the conduction system.

Two separate pathways are involved in the transmission of information involved in perception, arousal, and motor control. The **discriminative pathway** communicates sensory information, including discriminative touch and spatial orientation. This pathway integrates input from multiple receptors using the primary dorsal root ganglion neuron, the dorsal column neuron, and the thalamic neuron. Stimulation of this pathway results from vibration, touch, muscle, or joint movement. The discriminative pathway allows the identification of an object based on touch or the location of skin touch in two different areas, known as **two-point discrimination**. The **anterolateral pathway** involves both the anterior and lateral spinothalamic pathways and is characterized by multiple synapses and slow conduction. The sensations of pain, temperature, crude touch, and pressure not requiring the specific location of the origin of the stimulus are transmitted along this pathway. Increased wakefulness stimulated by a "startle" reaction exists due to the many fibers that travel to the reticular activating system by sensory conduction in this pathway. Autonomic responses, such as increased blood pressure and heart rate, activation of sweat glands, dilation of pupils, and constriction of blood vessels, are also stimulated when impulses are conducted along this pathway.

SOMATOSENSORY PROCESSING

The awareness, recognition, identification, and interpretation of stimuli involve processing. After stimuli reach the thalamus, further refinement occurs in the somatosensory cortex of the brain. The primary somatosensory cortex receives sensory information from the thalamus. This information is relayed to the somatosensory association areas, which interpret the stimuli into learned perceptions.

SOMATOSENSORY MODALITIES

Somatosensory modalities refer to the specific nature of the perception of various stimuli. The subjective interpretation of a stimulus, such as the difference between temperature and touch, is determined by the ability of a receptor to detect an impulse, the transmission of the impulse to the CNS, and the interpretation of the refined impulse.

Stimulus Discrimination

Acuity refers to the ability to locate the site of the initiation of a stimulus. High acuity allows for fine distinction and requires a greater density of neurons. Acuity reflects the threshold necessary for a neuron to achieve an action potential (see Chapter 10). Variations of acuity in sensory fields contribute to different levels of distinction between impulses.

Tactile Stimulation

Transmission of tactile stimuli usually occurs via large, myelinated nerve fibers. Touch, pressure, and vibration stimuli are recognized by receptors in and near the skin (Fig. 12.2) and include:

- Free nerve endings (detection of touch and pressure)
- Meissner corpuscle (highly developed sense of touch)
- Merkel disks (movement of light objects over skin, vibration)
- Pacinian corpuscle (detection of vibration)
- Hair follicle receptor (detection of movement on the surface of the body)
- Ruffini ending (detection of heavy and continuous touch and pressure)

Thermal Sensation

Thermoreceptors (receptors that recognize thermal sensation) are located under the skin and include cold, warmth, and pain receptors (discussed later in this chapter). Thermal (warm and cold) receptors are sensitive to the differences in the temperature of objects that contact the skin. Thermal pain receptors respond to extremes in temperature. Transmission of thermal sensation is much slower than tactile impulse conduction.

Position Sensation

Limb/body movement and position sensation, independent of vision, are mediated by proprioceptive receptors, muscle spindle receptors, and Golgi tendon organs. Stretch receptors in the skin (Ruffini endings, pacinian corpuscles, and Merkel cells) also assist in proprioception. Somatosensory signals are transmitted via the posterior column and the vestibular system, and they are processed in the thalamus and cerebral cortex.

Pain

The sensation of pain is disruptive to the quality of life. Determination of pain character provides clues to the underlying cause and provides a target for treatment.

CHARACTERIZATION OF PAIN

The sensation of pain is the result of a noxious stimulation of pain fibers. When the stimulus is initiated

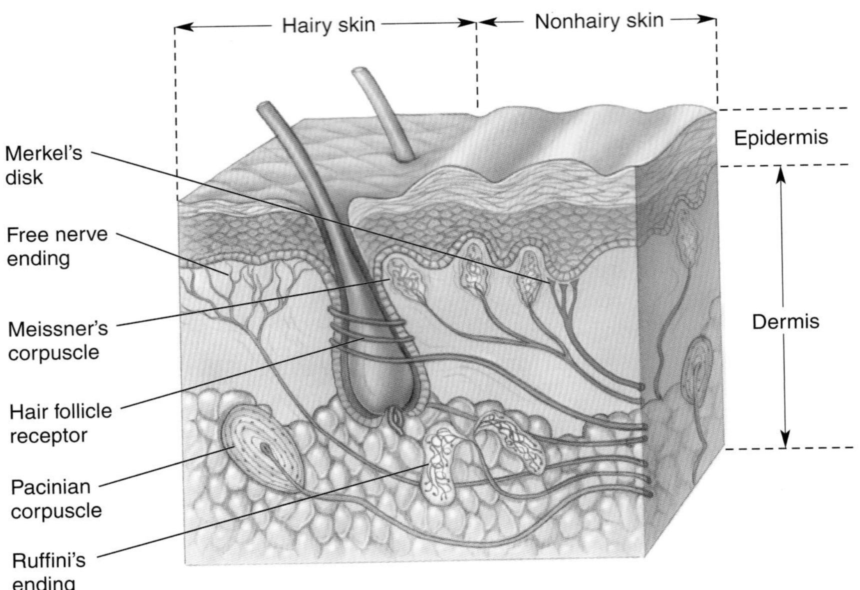

Figure 12.2. Cutaneous somatic sensory receptors. Distribution of sensory receptors in skin with and without hair. (Modified from Bear MF, Connors BW, Parasido MA. *Neuroscience: Exploring the Brain*. 3rd ed. Philadelphia, PA: Lippincott Williams & Wilkins; 2006.)

outside of the nervous system, the pain is characterized as **nociceptive**. Pain originating within the nervous system is termed **neurogenic** or **neuropathic**. Nociceptive pain involves specific receptors and pathways resulting in the sensation of pain. Neurogenic or neuropathic pain does not activate these receptors and does not follow a typical transmission pattern of impulse conduction.

CONDUCTION OF PAIN SENSATION

Nociception (pain sensation) involves free nerve endings stimulated by chemical, mechanical, or thermal stimuli, inducing autonomic and motor reflexes, which result in the interpretation of the stimuli as pain (Fig. 12.3). Events involved in this process include transduction, transmission, modulation, and perception. Box 12.1 summarizes these processes.

THEORIES OF PAIN

The theoretic origins of pain are based on an understanding of the neurophysiologic events associated with the initiation, transmission, and perception of pain. Two well accepted, traditional theories that attempt to explain the pain response include the pattern theory and the specificity theory, neither of which fully explains the origin, transmission, and perception of pain. The evolution of pain theory reflects the complexity of the pain sensation, incorporating the multiple dimensions and determinants of pain.

Pattern Theory

Pattern theory suggests that nerves transmitting pain impulses are shared with other senses. The perception of pain is derived from a specific pattern of neuronal impulse generation based on the type of stimulus and intensity, specifically the timing and location of impulse generation.[1] The shared pathways between pain and other somatosensory modalities influence the perceived sensation. The characteristics of receptor stimulation contribute to the specific somatosensory patterns, influenced by:

1. Duration of pain sensation
2. Quantity of tissue involved
3. The summation of impulses

An example of varying patterns of receptor stimulation and sensory perception includes the response of impulse generation through light touch and deep pressure. According to pattern theory, light, superficial skin pressure would generate low-frequency receptor firing and the perceived sensation of light touch. Conversely, deep skin pressure would generate high-frequency firing of the same receptor resulting in the perceived sensation of pain.

Specificity Theory

The **specificity theory** proposes that sensations of touch, warmth, cold, and pain involve distinct receptors and pathways unique to the specific sensation. The specific nature of impulse generation is proposed to begin in a specific pain receptor, transmitted along specific pathways leading to pain centers

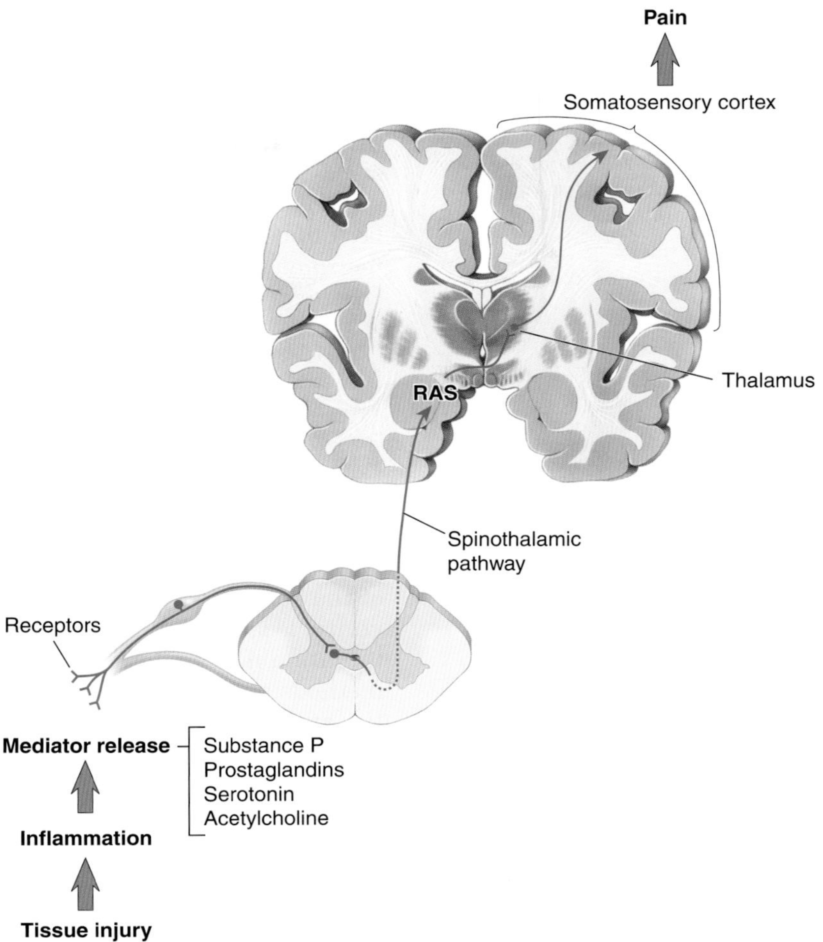

Figure 12.3. Mechanism of acute pain. Nociceptor stimulation is induced after tissue injury by release of inflammatory mediators. Impulses are transmitted to the dorsal horn of the spinal cord, synapsing with second-order neurons. Neurons cross and ascend via the spinothalamic pathway to the reticular activating system (RAS) and thalamus. The localization and perception of pain occurs in the somatosensory cortex.

in the brain where pain is perceived. Pain impulses travel from the periphery to the spinal cord, crossing to the opposite side at the synapses of the **substantia gelatinosa** (gray matter extending throughout the posterior horn of the spinal cord to the medulla oblongata). Impulses then ascend the specific pain pathways of the spinothalamic tract. The intensity of the pain is associated with the amount of tissue injured or damaged. For example, when the mechanoreceptor is stimulated, the impulse is transmitted on dedicated primary afferent neurons projecting to mechanoreceptor second-order neurons that synapse onto specific mechanoreceptive areas in the brain.[1]

Gate Control Theory

The **gate control theory** is one of the most well-known theories on the physiologic basis of pain, representing an explanation for pain that unites the contrasting principles underlying pattern and specificity theory. According to the gate control theory, peripheral receptors generating impulses along the primary afferent neurons enter the spinal cord in the substantia gelatinosa of the dorsal horn, serving as a gate, regulating the transmission of pain impulses.[1] The gate control theory proposes that stimulation of the large type A beta and alpha inhibitory fibers "close the gate" at the substantia gelatinosa, preventing crossover and inhibiting pain impulse conduction along type A delta and type C fibers, diminishing pain perception. Stimuli thought to promote transmission along type A beta and alpha fibers needed to close the gate include electrical stimulation, massage, scratching, or rubbing of the skin. Stimulation of small pain fibers promotes "opening the gate," activating neural transmission and perception of pain.

Intensity Theory

The intensity theory suggests that pain is an emotion that is the result of a stronger than usual stimulus.[1]

Box 12.1 Processes of Nociception

Transduction of noxious stimuli into a nerve impulse and depolarization of the nerve stimulates the conduction of the sensory impulse

- The electrical impulses promote the release of algesic (causing pain) substances, including substance P, hydrogen and potassium ions, serotonin, histamine, prostaglandins, and bradykinin

Transmission of nerve impulses from tissues to the CNS

- Occurs along type A (delta) and type C fibers
  - Rapidly conducting type A fibers
    - Produce sensations of sharp, stinging, or pin-prick–type local sensations
    - Induced by mechanical or thermal stimuli
  - Impulses along type C fibers producing a dull ache or burning general response
    - Induced by chemical stimuli
- Responses of the brain resulting from the transmission of impulses must be delivered back to the original site of stimulation.

Modulation of the pain occurs during transmission of the impulse

- Substances released in response to pain stimuli result from activation of inhibitory processes
  - Serotonin, norepinephrine, and endorphins
  - Inhibit the transmission of the pain impulse by slowing the release of nociceptive neurotransmitters

Perception of the pain response

- Involves the sensory (somatosensory cortex), emotional (limbic system), and subjective reactions to the stimuli
- Perception is varied among individuals because of the influence of
  - Pain threshold: the intensity of the pain required to achieve a response
  - Perceptual dominance: the existence of pain at another location which is given more attention
  - Pain tolerance: the degree to which pain is endured (duration or intensity) before initiating a response

Rather than a unique modality, this theory suggests that pain occurs as a result of intense stimulation of any sensory modality in the absence of distinct pathways for low- and high-threshold stimuli. An example of this type of pain generation is tactile stimulation that, as a single event, is not perceived as pain but when repeated a number of times achieves an intensity level that is perceived as painful.

Neuromatrix Theory

The **neuromatrix theory** suggests that pain is a multidimensional experience. Pain perception is the result of impulses generated along a widely distributed neural network in the brain (**body-self neuromatrix**), triggered either by sensory inputs or independent of identified stimulation.[1] The neuromatrix contains somatic, limbic, and thalamocortical components, integrating multiple sources of input resulting in the cognitive, affective, and sensory perceptions of pain.[2] Variations in the synaptic architecture of the neuromatrix are thought to be influenced by genetic, emotional, cultural, past experience, and stress regulation influences, contributing to individualized pain responses. Sensation patterns may be induced in the absence of a sensory trigger. The neuromatrix theory can help explain phantom and chronic pain.

Stop and Consider

Have you ever banged your head and began rubbing it in response to pain? How might this action decrease the pain sensation?

MANIFESTATIONS AND EVALUATION OF PAIN

Management of pain includes a careful evaluation of the subjective perception of pain. The nature, severity, location, initiating triggers, and patterns of radiation help to determine the cause and potential methods of treatment. Methods to objectively quantify an individual's pain, such as a pain drawing, can help determine severity of pain or evaluate pain control measures (Fig. 12.4). The classifications of pain are listed in Box 12.2.

TREATMENT OF PAIN

Pain relief, or analgesia, is the goal of pain treatment. Controlling pain to allow individuals to perform

Box 12.2 Classifications of Pain

Pain can be classified according to:

- Location
  - Cutaneous
  - Deep
  - Visceral
  - Referred
- Quality
  - Sharp
  - Burning
  - Diffuse
  - Throbbing
  - Stabbing
- Duration
  - Acute
    - Results from disease, inflammation, or injury to tissue
    - Sudden onset
    - Responsive to treatment
    - Self-limiting (lasting less than 3 months)
    - Associated with autonomic responses
  - Chronic
    - Persistent (lasting longer than 3 months)
    - Resistant to treatment
    - Associated with anorexia, insomnia, and depression

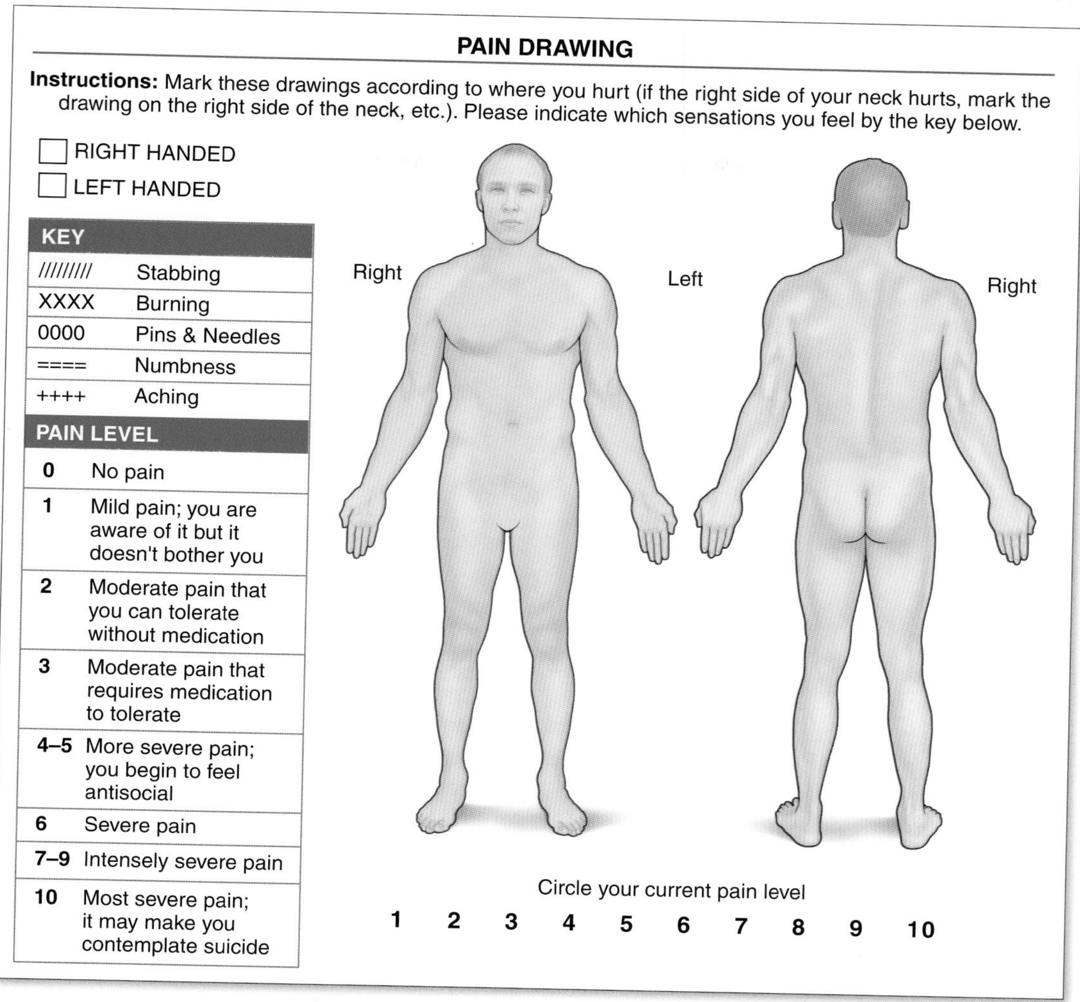

PAIN DRAWING

Instructions: Mark these drawings according to where you hurt (if the right side of your neck hurts, mark the drawing on the right side of the neck, etc.). Please indicate which sensations you feel by the key below.

☐ RIGHT HANDED
☐ LEFT HANDED

KEY	
/////////	Stabbing
XXXX	Burning
0000	Pins & Needles
====	Numbness
++++	Aching

PAIN LEVEL	
0	No pain
1	Mild pain; you are aware of it but it doesn't bother you
2	Moderate pain that you can tolerate without medication
3	Moderate pain that requires medication to tolerate
4–5	More severe pain; you begin to feel antisocial
6	Severe pain
7–9	Intensely severe pain
10	Most severe pain; it may make you contemplate suicide

Circle your current pain level

1 2 3 4 5 6 7 8 9 10

Figure 12.4. Tool for characterization of pain. Individuals are asked to mark body figures to identify location, severity, and character of pain. (Courtesy American Academy of Physical Medicine and Rehabilitation.)

activities of daily living is another goal of treatment. Several mechanisms of pain control are available. Box 12.3 lists available methods of pain control in adults. Newborns have complex behavioral, physiologic, and biochemical responses to pain and require special considerations in pain management. Infants are commonly subjected to painful procedures, such as heel lancing and circumcision. The nonpharmacologic interventions with the best evidence in the reduction of pain in infants include the behavioral strategies of nonnutritive sucking (e.g., pacifier), swaddling, rocking, and holding.[3]

Box 12.3 Methods of Pain Control

- Nonpharmacologic
  - Cognitive behavior interventions
    - Relaxation
      - Focus on lessening muscle tension
    - Distraction
      - Focus attention on stimuli not associated with pain
    - Cognitive reappraisal
      - Self-distraction
      - Focus on the positive aspects of the experience
    - Imagery
      - Use of imagination to develop a soothing mental picture
    - Biofeedback
      - Awareness of bodily function on a cognitive level
  - Physical agents
    - Heat
      - Increase in local circulation, reducing local ischemia and nociceptive stimulation
      - Modulation of pain
      - Release of endogenous opioids

- Cold
  - Vasoconstriction to decrease swelling and stimulation of nociceptive pain fibers
  - Reduced afferent activity
- Transcutaneous electrical nerve stimulation
  - Transmission of electrical impulses across the skin to peripheral nerve fibers
  - Stimulation of large fibers to modulate pain transmission
- Acupuncture
  - Insertion of needles at specific points on the body surface
  - Stimulate secretion of endorphins
  - Stimulate large fibers to modulate pain transmission

- Pharmacologic
  - Nonnarcotic analgesia (e.g., aspirin [acetylsalicylic acid], nonsteroidal anti-inflammatories, or acetaminophen)
    - Central and peripheral blockade of nerve impulses
    - Inhibition of cyclooxygenase enzymes, decreasing production of prostaglandins
    - Decreased sensitivity to bradykinin and histamine
  - Opioid analgesics (e.g., morphine, codeine)
    - Bind to mu, delta, and kappa receptors, modulating pain at the level of the spinal cord
    - Stimulate release of endogenous opioids, including enkephalins, endorphins, and dynorphins
  - Adjuvant analgesics (tricyclic antidepressants)
    - Block reuptake of serotonin from the synaptic cleft
    - Particularly useful in chronic pain

Module 2 Alterations in Vision

Vision is an important sensory function that informs us about the world around us. The processes resulting in sight are complex, involving the integration of eye structures, motor control, and neural control (Fig. 12.5).

Visual Structures and Function

Sight is achieved when light is reflected into the **cornea**, the clear, transparent structure that covers the exterior wall of the eye. Light then passes through the **pupil**, an opening in the **iris** (colored part of the eye). The pupil is able to control the amount of light that enters the eye, dilating to enhance light entry and constricting to decrease. Light entering the eye contacts the clear **lens**, responsible for fine-tuning of focus. The ability of the lens to change its shape, or **accommodate**, allows clear vision at a variety of distances. **Ciliary muscles** contract, promoting a rounder lens shape to focus an object at close range. Relaxation of ciliary muscles allows flattening of the lens and the ability to see objects at a distance.

Chambers are compartments in the eye. The anterior chamber sits behind the cornea. The lens and the iris are the remaining boundaries. The posterior chamber is positioned directly behind the iris, in front of the lens. The anterior chamber contains

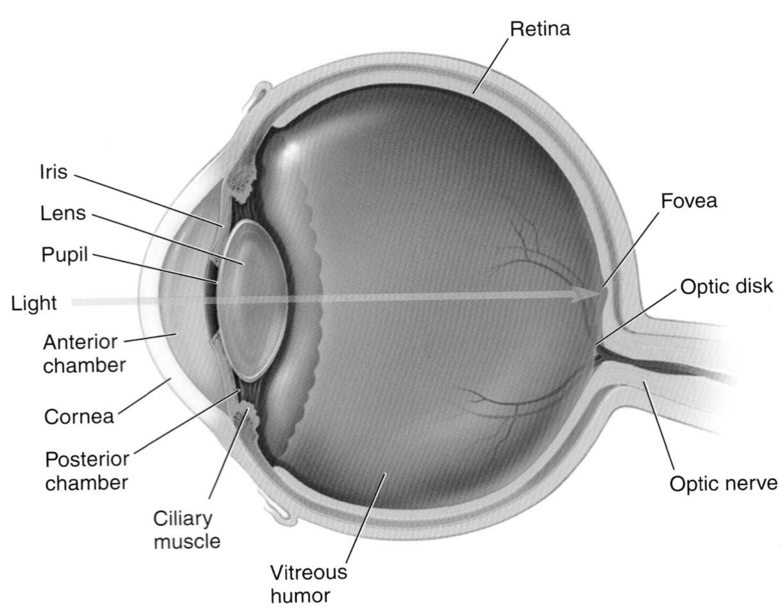

Figure 12.5. Structures of the eye.

the fluid, known as aqueous humor, that nourishes the lens and cornea. The vitreous body, a chamber containing clear, gelatinous fluid known as vitreous humor, is located behind the lens. The light that enters the eye passes through the lens and the vitreous humor where it is refracted, or bent, onto the retina.

Stop and Consider
Why is it necessary to control the amount of light entering the eye?

The **retina**, located over the posterior two-thirds of the eye, contains **photoreceptor** (receptor sensitive to light) cells called rods and cones. **Rods** produce a photopigment, **rhodopsin**, allowing vision in dim light. Opsin (a protein) and retinene (a vitamin A derivative) combine to form rhodopsin, which breaks down when in contact with light, stimulating a nerve impulse. Even low levels of light promote the breakdown of rhodopsin, allowing night vision.

Stop and Consider
Why does a vitamin A deficiency cause the development of night blindness?

The photoreceptors called **cones** provide the ability to see bright light and color; these cones are involved in visual acuity (clarity). The photopigments in cones also contain retinene and opsins differing from the type found in rods. In contrast to rods, cone photopigments require bright light for breakdown and generation of nerve impulse. There are three types of retinal cones. Each contains a different combination of retinene and opsin, which results in absorption of light of different wavelengths and colors.

1. Erythrolabe: red cone absorbs light at 625 nm wavelength
2. Chlorolabe: green cone absorbs light at 530 nm wavelength
3. Cyanolabe: blue cone absorbs light at 455 nm wavelength

Color vision is determined by the combination of cones stimulated by light from a particular image. The absence of a single group of color-receptive cones results in the inability to distinguish particular colors from others, a condition commonly known as color blindness. This condition is caused by a sex-linked recessive genetic trait, and it predominantly affects males.

The center of the retina, the **macula**, is the area responsible for central vision, color vision, and fine detail. The **fovea**, an area in the center of the macula, is the site at which the cones are most dense. Cones are the only photoreceptors located in the fovea, increasingly interspersed with rods toward the retina periphery. Rods are most highly concentrated in the peripheral retina, promoting peripheral and night vision. Rods and cones convert light into electrical impulses, which are transmitted first to the bipolar neurons, then to ganglion neurons. The axons of the ganglion neurons meet at the optic disk and exit the eye as the optic nerve (Fig. 12.6). The impulse continues to the optic chiasm where the medial halves of the retinal nerves crossover. The impulse travels to the optic tract, the thalamus, and the occipital lobe for processing. Each eye transmits a slightly different image, focused upside down on the retina. Mirror reversal also occurs because of light reflected from the right side of an object to the left side of the retina and vice versa. Visual images are coordinated in the brain during **visual processing**.

CONTROL OF EYE MOVEMENT

Extraocular muscles are responsible for the rotation, horizontal and vertical movement of the eyes (Fig. 12.7). A balance of contraction and relaxation of specific muscles allows controlled eye movement (Table 12.3). The six muscles that control eye movements are innervated by the oculomotor (III), trochlear (IV), and abducens (VI) cranial nerves. Eye movements can be described as follows:

- Saccades: looking from object A to object B
- Pursuit: smoothly following a moving object
- Convergence/divergence: both eyes turning inward/outward simultaneously
- Vestibular: eyes sensing and adjusting to head movement via connections with nerves in the inner ear
- Fixation maintenance: minute eye movements that position and accommodate both eyes

PROTECTIVE EYE STRUCTURES

The structures of the eye are protected by both physical and chemical barriers. Protective eye structures maintain function and promote optimal vision.

External Structures

Eyelids provide a protective barrier for the eye. Opening and closing of eyelids (blinking) promotes the removal of debris and provides moisture for the eye surface. Eyelashes also protect the eye and remove small particles of debris. The conjunctiva is a mucous membrane lining the undersurface of the eyelid and front of the eye.

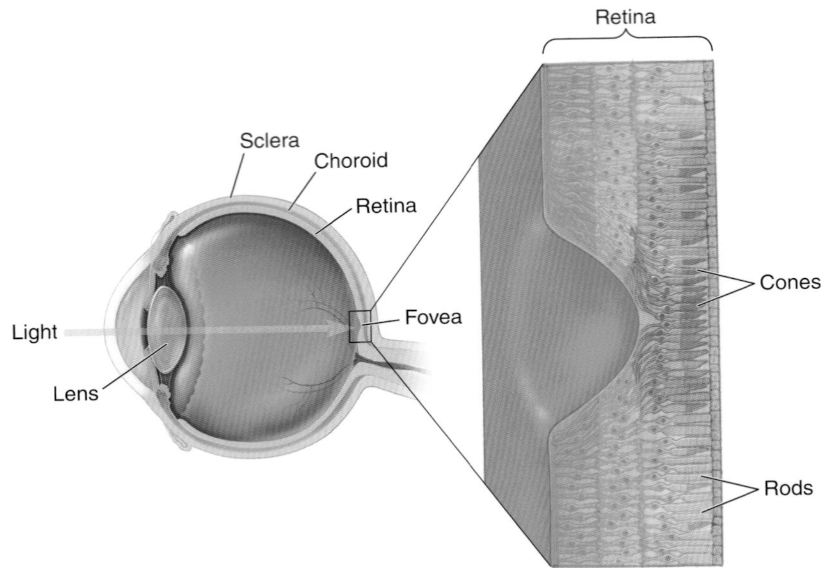

Figure 12.6. Lateral view of the eye. Impulses initiated in the photoreceptors, rods, and cones are transmitted by the bipolar cells to the ganglion cells of the retina. The fovea in the center of the macula is made entirely of cones. Surrounding tissue and blood vessels are displaced from the central area, fovea centralis, allowing light to pass unimpeded to the cones. (Modified from Bear MF, Connors BW, Parasido MA. *Neuroscience: Exploring the Brain*. 3rd ed. Philadelphia, PA: Lippincott Williams & Wilkins; 2006.)

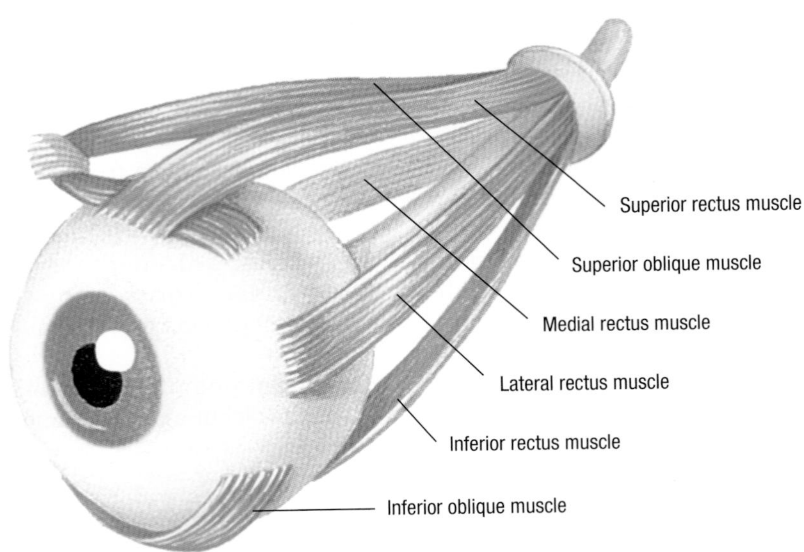

Figure 12.7. Extraocular eye muscles. Paired extraocular muscles control eye movement and include the superior/inferior rectus, medial/lateral rectus, and the superior/inferior oblique. The paired muscles have reciprocal responses, so that as one contracts, the other relaxes. (Courtesy Anatomical Chart Company.)

Tears

The **lacrimal glands** are the primary producers of tears. Tears protect the eyes by:

- Protecting against bacterial infection
- Providing nutrients and moisture
- Removing debris and waste from the eye

Closure of the eyelid forces tears downward, toward the nose, and into the puncta (openings in the upper and lower lids). Tears are forced into the lacrimal sac through narrow channels. Upon muscle relaxation and eye opening, tears move from the lacrimal sac to the nasolacrimal duct and into the nose.

Table 12.3 Extraocular Muscle Function

Extraocular Eye Muscle	Eye Movement
Lateral rectus	Outward, away from nose
Medial rectus	Inward, toward the nose
Superior rectus	Upward, slightly outward
Inferior rectus	Downward, slightly inward
Superior oblique	Inward and downward
Inferior oblique	Outward and upward

Stop and Consider
What is the most likely explanation for the runny nose that occurs during crying?

Aqueous Humor

The nutritive, watery fluid produced by the **ciliary body** is known as **aqueous humor** (Fig. 12.8). Released in the space between the iris and the lens (the posterior chamber), the aqueous humor maintains eye pressure and provides nutrients to the cornea and the lens. Movement of aqueous humor from the posterior chamber to the anterior chamber occurs by diffusion via the pupil, allowing reabsorption into the venous system for removal. The primary mechanism for reabsorption occurs through the **trabecular network** (a meshlike structure) into the canal of Schlemm, promoting movement into the venous system. A smaller quantity of aqueous humor is reabsorbed directly into larger blood vessels through the anterior ciliary body, known as the **uveal-scleral outflow pathway**.

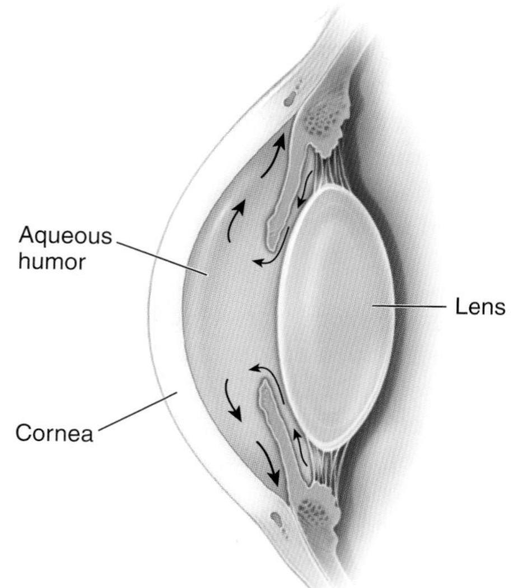

Figure 12.8. Aqueous humor. Aqueous humor flows from the posterior to the anterior chamber for reabsorption by the venous system to maintain eye pressure.

Alterations in Visual Function

Sight depends on the integration of multiple structures and processes within the eye and in surrounding tissues and organs. Alterations in vision can be induced by multiple causes, including damage to eye structures, motor dysfunction, and impaired neural conduction. Consequences can range from mild visual impairment amenable to correction or severe impairment, resulting in blindness.

ERRORS IN REFRACTION

Bending of light, or refraction, can be altered at any step from light entry into the eye through the contact of light onto the retina (Fig. 12.9). One common error in refraction is **myopia**, commonly known as nearsightedness. In myopia, the eye focuses an image in front of the retina due to lens thickness. **Hyperopia**, commonly referred to as farsightedness, is caused by the focusing of an image behind the retina, which alters the transmission of light. These conditions are easily corrected with the provision of a lens that regulates light rays. A biconcave lens causes light to diverge, providing correction of myopia. A biconvex lens is the necessary correction for hyperopia, promoting the convergence of light rays. **Astigmatism**, caused by irregular curvature of the cornea or lens, prevents the focusing of images, blurring vision. Correction of astigmatism can be accomplished through glasses, contact lenses, or refractive laser surgery, discussed in more detail later in the chapter. **Presbyopia**, a condition of farsightedness associated with aging, results from the inability of the ciliary muscle and lens to accommodate for near vision. This condition is easily corrected with bifocals.

ALTERATIONS IN EYE MOVEMENT

Strabismus is a term that describes the lack of coordinated extrinsic eye muscle function that prevents the eyes from lining up in the same direction. Known commonly as "crossed eyes," the misalignment of visual axes results in the inability to focus on a single object. **Amblyopia**, commonly known as "lazy eye," may result from strabismus, leading to the loss of visual detail from uncoordinated eye movement and focus. When visual axes are misaligned in children, the brain is able to suppress one of the images, resulting in visual impairment in the ignored eye.

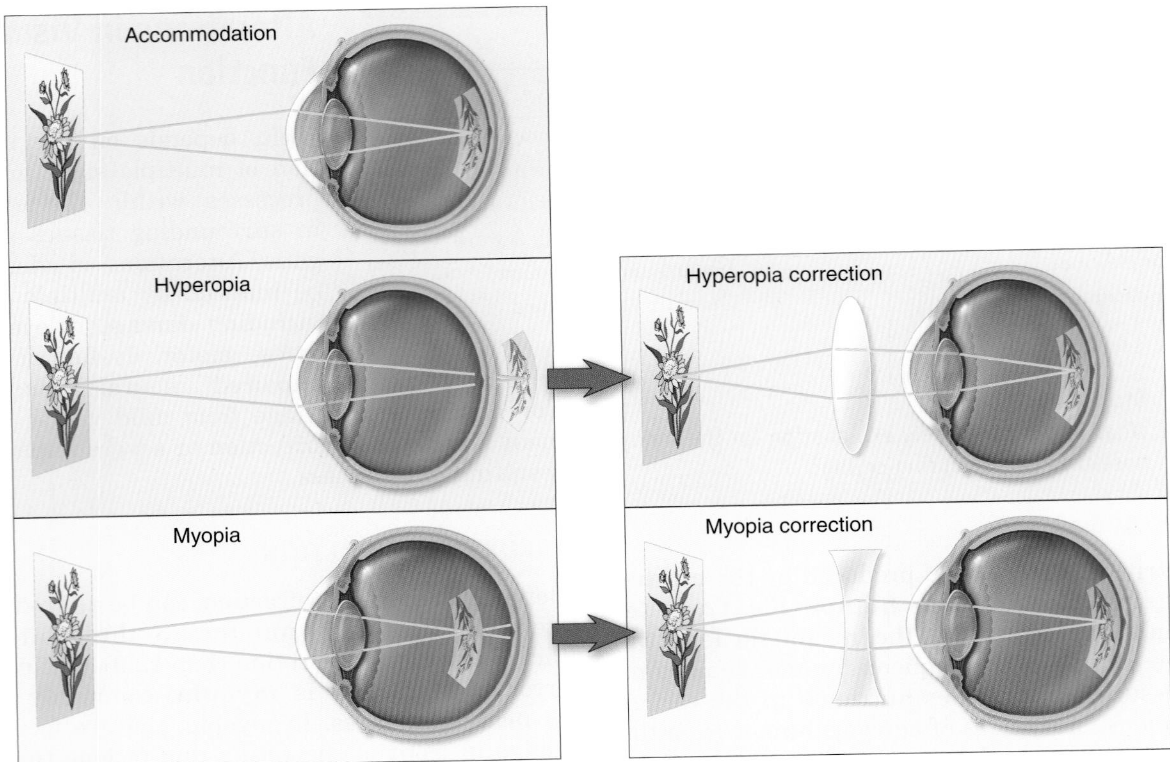

Figure 12.9. Error in refraction. Light entering the eye is focused onto the retina. Refraction errors misdirect light onto the retina, causing distortion of vision. (Modified from Bear MF, Connors BW, Parasido MA. *Neuroscience: Exploring the Brain*. 3rd ed. Philadelphia, PA: Lippincott Williams & Wilkins; 2006.)

The impairment may range from dimness of vision to the loss of permanent loss of vision in one eye. Visual impairment resulting from amblyopia may not be fully correctable.

Diplopia, a condition often resulting from a lack of coordination of the extraocular muscles, may result in double vision. Images fall on noncorresponding areas of the retina, causing the visual defect. Involuntary oscillations of the eye, known as **nystagmus**, result from abnormal function in the brain, labyrinth of the inner ear, and vestibular pathways responsible for controlling eye movement. Congenital nystagmus often results from oculo-motor abnormalities during neural development, manifesting at the age of 2 months. In the postnatal period, nystagmus can be acquired from a variety of visual input disruptions but is often the result of a head injury or space occupying lesion that interferes with vestibular pathways or cerebellar function. Other conditions known to contribute to the development of nystagmus include brainstem or cerebellar lesions, stroke, Ménière disease, multiple sclerosis, and drug or alcohol toxicity.

ALTERATIONS IN PROTECTIVE EYE STRUCTURES

Inflammation of the mucous membrane lining the eye, **conjunctivitis**, is commonly known as pink eye. Variations in categories of conjunctivitis are linked to the following causative factors:

- Viral conjunctivitis
  - Usually affects only one eye
  - Associated with excessive eye watering and a small amount of discharge
- Bacterial conjunctivitis
  - Usually affects both eyes
  - Associated with heavy discharge
- Allergic conjunctivitis
  - Usually affects both eyes
  - Associated with itching, redness, and excessive tearing

Cataracts result from the clouding of the lens, which alter vision focus by scattering the incoming light onto the retina (Fig. 12.10). Clouding often results from the clumping or aggregation of the protein component of the lens. As the size of the opaque area increases, vision is increasingly impaired. Cataracts are classified into three types:

1. Nuclear
   - **a.** Most common type
   - **b.** Forms in the center, or nucleus, of the lens
   - **c.** Distance vision affected more than near vision
   - **d.** Slow progression (years), associated with aging

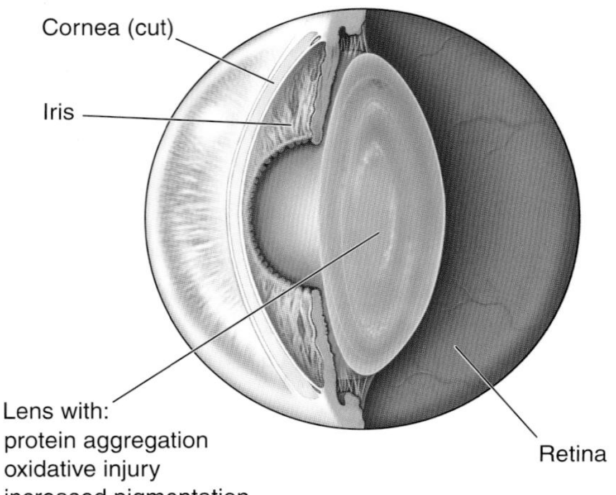

Figure 12.10. Cataract. Cross-section of the cornea showing cloudy lens. (Asset provided by Anatomical Chart Company.)

2. Cortical
   a. Forms in the lens cortex
   b. Extends from the outer lens toward the center
   c. Minimal vision impairment
3. Posterior subscapular
   a. Begins at the back of the lens
   b. Glare impaired vision
   c. Rapid progression (months)

MANIFESTATIONS AND EVALUATION OF ALTERATIONS IN VISION

Individuals often seek care when they notice that their vision has changed. Often, decreasing acuity or clarity of vision occurs over time. In the case of children, vision screening or change in academic performance may provide the impetus to seek further screening and diagnosis. A comprehensive vision screening is necessary to identify areas of deficit or dysfunction. The components of a vision screening are presented in Box 12.4.

Visual acuity, or sharpness, is commonly included in basic vision screening. It is important to evaluate both far and near vision. Evaluation of far distances is accomplished by using a standardized eye chart, such as the Snellen or E chart. The results are reported as a fraction, "20/X," with the numerator indicating what can be seen clearly at a 20-foot distance and the denominator indicating the distance at which the average eye can read the line. A report of 20/20 means that a person can see clearly at 20 feet what should be seen at 20 feet. A measurement of 20/40 means that what is seen clearly at 20 feet, the average person can read at 40 feet.

The results of a near vision test show a person's ability to see the details of near objects (within arm's distance from the body). Near vision is tested with a handheld card held at a comfortable distance. The patient reads the smallest line possible, which is recorded along with the distance. Some tests of near acuity use a standard handheld card at a prescribed distance. For example, when a Jaeger chart is used, it is placed 12 to 14 inches away. Individuals are asked to read the smallest of 10 available lines, ranging from 4- to 14-point type fonts, that they are able to read. The results are then converted to standards used in far vision evaluation.

Box 12.4 Components of Vision Screening

Vision evaluation often includes the following:

- Acuity-distance: visual acuity (sharpness, clearness) at 20 feet distance
- Acuity-near: clear vision for short distance (as in reading)
- Focusing skills: maintenance of clear vision at varying distances
- Eye tracking and fixation skills: the ability of the eyes to look at and accurately follow an object; a skill important in the process of reading
- Binocular fusion: the ability to use both eyes together at the same time
- Stereopsis: binocular depth perception
- Convergence and eye teaming skills: coordination of the eyes to aim, move, and work as a team
- Hyperopia: a refractive condition that causes difficulty in focus of near objects
- Color vision: the ability to distinguish colors
- Reversal frequency: confusing letters or words (b, d; p, q: saw, was)
- Visual memory: the ability to store and retrieve visual information
- Visual form discrimination: the ability to determine whether two shapes, colors, sizes, positions, or distances are the same or different
- Visual motor integration: the ability to combine visual input with other sensory input (e.g., hand and body movements, balance, and hearing); the ability to transform images from a vertical to a horizontal plane (such as from the blackboard to the desk surface)
- Intraocular pressure measurement: measurement of 10–21 mmHg considered normal

TREATMENT OF ALTERATIONS IN VISION

Treatment of alterations in vision is specific to the identified impairment. Muscle imbalances can be corrected by glasses, patching, or surgery, depending on the specific impairments identified. Errors in refraction may be corrected by glasses, contact lenses, or surgery. **Laser-assisted in situ keratomileusis (LASIK)** is a surgical procedure used to treat myopia, hyperopia, and astigmatism. Cataracts may also need to be surgically removed and replaced with a clear prosthetic lens. Glaucoma, covered in greater detail in the clinical model in this chapter, may require surgical or pharmacologic management.

Module 3 Alterations in Hearing and Balance

Hearing and balance involve a complex interaction between structural components of the ear and transmission of nerve impulses for sensory interpretation. The senses of hearing and balance are maximized by optimal function of both outer ear and inner ear structures.

Structural Components of the Ear

Structures of the outer, middle, and inner ear coordinate to funnel stimuli (sound) to the hearing receptors, initiating the signal that travels along the neural pathways to the brain. Figure 12.11 illustrates the structures of the ear.

OUTER EAR

The tissue that comprises what is viewed as the outer ear is known as the **pinna**. Composed of cartilage and soft tissue, the pinna maintains its shape, but it is also flexible and pliable. The pinna collects and funnels sound vibrations into the opening of the ear canal, or **external auditory meatus**. The ear canal is approximately 1 inch long in an adult and, similar to the pinna, is also comprised of cartilage. The ear canal is covered with small hairs and glands that secrete wax (**cerumen**). These structures in the ear canal serve as protection against foreign bodies and environmental debris. At the distal end, the ear canal becomes bony with a tight skin covering.

MIDDLE EAR

The **tympanic membrane**, or eardrum, is located at the end of the ear canal opposite the external auditory meatus, marking the boundary of the middle ear. The middle ear contains three bones, or **ossicles**, that form a connection between the eardrum and inner ear. Sound waves that contact the tympanic membrane cause a back and forth movement. Tympanic membrane movement causes repositioning of the ossicles, which changes sound waves into mechanical vibration (Fig. 12.12).

The three bones comprising the ossicles are the **malleus**, **incus**, and **stapes**. These bones are also known as the hammer, anvil, and stirrup, respectively. Connections between the tympanic membranes and ossicles promote transduction of the mechanical vibration, producing sound. The progressive connections between the tympanic membrane, malleus, incus, and stapes cause an in-and-out movement at the base of the stirrup, or the stapes footplate. These in-and-out movements represent patterns matching the initiating sound waves.

The middle ear is located in the air-filled mastoid portion of the temporal bone of the skull. The eustachian tube connecting the middle ear to the nasopharynx runs along the front wall of the middle ear to the back of the nose and throat, providing pressure equalization on both sides of the tympanic membrane. The eustachian tube is shorter and narrower in children, increasing the likelihood of eustachian tube blockage and pressure. The anatomic constraints in children may increase the risk of ear infection.

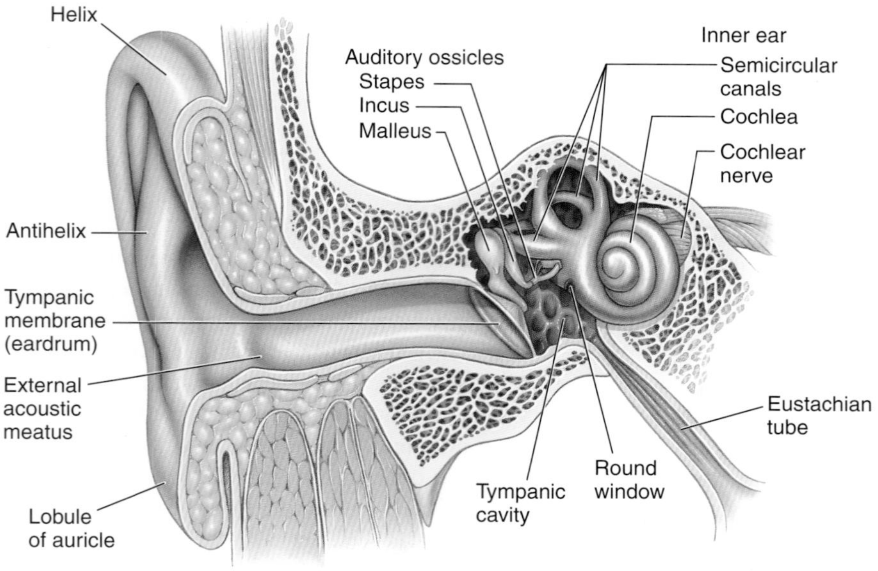

Figure 12.11. Structures of the ear. (Courtesy Anatomical Chart Company.)

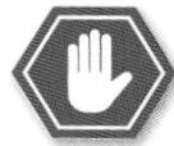

Stop and Consider
What are the ways that we can voluntarily manipulate pressure changes in the ear?

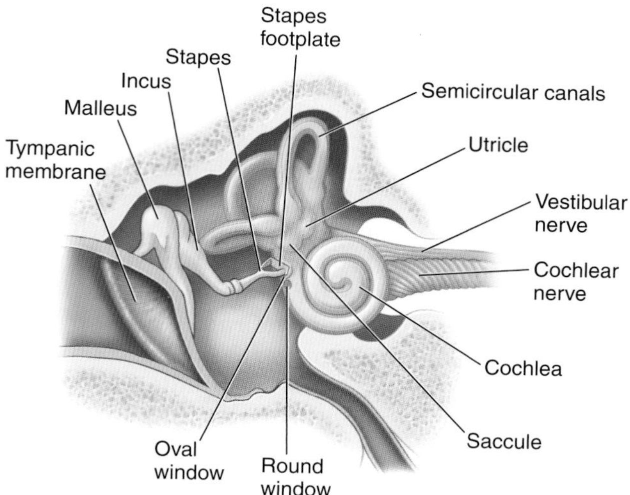

Figure 12.12. Vestibular structures of the ear. Sound vibrations contact the tympanic membrane, causing vibration of the ossicles and footplate of the stapes at the oval window. Movement of the oval window promotes fluid movement against the cochlea stimulating nerve impulses, which are transmitted to the brain via the cochlear nerve.

INNER EAR

The stapes footplate of the middle ear fits into the **oval window**, marking the boundary between the middle ear and the beginning point of the inner ear. The inner ear is comprised of the outer bony labyrinth and inner membranous labyrinth. Receptor stimuli results in signal transduction along the eighth cranial nerve (acoustic), comprised of the cochlear nerve (hearing) and the vestibular nerve (balance).

Hearing Processes

The perilymph-filled bony labyrinth contains the **cochlea**, important for hearing. Within the cochlea, the **Organ of Corti** contains hair cells, the receptors responsible for the neural impulse that allows hearing. The membranous labyrinth is a closed system of endolymph-filled canals lying within the cochlea. The ionic concentration difference between perilymph fluid outside the membranous labyrinth and the internal endolymph fluid creates an endolymphatic potential, generating a current that sensitizes the cochlear hair cells in the Organ of Corti to sound. Cochlear hair cells are innervated by the cochlear portion of the acoustic nerve. Impulses are then transmitted to the visual cortex in the occipital lobe, regulating hearing.

Mechanical energy from the ossicles forces the oval window into the cochlea. The motion of the

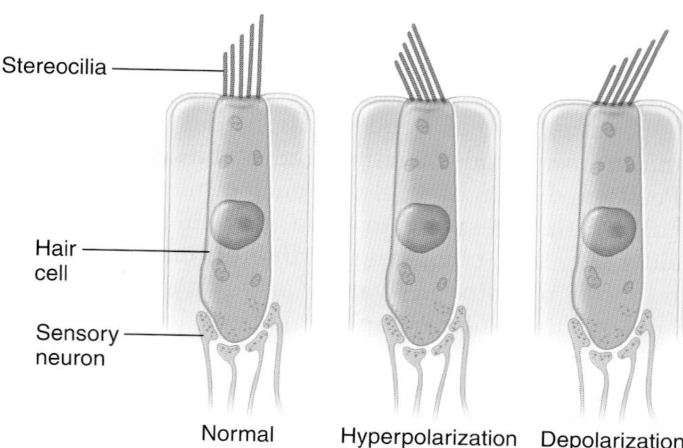

Figure 12.13. Hair cell. Hair cells hyperpolarize or depolarize depending on the direction in which the stereocilia bend.

cochlea's fluid stimulates hair cells. Sterocilia on each hair cell contribute to the ability to respond to unique sound frequencies, or pitches. Movement of stereocilia leads to hyperpolarization or depolarization (Fig. 12.13). Depolarization of hair cells causes impulse generation and transmission to the brain via the acoustic (vestibulocochlear) VIII cranial nerve to the relay center in the midbrain, the cochlear nucleus. At that point, nerve fibers from each ear divide into two pathways. One pathway ascends directly to the auditory cortex on the same side hemisphere, while the second pathway crosses over and ascends to the auditory cortex on the contralateral hemisphere. This mechanism allows impulses from each ear to reach both hemispheres.

The central auditory system processes auditory information, supporting the following functions:

- Sound localization
- Auditory discrimination (recognizing differences between different sounds)
- Sound pattern recognition
- Time, or temporal, aspects of hearing
- Integration of multiple auditory stimuli by reduction in the auditory performance of competing or incomplete signals

Balance Processes

The three semicircular canals and vestibule (containing the utricle and saccule, connected membranous sacs) are also located in the bony labyrinth and are important for balance and equilibrium. The perilymph in the semicircular canals senses motion caused by body movement, stimulating the hair cells lining the vestibular apparatus. Vestibular hair cells are innervated by the vestibular portion of the acoustic nerve. Impulses are then transmitted to the cerebellum via the vestibular branch of the acoustic nerve, regulating equilibrium and balance. The semicircular canals and vestibule (vestibular apparatus) detect head position and acceleration, maintaining body position and stable visual fields. Positioned at right angles to each other, the semicircular canals respond to head movement (up/down, side/side, tilt), triggering perilymph movement and hair cell receptor activation and generation of impulses. The semicircular canals provide information about head position to the vestibular apparatus through semicircular canal connection to the utricle and utricle-saccule connection. The utricle senses change in horizontal head position while the saccule is responsive to vertical acceleration.

Alterations in Hearing and Balance

Most disorders of the ear are not fatal, but they significantly affect an individual's daily functioning. Ear disorders can result in impaired hearing, altered balance, discomfort, and pain.

DISORDERS OF THE EXTERNAL EAR

Disorders of the ear canal are frequently caused by inflammation, drainage, or obstruction. Obstruction can result from the accumulation of cerumen or the presence of a tumor, diminishing the movement of sound to the middle ear. Cerumen may be removed by a process of **irrigation**, or rinsing the external canal with warm water, after it is determined that the tympanic membrane is intact. In the case of an obstructive tumor, surgical excision is usually the preferred treatment.

Stop and Consider
What are the risks to ear structures when the ears are irrigated?

Otitis externa, inflammation of the skin of the external ear, is a condition associated with pain and discomfort. Commonly known as "swimmer's ear," otitis externa often results from moisture in the ear canal or altered integrity of the skin in the ear canal. Manifestations include itching, redness, tenderness, and narrowing of tissues in the ear canal caused by swelling in response to inflammation. Mild hearing loss may result from drainage and from the reduced diameter of the ear canal.

ALTERATION IN MIDDLE EAR FUNCTION

Inflammation, trauma, and obstruction are often related to middle ear hearing loss. Eustachian tube dysfunction may lead to loss of hearing due to altered patency or obstruction, or as a contributing factor to other middle ear pathologies. Abnormally patent eustachian tubes promote movement of fluid from the nasopharynx into the middle ear. This particularly concerns infants and children because crying may precipitate the movement of secretions into the tube. Obstruction of the eustachian tube may promote the absorption of air from the middle ear, which is replaced by serous fluid escaping from surrounding capillaries. Hearing loss may result from the loss of mobility of the tympanic membrane caused by middle ear fluid, exudates compromising the conduction of vibration in the ossicles of the middle ear, or negative pressure in the middle ear resulting from eustachian tube obstruction.

Sudden changes in atmospheric pressure can result in **barotrauma**, or injury resulting from the inability of the ear to equalize barometric stress. Most commonly seen in air travel and sea diving, barotrauma results from middle ear pressure in parallel with atmospheric pressure. Persons at particular risk are those suffering from an upper respiratory infection with limited ability to normalize pressure in the eustachian tube.

Stop and Consider
What strategies can a person use to avoid barotrauma caused by air travel during an upper respiratory infection?

Otitis media, infection of the middle ear, is one of the most common disorders of the middle ear. Hearing loss may result from immobility of the tympanic membrane, fluid accumulation of the middle ear, and scarring from rupture of the tympanic membrane, altering function. Otitis media may be acute or recurrent, and it is associated with effusion (fluid) in the middle ear. This condition may be seen across all age groups but has the greatest prevalence in infants and children. The clinical model in this chapter provides a complete review of this condition. **Mastoiditis**, a bacterial infection causing inflammation of the air cells of the mastoid bone, may result as a complication of otitis media. Risks related to mastoiditis include meningitis, brain abscess, or facial palsy if it is not responsive to antibiotic therapy.

Otosclerosis, an autosomal-dominant condition, represents the most common cause of chronic, progressive, conductive hearing loss. Slow formation of spongy bone at the oval window immobilizes the footplate of the stapes, impairing the conduction of vibration. Most prevalent in females 15 to 30 years of age, affected individuals indicate a family history of this condition, consistent with the genetic basis of the disease. Surgical removal of the stapes with replacement of a prosthetic device restores partial or total hearing.

ALTERATION IN INNER EAR FUNCTION

Hearing loss caused by inner ear dysfunction is related to destruction of cochlear hair cells or damage to neural pathways. Tinnitus may be caused by noise-induced hearing loss, sensorineural hearing loss consistent with aging (**presbycusis**), hypertension, atherosclerosis, head injury, or cochlear infection/inflammation.

Balance and equilibrium are disturbed in altered function of the inner ear. **Ménière disease**, a condition associated with severe vertigo, sensorineural hearing loss, and tinnitus, is related to overproduction or decreased absorption of endolymph. Also known as endolymphatic hydrops or endolymphatic hypertension, hearing loss is caused by the progressive degeneration of vestibular and cochlear hair cells, described in greater detail in the clinical models. **Labyrinthitis**, or inflammation of the labyrinth of the inner ear, also precipitates severe vertigo and sensorineural hearing loss.

MANIFESTATIONS AND EVALUATION OF ALTERATIONS IN HEARING

Noticeable change in the ability to hear is commonly why individuals seek hearing evaluation. Difficulty hearing around groups of people, difficulty hearing competing sounds, or difficulty hearing specific types of pitches denotes a potential for hearing loss. Hearing screening is routine in particular groups of individuals, such as newborns or those individuals working in areas that increase risk for hearing loss. Hearing evaluation should include a thorough examination of all structural and functional auditory components. Deformities and lesions of the pinna and external auditory canal may indicate an acute, chronic, or congenital condition as the cause of hearing impairment. Audiometric testing can help determine the specific nature of hearing loss. Auditory acuity is the basic assessment of hearing, and provides a general sense of hearing sensation. Further testing can be pursued when evidence is present for hearing loss.

Screening procedures are performed to identify the type of loss (unilateral or bilateral, sensorineural, and/or conductive) and to quantify the degree of hearing loss. A thorough history should be completed to determine the duration, severity, and quality of the hearing loss. Associated symptoms should also be identified, such as pain or **tinnitus** (ringing or whistling in the ears).

Hearing Evaluation

The degree of hearing loss can be quantified using a unit of measure known as **decibels (dB)**. The frequency or pitch of the sound is referred to in **Hertz (Hz)**. Based on pure-tone average, hearing levels can be categorized based on frequencies from 500 to 4,000 Hz. Individuals who have normal hearing are able to detect sounds at a minimal frequency of −10 to +15 dB. Individuals who have hearing impairment require sounds with increasing decibels for detection. Minimal decibels needed for sound recognition may help determine the degree of hearing loss, described as follows:

1. Minimal hearing loss: 16 to 25 dB
2. Mild hearing loss: 26 to 40 dB
3. Moderate hearing loss: 41 to 55 dB
4. Moderate to severe hearing loss: 56 to 70 dB
5. Severe hearing loss: 71 to 90 dB
6. Profound hearing loss: 91 dB or more

The type of hearing loss can be determined based on the identification of the event or structure involved. **Conductive hearing loss** is localized to the outer or middle ear, and it may be temporary or permanent. **Sensorineural hearing loss** is often permanent, resulting from disease, trauma, or genetic inheritance of a defect in the cochlea nerve cells. The inner ear or the auditory nerve is usually involved in sensorineural hearing loss. **Mixed hearing loss** refers to a combination of both sensorineural and conductive hearing loss. **Central auditory processing disorder** is a disorder involving an alteration in auditory signal processing in the brain.

In addition to determining type and degree of hearing loss, auditory testing can determine whether the hearing loss is bilateral or unilateral, symmetric or asymmetric, or high frequency or low frequency. Specific tests included in hearing evaluation include an audiogram, with the following three components:

1. Pure-tone audiometry
   a. Recognition of faintest tones at selected pitches in the absence of background noise
   b. Results are graphed on an audiogram
2. Speech reception threshold
   a. Identification of the faintest level of speech heard, confirming pure-tone audiometry
   b. Minimal decibel measurement of the "loudness" of speech required for detection recorded
3. Speech discrimination score
   a. Recognition of words at a normal level of speech
   b. Measured by the percentage of spoken words identified when spoken at a hearing level above threshold

EVALUATION OF THE MIDDLE EAR

Tests that provide information about structures in the outer and middle ear are known as acoustic immittance measures. **Tympanometry** measures the degree of movement of the tympanic membrane to identify middle ear fluid, perforation, or cerumen blockage of the ear canal. **Acoustic reflex measurement** can be used to determine movement of the tympanic membrane in response to sound.

EVALUATION OF THE INNER EAR

The **pure-tone bone conduction** hearing test can be used to evaluate the inner ear, independent of middle and outer ear function. A small vibrator is placed on either the forehead or the mastoid bone, directly stimulating the auditory nerve. This test is limited to the identification of sensorineural hearing loss. Air conduction tests can be used to identify both conductive and sensorineural hearing loss.

The vestibular evoked myogenic potential (VEMP) test uses evoked potential techniques (see Chapter 10) to stimulate a sound-induced reflex. This test allows evaluation of the saccule (a sensory organ of the inner ear), the vestibular nerve, the medial vestibulospinal tract, and the spinal accessory nerve. Generation of a response to sound is caused by acoustical stimulation of the saccule, resulting in transduction of the impulse beneath the stapes footplate.

Individuals who experience acute or chronic exposure to environmental noise are at risk for hearing loss. Exposure to noise and high-level sound can cause damage to outside hair cells, the main targets of high-level sound. Tests specific to outer hair cell function include **otoacoustic emission (OAE)**. OAEs are faint sounds produced by the outer hair cells in the cochlea of the inner ear. Sound recordings, obtained by a small microphone placed in the ear canal, may identify the specific reason for hearing loss. OAEs may occur spontaneously or may be induced by a stimulus, such as a click or a pure-tone auditory stimulus.

Treatment of Alterations in Hearing

Alterations in hearing may be corrected by the use of hearing aids or assistive listening devices to amplify sound. When these devices provide little improvement in hearing, a cochlear implant may be considered. **Cochlear implants** are artificial devices surgically placed behind the ear. Using electrical stimulation of nerve endings, electrodes implanted in the cochlea transmit sounds to the auditory nerve, bypassing structures in the middle and outer ear. The device does not restore normal hearing, but it does provide a sense of sound that is processed into meaningful communication by the brain.

Hearing deficits in young children may be associated with impaired language and cognitive development. Early screening of hearing loss has provided an opportunity to treat loss at younger ages in an effort to promote language and cognitive development. Use of cochlear implants at younger ages has the potential to enhance cognitive development.[4]

Taste and Smell

The senses of taste and smell are linked such that if one is impaired, the other is also affected. While impairment of taste and smell is not life-threatening, alterations in these senses have the potential to negatively impact quality of life.

TASTE

The sensation of taste is also known as gustation. Taste is mediated by the chemoreceptors in the taste buds of the oral cavity. Taste or gustatory cells, one of the cell types that make up taste buds, are the sensory receptors responsible for triggering the impulse that is perceived as taste. Taste buds detect five types of basic tastes, including:

1. Sweet
2. Sour
3. Salty
4. Bitter
5. Savory

Substances must be dissolved in saliva to stimulate a taste response. Once dissolved, molecules released from food and drink by chewing, drinking or digesting food penetrate the taste buds, bind to the taste receptor on the gustatory hairs of the taste cell, and transmit the taste signal via action potentials along associated dendrites. Impulses travel primarily along the facial nerve (cranial nerve VII) and glossopharyngeal nerve (cranial nerve IX) where they synapse in the medulla and the thalamus, then proceed to the gustatory cortex in the parietal lobe.

Taste is also indirectly affected by other stimuli. Visual, thermal, scent, and even pain receptors are stimulated to enhance the taste sensation. Of these, the olfactory stimulation of the sense of smell has the greatest influence. Receptor sensitivity of taste cells may be altered by environmental factors (such as cigarette smoking), drug reactions (chemotherapy), and clinical conditions (chronic liver disease).

Taste disorders often involve smell. Conditions of taste disorders include phantom taste perception (lingering, unpleasant taste), reduced ability to taste one or all of the five basic tastes, or distortion of flavor such as persistent metallic taste.

SMELL

The sense of smell is often pleasurable, enhancing enjoyment of the food we eat and the world around us. An intact sense of smell can also be protective, warning us of potential threats such as gas leaks or environmental toxins. **Olfaction**, or the sense of smell, is regulated by olfactory receptors located in each nasal cavity. A second olfactory pathway is through the roof of the throat region to the nose. Olfactory hairs protrude from the receptor segments that extend through the nasal epithelium. Unmyelinated axons comprise the opposite end of the olfactory receptor, which merge with other olfactory axons to form the olfactory nerve (cranial nerve I). Afferent fibers ascend from the olfactory bulb to the olfactory cortex and are responsible for interpretation and processing of olfactory stimuli.

Alterations in olfactory sensation, while unpleasant, are not pathophysiologically significant. The most common smell disorders are associated with recent illness or injury. Conditions most frequently associated with smell disorders include upper respiratory infections, frontal head injuries, chemical exposure (including some medications), and smoking. Loss of smell acuity is also associated with aging.

Module 4 Clinical Models

The following clinical models have been selected to aid in the understanding and application of altered sensation. The student should pay attention to the commonalities and unique features of each condition when studying these models. Alterations in sensory functions often lead to physical and emotional distress and disruption of daily life (Fig. 12.14).

Fibromyalgia

Fibromyalgia, a condition of the soft tissues and muscles, is derived from the Latin words "fibro" for fibrous tissue and the Greek words "myo" for muscle and "algia" for pain. Estimated to affect 2% of the population, fibromyalgia is an increasingly recognized problem which has led to a renewed emphasis on improved management strategies. Fibromyalgia occurs in women seven times more frequently than in men. Women in the sixth or seventh decade of life have the highest prevalence of fibromyalgia.[5]

PATHOPHYSIOLOGY

Fibromyalgia causes significant pain and fatigue but is not linked to a well-defined pathogenesis. There is

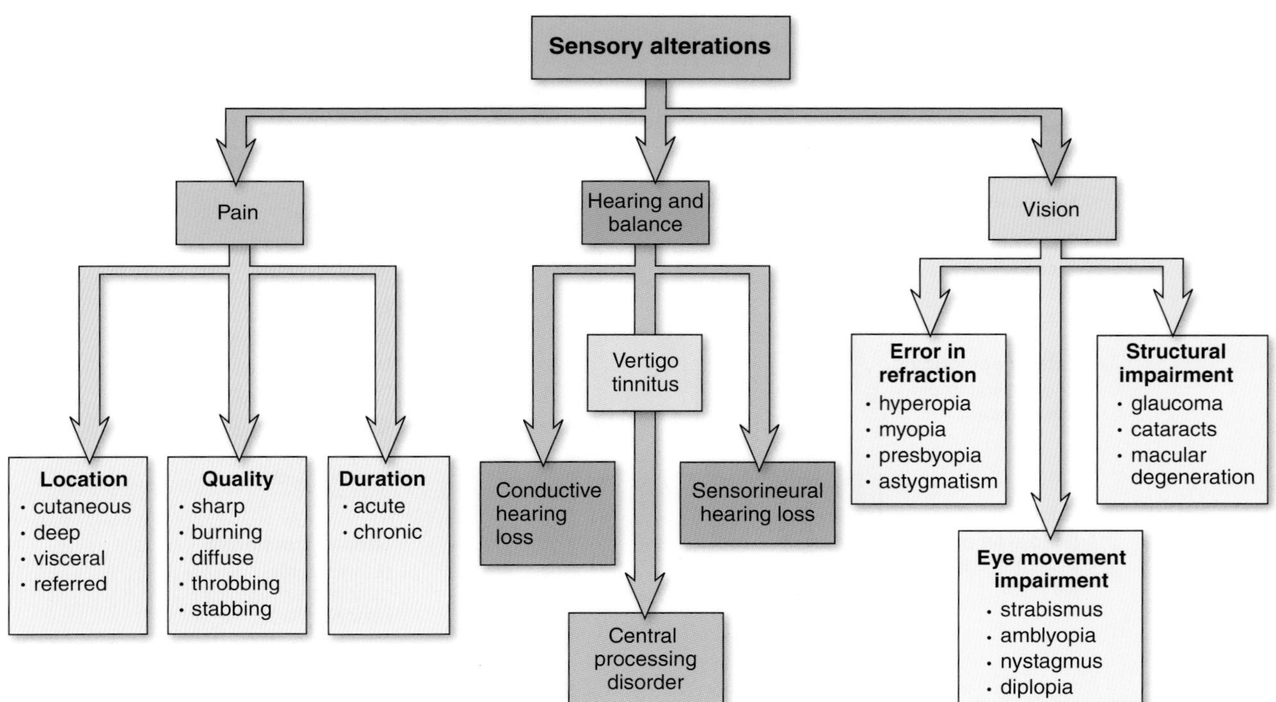

Figure 12.14. Concept map. Sensory alterations.

no definitive evidence of inflammation, muscle structural or functional alterations in fibromyalgia. The complexity of fibromyalgia pathogenesis involves genetics, developmental influences, triggering factors, and neurophysiologic and emotional variables.[5] Within families, the evidence of familial aggregation suggests a genetic predisposition to fibromyalgia. No reliable gene targets involving pain pathways have been identified though there is emerging evidence for alterations in DNA methylation in women with fibromyalgia indicating a potential epigenetic foundation.[6] Although there is no known cause or cure, research continues to determine the underlying mechanisms and effective treatments for the syndrome.

CLINICAL MANIFESTATIONS

Heightened sensitivity to noxious stimuli characterizes the clinical manifestations of fibromyalgia. A commonly diagnosed condition, fibromyalgia is characterized by disordered sleep, tenderness, stiffness and pain in the neck, shoulders, upper back, elbows, lower back, and hips.[7] Nonrestorative sleep, consistent with manifestations of fatigue, often accompany fibromyalgia.

Difficulty in concentration, depression and anxiety may coexist in individuals who have fibromyalgia. Serotonin levels are decreased in some individuals, consistent with symptoms of depression, pain, sleep alteration, anxiety, and altered muscle function. Alterations in brain structure and function including changes in brain matter volume and cerebral blood flow have been associated with fibromyalgia. It is not known if these alterations are causes of or responses to fibromyalgia.

DIAGNOSTIC CRITERIA

Diagnostic criteria include subjective findings of fatigue and chronic musculoskeletal pain of at least 3 months' duration. Eighteen areas of pain, or tender point sites, located in the neck, shoulders, rib junctions, joints, gluteus, trochanters, and knees have been identified in patients suffering from fibromyalgia (Fig. 12.15). Pain must be present in 12 of the 18 tender point sites for diagnosis.[7] Some people with fibromyalgia develop trigger points or ropy bands occurring throughout the body. The trigger points induce referred pain to other parts of the body, which is thought to be caused by pressure on blood vessels and nerves by fibrous bands causing tightening of **myofascia** (outer membrane of muscle tissue).

TREATMENT

Treatment of fibromyalgia is focused on symptom management, and it includes both nonpharmacologic and pharmacologic options.[8] Cognitive behavioral therapy, coupled with stress reduction methods and medication to promote sleep, are the most effective treatment regimens. Application of heat and cold, ultrasound, and deep massage may provide temporary relief of symptoms. Gentle exercise is

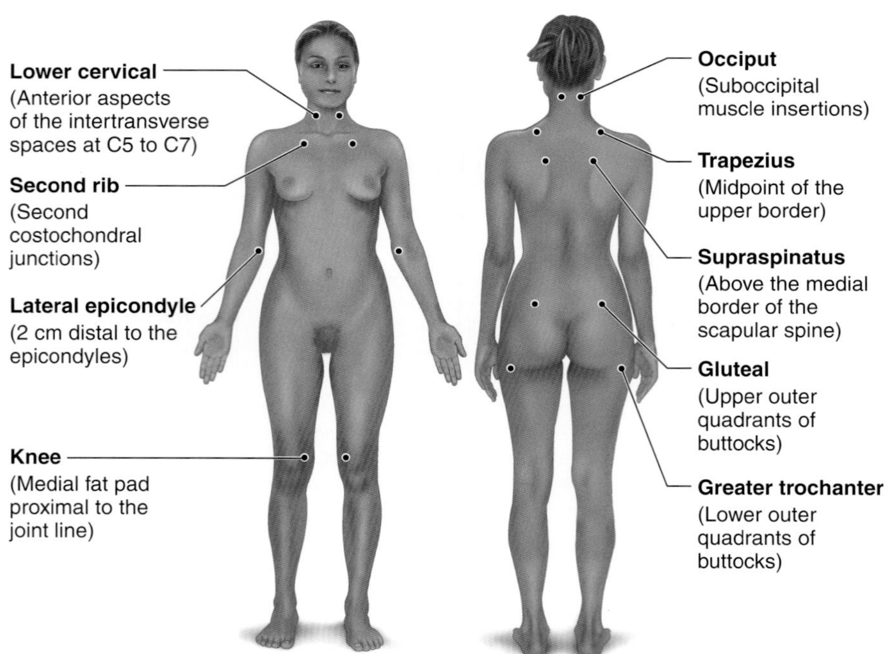

Figure 12.15. Tender points of fibromyalgia.

critical to maintaining muscle fitness. Stretching and exercise promote muscle strength and facilitate sleep. Alternative treatment options may include acupuncture, biofeedback, yoga, hypnosis, or other relaxation techniques.

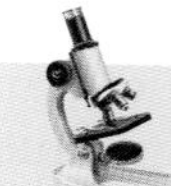

FROM THE LAB

No diagnostic tests exist to confirm fibromyalgia. It is a diagnosis of exclusion, meaning that tests to confirm other likely diagnoses (including hypothyroidism or hyperparathyroidism) rule out other possibilities, leaving fibromyalgia as the most likely diagnosis.

Treatment with analgesics, antidepressants, anticonvulsants and muscle relaxants are the mainstays of pharmacologic management of fibromyalgia.[5] Tricyclic antidepressants (e.g., amitriptyline, cyclobenzaprine) are used as first-line therapy to manage symptoms. Medications that block serotonin norepinephrine (SNRI) reuptake have also demonstrated effectiveness for relief of physical and emotional symptoms. Antiseizure medications (e.g., gabapentin, pregabalin) have been shown to have pain-relieving effects, reducing severity of stiffness and joint discomfort. Nonsteroidal anti-inflammatory medications may help reduce discomfort, particularly when combined with a tricyclic antidepressant.

Stop and Consider

Why aren't anti-inflammatory medications used as the primary pharmacologic treatment of fibromyalgia?

Migraine Headache

Migraines are characterized by neurologic dysfunction involving impairment of cortical, subcortical, and brainstem areas leading to altered autonomic, affective, cognitive, and sensory functions.[9] Migraines are recurrent, moderate to severe headaches that last 1 to 2 days and are often associated with nausea, vomiting, and sensitivity to noise and light. The manifestations of migraine may be severe, resulting in significant loss of productivity and quality of life. Migraine is reported to be more common in women.

PATHOPHYSIOLOGY

The precise cause of migraines is not clear. The genetic foundation of migraine is a current focus of investigation of this complex condition. Migraines are often initiated with a prodrome, early events that precede the classical migraine symptoms including aura and headache. A current phenomenon that may explain the pathophysiology of migraine is cortical spreading depression, a wave of depolarization that spreads across the cerebral cortex, leading to migraine aura.[9] Activation of nociceptors in the meninges and transmission along pain fibers in the trigeminovascular pathway to targets in the brain distinguishes pain originating in the cranial region from headaches stimulated by external events such as stress and tension. Over time, the neurons become sensitized to stimulation, contributing to the transformation of episodic to chronic migraines. Complex neurologic and biochemical events may initiate clinical symptoms. Primary factors implicated in migraine pathophysiology include serotonin, calcitonin gene-related peptide (CGRP). Decreased serotonin levels may precipitate the release of chemical mediators from the trigeminal nerve, altering blood vessel function.

CLINICAL MANIFESTATIONS

Migraines typically have four phases, each with distinctive clinical manifestations. Migraine phases include prodrome, aura, headache and postdrome. Affective symptoms (e.g., mood changes), food cravings, constipation, neck stiffness and yawning characterize the prodrome, occurring 24 to 48 hours before headache. Additional common manifestations of prodrome include:

- Increased energy
- Sweet cravings
- Fatigue
- Irritability

Classical or uncommon migraines affecting approximately 15% of individuals include aura approximately 15 to 30 minutes before the onset of the migraine. Migraine aura includes short-duration, focal neurologic events including visual, auditory, somatosensory, or motor symptoms. The characteristics of migraine headache pain are described as unilateral, pulsing, and throbbing. Nausea, vomiting, and photosensitivity are often associated with increasing migraine headache severity. With resolution of migraine headache, the postdrome period begins. During this period, head movement may precipitate the onset of pain in the area previously experienced during migraine headache. Other symptoms include fatigue and positive emotional feelings. Loss of productivity and reduction in work and leisure time may result.

DIAGNOSTIC CRITERIA

Migraines are often diagnosed based on a thorough review of history and physical examination. If headaches develop acutely, other tests, such as computed tomography or magnetic resonance imaging scan, may be done to rule out other pathology such as meningitis, tumor, or increased intracranial pressure. The diagnostic criteria for migraine headache without aura includes at least five migraine headache episodes meeting each of the following criteria[10]:

- Headache of 4 to 72 hours duration (untreated or treatment resistant)
- Headache characteristics of least two of the following:
  - Unilateral location
  - Pulsating quality
  - Moderate or severe intensity
  - Associated with routine physical activity
- Headache associated with at least one of the following:
  - Nausea, vomiting, or both
  - Sensitivity to light or sound

TREATMENT

Treatment of migraine headache includes nonpharmacologic and pharmacologic measures for prevention and treatment of existing pain. In susceptible people, migraines are often disabling and can be triggered by a variety of factors, including hormonal changes, anxiety, stress, and lack of food or sleep. Prevention may be indicated when an individual:

- Experiences two or more migraines each month
- Uses pain-relieving medications more than two times a week
- Does not get relief from analgesic treatments
- Has uncommon migraines

Nonpharmacologic strategies effective in preventing migraines included avoidance of triggers, regular exercise, smoking cessation, and stabilization of hormone levels with oral contraceptives or hormone replacement therapy.

Pharmacologic management for migraine headaches includes simple analgesics, triptans, and ergots.[11] Prodrome or aura, if present, signals the need for prompt and early treatment. Acute treatment is initiated during migraine to relieve symptoms and includes simple analgesics (e.g., acetaminophen, nonsteroidal anti-inflammatory drugs [NSAIDs], aspirin) as the first-line therapy for mild migraine headache.[12] If symptoms are unrelieved and are moderate to severe, triptans are recommended. Triptans mimic the action of serotonin, promoting constriction of blood vessels and interruption of pain pathways. The advantage of triptans is the rapid onset of action (within 15 minutes in the injectable form) and the high rate of effectiveness. Treatment effectiveness is increased when initiated early prior to the onset of moderate to severe symptoms. Antiemetic medications may also be needed to treat nausea and vomiting associated with migraine headache. Ergots (e.g., dihydroergotamine, DHE-45) may be used to abort migraine, working through serotonin receptors similar to the triptans. Novel pharmacologic treatments include the use of CGRP receptor antagonists for treatment of acute migraine.[13] Pharmacologic prevention for individuals with migraine headaches includes anticonvulsant therapy (e.g., topiramate).

Stop and Consider
What is the most likely mechanism for the prevention of migraines with antiseizure medications?

Otitis Media

Otitis media is a commonly diagnosed condition in children. A complete history of illness combined with physical examination is important in determining an accurate diagnosis. Otitis media is a condition commonly diagnosed in infants and young children, although adults can also be affected. According to the National Institute of Deafness and Other Communication Disorders, 75% of children experience at least one episode of otitis media by their third birthday. The high prevalence of otitis media is estimated to cost approximately $5 billion per year in the United States.

PATHOPHYSIOLOGY

Acute otitis media (AOM), infection in the middle ear, is the most frequent diagnosis in febrile children in the United States and the world.[14] Most antibiotic agents for children are prescribed for AOM. The course of infection is associated with a preceding respiratory infection, inflammation and accumulation of secretions produced by the middle ear mucosa. This environment presents an optimal medium for growth of upper airway viruses and bacterial pathogens in the middle ear, leading to AOM. Occlusion of the eustachian tubes caused by secretions and inflammation promotes development of negative pressure and serous effusion in the middle ear. Perforation of the tympanic membrane and spread of infection into the mastoid air cells are the most frequent complications. AOM is considered recurrent when three or more episodes occur over 6 months or four or more episodes occur over 1 year. Otitis media with effusion (OME) is more common than AOM and is characterized by fluid/effusion in the middle ear without infection. OME results from the trapping of fluid in the middle ear by obstruction in the eustachian tube.

CLINICAL MANIFESTATIONS

Clinical manifestations of otitis media include:

- Acute ear pain
- Enlarged periauricular lymph nodes
- Rhinorrhea (runny nose)
- Fever
- Impaired hearing

Examination of the ears using an otoscope may reveal gray or red tympanic membrane in OME and AOM, respectively (Fig. 12.16). Fluid may be visible behind the tympanic membrane, which may also appear to be bulging because of increased fluid volume. White areas on the tympanic membrane may be scarring from previous perforations. Discharge in the ear canal indicates possible acute perforation.

DIAGNOSTIC CRITERIA

Diagnosis of otitis media is usually made based on the history of symptoms and clinical findings, particularly those identified with otoscopic examination. It is important to distinguish OME from AOM for appropriate treatment. Criteria for diagnosis of AOM include[14]:

- Moderate to severe bulging of tympanic membrane
- Mild bulging of tympanic membrane **and** new onset ear pain or erythema of tympanic membrane
- New onset otorrhea (discharge in the ear canal)

TREATMENT

Management of AOM includes management of pain and treatment of infection.[14] Concerns about increasing rates of antibiotic resistance and lack of sound evidence for antibiotic effectiveness have encouraged a careful look at practice guidelines used in the treatment of AOM. As OME is not an infectious process, no antibiotic treatment is recommended though management of pain may be indicated. According to clinical practice guidelines published by the American Academy of Pediatrics,[14] the following recommendations for AOM treatment include:

- Antibiotic therapy in children ≥6 months of age with severe signs or symptoms
  - Moderate or severe ear pain for at least 48 hours
  - Fever with temperature ≥39°C (102.2°F)
- Antibiotic therapy in children ≥24 months of age without severe signs or symptoms
  - Mild ear pain for at least 48 hours
  - Temperature <39°C (102.2°F)
- Optional antibiotic therapy or observation based on joint parental/caregiver decision in children between 6 and 23 months of age without severe signs or symptoms
- Observation in children between ≥23 months of age without severe signs or symptoms

First-line antibiotic therapy includes amoxicillin if antibiotics are necessary and if not previously used in the past 30 days. Alternative antibiotic type is recommended if the infection is unresponsive to initial antibiotic therapy (after 48 to 72 hours).

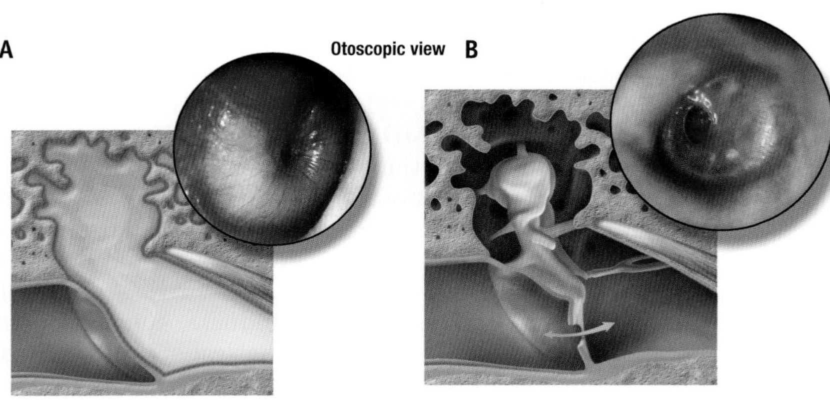

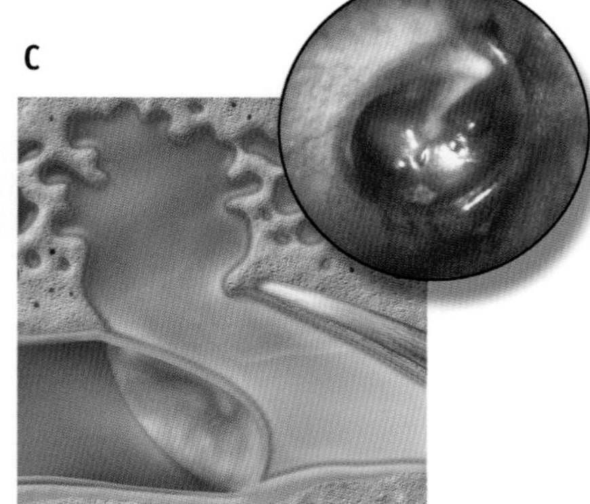

Figure 12.16. Classification of otitis media. **A:** Otoscopic examination in acute otitis media reveals infected fluid in the middle ear and a red tympanic membrane. **B:** Otitis media with effusion reveals middle ear fluid with a gray tympanic membrane. **C:** Tympanic membrane perforation reveals a hole in the tympanic membrane with possible fluid in the ear canal. (Courtesy Anatomical Chart Company.)

Ménière Disease

Ménière disease is a condition of altered vestibular function. The pathology is targeted to the labyrinth component of the inner ear, causing vertigo, tinnitus, hearing loss, pressure, and pain. Approximately 615,000 individuals are diagnosed with Ménière disease in the United States. Worldwide, the incidence of Ménière disease is estimated to range from 0.5 to 100 per 1,000, dependent on the diagnostic criteria applied. Age of onset is usually between 20 and 60 years,[15] and the condition is equally common between genders.

PATHOPHYSIOLOGY

The underlying etiology of Ménière disease is swelling of the membranous labyrinth in the cochlea and vestibular system of the inner ear. The labyrinth is composed of two parts: the body and membranous components. The increased volume of endolymph (endolymph hydrops) causes dilation of the membranous labyrinth, altering hearing and balance. Mild rupture of the membranous labyrinth reduces symptoms. Onset and duration of symptoms are unpredictable with debilitating effects. Symptoms can occur as often as daily or as infrequently as yearly.

CLINICAL MANIFESTATIONS

Manifestations of Ménière disease are related to vestibular dysfunction, often unilateral. Severity of symptoms can vary from mild to disabling. Vertigo, a feeling of spinning, is a hallmark of Ménière disease and is often associated with nausea and vomiting. Nystagmus and tinnitus may also develop. A feeling of fullness and pain in the ear and sensorineural hearing loss may also complicate the condition.

DIAGNOSTIC CRITERIA

The primary complaint of episodic dizziness prompts evaluation for Ménière disease. Hearing and balance assessment are important to the diagnosis of Ménière disease. Auditory examination can indicate the presence of sensorineural hearing loss. Auditory brainstem responses that measure electrical activity of the auditory nerve and the brainstem help to identify the type of hearing loss. Electrocochleography, a test that records sound-induced electrical activity in the inner ear, assists with diagnosis. Videonystagmography (VNG) determines communication between balance-related sensors and head movement on eye control.

TREATMENT

Treatment of Ménière disease is symptomatic. Regulation of body fluid through reduction in salt intake or diuretic therapy, smoking cessation, and stress reduction may reduce symptom occurrence. Antiemetics to prevent nausea and drugs to reduce vertigo are the main pharmacologic treatments. Treatment for acute symptoms includes vestibular suppressants. Betahistine, a histamine analog, is the first-line treatment in the reduction of the frequency and severity of symptoms. Destructive procedures may be attempted when medical therapy is not effective. Direct administration of the antibiotic gentamicin into the middle ear promotes ototoxicity, reducing vertigo though loss of hearing may result. Vestibular neurectomy, severing of the vestibular nerve, also helps reduce vertigo with no direct effect on hearing. Labyrinthectomy, or surgical removal of the labyrinth, may help reduce vertigo; however, loss of hearing may result. Nondestructive therapies include endolymphatic sac decompression or shunting, designed to improve drainage of endolymph.

Macular Degeneration

Degeneration of the central portion of the retinal macula, the fovea, is the central pathology of macular degeneration (MD). Factors contributing to the development of MD include aging, inflammation, injury, and infection. Gene–gene and gene–environment interactions influence susceptibility of MD.[16] According to the American Macular Degeneration Foundation, MD is the leading cause of blindness among older Americans in the United States. Overall, the prevalence among the US population is 9.2%.[17] Age-specific prevalence rates are comparable between races until age 75, when the prevalence increases significantly

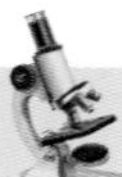

FROM THE LAB

Electronystagmography (**ENG**) is a group of tests that determine vestibular function based on eye movement. Nystagmus and other eye movements provide an evaluation of some brain functions. Eye movements are measured by small electrodes or are recorded by infrared video. Eye movements are evaluated as the eyes follow a target, when the head is positioned in different directions and during the caloric test. The caloric test uses warm and cool water or air irrigation to induce nystagmus, diagnostic of Ménière disease.

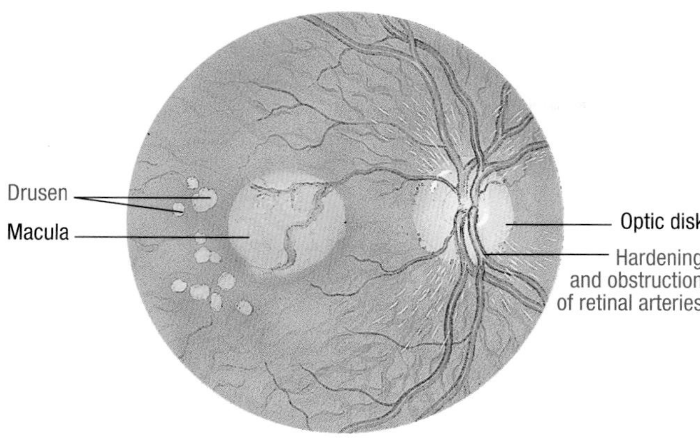

Figure 12.17. Retinal changes in macular degeneration. (Courtesy Anatomical Chart Company.)

among White individuals, according to the National Eye Institute and Prevent Blindness America.

PATHOPHYSIOLOGY

MD can be categorized into two forms: **dry (atrophic) MD** and **wet (exudative) MD**. Most cases of MD are of the dry variety, with retinal deterioration resulting from deposition of **drusen**, small yellow deposits, under the macula next to the basement membrane of the retinal pigment epithelium (Fig. 12.17). Drusen thins and dries out the macula, promoting loss of function. Loss of vision is correlated with increases in drusen deposits.

Wet or exudative MD is caused by the formation of new blood vessels under the retina and macula, known as **choroidal neovascularization** and causes far more vision loss than dry MD. Choroidal neovascularization may be a compensatory response to poor perfusion of the arteries of the retina because of obstruction. Leakage of fluid and bleeding from these new vessels alter the shape of the macula, distorting central vision. Once choroidal neovascularization occurs in one eye, it will likely develop in the other, especially when the risk factors of more than five large drusen, pigmental clumping, and hypertension are present. The two categories of choroidal neovascularization include classical and occult.

1. Classical
   a. Well defined
   b. Associated with more leakage than occult
   c. Vision ranges between 20/250 and 20/800
2. Occult
   a. Poorly defined
   b. Associated with less leakage than classical
   c. Vision ranges between 20/80 and 20/200

CLINICAL MANIFESTATIONS

Dry, atrophic MD is characterized by fluctuating vision, difficulty reading, and limited night vision. The progression of symptoms in the dry form of MD is usually slow. In wet, exudative MD, vision loss may be rapid and severe. Early symptoms are not always apparent, although some affected individuals may report a dark central spot. Consequences of MD include distortion of central vision; decreased ability to read, recognize faces or colors, or drive cars; and blindness.

Risk factors for development of MD include[18]:

1. Age older than 50 years
2. White race
3. Smoking
4. Diet low in antioxidants
5. Sun exposure

DIAGNOSTIC CRITERIA

Regular eye examinations by an ophthalmologist or an optometrist are important to identify MD early. An examination with an ophthalmoscope can determine if the characteristic changes associated with MD are present. Because symptoms are not always apparent, a thorough eye examination, including dilation of the eyes for visualization of the retina and macula, is necessary in at-risk individuals, especially older adults. Dilation of the eyes and visualization of the retina allow detection of leakage, bulging macula, and drusen deposition. This examination component should complement the routine screening eye examination. If MD is suspected, further evaluation may include:

- Amsler chart evaluation (see From the Lab)
  - Uses a grid (10 × 10 cm) containing 20.5-mm squares to a side, with white lines on a black background containing a central black spot
  - Evaluates changes in vision consistent with progressive MD
- Fluorescein angiography
  - Colored dye is injected into a peripheral vein
  - Pictures of the retina are taken as dye passes through it to detect the presence of abnormal fluid or progressive changes
- Optical coherence tomography
  - Imaging technique used to obtain detailed retinal images

TREATMENT

There are currently no treatment options for dry MD. Fortunately, dry MD is a slowly progressive condition. Treatment of wet MD is targeted toward limiting progression of retinal damage and loss of vision. In wet MD, the goal of therapy is to reduce choroidal neovascularization, reducing lesion size and leakage. Intraocular use of drugs that block vascular endothelial growth factor (VEGF) is the primary pharmacologic treatment effective in blocking the formation of new blood vessels.[19] Laser or conventional photocoagulation can be used to target neovascularization, though reduction in vision is a potential risk. Photodynamic therapy involves irradiation of retinal neovascularization through activation of an injected drug by laser.

Stop and Consider
Why do people with MD have difficulty with night vision and color differentiation?

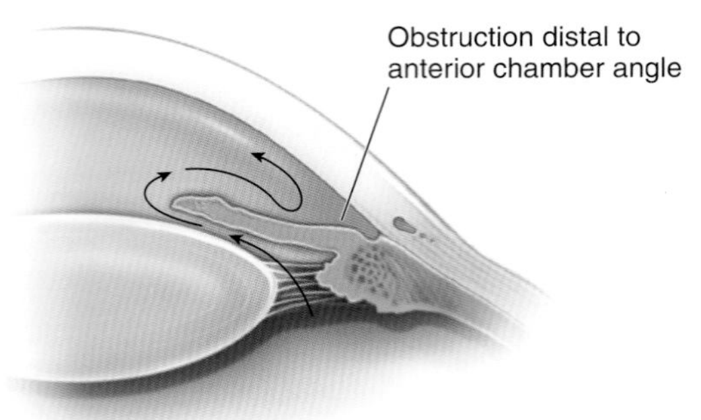

Figure 12.18. Open-angle glaucoma. Obstruction of the trabecular network leads to increased intraocular pressure.

Glaucoma

Glaucoma is the second leading cause of blindness among the elderly and the leading cause of preventable blindness in the United States. According to the National Eye Institute and Prevent Blindness America, 2.2 million Americans over age 40 (approximately 1.9% of the population) are affected by glaucoma. Prevalence is increased among Blacks, Hispanics, and the elderly. Gender differences are evident—women are affected at increased prevalence rates up through the age of 65 years, after which time rates become comparable. Prevalence rate for White females aged 65 to 69 years is 1.6%, compared with a rate of 4.8% among Black females at the same age. It is often silent, with damage resulting in the absence of warning signs.

PATHOPHYSIOLOGY

Glaucoma results in blindness, the result of progressive neurodegeneration of ganglion cells.[20] Vision loss is the result of damage to the optic nerve. Increased intraocular pressure (IOP) is a risk factor, although glaucoma may be present despite normal IOP. Primary open-angle glaucoma is the most common form of glaucoma, typically associated with increased IOP due to increased aqueous production and decreased outflow of aqueous humor (Fig. 12.18). Angle refers to the point where the iris and cornea meet. A chronic disease, primary open-angle glaucoma is likely hereditary. The trabecular network draining the aqueous humor becomes obstructed or "clogged," causing an increase in IOP in most cases. IOP of 22 mm Hg or more is considered abnormal, exceeding the expected normal pressure range of 14 to 16 mm Hg.

Angle-closure glaucoma, also known as acute or narrow angle, is characterized by a rapid rise in IOP caused by blockage of aqueous humor drainage due to narrowing or closure of the anterior chamber angle. Buildup of fluid and pressure promotes further narrowing of the angle. Complete closure is an acute crisis known as acute glaucoma. This form is more common in people of Asian descent and in people with hyperopia. Angle-closure glaucoma is an inheritable trait.

Normal- (or low-) tension glaucoma is characterized by normal IOP and progressive optical nerve damage with loss of visual fields. Approximately one-third of individuals with open-angle glaucoma have normal IOP. The underlying pathology is related to poor blood flow to the optic nerve or increased sensitivity of the retina to ocular pressure (Fig. 12.19). Management is focused on lowering ocular pressure to below "normal" to reduce retinal damage.

CLINICAL MANIFESTATIONS

Risk factors in the development of glaucoma include:

1. Age
2. Black race
3. Diabetes
4. Eye trauma
5. Long-term steroid use

In primary open-angle glaucoma, the cornea adapts to the increasing pressure without swelling, thereby not causing subjective symptoms. If untreated, open-angle glaucoma can result in gradual, but irreversible, loss of vision. Manifestations of vision loss include "blind spots" in the field of vision. Initially limited to the periphery, central vision is soon affected. This form of glaucoma responds well to pharmacologic management.

An acute episode of angle-closure glaucoma may be induced by increased pupil dilation caused by drugs or by being in a darkened room, such as a movie theater. Symptoms may include eye pain, headache, nausea, blurred vision, and "rainbows" around lights at night. Scarring of the trabecular network may result in chronic glaucoma and cataracts. Damage to the optic nerve may result in permanent loss of vision. Surgical management is often indicated.

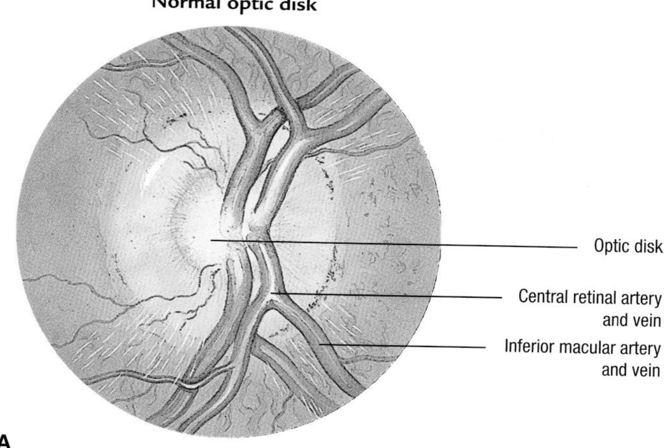

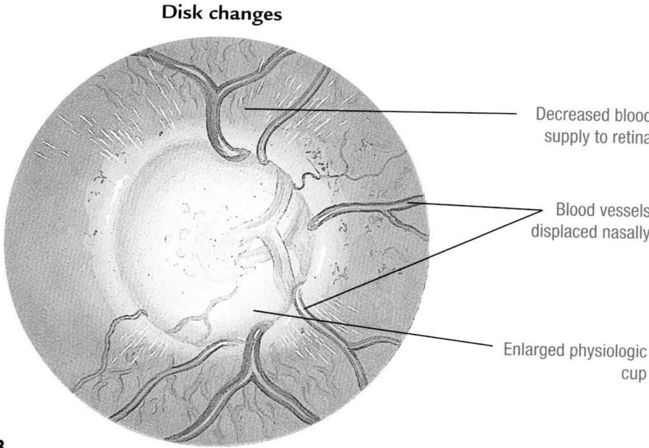

Figure 12.19. Glaucoma-induced changes in the optic disk **(A)**. Increased intraocular pressure reduces blood supply to the retina, leading to "blind spots" in the optic disk **(B)**.

DIAGNOSTIC CRITERIA

Early detection of glaucoma may promote effective treatment and management, decreasing associated loss of visual function. Efforts to determine the best screening type and frequency to detect early disease are ongoing. Pattern electroretinogram (PERG), electric potential derived from retinal ganglion cells, is used to evaluate IOP lowering after topical treatment in glaucoma patients with early visual field impairment. Function of retinal ganglion cells may be at least partially restored after IOP reduction in early disease.

Screening for glaucoma is completed in at-risk individuals as a component of comprehensive vision screening, usually by optometrists or ophthalmologists. Common screening tests for glaucoma include:

- Tonometry
  - Measure IOP
- Ophthalmoscopy
  - Detects changes in the optic nerve (cupping, pallor, hemorrhage) by using an ophthalmoscope in a funduscopic examination
- Visual field testing
  - Determines damage to the optic nerve
- Confocal laser optical coherence
  - Three-dimensional imaging to detect cupping and thickness of the retinal nerve

TREATMENT

The goal of glaucoma treatment is to lower IOP through decreased production and increased outflow of aqueous humor. Treatment of glaucoma may be pharmacologic or surgical.

- Pharmacologic
  - Miotics: increase the outflow of fluid
  - Epinephrine-based: increase the outflow of fluid
  - Beta blockers: decrease fluid levels
  - Carbonic anhydrase inhibitors: decrease fluid levels
  - Alpha-adrenergic agonists: decrease fluid levels
  - Prostaglandin analogs: increase fluid flow through secondary drainage
- Laser surgery
  - Trabeculoplasty: correction of the trabecular network to promote fluid outflow from the eye in open-angle glaucoma
  - Iridotomy: incision into the iris to promote fluid outflow in angle-closure glaucoma[21]
  - Cyclophotocoagulation: correction of ciliary tissue to decrease the production of fluid
- Conventional surgery
  - Trabeculectomy: surgical removal of a small portion of the trabecular meshwork under the lid to create new drainage

Stop and Consider
What are the implications for older Americans who develop glaucoma? What lifestyle changes can they expect to experience?

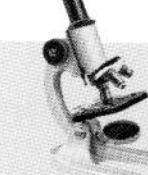

FROM THE LAB

Evaluation of the anterior chamber and angle can be accomplished by gonioscopy. Gonioscopy allows direct visualization of these structures via a special lens containing a mirror, eliminating the view-obstructing effects of the cornea and sclera. Indications for this evaluation include the need to visualize the anterior chamber, determine the angle, and classify glaucoma.

Retinopathy of Prematurity

Retinopathy of prematurity (ROP) is the leading childhood cause of blindness. As the name implies, infants born prematurely have the highest risk for developing ROP. Premature infants born at or less than 28 weeks gestation and those with low birth weight of less than 1,250 g (2.75 lb) are at highest risk for the development of ROP. In the United States, it is estimated that of the 10,000 infants born with a birth weight of less than 1,250 g, 68% of them will develop ROP, with approximately one-third progressing to severe ROP and nonreversible loss of vision.[21]

PATHOPHYSIOLOGY

The retina is one of the last organs to develop the vascular blood supply. In fetus, retinal development begins at 16 weeks gestation in a low-oxygen intrauterine environment and continues until birth. During that period, the retinal blood vessels grow out from the optic nerve toward the periphery, providing the retina with essential oxygen and nutrients. By the end of full term gestation at 38 to 40 weeks of pregnancy, fetal retinal vascularization is typically complete.

When retinal blood vessel growth is prematurely stopped with early delivery, retinal blood vessel growth is impaired. Further retinal blood vessel development must now occur in the high oxygen extra-uterine environment. As most infants at risk for ROP also have respiratory risks due to inadequately developed lungs, supplemental oxygen is provided to assure adequate ventilation and oxygen delivery to cells and tissues. The result is arrested growth of retinal blood vessels, the first phase of ROP.

The second phase of ROP is characterized by unregulated growth of retinal blood vessels into the vitreous cavity. The release of VEGF and other angiogenic factors promotes excessive growth of abnormal, leaky blood vessels. Hemorrhage and contraction of scarred, fragile blood vessels pulls the retina away, leading to retinal detachment and vision loss.

According to the National Eye Institute, ROP is classified in five stages based on disease severity. The stages are:

- Stage I: Mildly abnormal blood vessel growth
- Stage II: Moderately abnormal blood vessel growth
- Stage III: Severely abnormal blood vessel growth
- Stage IV: Severely abnormal blood vessel growth and partially detached retina
- Stage V: Completely detached retina

CLINICAL MANIFESTATIONS

The identification of clinical manifestations is challenging. Among infants at risk for ROP, a thorough ophthalmologic examination is necessary to detect the subtle changes associated with ROP. Manifestations of severe ROP may include:

- Leukocoria (white pupils)
- Nystagmus (abnormal eye movements)
- Strabismus (crossed eyes)
- Myopia (severe nearsightedness)

DIAGNOSIS

Ophthalmologic examination targets retinal blood vessels. In mild ROP, there may be evidence of normal growth of retinal blood vessels. Abnormalities of retinal blood vessels are evident in severe cases of ROP and include dilation, tortuosity and venous congestion of retinal blood vessels. Evidence of scarring and retinal detachment is observed in the most severe stages of ROP.

TREATMENT

The initial lessons about prevention of ROP came as a result of an epidemic that occurred in the 1940s and 1950s. At that time, hospital nurseries began using high concentrations of oxygen to manage the other critical problems of prematurity related to impaired ventilation. It is now recognized that delivery of high concentrations of oxygen to premature infants increases the risk of ROP. That risk for ROP must be balanced with the need to oxygenate other cells and tissues in the premature infant with impaired ventilation. Today, oxygenation of premature infants is monitored to provide concentrations of oxygen that do not exceed what is necessary to support the metabolic requirements of the infant, reducing risk for ROP.

In stages I and II, spontaneous resolution will result in children not requiring treatment. Children with stage I and stage II disease will likely develop normal vision. In stage III, some infants improve and develop normal vision without treatment. Others with abnormal growth patterns of enlarged or twisted retinal blood vessels require treatment, the stage referred to as stage III plus.

If initiated early, retinal detachment may be prevented. Retinal detachment in stages IV and V requires immediate treatment to increase potential for maximal vision. Treatment of infants with Stage III plus through stage V ROP involves invasive surgical intervention on the eye with either laser treatments or cryotherapy (freezing treatment). Later stages of ROP may require other treatments that are targeted toward correction of retinal detachment. Application of a scleral buckle, a silicone band tightened around the eye, reduces traction of the vitreous humor on the retina. The retina can relax onto the wall of the eye. A vitrectomy, replacement of the vitreous humor with saline, may also be done in stage V disease. The removal of retinal scar tissue during the procedure is done to promote flattening of the retina onto the eye wall.

SUMMARY

- Sensory systems relay information from the periphery to the CNS.
- The sensations of pain, touch, pressure, temperature, and proprioception are transmitted by the somatosensory system via specialized receptors and pathways.
- Vision results from light entry through the pupil, stimulating photoreceptors in the retina and generating a nerve impulse. Vision processing occurs in the occipital lobe of the brain, where visual images are coordinated.
- Hearing results from connections between the tympanic membrane and the ossicles, leading to the transduction of the mechanical vibration, producing sound.
- Balance and equilibrium are regulated by the semicircular canals of the ear, generating an impulse, which is then transmitted to the cerebellum via the vestibular branch of the acoustic nerve.
- Pain sensation is generated by stimulation of nociceptors, the impulse transmitted and modulated along pain fibers until it reaches the brain for processing.
- Alterations in vision may result from errors in injury or damage to visual structures, errors in refraction, impaired eye movement, and alterations in protective structures.
- Disorders of hearing are affected by outer, middle, and inner ear structural and functional integrity. Hearing loss may be conductive, sensorineural, mixed, or caused by a central auditory processing disorder.
- Pain can be characterized by location, quality, and duration. Management of pain is reflected by pain characteristics and is based on regulation of impulse inhibition. Options for pain treatment include nonpharmacologic and pharmacologic measures.
- Altered sensory transmission and conduction have implications for all body systems and whole body function. A thorough understanding of the concepts that govern neuronal transmission promotes the ability to apply knowledge in a variety of conditions and pathologies associated with sensory deficit.

CASE STUDY 12.1

A 75-year-old man discusses vision concerns with his ophthalmologist at his yearly visit. After a careful history and physical examination, he is diagnosed with bilateral cataracts.

1. What are the clinical manifestations associated with cataracts?
2. What is the underlying pathophysiology associated with cataracts?
3. How are cataracts diagnosed?
4. What are the possible treatments for cataracts?
5. What are the issues related to appropriate management of cataracts?

Log onto the Internet. Search for a relevant journal article or Web site that details cataract to confirm your predictions.

PRACTICE EXAM QUESTIONS

1. Which sensory receptor is responsible for impulses resulting in the sensation of touch?
   a. Mechanoreceptor
   b. Chemoreceptor
   c. Nociceptor
   d. Osmoreceptor

2. Which somatosensory neurons are responsible for communication of sensory information from the thalamus to the cerebral cortex and are present in the greatest quantity?
   a. First order
   b. Second order
   c. Third order
   d. Interneuron

3. The most likely site of pathology leading to alterations in balance is:
   a. The outer ear
   b. The middle ear
   c. The inner ear
   d. The tympanic membrane

4. Which type of pain involves a typical pattern of impulse conduction and originates outside of the nervous system?
   a. Neurogenic
   b. Nociceptive
   c. Neuropathic
   d. Analgesic

5. Hyperopia is a condition characterized by:
   a. Alterations in eye movement
   b. Infection of the conjunctiva
   c. Increased sensitivity to light
   d. Error in refraction

6. Infection of the middle ear is also known as:
   a. Mastoiditis
   b. Vestibulitis
   c. Otitis media
   d. Labyrinthitis

7. Sensorineural hearing loss is:
   a. Often permanent, resulting from disease, trauma, or genetic defect
   b. Localized to the middle ear and is often temporary
   c. Caused by alteration in auditory signal processing in the brain
   d. A response to immobility of the tympanic membrane

8. The mechanism of action of opioid analgesics is:
   a. Blockade of serotonin reuptake at the synaptic cleft
   b. Inhibition of cyclooxygenase enzymes and prostaglandin production
   c. Stimulation of large fibers to modulate pain transmission
   d. Modulate pain at the level of the spinal cord by binding to mu, delta, and kappa receptors

9. The mechanism of action of opiod analgesics is:
   a. Blockade of serotonin reuptake at the synaptic cleft
   b. Inhibition of cyclooxygenase enzymes and prostaglandin production
   c. Stimulation of large fibers to modulate pain transmission
   d. Modulate pain at the level of the spinal cord by binding to mu, delta, and kappa receptors

10. Which one of the following eye conditions is the result of increased intraocular pressure?
   a. Retinopathy of prematurity
   b. Glaucoma
   c. Wet macular degeneration
   d. Dry macular degeneration

11. Balance and body position are the function of
   a. Utricle
   b. Saccule
   c. Semicircular canals
   d. All of the above

12. Damage to the cochlear hair cells may result in
   a. Hearing loss
   b. Loss of balance
   c. Lack of proprioception
   d. None of the above

13. Fibromyalgia is diagnosed by
   a. Loss of bone mass
   b. Muscle inflammation
   c. Weight loss
   d. Multiple tender points

14. Which of the following is a symptom?
   a. Pain
   b. Hearing loss
   c. Loss of proprioception
   d. None of the above

15. Which of the following reports of pain level (0 to 10) is considered moderate, requiring medications?
   a. 1
   b. 2
   c. 3
   d. 4

16. Neuromatrix pain theory states
   a. Specific stimuli cause predictable pain responses
   b. Specific stimuli results in prevention of impulse crossing in spinal cord
   c. Neural network integration of multiple inputs determines pain perception
   d. Pain perception is determined by duration of impulse and amount of tissue involved

DISCUSSION AND APPLICATION

1. What did I know about pain and alterations in sensation before today?
2. What body processes are affected by pain and alteration in sensation? How do pain and alteration in sensation affect those processes?
3. What are the potential etiologies for pain and alteration in sensation? How do pain and alteration in sensation develop?
4. Who is most at risk for developing pain and alteration in sensation? How can these alterations be prevented?
5. What are the human differences that affect the etiology, risk, or course of pain and alteration in sensation?
6. What clinical manifestations are expected in the course of pain and alteration in sensation?
7. What special diagnostic tests are useful in determining the diagnosis and course of pain and alteration in sensation?
8. What are the goals of care for individuals with pain and alteration in sensation?
9. How does the concept of pain and alteration in sensation build on what I have learned in the previous chapters and in the previous courses?
10. How can I use what I have learned?

RESOURCES

National Pain Strategy: A Comprehensive Population Health-Level Strategy for Pain
http://iprcc.nih.gov/docs/HHSNational_Pain_Strategy.pdf

American Macular Degeneration Foundation:
https://www.macular.org/?gclid=CLPrw_L2hMwCFQkyaQodvnsFjQ

American Speech, Language and Hearing Association:
http://www.asha.org/public/hearing/disorders/types.htm
Information on types of hearing loss

National Eye Institute (NEI):
http://www.nei.nih.gov
Conducts and supports research on eye diseases and vision disorders.

National Institute for Deafness and other Communication Disorders (NIDCD):
http://www.nidcd.nih.gov/Pages/default.aspx
Information about hearing disorders

National Institute of Neurologic Disorders and Stroke:
http://www.ninds.nih.gov/disorders/chronic_pain/chronic_pain.htm
Information on chronic pain

Prevent Blindness America:
http://www.preventblindness.org

U.S. Food and Drug Administration, Center for Drug Evaluation and Research:
http://www.fda.gov/drugs/resourcesforyou/consumers/buyingusingmedicinesafely/understandingover-the-countermedicines/safeuseofover-the-counterpainrelieversandfeverreducers/default.htm
Information about over-the-counter analgesics

References

1. Moayedi M, Davis KD. Theories of pain: from specificity to gate control. *J Neurophysiol.* 2013;109:5–12. doi:10.1152/jn.00457.2012.
2. Melzack R, Katz J. Pain. *Wiley Interdiscip Rev Cogn Sci.* 2013;4(1):1–15. doi:10.1002/wcs.1201.
3. Pillai RRR, Racine NM, Gennis HG, et al. Non-pharmacologic management of infant and young child procedural pain. *Cochrane Database Syst Rev.* 2015;12:CD006275.
4. DeGiacomo A, Craig F, D'Elia A, et al. Children with cochlear implants: cognitive skills, adaptive behaviors, social and emotional skills. *Int J Pediatr Otorhinolaryngol.* 2013;77(12):1975–1990.
5. Borchers AT, Gershwin EM. Fibromylagia: a critical and comprehensive review. *Clinic Rev Allerg Immunol.* 2015;49:100–151.
6. Menzies V, Lyon DE, Archer KJ, et al. Epigenetic alterations and an increased frequency of micronuclei in women with fibromyalgia. *Nurs Res Pract.* 2013;2013:795784. doi:10.1155/2013/795784.
7. Wolfe F, Smythe HA, Yunus MB, et al. The American College of Rheumatology 1990 criteria for the classification of fibromyalgia. Report of the Multicenter Criteria Committee. *Arthritis Rheum.* 1990;33(2):160–172.
8. Peterson J. Understanding fibromyalgia and its treatment options. *Nurse Pract.* 2005;30(1):48–55.
9. Burstein R, Noseda R, Borsook D. Migraine: multiple processes, complex pathophysiology. *J Neurosci.* 2015;35(17):6619–6629.
10. Headache Classification Committee of the International Headache Society. The International Classification of Headache Disorders, 3rd edition. *Cephalalgia.* 2013;33(9):629–808.
11. Freitag FG, Schloemer F. Medical management of adult headache. *Otolaryngol Clin North Am.* 2014;46:221–237.
12. Forde G, Duarte RA, Rosen N. Managing chronic headache disorders. *Med Clin North Am.* 2016;100(1): 117–141. doi:10.1016/j.mcna.2015.09.006.
13. Mitsikostas DD, Rapoport AM. New players in the preventive treatment of migraine. *BMC Med.* 2015;13:279. doi:10.1186/s12916-015-0522-1.
14. Lieberthal AS, Carroll AE, Chonmaitree T, et al. The diagnosis and management of acute otitis media. *Pediatrics.* 2013;131(3):e964–e969. doi:10.1542/peds.2012-3488.
15. Harcourt J, Barraclough K, Bronstein AM. Meniere's disease. *BMJ.* 2014;349:g6544. doi:10.1136/bmj.g6544.
16. Katta S, Kaur I, Chakrabarti S. The molecular genetic basis of age-related macular degeneration: an overview. *J Genet.* 2009;88(4):425–449.
17. Klein R, Rowland ML, Harris MI. Racial/ethnic differences in age-related maculopathy. Third National Health and Nutrition Examination Survey. *Ophthalmology.* 1995;102:371–381. https://nei.nih.gov/eyedata/amd. Accessed December 6, 2015.
18. Mehta S. Age-related macular degeneration. *Prim Care.* 2015;42(3):377–391. doi:10.1016/j.pop.2015.05.009.
19. Garcia-Lavana A, Figueroa MS, Arias L, et al. Individualized therapy with ranibizumab in wet age-related macular degeneration. *J Ophthalmol.* 2015;2015:412903. doi:10.1155/2015/412903.
20. Tian K, Shibata-Germanos S, Pahlitzsch M, et al. Current perspective of neuroprotection and glaucoma. *Clin Ophthalmol.* 2015;9:2109–2118.
21. Penn JS, Madan A, Caldwell RR, et al. Vascular endothelial growth factor in eye disease. *Prog Retin Eye Res.* 2008;27(4):331–371.

Find additional resources for this chapter at http:thePoint.lww.com thePoint®

Chapter

13 Altered Hormonal and Metabolic Regulation

LEARNING OUTCOMES

1. Define and use the key terms listed in this chapter.
2. Identify features that characterize hormones.
3. Discuss the role of the hypothalamic–pituitary axis in regulating hormone levels.
4. Identify pathways for mediating cell-to-cell communication.
5. Describe the role of the neuroendocrine system in the stress response.
6. Analyze the mechanisms of impairment that can lead to altered hormonal and metabolic regulation.
7. Discuss common measures to diagnose and treat hormone dysfunction.
8. Apply concepts of altered hormonal and metabolic regulation to select clinical models.

INTRODUCTION

How many texts, e-mails, phone calls, and instant messages did you receive today? Communication between humans requires a sender, message, and receiver. Likewise, communication between cells relies upon neuronal and endocrine signals to regulate body functions. This chapter reviews basic mechanisms for cell-to-cell communication, particularly as it relates to hormone-driven messages. You are already familiar with this idea; all previous chapters in one way or another relied on the concept of sender, message, and receiver. This chapter builds on that learning. A basic understanding of communication mechanisms within the body will help to predict the impact of high or low hormone levels on the function of endocrine glands. Clinical models are presented to help understand specific disease conditions affected by hormone alterations.

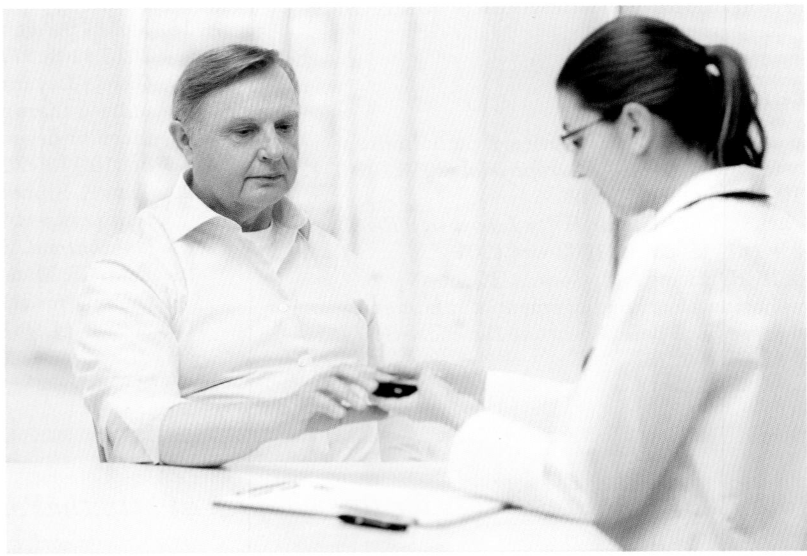

Healthcare practitioner measuring patient's blood sugar value. Image © Syda Productions.

Module 1 Function and Regulation of Hormones

Hormones are chemicals, formed originally in tissues or organs, which affect the growth and/or function of other target tissues or organs. The structure of hormones can vary in composition from a single amino acid, such as with thyroid hormone, to a complex combination of proteins, carbohydrates, or lipids, as occurs with cortisol. Hormones have many important regulatory functions, including metabolism, growth and development, muscle and fat distribution, fluid and electrolyte balance, sexual development, and reproduction. Hormones are also instrumental in the stress response. Table 13.1 outlines the functions specific to select hormones and should be referred to frequently as hormone processes are discussed.

Stop and Consider
In Table 13.1, hormones are organized alphabetically. How else could you organize this table? What type of organization is most useful to you as a learner?

Integrating Endocrine, Neuronal, and Defense Mechanisms in the Body

Hormones are commonly connected with the **endocrine system**, a collective group of tissues capable of secreting hormones (Fig. 13.1). The pancreas and thyroid are examples of endocrine glands. Note, however, that endocrine glands are not the only tissues capable of secreting hormones. Neurons can synthesize and release hormones. Neurotransmitters, such as epinephrine, dopamine, serotonin, and norepinephrine, are chemical messengers, synthesized by neurons, which rapidly stimulate a neuronal response. In this regard, neurotransmitters act as hormones. Inflammatory and immune cells release chemical mediators, such as cytokines, leukotrienes, and prostaglandins, which also function as hormones. The inflammatory and immune responses require these substances to trigger the mechanisms of defense. Some tumor cells also synthesize and release ectopic hormones, which ignore the body's control and feedback mechanisms and ultimately contribute to a loss of homeostasis.

Like an orchestra, the neurologic, inflammatory, immune, and endocrine systems collaborate in a unified symphony. Neurotransmitters act quickly, whereas endocrine hormones often take days to exert their maximum effect on target tissues. Yet these systems are highly dependent on one another. Regulatory processes integrate with an overall goal of protecting the body from injury and maintaining homeostasis.

Regulating Hormones

Several features are common to all hormones. Each of these features is discussed below.

- **Control:** hormone synthesis and release is controlled by tissues and organs; the hypothalamic–pituitary axis in the brain is an important control-center for many hormones
- **Patterns:** hormones exhibit predictable patterns of secretion, metabolism, and elimination
- **Feedback:** hormones listen and adjust based on negative or positive feedback loops
- **Action:** hormones exhibit two primary functions: (1) to act on target organs to achieve an effect or (2) to act on glands to produce another hormone
- **Receptor binding:** to exert an effect hormones must locate and attach onto target tissues

THE HYPOTHALAMIC–PITUITARY AXIS

The **hypothalamic–pituitary axis** controls the synthesis and secretion of many hormones. The *hypothalamus* contains neurons that synthesize prolactin, inhibiting hormones, and releasing hormones to act on the anterior pituitary gland. These include:

- Releasing hormones
  - Growth hormone-releasing hormone (GHRH)
  - Thyrotropin-releasing hormone (TRH)
  - Corticotropin-releasing hormone (CRH)
  - Gonadotropin-releasing hormone (GnRH)
- Inhibiting hormones
  - Somatostatin (inhibits growth hormone and thyroid-stimulating hormone)
  - Dopamine (inhibits prolactin)

The *pituitary* gland responds to these hypothalamic triggers and acts accordingly. It is important to understand that the pathways and hormones released from the *anterior* pituitary gland are different than the hormones released from the *posterior* pituitary. More specifically, to get from the hypothalamus to the anterior pituitary, prolactin, releasing, or inhibiting hormones (those listed above) travel through

Table 13.1 Functions of Select Hormones

Hormone	Source	Target	Function
Androgens	Testes	Reproductive organs	Control the development of reproductive organs, (testosterone) sperm production, and secondary sex characteristics and growth in males
Antidiuretic hormone (ADH)	Hypothalamus–posterior pituitary	Kidney	Promotes water reabsorption (retention of fluids)
Adrenocorticotropic hormone (ACTH)	Anterior pituitary	Adrenal cortex	Stimulates release of hormones from the adrenal cortex (primarily aldosterone and cortisol)
Corticotropin-releasing hormone (CRH)	Hypothalamus	Pituitary gland	Controls release of pituitary hormones
Epinephrine and norepinephrine	Adrenal medulla	Sympathetic nervous system	Transmits neural impulses
Estrogen	Ovaries	Reproductive organs	Promotes development of reproductive organs and secondary sex characteristics in women
Follicle-stimulating hormone (FSH)	Anterior pituitary	Reproductive organs	Stimulates growth of ovarian follicle and ovulation in women; stimulates sperm production in men
Glucagon	Pancreatic islet cells	Blood glucose	Stimulates glycogen breakdown in the liver to increase glucose in the blood
Glucocorticoids (cortisol)	Adrenal cortex	Multiple targets	Affects metabolism of all nutrients and growth; regulates blood glucose levels; has anti-inflammatory properties
Gonadotropin-releasing hormone (GnRH)	Hypothalamus	Pituitary gland	Controls release of pituitary hormones
Growth hormone-releasing hormone (GRHR)	Hypothalamus	Pituitary gland	Controls release of pituitary hormones
Growth hormone (GH)	Anterior pituitary	Bone, muscle, organs, and other tissues	Stimulates growth, protein synthesis, and fat metabolism; inhibits carbohydrate metabolism
Insulin	Pancreatic islet cells	Blood glucose	Facilitates glucose transport into the muscle, adipose, or liver cell to use for energy and growth
Luteinizing hormone (LH)	Anterior pituitary	Reproductive organs	Stimulates release of oocyte and production of estrogen and progesterone in women; stimulates secretion of testosterone in men
Mineralocorticosteroids (aldosterone)	Adrenal cortex	Kidney	Increases sodium reabsorption and potassium loss
Oxytocin	Hypothalamus–posterior pituitary	Uterus and breasts	Stimulates contraction of the uterus during labor and milk release from the breasts after childbirth
Parathyroid hormone (PTH)	Parathyroid glands	Bone, blood	Regulates calcium levels in the blood
Progesterone	Ovaries	Reproductive organs	Affects menstrual cycle; increases thickness of uterine wall; supports/maintains pregnancy
Thyroid hormones (TH): triiodothyronine (T_3) and thyroxine (T_4)	Thyroid gland	Multiple targets	Increases metabolic rate, needed for fetal and infant growth and development
Thyrotropin-releasing hormone (TRH)	Hypothalamus	Pituitary gland	Controls release of pituitary hormones
Thyroid-stimulating hormone (TSH)	Anterior pituitary	Thyroid gland	Stimulates synthesis and secretion of thyroid hormones (T_3 and T_4)

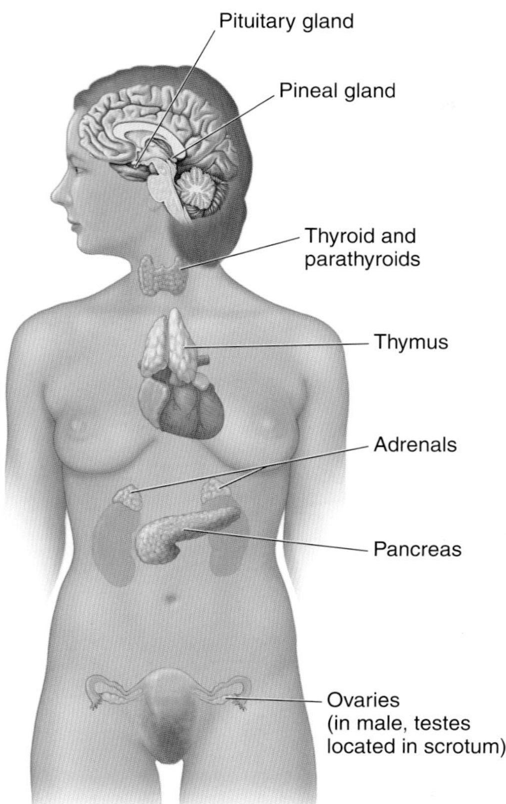

Figure 13.1. Organs of the endocrine system. (Courtesy Anatomical Chart Company.)

the hypophyseal portal system (blood vessels) to the anterior pituitary gland. Three possible scenarios that characterize release through the anterior pituitary are illustrated in Box 13.1. Each scenario demonstrates increasing complexity in the process and an example is provided. In contrast, the hypothalamus produces antidiuretic hormone (ADH) and oxytocin, which then travel along nerve axons to the posterior pituitary for unchanged release into the systemic circulation. This pathway through the posterior pituitary is not nearly as complicated as the anterior pituitary scenarios.

Stop and Consider

What are the major differences and similarities between the actions of the hypothalamus on the anterior pituitary gland versus the posterior pituitary gland? Why would this difference matter? What is an effective way to remember this difference?

A few hormones are secreted without initiation through the hypothalamus and come directly from the pituitary. One example is melanocyte-stimulating hormone, which is a hormone that regulates skin pigment. Pathways and actions for select hormones are depicted in Figure 13.2.

Box 13.1 Release of Hormones from the Hypothalamus to the Anterior Pituitary

Action 1:

- The hypothalamus produces the hormone.
- The hormone travels to the anterior pituitary.
- The hormone is released unchanged into the circulation.

Example: prolactin

Action 2:

- The hypothalamus produces a releasing hormone.
- The releasing hormone travels to and acts upon the anterior pituitary.
- The pituitary is stimulated to produce and release a different hormone into the circulation.

Example: growth hormone

Action 3:

- The hypothalamus produces a releasing hormone.
- The anterior pituitary is activated to release a stimulating hormone.
- The stimulating hormone acts on the gland to produce and secrete a final hormone that is released into the circulation.

Example: thyroid hormone

FEEDBACK MECHANISMS

What triggers the hypothalamus or pituitary to initiate a hormone release? Multiple mechanisms, such as neurotransmitters, injury and the resulting release of chemical mediators, and neuroendocrine signals provide input to the hypothalamus. This most commonly occurs through a **negative feedback loop** (Fig. 13.3). The mechanism of negative feedback is like an internal thermostat. When the temperature gets too hot, the thermostat shuts down the heat source; when the temperature is too cool, the furnace is activated to release heat. Amazingly, the hypothalamus and pituitary act as sensors that are constantly gauging the levels of hormones in the body. When levels rise above the expected range, the stimulation, production, or secretion of hormone is decreased. When levels fall, stimulation, production, or secretion of hormone is increased. The negative feedback mechanism is affected by environmental and body temperature, stress, nutrition, and the presence of specific body substances. For example, aldosterone levels adjust based on sodium and potassium levels in the body. Antidiuretic hormone is responsive to fluid levels in the body.

Although much less common, a few hormones are regulated by a **positive feedback loop**. In positive feedback, presence of the hormone stimulates increased production of the hormone until there is an interruption of the cycle. Oxytocin is one

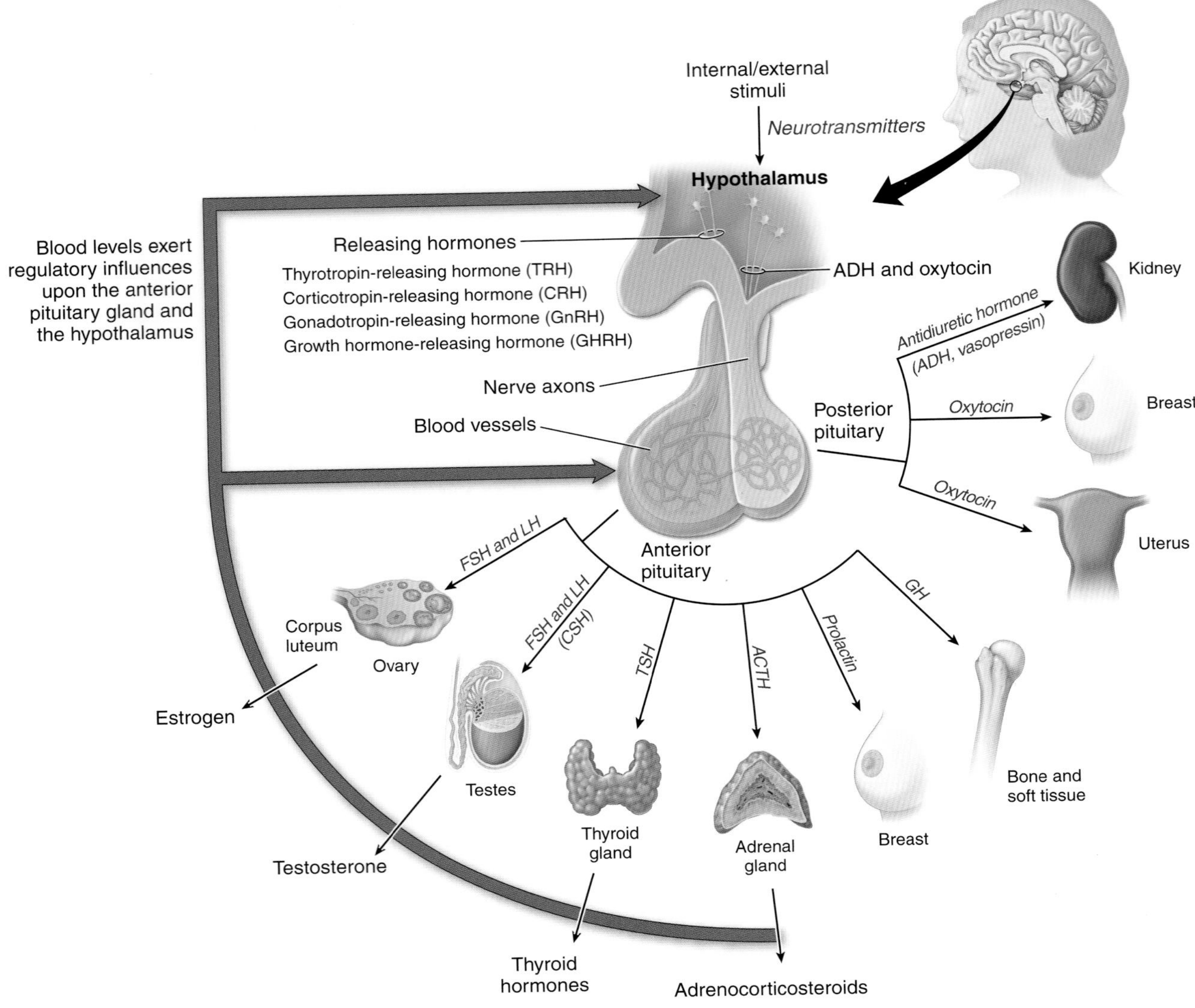

Figure 13.2. The hypothalamic–pituitary axis regulates the release of hormones. (Modified from Smeltzer SC, Bare BG. *Textbook of Medical-Surgical Nursing*. 10th ed. Philadelphia, PA: Lippincott Williams & Wilkins; 2003, with permission.)

example (Fig. 13.4). Specific feedback mechanisms for each hormone are discussed in depth within the clinical models.

HORMONE SECRETION, METABOLISM, AND ELIMINATION

Many hormones exhibit predictable patterns of secretion. For example, a 28-day cyclic secretion of estrogens, progesterone, luteinizing, and follicle-stimulating hormones regulates the female menstrual cycle. Some hormones have 24-hour diurnal patterns of secretion. For example, growth hormone levels increase during sleeping hours and decrease during waking hours. Secretion patterns highlight the complex, fluctuant, and responsive nature of hormones.

The accumulation of hormones is prevented through a process of inactivation and elimination. A common mechanism for inactivation is through enzymes that break down the hormone after attaching to the cell receptor and exerting an effect. Some hormones are also inactivated in the liver. Elimination commonly occurs through the urine or along with bile, via the feces.

RECEPTOR BINDING

Receptor binding allows hormones to act selectively on certain cells. The number of receptors on each cell can reach up to 100,000 or more. To access the cell, hormones seek out and attach to specific receptors, similar to a key that must fit a certain lock.

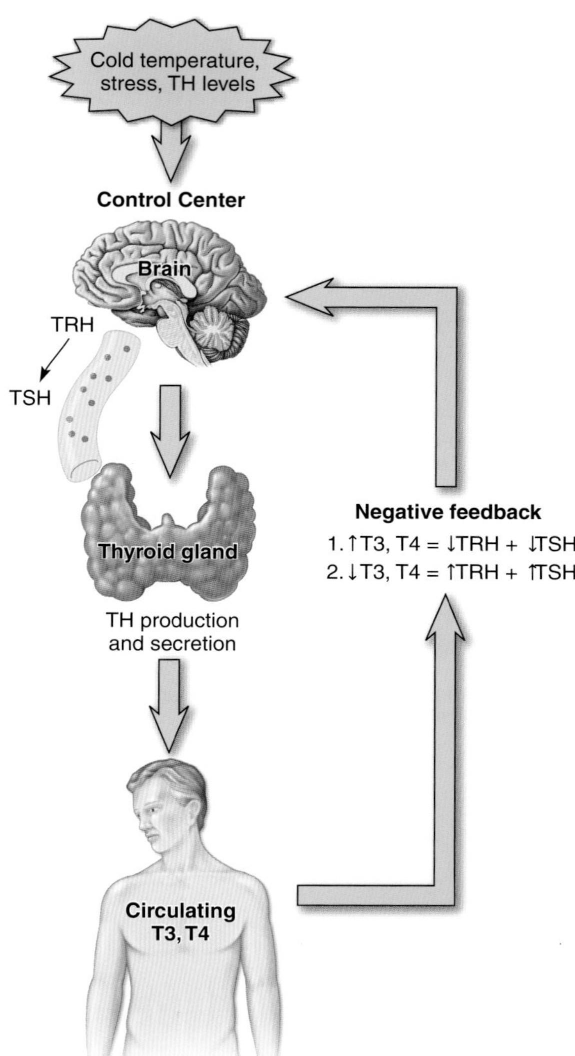

Figure 13.3. An example of a negative feedback loop. Circulating thyroid hormone (TH) levels ($T_3 + T_4$) alert the hypothalamus and anterior pituitary to increase or decrease thyrotropin-releasing hormone (TRH) and thyroid-stimulating hormone (TSH) secretion.

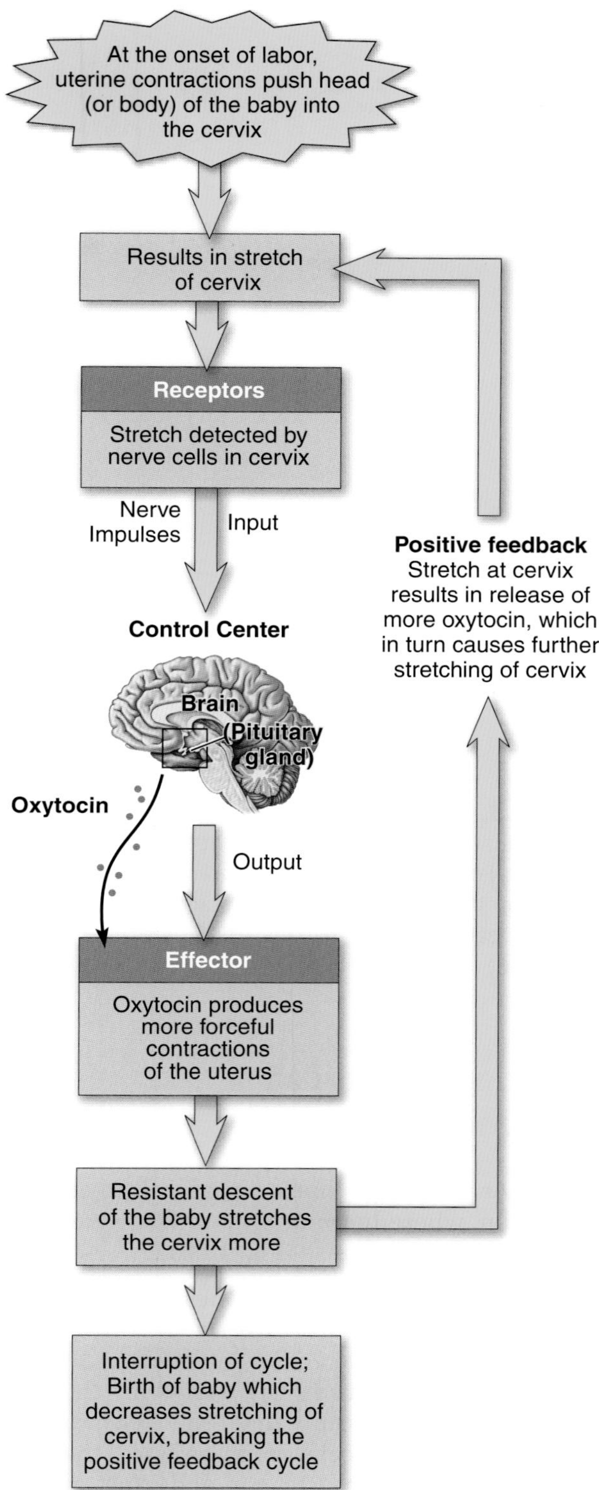

Figure 13.4. An example of a positive feedback loop. Oxytocin levels during labor and delivery increase release of additional oxytocin until the birth of the baby which decreases stretching of the cervix and the cycle is interrupted. (From Premkumar K. *The Massage Connection: Anatomy and Physiology*. Baltimore, MD: Lippincott Williams & Wilkins; 2004, with permission.)

Hormones can bind to a surface or inner receptor of a cell (Fig. 13.5). A surface receptor requires a second messenger to elicit a response from the cell. Without the appropriate receptor, the hormone moves along and has no impact on that cell. For example, skeletal muscle cells have receptors for growth hormone but are unresponsive to antidiuretic hormone. Receptor binding is altered when the number of receptors is reduced, as may occur with autoimmune conditions, or when the affinity, or attraction, for the hormone is reduced. The affinity can be reduced by many factors, such as genetics, hormone levels, and body fluid pH.

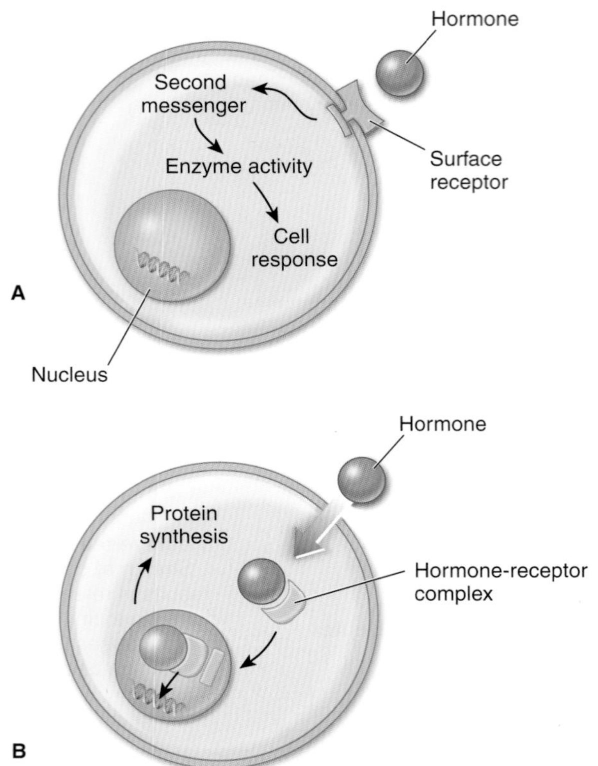

Figure 13.5. Two types of hormone–receptor interactions: the surface receptor **(A)** and the intracellular receptor **(B)**. (From Porth CM. *Essentials of Pathophysiology: Concepts of Altered Health States*. Philadelphia, PA: Lippincott Williams & Wilkins; 2003, with permission.)

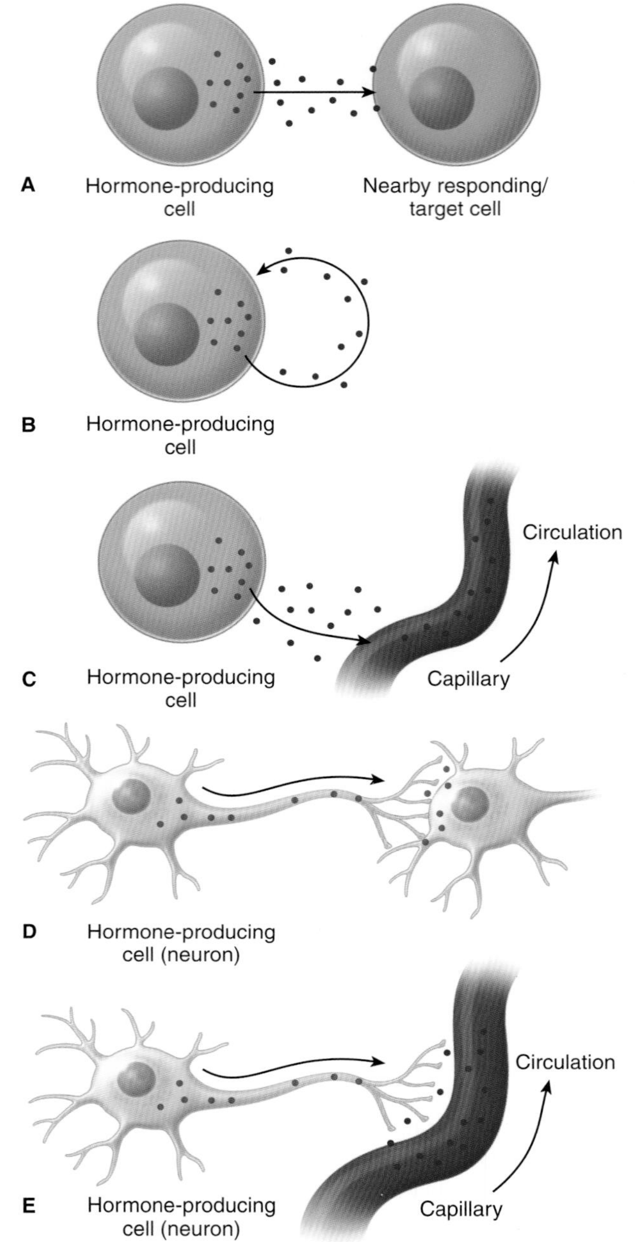

Figure 13.6. Hormonal mechanisms of mediating cell-to-cell communication. **A:** Paracrine pathway. **B:** Autocrine pathway. **C:** Endocrine pathway. **D:** Synaptic pathway. **E:** Neuroendocrine pathway.

Mediating Cell-to-Cell Communication

Five major pathways characterize cell-to-cell communication, where hormones move from production and secretion, to response (Fig. 13.6):

- **Paracrine pathway:** hormones are produced in a cell, secreted, and act directly on nearby receptive cells.
- **Autocrine pathway:** the same as the paracrine pathway except that the receptor cells are also secretory cells so, in essence, the cell is able to produce the hormone and exert an effect on itself.
- **Endocrine pathway:** hormones are produced in a cell, secreted, and travel through blood vessels to distant cells, attach to receptors, and act on that cell.
- **Synaptic pathway:** hormones are produced in the neuron, secreted, and travel along the axon to the synapse where they are released and taken up by a nearby neuron with the appropriate receptors to exert an effect.
- **Neuroendocrine pathway:** hormones are produced in a neuron, secreted, travel along the axon to the synapse, are released, are taken up into the vascular system, and travel to distant cells with the appropriate receptors to exert an effect.

Module 2 The Stress Response

Cell-to-cell communication is an integral part of the stress response. **Stress** is the body's reaction to harmful forces (stressors) capable of disturbing homeostasis. An individual's response depends on many factors such as age, general health, type of stressor, the persistence of the stressor, perception of the stressor, social support, and genetic influences. Homeostasis is dependent on an adequate response to stress through mobilizing energy, activating defense mechanisms, and repairing any damage. An inadequate or even excessive response to stress can result in destruction of body tissues. The neuroendocrine response and hormones play a vital role in this process. Figure 13.7 details how the stress response involves neurologic and hormonal influences.

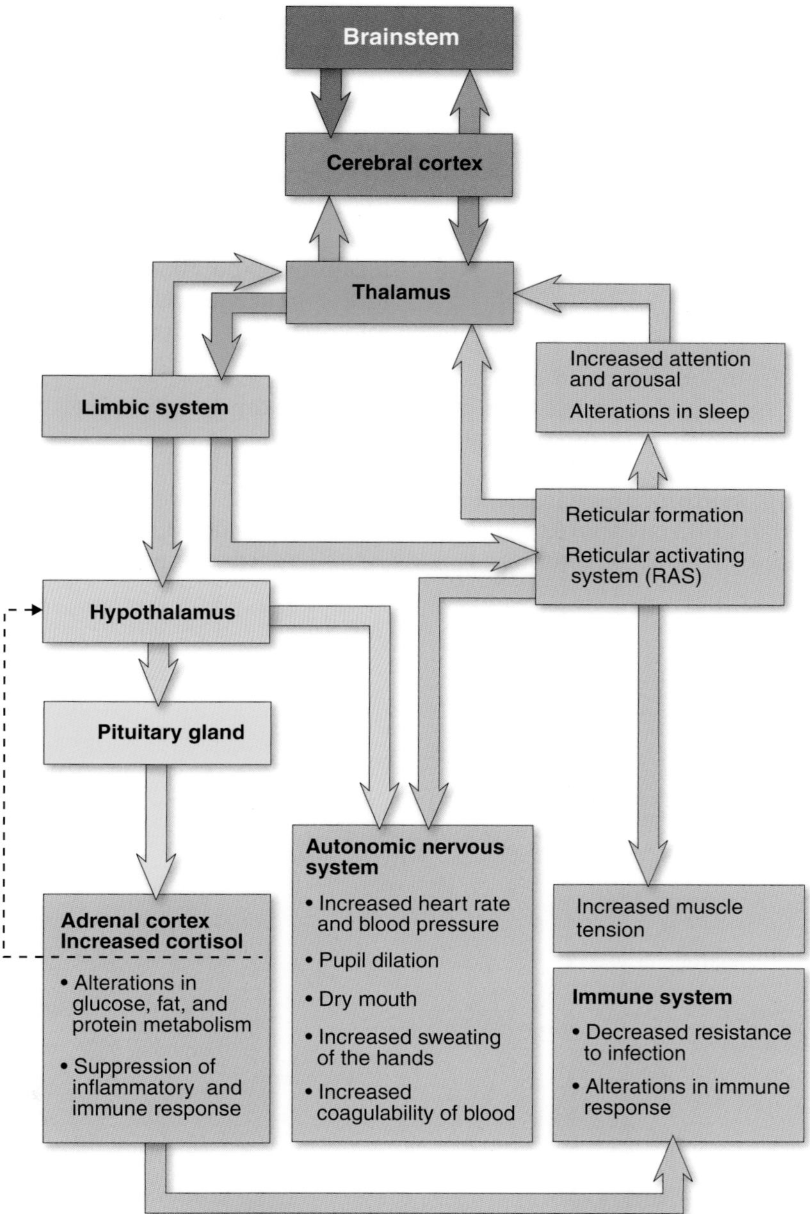

Figure 13.7. Concept map. Stress pathways. The broken line represents negative feedback. (Modified from Porth CM. *Essentials of Pathophysiology: Concepts of Altered Health States.* Philadelphia, PA: Lippincott Williams & Wilkins; 2003, with permission.)

Neurologic Response to Stress

Neurologic influences, particularly the central nervous system (CNS), are instrumental in the stress response. The brainstem coordinates the performance of the autonomic nervous system, cerebral cortex, limbic system, and hypothalamus and produces norepinephrine so the body can quickly defend against the stressor. Specific structures in the CNS that play a major role include:

- **Autonomic nervous system:** increases heart rate, blood pressure, respiratory rate, pupil dilation, and sweating. Blood flow is increased to the muscles, heart, and lungs in preparation of "fight or flight." Gastric function decreased to shunt blood to vital organs. Altered blood flow, decreased oxygenation to gastric tissues, and prolonged cortisol exposure may result in "stress ulcers" of the gastrointestinal tract.
- **Cerebral cortex:** regulates cognitive activities such as intense focus, planning, attention, and persistence.
- **Limbic system:** regulates emotional activities such as fear, anxiety, anger, and excitement, and stimulates the reticular activating system.
- **Thalamus:** intensifies sensory input related to the stressor such as vision, hearing, and smell.
- **Hypothalamus:** releases hormones to initiate the neuroendocrine response; acts on the autonomic nervous system.
- **Reticular activating system:** increases alertness and muscle tension and contributes to stimulation of the autonomic nervous system.

Hormonal Response to Stress

Four major hormones or groups of hormones are instrumental in the endocrine response to stress. First, stress stimulates the release of CRH from the hypothalamus. CRH stimulates the pituitary to secrete adrenocorticotropic hormone (ACTH), which in turn stimulates the adrenal glands to secrete cortisol. As depicted in Table 13.1, cortisol is needed to increase metabolism and regulate blood glucose levels for energy and also acts as a potent anti-inflammatory. Second, release of the catecholamines (epinephrine, norepinephrine, and dopamine) is triggered by the sympathetic nervous system, which also acts on the adrenal glands (Fig. 13.8). Catecholamines induce a neurologic response to receptive organs. For example, blood flow is shunted to vital organs, such as the heart, brain, and lungs. As a result, heart rate increases, blood pressure increases, respiratory rate increases, and the person becomes much more alert. The skeletal muscles also become activated to allow a rapid escape. Blood is shunted away from the skin and stomach. So, the person will look pale or ashen and digestion is decreased.

Stop and Consider
How do you usually respond to stress? Think about the last time you were in a haunted house or were really scared. How did your body respond? How does this correlate to the neuroendocrine response described in this section?

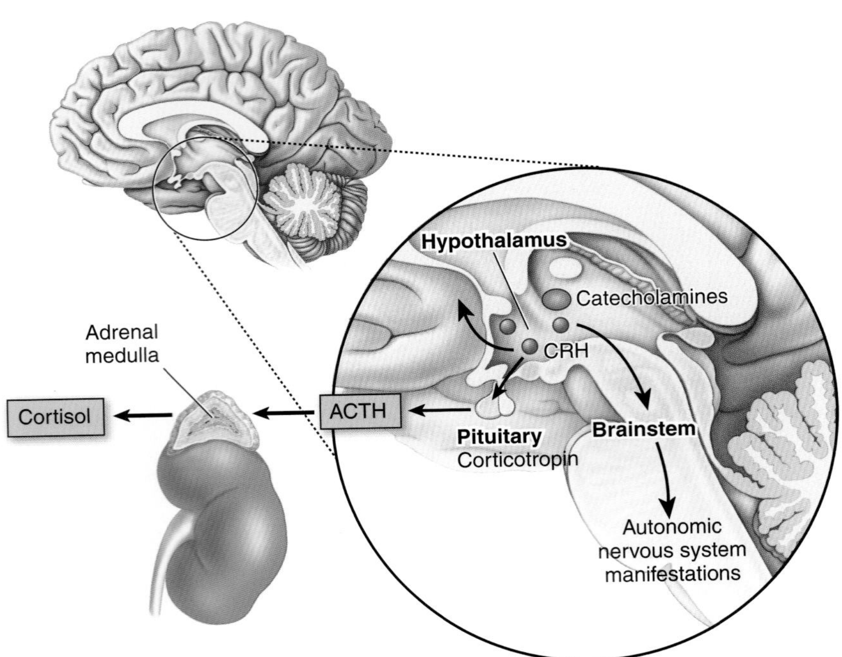

Figure 13.8. Stimulation of cortisol and catecholamines in the stress response. ACTH, adrenocorticotropic hormone; CRH, corticotropin-releasing hormone.

General Adaptation Syndrome

The neuroendocrine response is often initiated by a stressor. **General adaptation syndrome** is a term used to describe this neuroendocrine response and the corresponding physiologic changes. General adaptation syndrome is generally divided into three major stages: (1) the alarm stage; (2) the resistance stage; and (3) the exhaustion stage. In the alarm stage, catecholamines and cortisol are released in response to stimulation of the sympathetic nervous system, the hypothalamic–pituitary axis, and the adrenal glands. This stage is often referred to as the "fight or flight" stage. These hormones prepare the body for defense against the stressor. In short-term and mild stress situations, the response may resolve within the alarm stage and may be limited in intensity and duration.

Other hormones are also at play early in the stress response. Suppression of certain hormones, such as growth hormone, thyroid hormone, and the reproductive hormones, is necessary to conserve energy that will be needed to fend off the stressor. Antidiuretic hormone is increased to retain fluid thereby maintaining the blood pressure needed to perfuse vital tissues. Once the stress is resolved, prestress hormone levels are resumed.

Persistent stress is followed by the resistance stage, whereby cortisol levels decrease through negative feedback mechanisms. Excess cortisol is helpful in the early stages of stress to increase metabolism by breaking down proteins, releasing lipids, and increasing circulating glucose. This gives the body energy for fight or flight. However, over time, hypercortisolism is detrimental, leading to exhaustion of inflammatory and immune responses, excessive loss of body proteins and breakdown of tissues, and glucose intolerance. Therefore, cortisol secretion is not an effective method of adapting to prolonged stress. As indicated, some hormone levels are suppressed with stress and remain so during the resistance stage. This also has detrimental effects. Loss of circulating thyroid, growth, and reproductive hormones can have long-term effects on linear growth, metabolism, and reproduction. The persistent increase in antidiuretic hormone through prolonged stress is manifested by excessive fluid retention and subsequent hypertension (high blood pressure).

Chronic overwhelming stress leads to exhaustion. The exhaustion stage is characterized by energy depletion and degeneration of cells, tissues, organs, and organ systems. Severe, prolonged stress contributes to poor health and marks a significant loss to homeostasis.

Module 3 Altered Hormone Function

A number of mechanisms can impact hormones (Box 13.2). Most commonly, hormone excesses or deficits arise from impairment of the endocrine (secreting) gland, lack of hormone synthesis, excessive hormone synthesis, impaired receptor binding, impaired feedback mechanisms, or an altered cellular response to the hormone. Problems with hormone function can manifest through inadequate or excessive production, composition, secretion, receptor binding, uptake, metabolism, or elimination.

Damage to the Hypothalamic–Pituitary Axis

Damage to the hypothalamic–pituitary axis due to infection, inflammation, tumors, degeneration, hypoxia, hemorrhage, or genetic defects can lead to problems with the production and secretion of multiple hormones. Refer to Table 13.1 to review which hormones are synthesized and secreted through the hypothalamic–pituitary axis. **Hypopituitarism** is a generic term indicating decreased secretion of one or more pituitary hormones. **Hyperpituitarism** is an excess of pituitary hormone secretion. **Panhypopituitarism** indicates a decrease in pituitary hormones. Because the pituitary secretes

Box 13.2 Process of Altering Hormone Function

The following questions address the potential problems that can alter hormone function:

1. Is there impairment of the hypothalamic–pituitary axis?
2. Is there impairment of the endocrine gland?
3. Is there too little or too much hormone that is being produced and secreted?
4. Is the gland producing active hormone?
5. Is receptor binding adequate?
6. Is the target cell responding to the hormone?
7. Is the negative feedback loop impaired?
8. Is hormone being produced ectopically?
9. Is hormone metabolism (inactivation) and elimination impaired?

ACTH, thyroid-stimulating hormone (TSH), growth hormone (GH), follicle-stimulating hormone (FSH), luteinizing hormone (LH), and prolactin, damage to the pituitary has a broad range of clinical manifestations related to the loss of thyroid, adrenal, and reproductive glands and problems with growth.

Damage to Endocrine Glands

Destruction of endocrine glands or the lack of active hormone secretion can also lead to problems with target-tissue function. Endocrine glands can be impaired through genetic defects, autoimmune conditions, degeneration, atrophy, infection, inflammation, neoplastic growths, hypoxia, radiation, certain medications, and other types of injury. The gland becomes incapable of adequately responding to neuroendocrine messages, and hormone secretion is depressed or absent. Excessive stimulation of the endocrine gland can result in hyperplasia and an excessive amount of hormone production and secretion. In some cases, the endocrine gland is functioning appropriately, but the hormone may lack the necessary biologic activity to elicit the cellular response. This often occurs when antibodies destroy biologically active hormone even after the hormone is secreted from the gland.

Damage to Cell Receptors

Receptor binding and cell-to-cell communication are required to elicit a cellular response. Disorders of receptor binding may involve one or more of the following:

1. A decreased number of receptors
2. The lack of receptor sensitivity to the hormone
3. The presence of antibodies that block receptor sites or occupy the receptor site and mimic the hormone
4. The presence of tumor cells with receptor activity that deprives the unaffected cells of the hormone

Impaired receptor binding is manifested through circulating levels of hormones that are incapable of eliciting an appropriate cellular response. Likewise,

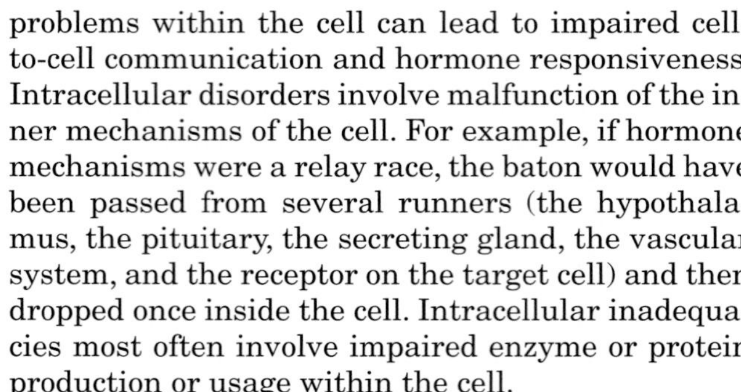

problems within the cell can lead to impaired cell-to-cell communication and hormone responsiveness. Intracellular disorders involve malfunction of the inner mechanisms of the cell. For example, if hormone mechanisms were a relay race, the baton would have been passed from several runners (the hypothalamus, the pituitary, the secreting gland, the vascular system, and the receptor on the target cell) and then dropped once inside the cell. Intracellular inadequacies most often involve impaired enzyme or protein production or usage within the cell.

Damage to Feedback Mechanisms

Feedback mechanisms may fail to respond to hormone levels and continue to suppress or stimulate hormone production and secretion. This impairment can occur at any point along the hypothalamic–pituitary axis, at the level of the secreting gland, the receptors, or target tissues. Impairment of feedback mechanisms may be a problem of ectopically produced hormone. Some neoplasms are capable of producing and secreting ectopic hormones. The tumor is not part of the negative feedback mechanism and continues to produce and secrete excessive hormones despite high serum levels. Removal of the tumor will often result in resolution of hormone hypersecretion. The most common ectopically produced hormones are ADH and ACTH.

Damage to Metabolism and Elimination Mechanisms

The metabolism (inactivation) and elimination of hormones is essential to maintaining homeostasis. The impaired ability to metabolize or eliminate hormones, such as that which may occur with liver or kidney disease, will result in excess circulating hormone.

General Manifestations of Altered Hormone Function

Hypopituitarism, a deficit of one or more pituitary hormones, usually has a gradual onset, and clinical manifestations are not evident until most of the pituitary gland has been destroyed. The general manifestations are often vague and may include fatigue, weakness, anorexia, sexual dysfunction, growth impairment,

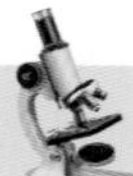

FROM THE LAB

Hormone function is measured directly or indirectly. Current detection of hormone activity is assayed with nonradioactive immunoassays with fluorescence labels, enzymes, and other techniques. Chemiluminescence is one such technique that uses light-producing chemical reactions to detect amounts of hormone in ligand-binder assays.

Table 13.2 General Manifestations of Select Hormone Excesses and Deficits

Hormone	Excess	Deficit
Antidiuretic hormone	Fluid retention, low urine output, hyponatremia	Excessive water losses through the urine, leading to nausea, vomiting, fatigue, muscle thirst, dehydration, can progress to shock twitching; can progress to convulsions and death
Glucocorticoids (cortisol)	Truncal obesity, moon face, buffalo hump, glucose intolerance, atrophic skin, striae, osteoporosis, psychological changes, poor wound healing, increased infections	Hypoglycemia, anorexia, nausea, vomiting, fatigue, weakness, weight loss, poor stress response
Growth hormone	Before puberty (called gigantism): excessive skeletal growth. After puberty (called acromegaly): bony proliferation of spine, ribs, and face, hands, and feet, enlarged tongue, edema, overactive sebaceous glands, coarse skin and body hair, pain, weakness, and inflammation related to excessive growth; hypertension and left heart failure may also occur	Short stature, obesity, immature facial features, delayed puberty, hypoglycemia, seizures in children; obesity, insulin resistance, and high circulating lipids in adults
Mineralocorticoids (aldosterone)	Hypertension, hypokalemia, hypernatremia, muscle weakness, fatigue, polyuria, polydipsia, metabolic alkalosis	Weakness, nausea, anorexia, hyponatremia, hyperkalemia, dehydration, hypotension, shock, death
Thyroid hormone	Hypermetabolism, weight loss, diarrhea, exophthalmos, anxiety, goiter	Hypometabolism, weight gain, constipation, goiter, dry skin, coarse hair
Parathyroid hormone	Hypercalcemia, excessive osteoclastic activity and bone resorption, pathologic fractures, formation of renal calculi	Hypocalcemia, muscle spasms, hyperreflexia, seizures, bone deformities

dry skin, constipation, and cold intolerance. Hyperpituitarism, an excess of one or more pituitary hormones, also has a wide range of manifestations depending on which hormones are elevated. Table 13.2 details general manifestations of specific hormones excesses and deficits.

Diagnosing and Treating Altered Hormone Function

Diagnosing alterations in hormonal or metabolic function begins with a complete patient history and physical examination and often relies on measuring hormone levels or other indicators in the blood or urine. Hormone suppression or stimulation tests can be used to detect hormone responses. Because secretion rates can fluctuate over time, urine hormone levels are often collected over a 24-hour period. Serum electrolyte, glucose, calcium, and other lab tests may provide indirect information on hormone functioning. Imaging studies, such as computed tomography (CT) or magnetic resonance imaging (MRI) scans, may be needed to locate a tumor that could be suppressing or stimulating hormone secretion. Genetic testing may also be needed to identify a genetic alteration that is affecting hormone function.

Treating hormone alterations varies depending on the cause. Hormone elevations require eliminating the excess hormone. This often occurs by removing tumors that may be secreting ectopic hormone, removing all or part of the corresponding endocrine gland, or administering medications that block the effects of the hormone. Low hormone levels often require lifelong replacement through pharmacotherapy.

Module 4 Clinical Models

The following clinical models have been selected to aid in the understanding and application of altered hormonal processes and effects. The structure, function, and altered function of the reproductive organs and the endocrine pancreas have been reserved for Chapters 14 and 20, respectively.

Syndrome of Inappropriate Antidiuretic Hormone Secretion

ADH is produced in the hypothalamus, travels to the posterior pituitary, and is released into the circulation. ADH controls fluid balance by regulating reabsorption of water by the kidneys (Fig. 13.9). Secretion rates of ADH are based on serum osmolality and extracellular fluid volume. The hypothalamus senses changes in serum osmolality and alters secretion of ADH. Similarly, sensors in the blood vessels recognize changes in blood volume and can affect ADH secretion. High levels of ADH stimulate water retention; low levels of ADH trigger water loss through urination.

The **syndrome of inappropriate antidiuretic hormone (SIADH)** secretion is a condition of excessive production and release of ADH despite changes in serum osmolality and blood volume. Although ADH levels can transiently increase with certain medications and stressful stimuli, such as trauma, exposure to temperature extremes, pain conditions, surgery, or infection, the diagnosis of SIADH is typically reserved for those without such stimuli to explain excessive ADH release. The most common cause of SIADH is a tumor, somewhere in the body, which is secreting ectopic ADH.

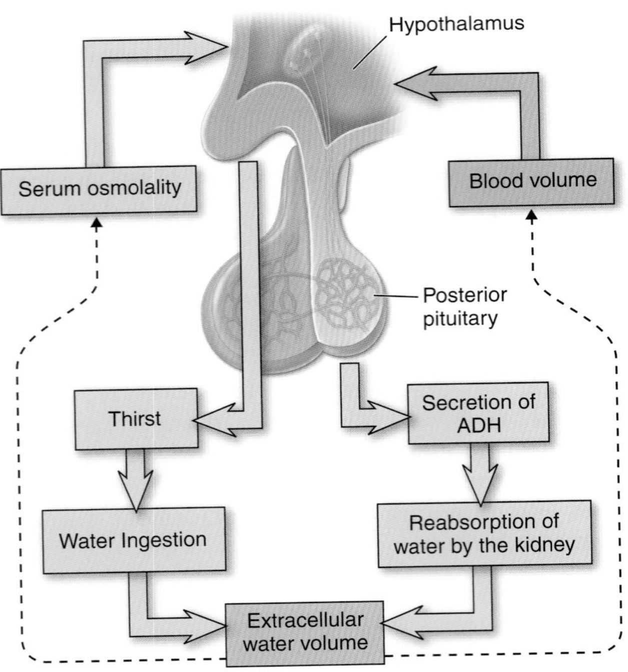

Figure 13.9. Pathways for regulation of extracellular fluid volume by thirst and antidiuretic hormone. ADH, antidiuretic hormone. (Modified from Porth CM. *Essentials of Pathophysiology: Concepts of Altered Health States.* Philadelphia, PA: Lippincott Williams & Wilkins; 2003, with permission.)

PATHOPHYSIOLOGY

Antidiuretic hormone promotes water retention by increasing the permeability of the nephrons in the kidneys. Most of the body water accumulates intracellularly and alters cell function. The CNS is most sensitive to these changes. Because water initially accumulates intracellularly, edema or fluid overload in the vascular system is uncommon. The excess circulating fluid within cells increases total body water concentration and eventually dilutes the sodium concentration in the extracellular space.

CLINICAL MANIFESTATIONS

Clinical manifestations are related to hypotonic hyponatremia and include a decreased and concentrated urine output. The severity of symptoms depends on the serum sodium level and the rate of onset. Significant symptoms usually do not manifest until serum sodium is less than 115 to 120 mEq/L. A more rapid onset of hyponatremia leads to greater severity of symptoms. Initially, these symptoms include anorexia, nausea, vomiting, headache, irritability, disorientation, muscle cramps, and weakness. As the serum sodium level drops below 110 mEq/L, additional symptoms emerge, including psychosis, gait disturbances, seizures, or coma.

DIAGNOSTIC CRITERIA

Diagnosis is based on the following clinical and laboratory findings:

- Hyponatremia (serum sodium less than 135 mEq/L)
- Hypotonicity (plasma osmolality less than 280 mOsm/kg)
- Decreased urine volume
- Highly concentrated urine with a high sodium content
- Absence of renal, adrenal, or thyroid abnormalities

TREATMENT

Treatment focuses on removing the cause of SIADH if possible. For patients with mild symptoms of hyponatremia, water restriction is often the only necessary therapy. Severe hyponatremia generally requires isotonic or hypertonic saline administered intravenously. Hypertonic intravenous (IV) solutions are reserved for those individuals with severe hyponatremia who display alterations in mental status. Medications may be administered to block the effects of ADH or to increase urine output if removing the cause is not feasible.

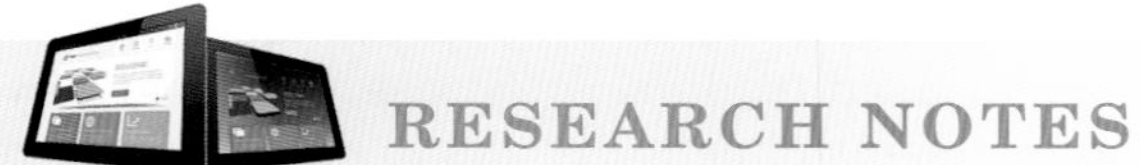

Like dominoes, clinical manifestations of endocrine disorders can have a direct effect on many other aspects of homeostasis. For example, a recent large study confirmed that hyponatremia, a common clinical manifestation of SIADH, was associated with subsequent development of osteoporosis and fractures due to bone fragility in a matched case-control study of over 80,000 patients. In addition, the odds of developing osteoporosis or fragility fracture increased incrementally with each reduction in serum sodium level.[1]

Diabetes Insipidus

Diabetes insipidus (DI) is a condition of insufficient ADH that results in the inability of the body to concentrate or retain water (Fig. 13.10). The prevalence has been estimated at 3 per 100,000 population.[2] Three major causes of DI include:

- Insufficient production of ADH by the hypothalamus or ineffective secretion by the posterior pituitary
- Inadequate kidney response to the presence of ADH, also called nephrogenic DI
- Ingestion of extremely large volumes of fluids and decreasing ADH levels; water intoxication can sometimes be attributed to a psychiatric disturbance

PATHOPHYSIOLOGY

Impairment of hypothalamic osmoreceptors after trauma or surgery to a region at or near the hypothalamus is the most common cause. Nephrogenic DI can be observed in those with chronic renal insufficiency, lithium (a drug used to treat manic-depressive disorder) toxicity, hypercalcemia, hypokalemia, or with disease of the renal tubules. Rarely, nephrogenic DI is inherited as an X-linked disorder.

Stop and Consider
What effect would drinking alcohol have on ADH levels?

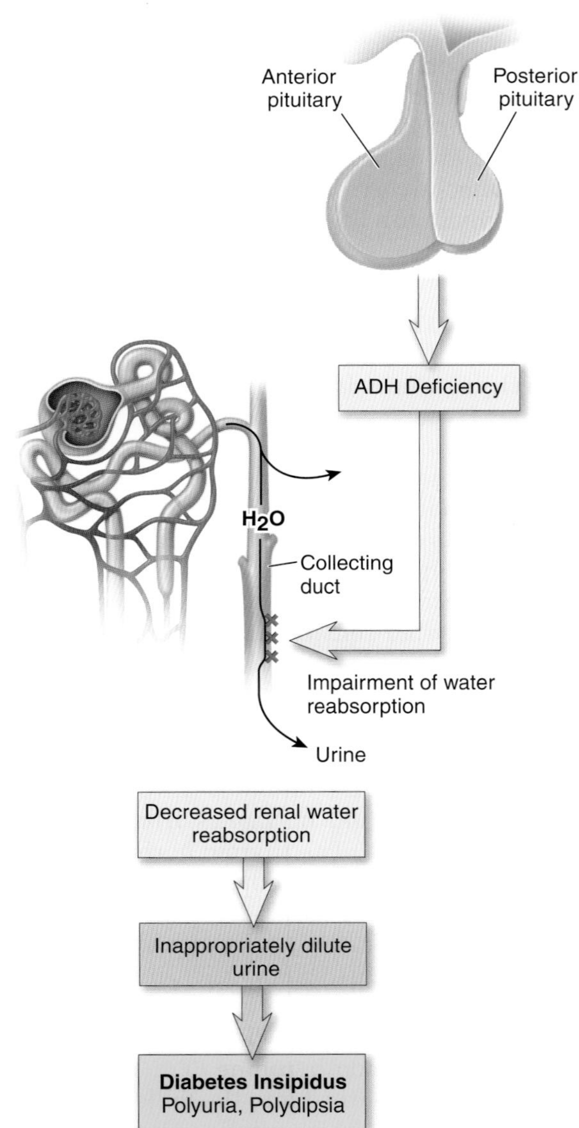

Figure 13.10. The mechanism of diabetes insipidus. ADH, antidiuretic hormone. (Modified from Rubin E, Farber JL. *Pathology*. 4th ed. Philadelphia, PA: Lippincott Williams & Wilkins; 2005, with permission.)

CLINICAL MANIFESTATIONS

Manifestations depend on the severity of DI. Loss of ADH or inadequate kidney response to ADH results in **polyuria** (large volume urine output) and excessive thirst. The urine is highly dilute with a low specific gravity. Loss of fluids leads to serum hyperosmolality and severe dehydration. Shock and death can occur if untreated.

DIAGNOSTIC CRITERIA

Diagnosis is made through a careful patient history and physical examination. The patient history often includes recent surgery to remove a tumor of the brain, or other cranial surgery, or head trauma. The physical examination may detect signs of dehydration and possibly an enlargement of the bladder due to constant over-filling. Laboratory measurement of serum solute concentration, ADH levels, and urine-specific gravity is used to confirm the diagnosis. A urine-specific gravity of 1.005 or less and a urine osmolality less than 200 mOsm/kg are often found in DI.

TREATMENT

Except for those without access to water, most patients can drink enough fluid to replace urine losses. Hydration is an important aspect of treatment. In some cases, particularly in those with inadequate thirst, IV hydration with a hypotonic solution is required. Pharmacologic treatment may include the use of desmopressin (DDAVP), a synthetic vasopressin analog, which acts as a potent antidiuretic. If the cause cannot be corrected, this drug may be required for the individual's lifetime.

Hyperthyroidism

Hyperthyroidism is a state of excessive thyroid hormone. Hyperthyroidism can result from excessive stimulation to the thyroid gland, diseases of the thyroid gland, or excess production of TSH by a pituitary adenoma. Certain medications contain large amounts of iodine, such as cough expectorants, health food supplements that contain seaweed, and iodinated contrast dyes, which can induce hyperthyroidism in thyroid-sensitive individuals.

The production of thyroid hormone is a multistep process. Thyrotropin-releasing hormone from the hypothalamus triggers the release of thyroid-stimulating hormone from the anterior pituitary, which in turn stimulates the production and release of the thyroid hormones from the thyroid gland (see Fig. 13.3). The thyroid hormones are produced in the follicular (epithelial) cells of the thyroid. The follicles use iodide from dietary intake of iodized salt, combine this with tyrosine (an amino acid) and secrete this combination into the central colloid portion of the follicle to form the thyroid hormones: tetraiodothyronine (T_4), also referred to as thyroxine, and triiodothyronine (T_3). When needed, T_3 and T_4 are reabsorbed into the follicular cells and then released into the circulation. T_4 is reduced by deiodination in the peripheral tissues to T_3, the active form of the hormone. Circulating thyroid hormone provides feedback to the hypothalamus and pituitary gland. TSH is suppressed or activated depending on circulating thyroid hormone levels. Stress and cold environmental temperatures also act to stimulate thyroid hormone production.

Stop and Consider
What would happen if you had a diet that did not include iodized salt?

Thyroid hormone has an impact throughout the body and plays a critical role in stimulating metabolism. Other functions include facilitating the breakdown of carbohydrates, proteins, and fats for energy, stimulating heat and glucose production, producing structural proteins, enzymes, and other hormones, and promoting growth and development in children. As a result of thyroid hormone release, there is:

- Increased glucose absorption
- Release of lipids from adipose tissue
- Metabolism of proteins from muscle tissue
- Increased cholesterol breakdown in the liver
- Increased production of metabolic by-products
- Increased oxygen consumption
- Increased body heat production
- Increased cardiac output
- Increased gastric motility
- Increased muscle tone and reactivity
- Increased activation of cognitive processes

PATHOPHYSIOLOGY

Graves disease, an excessive stimulation of the thyroid gland, is the most common cause of hyperthyroidism and is the most common autoimmune condition in the United States. Prevalence is estimated at 0.5 per 1,000 population. Women are 7 to 10 times more likely to develop Graves disease than men.[3] As with many autoimmune conditions, the triggering event is often unknown; genetic (e.g., family history or gender) and environmental (e.g., stress or smoking) factors are implicated. In Graves disease, IgG antibodies bind to the TSH receptor on thyrocytes (thyroid cells) and stimulate excessive thyroid hormone secretion, causing a state of **thyrotoxicosis**. Chronic thyrotoxicosis can be complicated by progressive thyroid failure and result in hypothyroidism. The thyroid gland undergoes hyperplasia due to excessive stimulation. **Thyrotoxic crisis**, or thyroid storm, is a sudden, severe worsening of hyperthyroidism that may result in death.

CLINICAL MANIFESTATIONS

Major clinical manifestations are related to enlargement of the thyroid gland and the excessive metabolic rate of the body (Fig. 13.11). Weight loss, agitation, restlessness, sweating, heat intolerance,

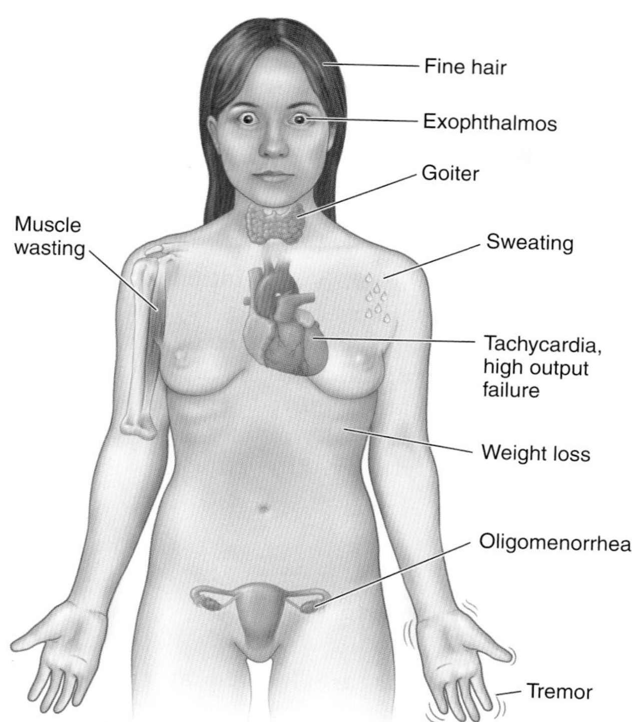

Figure 13.11. Major clinical manifestations of Graves disease.

diarrhea, tachycardia, palpitations, tremors, fine hair, oily skin, irregular menstrual cycle in women, and weakness are common findings. The development of a **goiter** (enlargement of the thyroid gland) may occur because of follicular epithelial cell hyperplasia. **Exophthalmos** (a protrusion of the eyeballs) is also characteristic of Graves disease. This protrusion is usually bilateral and results from the interaction of TSH-sensitized antibodies interacting with fibroblast antigens found in extraocular muscles and tissues. The interaction results in lymphocyte infiltration, edema, and fibroblast accumulation, which displaces the eyeballs forward. Exophthalmos often persists despite treatment of hyperthyroidism.

DIAGNOSTIC CRITERIA

Diagnosis of Graves disease is based on the patient history and physical examination; common clinical manifestations are noted. The patient history may be significant for a family history of autoimmune disease, thyroid disease, or emigration from an iodine-deficient location. The physical examination often reveals an enlarged and slightly firm thyroid gland as well as protrusion of the eyes. Measurement of serum TSH level is a useful screening test for the presence of hyperthyroidism; however, the diagnosis of hyperthyroidism must be confirmed by the measurement of serum-free thyroxine. In thyrotoxicosis, TSH levels are greatly suppressed. This is caused by the negative feedback loop, which communicates high thyroid hormone levels to the hypothalamic–pituitary axis and causes suppression of TSH. Laboratory studies may also reveal elevated serum levels of T_3 and T_4. Increased uptake of radioactive iodine by the thyroid gland confirms the diagnosis.

TREATMENT

Treatment measures are based on reducing thyroid hormone levels often through gland destruction via radioactive iodine, medications that block thyroid hormone production, or, less commonly, surgical removal of all or part of the gland. Full ablation (removal) of the thyroid gland requires lifelong supplementation with oral thyroid hormone replacement therapy.

Hypothyroidism

Hypothyroidism is a state of deficient thyroid hormone. Prevalence is estimated at 3.7% of the population with a five times greater risk in those older than age 80.[4] Hypothyroidism can be congenital or acquired. Congenital hypothyroidism occurs during fetal development and results in a lack of thyroid gland development, a lack of appropriate synthesis of thyroid hormone, or problems with TSH secretion. In utero, maternal T_4 crosses the placenta; therefore, the newborn appears unaffected at birth. If the child is untreated after birth, the lack of thyroid hormone production and secretion results in mental retardation and impaired growth, a condition referred to as **cretinism**. Neonatal screening, when instituted, detects congenital hypothyroidism, allowing treatment with thyroid hormone replacement to be initiated.

PATHOPHYSIOLOGY

Acquired hypothyroidism can result from (1) deficient thyroid hormone synthesis; (2) destruction of the thyroid gland; or (3) impaired TSH or TRH secretion. Common causes of acquired hypothyroidism include autoimmunity, iodine deficiency, surgical removal of or radiation therapy to the thyroid gland, medications that destroy the thyroid gland, and genetic defects that affect the thyroid hormones. Autoimmune processes attack the thyroid gland or may block TSH or the TSH receptor without activating the thyroid gland, as in hyperthyroidism. Hashimoto thyroiditis is an autoimmune hypothyroidism that can result in total destruction of the thyroid gland.

This condition affects women up to 10 times more frequently than men.[5]

CLINICAL MANIFESTATIONS

Clinical manifestations are often gradual and include fatigue, cold intolerance, weakness, weight gain, dry skin, coarse hair, constipation, lethargy, impaired reproduction, and impaired memory (Fig. 13.12). Goiter may also be present in hypothyroidism as the gland enlarges in an effort to increase function. Dietary iodine deficiency, excess, or the use of medications that suppress thyroid hormones can stimulate the development of hypothyroid goiter. **Myxedema** is a unique characteristic finding of hypothyroidism. Protein–carbohydrate complexes accumulate in the extracellular matrix drawing water into the tissues, resulting in boggy, nonpitting, edematous tissues especially of the face and mucous membranes, hands, and feet.

DIAGNOSTIC CRITERIA

Diagnosis of hypothyroidism is based on patient history and physical examination, during which characteristic clinical manifestations are noted. Laboratory studies include the sensitive TSH assay, free T_4, total T_4, and T_3 uptake, thyroid autoantibodies, and antithyroglobulin tests to confirm the diagnose and provide evidence as to causality. Serum thyroid hormones may be decreased, and TSH is often elevated.

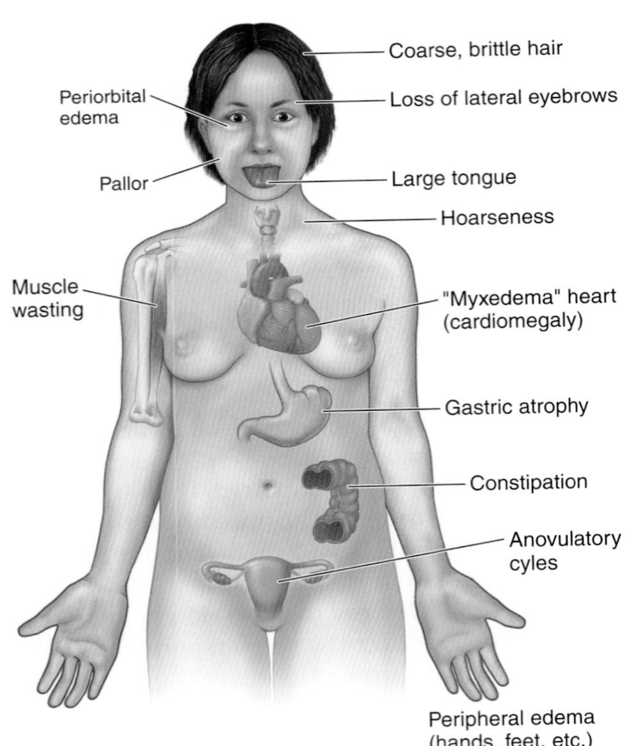

Figure 13.12. Major clinical manifestations of hypothyroidism.

TREATMENT

Treatment focuses on replacing the deficient hormone with the goals of normalization of TSH, T_4, and T_3 levels, along with alleviation of the clinical signs and symptoms. Lifelong thyroid hormone replacement therapy is initiated and increased gradually until optimal hormone levels and clinical improvement are achieved. The most common drug used to treat hypothyroidism is levothyroxine (Synthroid, Levoxyl). Levothyroxine is a synthetic form of T_4.

Cushing Syndrome

The adrenal glands are located at the apex of the kidneys and contain two distinct parts: (1) an outer adrenal cortex and (2) an inner adrenal medulla (Fig. 13.13). The adrenal hormones play a critical role in the stress response. The adrenal medulla secretes epinephrine and norepinephrine. Table 13.3 illustrates the three categories and functions of steroid hormones secreted by the adrenal cortex.

Stop and Consider
Would loss of the adrenal cortex or the adrenal medulla be more problematic?

Cushing syndrome refers to a condition of prolonged exposure to elevated levels of either endogenous (from the adrenal cortex or cortisol-producing tumors) or exogenous glucocorticoids (as when taking glucocorticoid drugs). Glucocorticoids contribute to metabolic function, the inflammatory and immune

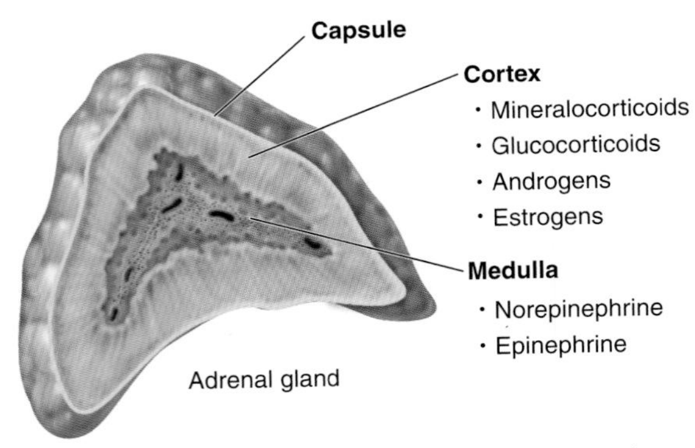

Figure 13.13. Hormone secretion from the adrenal cortex and adrenal medulla.

Table 13.3 Categories of Steroid Hormones Secreted by the Adrenal Cortex

Category	Major Example	Functions
Mineralocorticoids	*Aldosterone* (secretion stimulated by the renin–angiotensin system and serum potassium levels)	Regulates sodium and potassium levels; regulates water balance and blood pressure
Glucocorticoids	*Cortisol* (secretion stimulated by corticotropin-releasing hormone from the hypothalamus and adrenocorticotropic hormone from the anterior pituitary)	Regulates metabolism, inflammatory/immune responses, and the stress response
Adrenal sex	*Androgens* (secretion; see cortisol)	Contribute to pubic and axillary hair growth hormones in women; minimally impact sexual function

responses, and the stress response. More specifically, glucocorticoids function to:

- Stimulate glucose production
- Decrease tissue glucose utilization
- Increase breakdown and circulation of plasma proteins
- Increase mobilization of fats
- Prevent the release of chemical mediators that trigger the inflammatory response
- Decrease capillary permeability and inhibit edema formation
- Inhibit the immune response
- Inhibit bone formation
- Stimulate gastric acid secretions
- Contribute to emotional behavior
- Contribute to an effective stress response

PATHOPHYSIOLOGY

Four major processes can lead to Cushing syndrome:

1. Long-term administration of corticosteroid medications (such as prednisone)
2. Tumors of the pituitary gland that stimulate excess ACTH production
3. Tumors of the adrenal gland that stimulate excess cortisol production
4. Ectopic production of ACTH or CRH from a tumor at a distant site, such as small cell carcinoma of the lung

Long-term administration of corticosteroid medications is indicated for a wide variety of chronic inflammatory and autoimmune conditions. Exogenous corticosteroids suppress the inflammatory and immune responses and can decrease the deleterious effects of chronic inflammation. Long-term use of these medications will result in suppression of cortisol production by the adrenal cortex and should not be discontinued abruptly.

Stop and Consider
You are on a 1-week hiking trip and one of your friends forgets her glucocorticoid medication that she takes for severe asthma. Should she go back and get the medication or is she okay without it for that week?

Excessive ACTH production, through pituitary or ectopic tumors, overstimulates the adrenal cortex. This results in adrenal hyperplasia and excess cortisol production. This form of hypercortisolism depends on ACTH, and reduction of cortisol levels may require removal of the ACTH-secreting tumor or CRH-secreting tumor if this is stimulating the excess ACTH production. Adrenal tumors, however, hypersecrete cortisol directly and are not directed by ACTH.

Stop and Consider
Map out how the negative feedback loop is impacted by an ACTH-dependent hypercortisolism versus a non–ACTH-dependent hypercortisolism.

CLINICAL MANIFESTATIONS

Excess secretion of glucocorticoids can result in metabolic alterations, excessive circulating glucose and subsequent glucose intolerance, suppression of the inflammatory and immune responses, behavioral changes, and an impaired stress response. Mobilization of fats and changes in fat metabolism lead to obesity of the trunk, face, and upper back. Obesity of the face and posterior neck and back has been characterized by the terms "moon face" and "buffalo hump" (Fig. 13.14). Striae, or stretch marks, can develop from truncal obesity. Protein degradation results in extremity weakness and muscle wasting. The skin becomes atrophic and thin. Bones exhibit osteoporosis. Suppression of the inflammatory and immune responses leads to increased infections, skin ulcerations, and poor wound healing. Glucose intolerance, from excess circulating glucose and loss of tissue utilization, can lead to diabetes mellitus. Changes in behavior can range from euphoria to minor emotional disturbances to psychosis.

Stimulation of the adrenal cortex to overproduce cortisol can also stimulate the production of the other adrenal cortex hormones, primarily androgens and aldosterone. Clinical manifestations can reflect

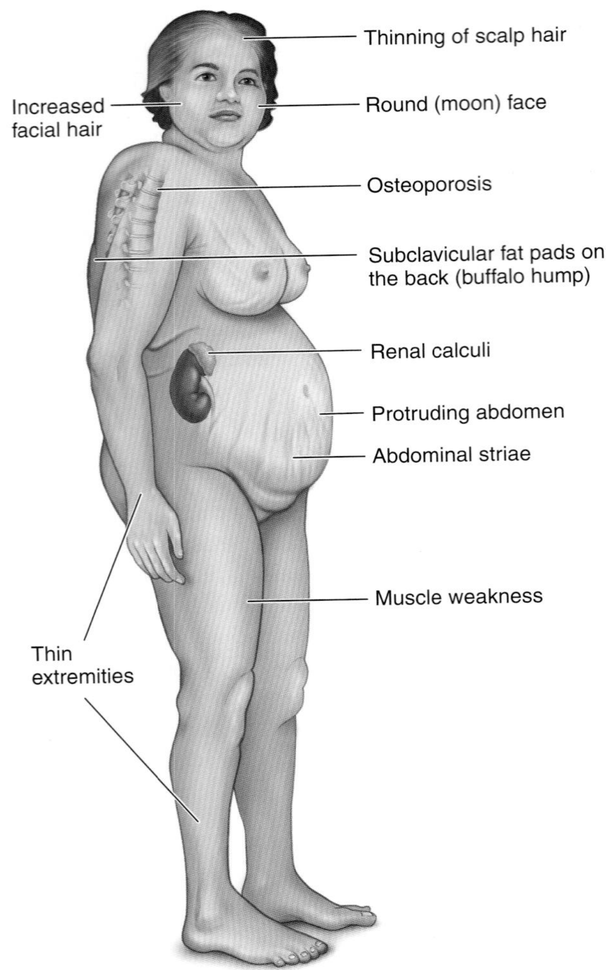

Figure 13.14. Dominant features of Cushing syndrome.

elevations of these hormones. Excess aldosterone results in hypertension and hypokalemia. Excess androgens can result in **hirsutism**, the development of excessive body and facial hair, or changes in patterns of pubic and axillary hair growth (primarily in women).

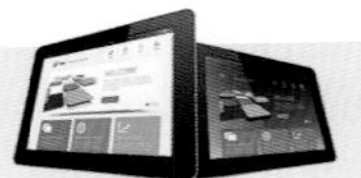

RESEARCH NOTES

Scientists have noted that somewhere between 5% and 13% of cases of hypertension are caused by abnormally high aldosterone levels. Research continues to explore the long-term effects of excess aldosterone, particularly on cardiovascular function. Improved treatment of hypertension may rely on blocking aldosterone when indicated, preventing hypertension, and limiting harmful cardiovascular effects of hyperaldosteronism. The high prevalence of hypertension in Black individuals may be explained, in part, by the role of aldosterone in maintaining the antioxidant–oxidant balance. Aldosterone decreases the activity of the enzyme glucose-6-phosphate dehydrogenase (G-6-PD). This enzyme has a role in antioxidant defenses. A deficiency of G-6-PD is seen in 10% to 15% of Black people, perhaps related to high aldosterone levels. This may also explain the levels of high blood pressure in this population.[6]

DIAGNOSTIC CRITERIA

Diagnosis of Cushing syndrome is often based on a 24-hour urine collection during which elevations in cortisol excretion are noted. False-positive tests may result in those with obesity, alcoholism, chronic renal failure, anorexia, or bulimia, because these also raise cortisol secretion. Imaging studies are needed to locate tumors that may be secreting excess ACTH or cortisol.

TREATMENT

Treatment is focused on removing the cause of excess hormone production. Surgery or radiation may be needed to remove tumors. Corticosteroid medications may be needed to avert an adrenal crisis during acute illness and then they must be gradually withdrawn.

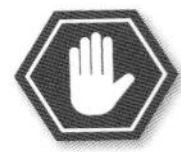

Stop and Consider
How would a deficiency of cortisol present in terms of clinical manifestations?

Addison Disease

Although rare, acute ACTH deficiency is considered one of the most serious endocrine disorders because it can lead to severe hypotension, shock, and death. Adrenal cortical insufficiency can result from lack of CRH or ACTH, or lack of secretion of hormones from the adrenal cortex. Disease typically presents when 90% or more of the adrenal cortices are destroyed or nonfunctional.

PATHOPHYSIOLOGY

Lack of ACTH production from the pituitary is most often caused by destruction of the pituitary gland from tumors, hemorrhage, trauma, radiation, or surgical removal. Adrenal cortical insufficiency can also result from lack of hormones secreted from the adrenal cortex. Autoimmune destruction of the layers of the adrenal cortex is the most common cause of **Addison disease**. This destruction leads to the inability of the adrenal gland to produce any glucocorticoids, mineralocorticoids, or androgens. As a result, ACTH levels are elevated to increase the secretion of these three major steroid hormones from the adrenal glands.

CLINICAL MANIFESTATIONS

Clinical manifestations are based on insufficient levels of the steroid hormones as depicted in Table 13.4. Elevations in ACTH levels stimulate skin melanocytes, resulting in a characteristic hyperpigmentation, or darkening, of the skin and mucous membranes.

Table 13.4 Clinical Manifestations of Addison Disease

Deficient Hormones	Clinical Manifestations
Glucocorticoids	Hypoglycemia, weakness, poor stress response, fatigue, anorexia, nausea, vomiting, weight loss, personality changes
Mineralocorticoids	Dehydration, hyponatremia, hyperkalemia, hypotension, weakness, fatigue, shock
Androgens	Sparse axillary and pubic hair in women

DIAGNOSTIC CRITERIA

Diagnosis of Addison disease is based on the clinical presentation and laboratory analysis of electrolyte levels demonstrating hyponatremia and hyperkalemia. Serum corticosteroid levels can also be measured, and results will show corticosteroid levels that remain depressed after administration of ACTH.

TREATMENT

In acute illness, isotonic IV fluid replacement is infused along with hydrocortisone sodium succinate or phosphate. Improvement in blood pressure should occur within 4 to 6 hours. Gradually, the IV infusion of hydrocortisone is tapered and oral replacement of glucocorticoid and mineralocorticoid hormones ensues for the remainder of the individual's life. Because of elevations in sodium excretion, salt intake may need to be increased in hot weather. The exception to this is for those patients with Addison disease caused by tuberculosis. The tuberculosis bacteria can also destroy the adrenal gland. Treatment of the bacteria with antibiotics is required, and adrenal function resumes without lifelong glucocorticoid and mineralocorticoid replacement.

SUMMARY

- Hormone messengers have many important regulatory functions, including energy metabolism, growth and development, muscle and fat distribution, fluid and electrolyte balance, sexual development, and reproduction.
- Hormones are instrumental in the stress response and are essential for maintaining homeostasis.
- The initiation of hormone secretion and regulation for many hormones relies on neuronal control through the hypothalamic–pituitary axis, receptor binding, intracellular communication, and feedback mechanisms.
- Functional deficits usually arise from impairment of the endocrine (secreting) gland, lack of, or excessive hormone synthesis, impaired receptor binding, impaired feedback mechanisms, or an altered cellular response to the hormone.
- Problems with hormone function can manifest through inadequate or excessive production, composition, secretion, receptor binding, uptake, metabolism, or elimination of hormones.
- The general manifestations of hypopituitarism are often vague and may include fatigue, weakness, anorexia, sexual dysfunction, growth impairment, dry skin, constipation, and cold intolerance; likewise, hyperpituitarism also has a wide range of manifestations depending on which hormones are elevated.
- Diagnosing alterations in hormonal or metabolic function begins with a complete patient history and physical examination and often relies on measuring hormone levels or other indicators in the blood or urine; imaging studies, such as CT or MRI scans, may be needed to locate a tumor that could be suppressing or stimulating hormone secretion. Genetic testing may also be needed to identify a genetic alteration that is affecting hormone function.
- Treating hormone alterations varies depending on the cause; hormone deficits often require exogenous replacement and hormone elevations require eliminating the excess hormone. This often occurs by removing tumors that may be secreting ectopic hormone, removing all or part of the corresponding endocrine gland, or administering medications that block the effects of the hormone.

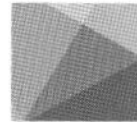

CASE STUDY 13.1

A 43-year-old male is diagnosed with a somatotrope adenoma. Somatotropes are pituitary cells that secrete growth hormone. As a result, he is diagnosed with **acromegaly**, or an excess of growth hormone that occurs after puberty.

1. Outline the process that is most likely occurring in this man's body.
2. What hormone is altered?
3. What would you expect for clinical manifestations?
4. What diagnostic tests could be used?
5. What treatment measures would you anticipate?

Log on to the Internet. Search for a relevant journal article or Web site (such as http://www.emedicine

.com/med/topic27.htm) that details acromegaly, and confirm your predictions.

CASE STUDY 13.2

A father has noticed that his child is quite a bit shorter than the other kids his age. The child, now 2 years old, was of normal birth length. Over time, though, he has not kept up with the linear growth of other children his age. He appears to learn new things without difficulty but is overweight and has immature facial features. He does have a history of hypoglycemia and seizures. He is diagnosed with congenital growth hormone deficiency.

1. Outline the process that is most likely occurring in this child's body.
2. What hormone is altered?
3. What would you expect for clinical manifestations?
4. What diagnostic tests could be used?
5. What treatment measures would you anticipate?

Log on to the Internet. Search for a relevant journal article or Web site that details congenital growth hormone deficiency (such as: http://emedicine.medscape.com/article/117012-clinical) and confirm your predictions.

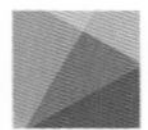

CASE STUDY 13.3

A 4-year-old boy presents with symptoms of androgen excess, including rapid growth, pubic hair, and aggressive behavior. His bone age was determined to be advanced. The child was also found to have significant hypertension. He is diagnosed with congenital adrenal hyperplasia.

1. Outline the process that is most likely occurring in this child's body.
2. What hormone is altered?
3. What would you expect for clinical manifestations?
4. What diagnostic tests could be used?
5. What treatment measures would you anticipate?

Log on to the Internet. Search for a relevant journal article or Web site, such as http://emedicine.medscape.com/article/117012-clinical, that details congenital adrenal hyperplasia, and confirm your predictions.

PRACTICE EXAM QUESTIONS

1. Which of the following is *not* a major role of hormones?
   a. Growth stimulation
   b. Erythrocyte synthesis
   c. Fluid balance and regulation
   d. Metabolic rate regulation

2. The release of hormones from glands is most often controlled by:
   a. Negative feedback mechanisms
   b. Nephrogenic mechanisms
   c. Ectopic hormone production
   d. Active transport

3. The most common cause of endocrine disorders is:
   a. Surgical removal of endocrine glands
   b. Infection
   c. Adenomas
   d. Immunodeficiency

4. Excess cortisol is represented by which condition?
   a. Addison disease
   b. Cushing syndrome
   c. Diabetes insipidus
   d. Hyperthyroidism

5. Diabetes insipidus, if left untreated, will rapidly develop into:
   a. Malignant hypertension
   b. Diabetic coma
   c. Dehydration
   d. Metabolic alkalosis

6. A patient is asked to collect a 24-hour urine test to check a hormone level. Why is the 24-hour urine needed?
   a. To measure female reproductive hormone levels
   b. To obtain a measurement of hormone secretion over time
   c. It is easier than obtaining a blood sample
   d. Urine is not an effective method of measuring hormone levels

7. You are experiencing constipation, dry skin, weight gain, and cold intolerance. Which condition are you most likely experiencing?
   a. Hyperthyroidism
   b. Addison disease
   c. Cushing syndrome
   d. Hypothyroidism

8. Which of the following occurs with elevated levels of cortisol?
   a. Fatty acids are mobilized
   b. Glucose levels are suppressed
   c. Plasma protein levels increase
   d. Inflammation increases

9. Which type of hormone is not produced in the adrenal cortex?
a. Mineralocorticoids
b. Glucocorticoids
c. Adrenal sex hormones
d. Neurotransmitters

10. Diagnosis of SIADH is based on which of the following?
a. Hyponatremia
b. Hypertonicity
c. Increased urine volume
d. Dilute urine with a low sodium content

11. Release of hormones from the anterior pituitary differs from those released by the posterior pituitary. What is the major way in which these are different?
a. The posterior pituitary is much less complicated
b. The anterior pituitary releases only two hormones
c. The posterior pituitary follows the positive feedback loop
d. The anterior pituitary is controlled by the hypothalamus

12. Which of the following major pathways occurs when a hormone is produced in a cell and can have an impact on neighboring cells and on its own cell?
a. Paracrine pathway
b. Autocrine pathway
c. Synaptic pathway
d. Neuroendocrine pathway

13. A patient presents with SIADH and a serum sodium level of 100 mEq/L. What would you expect for clinical manifestations for this patient?
a. Polyuria, polydipsia, polyphagia
b. Nausea, vomiting, headache
c. Muscle cramps, weakness, irritability
d. Seizures, psychosis, gait disturbances

14. A patient presents with exophthalmos. What condition is she likely experiencing?
a. Addison disease
b. Cushing disease
c. Graves disease
d. Diabetes insipidus

DISCUSSION AND APPLICATION

1. What did I know about altered hormonal and metabolic regulation prior to today?

2. What body processes are affected by altered hormonal and metabolic regulation? What are the expected functions of those processes? How does altered hormonal and metabolic regulation affect those processes?

3. What are the potential etiologies for altered hormonal and metabolic regulation? How does altered hormonal and metabolic regulation develop?

4. Who is most at risk for developing altered hormonal and metabolic regulation? How can altered hormonal and metabolic regulation be prevented?

5. What are the human differences that affect the etiology, risk, or course of altered hormonal and metabolic regulation?

6. What clinical manifestations are expected in the course of altered hormonal and metabolic regulation?

7. What special diagnostic tests help determine the diagnosis and course of altered hormonal and metabolic regulation?

8. What are the goals of care for individuals who have altered hormonal and metabolic regulation?

9. How does the concept of altered hormonal and metabolic regulation build on what I have learned in the previous chapters and in previous courses?

10. How can I use what I have learned?

RESOURCES

The Hormone Health Network is an international resource clinical and scientific expertise in endocrinology:
http://www.hormone.org/

References

1. Usala RL, Fernandez SJ, Mete M, et al. Hyponatremia is associated with increased osteoporosis and bone fractures in a large US health system population. *J Clin Endocrinol Metab*. 2015;100(8):3021–3031.
2. Khardori R. Diabetes insipidus. 2015. http://emedicine.medscape.com/article/117648-overview#a6
3. Lee S. Hyperthyroidism. 2015. http://emedicine.medscape.com/article/121865-overview#a6
4. Orlander P. Hypothyroidism. 2015. http://emedicine.medscape.com/article/122393-overview#a5
5. Rubin E, Gorstein F, Rubin R, et al. *Rubin's Pathology: Clinicopathologic Foundations of Medicine*. 4th ed. Baltimore, MD: Lippincott Williams & Wilkins, 2005.
6. Mikta M. Scientists probe aldosterone's role in hypertension and heart disease. *JAMA*. 2004;292:2704–2705.

Find additional resources for this chapter at http:thePoint.lww.com thePoint®

Chapter 14

Altered Reproductive Function

LEARNING OUTCOMES

1. Define and use the key terms listed in this chapter.
2. Identify structures and processes required for effective reproductive function.
3. Analyze the mechanisms of impairment that can lead to altered reproductive function.
4. Discuss common measures to diagnose and treat altered reproductive function.
5. Apply concepts of altered reproductive function to select clinical models.

INTRODUCTION

Consider the complexity of creating a new human being. Reproductive function is reliant upon structural integrity, neurologic, and hormonal processes of males and females. Both are needed, and they must work together in order to be successful. This chapter focuses on structural and functional expectations in order to reproduce and processes that can alter reproductive function.

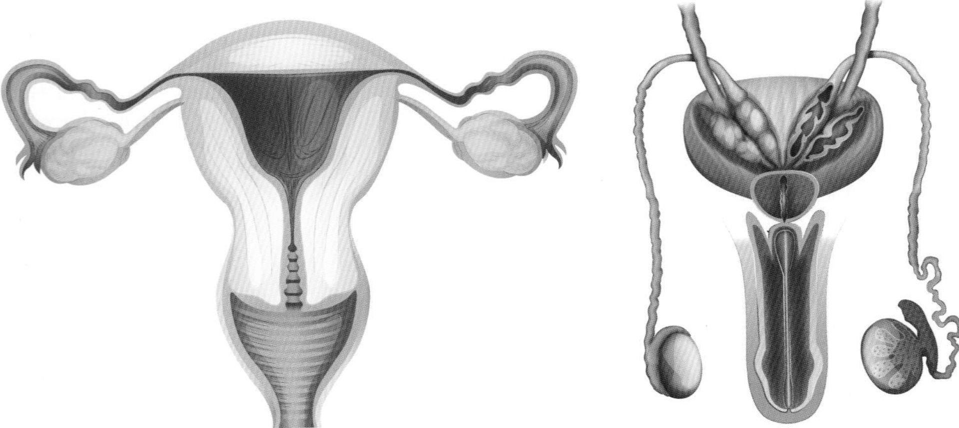

Female and male reproductive systems. Image © BlueRingMedia

Module 1 Regulation of Reproduction

Female Reproductive Hormone Function

Structural integrity is required to achieve reproduction. For females, this includes the external genitalia and internal reproductive structures. External genitalia features the mons pubis, labia majora, vestibule, Bartholin glands, labia minora, clitoris, Skene glands at the urethral opening, and the vaginal orifice (Fig. 14.1). The primary purpose of external structures is protection and lubrication. The clitoris, analogous to the male penis, is highly sensitive and distends during sexual stimulation.

Internal reproductive structures include the vagina, uterus, fallopian tubes, and ovaries, located in the pelvic cavity (Fig. 14.2). The vagina is needed as an outlet for menses and other secretions and also serves the function of sexual fulfillment and entry for sperm from the male penis. The cervix forms the inlet to the uterus. Secretions from the cervix offer some protection from infection and allow increased or decreased receptivity to sperm depending on hormone influences. The uterus, a muscular organ, has three layers: an inner endometrium, a middle myometrium, and an outer perimetrium. The functional layer of the endometrium proliferates as the uterine lining builds and sloughs as menses each month. The muscular myometrium contracts to expel menses and provides uterine contractions during childbirth.

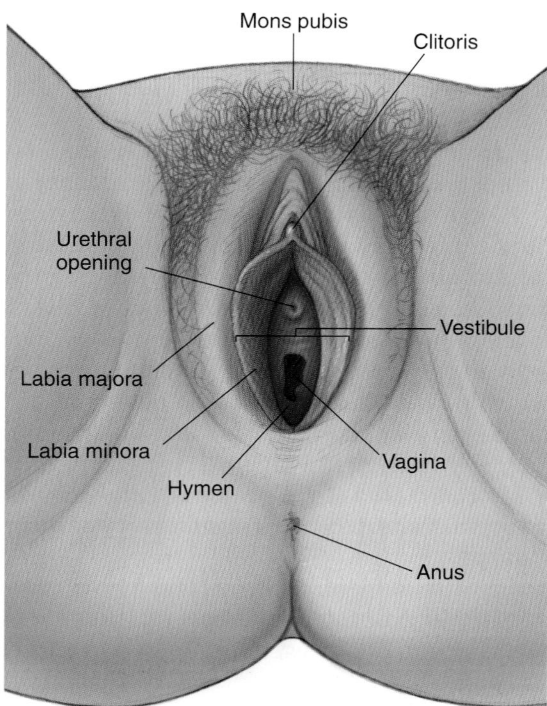

Figure 14.1. Female external genitalia. (From Westheimer R, Lopater S. *Human Sexuality*. Baltimore, MD: Lippincott Williams & Wilkins; 2003.)

Fallopian tubes extend from the uterus to a funnel-shaped opening with finger-like projections toward the ovaries to attract the ovum (Fig. 14.3). The fallopian tubes form an important connective passageway for the ova and sperm. The almond-shaped ovaries have four parts:

- Stroma, the supporting tissue
- Interstitial cells, which secrete estrogen
- Follicles, which contain the ova (germ cells)
- Corpus luteum, forms after the ovum has been released from the ovarian follicle

Led by the hypothalamus, pituitary, and ovaries, hormonal processes are also needed to facilitate reproduction (Fig. 14.4). The ovaries produce the female sex hormones: estrogens, progesterone, and androgens. These hormones are secreted in a monthly cyclical pattern under the direction of the hypothalamus (gonadotropin-releasing hormone [GnRH]) and the anterior pituitary (follicle-stimulating hormone [FSH], luteinizing hormone [LH]).

If pregnancy occurs, three additional hormones come into play. Human chorionic gonadotropin (hCG) appears within 2 to 3 days after the zygote implants into the endometrium. hCG is produced by the zygote and acts on the corpus luteum to maintain its estrogen and progesterone-secreting function. Home pregnancy tests measure the presence of hCG in the urine. The anterior pituitary also secretes prolactin during and after pregnancy to allow lactation to occur. Oxytocin is a hormone secreted from the posterior pituitary that stimulates contractions during labor and milk ejection during lactation.

As indicated, the interstitial cells of the ovary secrete estrogens. The estrogens (estradiol, estrone, and estriol) are the primary female sex hormones. These are secreted throughout the monthly menstrual cycle and dominate from the end of menses to ovulation. The major actions of the estrogens include:

- Female reproductive organ development
- Female body fat contour distribution
- Breast development and skeletal growth during puberty

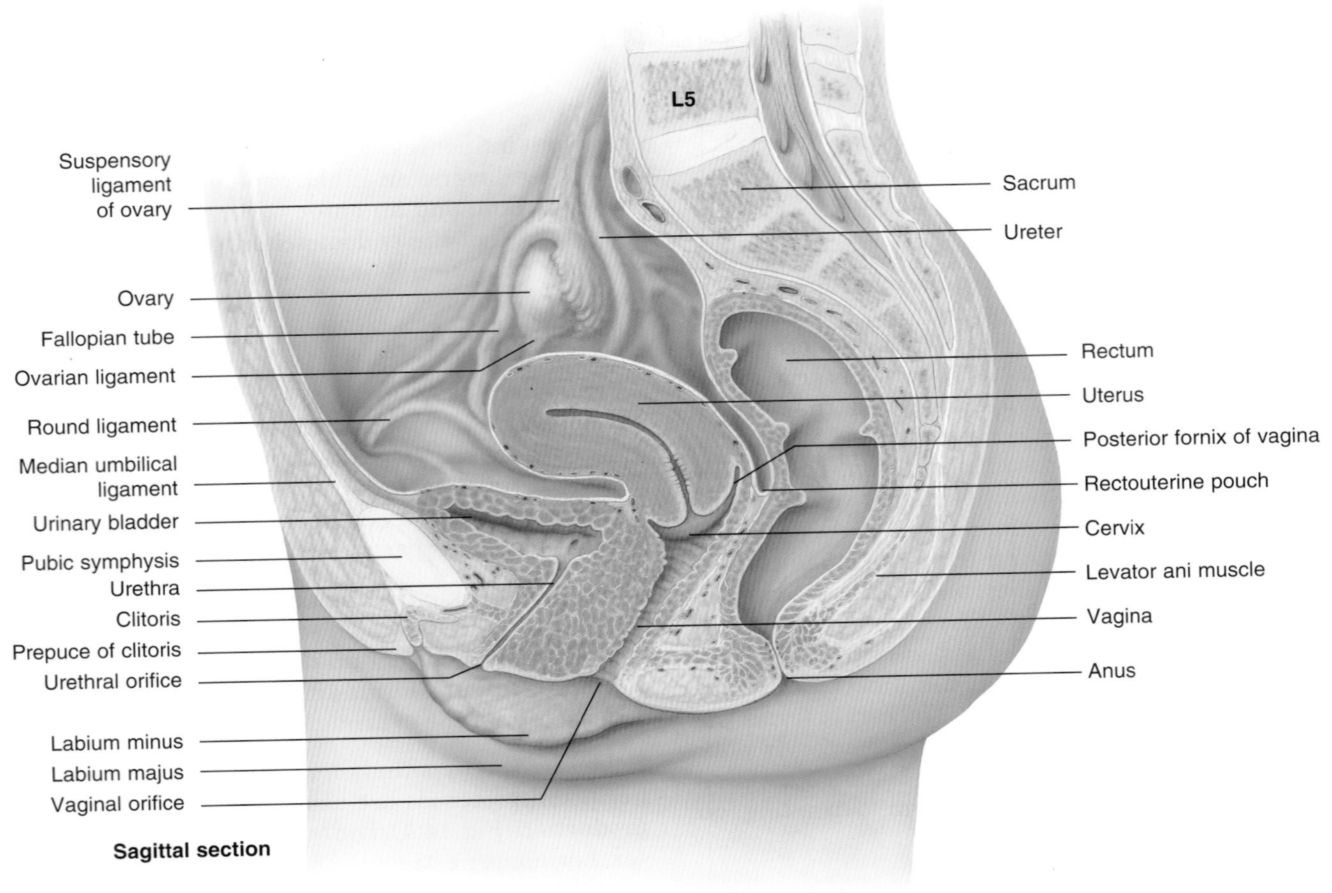

Figure 14.2. Female reproductive structures.

- Ovulation and support of pregnancy and lactation
- Cervical mucus alterations (copious, thin, watery, and more receptive to sperm)
- Axillary and pubic hair growth
- Female skin maintenance
- Decreased bone resorption; maintenance of bone integrity
- Retention of sodium and water

Progesterone is another important female sex hormone, secreted in large amounts from ovulation to the onset of menstruation. The corpus luteum of the ovary secretes progesterone and estrogen. Progesterone thickens the lining of the uterus to support implantation and nourishes the embryo in early pregnancy. Progesterone also helps to maintain the pregnancy by relaxing smooth muscles in the uterus to avoid expulsion of the embryo. Progesterone elevates the core body temperature slightly and can induce nausea, headaches, constipation, indigestion, and swelling in pregnancy.

Ovulation is the process of releasing an oocyte from an ovarian follicle. Ovulation occurs once every 21 to 40 days for most women (the average is approximately 28 days). Ovulation relies on hormone regulation and is typically divided into two parts: (1) the follicular phase in the first half of the ovulatory cycle; and (2) the luteal phase in the second half of the ovulatory cycle (Fig. 14.5). Follicles are epithelial capsules that hold oocytes. Follicles are further distinguished as primary and secondary follicles. Primary follicles are inactive. During each ovulatory cycle, approximately 10 primary follicles are stimulated by FSH and LH and become secondary, or active, follicles.

During the follicular phase, secondary follicles enlarge, further develop, and become capable of secreting estrogen and progesterone. In a process that is not completely understood, one of these follicles becomes dominant by secreting large amounts of estrogen, and the remaining follicles subsequently become **atretic** (atrophic). The dominant follicle

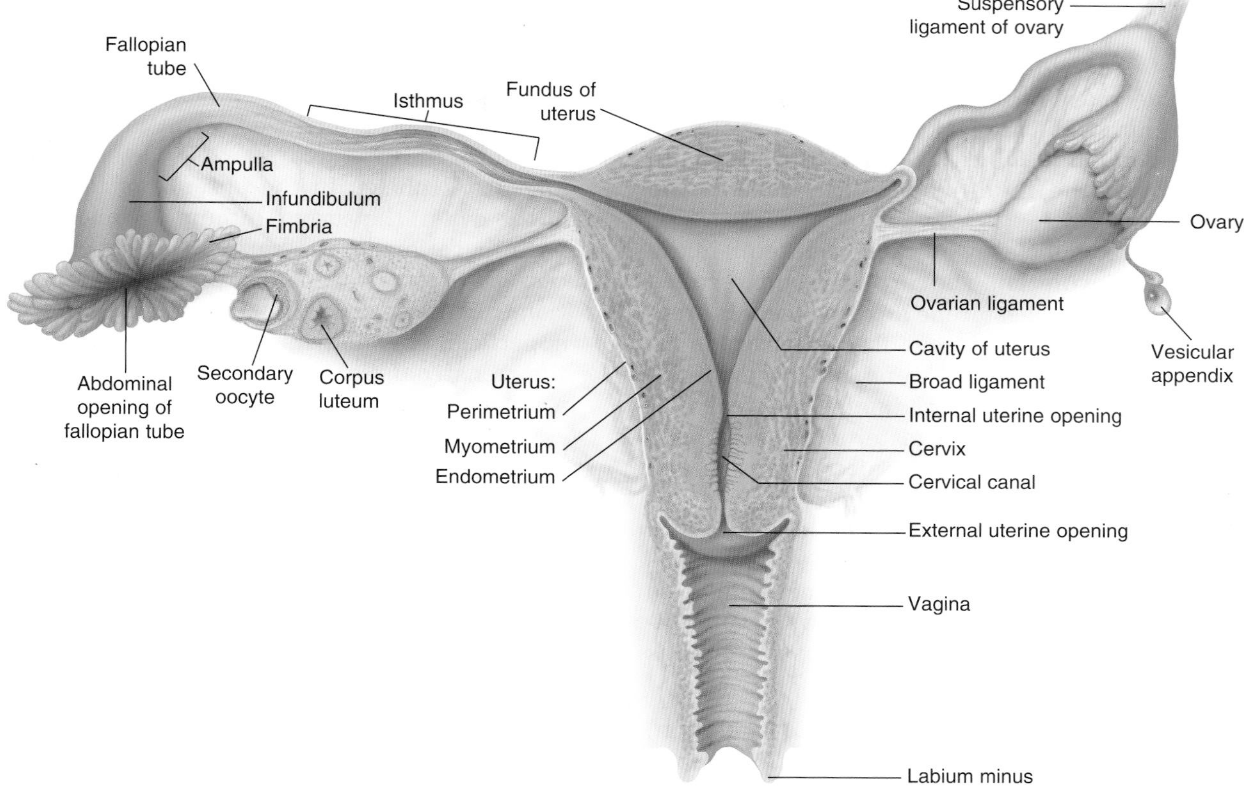

Figure 14.3. Cross-section of ovaries, fallopian tubes, uterus, and vagina.

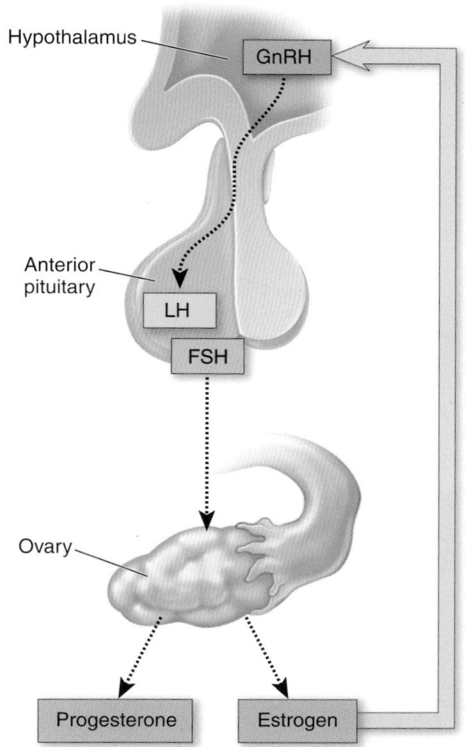

Figure 14.4. Feedback regulation of ovarian function. FSH, follicle-stimulating hormone; GnRH, gonadotropin-releasing hormone; LH, luteinizing hormone. (Modified from Premkumar K. *The Massage Connection: Anatomy and Physiology*. Baltimore, MD: Lippincott Williams & Wilkins; 2004.)

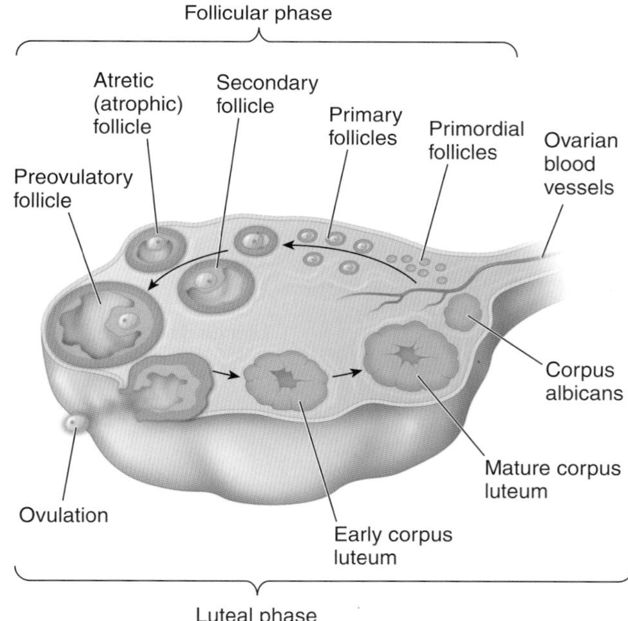

Figure 14.5. Sequence of ovulatory events showing ovarian follicle origin, growth, and rupture and the formation and degradation of the corpus luteum. The atretic (atrophic) follicle was one that did not fully mature.

continues to secrete estrogen, which alerts the pituitary to decrease FSH. LH levels remain elevated and then surge at the peak of estrogen secretion from the dominant follicle, causing the oocyte to break through the fluid-filled follicle. This is the point of ovulation.

The ruptured follicle forms a corpus luteum in the luteal phase of ovulation. The corpus luteum secretes large amounts of progesterone and estrogen. If pregnancy occurs, the progesterone from the corpus luteum hormonally supports the pregnancy until the placenta has developed (approximately 14 weeks). If pregnancy does not occur, progesterone and estrogen levels drop within about 14 days after ovulation and menstruation begins.

Corresponding to the ovulatory cycle is the growth of the endometrium, or lining of the uterus (Fig. 14.6). The growth of the endometrium, also under the direction of hormones, allows zygote implantation and nourishment. Endometrial growth is divided into three phases:

- *Proliferative* (end of menstruation to ovulation) phase: At the end of menstruation, the endometrium is thin. Estrogen acts to support growth (proliferation) of the superficial layer of the endometrium. The endometrium thickness increases to six to eight times greater than that found at the end of menstruation.
- *Secretory* (ovulation to the beginning of menstruation) phase: Progesterone, in addition to estrogen, further supports proliferation of the endometrium. The lining becomes thick, vascular, and swollen. The fertilized ovum can embed into this thick lining.
- *Menstrual* phase: In the absence of fertilization of the ovum, the corpus luteum becomes useless. Disintegration of the corpus luteum results in cessation of estrogen and progesterone production from these cells. This leads to shedding of the superficial endometrial layer, which is also called the menstrual period.

Male Reproductive Hormone Function

The male reproductive organs and tissues include the testes, epididymis, vas deferens, seminal vesicles, prostate, and penis (Fig. 14.7). The male genitourinary system is responsible for urine elimination, sexual function, and reproduction. Androgens, the male sex hormones, promote metabolism and growth. The pattern of male sex hormone secretion does not follow a cyclical pattern as seen with females; the hormone secretion rates remain fairly constant throughout the male's adult life.

Stimulation of androgen production and release begins in the hypothalamus (Fig. 14.8). The hypothalamus releases GnRH, which stimulates the anterior pituitary to release LH and FSH. LH acts on the Leydig cells in the testes to produce testosterone,

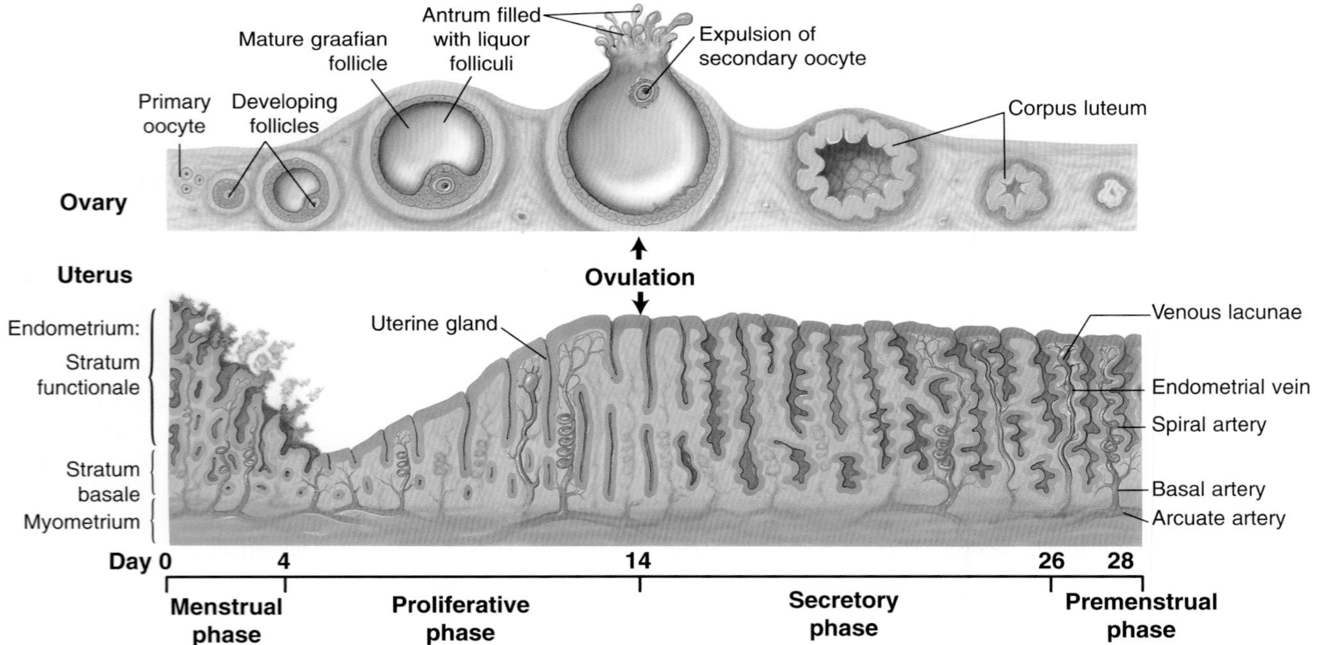

Figure 14.6. Corresponding ovulatory cycle and growth of the endometrium.

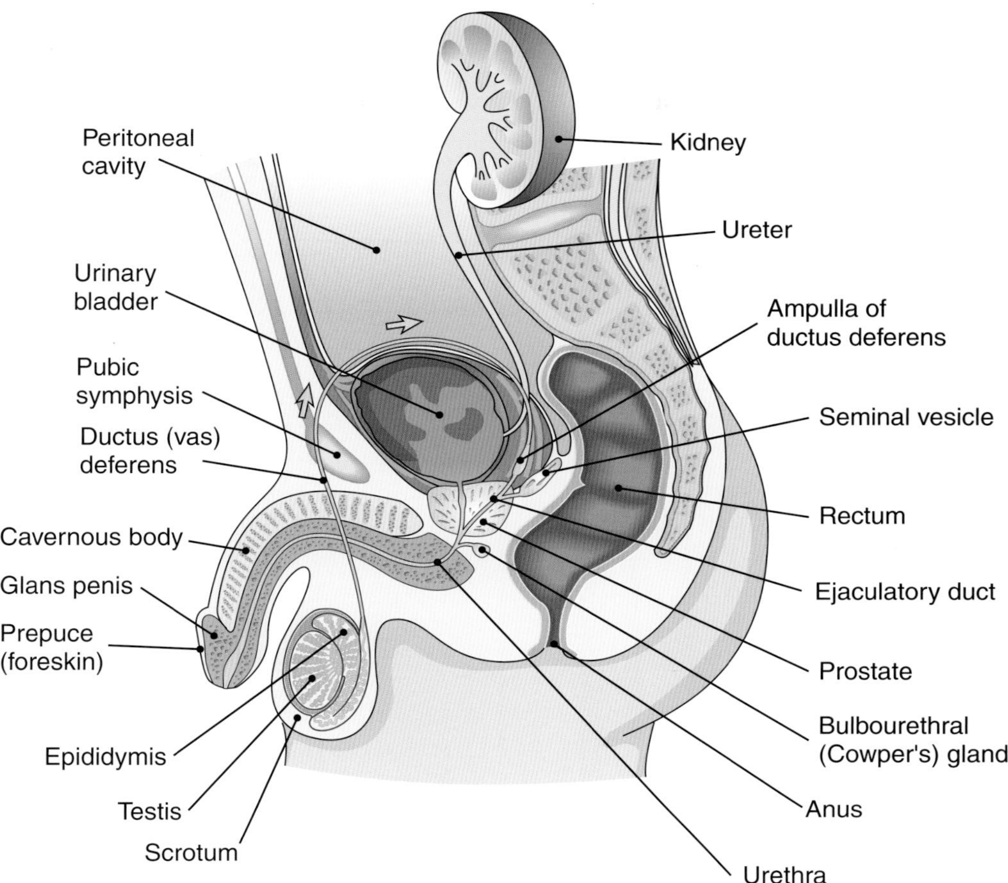

Figure 14.7. Male reproductive structures.

the primary male sex hormone. Testosterone has multiple effects, including:

- Development and function of male reproductive organs
- Sperm production and maturation
- Protein metabolism
- Muscle mass promotion
- Skin thickness promotion
- Sebaceous gland activity
- Growth of pubic, chest, and facial hair
- Maturation of the larynx, resulting in a deeper voice tone

Excess testosterone levels alert the hypothalamus to decrease secretion of GnRH and the pituitary to decrease production of LH.

The second major sex hormone secreted from the pituitary is FSH. When gonadotropin (FSH, LH) levels increase, FSH acts on the Sertoli cells within the seminiferous tubules to secrete inhibin, a hormone that alerts the pituitary to suppress secretion of the gonadotropins. Sertoli cells also play a role in spermatogenesis.

Spermatogenesis occurs in the seminiferous tubules of the testes. Spermatozoa are released from the epithelial lining of the tubules into the lumen. Sertoli cells play an active role in releasing sperm into the lumen. Spermatogenesis requires a 2° to 3° cooler scrotal temperature than that found with the core body temperature. Failure of the testes to descend into the scrotum or excessive heat to the scrotum, such as occurs when sitting in a hot tub, can impair spermatogenesis. Testosterone production is not affected by temperature. Maturation of the sperm takes place within approximately 60 days. Spermatozoa then transit to the epididymis (the reservoir), then eventually to the vas deferens, and then exit the body through the urethra (Fig. 14.9). The accessory glands, seminal vesicles, prostate, and Cowper glands facilitate the transport of spermatozoa during the ejaculatory process and aid in spermatozoa survival.

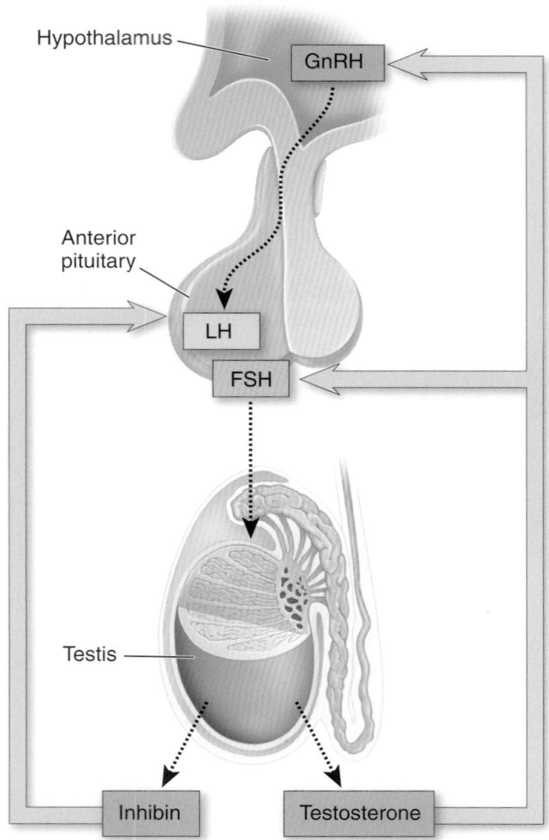

Figure 14.8. Feedback regulation of testicular function. FSH, follicle-stimulating hormone; GnRH, gonadotropin-releasing hormone; LH, luteinizing hormone. (From Premkumar K. *The Massage Connection: Anatomy and Physiology*. Baltimore, MD: Lippincott Williams & Wilkins; 2004.)

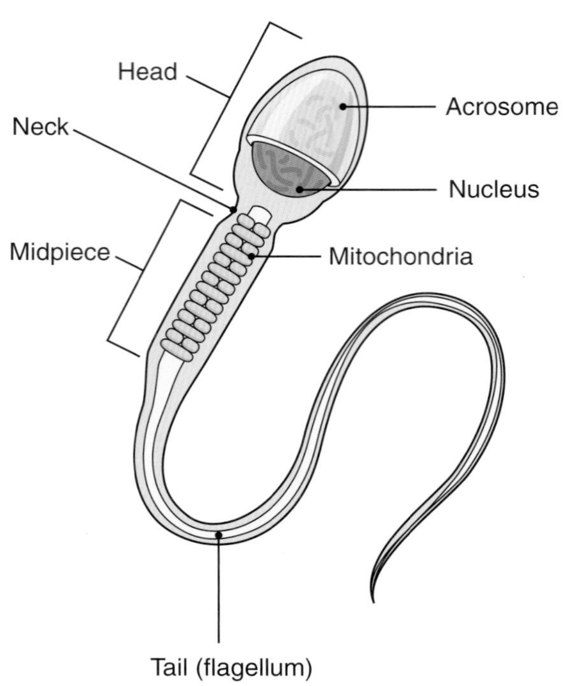

Figure 14.9. Structure of spermatozoa.

Module 2 Altered Reproductive Function

Achieving pregnancy is a complex interaction of ovulation, spermatogenesis, intercourse, ejaculation, conception, implantation, and embryo growth. Infertility, defined as the inability to achieve pregnancy after 1 year of unprotected intercourse, can result from problems in any of these steps. About 10% to 15% of couples are infertile. In many cases, the exact cause of infertility is not identified.

Altered reproduction can result from a functional impairment in the male or female partner, or both. Figure 14.10 illustrates causes of acquired infertility impacting females. Factors involved with altered reproduction may include:

- *Hormonal* imbalance causing the absence of, or infrequent, ovulation, which impairs oocyte development and release; testosterone losses result in impaired sperm production.
- *Motility* impairment caused by adhesions or obstruction in the pathway from the cervix to the ovary, which results in problems with oocyte or sperm transit and block the joining of these cells. Examples include inhospitable cervical mucus that blocks sperm from entering the uterus or previous or current infection that results in adhesions and obstruction of reproductive structures. **Leiomyomas**, fibrous tumors that may form in the uterus, distort the endometrial cavity.
- *Immune* problems caused by antibodies to the male sperm, which quickly destroy sperm, rendering it unable to reach the oocyte.

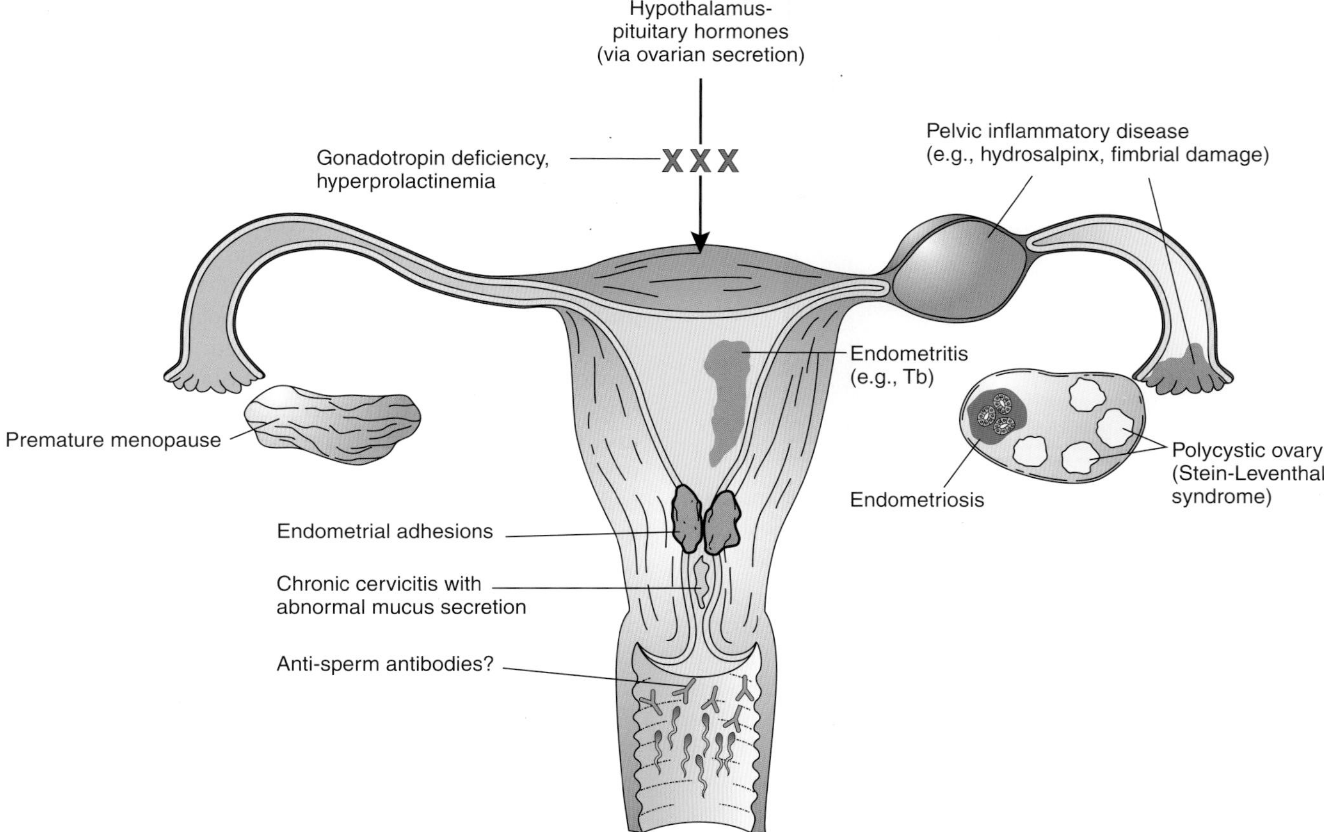

Figure 14.10. Causes of acquired infertility in females. (From Rubin E, Farber JL. *Pathology*. 3rd ed. Philadelphia, PA: Lippincott Williams & Wilkins; 1999.)

General Manifestations of Altered Reproductive Function

The inability to conceive and maintain a pregnancy is a universal clinical manifestation for infertility. In many cases, particularly in men, there are no other signs or symptoms. With hormone alterations, irregular menstrual periods or **amenorrhea** (absent menstrual periods) may be reported. This often signifies **anovulation**, the absence of ovulation manifested by the excess or deficit of one or more reproductive hormones. Amenorrhea can also result from emotional stress, or prolonged strenuous exercise. With the exception of pregnancy-induced amenorrhea, absent menstrual periods is often the result of central nervous system (CNS) alterations that affect the release of GnRH from the hypothalamus and therefore suppress or overstimulate the production of reproductive hormones. For example, a pituitary adenoma may induce hyperprolactinemia, a condition that results in anovulation and subsequently produces amenorrhea.

Pain is another possible clinical manifestation. Testicular/scrotal pain in men or pelvic pain in women may occur with infection or inflammation of reproductive structures. **Dysmenorrhea**, or severe pain with menstrual periods, **dyspareunia**, or pain with intercourse, and other forms of pelvic pain may be present with infections or structural impairment in women. **Endometriosis**, a condition involving endometrial tissue that is located outside of the uterus, can result in pelvic adhesions, distortion of pelvic structures, and dysmenorrhea (Fig. 14.11).

Diagnosing and Treating Altered Reproductive Function

The diagnosis of altered reproduction is based on the couple's inability to conceive or the presence of clinical manifestations described above. Determining the cause requires a systematic history, physical examination, and specialized diagnostic tests. Initially, a semen analysis must be completed in the male along

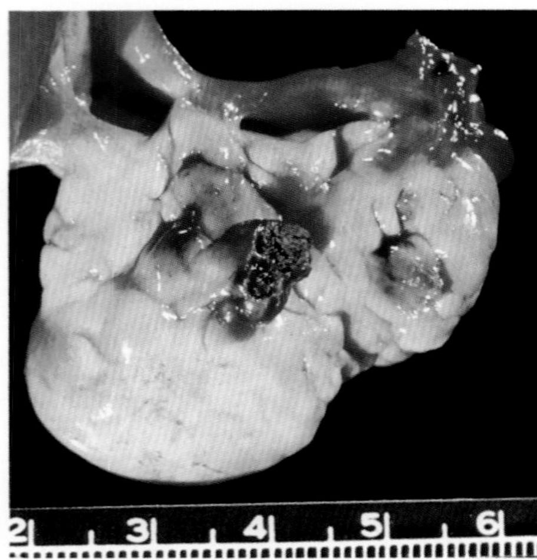

Figure 14.11. Endometriosis implants on the ovary appear as red-blue nodules. (From Rubin E, Farber JL. *Pathology*. 3rd ed. Philadelphia, PA: Lippincott Williams & Wilkins; 1999.)

with an analysis of ovulation in the female. Determination of ovulation can involve observing for cervical mucus changes at the time of ovulation, measuring the basal body temperature over 2 to 3 months (noting the 0.5°F increase at the time of ovulation as progesterone levels rise), or using a home ovulation predictor kit, which measures the LH surge just prior to ovulation. Figure 14.12 illustrates a pathway for diagnosis for those with amenorrhea.

Patency of the reproductive structures can be visualized using hysterosalpingography (Fig. 14.13). This procedure involves injecting a radiopaque material into the uterus and fallopian tubes, then using a fluoroscope and radiograph to determine the presence of obstructions through the reproductive pathway. Laparoscopy, a scope placed through an incision in the abdomen, can view peritoneal and abdominal structures outside of the uterus and fallopian tubes.

General treatment involves supportive counseling, education about intercourse frequency, avoidance of lubricants, which can act as a spermicide, and basic health maintenance. Focused treatment is aimed at the cause, if identified. Sexually transmitted or other pelvic infections place the female at high risk for infertility and must be treated quickly and completely. Obstructive processes, such as leiomyomas, endometriosis, or pelvic adhesions, may require surgical intervention. Ovulatory failure requires a determination of the endocrine problem and a corresponding treatment. Some individuals may require clomiphene citrate, a medication that induces ovulation. In those with hyperprolactinemia, medications may be needed to reduce prolactin and therefore induce ovulation. Artificial insemination may be used to inject sperm into the uterus if cervical mucus is thick or if the sperm quantity or quality is compromised. Some couples seek advanced reproductive technologies such as in vitro fertilization. The evaluation and treatment of infertility is highly complex and emotionally charged. Sensitivity to the range and intensity of emotions is an important aspect of care.

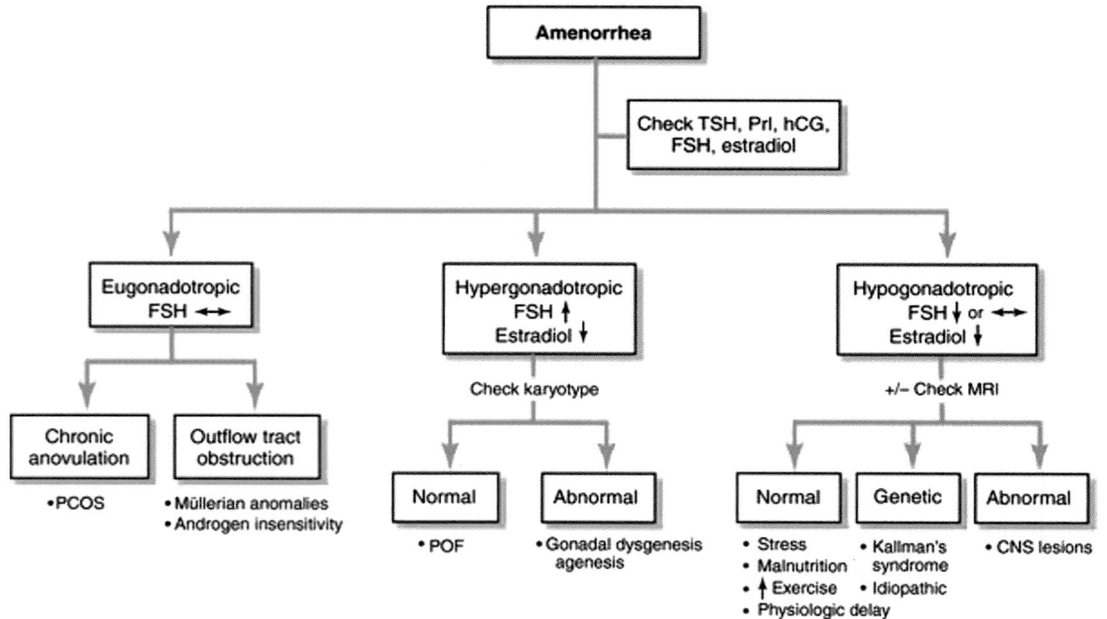

Figure 14.12. The evaluation of amenorrhea. CNS, central nervous system; FSH, follicle-stimulating hormone; hCG, human chorionic gonadotropin; MRI, magnetic resonance imaging; PCOS, polycystic ovary syndrome; POF, premature ovarian failure; Prl, prolactin; TSH, thyroid-stimulating hormone.

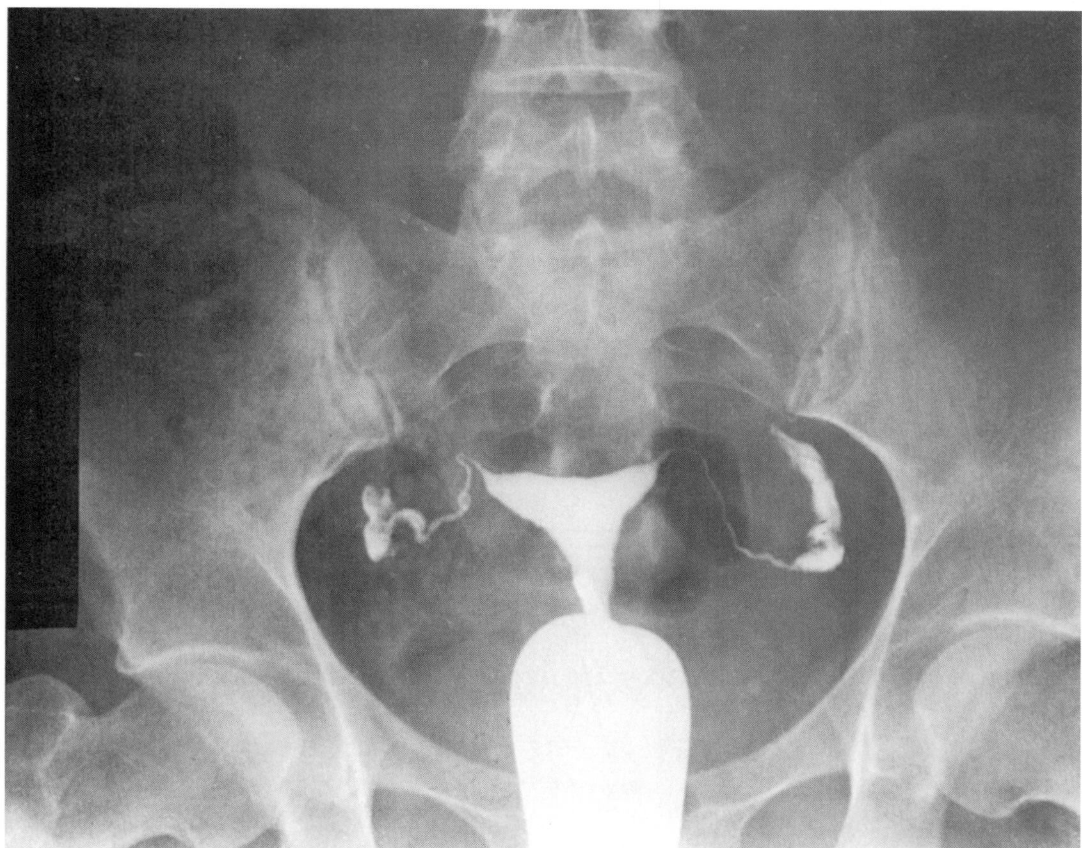

Figure 14.13. Anteroposterior radiograph of the female pelvis after injection of radiopaque compound into the uterine cavity (hysterosalpingogram). (From Snell RS. *Clinical Anatomy*. 7th ed. Philadelphia, PA: Lippincott Williams & Wilkins; 2003.)

Module 3 Clinical Models

Pelvic Inflammatory Disease

Pelvic inflammatory disease (PID) is the result of a sexually transmitted infection of the reproductive tract (Fig. 14.14). The most frequent cause is a combination of sexually transmitted microorganisms including *Chlamydia trachomatis* and *Neisseria gonorrhoeae*. In women, sexual intercourse propels microorganisms into the vagina where the infection then ascends into the cervix, uterus, fallopian tubes, ovaries, and even into the peritoneal cavity.

PATHOPHYSIOLOGY

After attaching to the epithelial cells lining the reproductive tract, the offending microorganisms elicit acute inflammatory and immune responses. The reproductive tract becomes hyperemic and edematous. The fallopian tubes become obstructed with purulent exudate. Repeated or chronic infection results in scar formation. This scarring is particularly problematic in the fallopian tubes and ovaries, where ovulation and free movement of the ovum to the uterus is prohibited. Ectopic pregnancy, tubo-ovarian abscess, pelvic adhesions, and infertility are potential complications of PID. In the male reproductive tract, sexually transmitted infections can result in a similar problem in the urethra, epididymis, and testes.

CLINICAL MANIFESTATIONS

Early infection is often asymptomatic, increasing the likelihood of transmission to others. As the infection ascends and the inflammatory and immune responses become more intensified, common clinical manifestations include pelvic and lower abdominal pain, purulent cervical discharge, cervical motion tenderness, fever, and malaise.

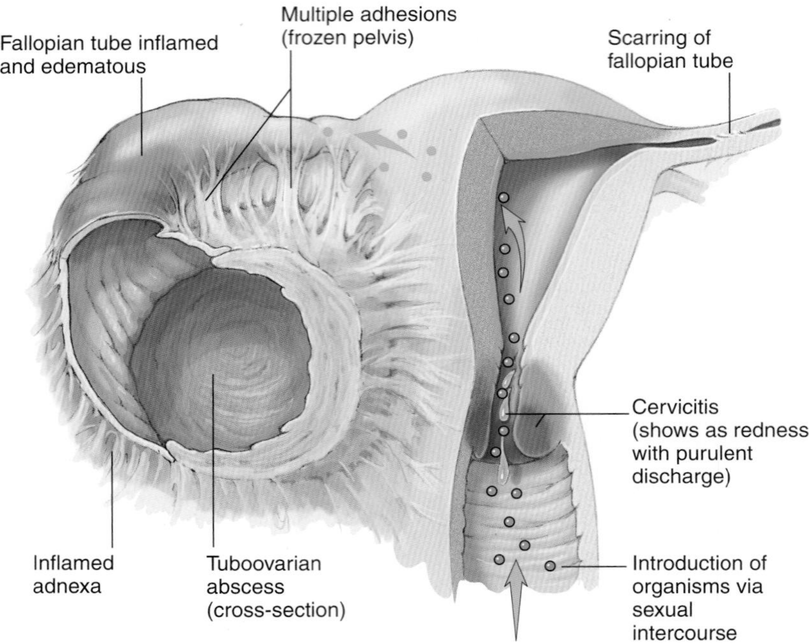

Figure 14.14. Clinical manifestations and complications of pelvic inflammatory disease.

DIAGNOSTIC CRITERIA

Diagnosis of PID is based on history, physical examination, and laboratory studies. The minimum criteria for the diagnosis of PID include lower abdominal tenderness on palpation, adnexal (tissues supporting the uterus) tenderness, and cervical motion tenderness. Cervicitis and a purulent discharge from the cervix may be visualized during pelvic examination. The presence of fever, elevation in the erythrocyte sedimentation rate or C-reactive protein (nonspecific tests of inflammation), and positive bacterial cultures of infected genitourinary secretions provide additional clues for diagnosis. Laparoscopy may be used to confirm the diagnosis as needed.

TREATMENT

Treatment of PID requires an immediate and often prolonged course of oral or intravenous antibiotics. Hospitalization with intravenous antibiotics and fluids is required if the patient is:

- Pregnant
- Immunodeficient
- Presenting with severe illness, nausea, vomiting, or a high fever
- Unable to follow or tolerate the outpatient treatment with oral antibiotics
- Potentially in need of emergency surgery, such as if appendicitis cannot be excluded
- Diagnosed with a tubo-ovarian abscess

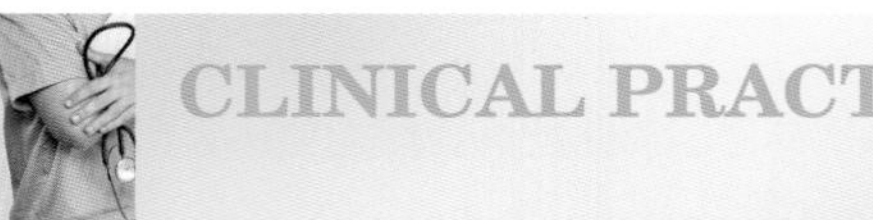

Treatment of sexual contacts for those with sexually transmitted infections is important to avoid reinfection. The patient must abstain from intercourse during the treatment regimen and until partners are treated and cure is achieved.

The goal of treatment is to prevent complications such as pelvic adhesions, ectopic pregnancy, abscesses, and infertility.

Polycystic Ovarian Syndrome

Polycystic ovary syndrome (PCOS) is a condition of excess androgen production from the ovaries and occurs in about three-quarters of women with anovulatory infertility (Fig. 14.15).

In PCOS, excess androgen exposure results in:

- Multiple immature ovarian follicles
- Decreased progesterone production
- Increased acyclic (constant) estrogen production
- Anovulation
- **Hirsutism** (abnormal growth of hair on face and body, see Fig. 14.16)

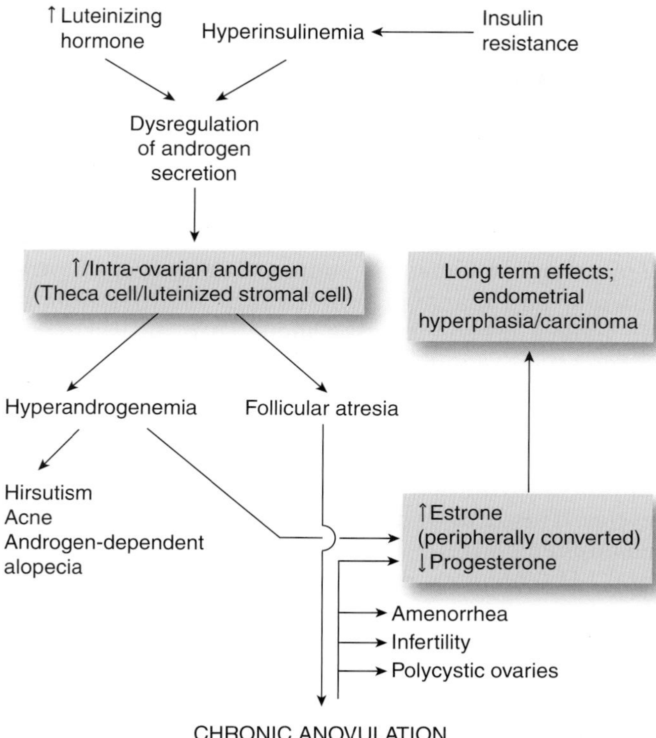

Figure 14.15. Concept map. Pathogenesis of polycystic ovary syndrome. (From Rubin E, Farber JL. *Pathology*. 3rd ed. Philadelphia, PA: Lippincott Williams & Wilkins; 1999.)

- Acne
- Obesity from conversion of androgens to estrogen in adipose tissues
- Hypertension
- Diabetes
- Obstructive sleep apnea

PATHOPHYSIOLOGY

The exact cause of PCOS is unknown. A genetic cause has been suggested and those with PCOS are more likely to have a mother or sister also with PCOS. The reproductive cycle is regulated by changing hormone levels produced by the pituitary and by the ovaries. In PCOS, the pituitary gland secretes high levels of LH and the ovaries make excess androgens. The continued presence of FSH allows for follicle development but maturation of the follicles does not occur. In the absence of ovulation, estrogen alters GnRH resulting in high LH levels with elevation of androgen release and suppression of FSH. The menstrual cycle is disrupted. Chronic anovulation produces bilaterally distended and cystic ovaries. A relationship has been noted between high androgen levels and insulin resistance, where insulin excess promotes excessive androgen production by the ovaries. Insulin sensitizing drugs have been

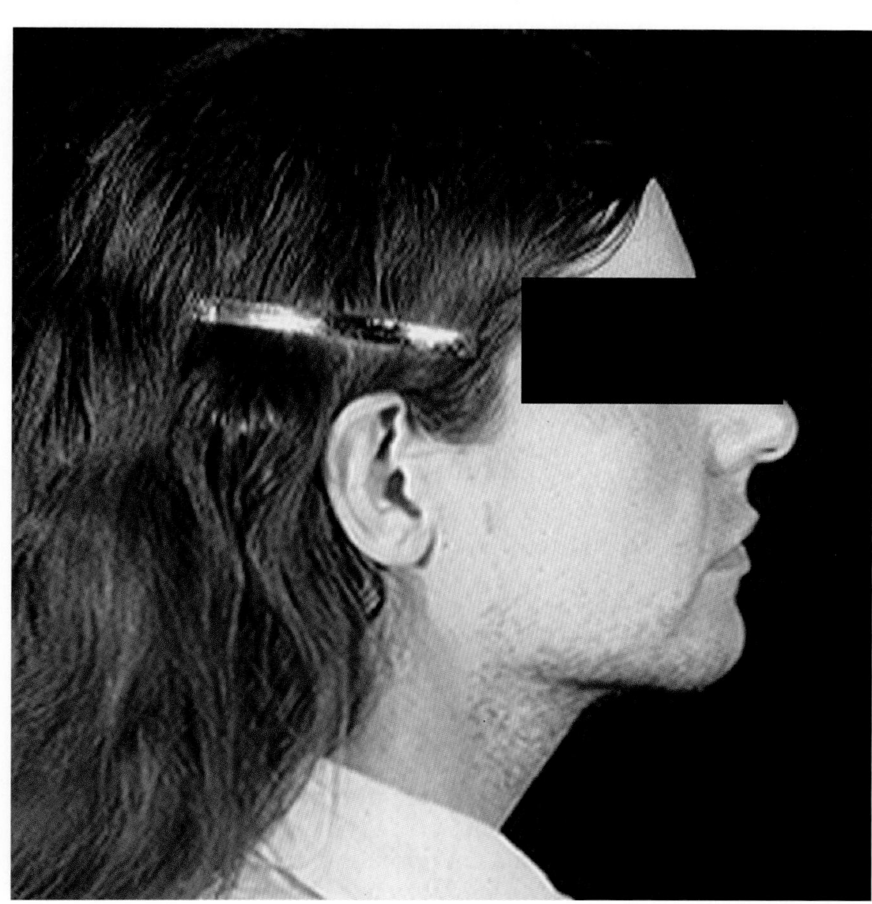

Figure 14.16. Typical facial hirsutism in polycystic ovarian syndrome. (From Berek JS. *Berek & Novak's Gynecology*. 15th ed. Philadelphia, PA: Lippincott Williams & Wilkins; 2012.)

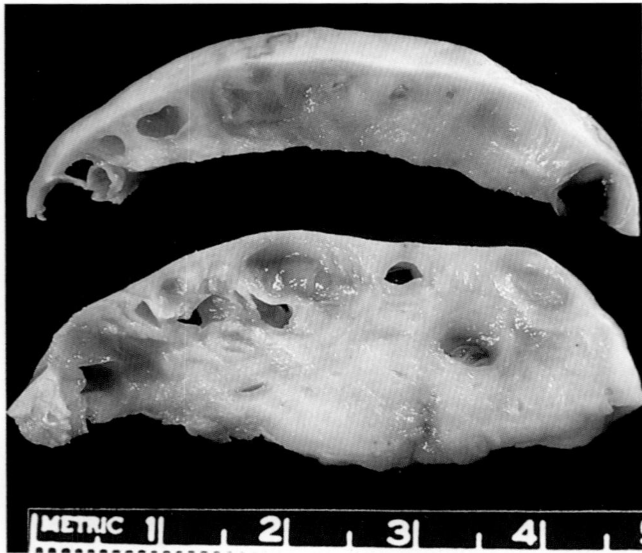

Figure 14.17. Polycystic disease of the ovary. Cut sections of an ovary show numerous cysts embedded in a sclerotic stroma. (From Rubin E, Farber JL. *Pathology*. 3rd ed. Philadelphia, PA: Lippincott Williams & Wilkins; 1999.)

shown to promote ovulation and, ultimately, pregnancy in some cases.

CLINICAL MANIFESTATIONS

Clinical manifestations with PCOS are associated with menstrual irregularities, excess androgen production, and, in many cases, polycystic ovaries (Fig. 14.17). Prolonged menstrual periods and menstrual intervals longer than 35 days or fewer than eight menstrual cycles per year are not uncommon. Excess androgen production may result in physical signs, such as hirsutism (excess facial and body hair), acne, and male-pattern baldness, with some variability based on ethnicity. Obesity is present in about half of women with PCOS. Acanthosis nigricans (darkened, velvety skin) on the nape of the neck, armpits, inner thighs, vulva, or under the breasts can occur as a result of insulin resistance. In some cases, PCOS is only identified when fertility is desired and not achieved.

DIAGNOSTIC CRITERIA

In 2013, the Endocrine Society released practice guidelines for the diagnosis and treatment of PCOS.[1] In those guidelines, the Rotterdam criteria should be used for diagnosis. These criteria require the presence of two of the following: androgen excess, ovulatory dysfunction, and/or polycystic ovaries. Laboratory tests are used to identify hormone alterations and rule out hyperprolactinemia and ovarian or adrenal tumors. Enlarged ovaries containing numerous small cysts can be detected by transvaginal ultrasound. Additionally, fasting cholesterol and triglyceride levels are needed to determine hypercholesterolemia and a glucose tolerance test is needed to determine insulin resistance.

TREATMENT

Treatment is aimed at suppressing androgen production and managing the clinical manifestations. To induce pregnancy, treatment with antiestrogen medications to induce ovulation, such as clomiphene citrate, is needed. Caution must be used because of the risk for ovarian hyperstimulation. Metformin is an oral medication that lowers insulin levels and improves ovulation thereby regulating menstrual cycles. This drug is often used in combination with clomiphene citrate. If unsuccessful, injectable FSH and LH (gonadotropins) may be used. Laparoscopic laser surgery to puncture the multiple ineffective follicles may improve follicular function.

If pregnancy is not desired, low-dose birth control pills decrease androgen production and correct irregular bleeding. Progesterone can also be taken for 10 to 14 days each month to regulate menstrual periods but does not improve androgen levels. Managing obesity, high cholesterol, diabetes, and hypertension are important to prevent long-term cardiovascular risks. Spironolactone may be used to block the skin effects of androgens, including the reduction of excessive hair growth and acne. Shaving, waxing, depilatory creams, laser hair removal, and even electrolysis are also used to reduce excessive hair.

Ovarian Cancer

Neoplasia can occur anywhere throughout the reproductive tract. Uncommonly, women can develop cancer of the vulva or vagina. More commonly, neoplasias can be found in the cervix, uterus, and ovaries. Endometrial cancer of the uterus is the most common invasive cancer in the reproductive tract for women. Epithelial carcinoma of the ovary is the second most common genitourinary cancer (70% to 90% of all ovarian malignancies) and the fifth most frequent cause of death in women. More than 48% of all cases occur in women over the age of 65.[2]

PATHOPHYSIOLOGY

Ovarian cancer arises due to a combination of genetic and environmental risk factors. Family history has an important role in the development of ovarian cancer. Approximately 5% to 10% of ovarian cancers are hereditary, presenting as one of three patterns: ovarian cancer alone, ovarian-breast cancer, or ovarian-colon cancer. In these types, the most important risk factor is a family history of a first-degree relative (mother, daughter, or sister) with the disease. This risk increases in women with two or more first-degree relatives with ovarian cancer. The *BRCA1* gene, located on chromosome 17q21, has been linked to families affected with ovarian cancer and in the breast-ovarian cancer combination. The risk has been reported at 15% to 45% in those with the *BRCA1* mutation. *BRCA2*, located on chromosome 13q14, is also responsible for some instances of inherited ovarian and breast cancer. Both follow an autosomal dominant pattern. Gene mutations, implicated in almost all high grade serous ovarian cancer, occur at *TP53* and with over 100 significant foci. Those with breast cancer also have a significant risk of developing epithelial ovarian cancer.

Environmental factors also play a significant role. For example, ovarian cancer development appears correlated with increased trauma to the ovaries. Monthly ovulation results in the ovum breaking through the epithelial surface of the ovary, causing an inflammatory response and requiring tissue repair. Over time with repeated ovulation, the risk for ovarian cancer increases. Pregnancy, the use of contraceptives, and other events that suppress ovulation may have a protective effect. Also, risk for ovarian cancer has been shown to increase with postmenopausal use of hormone therapy.

The pathophysiology of ovarian cancer follows that of other alterations in cellular proliferation and differentiation. Classification of ovarian cancer is based on tissue of origin and includes:

- **Epithelial tumors:** Arise from the surface of the ovary. Serous adenocarcinoma, an epithelial tumor that resembles the epithelial tissue of the fallopian tube, is the most common type.
- **Germ cell tumors:** Comprise 25% of ovarian tumors but are mostly benign in adult women. Germ cell tumors can also occur in children but are more often malignant in children and young adults. Germ cell tumors resemble embryonic tissues. Development is similar to that of testicular cancer.
- **Sex cord tumors:** Comprise 10% of ovarian tumors. These tumors arise from primitive sex cord or connective tissue of the developing ovary.

The spread of ovarian cancer occurs via local shedding into the peritoneal cavity with seeding and implantation on the peritoneum. This is followed by local invasion of the bowel and bladder. Infiltration of the pelvic lymph nodes is common, and its incidence increases with greater severity of disease. At the time of diagnosis, ovarian cancer is staged from I to IV:

I. Limited to one or both ovaries
II. Extends into pelvis
III. Metastases in peritoneum outside the pelvis
IV. Distant metastases

As with other types of cancer, metastases can relocate in the ovaries from a primary tumor that originates elsewhere. Ovarian cancer is curable in a high percentage of patients if detected in the early stages. Unfortunately, at the time of diagnosis, three of every four women have local spread to the pelvis or distant metastases, making ovarian cancer one of the most lethal female reproductive cancers (Fig. 14.18). More than half of these individuals are at a stage III or greater at diagnosis. For stage III or IV tumors that cannot be removed adequately via surgery, the 5-year survival rate is less than 10%. The composite 5-year survival rate for all patients diagnosed with ovarian cancer is 35%.[3]

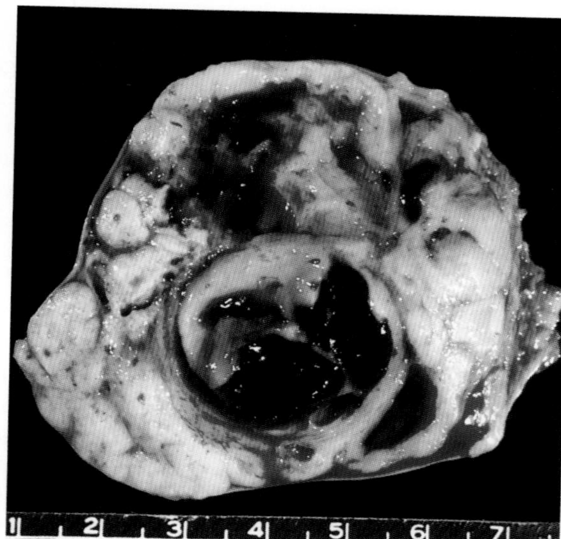

Figure 14.18. Ovarian cancer. A cross-section of the enlarged ovary shows a solid tumor with focal hemorrhages. (Modified from Rubin E, Farber JL. *Pathology*. 4th ed. Philadelphia, PA: Lippincott Williams & Wilkins; 2005.)

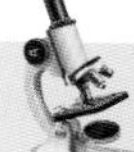

FROM THE LAB

The serum CA-125 level, a tumor marker (antigen), indicates a high probability of epithelial ovarian cancer. However, CA-125 has no prognostic significance when measured at diagnosis. This tumor marker has greater utility in monitoring treatment efficacy and determining recurrence of disease in those with an elevated CA-125 at diagnosis. This test can also be elevated in other malignant and nonmalignant conditions, such as endometriosis.

CLINICAL MANIFESTATIONS

Ovarian cancer is often asymptomatic in the early stages. Vague abdominal bloating may be noticed in some. As with pregnancy, the peritoneum allows for growth of tumors without immediate obstruction on other nearby structures. Therefore, most patients have widespread disease at the time of diagnosis. Large tumors may manifest as abdominal distention, pressure, or pain.

DIAGNOSTIC CRITERIA

Diagnosis is based on patient history, physical examination (bimanual palpation of the ovaries), laparoscopic or other surgical exploration of the peritoneal cavity, and cytologic examination of ovarian epithelial cells. If the tumor appears to be isolated to the ovary or pelvis, laparotomy is used to examine the peritoneum and obtain ovarian, lymph, and surrounding tissues for analysis. Serum tumor marker levels are also obtained at diagnosis.

TREATMENT

Treatment is based on the stage of ovarian cancer at diagnosis. For those diagnosed at stages I or II, a tumor that is well differentiated or moderately well differentiated is treated through surgical (debulking) removal of the uterus, both ovaries, and surrounding omentum. The diaphragm is biopsied along with multiple lymph nodes to detect spread. In those patients considering childbearing with stage I well-differentiated tumors, the removal of reproductive organs may be limited to the affected ovary and fallopian tube. In all stages with a less-differentiated tumor and greater spread, surgery is accompanied by extensive internal and external radiation therapy and local and systemic combination chemotherapy. The goal of therapy is to remove all neoplastic cells and induce complete remission.

Menopause

Menopause, the complete cessation of ovarian activity, is an expected biological stage marking the end of a woman's reproductive life. This occurs generally around 48 to 55 years of age. **Perimenopause** is the 4- to 5-year gradual transition between predictable reproductive cycles and menopause. Subtle changes in bleeding patterns are the earliest manifestation of the perimenopausal period.

PATHOPHYSIOLOGY

From **menarche** (the time leading to the first menstrual period) onward, the cells of the reproductive system respond to trophic signals produced by the ovarian steroid hormones, estrogen and progesterone. The feedback mechanisms of the hypothalamus–pituitary axis acting upon the ovaries regulate both the stimulation and suppression of estrogen to allow for adequate physiologic functioning. The loss of hormones associated with ovarian cycles precipitates atrophic changes in the cells of the reproductive organs and the symptoms commonly associated with menopause.

As the ovaries age, the follicles become exhausted and unable to respond to functional demands despite adequate stimulation. Reduced release of ovarian hormones triggers the hypothalamus to increase secretion of GnRH. As a result, the anterior pituitary secretes additional FSH and LH yet this activity is ineffective in producing the desired effect because the aging ovaries are no longer able to produce estrogen and progesterone.

CLINICAL MANIFESTATIONS

The clinical manifestations occur as a result of loss of the estrogen effect on cells of target organs. Estrogen deprivation can cause obvious effects leading to acute symptoms, and can also cause changes that are not detected until much later. The full effects of estrogen deprivation may not be detected for many years but includes cessation of the menstrual cycle, effects on internal and external genitalia and sexual functioning, breasts, vasomotor response, mood, sleep, and bone mineralization (Fig. 14.19).

Atrophic changes occur in other estrogen-stimulated tissues. Breast size is decreased because of atrophy of internal breast structures, including the ducts and lobes. Skin elasticity reduces. Body hair and subcutaneous fat levels decrease. The ovaries and uterus atrophy. The walls of the vagina become thin. Dyspareunia (painful intercourse) is often a consequence of vaginal atrophy because these cells can no longer produce adequate amounts of lubrication for comfort. Urinary difficulties, such as urgency and stress incontinence, can be attributed to atrophy of bladder cells as a result of the loss of hormonal stimulation necessary for optimal cell functioning.

Hot flashes or flushes are the common description of the vasomotor symptoms associated with menopause. Localized in the upper half of the body, hot flashes are described as a sudden feeling of warmth and are associated with reddened skin and sweating. Vasomotor symptoms are brief, lasting between 30 seconds and 5 minutes. Frequency and severity can vary from mild to severe and can be quite disruptive. Although the physiologic explanation is not completely understood, vasomotor symptoms are likely the result of altered thermoregulation.

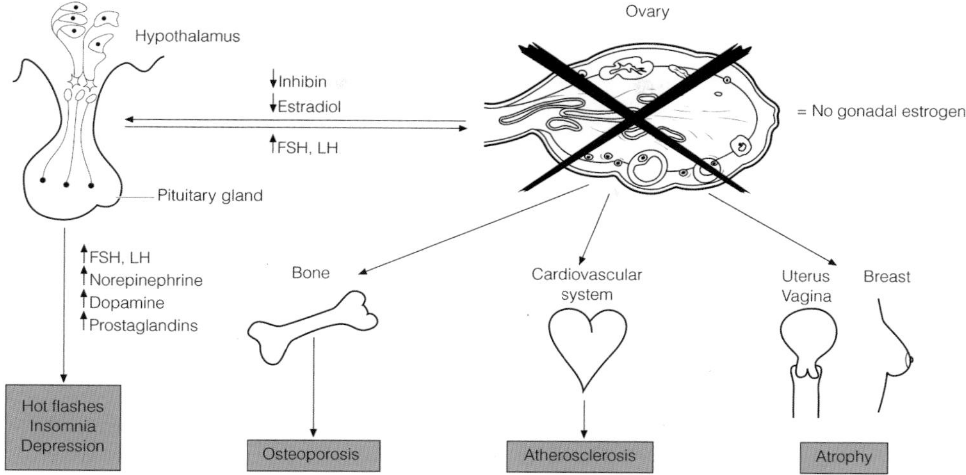

Figure 14.19. Changes in both the ovary and the hypothalamus contribute to the physiologic changes of menopause.

Alterations in sleep and mood, including symptoms of depression and fatigue, have been associated with menopause. Although this is not a universal manifestation, women with a prior history of depression are more likely to develop symptoms, especially in early perimenopause. Irritability, mood lability, and anxiety are also common. Trouble falling asleep or disrupted sleep may be a response to hot flashes, depression and other mood changes, or chronic pain and lead to severe fatigue.

Sexual functioning may be affected by the hormonal changes of menopause. In addition to the physical changes of the reproductive organs described previously, motivation to engage in sexual activities (libido) may be affected. Women report less frequent sexual activity and less satisfaction during this developmental period.

Bone demineralization occurs with advancing age but is more rapid after menopause. Menopausal bone loss, the manifestation of bone atrophy, results from the effects of cytokines in the absence of the protective effects of the ovarian hormones. This imbalance promotes delayed apoptosis of cells that breaks down bone (osteoclasts) and enhances apoptosis of cells favoring bone growth (osteoblasts).

Cardiovascular disease is a significant cause of mortality in women older than 50 years. Markers of cardiovascular disease are altered after menopause, increasing risk of stroke and heart attack. Cholesterol levels, including the components high-density lipoprotein (HDL) and low-density lipoprotein (LDL), are altered in favor of an increased ratio of LDL:HDL, increasing cardiovascular risk.

DIAGNOSTIC CRITERIA

The diagnosis of menopause is based on history of amenorrhea for at least 12 months in the absence of any other causes, such as pregnancy. There is no single, reliable diagnostic test. Laboratory markers for menopause include an increase in serum FSH; this is the most significant marker for ovarian failure. FSH levels rise higher than LH levels; however, both increase at a rate greater than seen during the surge of the menstrual cycle. Also noted are decreases in estradiol and inhibin, which no longer demonstrate large cyclical variations as seen during the menstrual years.

TREATMENT

Although many women do not require treatment, others rely on pharmacologic and nonpharmacologic treatment for the management of disruptive symptoms, such as hot flashes or mood swings. Treatment is best when individualized and targeted toward the specific concern.

Until 2002, hormone replacement therapy (HRT) with estrogen was the standard treatment for women to ameliorate symptoms and prevent long-term health risks associated with menopause, including cardiovascular disease. Research has since shown a lack of evidence to support the use of estrogen alone for the expected protective effects, and a higher risk for morbidity, such as the development of endometrial cancer.

Most recently in May 2013, the British Menopause Society and Women's Health Concern issued updated guidelines on the use, benefits, and risks of HRT.[4] In these recommendations, HRT using a combination of estrogen and progesterone can be administered to synthetically increase ovarian hormone levels, reverse the atrophic changes, and decrease symptoms associated with menopause using the following criteria:

- Severe symptoms requiring treatment
- Short-term duration

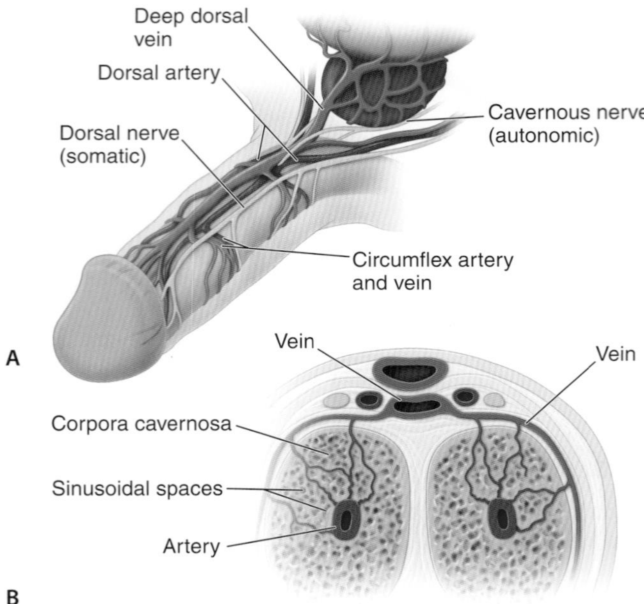

Figure 14.20. Anatomic depiction of penile erection. **A:** Innervation and arterial and venous blood supply to the penis. **B:** Cross-section of corpora cavernosa.

- Lowest effective dose
- Topical application (such as with a vaginal cream) to avoid systemic effects

Initiation of HRT in women older than 65 years is not recommended because of the increased associated risk of dementia in this age group.

Tissue-targeted therapies are also useful when managing specific manifestations. Because of the specificity of hormone binding to selective receptors, drug effects can be modulated based on the targeting of specific receptors located predominantly in a certain tissue type. Selective estrogen receptor modulators (SERM) are drugs designed to capitalize on these pharmacologic principles. The drug raloxifene is often used for prevention of osteoporosis in postmenopausal women. Raloxifene binds to specific receptors and results in antagonist effects in the endometrium and breast tissue, decreasing bone breakdown, total cholesterol, and LDL levels.

Nonpharmacologic strategies should be considered in the management of menopausal symptoms. The following measures may help minimize the discomfort and unpleasantness associated with many common menopause-related concerns:

- Dress in layers
- Avoid spicy foods
- Avoid caffeine and alcohol
- Initiate deep breathing measures at the start of a hot flash
- Use relaxation techniques
- Incorporate soy products containing phytoestrogens in the diet
- Perform pelvic floor exercises to strengthen muscles of the pelvis and vagina
- Use water-based lubricants during intercourse

Erectile Dysfunction

Sexual dysfunction is one of the most common health problems affecting men and includes such problems as low sexual interest, erectile dysfunction, premature ejaculation, and structural abnormalities of the penis. **Erectile dysfunction (ED)** is the inability to achieve or maintain an erection sufficient for satisfactory sexual performance. ED is one of the main types of sexual dysfunction in men, and the prevalence increases with age. In one US study, around 51% of men between the ages of 40 and 70 years reported experiencing ED. Other countries throughout the world have demonstrated a similar prevalence.[5]

PATHOPHYSIOLOGY

Achieving an erection is a complex interaction of arousal and parasympathetic nervous stimulation at the S2-S4 level, signaling increased blood flow that becomes trapped in the corpora cavernosa of the penis (Fig. 14.20). This trapping of blood in the corpora cavernosa depends on smooth muscle relaxation that occludes the veins and does not allow blood flow out. The erection is reversed under the influences of the sympathetic nervous system. All of these activities are facilitated by androgen activity on the hypothalamus and anterior pituitary.

CLINICAL MANIFESTATIONS

The inability to achieve and maintain an erection is the primary clinical manifestation. The complexity of ED is illustrated by several causes that may lead to other manifestations. These causes include:

- **Hormonal factors:** Hypogonadism, hypothyroidism, or adrenal cortical hormone dysfunction, resulting in inadequate hormonal "priming" of the sexual centers of the brain
- **Neurological factors:** Spinal cord or perineal nerve injury resulting in inadequate nerve signaling to the penile vessels
- **Psychological factors:** Anxiety, low self-esteem, or depression resulting in inadequate arousal
- **Vascular obstruction:** Hypertension, atherosclerosis, vascular obstruction, and smoking disallow blood flow to the corpora cavernosa and spongiosa, thereby preventing erection from occurring

- **Impaired veno-occlusive ability:** The inability to trap blood within the corpora cavernosa
- **Certain medications:** Antihypertensives, can inhibit hormone and erectile function

DIAGNOSTIC CRITERIA

Diagnosis of ED is based on a comprehensive history and physical examination to identify the potential cause. Laboratory measurement of testosterone, LH, thyroid, and prolactin levels may suggest a hypothalamic, pituitary, or hormonal problem. Hypogonadism—specifically, a reduction in the levels of testosterone—can contribute to ED.

TREATMENT

Treatment is individualized and directed by the etiology (physical, psychological, or both). Testosterone replacement therapy, or other hormone intervention, may be indicated. Psychological influences may be addressed and treated by a mental health professional. Medications, such as sildenafil (Viagra), vardenafil, and tadalafil, are often prescribed for men with ED. These drugs act to promote smooth muscle relaxation and vascular congestion in the corpora cavernosa, thereby maintaining an erection. Penile implants or other devices may be used to help maintain an erection.

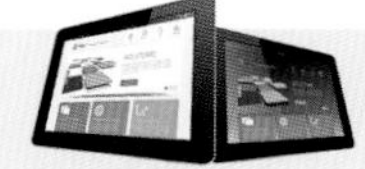

RESEARCH NOTES

Lifestyle, most notably obesity, smoking, and alcohol use, affects the development of ED. One study aimed to determine the impact of lifestyle changes (weight loss and physical activity) on male erectile function. After a 2-year diet and exercise intervention, those men who had significant decreases in body weight, body mass index, waist–hip ratio, blood pressure, glucose levels, and total cholesterol demonstrated a statistically significant improvement in sexual function. The researchers suggested that obesity resulted in a state of chronic oxidative stress and inflammation throughout the body. The inflammation was responsible for blood vessel lining obstruction. Weight reduction saw a corresponding decrease in inflammatory markers and a subsequent improvement in sexual function.[6]

Benign Prostatic Hyperplasia

The prostate gland is a small organ about the size of a walnut, which lies below the bladder and surrounds the urethra. The prostate tissue produces prostate-specific antigen and prostatic acid phosphatase, an enzyme found in seminal fluid. The major role of the prostate is to secrete a fluid, which combines with semen, to increase sperm motility and decrease vaginal acidity. Benign prostatic hyperplasia (BPH) affects more than 50% of men over age 60 and as many as 90% of men over age 70.[7] BPH is a condition of aging; nearly all men over the age of 50 have some level of enlargement of the prostate.

PATHOPHYSIOLOGY

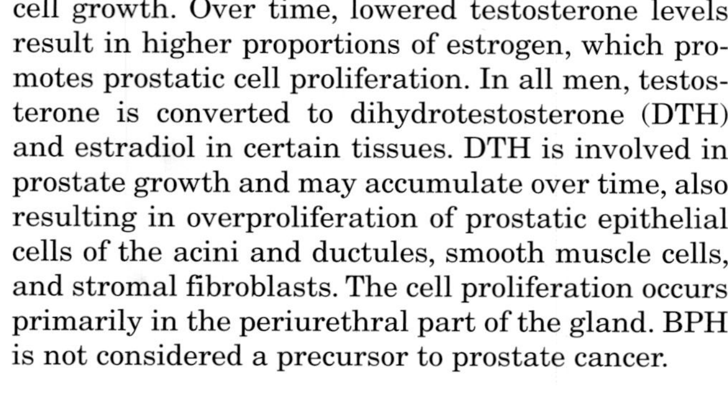

The cause of BPH is unknown. Hormone changes associated with aging have an impact on prostatic cell growth. Over time, lowered testosterone levels result in higher proportions of estrogen, which promotes prostatic cell proliferation. In all men, testosterone is converted to dihydrotestosterone (DTH) and estradiol in certain tissues. DTH is involved in prostate growth and may accumulate over time, also resulting in overproliferation of prostatic epithelial cells of the acini and ductules, smooth muscle cells, and stromal fibroblasts. The cell proliferation occurs primarily in the periurethral part of the gland. BPH is not considered a precursor to prostate cancer.

CLINICAL MANIFESTATIONS

Clinical manifestations of BPH are related to urethral obstruction from the enlarged prostate, which impedes the flow of urine from the bladder to the urinary meatus. This results in urinary frequency, dribbling, hesitancy, incontinence, urgency, and retention. Complete obstruction leads to acute urinary retention and an absolute inability to urinate. This leads to severe pain and can progress to renal failure and death if not treated.

DIAGNOSTIC CRITERIA

Diagnosis is based on patient history, physical examination, laboratory tests, and evaluation of symptoms. The physical examination includes a digital rectal examination. This procedure allows the health practitioner to determine the size, shape, and consistency of the prostate gland, as palpated through the rectal wall (Fig. 14.21). Benign enlargement of the prostate tissue is soft; malignant tissue is hard, asymmetrical, and often has a cobblestone texture. Prostate-specific antigen (PSA) is often measured to determine elevations that may indicate prostate hyperplasia or dysplasia. Elevations in PSA are followed by a biopsy to confirm or rule out malignancy. The American Urological Association (AUA) Symptoms Index may be used. This index is a 7-question survey on a 1 to 5 scale related to presence and

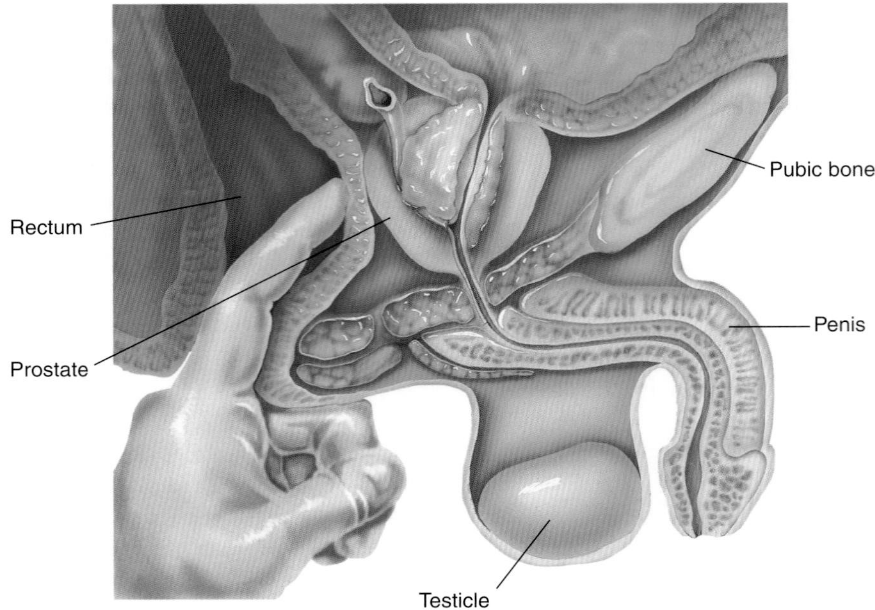

Figure 14.21. Digital rectal examination of the prostate. (Nath JL. *Using Medical Terminology: A Practical Approach*. Baltimore, MD: Lippincott Williams & Wilkins; 2005.)

frequency of symptoms related to BPH. A higher point total (i.e., 20 to 35) equates to greater severity of symptoms. Urodynamic tests can be used to measure the volume and pressure of urine in the bladder and to evaluate the flow of urine.

TREATMENT

Treatment is reserved for those men with significant symptoms. Pharmacologic treatments may be prescribed that relax the smooth muscles of the arteries, prostate, and bladder neck to relieve urinary obstruction. Because the prostate also depends on hormonal stimulation, drugs may be prescribed that inhibit the action of testosterone by restricting conversion to DTH. The lack of hormonal stimulation results in prostate atrophy. Laser or other heat-based treatments may also be applied to destroy all or part of the prostate gland. Surgical intervention may also be included in the treatment regimen, depending on the severity of symptoms and potential risks to the patient. The most common procedure is the transurethral resection of the prostate (TURP). In this procedure, part of the prostate is removed using a surgical instrument placed into the urethra via the penis. For patients who are not appropriate candidates for pharmacologic, laser, or surgical treatments, a stent may be placed in the urethra. A stent is a small, rigid tube that holds the urethra open and allows urine to drain. The disadvantages to stents are that they can illicit irritation, frequent urination, pain, and incontinence, and they are difficult to remove if removal is necessary.

Prostate Cancer

During a man's lifetime, the risk of developing prostate cancer is one in six, making it the second leading cause of cancer death in men after lung cancer. About 85% of men with prostate cancer are diagnosed after the age of 65.[8]

PATHOPHYSIOLOGY

Similar to BPH, carcinoma of the prostate is predominately a disease of older men. The exact cause is often unknown. Risk factors for the development of prostate cancer include advancing age, family history of prostate cancer, Black race, smoking, and nutritional factors, such as high intake of fats and meat, low intake of lycopene (found primarily in tomato-based products) and fruit, and high dietary calcium.

The malignant transformation of prostate epithelial cells, as with other forms of cancer, is a result of a complex series of initiator and promoter events with genetic and environmental influences. Approximately 5% to 10% of prostate cancer cases are estimated to be related to inherited genetic factors or prostate cancer susceptibility genes.[8] One major locus of susceptibility is found at chromosome 1q24, designated as *HPC1* (hereditary prostate cancer). This mutation is associated with a younger age at diagnosis, a higher tumor grade, and more advanced stage at diagnosis. Several other chromosome regions, which have been linked to susceptibility in inherited and sporadic forms of prostate cancer, have also been identified.

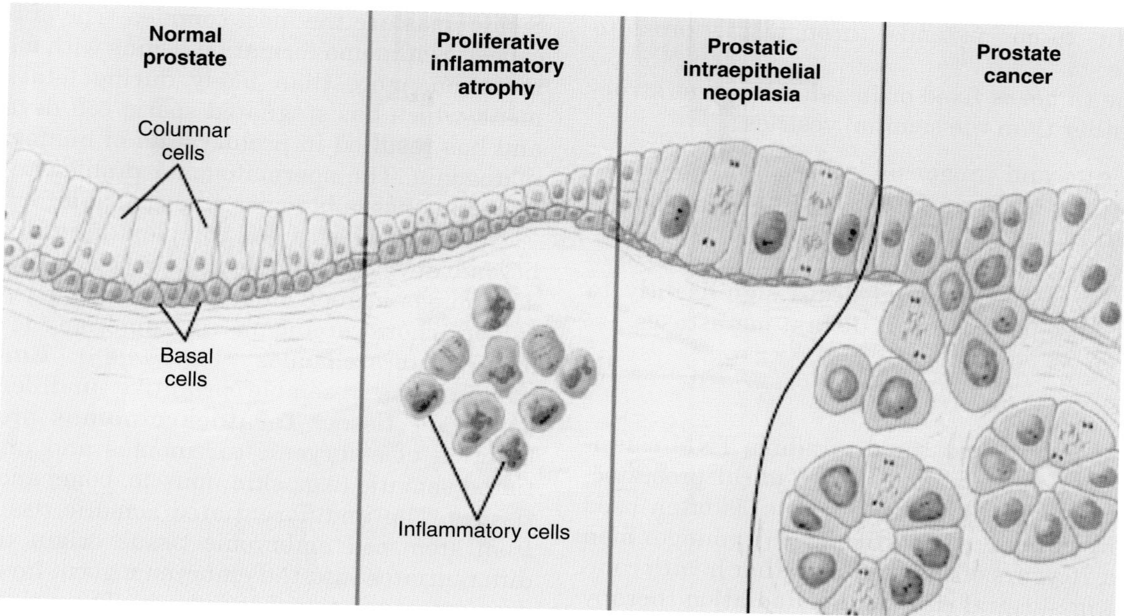

Figure 14.22. Proliferative inflammatory atrophy is hypothesized to be a precursor to prostatic intraepithelial neoplasia, which in turn is the precursor of prostate cancer. (From Nelson WG, De Marzo AM, Isaacs WB. Prostate cancer. *N Engl J Med*. 2003;349:366, with permission.)

More than 95% of primary prostate cancers are classified as adenocarcinomas. Androgens and estrogens are two hormones that appear to support carcinogenesis by influencing prostate epithelial proliferation, although elevations in androgens are not found universally in those with prostate cancer. Premalignant changes in patients with prostate cancer are designated as prostatic intraepithelial neoplasia and are characterized by atypical lumen cells lining the prostatic ducts (Fig. 14.22). These lesions are believed to progress to prostate adenocarcinoma, with the neoplasm arising in the peripheral portion of the gland. This peripheral location is clinically significant in that the tumor does not compress the urethra until later in its progression.

CLINICAL MANIFESTATIONS

Prostate cancer is often asymptomatic and is found incidentally after a digital rectal examination and PSA screening. When clinical manifestations are present, the tumor has often expanded and is obstructing the urethra. In this case, the manifestations are identical to that of BPH and include urinary frequency, dribbling, hesitancy, incontinence, urgency, and retention. Common systemic manifestations, paraneoplastic syndromes, and manifestations significant for metastatic spread, such as pain as the tumor spreads to the bone, also apply to prostate cancer.

DIAGNOSTIC CRITERIA

Digital rectal examination, transrectal ultrasound, and PSA levels are used to screen for prostate cancer. Diagnosis is confirmed through a cytologic analysis of prostate tissue (biopsy) via fine needle aspiration usually performed transrectally. Pelvic lymph node dissection during surgical treatment for those undergoing radical prostatectomy is often required to determine lymph node involvement. Radionucleotide bone scans are used to detect metastases to the bone, the most common site of distant spread. Once diagnosed, prostate cancer is staged using the TNM classification system, with slight modifications in the tumor designation:

- **T1:** The tumor is clinically inapparent, not palpable or visible by imaging.
- **T2:** The tumor is confined to the prostate.

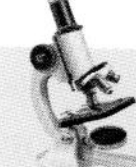

FROM THE LAB

PSA in the blood may be bound to proteins or may exist in an unbound state. Total PSA is the sum of levels of both forms. Free PSA measures only the levels of unbound PSA. Some studies suggest that malignant prostate cells produce more *bound* PSA; therefore, a low level of free PSA compared to total PSA may indicate malignant prostatic neoplasia. A high level of free PSA compared to total PSA might indicate BPH or an inflammatory condition of the prostate.

- **T3:** The tumor extends through the prostate capsule.
- **T4:** The tumor is fixed or invades adjacent structures other than the seminal vesicles.

Survival rate and prognosis is based on the histologic features (differentiation and distribution) of the tumor and staging. The 5-year survival is more than 99% for patients with local or regional disease spread. The 5-year survival drops significantly to 33.5% in those patients with distant metastases.[8]

TREATMENT

Treatment is based on tumor grading, TNM classification, age, and health status. Radical prostatectomy (removal of the entire prostate) is often used to treat prostate cancer, particularly in younger men (less than 70 years of age) without other health complications or surgical risk factors. Radiation therapy and chemotherapy may be used as a surgical adjunct or for those who are not surgical candidates. Androgen-deprivation hormone therapy may also be used to decrease prostate cell proliferation. Because prostate cancer is considered a slow-growing tumor and is typically diagnosed later in life, "watchful waiting" may be the treatment of choice in those without clinical symptoms. This approach avoids the complications inherent with surgical, radiation, and chemotherapeutic interventions, and it appreciates the reality that many men with clinically undetectable prostate cancer die from other causes.

Testicular Cancer

Testicular cancer is a highly treatable and often curable cancer, which is most commonly found in men between 20 and 40 years of age. Approximately 90% of tumors arise from germ cells. The remaining tumors are of sex cord cell origin or metastases from other sites.

PATHOPHYSIOLOGY

Germ cell tumors are classified according to cell origin and include the following:

- Seminomas—Malignant germ cells that resemble primitive sperm cells
- Nonseminomas—Malignant germ cells that do not resemble primitive sperm cells and actually appear as embryonic or undifferentiated somatic (e.g., skin, muscle, glands, etc.) components

The germ cell divides through mitosis and differentiates into a primitive sperm cell, called a **spermatogonia**, and finally into a mature spermatocyte. Seminomas are the most common type of testicular cancer. Seminoma formation begins with a germ cell mutation, more than likely during fetal development, which has stagnated sperm cell development and has resulted in proliferation of immature spermatogonia. The spermatogonia proliferate and the testicular tissue becomes enlarged and fibrotic.

Nonseminomas are a complex derivative of embryonic development. Notable subcategories of nonseminomas include embryonal carcinomas, yolk sac tumors, choriocarcinomas (arising from the chorion), and teratocarcinomas (Fig. 14.23). **Embryonic carcinomas** resemble primitive undifferentiated embryonic tissue. **Teratocarcinomas** are a combination of embryonic carcinomas and undifferentiated somatic (e.g., skin, muscle, bone, and glands) tissues. The undifferentiated somatic tissue arises from stem cell embryonic tissue origin that then differentiates into the embryonic germ layers (ectoderm, mesoderm, and endoderm). These tissues then further differentiate into various somatic tissues. In other words, teratocarcinomas appear as undifferentiated embryonic tissue and skin or bone cells where mature spermatocytes should be found. The origin of some nonseminomas may result from misplaced fetal germ cells that did not migrate to seminiferous tubules during fetal testicular organogenesis. The nonseminomas grow faster, are more invasive, and are more likely to metastasize than the seminomas.

Although the exact cause is often unknown, an alteration in chromosome 14 may be implicated in those with testicular cancer. A major risk factor is **cryptorchidism**, or undescended testis, and other problems with testicular development. Those with cryptorchidism are 20 to 40 times more likely to develop testicular cancer. One theory of carcinogenesis indicates that an initiating event and mutation occurs during fetal development. Autonomy and anaplasia are then promoted through hormonal stimulation during puberty. Tumor development often progresses through two major stages: (1) carcinoma in situ and (2) invasive carcinoma. The carcinoma in situ common with testicular cancer is confined to the seminiferous tubules. Testicular cancer is often malignant at diagnosis.

Although testicular cancer is highly treatable and curable, the prognosis for testicular cancer is less favorable when the following factors exist:

- The presence of bone, liver, or brain metastases
- High serum tumor markers
- The presence of a primary mediastinal nonseminoma
- A large number of lung metastases

The largest proportion of patients with seminomas (90%) is diagnosed with primary tumors without metastases or elevations in tumor markers. Patients with seminomas at a primary site without

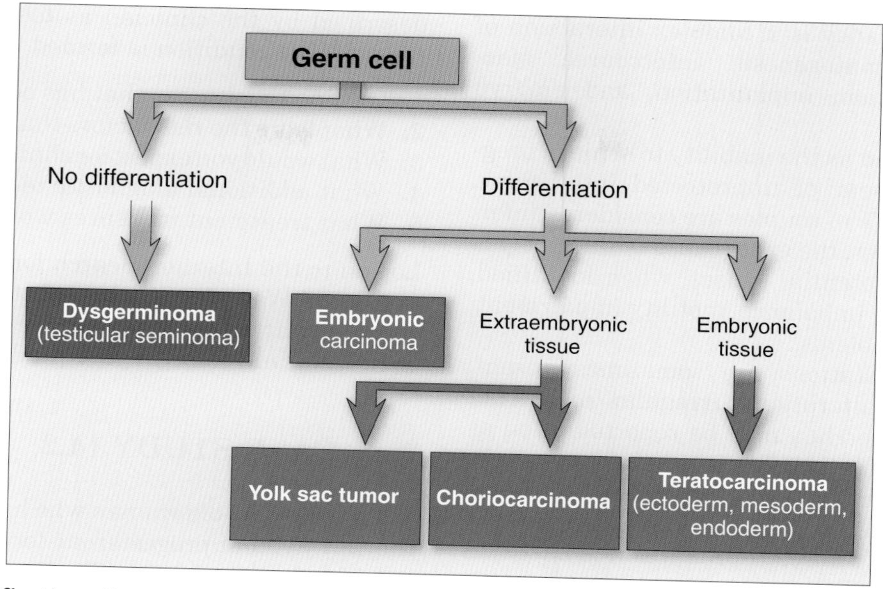

Figure 14.23. Classification of germ cell tumors of the testes. (Modified from Rubin E, Farber JL. *Pathology*. 4th ed. Philadelphia, PA: Lippincott Williams & Wilkins; 2005.)

metastases or elevations in tumor serum markers demonstrate a 5-year survival of 95%.[9] In contrast, those patients with mediastinal nonseminomas with metastasis or elevated tumor markers have a 73% 5-year survival. Even with widespread metastases, those with primary testicular cancer may also be cured and should be treated as such.

CLINICAL MANIFESTATIONS

Common clinical manifestations include a small painless testicular mass, slight enlargement of the testicle, heaviness or enlargement of the scrotum, and mild testicular discomfort.

DIAGNOSTIC CRITERIA

Self-testicular examination is an important aspect of early detection and should be practiced by all men on a monthly basis. Diagnosis of the primary tumor is through physical examination and radical orchiectomy (removal of the testicle). Transscrotal biopsy is not recommended because it may result in seeding of the tumor into the scrotum or spread to inguinal lymph nodes. Tumor markers provide additional clues to the diagnosis and treatment efficacy. Imaging studies, such as ultrasound, CT scan, and MRI, can identify the tumor location and spread.

TREATMENT

Treatment of testicular cancer involves surgical removal of the tumor and affected testicle or testicles. Radiation and chemotherapy may also be used in treatment. The risks involved with radiation and chemotherapeutic treatment in testicular cancer include infertility, secondary leukemias (or other types of cancer), and possible renal function impairment. This type of cancer is often curable.

SUMMARY

- Reproductive function is reliant upon structural integrity, neurologic, and hormonal processes of males and females.
- Female reproductive organs include the vagina, uterus, fallopian tubes, and ovaries. The ovaries produce the female sex hormones: estrogens, progesterone, and androgens. These hormones are secreted in a monthly cyclical pattern under the direction of the hypothalamus (GnRH) and the anterior pituitary (FSH, LH).
- The male reproductive organs and tissues include the testes, epididymis, vas deferens, seminal vesicles, prostate, and penis. Androgens, the male sex hormones, promote metabolism and growth. The pattern of male sex hormone secretion does not follow a cyclical pattern as seen with females; the hormone secretion rates remain fairly constant throughout the male's adult life.
- Stimulation of androgen production and release in males begins in the hypothalamus. The hypothalamus releases GnRH, which stimulates the anterior pituitary to release LH and FSH. LH acts on the Leydig cells in the testes to produce testosterone, the primary male sex hormone.

- Achieving pregnancy is a complex interaction of ovulation, spermatogenesis, intercourse, ejaculation, conception, implantation, and embryo growth.
- Infertility, defined as the inability to achieve pregnancy after 1 year of unprotected intercourse. About 10% to 15% of couples are considered infertile. In many cases, the exact cause of infertility is not identified. Potential causes, when identified, include hormone imbalance, motility impairment, and immune problems.
- Clinical manifestations are sometimes absent. With hormone alterations, irregular menstrual periods or amenorrhea may be reported often as a result of anovulation. Testicular/scrotal pain in men or pelvic pain in women may occur with infection or inflammation of reproductive structures.
- The diagnosis of altered reproduction is based on the couple's inability to conceive or the presence of clinical manifestations. Initially, a semen analysis must be completed in the male along with an analysis of ovulation in the female. Patency of the female reproductive structures can be visualized using hysterosalpingography or laparoscopy.
- Treatment involves supportive counseling, education about intercourse frequency, avoidance of lubricants that can act as a spermicide, and basic health maintenance. Sexually transmitted or other pelvic infections place the female at high risk for infertility and must be treated quickly and completely. Obstructive processes, such as leiomyomas, endometriosis, or pelvic adhesions, may require surgical intervention.
- Some individuals may require clomiphene citrate, a medication that induces ovulation. In those with hyperprolactinemia, medications may be needed to reduce prolactin and therefore induce ovulation. Artificial insemination may be used to inject sperm into the uterus if cervical mucus is thick or if the sperm quantity or quality is compromised. Some couples seek advanced reproductive technologies such as in vitro fertilization.
- The evaluation and treatment of infertility is highly complex and emotionally charged. Sensitivity to the range and intensity of emotions is an important aspect of care.

CASE STUDY 14.1

A couple seeks reproductive counseling for inability to achieve a pregnancy after 14 months of unprotected intercourse. After multiple diagnostic tests with both individuals, the male partner is determined to have a moderately decreased sperm count and motility. Upon physical examination of the scrotum, enlargement of scrotal veins is determine, described by the clinician as feeling like "a bag of worms." The condition is termed varicocele.

1. Outline the process that has occurred in his body.
2. What were the risk factors that he demonstrated?
3. What would you expect for clinical manifestations?
4. What additional diagnostic tests could be used?
5. What treatment measures would you anticipate?

Log on to the Internet. Search for a relevant journal article or Web site (such as http://emedicine.medscape.com/article/438591-overview), which details varicocele, and confirm your predictions.

CASE STUDY 14.2

J.T. is a 62-year-old woman who has been on estrogen therapy without progesterone for menopausal symptoms for the past 6 years. She is seeking medical care for unexplained vaginal bleeding. She is obese and has been menopausal for 8 years and has not had any menstrual bleeding until a week ago. She does not have any pelvic discomfort. After examination, she is scheduled for a dilatation and curettage (D&C) with biopsy. The biopsy reveals endometrial cancer.

1. Outline the process that has mostly likely occurred in her body.
2. What would you notice for clinical manifestations?
3. What diagnostic tests were used and what do these tell you?
4. What treatment measures would you anticipate?

Log on to the Internet. Search for a relevant journal article or Web site (such as http://www.cancer.gov/cancertopics/types/endometrial/), which details endometrial cancer, and confirm your predictions.

PRACTICE EXAM QUESTIONS

1. Your patient is complaining of menopausal hot flashes and other symptoms. Which of the following would you recommend as a nonpharmacologic method for relief of these symptoms?
   a. Increase spicy foods
   b. Increase caffeine intake
   c. Use relaxation techniques
   d. Avoid soy products containing phytoestrogens

2. Your neighbor is taking an anatomy and physiology course and asks you what would happen if a person did not have ovarian interstitial cells. What would you say?
   a. The person would be lacking ovarian support structures
   b. The person would not be able to secrete estrogen

c. The person would not have a place to house germ cells
d. The person would have no difficulties as interstitial cells are not located in the ovaries

3. Your family is worried because your cousin has a testosterone deficiency. What would you notice for clinical manifestations?
a. Increased skin thickness
b. Clear skin, free of acne
c. Excessive chest and facial hair
d. Bulky skeletal muscle development

4. Your pregnant friend is complaining of nausea, headaches, constipation, indigestion, and swelling. What hormone is wreaking havoc in her body?
a. Progesterone
b. Estrogen
c. Thyroid-stimulating hormone
d. Human chorionic gonadotropin hormone

5. Which of the following would be illustrative of a mobility impairment leading to infertility?
a. Anovulation
b. Presence of leiomyomas
c. Low sperm production
d. Menopause

6. Your 16-year-old niece confides in you that she has not had a period for 2 months. She does not think she is pregnant and denies having sexual intercourse. What is another likely explanation?
a. Endometrial cancer
b. Severe emotional stress
c. Lack of physical activity
d. FSH deficiency

7. Dave and his wife have been trying to conceive for the past 2 years. They go on a long awaited vacation and he wants to sit in the hot tub. Why is this not recommended for men who are trying to conceive?
a. LH and FSH release are inhibited with exposure to chlorinated water
b. Temperature does not make a difference; he can freely enjoy the hot tub
c. Spermatogenesis requires a higher body temperature than that found with the core body temperature
d. Spermatogenesis requires a cooler body temperature than that found with the core body temperature

8–15. Match the clinical model with the type of altered reproductive function:

8. Pelvic inflammatory disease	a. Hormonal imbalance
9. Ovarian cancer	b. Motility problem
10. Polycystic ovarian syndrome	c. Immune problem
11. Menopause	
12. Erectile dysfunction	
13. Benign prostatic hypertrophy	
14. Prostate cancer	
15. Testicular cancer	

DISCUSSION AND APPLICATION

1. What did I know about altered reproduction function prior to today?
2. What body processes are affected by altered reproduction function?
3. What are the potential etiologies for altered reproduction function? How does altered reproduction function develop?
4. Who is most at risk for developing altered reproduction function? How can altered reproduction function be prevented?
5. What are the human differences that affect the etiology, risk, or course of altered reproduction function?
6. What clinical manifestations are expected in the course of altered reproduction function?
7. What special diagnostic tests are useful in determining the diagnosis and course of altered reproduction function?
8. What are the goals of care for individuals with altered reproduction function?
9. How does the concept of altered reproduction function build on what I have learned in the previous chapters and in previous courses?
10. How can I use what I have learned?

RESOURCES

American Cancer Society:
http://www.cancer.org/

American Society for Reproductive Medicine (ASRM):
http://www.asrm.org

The Menopause Society:
http://www.menopause.org/for-professionals

References

1. Legro RS, Arslanian SA, Ehrmann DA, et al. Diagnosis and treatment of polycystic ovary syndrome: an Endocrine Society clinical practice guideline. *J Clin Endocrinol Metab*. 2013;98(12):4565–4592.
2. National Cancer Institute Surveillance, Epidemiology, and End Results Program. SEER stat fact sheets: ovary cancer. Bethesda, MD: National Cancer Institute. http://seer.cancer.gov/statfacts/html/ovary.html. Accessed November 11, 2015.
3. American Cancer Society. Cancer facts & figures 2015. Atlanta, GA: American Cancer Society. http://www.cancer.org/acs/groups/content/@editorial/documents/document/acspc-044552.pdf. Accessed November 11, 2015.
4. Barclay L. HRT use: new guidelines from the British Menopause Society. *Medscape Medical News*. http://www.medscape.com/viewarticle/804778. Accessed November 11, 2015.
5. Selvin E, Burnett AL, Platz EA. Prevalence and risk factors for erectile dysfunction in the US. *Am J Med*. 2007;120(2):151–157.
6. Esposito K, Giugliano F, DiPalo C, et al. Effect of lifestyle changes on erectile dysfunction in obese men: a randomized control trial. *JAMA*. 2004;291:2978–2987.
7. National Kidney and Urologic Diseases Clearinghouse. Prostate enlargement: benign prostatic hyperplasia. 2014. http://www.niddk.nih.gov/health-information/health-topics/urologic-disease/benign-prostatic-hyperplasia-bph/Pages/facts.aspx#9. Accessed November 12, 2015. NIH publication no. 14-3012.
8. National Cancer Institute. Genetics of prostate cancer. http://www.cancer.gov/types/prostate/hp/prostate-genetics-pdq. Accessed November 12, 2015.
9. Cancer.Net. Testicular cancer statistics. 2015. http://www.cancer.net/cancer-types/testicular-cancer/statistics. Accessed November 12, 2015.

Find additional resources for this chapter at http:thePoint.lww.com thePoint®

Altered Ventilation and Diffusion

Chapter 15

LEARNING OUTCOMES

1. Define and use the key terms listed in this chapter.
2. Explain the role of ventilation and diffusion in oxygen/carbon dioxide gas exchange.
3. Describe the processes that can impair ventilation and diffusion.
4. Recognize the effects of impaired ventilation and diffusion.
5. Identify the common signs and symptoms of altered ventilation and diffusion.
6. Describe diagnostic tests and treatment strategies relevant to disordered ventilation and diffusion.
7. Apply the concepts of altered ventilation and diffusion to select clinical models.

INTRODUCTION

Take a deep breath. Exhale. Oxygen from the air goes in; carbon dioxide goes out. When you breathe, four major processes are occurring as your chest rises and falls: ventilation, diffusion, perfusion, and respiration. **Ventilation** is the process of moving air into and out of the trachea, bronchi, and lungs. **Diffusion** is the process of moving and exchanging the oxygen acquired during ventilation and carbon dioxide waste across the alveolar capillary membranes. **Perfusion** is a process of supplying oxygenated blood to the lungs and organ systems via the blood vessels. **Respiration** is a process in which cells throughout the body use oxygen aerobically to make energy. As a health care provider, it is critically important to recognize problems associated with altered ventilation and diffusion.

Module 1 Pulmonary Structure and Function

The pulmonary, or respiratory, system is responsible for ventilation and diffusion. The major function is the exchange of gases between the environment and the blood. The pulmonary system comprises the lungs, airways, chest wall, and pulmonary circulation (Fig. 15.1). The structural path of the pulmonary system is often divided into the upper and lower airways. The upper airway comprises the nose or mouth, nasopharynx, and oropharynx. The laryngeal pharynx connects the upper and lower airways. The lower airway comprises the trachea, bronchi, and bronchioles. The branching anatomic structure

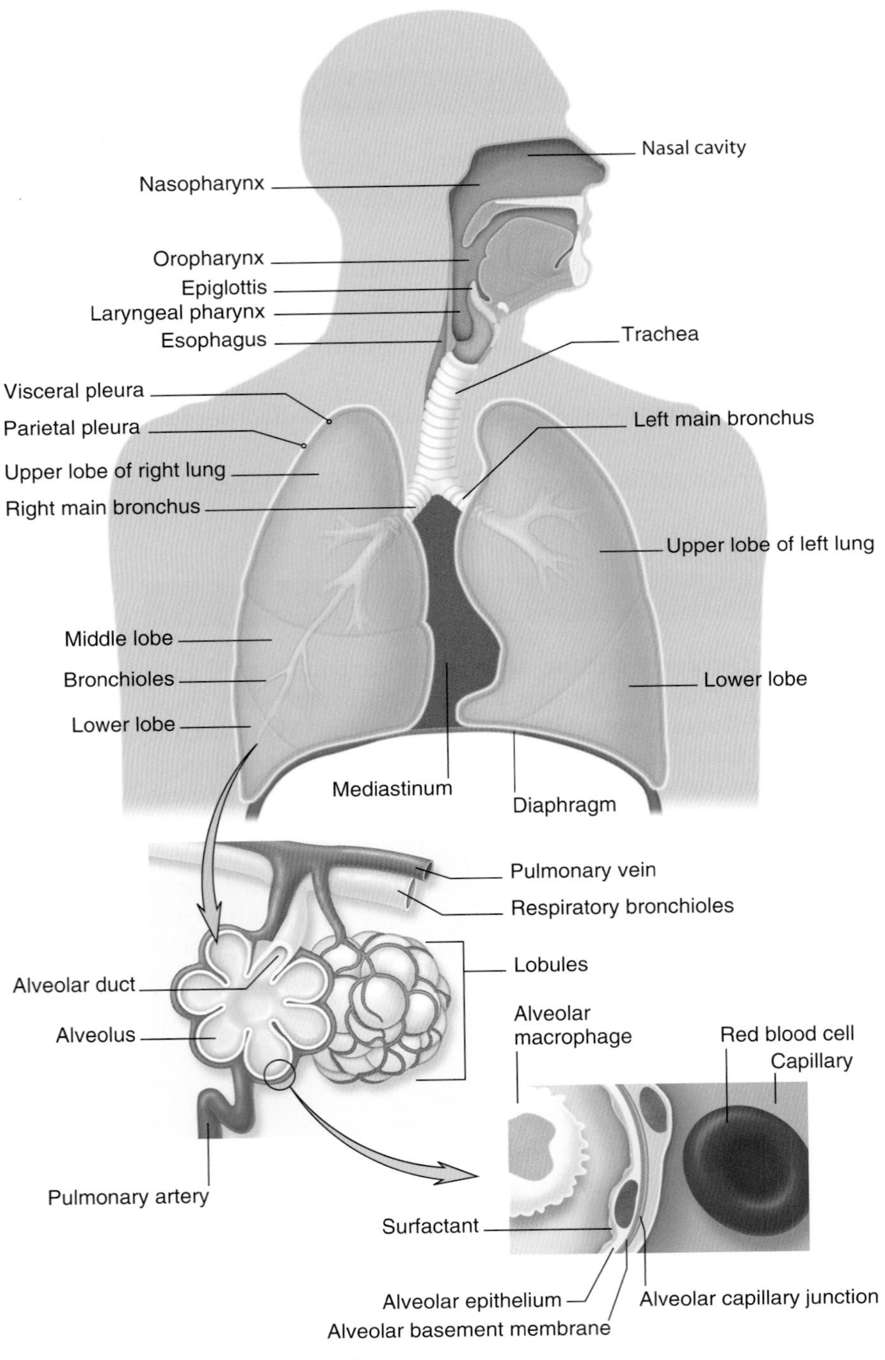

Figure 15.1. Anatomy of the airways.

of the pulmonary system is ideal for maximizing surface area to allow for optimal gas diffusion, or movement of gases across the alveoli.

Because the pulmonary system is vulnerable to the external environment, defense mechanisms are needed to protect the lungs from environmental injury. These defense mechanisms are highly effective and include:

- *Protective structures,* such as hairs and turbinates (shell-shaped structures) in the nose and cilia in the upper and lower airways, which trap and remove foreign particles from the air
- *Mucosal lining* of the upper and lower airways, which warms and humidifies air
- *Irritant receptors* throughout the nose and airways, which recognize injurious agents and respond by triggering a sneeze or cough reflex to remove foreign particles
- *Immune protections*, such as an immune coating in the respiratory tract mucosa and macrophages in the alveoli, which ingest and remove bacteria and other foreign materials via phagocytosis

Stop and Consider
How are defense mechanisms and the body protections affected in the person who is a mouth breather?

Intercostal muscles, ribs, and skin surround the lungs and provide protection against injury. The muscles of the chest cavity and the diaphragm perform the muscular work of breathing. Two major membrane layers line the lungs and chest cavity: the (outer) parietal pleura and (inner) visceral pleura. These layers are separated by a pleural space, which is filled with a lubricating fluid, secreted by the pleura, that allows the two layers to slide over each other with minimal friction.

The pulmonary circulation is responsible for the delivery of oxygen and other nutrients to the lung tissues. It is also responsible for the filtration of clots, air, or other foreign materials from the circulation. The capillaries of the lungs near the alveoli facilitate the exchange of oxygen and carbon dioxide. The pulmonary circulation is discussed further in Chapter 16.

Ventilation

The process of ventilation involves both acquiring oxygen (inspiration) and removing carbon dioxide (expiration) from the blood. The transport of oxygen through the lungs is the *only* mechanism for acquiring oxygen. Oxygen is necessary for cellular metabolism, which means that for the cell to expend energy efficiently and perform its designated function, there must be oxygen present. The release of carbon dioxide is equally as important. Optimal cell functioning occurs within a very narrow pH range. The release and retention of carbon dioxide is one mechanism for maintaining this balance.

The rate and volume of ventilation is regulated by the following components:

- A functioning respiratory control center in the brain
- Lung receptors
- Chemoreceptors

The drive to ventilate is stimulated by the respiratory control center in the brainstem in response to chemical messages in the body. The respiratory control center comprises neurons in the pons and medulla. It sends neuronal impulses to the diaphragm, intercostal muscles, sternocleidomastoid muscles, and other accessory muscles and causes them to contract or relax. The autonomic nervous system (ANS) also innervates the lungs and acts on the smooth muscles of the conducting airways to promote airway constriction (parasympathetic division) or dilation (sympathetic division). The activity of the ANS will increase or decrease the diameter of the airways and affect the amount of air that is able to get in and out of the lungs.

Neuronal impulses are directed by lung receptors that map the current state of breathing and lung function. Lung receptors are located in the epithelium and smooth muscle of the airways, and they are near the alveolar capillary junctions. Specific lung receptors have particular roles. For example, lung receptors located in the epithelium of the conducting airways are responsible for sensing irritants in the lungs and stimulating the cough reflex. Lung receptors in the smooth muscles of the airways are activated to promote expiration in order to prevent excessive lung inflation. Lung receptors in the capillaries detect increases in capillary pressure and stimulate a reduction in this pressure.

Chemoreceptors detect gas exchange needs based on the $Pa{O_2}$, $Pa{CO_2}$, and pH levels in the blood and cerebrospinal fluid (CSF). Central chemoreceptors are located near the respiratory control center and respond to pH changes in the CSF. Because CO_2 diffuses across the blood–brain barrier until both the arterial $Pa{CO_2}$ and CSF $Pa{CO_2}$ are equal, the CO_2 levels detected by the central chemoreceptors reflect that in the blood. The central chemoreceptors then alter the rate of breathing to adapt to the higher or lower levels of CO_2 in the body. Recall that carbon dioxide is acidic. If the blood is more acidic, the respiratory center increases the rate and depth of breathing to release or "blow off" excess carbon dioxide. If the blood is more alkaline, the respiratory center decreases the rate and depth of breathing to retain carbon dioxide. Peripheral chemoreceptors, which are most sensitive to oxygen levels in the arterial blood (PaO_2), are located in the aorta and carotid arteries. Peripheral chemoreceptors trigger an increase in ventilation in response to low oxygen levels in the blood. Cervical and thoracic nerves are then stimulated accordingly to conduct the specified breathing adaptation.

Stop and Consider
How does your breathing change when you exercise? Why do you think this happens?

The messages sent by the lung and chemoreceptors are ultimately sent to the cervical and thoracic nerves, which act on the pulmonary system to adapt the breathing pattern to maintain homeostasis. The work of breathing is improved with functional and strong muscles of ventilation, such as the intercostal muscles, diaphragm, and sternocleidomastoid muscles, along with proper lung compliance (allows maximal inspiration), elastic recoil (promotes expiration), and low airway resistance. **Compliance** is the expected distensibility, or expandability, of the lung tissue and chest wall. Airway resistance is based on the area of the inner lumen of the airway and on properties, such as viscosity and velocity, of the gas moving through that airway.

INSPIRATION

Inspiration is the process of breathing in to acquire oxygen. Similar to inflating a balloon, movement of air is always unidirectional and travels from an area of high pressure to low pressure. In this example, the pressure inside the balloon (the "lungs") is lower than that of the person blowing air into the balloon (the "atmosphere"). A major difference is that the *chest cavity changes size to alter the pressure gradient*, thereby drawing air into the lungs, as opposed to the air moving in and changing the size, as you would see with a balloon. Neuronal stimulation and the movement of the diaphragm downward and external intercostal muscles outward allow this increase in chest cavity size, reduce pressure inside the lungs, and pull air into the lungs.

EXPIRATION

Expiration, the process of removing carbon dioxide out of the body through the lungs, is also regulated within the respiratory center of the brain. In expiration, the diaphragm and external intercostal muscles relax. The chest wall moves inward and the diaphragm moves upward. The intrathoracic (inside the thoracic cavity) pressure becomes greater than the atmospheric pressure. This stimulates air to flow passively out into the atmosphere. Exhalation can also be forced if the abdominal and intercostal muscles are contracted voluntarily, thereby increasing pressure to move the diaphragm upward and pull the ribs inward. The idea is to compress the lungs and increase the pressure inside the airways. Air then moves from the region of higher to lower pressure, or, in this example, from the lungs to the atmosphere.

MEASUREMENT OF VENTILATION

The measurement of lung volumes can determine the effectiveness of inspiration and expiration. Measurements are completed by breathing in or out through a spirometer where measurement of air volume occurs. Changes in lung volumes or pulmonary function can be an early sign of impaired ventilation. Predicted values (the measurement readings that are expected) vary based on age, height, and gender. The following are examples of major measurements of ventilatory capacity:

- **Tidal volume (TV)** is the amount of air that is exhaled after passive inspiration; this is the volume of air going in and out of the lungs at rest; in adults, this volume is approximately 500 mL.
- **Vital capacity (VC)** is the maximal amount of air that can be moved in and out of the lungs with forced inhalation and exhalation.
- **Forced vital capacity (FVC)** is the maximal amount of air that is exhaled from the lungs during a forced exhalation.
- **Forced expiratory volume in 1 second (FEV_1)** is the maximal amount of air that can be expired from the lungs in 1 second.
- **Residual volume (RV)** is the volume of air that remains in the lungs after maximal expiration.
- **Total lung capacity (TLC)** is the total amount of air in the lungs when they are maximally expanded and is the sum of the VC and RV.

Diffusion

Oxygen and carbon dioxide are exchanged at the alveolar capillary junctions in the process of diffusion. The alveolar capillary junction is a thin membrane composed of a layer of alveolar epithelial cells with a basement membrane and the capillary epithelium with a basement membrane. These are separated by a narrow interstitial space and are supported by connective tissue. Between the alveolus and capillary, oxygen moves in to the circulation and carbon dioxide moves out to the atmosphere. Figure 15.1 depicts the proximity of the alveolus and capillary. The alveoli that comprise the alveolar portion of this junction are commonly designated type I alveolar cells (those that provide structure and air exchange) or type II (those that are active in secreting **surfactant**, a lipoprotein lubricant that coats the inner portion of the alveolus, promotes ease of expansion, and repels fluid accumulation). Surfactant is essential to maintain the integrity, air exchange, and diffusion function of the pulmonary system. Without surfactant, inflation of the alveoli would be almost impossible and would make breathing difficult.

During diffusion, two major processes are occurring simultaneously: (1) oxygen is trying to get to all cells and (2) carbon dioxide is trying to escape the body through the lungs. The effectiveness of this transaction depends on:

- Pressure: The amount of partial pressure of the oxygen or carbon dioxide in the blood
- Solubility: Carbon dioxide is much more soluble than oxygen; therefore, carbon dioxide is able to diffuse at a greater rate than oxygen.
- Membranes: The thickness and surface areas of the alveolar and capillary membranes

PARTIAL PRESSURE

Oxygen and carbon dioxide are composed of countless particles in constant collision. The force of these collisions results in the formation of pressure. With oxygen, approximately 1% to 13% is carried in the circulation as a dissolved gas in the plasma. This portion creates a pressure in the plasma, which is referred to as the **partial pressure** and is reported in mm Hg. The symbol for the partial pressure of oxygen in the arterial blood is **Pao_2**. Pao_2 is measured as part of the arterial blood gas panel by drawing blood from a small artery. Because there is no direct method to measure oxygen concentrations in the body, the Pao_2 gives a reasonable estimate of the presence of oxygen in the blood based on the pressure exerted by this gas. Pao_2 is influenced by several factors, such as the presence and concentration of oxygen, altitude, or even aging. Similar to oxygen, the dissolved CO_2 in the plasma forms a partial pressure. The symbol for the partial pressure of carbon dioxide in arterial blood is **$Paco_2$**. $Paco_2$ is also part of the arterial blood gas panel. It is measured through an arterial blood sample and is reported in mm Hg.

OXYGEN DIFFUSION AND TRANSPORT

After inspiration and diffusion across the alveolar capillary junction occur, oxygen dissolves in the plasma, forming a partial pressure (Pao_2). As the Pao_2 increases, oxygen dissociates from the plasma and connects with hemoglobin molecules on red blood cells. The oxygen–hemoglobin combination is now called **oxyhemoglobin (Hbo_2)**. The connection to hemoglobin is based on oxygen's attraction to iron. Iron is the magnet that pulls oxygen onto the hemoglobin molecule. The oxygen then circulates throughout the body. When the oxygen is on the hemoglobin, it is *not* accessible to the cell.

Stop and Consider

What happens to your oxygen-attracting ability if you eat a diet low in iron?

This binding by attraction to hemoglobin continues until the hemoglobin molecules are completely saturated with oxygen. **Oxygen saturation (Sao_2)** refers to the amount of oxyhemoglobin; that is, the amount of hemoglobin that is combined, or saturated, with oxygen. Four oxygen molecules can ride on each hemoglobin vehicle. When all four seats are filled, the hemoglobin is termed **fully saturated** or 100% saturated. Less than this amount indicates a reduction in the presence of oxygen or carrying capacity of the hemoglobin vehicle. Sao_2 is *not* affected by blood volume or hemoglobin level. The Sao_2 is simply saying that for the hemoglobin present, this percent is saturated with oxygen. Feasibly, an individual could have a severe hemorrhage and still measure an Sao_2 of 100%.

Once saturation has been achieved, oxygen continues to diffuse and dissolve in the plasma until the partial pressure in the arteries is equal to that of the partial pressure of the oxygen in the alveoli. Diffusion across the alveoli ceases until the need for oxygen is again detected by changes in the Pao_2. The dissolved oxygen in the plasma is diffused into and used by the cells for cellular metabolism. Oxygen is much less soluble than carbon dioxide; therefore, at any time, approximately 87% to 99% of the oxygen is combined with hemoglobin; the remainder is found dissolved in the plasma of the blood.

CARBON DIOXIDE DIFFUSION AND TRANSPORT

A major waste product of cellular function and respiration is carbon dioxide. If the cell is forced into anaerobic respiration, acidic metabolic wastes are produced in addition to CO_2. One mechanism for ridding the body of this excess acid is to free the CO_2 into the circulation, where it then travels to the alveoli and through the lungs for exhalation. Carbon dioxide diffuses much more readily than oxygen and moves easily across the alveolar capillary junctions. Once released from the cells, carbon dioxide is transported through the circulation similar to oxygen in that it is:

- *Dissolved* in the plasma (approximately 10% of the CO_2)
- *Bound* to hemoglobin (approximately 20% to 30% of the CO_2)
- *Diffused* into the red blood cells as bicarbonate (approximately 60% to 70% of the CO_2)

Stop and Consider
What happens to oxygen and carbon dioxide transport if there is a lack of red blood cells, such as occurs in severe hemorrhaging?

The major portion of the CO_2 found diffused into the red blood cell is converted through the buffering systems to either carbonic acid or bicarbonate ions. Next, the carbonic acid or bicarbonate continues in the plasma to help regulate blood pH. Excess CO_2 is released easily from the hemoglobin, diffuses readily through alveolar capillary junction, and is exhaled through the lungs. Conditions that can decrease expiratory efficiency, such as fibrosis and air trapping in the alveoli, greatly affect CO_2 transport. The CO_2 will not be able to cross the alveolar membrane, will be retained in the body, and will lead to acidosis.

DIFFUSING CAPACITY

The ability of the alveolar capillary junction to exchange oxygen and carbon dioxide between the atmosphere and the blood can be measured quantitatively. The **diffusing capacity** is defined as a measurement of carbon monoxide (CO), oxygen, or nitric oxide transfer from inspired gas to pulmonary capillary blood and reflects the volume of a gas that diffuses through the alveolar capillary membrane each minute. This volume is determined most commonly by comparing how much carbon monoxide (CO) at nontoxic levels is taken up by the blood and dividing this by the pressure across the alveolar capillary membrane. Individuals with alveolar fibrosis or obstruction would be appropriate candidates for undergoing an analysis of diffusing capacity. During the test, the individual breathes in a gas containing CO and one or more tracer gases to allow determination of the gas-exchanging capability of the lungs. For example, the oxygen-diffusing capacity in a state of rest averages about 21 mL per minute per mm Hg. If the average pressure difference between the alveoli and arterial blood is 11 mm Hg, the amount of oxygen that diffuses per minute would average $21 \times 11 = 230$ mL.

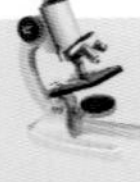

FROM THE LAB

Oxygen saturation (oxyhemoglobin) (Sa_{O_2}) is often measured using pulse oximetry, a noninvasive method of determining hypoxemia even before clinical signs and symptoms are noted. The principle of pulse oximetry is based on red (600 to 750 nm wavelength) and infrared (850 to 1,000 nm wavelength) light absorption levels for oxygenated and deoxygenated hemoglobin. Oxygenated hemoglobin absorbs more *infrared* light and allows more red light to pass through. Deoxygenated hemoglobin absorbs more *red* light and allows more infrared light to pass through. A sensor is placed on the finger, toe, nose, earlobe, or forehead. Both red and infrared light are transmitted to a photo detector. The sensor measures the amount of red and infrared light absorbed by hemoglobin. The expected range of Sa_{O_2} is generally 95% to 100%. An Sa_{O_2} below 70% may be life-threatening.

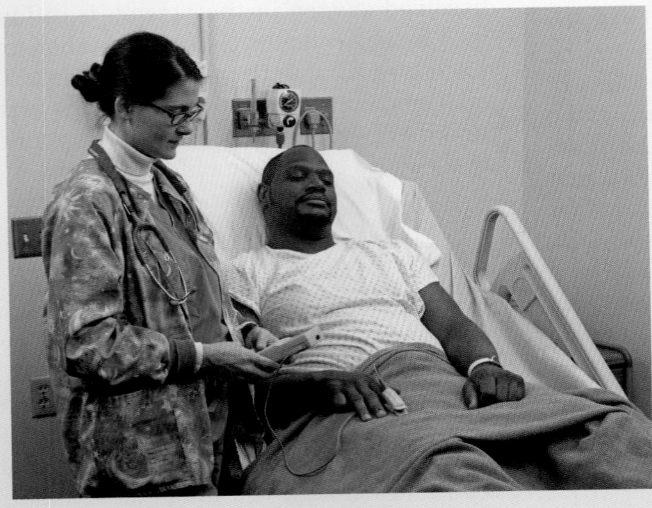

A fingertip oximeter sensor (adult). (From Evans-Smith P. *Taylor's Clinical Nursing Skills*. Philadelphia, PA: Lippincott Williams & Wilkins; 2004.)

Stop and Consider
Based on what you know about why and how Sa_{O_2}, Pa_{O_2}, and Pa_{CO_2} are measured, what factors do you think would affect these readings?

Module 2 Impaired Ventilation

Impaired ventilation is a problem of blocking airflow in and out of the lungs, thereby restricting oxygen intake and carbon dioxide removal from the body. Two major mechanisms are implicated: (1) compression or narrowing of the airways and (2) disruption of the neuronal transmissions needed to stimulate the mechanics of breathing. Compression or narrowing of the airways anywhere from the nose or mouth to alveoli increases airway resistance and leads to difficulties with airway clearance. This occlusion can be partial or complete. Examples of processes that contribute to ineffective airway clearance include inflammation, edema, and exudate accumulation from an infectious process, a structural narrowing of the passageway, strangulation, or the presence of a foreign body. In these cases, air is restricted from moving in and out of the body.

Disruption of neuronal transmission to the lungs also alters ventilatory capacity by ignoring the messages sent by chemoreceptors and lung receptors and interrupting the mechanics of breathing. Oversedation during a surgical procedure or a drug overdose can promote a loss of neurologic stimulation on the respiratory center. Damage to the respiratory center of the brain, cervical nerves, or thoracic nerves leads to an unresponsive or ineffective breathing pattern that does not adapt to oxygen intake needs and carbon dioxide removal needs of the body. For example, severing the cervical nerves results in cessation of spontaneous lung function and requires external mechanical ventilation. Table 15.1 highlights effective and ineffective breathing patterns related to select physiologic and pathophysiologic processes. When a person's breathing pattern is responsive, the rate, depth, and rhythmic pattern of breathing adapt to physiologic changes occurring in the body. Breathing patterns become ineffective when these qualities (rate, depth, and rhythm) do not successfully maintain homeostasis, particularly in maintaining acid–base balance. All of the clinical models in this chapter demonstrate some level of ineffective airway clearance and modification in breathing patterns related to obstructive, restrictive, or altered neuronal processes.

Stop and Consider
How long can you hold your breath? How do you feel while you are holding your breath? When you cannot hold your breath any longer and you start to breathe, how does your body respond?

Table 15.1 Adaptations in Breathing Patterns

Type of Breathing Pattern	Description of Pattern	Diagram of Pattern	Reason for Occurrence
Eupnea	The expected pattern of breathing characterized by a rate between 10 and 20 breaths/min in adults, 500 and 800 mL in depth, and a regular rhythm	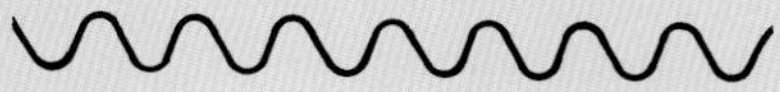	Effective and responsive gas exchange
Tachypnea	Rapid, shallow breathing characterized by a rate of breathing above 24 breaths/min in adults	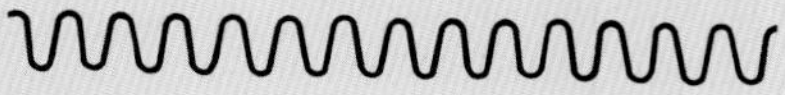	The body needs to release excess carbon dioxide and responds by increasing the rate of breathing. This is an expected response to fever, fear, or exercise; can also occur with respiratory insufficiency pneumonia, or injury to respiratory center.
Apnea	Cessation of breathing for 10 seconds or longer, usually interspersed with another breathing pattern described in this table	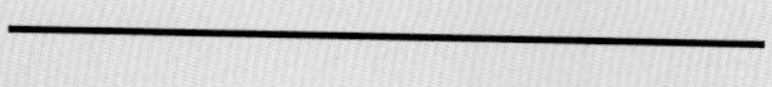	Can result from brain injury, premature birth, or as an obstructive process during sleep

(continued)

Table 15.1 Adaptations in Breathing Patterns (*continued*)

Type of Breathing Pattern	Description of Pattern	Diagram of Pattern	Reason for Occurrence
Hyperpnea (Kussmaul respirations), hyperventilation	Increase in the rate and the depth of breathing. Hyperpnea is responsive to Pa_{O_2}/Pa_{CO_2} requirements; hyperventilation occurs in excess of what is needed to maintain Pa_{CO_2}.		Excess carbon dioxide needs to be released. This can occur with extreme exertion, fear, or anxiety, or with diabetes ketoacidosis, aspirin overdose, or brain injury. Hyperventilation blows off excessive CO_2, causing a decreased level in the blood.
Bradypnea, hypoventilation	Slow breathing with regular depth and rate. Hypoventilation refers to decreased and inadequate ventilation.		Drug-induced depression of the respiratory center, increased intracranial pressure, diabetic coma
Cheyne–Stokes	A breathing pattern that alternates hyperpnea in a crescendo–decrescendo pattern and periods of apnea		Increased intracranial pressure, breathing bilateral damage to cerebral hemispheres or diencephalons, drug-induced respiratory depression, heart failure, uremia
Ataxic breathing	A breathing pattern of unpredictable irregularity. Can combine any or all breathing patterns above.		Severe head trauma and damage to respiratory center, brain abscess, heat stroke, spinal meningitis, encephalitis
Obstructive breathing	Prolonged and incomplete expiration to overcome increased airway resistance and air trapping		Chronic obstructive lung disease, asthma, chronic bronchitis

Eupnea, tachypnea, apnea, bradypnea, and Cheyne–Stokes from *Nursing Procedures*. 4th ed. Ambler, PA: Lippincott Williams & Wilkins; 2004; Hyperpnea, ataxic breathing, and obstructive breathing from Bickley LS, Szilagyi P. *Bates' Guide to Physical Examination and History Taking*. 8th ed. Philadelphia, PA: Lippincott Williams & Wilkins; 2003.

IMPAIRED VENTILATION–PERFUSION MATCHING

A second mechanism for impairing gas exchange is termed ventilation–perfusion (V/Q) mismatching. This means either that areas of the lung are ventilated but not perfused or that the lung is perfused but not ventilated. Examples of problems that can impair ventilation are described in the previous section. With impaired ventilation, inadequate oxygen comes into the lungs even though the blood flow is ready and able to carry the oxygen that is present. If the perfusion aspect is impaired, the blood flow to the lungs is restricted in one or more areas. Oxygen may be coming into the body but there is no blood flow to carry this away to other body cells. A more complete discussion of ventilation–perfusion mismatching is reserved for Chapter 16.

IMPAIRED DIFFUSION

Impaired diffusion is a process of restricting the transfer of oxygen or carbon dioxide across the alveolar capillary junction. Because the rate of diffusion depends on the solubility and partial pressure of the gas, *and* on surface area and thickness of the membrane, impaired gas exchange can occur with changes in any of these properties. All of the clinical models in this chapter demonstrate some level of impaired gas exchange related to a decrease in the functional alveolar capillary junction surface area.

Partial pressure is increased when more molecules are packed into a space, when the temperature increases (promoting an increase in particle collisions), and when the barometric pressure increases. A loss of partial pressure, and subsequent decrease in oxygen presence, can occur during a state of oxygen deprivation, during hypothermia, or when the body is responding to changes in atmospheric pressure (high altitude). The partial pressure of oxygen generally increases during the administration of high concentrations of oxygen and potentially during a fever. The partial pressure of carbon dioxide is increased during states of greater tissue metabolism, such as occurs with fever or strenuous exercise. This results in higher levels of carbon dioxide in the blood.

Changes in the alveolar capillary membrane also impair diffusion. Damage to the alveoli or capillaries limits the accessible and usable surface area and restricts oxygen and carbon dioxide transport. Many disease processes, such as pneumonia, pulmonary edema, and acute respiratory distress syndrome (ARDS), fill the alveolar capillary junction with the products of inflammation or infection. This obstructs the passage of gases needed for cell function and for the maintenance of optimal pH in the blood. Chronic injury to the alveoli, such as with emphysema, can lead to fibrosis, or thickening of the alveolar capillary membrane, and can also impair gas exchange.

THE EFFECTS OF IMPAIRED VENTILATION AND DIFFUSION

Many conditions, even diseases outside of the "respiratory" system, can challenge the ventilatory and diffusion capabilities of the body. Any situation that presents a demand for higher levels of oxygen or an increase in cellular metabolism requires pulmonary adaptation to maintain homeostasis. For example, strenuous exercise requires extensive adaptation to provide adequate oxygen to cells and to remove the excess carbon dioxide (as a by-product of cellular metabolism). When the body is unable to keep up with the demands, either because the demands are too great or the ventilation or diffusion capabilities are restricted, this can lead to:

1. Hypoxemia
2. Hypoxia
3. Hypercapnia

These three effects directly result from decreased oxygen presence or utilization, or the retention of carbon dioxide. Basically, the body is unable to take in enough oxygen or is unable to release enough carbon dioxide. These basic effects directly apply to the selected clinical models in this chapter and all other conditions that affect ventilation and diffusion.

Hypoxemia and Hypoxia

Hypoxemia is decreased oxygen in the arterial blood leading to a decrease in the partial pressure of oxygen (Pa_{O_2}). The major causes of hypoxemia include oxygen deprivation, hypoventilation, problems with adequate diffusion, and inadequate uptake of oxygen in the blood. Hypoxemia can range from mild to severe and becomes problematic when cells are deprived of adequate oxygen, a condition referred to as **hypoxia**. When hypoxemia leads to hypoxia, the effects are widespread. All cells that depend on oxygen for efficient cellular metabolism are vulnerable, particularly cells within the vital organs (the brain, heart, and lungs). The brain has an incredibly high demand for oxygen and has minimal storage capacity. Oxygen deprivation throughout the body results in reduced cell metabolism and function. This, in turn, forces the cell to use anaerobic metabolism. Anaerobic metabolism leads to the rapid development of metabolic acidosis. The body needs to maintain a relatively constant pH for optimal cell functioning. Cellular death results from extreme or prolonged hypoxia. The cerebral effects of chronic hypoxia can range from restlessness (an early sign, particularly in children) to lethargy, coma, and eventually, death.

Although hypoxemia can lead to hypoxia, hypoxia can result even when there is adequate arterial oxygen. For example, a reduction in circulation caused by an arterial blockage can deprive the cells distal to the blockage of oxygen even though the total amount of circulating oxygen is adequate. In this case, cell death results only in those cells deprived of oxygen.

Hypercapnia

Hypercapnia refers to a state of increased carbon dioxide in the blood. Carbon dioxide is much more easily diffused than oxygen; therefore, hypercapnia presents only in cases of severe alveolar hypoventilation and subsequent hypoxia. Conditions that inhibit ventilation or promote trapping of air in the alveoli contribute to the development of hypercapnia. The major effect is respiratory acidosis caused by CO_2 retention. This can lead to electrolyte disturbances, which can alter cardiac conduction and brain function, resulting in an ineffective heart rhythm, coma, and death. The determination of the level of hypercapnia requires measurement of arterial blood gases. Figure 15.2 summarizes the processes from ventilation and diffusion to hypoxemia, hypoxia, and hypercapnia.

Stop and Consider
How does the body respond to low oxygen or increased carbon dioxide in the blood or tissues?

GENERAL MANIFESTATIONS OF IMPAIRED VENTILATION AND DIFFUSION

Although some subtle variations in manifestations exist across conditions, the local and systemic clinical manifestations of altered ventilation and diffusion have many commonalities. Local manifestations (those triggered in the airways and lung tissues) are most often related to inflammatory processes in response to injury. The injury triggers vasodilation,

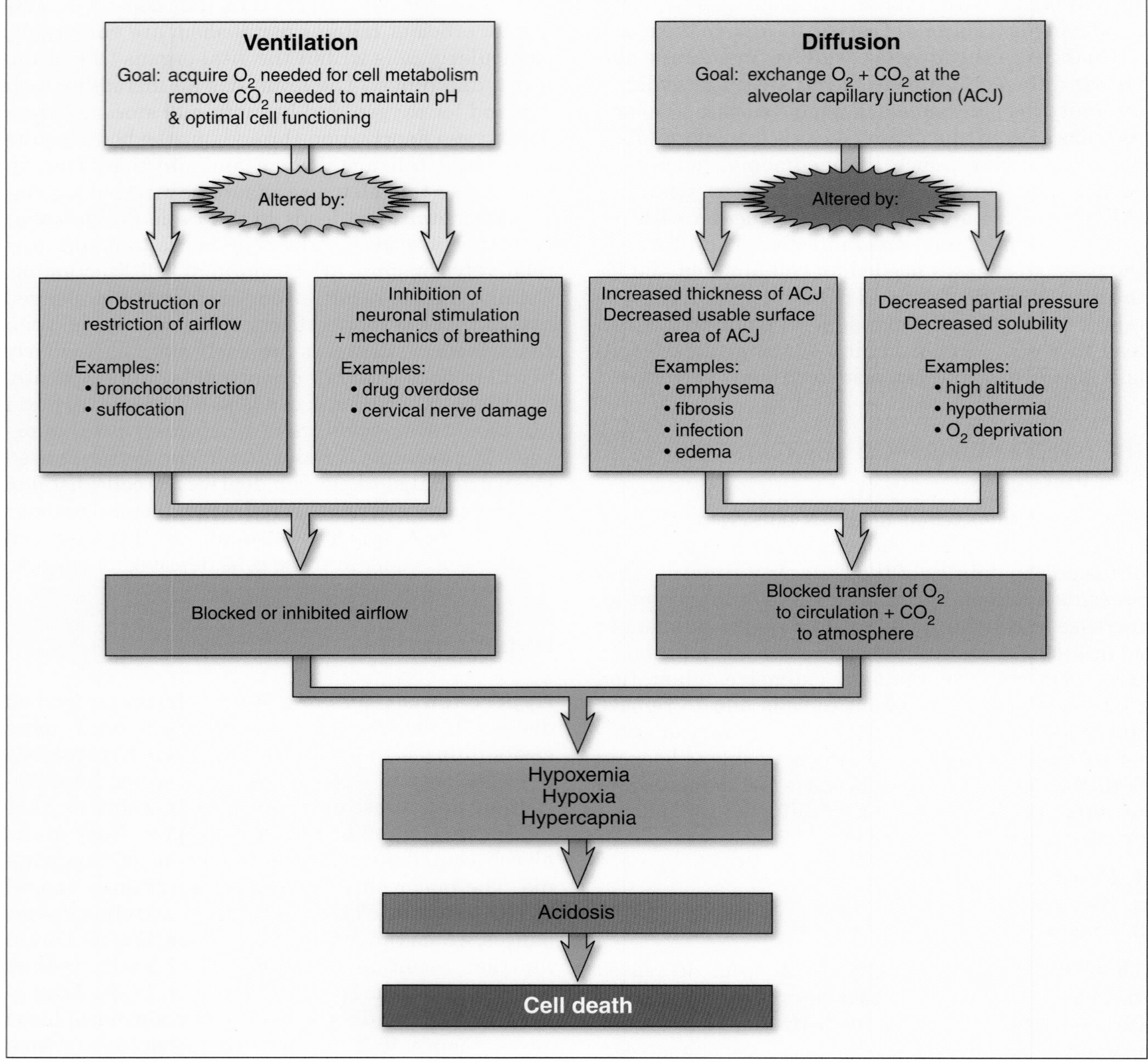

Figure 15.2. Concept map. Altered ventilation and diffusion.

increased capillary permeability, exudate formation, and pain in the affected region of the airways, lungs, or chest cavity. Potent chemical mediators regulate these inflammatory processes and are responsible for many of the local and systemic manifestations.

The following are potential local manifestations:

- Cough
- Excess mucous production
- Hemoptysis
- Dyspnea
- Use of accessory muscles
- Chest pain
- Barrel chest

A cough with or without excessive sputum production is a common clinical manifestation of altered ventilation and diffusion. The cough reflex is a protective mechanism that is triggered to rid the airways of an irritating agent. An acute cough typically lasts less than 3 to 8 weeks and is commonly associated with viral infections, seasonal allergies, **aspiration** (inhaling a foreign substance into the lungs), or pulmonary embolus (a blockage that occludes a pulmonary blood vessel). A chronic cough is one that extends beyond 8 weeks and is commonly associated with asthma, gastroesophageal reflux (gastric contents back up into the esophagus and stimulate the cough reflex), or chronic postnasal drainage.

In smokers, chronic cough is a common manifestation of chronic bronchitis or lung cancer.

Excess mucous production of the airways is related to the inflammatory response. This mucus is often the irritating agent that triggers the cough reflex and often provides clues to the offending agent or process. This condition can be observed by having the individual **expectorate**, or spit out, the mucus that is ejected during the cough. **Sputum** refers to this expectorated material. **Phlegm** is a term that describes large amounts of sputum expectorated from the oropharynx. Specific pathogens may produce sputum with a distinct color or odor. For example, bacterial infections are often characterized by thick, purulent sputum. Pneumococcal pneumonia may lead to a rust-colored, dark sputum. Typically, the onset of a viral acute upper respiratory infection (a common cold) begins with clear, thin mucus. As phagocytes move into the area of inflammation to ward off any infection, these cells then die and are shed off as yellow or green mucus. **Hemoptysis** (coughing up blood from the respiratory tract) is defined by the presence of red blood cells in the sputum. Blood in the sputum is often significant and can be caused by heavy exertion during coughing (blood streaking within the mucus) or from tuberculosis, a tumor, or more severe trauma. When combined with edema in the lung tissues (pulmonary edema), the sputum often becomes not only blood-tinged but also frothy or foamy.

Difficulty breathing is a common report in individuals with altered ventilation or diffusion. **Dyspnea** is the subjective feeling of shortness of breath or the inability to get enough air. The stimulus is based on the presence of hypoxemia, hypercapnia, and the subsequent reduction in pH; however, the exact mechanism is often unknown. One theory is that lung receptors or chemoreceptors act on the brain and muscles active in breathing to stimulate this sensation. Dyspnea often leads to certain physical and emotional responses, such as the physical need to sit in an upright or standing position, a condition called **orthopnea**, to maximize lung expansion. An individual may also use accessory muscles and demonstrate nasal flaring to promote the work of breathing. **Retractions** are the pulling in of accessory muscles usually in the intercostal, substernal, and supraclavicular spaces to promote more effective inspiration. Along with position and effort changes, individuals experiencing air trapping may perform **pursed lip breathing**, a process of holding the lips puckered tightly together while slowly exhaling, to maintain positive airway pressure in the alveoli to minimize air trapping and promote expiration of carbon dioxide. Emotional manifestations of dyspnea include anxiety, a sense of panic, frustration, and anger.

Chest pain can originate in the visceral and parietal pleura, the airways, or the chest wall. Inflammatory processes within the pleura often lead to pleural pain, which increases with deep inspiration, and is often described as sharp or stabbing pain. **Auscultation** (listening with a stethoscope) will reveal a grating, scratching sound (called a pleural friction rub) with inspiration. Costochondritis, inflammation of one or more costal cartilages, is also characterized by pain in the anterior chest wall and may be triggered by coughing. Similarly, inflammation of the airways, intercostal muscles, or accessory muscles can also present as localized pain and be triggered by coughing. Chest pain, although frequently of pulmonary origin, must be differentiated from cardiac pain because of the possibility of the individual experiencing a myocardial infarction.

Changes in the shape of the chest wall, known as barrel chest, can also occur with chronic lung disease. Typically, the chest wall shape is an oval, in which the anterior–posterior (AP) plane is narrower than the transverse (T) plane (an AP:T ratio of approximately 1:2). Chronic dilation and distention of the alveoli, as seen in emphysema, often results in a barrel chest appearance, in which the AP:T ratio becomes 1:1 (Fig. 15.3).

Changes in breathing patterns (see Table 15.1) and in the characteristics of breath sounds are also common local manifestations of altered ventilation and diffusion. The sounds emitted by the lungs during inspiration and expiration also give clues to the presence and extent of altered ventilation and diffusion. **Adventitious**, or altered, breath sounds are typically the result of either airway constriction or fluid accumulation (Box 15.1). Airway constriction results in wheezing breath sounds. Fluid accumulation leads to fine or course crackles. The characteristics of these sounds vary based on anatomic location (larger vs. smaller airways) or type of secretions (thin, watery vs. thicker mucus).

Systemic manifestations of altered ventilation are caused by the effects of hypoxemia, hypoxia, and hypercapnia. In the presence of inflammation, systemic manifestations, such as fever, malaise, leukocytosis, and higher levels of circulating plasma proteins, can apply to problems of altered ventilation and diffusion. The intensity of the hypoxic or hypercapnic response is variable depending on the extent of oxygen deprivation and carbon dioxide retention. Responses may include:

- Dusky or cyanotic mucous membrane color
- Changes in arterial blood gases
- Mental status changes
- Finger clubbing

Changes in arterial blood gases, pH, PaO_2, and $PaCO_2$, and mental status changes are discussed above as

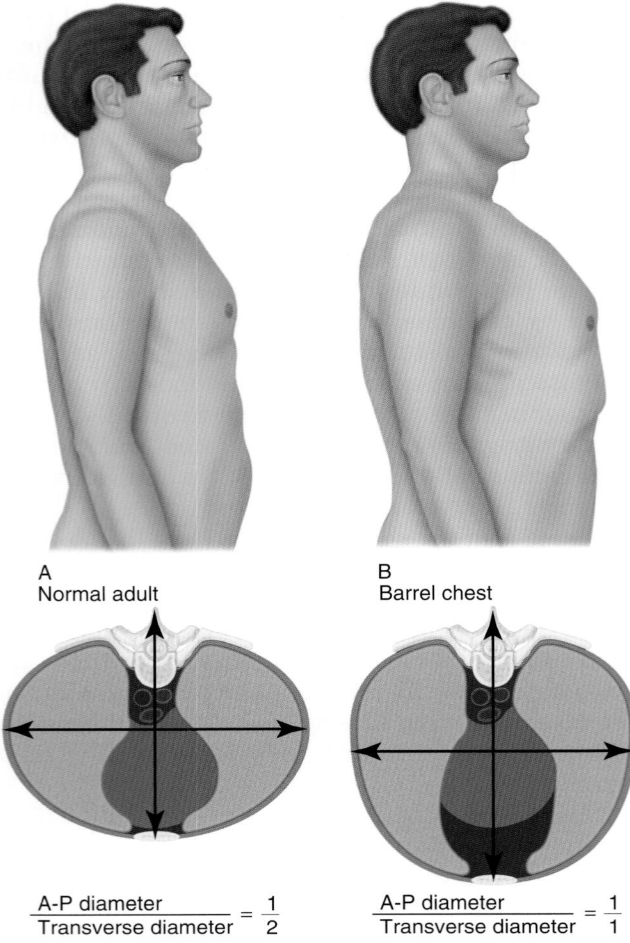

Figure 15.3. Comparison of expected anatomy and barrel chest alteration that occurs with emphysema. **A:** The expected chest cross-section. **B:** The barrel chest.

effects of hypoxemia, hypoxia, and hypercapnia. Changes in skin and mucous membrane color can also result from severe hypoxemia. **Cyanosis** is caused by a greater proportion of desaturated hemoglobin in the blood, which gives the blood a bluish hue. Central cyanosis, a problem of low oxygen saturation in the arterial blood, often presents as color changes in the skin and mucous membranes. In individuals with dark skin, the skin color change is often described as ashen or dusky. In light skin, the color is often described as pale or bluish. Because skin color varies among individuals, the most reliable indicator of central cyanosis on examination is the finding of a bluish color of the mucous membranes. Individuals with peripheral cyanosis, a problem of sluggish blood flow in the fingers and toes, often present with sluggish capillary refill (demonstrated by a slow return of blood when the nail bed is compressed and then released) and a pale or bluish hue in the nail beds.

Box 15.1 Adventitious Breath Sounds

Crackles are snapping, popping, or bubbling sounds emitted during inspiration and expiration and caused by fluid accumulation in the airways; fine crackles are higher pitched with a shorter duration and signify fluid in smaller airways; coarse crackles are louder and lower pitched and signify fluid in the larger airways.

Rales is a previously used term to describe fine crackles from fluid secretions in the airways; the term rales has been replaced with crackles.

Wheezing is a continuous, high-pitched, whistling sound; it is significant for obstruction or tightness in the small airways.

Rhonchi is a term used to describe both low-pitched wheezing sounds with a snoring quality (sonorous wheezing) when the airway narrowing is in the larger airways, and high-pitched wheezing sounds with a squeaking quality (sibilant wheezing) when the airway narrowing is in the smaller airways. Rhonchi occur when thick mucus partially blocks the airways.

Stridor is a harsh, high-pitched, creaking sound, which is significant for obstruction in the upper airway, especially of the trachea or larynx.

Diminished breath sounds is a term used to describe quieter breath sounds that are barely audible; this is significant for complete obstruction in one or more airways.

Absent breath sounds signifies no air movement through the lungs.

Chronic problems with ventilation and diffusion may result in clubbing of the fingers. **Clubbing** is a painless enlargement and flattening of the tips of fingers or toes caused by chronic hypoxia (Fig. 15.4). Although the exact mechanism is unknown, clubbing is consistently associated with chronic conditions that disturb oxygenation, such as prolonged obstruction or fibrosis of the airways.

LABORATORY AND DIAGNOSTIC TESTS

Detection of altered ventilation and diffusion is based on a thorough patient history and physical examination supported by relevant diagnostic and

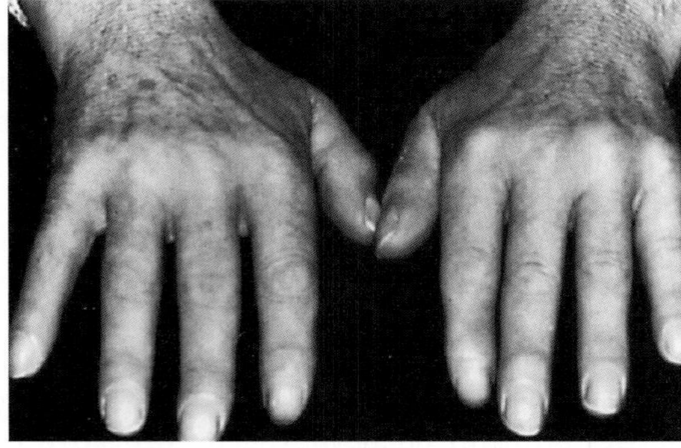

Figure 15.4. Clubbing of the fingers. (From Crapo JD, Glassroth J, Karlinsky JB, et al. *Baum's Textbook of Pulmonary Diseases*. 7th ed. Philadelphia, PA: Lippincott Williams & Wilkins; 2004.)

laboratory tests. Table 15.2 presents common laboratory and diagnostic tests performed when an individual has a suspected alteration in ventilation and diffusion.

Table 15.2 Laboratory and Diagnostic Tests Performed to Determine Altered Ventilation and Diffusion

Lab or Diagnostic Test	Purpose of the Test
Pulmonary function tests (PFTs)	Broad range of noninvasive tests including spirometry, lung volume measurements, and diffusion capacity that involve breathing into a tube that measures the pressure exerted during ventilation. Spirometry is useful in detecting obstructive lung disease by monitoring how well the lungs exhale.
Arterial blood gases (ABGs)	Determines presence of acid–base imbalances and degree of hypoxemia and hypercapnia from an arterial blood sample
Pulse oximetry	Noninvasive test that measures oxygen saturation (see From the Lab)
Bronchoscopy	Direct visualization of bronchioles; can be used to take biopsy, take sputum samples, or remove foreign objects from airway
Radiograph, CT, MRI	Used to detect structural problems, presence of consolidation, obstruction, or cavitation in the airways and lung tissue
Nuclear (V/Q) lung scan	Detects pulmonary embolism (lung blockage) and lung disease, such as emphysema and chronic obstructive pulmonary disease, by using a nuclear medicine camera and computer imaging to visualize the amount and distribution of minute amounts of radioactive materials inspired into the lungs (V) or injected into a vein (Q) that then flows to and perfuses the lung
Culture and sensitivity tests	Determines presence and type of microorganisms in the blood and/or sputum; the results dictate the appropriate antibiotic treatment if indicated
Thoracentesis	Determines the presence of a pleural effusion (excess fluid in the pleural space) by inserting a needle from the chest or back into the lung pleural space; the fluid is examined to determine the cellular and chemical composition, the presence of malignant cells, and the presence of microorganisms

V, ventilation (airflow in and out of the lungs); Q, perfusion (blood flow to the lungs); CT, computed tomography; MRI, magnetic resonance imaging.

TREATING IMPAIRED VENTILATION AND DIFFUSION

The treatment of any health condition is based on determining the cause. Occasionally, in conditions of altered ventilation and diffusion, the cause cannot be reversed. The principles that guide improving ventilation are based on:

1. Removing obstructions (i.e., foreign body, tumor, edema)
2. Restoring the integrity of the chest wall, lungs, and other respiratory structures
3. Decreasing inflammation
4. Decreasing, thinning, and moving mucus out of the airway
5. Opening and maintaining integrity of the airways
6. Supplementing oxygen
7. Controlling infectious processes
8. Using mechanical ventilation, as indicated

Table 15.3 outlines common treatment modalities for impaired ventilation and diffusion.

Table 15.3 Altered Ventilation and Diffusion Treatment Principles

Treatment	Mechanism of Action	Appropriate Uses
Anti-inflammatory medications	Reduces inflammatory response by acting on chemical mediators to decrease excess blood flow, swelling, heat, redness, and pain to the affected area	Inflammation that impinges on ventilatory function such as with asthma
Humidification	Moistens and liquefies secretions to aid in expectoration	Use in the presence of excessive, thick, or sticky mucus
Decongestants	Decreases nasal congestion through vascular vasoconstriction, which decreases blood flow, reduces exudate, and shrinks swollen mucous membranes	Use in the presence of excessive, thick, or sticky mucus
Antitussives	Suppresses cough by inhibiting cough receptors in the medulla (some have local effects as well)	Use when cough is excessive and interferes with sleep
Bronchodilators	Opens airways by relaxing bronchial smooth muscles	Conditions that cause bronchoconstriction: asthma, COPD

(continued)

Table 15.3 Altered Ventilation and Diffusion Treatment Principles (*continued*)

Treatment	Mechanism of Action	Appropriate Uses
Chest physiotherapy	Using a pounding motion or vibration on the chest to physically loosen thick secretions	Conditions that result in thick, tenacious secretions such as in cystic fibrosis
Antimicrobials	Antibiotics have a range of mechanisms focused on destroying or reducing impact of bacteria; antivirals may also be prescribed as appropriate	Bacterial infection (antibiotics) such as bacterial pneumonia
Oxygen therapy	Provides direct oxygen supplementation	Hypoxia
Mechanical ventilation	Life support measure that provides the work of breathing	Respiratory failure
Surgery	Surgical removal of abnormal tissues or structures within the chest (thoracotomy)	Multiple uses, including confirmation of the diagnosis of lung disease, repair of the lung, removal of lung tumors, or removal of pus from pleural space (empyema)

COPD, chronic obstructive pulmonary disease.

Module 3 Clinical Models

The following clinical models have been selected to aid in the understanding and application of altered ventilation and diffusion processes and effects. Commonalities and unique features of each clinical model should be noted when reading this section.

Pneumonia

Pneumonia is selected as a clinical model to demonstrate the impact of a common acute infectious process on ventilation and diffusion. **Pneumonia** refers to inflammation of the lungs occurring commonly in the bronchioles, interstitial lung tissue, or the alveoli. The elderly, the very young, and those individuals who smoke or are immunosuppressed or hospitalized are most at risk for developing pneumonia. It is in the top 10 leading causes of death in the United States.

PATHOPHYSIOLOGY

Microorganisms, including bacteria, viruses, and fungi, spread by respiratory droplets, are the most common cause of pneumonia. Pneumonias are often distinguished as either community acquired or hospital acquired (nosocomial) depending on where the disease was contracted. Nosocomial pneumonias, particularly in the immunosuppressed individual, tend to be more severe and lead to a less favorable prognosis than community-acquired pneumonias. Typical community-acquired pneumonia is most commonly caused by *Streptococcus pneumoniae, Haemophilus influenzae,* and *Staphylococcus* species. Atypical forms of community-acquired pneumonia are caused by *Mycoplasma pneumoniae, Legionella,* and *Chlamydia* species. The influenza virus is the most common viral pathogen known to cause pneumonia. Nosocomial, or hospital-acquired, pneumonia is most commonly caused by infection with *Pseudomonas aeruginosa* or *Staphylococcus aureus*. Infection with an opportunistic fungal infection in the lungs, such as with *Candida albicans* or *Pneumocystis carinii,* indicates immunosuppression or immunodeficiency. Pneumonia can also occur when breathing in items not intended for the lungs, such as foods, fluids, and stomach contents, a condition called aspiration pneumonia.

In many cases, the defense mechanisms in the nasopharynx and oropharynx of the upper respiratory tract effectively trap and expel microorganisms before causing infection. For pathogens that happen to escape the cough reflex and mucociliary blanket, macrophages located in the alveoli are often adequate to engulf and destroy the offending microorganism. When these defense mechanisms are inadequate, the inflammatory and immune responses are triggered, particularly in the interstitial lung tissue and alveoli. The inflamed alveoli fill with exudate. Other products of inflammation (red blood cells [RBCs], white blood cells [WBCs], and fibrin) accumulate as well and cause **consolidation**, or a solid mass in the lung tissue. These areas of consolidation are evident on radiograph and are often the key diagnostic feature of typical pneumonia (Fig. 15.5).

With typical pneumonia, the presence of another viral infection, such as influenza, promotes attachment of the pneumococcal bacteria to the receptors

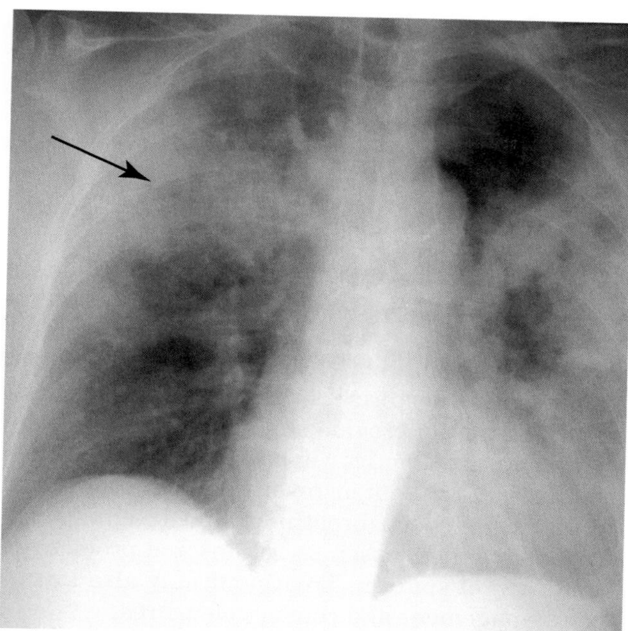

Figure 15.5. Chest radiograph in a 50-year-old patient with pneumonia shows opacity characteristic of lung consolidation. (From Crapo JD, Glassroth J, Karlinsky JB, et al. *Baum's Textbook of Pulmonary Diseases*. 7th ed. Philadelphia, PA: Lippincott Williams & Wilkins; 2004.)

on the respiratory epithelium. The bacteria can then infect the type II alveolar cells. The pneumococci multiply along the alveolus and penetrate the alveolar epithelium, thereby moving across to infect adjacent alveoli. In contrast, atypical pneumonia causes damage often through immune-mediated mechanisms rather than direct damage cause by the bacteria. The spread of infection with atypical pneumonia is more likely to spread beyond the lobar boundaries and is often bilateral.

Histologic changes in the lungs during the progression of pneumonia can be categorized in three stages:

1. Recent infection shows rapid filling of the alveolar capillaries with a frothy, serous, and blood-tinged fluid.
2. A "red hepatization" stage follows and is marked by the filling of alveoli with fibrinous exudates, which appear as areas of dry, granular, dark-red lung tissue.
3. Within 72 hours, the "gray hepatization" stage occurs marked by WBCs packing into the alveoli as RBCs and epithelial cells degenerate. The pneumococcal bacteria release toxins that contribute to cell death. Eventually the bacteria are opsonized by WBCs, a yellow exudate forms, these exudates are then absorbed, and resolution begins.

Box 15.2 Potential Causes of Respiratory Failure

Respiratory failure can be a life-threatening consequence of:

- Impaired ventilation
  - Total airway obstruction
  - Head injury leading to severe hypoventilation
  - Weakness or paralysis of respiratory muscles
  - Chest wall injury
- Impaired matching of ventilation and perfusion
- Chronic obstructive pulmonary disease
  - Atelectasis
  - Severe infection
- Impaired diffusion
  - Pulmonary edema
  - Acute respiratory distress syndrome

The general effects of altered ventilation and diffusion apply to pneumonia: oxygen diffusion is greatly impaired, hypoxia sets in, metabolic acidosis occurs, and dehydration may result. Dehydration is related to fluid losses through hyperventilation and fever, and it is exacerbated by inadequate fluid intake. Although most cases of pneumonia resolve within 2 weeks with appropriate treatment, individuals with preexisting respiratory disease are more likely to experience a deterioration of respiratory status, leading to respiratory failure and death.

Respiratory failure can result from any problem that severely affects ventilation, ventilation-perfusion matching, or diffusion. It can occur quickly or insidiously. Box 15.2 outlines major causes of respiratory failure and relevant examples. Respiratory failure represents the failure of the lungs to adequately oxygenate the cells of the body and remove carbon dioxide. It is a life-threatening emergency. Respiratory failure can lead to a state of **anoxia**, a

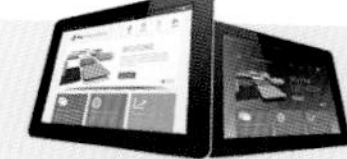

RESEARCH NOTES

Mechanical ventilation with gas has been a mainstay of treatment for severe altered ventilation. This approach can sometimes cause more harm than good by exacerbating lung injury through structural damage and release of inflammatory chemical mediators within the lung. For more than 40 years, researchers have been investigating methods to reduce a patient's time on a mechanical ventilator without risking reintubation. In a recent Cochrane review, researchers found that using noninvasive positive pressure ventilation (such as with a CPAP) as a weaning strategy for intubated adults with respiratory failure was an effective way to reduce mechanical ventilation time and prevented reintubation.[1]

total lack of oxygenation. The cells quickly become hypoxic and the blood can become acidotic. If not reversed, death can ensue within minutes.

CLINICAL MANIFESTATIONS

Clinical manifestations relevant to pneumonia include sudden onset of fever, chills, cough, sputum production, fatigue, loss of appetite, dyspnea, tachypnea, tachycardia, pleuritic pain, and adventitious breath sounds caused by fluid accumulation in the lungs (crackles). These manifestations are related to the inflammatory and infectious processes. In adults (particularly in the elderly), headache and even confusion can occur.

DIAGNOSTIC CRITERIA

Diagnosis is based on a thorough patient history and physical examination, noting the characteristic clinical manifestations. A complete blood count is performed to determine an elevation in the WBC count, which suggests bacterial infection. A chest radiograph or possibly a thoracic CT scan is also needed to identify areas of consolidation and to rule out other diseases or complications that may present with similar symptoms, such as **bronchiectasis** (irreversible dilation and destruction of the bronchial tree most often caused by chronic obstruction or infection), lung tumors, or heart failure.

Identifying the causative microorganism is important for directing the treatment regimen and for predicting the severity of disease and prognosis. This is completed through a Gram stain and culture and sensitivity tests of expectorated sputum. In addition, certain characteristics of sputum may suggest a specific pathogen. For example, individuals with pneumococcal pneumonia often present with bloody or rust-colored, dark sputum. Individuals with infections caused by *Haemophilus* or *Pseudomonas* are likely to expectorate green sputum. Anaerobic infections are typically foul smelling. Pleural fluid may also be aspirated via thoracentesis and tested if there is a pleural effusion (fluid in the pleural space) or empyema (lung abscess).

Monitoring the ventilation and perfusion status of the individual with pneumonia requires measurement of oxygenation through the use of pulse oximetry and arterial blood gases. A nuclear (V/Q) lung scan may also be necessary to determine ventilation and perfusion efficacy.

TREATMENT

The goal of treatment for pneumonia is to restore optimal ventilation and diffusion. The plan of care, particularly the location of treatment (hospital or home) and the appropriate antibiotic, depends on the type of pneumonia (community or hospital acquired), the severity of disease, the presence of comorbid conditions, and the type of pathogen. For example, the initial antibiotic to treat community-acquired pneumonias in low-risk patients is a macrolide, such as azithromycin. Macrolides help to eradicate gram-positive microorganisms, along with *Mycoplasma* and *Legionella* species. Community-acquired pneumonias in high-risk individuals (those older than 60 or with a comorbid condition) would be prescribed a macrolide along with an antibiotic that provides coverage of gram-negative bacteria. Severe pneumonia requires hospitalization to provide adequate oxygen therapy, intravenous antibiotics (if bacterial), and intravenous fluids to prevent or reverse dehydration. Chest physiotherapy, deep breathing, and coughing may be needed to help loosen secretions and promote expectoration of sputum. Treatment may also involve fever management and comfort measures.

Chronic Obstructive Pulmonary Disease

Chronic obstructive pulmonary disease (COPD) is a generic term that describes all chronic obstructive lung problems, including asthma, emphysema, and chronic bronchitis, separately or in combination. COPD is one of the leading causes of death worldwide.

COPD is primarily used to denote the presence of both emphysema and chronic bronchitis (and, to some extent, asthma). Inflammatory processes in both the alveoli and in the bronchi/bronchioles characterize COPD. The disease is progressive, unremitting, and irreversible, although progression can be slowed if treatment is implemented early in the course of the disease. Although smoking has been implicated in the development of COPD, approximately 10% to 20% of those affected have never smoked. Because of significant lung reserves, symptoms may only become apparent when lung function is at or below 50%. In this section, emphysema, chronic bronchitis, and asthma are discussed separately.

Emphysema

Emphysema is an irreversible enlargement of the air spaces beyond the terminal bronchioles, most notably in the alveoli, resulting in destruction of the alveolar walls and obstruction of airflow. The most notable cause of emphysema is chronic smoking, although in nonsmokers, development of emphysema is often due to the genetically inherited deficiency of alpha$_1$-antitrypsin (AAT). Less commonly, pulmonary vascular damage from the insoluble fillers (e.g., cornstarch or cotton fibers) found in intravenous drugs (such as methadone or cocaine), immune deficiency syndromes, or connective tissue disorders (such as Marfan syndrome) can lead to the development of emphysema.

PATHOPHYSIOLOGY

In early or mild emphysema, the primary source of obstruction is the development of inflammation in the small airways distal to the respiratory bronchioles. If diagnosed early, the inflammation in the small airways can be reduced, thereby providing some relief from airway obstruction. In moderate-to-severe disease, the loss of elastic recoil in the alveoli is the primary mechanism of airflow obstruction. This is not reversible. Vascular changes in the lungs develop simultaneously along with the airway obstruction. The inner lining of the arteries and arterioles that perfuse the lungs become thick and fibrotic. This further contributes to alveolar and capillary destruction. Patterns of alveolar destruction can occur in the respiratory bronchioles and spread peripherally, termed *centriacinar*, or uniformly destroy the entire alveolus, termed *panacinar*. Centriacinar emphysema is typically associated with chronic smoking and primarily affects the upper half of the lungs, whereas panacinar emphysema occurs in those with AAT deficiency (Fig. 15.6).

Chronic smoking impairs alveolar function through the following cascade of events:

1. Inhalation of smoke triggers the inflammatory response.
2. Neutrophils and later macrophages are activated and retained in the lung tissue.
3. Neutrophils and macrophages release proteolytic enzymes, such as proteinases and elastases, that destroy components of the extracellular matrix, such as elastin, in the lungs.
4. The elasticity of the lung is significantly reduced leading to the inability of the alveoli to recoil and release CO_2 into the atmosphere.

Elasticity is essential in the alveoli. Loss of elasticity affects the ability of the alveoli to contract and move air back out of the body. The airspaces become enlarged and ineffective. If the alveolar walls collapse, air remains trapped in the alveoli (Fig. 15.7). **Air trapping** decreases effective O_2 intake and especially CO_2 release. The experience of air trapping is demonstrated through taking a full breath and releasing half of the air and then again taking a full deep breath and releasing half of the air. When a person takes a deep breath and releases only half of the air, hyperinflation occurs in the lungs. The alveoli become further stretched and continue to lose elasticity. CO_2 is retained and blood pH is reduced.

The lungs require protection against the destruction imposed by proteolytic enzymes. This is the

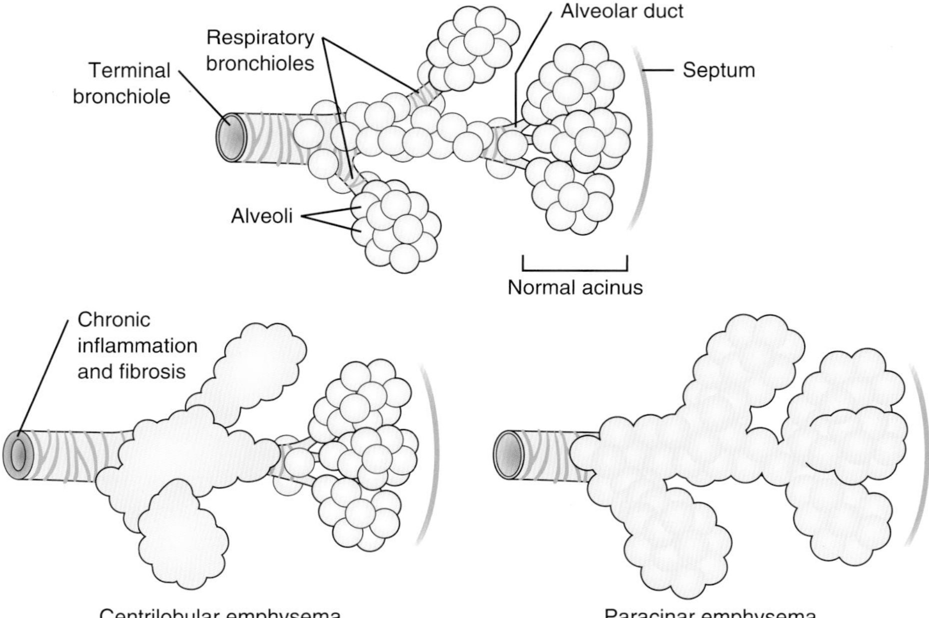

Figure 15.6. Types of emphysema. The acinus, the gas-exchanging structure of the lung distal to the terminal bronchiole, consists of the terminal bronchiole, respiratory bronchioles, alveolar ducts, alveolar sacs, and alveoli. In centrilobular (proximal acinar) emphysema, the respiratory bronchioles are mainly involved. In paraseptal (distal acinar) emphysema, the alveolar ducts are mainly affected. In panacinar (panlobular) emphysema, the acinus is uniformly damaged.

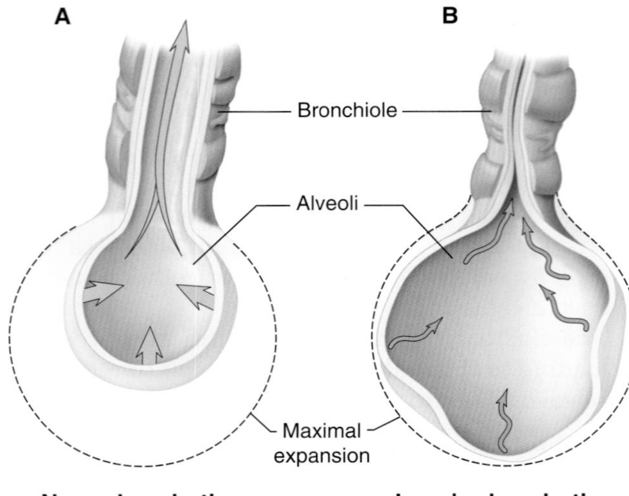

Figure 15.7. Elastic recoil in the alveoli. **A:** Unaffected alveolus. **B:** Air trapping seen in emphysema caused by the loss of alveolar elastic recoil.

primary role of antiprotease enzymes, particularly AAT, an enzyme that is synthesized by cells in the lungs. This enzyme works to combat the destructive enzymes from digesting structural proteins and helps to maintain the integrity of the lungs. With emphysema, an imbalance of the destructive (proteolytic) and protective (antiproteolytic) enzymes exists, favoring the destructive. In smokers, lung destruction is a manifestation of excess proteinase release and a loss of antiproteinase defenses within the lungs.

The development of emphysema in nonsmokers is most often related to the manifestation of a genetic disorder attributed to a reduction or absence of antiprotease enzymes. In AAT deficiency, the affected individual has inherited an autosomal-codominant disorder located on the long arm of chromosome 14. In codominant disorders, the phenotype is expressed in the individual who has inherited two equally dominant genes. This genetic defect causes an acceleration of the breakdown of cells and tissues in the lungs with the early onset of panacinar emphysema.

CLINICAL MANIFESTATIONS

Clinical manifestations are related to obstruction of the small airways and alveoli, chronic hypoxemia, and hypercapnia. Most patients with emphysema have smoked heavily for 20 or more years and present with a chronic productive cough, most notable upon waking in the morning. Dyspnea and wheezing may occur with minimal exertion. As the disease progresses, a barrel chest develops because of chronic hyperinflation of the airways. Patients with emphysema commonly perform pursed lip breathing to increase the pressure in the airways, to prevent alveolar wall collapse, and to allow the air to escape the alveoli. In severe disease, simple activities, such as brushing one's teeth, can cause tachypnea and respiratory distress.

DIAGNOSTIC CRITERIA

Diagnosis of emphysema is based on a thorough patient history and physical examination, noting a significant smoking history and characteristic clinical manifestations. Expiratory airflow should be measured using pulmonary function tests. In nonsmokers who have suspected emphysema, AAT levels can be measured and will be found to be well below the expected range. In general, individuals with AAT deficiency and an increased risk for the development of emphysema will have 10% to 15% of the expected AAT level. Physical examination includes auscultation of lung sounds and observation of expiratory effort with simple activities. The respiratory rate tends to increase in proportion to disease severity. Cyanosis and peripheral edema may also be observed. Chest radiograph will show signs of hyperinflation.

Pulmonary function tests are critical in the diagnosis of emphysema and the level of airflow obstruction. Spirometry allows a determination of disease progression and the response to treatment. FEV_1 is the most common test to determine airflow obstruction; a prolonged forced expiratory time (FET) greater than 6 seconds indicates severe disease. Hypercapnia, measured in the arterial blood gas panel, is commonly observed when the FEV_1 falls below 30% of the predicted volume. For example, if a patient (based on age, gender, and height) is expected to forcefully exhale 4 L of air per second, hypercapnia will present when forced exhalation expels less than 1.2 L of air per second. This indicates severe outflow obstruction. Hypoxemia is often present in early disease and continues throughout the disease progression; however, hypercapnia predominates as the disease progresses.

TREATMENT

Because emphysema is irreversible, the goals of treatment are to maintain optimal lung function in order to allow the individual to perform the desired activities of daily living. Treatment begins with smoking cessation and may also include drug therapy (with danazol or tamoxifen) to increase production of AAT by the liver or by administering exogenous AAT via intravenous infusion or inhalation. Bronchodilators, steroid anti-inflammatory drugs, mucolytic agents (to reduce thickness and promote clearance of sputum), and antibiotics are the mainstays of therapy for individuals with emphysema. Supplemental oxygen is often required. Lung volume reduction or lung transplant are possible surgical treatment measures.

Chronic Bronchitis

Chronic bronchitis is defined by the presence of a persistent, productive cough with excessive mucous production that lasts for 3 months or longer for two or more consecutive years. The chronic bronchitis label is applied only after all other potential causes of chronic cough are excluded. The cause of chronic bronchitis is most commonly chronic smoking or exposure to environmental pollutants that irritate the airways.

PATHOPHYSIOLOGY

Chronic bronchitis results from several changes in the bronchi and bronchioles of the lungs in response to chronic injury including (Fig. 15.8):

- Chronic inflammation and edema of the airways
- Hyperplasia of the bronchial mucous glands and smooth muscles
- Destruction of cilia
- Squamous cell metaplasia
- Bronchial wall thickening and development of fibrosis

The chronic inflammatory process, metaplasia, fibrosis, and mucous gland hyperplasia cause airway deformities and obstruct airflow by narrowing the airway lumen and further occluding this narrowed lumen through overproducing mucus. This is particularly problematic in the smaller airways and

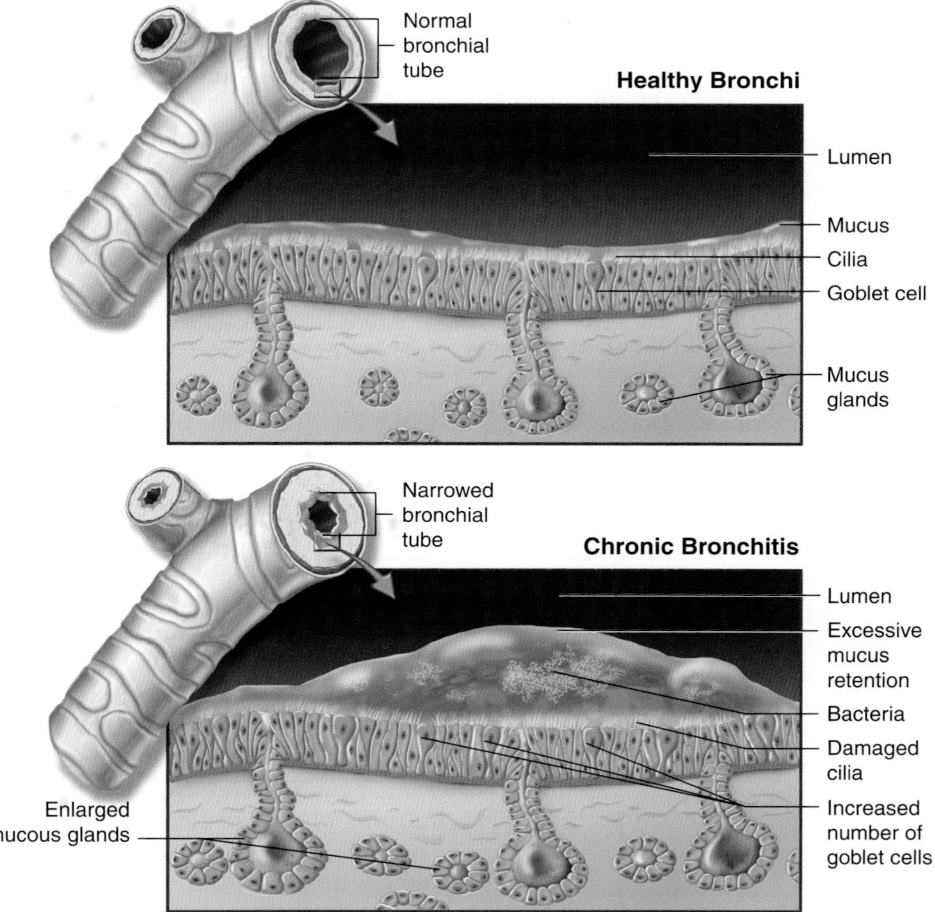

Figure 15.8. In chronic bronchitis, irritants inhaled for a prolonged period inflame the tracheobronchial tree. The inflammation leads to increased mucus production and a narrowed or blocked airway. As inflammation continues, the mucus-producing goblet cells undergo hypertrophy, as do the ciliated epithelial cells that line the respiratory tract. Hypersecretion from the goblet cells blocks the free movement of the cilia, which normally sweep dust, irritants, and mucus.

accounts for most airway obstructions. The loss of ciliated epithelium allows fine particles to enter the airway easily and predispose the individual to infection.

CLINICAL MANIFESTATIONS

The clinical manifestations of chronic bronchitis are often similar to that of emphysema because the two conditions often occur simultaneously. A chronic productive cough, often with purulent sputum, is frequent. Dyspnea occurs with minimal exertion. Chronic bronchitis leads to a prolonged expiratory phase along with wheezing and crackles upon auscultation of the lungs. Hypoxemia, hypercapnia, and cyanosis are more commonly found in those with chronic bronchitis compared with individuals with emphysema because of the presence of excessive bronchial mucus and obstructed ventilation.

DIAGNOSTIC CRITERIA

The diagnosis of chronic bronchitis is based on the clinical presentation of a persistent, productive cough over a period of 3 months or more within two consecutive years. A history of smoking is often present along with recurrent upper and lower respiratory infections. Arterial blood gases may be significant for hypoxemia and hypercapnia. Laboratory tests may indicate polycythemia (the overproduction of RBCs) as a compensatory measure to combat chronic hypoxemia. As with emphysema, pulmonary function tests are performed and demonstrate a reduction in FEV_1 and prolonged FET. Sputum specimens are often examined and tested for the presence of pathogens.

TREATMENT

As with emphysema, treatment of chronic bronchitis is aimed at alleviating symptoms, improving airway and lung function, slowing the progression of the disease, and improving overall quality of life. Treatment strategies are most effective when implemented early in the course of the disease. Smoking cessation is a critical component of success, as are pulmonary rehabilitation, bronchodilator therapy, steroid anti-inflammatory drugs, mucolytic agents, supplemental oxygen when indicated, and antibiotic therapy and immunizations to treat and protect against infection.

Asthma

Asthma is a chronic inflammatory disorder of the airways that results in intermittent or persistent airway obstruction because of bronchial hyperresponsiveness, inflammation, bronchoconstriction, and excess mucous production. The development of asthma often occurs in childhood, but the condition can emerge at any point in the life span. Worldwide, around 18.7 million adults have asthma.[2] Individuals most likely to develop asthma include those considered **atopic**, or having a genetic predisposition to developing hypersensitivities.

PATHOPHYSIOLOGY

Although the exact cause is unknown, asthma is increased in individuals who are frequently exposed to environmental allergens, such as cigarette smoke or dust mites. This discussion of asthma combines what is known about hypersensitivity reactions and the inflammatory process, because both of these concepts play a major role.

The inflammatory and immune response is often stimulated through exposure to an allergen. This allergen varies based on the individual and is often referred to as the asthma "trigger." Common environmental exposures that are known to result in hypersensitivity reactions and trigger the inflammatory response include smoke, dust, dust mites, mold, or animal hair. Other common triggers that can result in bronchospasm include exercise, temperature extremes, illness, and anxiety. Exercise-induced asthma (EIA) is a condition in which exercise or vigorous physical activity triggers acute bronchospasm, coughing, and wheezing in susceptible persons.

After an individual is exposed to the trigger, an IgE-mediated hypersensitivity reaction is immediate (Fig. 15.9A). IgE mast cells are stimulated to release chemical mediators. These chemical mediators promote increased edema and subsequent bronchoconstriction in the airways. Further products of inflammation then move into the area. Mast cells call forth additional chemical mediators, such as histamine and prostaglandins. Hours later, leukotrienes are released. These chemical mediators stimulate further bronchospasm, swelling, and excessive mucous production in the airways (Fig. 15.9B). The late inflammatory response occurs approximately 6 to 24 hours after exposure to the trigger and is marked by airway edema and the formation of mucous plugs from exudate and cell debris in the airways. The mucous plugs can take weeks to resolve. Over time, the cells of chronic inflammation, along with eosinophils, infiltrate the airways and cause destruction of the respiratory epithelium, smooth muscle hyperplasia, and narrowing of the airways. These structural changes, called airway remodeling, strongly affect the irreversibility of the condition.

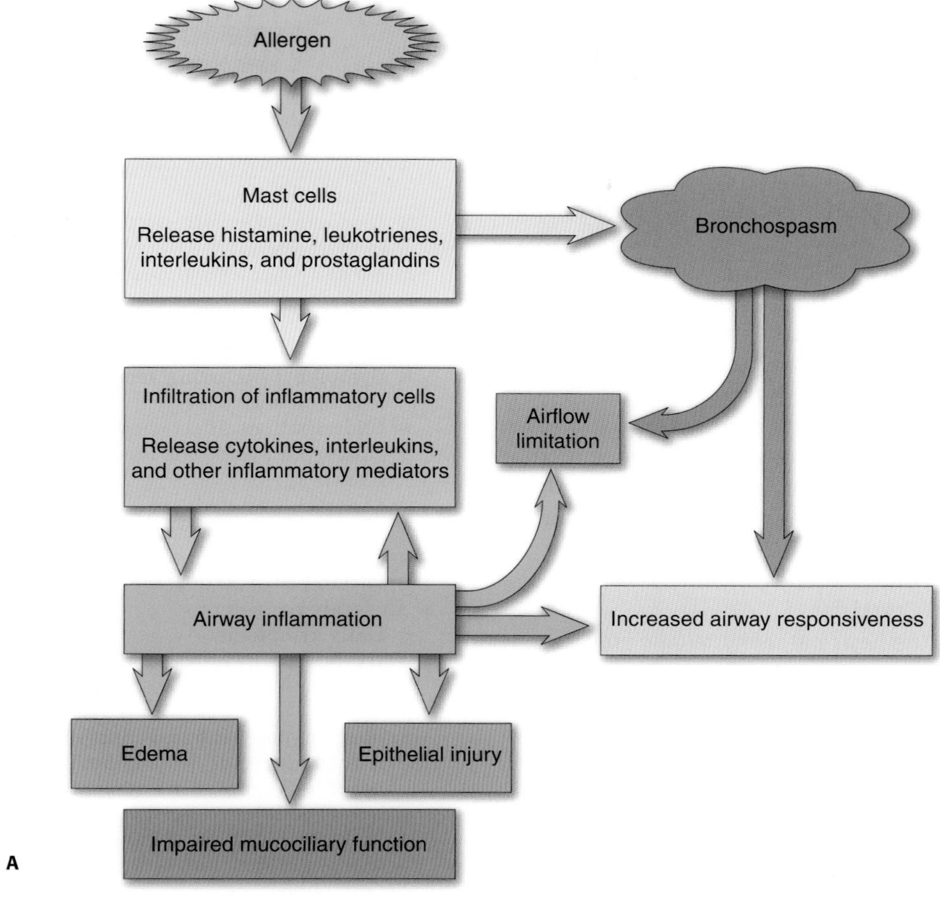

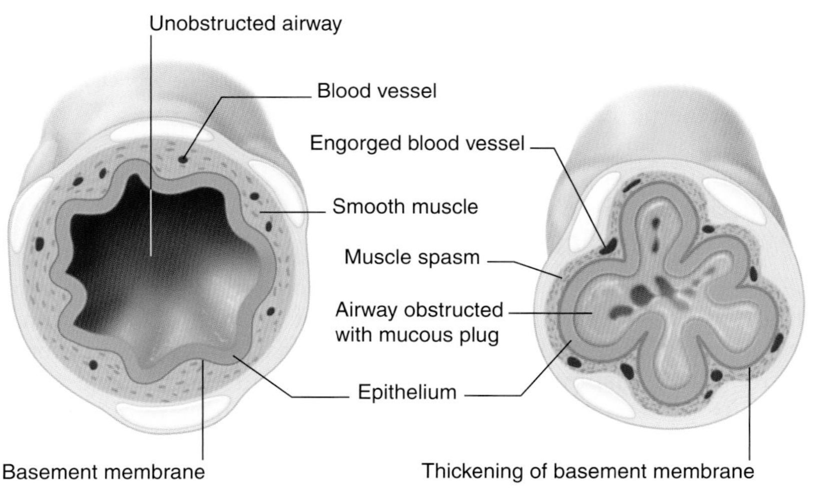

Figure 15.9. Asthma. **A:** Pathogenesis. (Modified from Porth CM. *Pathophysiology: Concepts of Altered Health States*. 7th ed. Philadelphia, PA: Lippincott Williams & Wilkins; 2004.) **B:** Narrowed bronchiole.

CLINICAL MANIFESTATIONS

Clinical manifestations depend on the state of airway hyperreactivity and inflammation. In periods of remission, the individual is symptom free. As an exacerbation is emerging, the individual may not notice any symptoms, although pulmonary function tests begin to decline. In times of exacerbation, hyperreactivity and inflammation in the airways causes wheezing, breathlessness, chest tightness, excessive sputum production, and coughing, particularly at night or in the early morning. During an asthma episode, the individual may exhibit anxiety, tachypnea, and the use of accessory muscles. Hyperventilation initially leads to respiratory alkalosis; however, compensation is usually temporary, and acidosis develops because of ineffective expiration. Even with a partial airway obstruction, hypoxia quickly results.

Stop and Consider

Based on the basic pathophysiologic processes, construct a treatment plan for a person with asthma. What environmental modifications would you make? What would be the goals of pharmacologic therapy?

DIAGNOSTIC CRITERIA

The patient may request an evaluation for asthma during a time of remission or may present to the health professional in acute distress. The diagnosis includes evaluating signs and symptoms and determining the triggers to determine the likelihood that the manifestations are actually attributable to asthma. The patient history is often significant for atopy or asthma in the family. The patient may or may not be currently experiencing the characteristic clinical manifestations. Physical findings indicative of asthma include:

- Evidence of respiratory distress
- Pulsus paradoxus, an exaggerated decrease in systolic blood pressure during inspiration
- Wheezing breath sounds
- A prolonged expiratory phase
- Atopic dermatitis, eczema, or other allergic skin conditions that may indicate hypersensitivities

Laboratory findings may reveal eosinophilia (indicating allergy) and arterial blood gases indicative of hypoxemia and hypercapnia. Pulse oximetry is useful in screening for hypoxemia and may be used to grade asthma severity. Spirometry is used to determine the effectiveness of airflow. The peak expiratory flow rate (PEFR) is a common measure used to track forced expiration. The peak flow meter is a convenient, portable, inexpensive tool. Measurements over time can provide information about the patient's response to therapy and can indicate the emergence of an asthma exacerbation. Chest radiograph may demonstrate hyperinflation or infiltrates of the lung fields and can be used to rule out other sources of pleuritic chest pain, such as pneumonia or **pneumothorax** (the presence of air in the pleural space that causes the lung to collapse). Once diagnosed, asthma can then be classified based on severity, frequency, and duration of disease. The classification guides treatment measures are found in Box 15.3.

Box 15.3 Asthma Classification and Treatment Based on Severity

- Mild intermittent
  - Intermittent symptoms occurring less than once a week with brief exacerbations
  - Nocturnal (nighttime) symptoms occurring less than twice a month
  - Asymptomatic with normal lung function between exacerbations
  - No daily medication needed
  - FEV_1 or PEFR greater than 80%, with less than 20% variability
- Mild persistent
  - Symptoms occurring more than once a week but less than once a day
  - Exacerbations affect activity and sleep
  - Nocturnal symptoms occurring more than twice a month
  - Low-dose inhaled anti-inflammatory one to four times per day and inhaled bronchodilator as needed
  - FEV_1 or PEFR greater than 80% predicted, with variability of 20 to 30%
- Moderate persistent
  - Daily symptoms
  - Exacerbations affect activity and sleep
  - Nocturnal symptoms occurring more than once a week
  - Medium-dose inhaled anti-inflammatory one to four times per day, a long-acting bronchodilator, especially for nighttime symptoms, and short-acting bronchodilator as needed
  - FEV_1 or PEFR 60 to 80% of predicted, with variability greater than 30%
- Severe persistent
  - Continuous symptoms with frequent exacerbations, nocturnal asthma symptoms
  - Physical activities limited by asthma symptoms
  - High-dose inhaled and oral anti-inflammatory, a long-acting bronchodilator, and short-acting bronchodilator as needed
  - FEV_1 or PEFR less than 60%, with variability greater than 30%

TREATMENT

The treatment of asthma is comprised of four major components:

1. Monitoring lung function through peak flow testing

2. Controlling environmental triggers
3. Pharmacologic therapy to reverse inflammation, bronchoconstriction, and mucous secretion
4. Patient education to facilitate adherence to the treatment plan

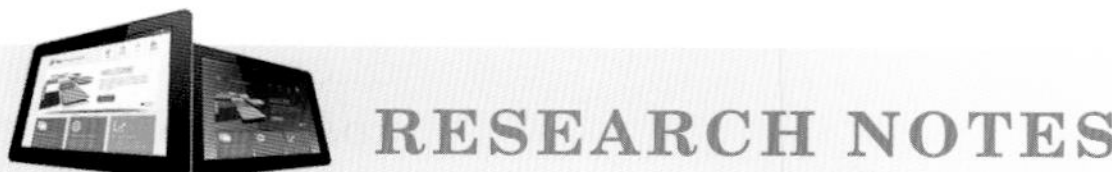

RESEARCH NOTES

Alternative and complementary therapies have been implemented as possible treatments for conditions of altered ventilation and diffusion. One group of researchers explored the effectiveness of acupressure in promoting relaxation, decreasing anxiety, and alleviating dyspnea in patients with COPD. In this randomized clinical trial, patients were either provided true acupoint acupressure or a sham treatment. Those patients undergoing true acupoint acupressure demonstrated significant improvements in pulmonary function, dyspnea scores, 6-minute walking distance measurements, and state anxiety scale scores.[3]

A written action plan is an essential aspect of care for the individual with asthma. The action plan outlines methods for avoiding triggers and describes what to do when an asthma exacerbation is occurring. The plan is based on the measurement of the PEFR using a peak flow meter. The individual determines his or her highest PEFR, or "personal best," over a symptom-free period of 1 to 3 weeks. The inability to expire at or above 80% of the personal best requires attention because an asthma exacerbation may be occurring.

Pharmacologic treatments are prescribed based on the classification of asthma severity. Medications used to treat asthma are divided into two major categories: bronchodilators and anti-inflammatory drugs. Inhaled beta$_2$-adrenergic agonists (bronchodilators), such as albuterol, provide quick relief of bronchoconstriction and can prevent EIA. Anticholinergics and methylxanthines are other drug categories used to promote bronchodilation. These medications relax the smooth muscles of the airway but do not effectively reduce airway inflammation. Long-term control medications, such as glucocorticoids, cromolyn, and leukotriene modifiers, are needed to prevent the frequency and severity of the inflammatory component of asthma. These medications also prevent chronic damage to the airways. For example, inhaled glucocorticoids suppress the activation of mast cells and other components active in inflammation and decrease airway hyperreactivity.

Asthma, although most often reversible, can lead to total airway obstruction if the inflammation is severe. In **status asthmaticus**, or intractable asthma, bronchospasm is not reversed by the patient's medications or other measures. Obstruction leads to decreased expiration, air trapping, hypoxemia, hypercapnia, and acidosis. Absent lung sounds and significant elevations in the $Pa{CO_2}$ (above 70 mm Hg) indicate a poor prognosis. Status asthmaticus is life-threatening and requires immediate emergency treatment.

Cystic Fibrosis

Cystic fibrosis (CF) is an autosomal recessive disorder of electrolytes and subsequently water transport that affects certain epithelial cells, such as those lining respiratory, digestive, and reproductive tracts. CF most commonly affects Caucasians of European descent and is the most common lethal inherited disease in that group. Incidence appears greatest in homogenous populations. This disorder leads to the production of excessive and thick exocrine secretions (e.g., mucus) leading to obstruction, inflammation, and infection. CF is also associated with impaired local immune defenses in the lungs as well as pancreatic insufficiency. Most affected individuals are diagnosed by 1 year of age. A small percentage of individuals exhibit a mild presentation and are not diagnosed until after 10 years of age. End-stage lung disease is the most common cause of death.

PATHOPHYSIOLOGY

Cystis fibrosis is caused by a mutation of the CF (also called the cystic fibrosis transmembrane conductance regulator, or CFTCR) gene located on the long arm of chromosome 7. Because CF is an autosomal recessive disease, a deleterious mutation is required on both inherited CFTCR alleles for development of the disease. More than 1,000 possible CFTCR mutations, if found on both alleles in any combination, have been identified. Consistent with autosomal recessive inheritance, those with one mutated allele and one nonmutated allele are considered carriers and have no symptoms of the disease.

The CFTCR mutation leads to impaired electrolyte transportation across epithelial cells on mucosal surfaces (Fig. 15.10). For example, the effective functioning of chloride ion channels depends on CFTCR, which encodes for a protein that serves as a chloride channel and is regulated by cyclic adenosine monophosphate (cAMP). Mutations in the gene for CFTCR lead to impairment in the cAMP-regulated chloride transport across many different types of epithelial cells on mucosal surfaces, such as those found lining the respiratory tract, pancreas, bile ducts, sweat ducts, and vas deferens. The inability of these epithelial cells to conduct chloride and therefore transport water across the mucosal surfaces leads to thick

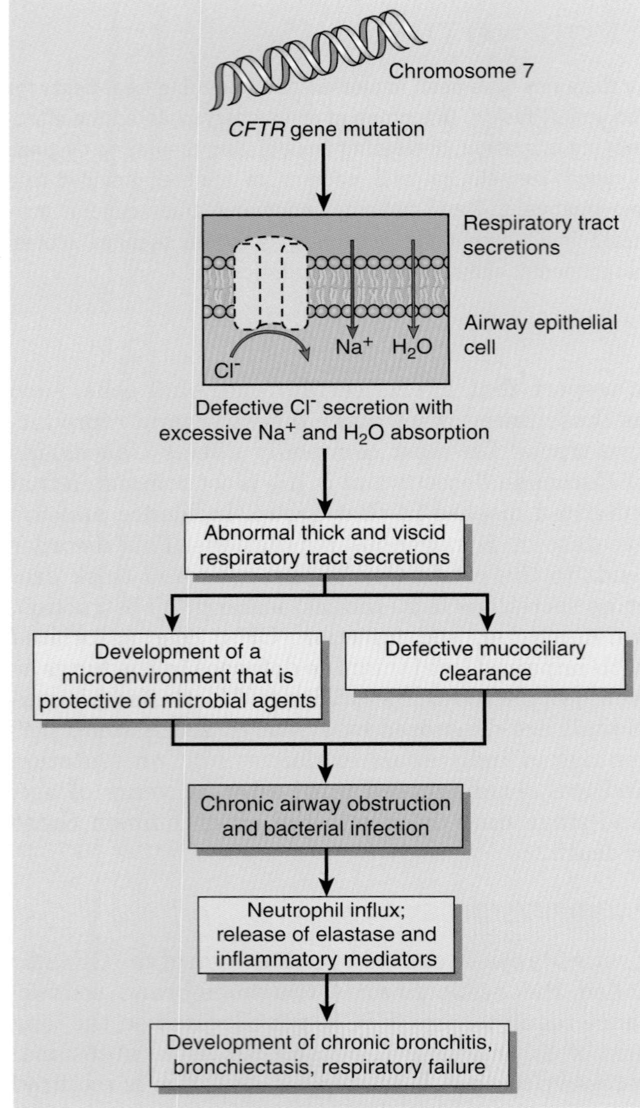

Figure 15.10. Pathogenesis of cystic fibrosis.

secretions and obstruction in the respiratory tract, pancreas, gastrointestinal tract, sweat glands, and other exocrine tissues. Although the manifestations appear mostly related to impaired transport of electrolytes, the complete mechanism of disease, particularly those leading to the complications associated with the lungs, is unknown.

CF is most strongly associated with mucous plugging, inflammation, and infection in the lungs with respiratory failure as the most common cause of death. Mucous plugging is a result of:

- A greater volume of mucus produced by a larger number of mucous-secreting cells in the airways
- Airway dehydration and thickened mucus caused by impaired chloride secretion, excessive sodium absorption, and decreased water content in the airway tissues
- Adherence of the mucus to the epithelium with impaired ciliary action required to clear the mucus from the airways

Mucous plugging, the formation of tenacious secretions, and a reduced ability to clear the secretions are optimal conditions for the growth and retention of bacteria. Progressive lung disease often begins shortly after birth with the emergence of a persistent respiratory infection. Impairment of local immune function leads to failure of opsonization and phagocytosis and contributes to this persistent lung infection with distinctive bacteria, such as *Staphylococcus aureus* and *Pseudomonas aeruginosa*. The progression from bronchitis to bronchiolitis, to bronchiectasis, and eventually to permanent lung damage largely depends on an intense, chronic inflammatory response dominated by neutrophils. The significance of the excessive presence of neutrophils is the release of proteases by these cells. Proteases promote an intense inflammatory response, cause destruction of lung tissue, inhibit destruction or neutralization of bacteria, and promote additional mucous production. Over time, the airways and lung tissue in CF are characterized by air trapping, hyperinflation, abscess formation, lung tissue consolidation, persistent pneumonia, lung tissue fibrosis, and cyst formation, hence the name CF. Erosion of lung tissues and nearby bronchial arteries can lead to hemoptysis. Eventually, pulmonary involvement can lead to right-sided heart failure (cor pulmonale) and end-stage lung disease.

CF also has effects that go beyond ventilation and diffusion. Reduced chloride secretion and restricted water into the intestinal tract (along with inflammation, scarring, and strictures) lead to obstruction of intestinal contents. Along with intestinal motility problems, most individuals with CF (90% to 95%) have pancreatic insufficiency. Pancreatic insufficiency decreases digestion and the absorption of intestinal contents. The role of pancreatic enzymes, digestion, and absorption is described in detail in Chapter 17. The liver may also be affected in CF because the mutation of CFTCR leads to impairment of passive transport of chloride and water across the epithelial cells that line the biliary ductules. This leads to an increased viscosity of bile. Biliary obstruction can lead to obstructive cirrhosis.

CLINICAL MANIFESTATIONS

The presenting clinical manifestations, age at diagnosis, symptom severity, and rate of disease progression vary widely among individuals with CF. Clinical manifestations are associated with tenacious (thick) secretions leading to respiratory and gastrointestinal impairment. Recurrent respiratory infections, along with a chronic cough often accompanied by mucoid or purulent sputum, are common manifestations of CF. Coughing can be forceful and can lead to vomiting. Other respiratory manifestations include tachypnea, recurrent wheezing or crackles, hemoptysis, dyspnea on exertion, chest pain, and respiratory distress with chest retractions, cyanosis, barrel chest, recurrent sinusitis, and the development of nasal polyps. Finger clubbing can also be caused by chronic hypoxia.

Newborns may present with intestinal obstruction (a meconium ileus) at birth with a delayed or absent passage of meconium stool. Infants and children most commonly demonstrate increased frequency of large, greasy, malodorous stools, which indicate fat malabsorption. This condition can be accompanied by recurrent abdominal pain, distention, and poor absorption of fat-soluble vitamins. Weight loss or poor weight gain is common. Additional clinical manifestations include sweat abnormalities and excessive salt depletion. A child, when kissed by a caregiver, may have a salty taste to the skin. Jaundice, gastrointestinal bleeding, and rectal prolapse may occur.

Males with CF are frequently sterile because of an absence of the vas deferens. The male child may also have undescended testicles or hydrocele. Secondary sexual development is often delayed in females with CF, although fertility is maintained or somewhat decreased.

DIAGNOSTIC CRITERIA

The diagnosis of CF is based on a thorough patient history and physical examination, noting the characteristic clinical manifestations. The diagnosis can be confirmed by a sweat test, which will reveal a sweat chloride concentration of 60 mEq/L or greater. Values of 40 to 60 mEq/L are considered borderline, and the test must be repeated because values in this range can be inconsistent with the diagnosis in some patients with typical features. Genetic testing may be performed to detect certain CFTCR mutations. The identification of two CFTCR mutations with associated clinical symptoms is diagnostic; however, negative results on genotype analysis do not exclude the diagnosis. The ability to sequence the entire gene will enable clinicians to detect all known mutations in any given individual and will have greater reliability in diagnosing CF. Other diagnostic tests, such as chest and sinus radiography and sputum analysis, can also contribute to the diagnosis. Chest radiography will reveal hyperinflation and peribronchial thickening. Sinusitis throughout all sinuses is uncommon in children and young adults, and its presence strongly suggests CF. The fluid obtained from a bronchoalveolar lavage usually shows a high percentage of neutrophils and the detection of *Pseudomonas aeruginosa* supports the diagnosis of CF in an individual without the typical presentation. Because early detection and treatment is critical in the course and prognosis of disease, newborn screening has been recommended in many developed countries.

TREATMENT

Treatment goals for CF involve maximizing ventilation, diffusion, and nutrition through:

- Liquefying and clearing the airways of mucus
- Avoiding and controlling respiratory infections
- Reducing inflammation and promoting bronchodilation in the airways
- Providing or encouraging optimal nutrition through the use of enzyme supplements to reduce malabsorption, multivitamin and mineral supplements, and a high-calorie diet
- Managing disease complications, such as diabetes mellitus, bowel obstruction, fatty liver, biliary cirrhosis, and portal hypertension

Individuals with end-stage lung disease may consider lung transplantation. Currently, the median age of survival is 30 years; males survive significantly longer than females, although many individuals with CF are living into their 40s and 50s.

Acute Respiratory Distress Syndrome

ARDS is a condition of severe acute inflammation and pulmonary edema without evidence of fluid overload or impaired cardiac function (Fig. 15.11). This condition was previously referred to as adult respiratory distress syndrome, but ARDS does occur in children.

PATHOPHYSIOLOGY

Damage to the alveolar epithelium and vascular endothelium triggers the onset of severe inflammation. Injury can result from inhalation of excessive smoke or toxic chemicals, overwhelming lung infections, aspiration of gastric contents into the lungs, lung trauma, anaphylaxis, lack of pulmonary blood flow, and other conditions that impair the alveoli. The presence of sepsis (bacterial infection in the blood) and the systemic inflammatory response syndrome (SIRS) are clinical conditions associated with the development of ARDS. In ARDS, the time from lung injury to respiratory distress is about 24 to 48 hours.

The inflammatory response is consistent with the process discussed in Chapter 3. Chemical mediators promote vasodilation and increased capillary permeability in the lungs. Inflammatory cells, proteins,

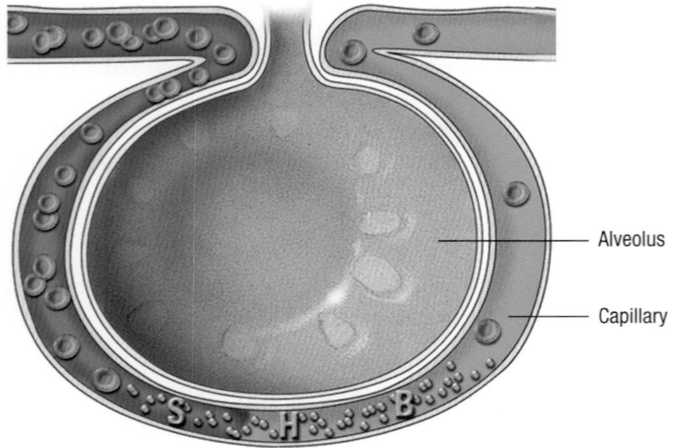

Phase 1. Injury reduces blood flow to the lungs. Platelets aggregate and release histamine (H), serotonin (S), and bradykinin (B).

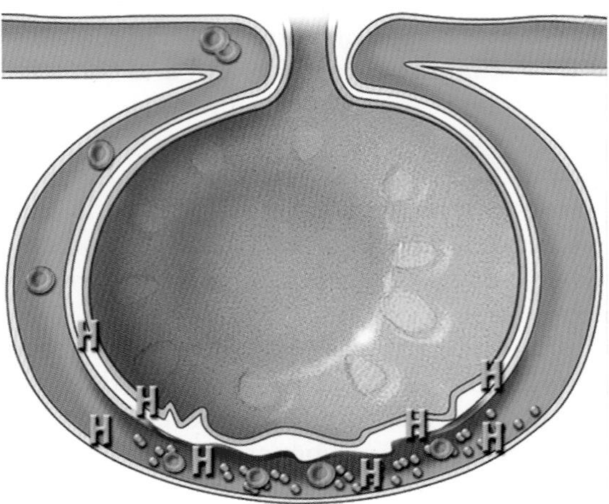

Phase 2. Those substances, especially histamine, inflame and damage the alveolocapillary membrane, increasing capillary permeability. Fluids then shift into the interstitial space.

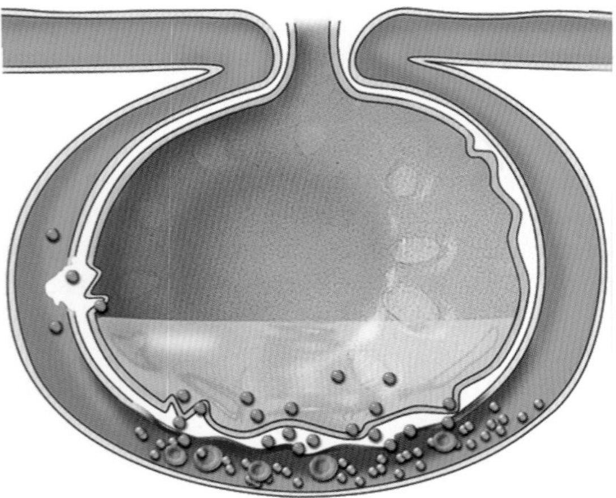

Phase 3. As capillary permeability increases, proteins and fluids leak out, increasing interstitial osmotic pressure and causing pulmonary edema.

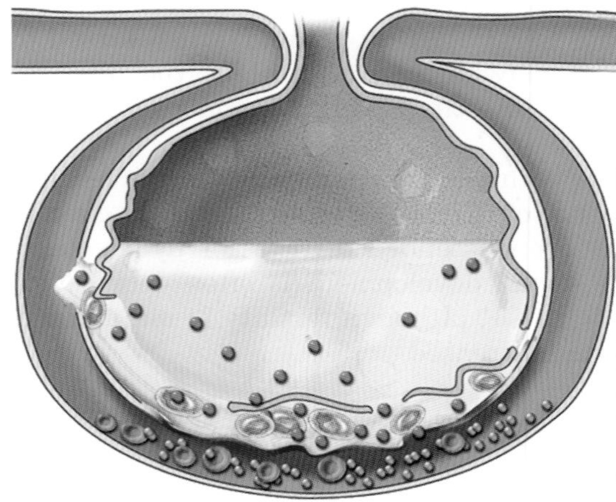

Phase 4. Decreased blood flow and fluids in the alveoli damage surfactant and impair the cell's ability to produce more. As a result, alveoli collapse, impeding gas exchange and decreasing lung compliance.

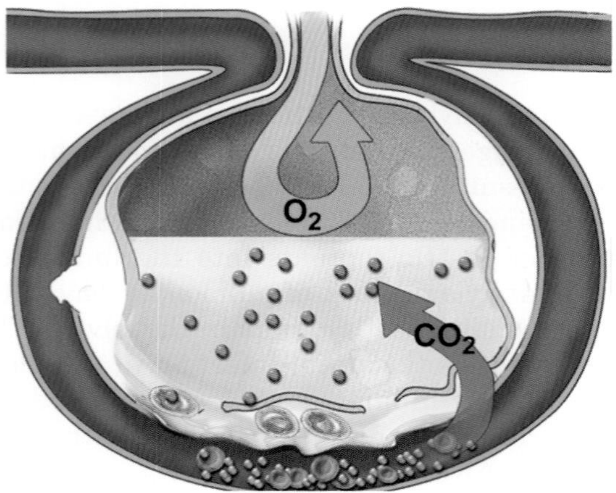

Phase 5. Sufficient oxygen can't cross the alveolocapillary membrane, but carbon dioxide (CO_2) can and is lost with every exhalation. Oxygen (O_2) and CO_2 levels decrease in the blood.

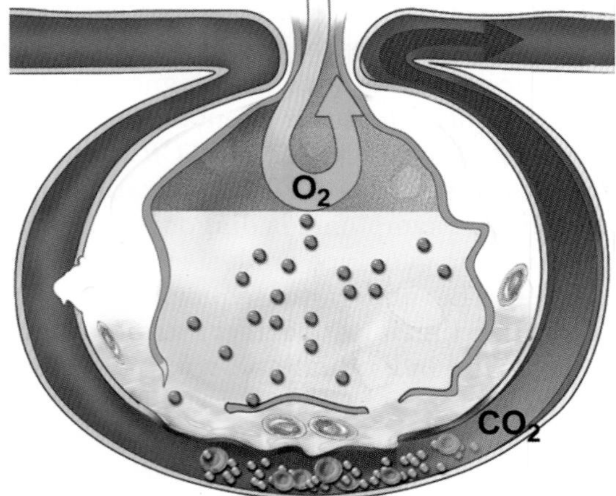

Phase 6. Pulmonary edema worsens, inflammation leads to fibrosis, and gas exchange is further impeded.

Figure 15.11. Phases of acute respiratory distress syndrome. (Courtesy Anatomical Chart Company.)

Box 15.4 Potential Causes of Atelectasis

Atelectasis, a condition of collapse and nonaeration of the alveoli can have a number of causes, including:

- *Compression* of the alveoli by a mass or fluid accumulation, such as with a tumor or pleural effusion, which exerts pressure on the lung and prevents air from entering the alveoli
- *Obstruction*, which prevents air from entering the airways and alveoli; existing air is reabsorbed into the tissues and the alveoli become empty
- *Destruction* of surfactant, as with the inflammatory response, increases surface tension in the alveoli and promotes collapse
- *Fibrosis*, such as with emphysema, restricts alveolar expansion and promotes collapse

and fluids escape the intravascular space and leak into the interstitium (lung tissues) and alveolar space, resulting in pulmonary edema, which damages the alveolar capillary junction. Damage to type II alveolar cells, increased protein, and fluid accumulation disrupts the production of surfactant resulting in **atelectasis** (alveolar nonaeration and collapse). Other potential causes of atelectasis are summarized in Box 15.4. Initially, oxygen diffusion is greatly impaired, but CO_2 is still able to cross the alveolar capillary junction to be expired. As the process of alveolar impairment advances, a hyaline membrane forms, and CO_2 release is also interrupted. The hyaline membrane is a thin, clear-basement membrane that is impervious to gases. This leads to a state of impaired ventilation and diffusion marked by poor lung expansion, hypoxemia, hypercapnia, and acidosis.

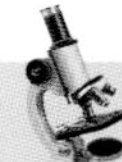

FROM THE LAB

Arterial blood gas analyses are the method of measuring arterial blood and determining levels of pH, Pao_2, and $Paco_2$. In respiratory failure, pH falls below 7.3, Pao_2 falls below 50 mm Hg (the expected range is 80 to 100 mm Hg), and $Paco_2$ rises above 50 mm Hg (the expected range is 35 to 45 mm Hg).

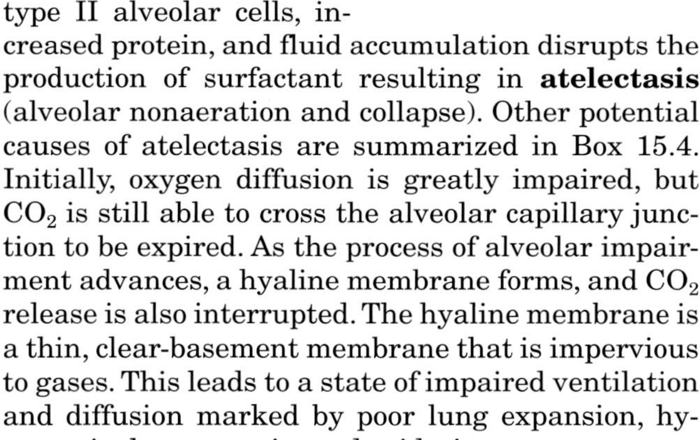

ARDS can be reversed if the symptoms are identified early. Healing involves reabsorption of the alveolar edema, regeneration of the epithelial cells and type II alveolar cells, and structural remodeling of the airway. In some cases, the patient has an uncomplicated acute inflammatory response with rapid resolution. Other patients experience a permanent loss of lung volume and function attributed to lung tissue edema, necrosis, and alveolar fibrosis in affected areas. If untreated, death can ensue within 48 hours. The mortality rate, as a result of multisystem organ failure, is approximately 30% to 40%.

CLINICAL MANIFESTATIONS

Early clinical manifestations include tachypnea, dyspnea, retractions, crackles caused by fluid accumulation, and restlessness. Some patients may present in the course of disease without any signs or symptoms except for mild tachypnea. Within 48 hours, severe respiratory distress becomes apparent.

DIAGNOSTIC CRITERIA

The diagnosis of ARDS is based on a careful patient history, physical examination, laboratory, and imaging studies. A high index of suspicion is required when encountering any individual who has lung injury. Arterial blood gases often depict hypoxemia with early respiratory alkalosis quickly progressing to hypercapnia and respiratory alkalosis. Blood cultures may be needed to detect sepsis, the most common cause of ARDS. Chest radiograph is often normal early in the course of disease but then reveals bilateral diffuse infiltrates advancing to total opacity as the disease progresses.

TREATMENT

Treatment strategies are supportive and focused on removing the causative factors triggering the inflammatory response. Administration of 100% oxygen is often warranted to keep oxygen saturations above 90%. If the oxygen saturations remain below this level and the patient becomes fatigued or acidotic, intubation with mechanical ventilation may be necessary. If mechanical ventilation is ineffective in maintaining oxygen saturations above 90%, positive end-expiratory pressure (PEEP) is instituted to maintain pressure in the airways during expiration and promote reinflation of alveoli. In patients with ARDS, maintenance of adequate alveolar ventilation is an important marker for survival.

SUMMARY

- The process of ventilation involves both acquiring oxygen (inspiration) and removing carbon dioxide (expiration) from the blood.
- The transport of oxygen through the lungs is the *only* mechanism for acquiring oxygen.
- Oxygen is necessary for cellular metabolism, which means that for the cell to expend energy

efficiently and perform its designated function, oxygen must be present.

- Optimal cell functioning occurs within a narrow pH range, and the release and retention of carbon dioxide is one mechanism for maintaining this balance.
- Oxygen and carbon dioxide are exchanged at the alveolar capillary junctions in the process of diffusion.
- Impaired ventilation is a problem of blocking airflow in and out of the lungs, thereby restricting oxygen intake and carbon dioxide removal from the body. Two major mechanisms are implicated: (1) compression or narrowing of the airways and (2) disruption of the neuronal transmissions needed to stimulate the mechanics of breathing.
- Impaired diffusion is a process of restricting the transfer of oxygen or carbon dioxide across the alveolar capillary junction. Because the rate of diffusion depends on the solubility and partial pressure of the gas, *and* surface area and thickness of the membrane, impaired gas exchange can occur with changes in any of these properties.
- Any situation that presents a demand for higher levels of oxygen or an increase in cellular metabolism requires pulmonary adaptation to maintain homeostasis, because oxygen deprivation and carbon dioxide retention affect all cells in the body.
- The major implications of altered ventilation and diffusion include hypoxemia, hypoxia, hypercapnia, and acidosis.
- Local manifestations of impaired ventilation and diffusion include cough, mucous production, sputum changes, dyspnea, use of accessory muscles, adventitious lung sounds, chest pain, barrel chest, and pursed lip breathing.
- Systemic manifestations of altered ventilation are caused by the effects of inflammation, hypoxemia, hypoxia, and hypercapnia. These manifestations include fever, malaise, leukocytosis, cyanosis, changes in arterial blood gases, mental status changes, and finger clubbing.

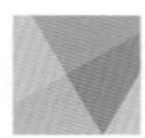

CASE STUDY 15.1

A 6-month-old child has an acute respiratory syncytial virus (RSV) infection, which is an acute viral infection in the lungs. Think about which clinical model discussed in this chapter is most related to this process. From your reading and experience regarding infectious processes and now altered ventilation and diffusion, answer the following questions:

1. What process is most likely occurring in this child's body?
2. What are the probable ventilation and diffusion effects of exposure to this virus?
3. What would you expect for clinical manifestations?
4. What diagnostic tests could be used?
5. What treatment measures would you anticipate?

Log on to the Internet. Search for a relevant journal article or Web site, such as http://emedicine.medscape.com/article/971488-overview, that details RSV, and confirm your predictions.

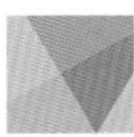

CASE STUDY 15.2

Joan accompanies her husband Dan to the clinic and reports to the nurse that Dan's snoring seems to be getting worse over the past year. She has resorted to sleeping in a nearby bedroom with earplugs. Dan states that when he wakes up he doesn't feel that rested, although he does refer to himself as a "good sleeper" and states he is "able to fall asleep easily." Dan undergoes a sleep study and is diagnosed with obstructive sleep apnea. Think about which clinical model discussed in this chapter is most related to this process. From your reading and experience regarding obstructed ventilation, answer the following questions:

1. What process is most likely occurring in this man's body?
2. What are the probable ventilation and diffusion effects from obstructive sleep apnea?
3. What would you expect for clinical manifestations?
4. What diagnostic tests could be used?
5. What treatment measures would you anticipate?

Log on to the Internet. Search for a relevant journal article or Web site, such as http://emedicine.med scape.com/article/295807-overview, that details obstructive sleep apnea, and confirm your predictions.

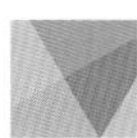

CASE STUDY 15.3

Patty has just undergone abdominal hysterectomy and, due to complications, has been bed-bound for a week. She develops an abrupt onset of chest pain and shortness of breath. She is taken to the emergency department and diagnosed with a pulmonary embolism, which is a blockage in one of her blood vessels in the lungs, most likely from a thrombus that traveled from her legs. Think about which clinical model discussed in this chapter is most related to this process. From your reading and experience regarding ventilation and diffusion, answer the following questions:

1. What process is most likely occurring in this woman's body?

2. What are the probable ventilation and diffusion effects from a pulmonary embolism?
3. What would you expect for clinical manifestations?
4. What diagnostic tests could be used?
5. What treatment measures would you anticipate?

Log on to the Internet. Search for a relevant journal article or Web site, such as http://emedicine.medscape.com/article/300901-overview, that details pulmonary embolism, and confirm your predictions.

PRACTICE EXAM QUESTIONS

1. Which of the following does *not* affect diffusing capacity?
   a. The partial pressure of oxygen and carbon dioxide
   b. The alveolar surface area
   c. The density of the alveolar membrane
   d. The volume of air in the atmosphere

2. *Total* obstruction of the airway by aspirated material is manifested by:
   a. Hoarse cough
   b. Rapid loss of consciousness
   c. Dyspnea
   d. Inflammation of the mucosa

3. A reduced number of erythrocytes (RBCs) in the blood results in the following change in the oxygen saturation ($Sa{O_2}$) of the blood:
   a. The $Sa{O_2}$ would increase
   b. The $Sa{O_2}$ would decrease
   c. The number of RBCs will not affect the $Sa{O_2}$
   d. There will be a decrease only if the osmotic pressure of the blood is also decreased

4. Which is a major cause of respiratory failure?
   a. Aspiration
   b. Atelectasis
   c. Sepsis
   d. All of these

5. Emphysema differs from chronic bronchitis in that emphysema:
   a. Is characterized by mucous production and inflammation
   b. Obstructs the large airways
   c. Obstructs the alveoli
   d. There are no differences between the two conditions

6. You have admitted a 20-year-old male to the emergency room with a history of asthma. He is having an acute asthma attack and is wheezing, fighting for air, hypoxic, and afraid. What is causing these acute symptoms?
   a. Relaxation of bronchial smooth muscle with dry mucous membranes
   b. Constriction of the bronchial smooth muscle and air trapping
   c. Acute destruction of lung tissue
   d. Contraction of the elastic fibers of the lung

7. Which of the following clinical manifestations are related to hypoxemia?
   a. Cyanosis
   b. Cough
   c. Chest pain
   d. Hemoptysis

8. How would you know you have hypoxemia?
   a. Radiograph
   b. Measure the partial pressure of oxygen in blood
   c. Measure the partial pressure of carbon dioxide in blood
   d. All of these detect hypoxemia

9. Which of the following can trigger acute respiratory distress syndrome?
   a. Severe lung infection
   b. Inhaling toxic fumes
   c. Aspirating stomach contents into the lungs
   d. All of these

10. What is the major problem in cystic fibrosis?
    a. Formation of cysts in fibrotic tissues
    b. Pancreatitis
    c. Lung injury
    d. Electrolyte and water transport

11. Which of the following diseases is most likely the cause of your patient's barrel chest?
    a. Emphysema
    b. Pneumonia
    c. Tuberculosis
    d. Acute respiratory distress syndrome

12. Which of the following is least likely to be a part of the daily routine for a patient with severe asthma?
    a. Inhaled bronchodilators
    b. Inhaled corticosteroids
    c. Oxygen therapy
    d. Avoiding triggers

13. If a patient gets air in his or her pleural space, this results in:
    a. Pneumonia
    b. Pneumothorax
    c. Pleuritis
    d. Plethora

14. Which of the following pathways best describes the pathophysiology of acute respiratory distress syndrome?
    a. Injury–inflammation–pulmonary edema–alveolar collapse–hypoxemia–fibrosis
    b. Infection–edema–fibrosis–hypoxemia–alveolar collapse–pulmonary edema
    c. Genetic mutation–sodium transport impaired–mucous stasis–infection–hypoxemia
    d. Trigger–inflammation–airway constriction–alveolar collapse–hypoxemia–fibrosis

DISCUSSION AND APPLICATION

1. What did I know about altered ventilation and diffusion prior to today?
2. What body processes are affected by altered ventilation and diffusion? What are the expected functions of those processes? How does altered ventilation and diffusion affect those processes?
3. What are the potential etiologies for altered ventilation and diffusion? How does altered ventilation and diffusion develop?
4. Who is most at risk for developing altered ventilation and diffusion? How can altered ventilation and diffusion be prevented?
5. What are the human differences that affect the etiology, risk, or course of altered ventilation and diffusion?
6. What clinical manifestations are expected in the course of altered ventilation and diffusion?
7. What special diagnostic tests help determine the diagnosis and course of altered ventilation and diffusion?
8. What are the goals of care for individuals with altered ventilation and diffusion?
9. How does the concept of altered ventilation and diffusion build on what I have learned in the previous chapters and in previous courses?
10. How can I use what I have learned?

RESOURCES

The American Lung Association is an important source of information related to several types of lung diseases and includes current research updates at: http://www.lung.org

The Cystic Fibrosis Foundation provides guidelines, reports, and other resources at: https://www.cff.org/

The Global Initiative for Asthma provides guidelines, reports, and other resources at: http://www.ginasthma.org/GuidelinesResources.asp?l1=2&l2=0

References

1. Burns KE, Meade MO, Premji A, et al. Noninvasive positive-pressure ventilation as a weaning strategy for intubated adults with respiratory failure. *Cochrane Database Syst Rev*. 2013;12:CD004127. doi:10.1002/14651858.CD004127.pub3.
2. Center for Disease Control and Prevention, National Center for Health Statistics. FastStat Health Statistics 2015. http://www.cdc.gov/nchs/fastats/asthma.htm. Accessed December 19, 2015.
3. Wu H, Wu S, Lin J, et al. Effectiveness of acupressure in improving dyspnea in chronic obstructive pulmonary disease. *J Adv Nurs.* 2004;45(3):252–259.

Find additional resources for this chapter at http:thePoint.lww.com thePoint®

Altered Perfusion

Chapter

16

LEARNING OUTCOMES

1. Define and use the key terms listed in this chapter.
2. Explain the role of perfusion in maintaining health.
3. Identify the key requirements for effective perfusion.
4. Determine processes that can alter perfusion.
5. Identify the common signs and symptoms of altered perfusion.
6. Describe diagnostic tests and treatment strategies relevant to altered perfusion.
7. Apply concepts of altered tissue perfusion to select clinical models.

INTRODUCTION

Think for a moment about the magnitude of a beating heart. Your heart beats about 70 times a minute, every minute of every day of every year of every decade of your life. Without fail, the heart beats, for without it we would die. What is it about the beating heart that keeps us alive? What other factors play a role in perfusing the body? What effect does reduction in perfusion have on the body? This chapter takes a careful look at these questions.

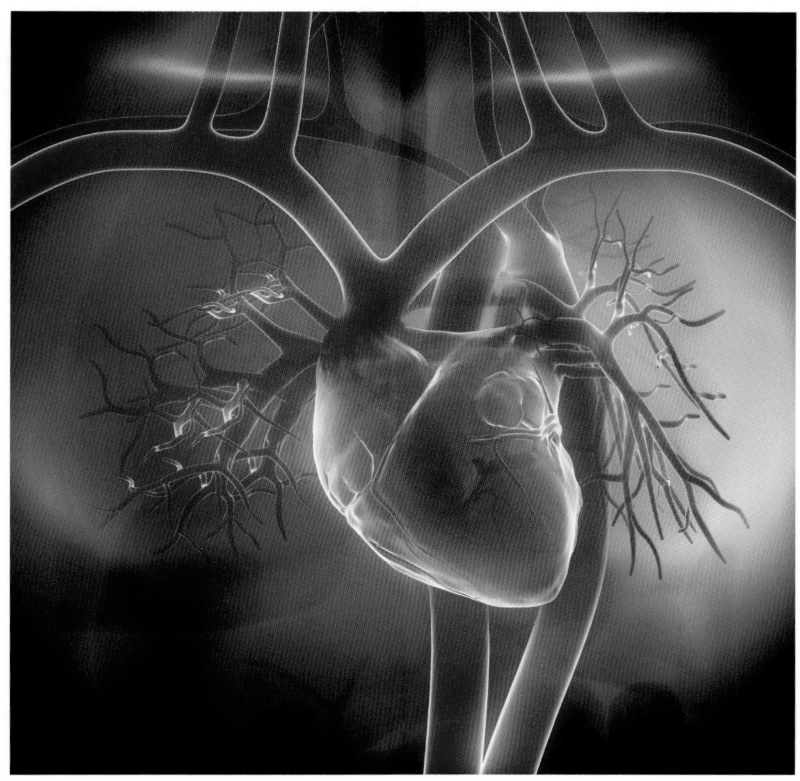

Pulmonary trunk, vein, and aorta in heart. Image © CLIPAREA

Module 1 Perfusion

Perfusion is the process of forcing blood or other fluid to flow through a vessel and into the vascular bed of a tissue to provide oxygen and other nutrients. Requirements for effective perfusion include:

- **Adequate ventilation and diffusion:** The ability to breathe in and transport oxygen across the capillaries is mandatory for effective distribution of oxygen to the tissues.
- **Intact pulmonary circulation:** Pulmonary circulation is required for the uptake of oxygen from inspired air.
- **Adequate blood volume and components:** An expected blood volume is required to carry oxygen (on hemoglobin) and maintain blood pressure. The role of hemoglobin and oxygen saturation in the blood is discussed in Chapter 15.
- **Adequate cardiac output:** An optimal stroke volume, an optimal heart rate, and an efficient heart rhythm are needed to maximize perfusion to the tissues.
- **Intact cardiac control center in the medulla of the brain:** The cardiac control center is needed to regulate heart rate and force of cardiac contractions, and to detect and respond to changes in blood pressure.
- **Intact receptors:** Receptors play a major role in sensing changes in cardiac function and blood pressure, and they provide feedback to the cardiac control center in the brain.
- **Intact parasympathetic and sympathetic nervous systems:** The autonomic nervous system is responsible for mediating changes in the cardiovascular system based on demands.
- **Intact cardiac conduction:** Conduction of impulses is essential in stimulating cardiac contractility.
- **Intact coronary circulation:** Coronary circulation maintains perfusion to cardiac structures, enabling the heart to distribute oxygenated blood to the remainder of the body.
- **Intact systemic circulation:** The coronary and systemic circulation is designed to distribute oxygenated blood to tissues and organs.
- **Adequate tissue uptake of oxygen:** Oxygen-dependent cells and tissues must be receptive to oxygen and nutrients to survive.

From Ventilation to Perfusion

Adequate ventilation and diffusion are required for intake and transport of oxygen and the removal of carbon dioxide. Perfusion with oxygenated blood cannot occur without the inhalation and diffusion of oxygen. Once oxygen enters the lungs and moves across the alveolar–capillary junction, the pulmonary circulation is crucial in taking up and distributing the oxygen. Therefore, effective gas exchange relies on a reasonably equal intake of oxygen (ventilation) and the movement of this oxygen (perfusion) from all areas of the lungs to the blood (Fig. 16.1).

The relationship between ventilation and perfusion is expressed as the **ventilation–perfusion**

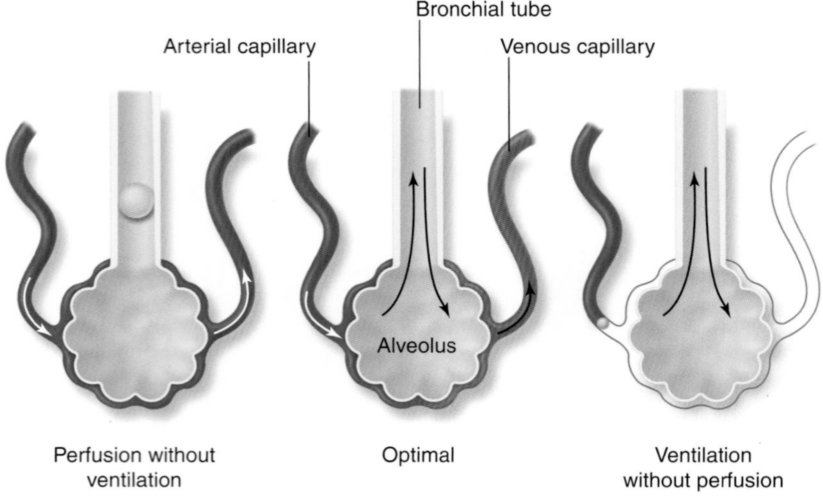

Figure 16.1. Matching ventilation and perfusion. Optimal matching of ventilation and perfusion **(Center)**. Perfusion without ventilation **(Left)**. Ventilation without perfusion **(Right)**.

ratio, which is typically 0.8:0.9. This means that the rate of ventilation is usually slightly less than the rate of perfusion. The largest volume of ventilation and perfusion is performed in the lower lobes of the lungs. In the lower lobes:

1. Ventilation is optimal because the surface tension for the alveoli is lowest and the lungs are most easily inflated.
2. Perfusion is optimal as the blood pressure through the lower lobes allows maximal blood flow.

Ventilation–perfusion is also affected by gravity. The lung tissues that are most dependent, or closest to the ground, are the most ventilated and perfused.

Stop and Consider
Given that ventilation–perfusion is gravity dependent, how does your body position impact where the greatest volume of ventilation–perfusion occurs?

Circulation

For effective perfusion, blood vessels must deliver oxygen and nutrients to tissues and remove waste. These steps occur through a process of circulation. In this chapter, circulation is discussed based on three critical, but interconnected, pathways:

- The pulmonary circulation, where circulation through the lungs provides the ability to transfer oxygen from the atmosphere into the body
- The cardiac circulation, where blood flow to the heart muscle supports the heart's work in pumping oxygenated blood to the body
- The systemic circulation, where oxygen and nutrients are distributed to other body tissues

Effective circulation depends on the patency of blood vessels and on the adjustment of the microcirculation to meet the demands of tissues. Arteries transport oxygenated and nutrient-rich blood to tissues; veins transport deoxygenated blood and waste products away from tissues for removal out of the body. Arterioles, capillaries, and venules form the microcirculation are the primary locale for exchange of nutrients at the cellular level. A large network of capillaries in a tissue or organ increases the surface area for exchange of nutrients and wastes and allows for increased perfusion. For example, the heart, an organ that requires high levels of oxygen, has an extensive capillary network. When demands on the heart increase, vasodilation occurs and more blood flow is channeled to this organ. Similarly, oxygen transport to other organs adjusts related to demands, such as skeletal muscles during exercise. Cellular demands, measured by increased cell metabolism or energy expenditure, increase perfusion to the cells. This process involves a complex interaction of chemical mediators, metabolic waste products, and nucleotides that act on the blood, endothelial cells of the vessels, smooth muscle cells, and the extracellular matrix to open and widen capillary channels.

PULMONARY CIRCULATION

The pulmonary circulation forms the conduit by which oxygen and carbon dioxide can be exchanged between the atmosphere and the body. The pulmonary circulation comprises the right side of the heart and the pulmonary artery, capillaries, and veins. Note that the pulmonary artery carries deoxygenated blood to the lungs and that the pulmonary veins carry oxygenated blood to the left side of the heart. This portion of the circulation functions at a much lower pressure than the systemic circulation. Blood moves slowly past the lungs to allow maximum gas exchange.

Stop and Consider
How would an ineffective right ventricle affect the pulmonary and systemic circulation?

SYSTEMIC CIRCULATION

The systemic circulation comprises all arteries, capillaries, and veins except those of the pulmonary circulation. The systemic circulation functions at a much higher pressure than the pulmonary circulation, because blood must work against resistance to get to peripheral tissues. The systemic circulation is motored by the left side of the heart, particularly the left ventricle, which is the strongest pumping chamber.

CORONARY CIRCULATION

The coronary circulation is considered part of the systemic circulatory network but is singled out primarily because the heart is the pump that pushes oxygenated blood to the rest of the body. The heart is therefore considered a vital organ, and perfusion of this organ is essential for life. Cardiac muscle cells require a constant supply of oxygen and nutrients; these cells have little storage capacity. Perfusing the heart, by continuously providing oxygen and nutrients, occurs via the coronary circulation. Two major vessels, the right and left coronary artery, branch directly off the aorta to perfuse the right and left side of the myocardium (muscle) of the heart. The heart is also perfused by extensive collateral circulation (accessory arterial and venous branches) stemming from these major vessels. Additional collateral

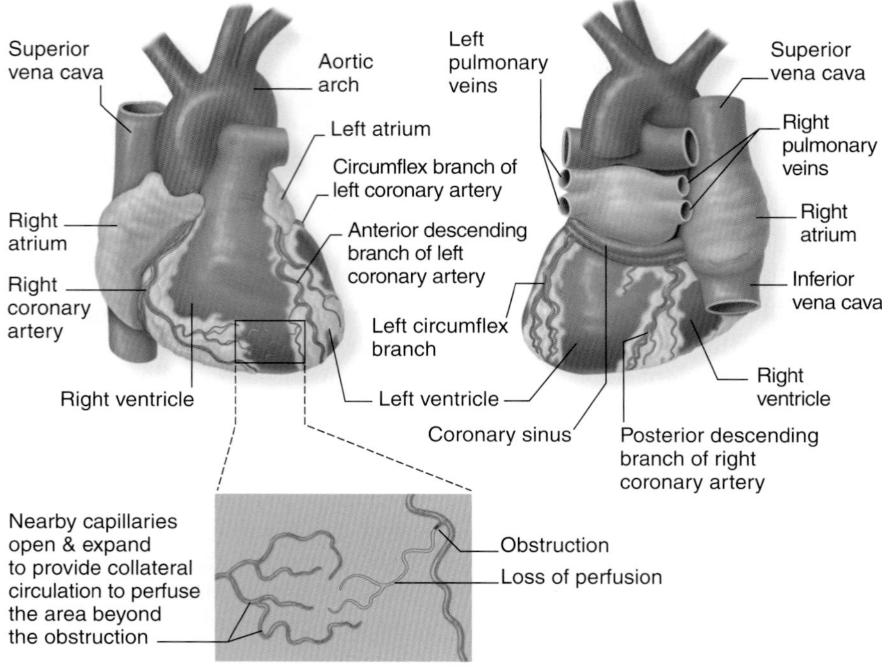

Figure 16.2. Coronary circulation and the development of collateral circulation.

circulation develops when an increased need exists for blood flow to a specific area of the heart, such as with greater cardiac demands or obstruction of blood flow to heart tissues (Fig. 16.2).

Stop and Consider
How would moderate-to-heavy aerobic exercise affect the development of collateral circulation of the heart?

Movement of Blood Through the Circulation

The unique structural design of the heart promotes the movement of blood through the arteries to the capillaries (Fig. 16.3). The heart has three distinct layers:

- **Pericardium:** The outer covering of the heart, which holds the heart in place in the chest cavity, contains receptors that assist with the regulation of blood pressure and heart rate, and forms a first line of defense against infection and inflammation. Pericardial fluid is found between the layers of the pericardium, providing a cushion and lubricant to minimize friction as the heart beats.
- **Myocardium:** The thick muscular layer of the heart. The thickness of the myocardium varies depending on location. The left ventricle often has the thickest myocardial area, because this ventricle works harder than other heart chambers to overcome the resistance of pumping blood to the aorta and to the systemic circulation. The myocardium undergoes hypertrophy if the heart workload increases.

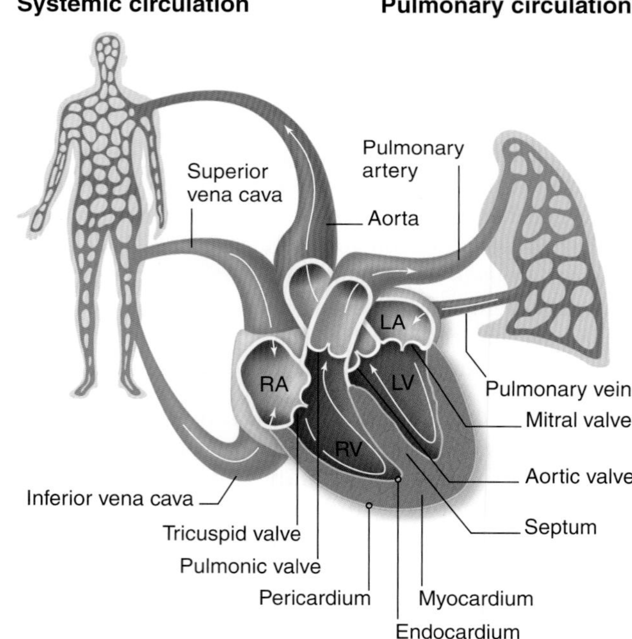

Figure 16.3. Layers of the heart and direction of continuous blood flow through the valves and heart chambers. LA, left atrium; LV, left ventricle; RA, right atrium; RV, right ventricle.

- **Endocardium:** The inner lining of the heart that forms a continuous layer of endothelium that joins the arteries and veins to the heart, forming a closed circulatory system.

Stop and Consider
What is pericarditis? What would be the problem with this condition? What clinical manifestations do you think would be present?

The heart has four chambers: a right and left atrium and a right and left ventricle. The left and right sides of the heart are separated by a septum. Blood passes through valves that separate the atria from the ventricles, and the ventricles from the pulmonary artery and the aorta. The locations and characteristics of heart valves are depicted in Figures 16.3 and 16.4. These one-way valves are needed to promote forward movement of blood.

The movement of blood follows a predictable, continuous path. This discussion starts with the return of venous blood to the heart, which depends on skeletal muscle contractions and one-way valves within the veins that prevent backflow of blood. Blood that is returned from the head and arms travels through the superior vena cava, and blood that is returned from the trunk and legs travels through the inferior vena cava. Both paths lead to the right atrium. From here, the blood goes through the tricuspid valve to the right ventricle, through the pulmonic valve to the pulmonary artery and to the lungs. This deoxygenated blood becomes oxygenated through the ventilation–perfusion exchange. The blood returns to the heart via the pulmonary vein to the left atrium, through the bicuspid (mitral) valve to the left ventricle, through the aortic valve to the aorta, then to the systemic circulation, and again returning via venous return to the right side of the heart.

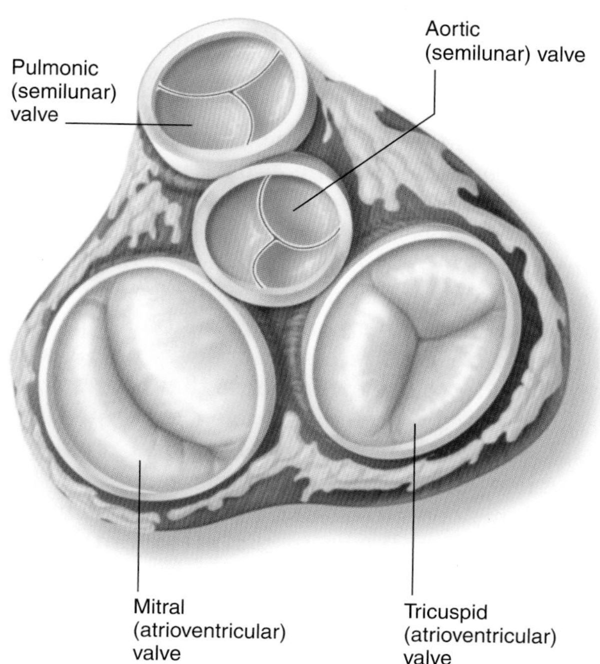

Figure 16.4. Superior view of the heart. Characteristics of semilunar versus atrioventricular valves.

CARDIAC CYCLE

The myocardium of the heart contracts and relaxes, forming the pumping action of the heart that promotes perfusion. The **cardiac cycle** refers to one contraction and one relaxation phase. Contractions, called **systole**, forcefully move blood out of the ventricles. Relaxation, referred to as **diastole**, allows blood to fill the ventricles. After the ventricles fill, systole begins with the closure of atrioventricular (AV) valves. The AV valves are the bicuspid (mitral) valve and the tricuspid valve. AV valve closures correspond to the first heart sound. Traditionally, heart sounds are described as "lub dub." AV valve closures are the first part ("lub") of this description. The first heart sound is also referred to as S_1.

After AV valve closure, the ventricles contract, and pressure in the ventricles then becomes greater than that in the aorta and pulmonary artery. The semilunar valves, composed of the aortic and pulmonic valves, open to eject blood from the ventricles. Once the blood is ejected and at the end of systole, the ventricles relax. Pressure is now greater in the aorta and pulmonary artery. The valves prevent blood from flowing back into the ventricles. Rapid closure of the aortic and pulmonic valves prevents backflow of blood. Closure of these valves corresponds to the second heart sound ("dub" of lub dub). This second heart sound is also referred to as S_2.

During diastole, pressure again directs the valves. The ventricles are now relaxed and empty. Blood flow is accumulating, and pressure becomes greater in the atria. The AV valves open and the blood moves into the ventricles. Additional heart sounds can sometimes be heard during this time. S_3 might be heard if there is rapid filling of the ventricle and the ventricle is weak, distended, or otherwise impaired. S_4 may be heard during atrial contraction.

CONDUCTION OF IMPULSES

Cardiac contractions rely on the passage of ions and electrical impulses from one myocardial cell to another. These impulses are generated and conducted as a weak electrical current within the heart itself. This process is generated through action potentials, or electrical currents moving charged ions (specifically, sodium, calcium, and potassium) along the cell membrane through channels. General action potentials and conduction are discussed in Chapter 10. In the cardiac cycle, two major types of action potentials (slow or fast responses) stimulate cardiac contraction and relaxation. These types of action potentials work in an organized manner to induce:

1. Rapid depolarization
2. Early repolarization
3. Plateau
4. Rapid repolarization
5. A resting phase

The cell membrane is typically found to have a positive net charge on its outer surface and negative charge on its inner surface. Depolarization is a change in polarity, in which ions shift, resulting in a sudden change in voltage. In depolarization, fast sodium channels open, allowing a rapid influx of sodium (positively charged) ions into the cell. As the cell voltage peaks, the fast sodium channel closes and the cell moves into the early stage of repolarization. This early repolarization is followed by a plateau phase, in which calcium and sodium ions slowly enter the cell through slow calcium–sodium channels. This calcium influx facilitates the prolonged contraction of cardiac muscle fibers. The cell then moves into rapid repolarization. Repolarization is basically a regrouping phase, in which the cell membrane becomes polarized again with a positive charge on the outer and a negative charge on the inner surface of the cell membrane. In the case of cardiac myocytes, the sodium and calcium channels close and sodium and calcium no longer move into the cell. To reestablish the polarity within the cell, the cell membrane becomes more permeable to potassium. This positively charged ion (K^+) exits the cell. This process is repeated again and again to produce cardiac contraction and relaxation that is characteristic of the heart.

The electrical activity imposed by ions on cardiac cells can be measured by using an electrocardiogram (ECG, also referred to as an EKG). Electrodes are placed on the body in designated areas and the electrical activity is transmitted to a screen. Figure 16.5 illustrates the ECG output and how this measurement corresponds to the action potential. It also demonstrates how the letters P, Q, R, S, and T represent certain points on the ECG. These letters correspond to the following aspects of the action potential:

- P wave = the depolarization of the atria via the sinoatrial node
- P–Q interval = the depolarization of the AV node and bundle fibers
- QRS = depolarization of the ventricles
- T = repolarization of the ventricles
- U = repolarization of Purkinje fibers

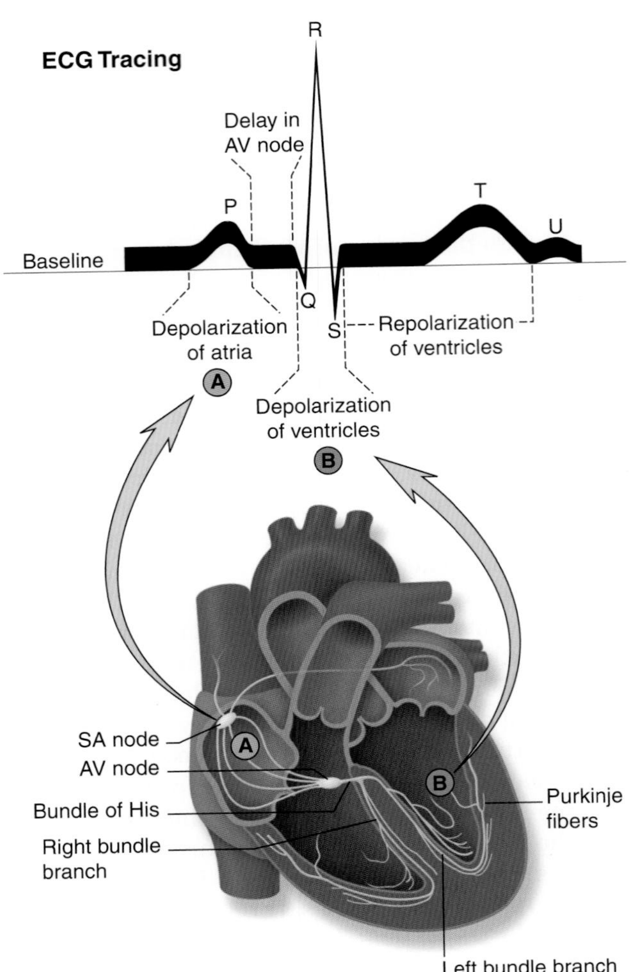

Figure 16.5. Conduction system of the heart and action potentials represented in the electrocardiogram (ECG) tracing. **A:** Depolarization of the atria. **B:** Depolarization of the ventricles. AV, atrioventricular; SA, sinoatrial.

An important parallel process to the formation of action potentials is the orderly conduction of impulses through the heart. The conduction system involves specialized myocardial cells in the **sinoatrial (SA) node**, or pacemaker, which generate a rhythmic impulse in the atria (see Fig. 16.5). As mentioned previously, action potentials consist of two types of responses: fast and slow. The SA node is stimulated by the slow response that occurs when the calcium–sodium channels open. As stated previously, this was where stimulation of a prolonged contraction phase of the heart was generated. The electrical message to contract then passes along the myocardial cell pathway to the **atrioventricular (AV) node**. The AV node, as its name suggests, connects the conduction of impulses between the atria and ventricles. The impulse is slowed upon reaching the AV node to allow the atria to empty blood completely into the ventricles before stimulating the ventricles to contract. The AV node generates the impulse that travels along specialized fibers, known as the AV bundle at the bundle of His, forming the left and right bundle branches and culminating into Purkinje fibers. These fibers conduct electrical impulses that stimulate the ventricle to contract. Blood is then ejected from the ventricles.

Stop and Consider

What would happen if the AV node conduction was blocked? What would happen if the bundle branch conduction was blocked?

CARDIAC OUTPUT

Measurement of the heart's efficiency to pump optimal amounts of blood is referred to as cardiac output. **Cardiac output (CO)** depends on stroke volume (SV) and heart rate (HR) and is expressed as: CO = SV × HR. **Stroke volume** is the amount of blood pumped out of one ventricle of the heart in a single beat. **Heart rate** is the number of heartbeats that occur in 1 minute. Cardiac output varies with age, body size, and metabolic needs of body tissues. The average cardiac output in adults is about 3.5 to 8.0 L/min. This means that every minute, up to 8 L of blood moves through the heart. During exercise, when metabolic needs increase, cardiac output can increase fourfold. Responsive cardiac output is based on five major factors, outlined in Box 16.1.

Stop and Consider

What happens to preload when venous return is diminished? What happens to preload when venous return is excessive and cardiac muscle fibers get stretched too far?

BLOOD PRESSURE

Blood pressure is the pressure or tension of the blood within the systemic arteries. Blood pressure is needed to continuously perfuse vital organs. Pressure in the arteries is maintained by:

1. Contraction of the left ventricle
2. Peripheral vascular resistance
3. Elasticity of the arterial walls
4. Viscosity and volume of the blood

In other words, blood pressure is a product of cardiac output and the amount of resistance in the arteries.

Stop and Consider

What would your body need to do to maintain optimal blood pressure if you had increased peripheral vascular resistance as may occur with arteriosclerosis (a condition of stiffening of the arteries)?

Box 16.1 Major Factors Impacting Cardiac Output

- Preload
  - Work imposed on the heart just before contraction
  - Also called ventricular end-diastolic volume because it represents the pressure in the ventricles just before systole
  - Optimal preload depends on adequate venous return to fill the heart with blood and adequate cardiac muscle stretching to promote a strong contraction
  - An indicator of the filling and muscle stretching needed to eject an optimal amount of blood from the ventricles
- Cardiac contractility
  - The ability of the heart to increase the force of the contraction without changing the diastolic, or resting, pressure
  - Affected by calcium ions that aid in muscle contractions
- Afterload
  - The amount of pressure in the ventricle toward the end of the cardiac contraction
  - The cardiac muscle fibers are shortened and contracted and the ventricles have been emptied
  - Squeezing pressure against the resistance of blood trying to back up into the ventricles
  - Affected by increased resistance from the aorta and pulmonary artery
  - Increases when valves are impaired
- Heart rate
  - Part of the equation that predicts cardiac output
  - Must also respond to changes in demands to maximize perfusion
  - Slower heart rate equals greater diastolic filling
  - Excessively rapid heart rate can move blood quickly but does not allow maximal amounts of blood to be moved with each contraction
- Blood volume
  - Quantity and quality of blood affect the workload on the heart
  - Excessive blood increases pressure; deficient blood lowers pressure
  - Increased blood viscosity (thickness) increases pressure; thinner blood viscosity lowers vascular resistance and blood pressure
  - The heart must adjust to these pressures to maintain an optimal stroke volume

Blood pressure is measured in millimeters of mercury (mm Hg). The average blood pressure for adults is about 120/80. The first number (120 in the example) is called the systolic blood pressure. The second number (80 in the example) is called the diastolic blood pressure. Figure 16.6 illustrates the factors involved in blood pressure. **Systolic blood pressure** is the amount of pressure exerted during contraction of the left ventricle and ejection of blood into the aorta. The stroke volume, heart rate, and resistance in the aorta affect systolic blood pressure. Specific activities that can elevate systolic blood pressure include exercise, smoking, cardiovascular disease, and

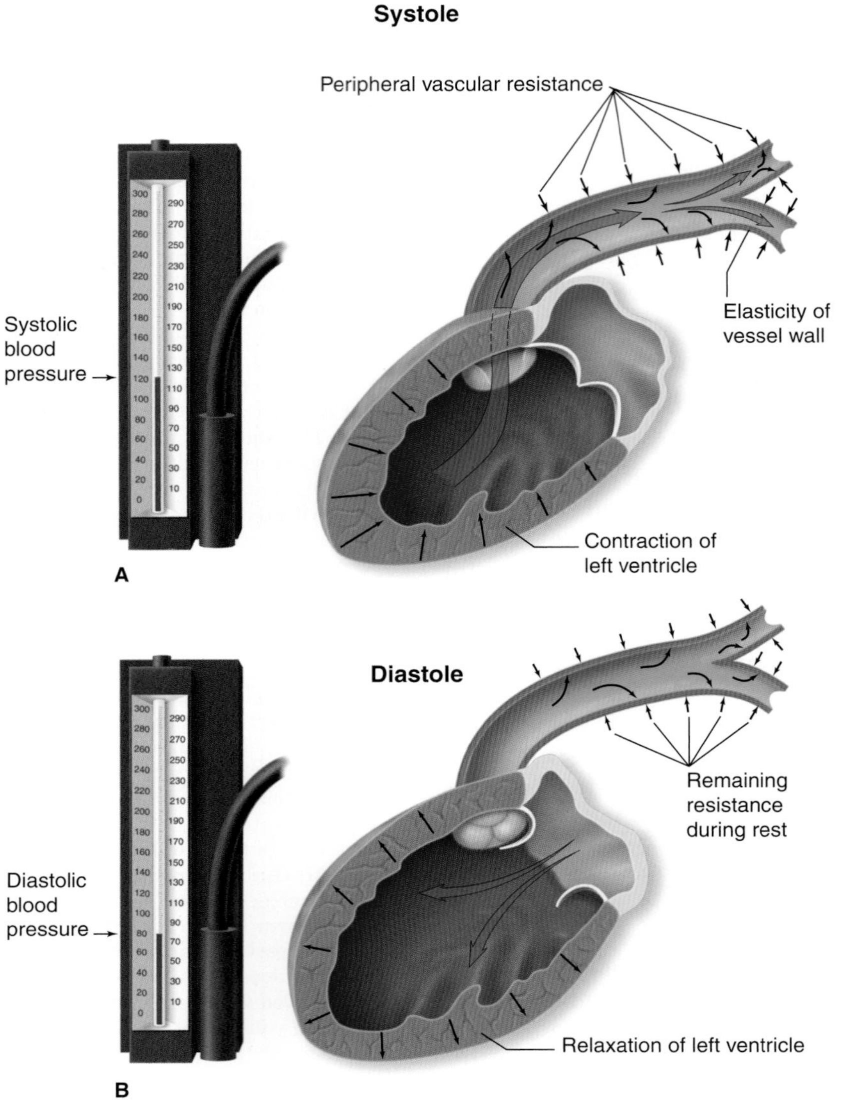

Figure 16.6. Factors involved with systolic and diastolic blood pressure. **A:** Systolic blood pressure represents the ejection of blood into the aorta during systole, or contraction of the left ventricle. **B:** Diastolic blood pressure represents the pressure in the arterial system during diastole, or resting of the left ventricle.

stress. **Diastolic blood pressure** is the amount of pressure that remains in the aorta during the resting phase of the cardiac cycle. Elevations in diastolic blood pressure may indicate that the arteries are not allowed to appropriately rest between cardiac contractions. Depressions in diastolic blood pressure are related to either lack of adequate resistance in the aorta or backflow of blood (and subsequently a loss of baseline pressure) through the aortic valve. The difference between the systolic and diastolic blood pressure is called the **pulse pressure**. Convergence, or narrowing, of the systolic and diastolic pressure often reflects a loss of systolic pressure rather than an elevation in diastolic pressure. For example, extensive blood loss decreases systolic pressure while diastolic pressure remains unchanged. The **mean arterial pressure**, considered an adequate measure of *systemic* tissue perfusion, is one-third the pulse pressure plus diastolic pressure.

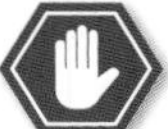

Stop and Consider

Do you think that it is more problematic to have persistent elevations in systolic or diastolic blood pressure?

NEURONAL CONTROL OF BLOOD PRESSURE AND CARDIOVASCULAR ADAPTATION

How does the cardiovascular system adjust to the variable perfusion demands of the cells and tissues?

Regulation and adaptation of cardiac and vascular function are controlled by neurons in the medulla and pons, which act on the autonomic nervous system (ANS). The sympathetic division of the ANS stimulates increased heart rate, cardiac contractility, and the tension or resistance of blood vessels. The parasympathetic division of the ANS also acts on the heart to decrease heart rate. All of these adaptations are in response to multiple signals in the brain and cardiovascular system.

Blood pressure regulation requires adjustment in cardiac output (the pushing pressure) and peripheral vascular resistance (the resisting pressure) primarily through neuronal and hormonal mechanisms (Fig. 16.7). Similar to regulation of cardiac conduction, the ANS adjusts blood pressure. The sympathetic nervous branch increases heart rate and cardiac contractility and can selectively produce artery and arteriole vasoconstriction to increase peripheral vascular resistance. Changes in blood pressure occur in response to:

1. Baroreceptors and chemoreceptors in the arteries
2. The renin–angiotensin system
3. The kidneys

Baroreceptors, located throughout the blood vessels and the heart, sense pressure changes in the arteries. For example, when the resistance, or stretch, of the artery decreases (the blood pressure is sensed as low), the baroreceptors alert the cardiac control center in the brainstem. The brainstem acts on the sympathetic nervous system to stimulate beta-1 receptors in the heart. Beta-1 receptors increase cardiac output. Simultaneously, alpha-1 receptors in the blood vessels are stimulated, causing vasoconstriction. These receptors are mentioned because they are major targets of pharmacologic treatment with hypertension. Blocking these receptors reduces cardiac output and reduces vascular vasoconstriction. When optimal blood pressure is achieved, sympathetic stimulation by the baroreceptors subsides. Chemoreceptors in the aorta and carotid arteries

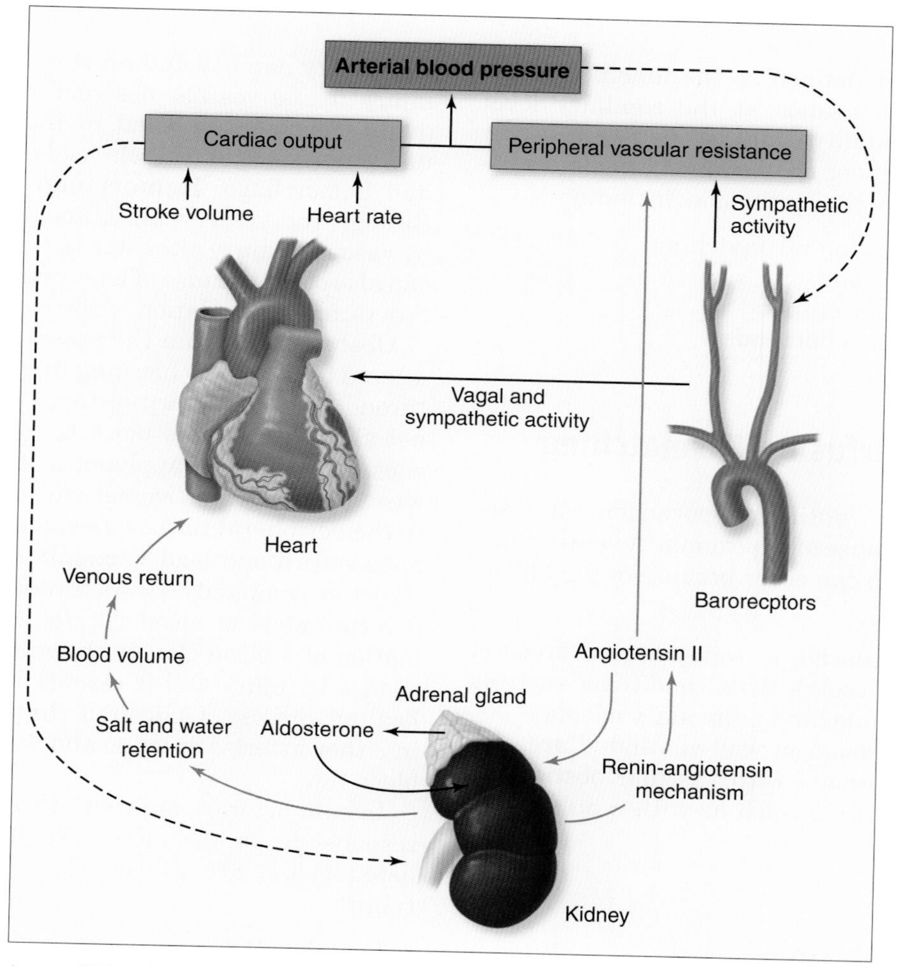

Figure 16.7. Mechanisms of blood pressure regulation. Dashed lines represent stimulation of blood pressure regulation. Solid lines represent response to stimulation of kidneys and baroreceptors. (From Porth CM. *Essentials of Pathophysiology: Concepts of Altered Health States*. Philadelphia, PA: Lippincott Williams & Wilkins; 2003.)

also play a vital role in blood pressure regulation by detecting changes in oxygen, carbon dioxide, and pH of the blood. Chemoreceptors then provide feedback to alter ventilation and promote vasoconstriction as needed to maximize oxygenation of vital organs.

Circulating enzymes, hormones, plasma proteins, and neurotransmitters also affect blood pressure regulation. Renin, an enzyme produced and secreted from the kidneys, converts the plasma protein angiotensinogen to angiotensin I. Angiotensin I is converted to angiotensin II by an enzyme in the lungs. Angiotensin II is a potent circulating vasoconstrictor. Angiotensin II therefore works to promote an increase in blood pressure when acting on the arteries and arterioles. Angiotensin II also stimulates the adrenal cortex to increase production and secretion of aldosterone (Chapter 8). Aldosterone increases salt and water retention by the kidneys and can contribute to expanding blood volume. Antidiuretic hormone (vasopressin) also plays a role in blood pressure regulation. In high doses, antidiuretic hormone, secreted from the posterior pituitary, is a potent vasoconstrictor. Antidiuretic hormone also promotes retention of fluids, which can enhance blood volume. Epinephrine, a neurotransmitter, acts to promote blood pressure directly by stimulating heart rate and cardiac contractility and promoting tension in the vessels.

Stop and Consider

Think back to the last time that you felt dizzy when you stood up too fast. Why do you think this occurred? How did the baroreceptors respond?

Module 2 Altered Perfusion

Altered perfusion is defined as the inability to adequately oxygenate tissues at the capillary level (Fig. 16.8). This inability could be the result of low oxygen presence or poor utilization of oxygen.

Many factors can alter perfusion, including:

- Ventilation–perfusion mismatching
- Impaired circulation
- Inadequate cardiac output
- Excessive perfusion demands

Ventilation–Perfusion Mismatching

Problems with the ventilation–perfusion ratio are the most common cause of hypoxemia. A ventilation–perfusion mismatch can occur because of the following conditions:

- Inadequate ventilation in well-perfused areas of the lungs. This occurs with conditions such as asthma, pneumonia, and pulmonary edema.
- Inadequate perfusion in well-ventilated areas of the lungs. This occurs with vascular obstructive processes in the lung, such as with a pulmonary embolus.

Impaired Circulation

Problems with circulation lead to inadequate or excess blood flow to tissues or organs. Impaired circulatory patency and functioning can result from injury to the vessels, obstructive processes, inadequate movement of blood, or inadequate blood volume. Injury to the vessels leads to loss of integrity and hemorrhage. **Hemorrhage**, the loss of blood through the vessel wall, is most commonly caused by vascular injury often due to trauma. Hemorrhage can also occur because of aneurysms, coagulation disorders, and degradation of the vessel by neoplasms.

Obstruction within the vessel also contributes to altered perfusion by blocking free movement of blood through the circulatory system. Occluded arteries do not allow oxygenated blood to reach peripheral tissues. For example, applying a tourniquet or otherwise compressing a vessel will disallow blood flow to the peripheral tissues. Occluded veins restrict venous return and lead to circulatory congestion. Obstruction commonly occurs through the development of a thrombus, or blood clot. Remember that the formation of a blood clot, or **thrombosis**, occurs in response to injury and is essential during the wound healing process. Undesired thrombi can also form in either arteries or veins and subsequently occlude blood flow.

In both arteries and veins, three major factors are responsible for thrombus formation. These factors, listed below, are collectively known as **Virchow triad**:

1. Vessel wall damage
2. Excessive clotting
3. Alterations in blood flow, such as turbulence or sluggish blood movement

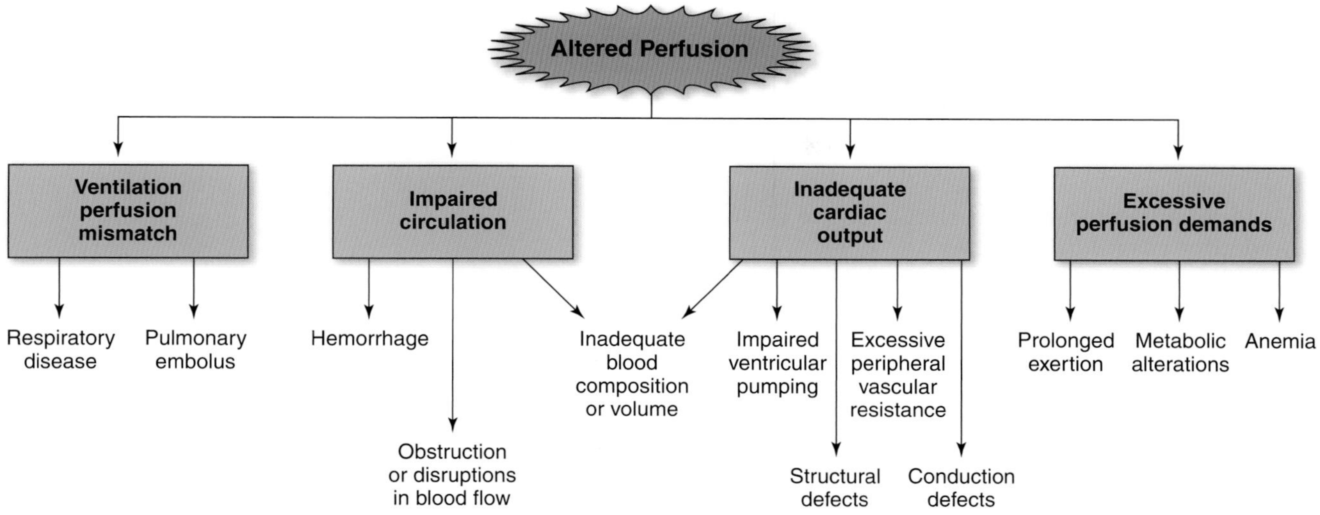

Figure 16.8. Concept map. Altered perfusion.

Injury to vessel endothelium, followed by the formation of atherosclerosis, is the most common cause of thrombus formation in arteries and also contributes to venous thrombosis.

Atherosclerosis is a condition of irregularly distributed lipid deposits in the inner lining, or intima, of large or medium arteries. The onset of atherosclerosis is theorized to begin as a process of injury to the intima (inner lining of the vessel), perhaps from hypertension, smoking, or environmental exposures. Low-density lipoprotein (LDL) filters into the lining of the artery and becomes trapped along the injured intima. The lipoprotein becomes oxidized and engulfed by macrophages, producing foam cells. Foam cells accumulate and combine with additional lipids to form fatty streaks. These fatty streaks gradually become fibrous plaques. Fibrous plaques accumulate at the sites of injury covered by platelet caps that continue to expand. These areas of atherosclerosis may eventually occlude the artery.

Turbulent or stagnant blood flow also contributes to thrombus formation. Bifurcations, aneurysms, and areas of venous stasis are common sites of altered blood flow. **Bifurcations** are regions wherein a vessel branches. Blood flow slows or backs up in an effort to negotiate the narrowed pathway. Arterial **aneurysms** are local outpouchings caused by weakness in the vessel wall (Fig. 16.9). Damage to the vessel wall, as may occur with atherosclerosis, promotes the development of aneurysms. The loss of vessel wall pressure allows slower transit of blood. **Venous stasis** occurs in veins with reduced venous return. Situations that promote venous stasis include heart failure, varicose veins, or prolonged bed rest or immobilization. Venous stasis is most commonly found in the legs, where blood pools in the extremities. These three situations (bifurcations, aneurysms, and venous stasis) all impede forward movement of blood. This allows the accumulation of clotting factors needed to form thrombi.

Stop and Consider

What is the mechanism for development of venous thrombi formation in an individual on bed rest?

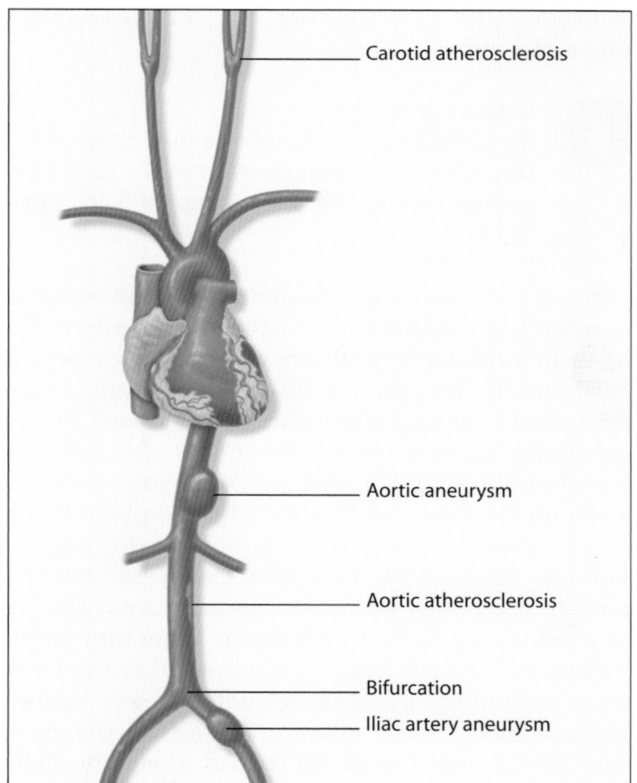

Figure 16.9. Bifurcation, aneurysm, and atherosclerosis. These conditions cause turbulent blood flow.

Disorders of excess clotting allow unregulated formation of thrombi throughout the body. Hypercoagulability can be congenital or acquired. Genetic mutations can result in excess coagulant factors or deficient anticoagulant mechanisms. Acquired causes of hypercoagulability include:

- Autoimmune mechanisms that activate platelets and alter coagulation factors
- Certain types of cancer, or myeloproliferative disorders, such as **thrombocythemia** (excess platelets)
- Sickle cell anemia
- Polycythemia vera
- Use of oral contraceptives
- Vascular changes in the late stage of pregnancy

The following outcomes may potentially occur with thrombus formation:

1. The thrombus continues to grow and occlude the vessel completely
2. The thrombus is degraded by enzymes and decreases in size
3. All or part of the thrombus breaks off and travels through the circulation (Fig. 16.10)

Once a thrombus breaks off and travels, it is referred to as a **thromboembolus**, or simply an embolus. An **embolus** is any plug of material, such as thrombi, air, neoplasms, microorganisms, or amniotic fluid, that travels in the circulation and can obstruct the lumen of a vessel.

Stop and Consider
When preparing an intravenous fluid or medication, all air must be removed from the tubing or syringe. Describe the consequence of being careless in air removal.

When a vessel becomes obstructed, it can result in an infarct. An **infarct** is an area of necrosis resulting from a sudden insufficiency of arterial or venous blood supply. The process of obstructing the vessel is referred to as an **infarction**. Loss of blood supply and necrosis formation results in loss of function of the affected tissue. The severity of the infarction depends on the size and location of the emboli. Small emboli result in small and less significant areas of necrosis. Areas with extensive collateral circulation are capable of perfusing tissue around the obstructed vessel. Larger emboli can lodge into larger vessels, occlude the large vessel and all of the large vessel's tributaries, and cause sudden death. Venous thromboemboli most often originate in the deep veins of the legs, break off, travel along the vein, and lodge in the pulmonary arteries where the vessels narrow and bifurcate. Arterial thromboemboli most often originate in the heart as atherosclerotic plaques, and they can travel to the brain, intestines,

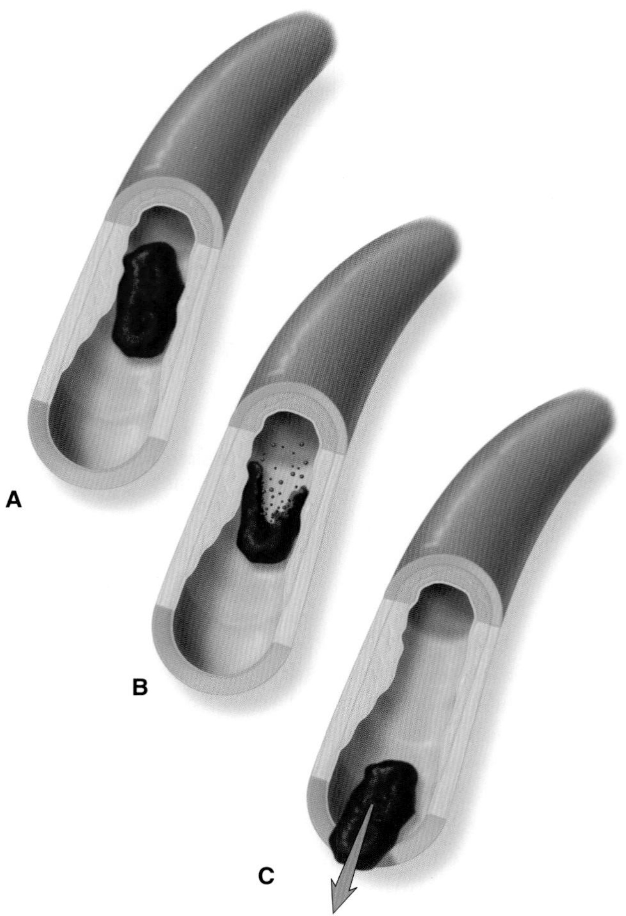

Figure 16.10. Potential outcomes of thrombus formation. **A:** Partial or total occlusion of the vessel. **B:** Enzymes degrade thrombus. **C:** The thrombus dislodges, forming an embolus, which travels within the vessels and occludes a smaller blood vessel at a distant site.

lower extremities, or kidneys. Myocardial infarction (MI) and stroke are two clinical models that are presented in this chapter to illustrate the impact of infarction on vital organs.

Inadequate Cardiac Output

Cardiac output is inadequate when the heart is unable to successfully eject the necessary amount of blood to the pulmonary and systemic circulation. Major categories of problems leading to inadequate cardiac output include:

- Changes in blood volume, composition, or viscosity
- Impaired ventricular pumping
- Structural heart defects, such as valve defects that allow leaking or regurgitation of blood
- Conduction defects that lead to an unresponsive heart rate and rhythm
- Excessive or significantly reduced peripheral vascular resistance

Changes in blood volume, composition, or viscosity can affect cardiac output and result in altered perfusion. Blood volume and viscosity is altered with such conditions as hypercoagulation, dehydration, or hemorrhage. Disseminated intravascular coagulation is a clinical model in this chapter used to illustrate the impact of coagulation disorders and hemorrhage on cardiac output and perfusion. Basically, blood outside of the circulation is not accessible to tissues. Blood composition, particularly with anemia, alters oxygen transport. In anemia, in which there are not enough red blood cells to carry oxygen, the heart tries to move the small number of cells at a faster heart rate and becomes overtaxed.

Impaired ventricular pumping is a second major category of problems that lead to impaired cardiac output. The heart is a muscle. Loss of muscle activity leads to the inability to move blood effectively forward through the arterial circulation. This leads to congestion of venous blood and impaired venous return. Heart failure is a clinical model selected to further illustrate problems with impaired ventricular pumping and venous insufficiency.

Structural heart defects are a third category of problems leading to impaired cardiac output. Several potential structural heart defects exist that can affect cardiac output. Structural heart defects basically impair the smooth, directional flow of blood through the heart chambers (Fig. 16.11). Heart defects can involve:

- Openings between the chamber septa, such as with an atrial septal defect (ASD) or ventricular septal defect (VSD)

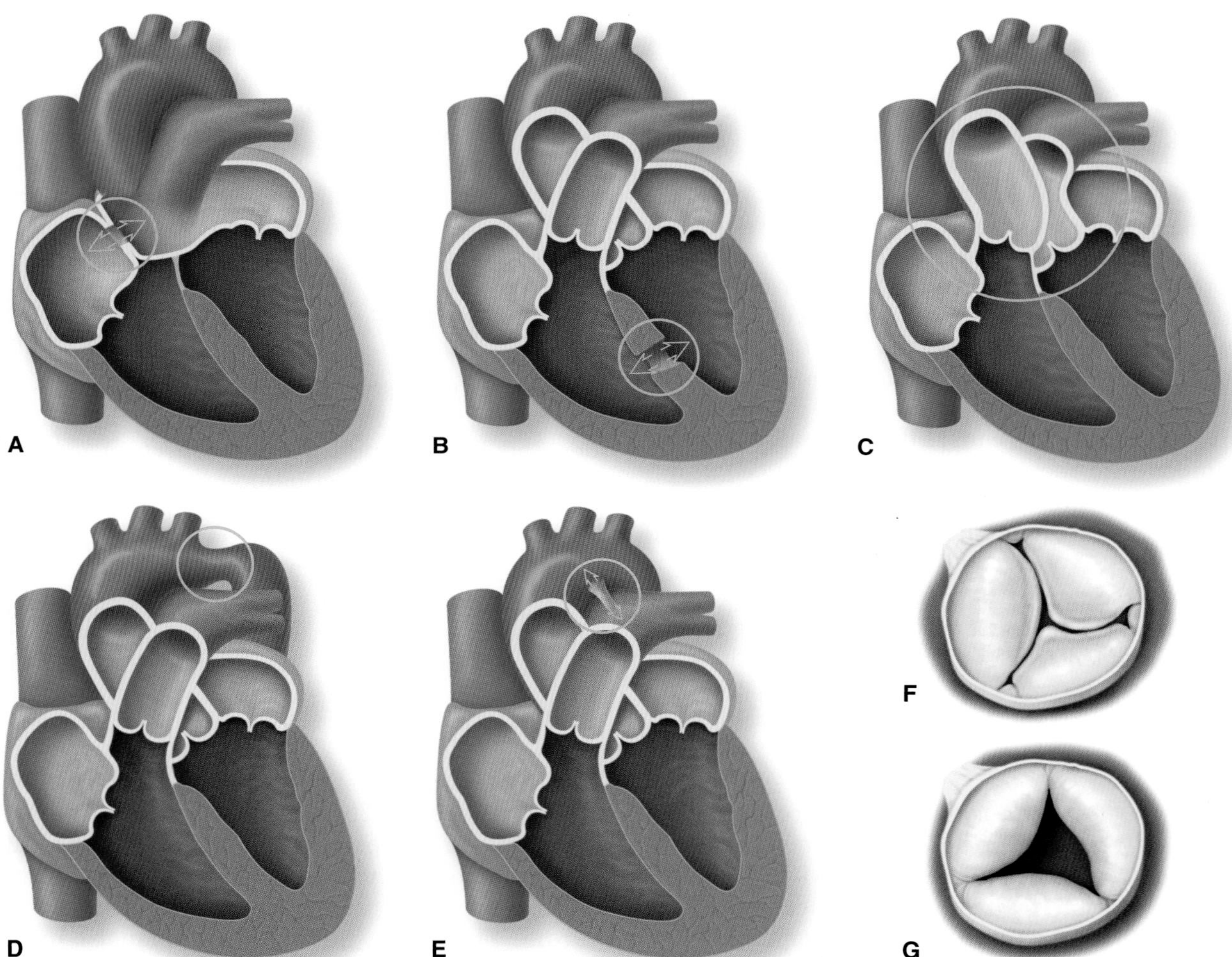

Figure 16.11. Examples of structural heart defects. **A:** Atrial septal defect. Blood is shunted from the higher pressure left atria to the lower pressure right atria. **B:** Ventricular septal defect. Blood is shunted from the higher pressure left ventricle to the lower pressure right ventricle. **C:** Transposition of the great vessels. The pulmonary artery is attached to the left side of the heart and the aorta to the right side. **D:** Coarctation (narrowing) of the aorta. **E:** Patent ductus arteriosis. The high pressure blood of the aorta is shunted back to the pulmonary artery. **F:** Thickened and stenotic valve leaflets. **G:** Regurgitant valve that does not completely close.

- Transposition or coarctation (narrowing) of the great vessels
- Lack of closure of the ductus arteriosis at or shortly after birth
- Valve defects such as stenosis, regurgitation, or prolapse

Openings between the atria and ventricles allow blood to move between the right and left side of the heart. Atrial septal defect is an opening between the left and right atria. Ventricular septal defect is an opening between the left and right ventricle. Two major problems with septal defects are (1) the co-mingling of oxygenated and deoxygenated blood within the heart chambers and (2) changes in blood flow volume and subsequent cardiac output.

Blood movement across the chambers is referred to as **shunting**. The direction of blood movement across chambers will go from the area of greater to lesser pressure. A left-to-right shunt is the movement of blood from the left side (oxygenated) of the heart to the right side (deoxygenated). The pressure on the right side of the heart and in the pulmonary circulation becomes greater. Larger defects allow greater volumes of blood to move left to right, leading to excessive pressure in the right ventricle and pulmonary edema. Cardiac output from the left ventricle to the systemic circulation is compromised because of loss of blood from the left side of the heart through the defect. A right-to-left shunt is the movement of blood from the right side (deoxygenated) of the heart to the left side (oxygenated). Movement of blood from right to left causes deoxygenated blood to be pumped into the systemic circulation. Small defects can be asymptomatic. Larger defects can lead to an overtaxed left ventricle and severe hypoxemia.

Stop and Consider

Based on the pressure differential between the right and left sides of the heart, do you think it is more common to have a left-to-right or right-to-left shunt? Which one would most likely result in cyanosis?

Valvular defects are congenital or acquired. The bicuspid (mitral) and aortic valves are most often affected. Acquired causes of these defects include infection, inflammation, trauma, and degeneration. Such problems cause the valve to open or close improperly. **Stenosis** is a problem in which narrowing of the valve occurs, making the valve unable to open adequately. This narrowing causes increased resistance and turbulence as the blood moves past the valve. The heart ventricle must work harder to pump blood past the stenotic valve. **Regurgitation** is a problem of incompetence of the valve, in which it is unable to properly close, allowing reflux of blood. Again, the heart chambers must work harder against the constant backflow of blood.

A fourth problem of cardiac output, conduction defects alter an optimal heart rate and rhythm. **Cardiac dysrhythmias** are indicative of problems with maintaining an efficient heart rhythm. Dysrhythmias can stem from problems with the SA node, AV node, cardiac cells that join the SA and AV nodes, or conduction systems in the atria or ventricles. Without a regular, productive, efficient heart rhythm, the heart is unable to perfuse body tissues adequately. The most problematic dysrhythmias are found with the ventricular conduction system, which restricts the heart's ability to pump blood to the aorta or pulmonary artery. One example is ventricular **fibrillation**, which is a problem of the heart ventricle vibrating instead of effectively pumping. This problem can also occur in the atria and is then referred to as atrial fibrillation. A defibrillator uses an electrical current to shock the heart in an attempt to reestablish the efficient heart rhythm. Another potential problem that results in dysrhythmias is obstruction of cardiac conduction, often at the AV node, a condition referred to as **heart block**. Without coordination of the atria and ventricles, the movement of blood through the heart is uncoordinated and inefficient.

Excessive Perfusion Demands

Altered, or excessive, tissue metabolism can lead to altered perfusion from lack of meeting this excessive demand. Even though all other aspects of ventilation and diffusion are functioning optimally, the tissues are asking too much. This can result from extreme and prolonged exertion or metabolic alterations, as with hyperthyroidism (Chapter 13).

General Manifestations of Altered Perfusion

The general manifestations of altered perfusion depend on the cause. The effects of chronic hypoxia were discussed in Chapter 15. Impaired cardiac output produces clinical manifestations, such as cyanosis, edema, shortness of breath, impaired growth, tachycardia, tachypnea, and fatigue. Changes in blood volume or peripheral vascular resistance can lead to hypotension or hypertension. Obstructive processes, such as myocardial or cerebral infarction, generally result in loss of function of that organ because of ischemia, along with pain and edema. The formation of deep vein thrombosis, also an obstructive process, may manifest as tenderness in the calf, especially with dorsiflexion of the foot, called **Homans sign**.

Total occlusion of veins leads to edema, coolness, pallor, and cyanosis of the lower extremity. Hemorrhage also leads to altered perfusion. Skin manifestations of hemorrhage are **ecchymoses**, bruises from superficial bleeding into the skin, **petechiae**, pinpoint hemorrhages, or **purpura**, diffuse hemorrhages of the skin or mucous membranes. Larger accumulations of blood in the tissue form a **hematoma**. Heart murmurs are a diagnostic clue to the presence of valve or septal defects.

Diagnosing and Treating Altered Perfusion

Multiple diagnostic aids are available to identify altered perfusion. Treatment measures are aimed at improving cardiac output and maintaining the integrity of circulation. Tables 16.1 and 16.2 illustrate select diagnostic tools and treatment measures indicated in altered perfusion.

Table 16.1 Select Diagnostic Aids to Detect Altered Perfusion

Diagnostic Test	Type of Test	Rationale for Use
Echocardiography (cardiac ultrasound)	Ultrasound picture of cardiac structures and great vessels	Detects cardiovascular and valvular lesions, changes in heart size, changes in heart position, and wall motion abnormalities; transesophageal echocardiography provides a clearer view of heart and great vessel structures with a probe that is positioned in the esophagus
Cardiac catheterization	Insertion of a catheter (small tube) that is passed into the heart from a vein or artery	Used to withdraw blood samples, measure pressures, or inject contrast media to detect functional and structural defects (coronary angiography); also used to surgically correct certain cardiac defects
Chest radiograph	Radiographic picture of chest	Shows heart borders; detects changes in heart size and position; detects pulmonary congestion and pleural effusion
Electrocardiography (ECG)	Measurement of electrical impulses in the heart	Detects disturbances in cardiac conduction and increases in chamber size, the presence of ischemia, or myocardial infarction; a Holter monitor is a portable device that records 24-hour ECG activity as a patient performs his or her usual daily activities
Pressure measurements	Sphygmomanometry is an indirect, noninvasive measurement of systolic and diastolic blood pressure using a blood pressure cuff and sphygmomanometer; invasive pressure measurements involve directly threading a catheter (often from the femoral artery) into the structure of interest	Determines hypotension or hypertension; cardiac catheterization measures pressure in the arteries, veins, and heart chambers
Stress test	Treadmill or bicycle exercise is used in conjunction with ECG, blood pressure monitoring, or other imaging studies; stress can also be induced through pharmacologic agents and is typically used in combination with imaging studies, such as radionucleotide imaging and echocardiography	Determines elicitation of chest pain, ECG, or imaging study changes significant for myocardial ischemia
Cardiac nuclear scanning	Uses intravenous radioactive compounds, which collect in the heart, and a gamma camera to produce diagnostic images; myocardial perfusion scanning allows the visualization of blood flow patterns to the myocardium; cardiac gating synchronizes images of the heart with cardiac conduction based on the ECG output	Indicated for individuals with unexplained or exercise-induced chest pain to permit the early detection of heart disease or to determine the effective revascularization of the heart after PTCA or bypass surgery; detects myocardial activity and blood flow; may be used in combination with a stress test
Doppler ultrasonography	A noninvasive form of ultrasound that measures the changes in sound frequencies to detect movement, most commonly of red blood cells	Measures aortic and other blood vessel flow velocities; can be used to augment echocardiography to determine flow velocities within the echocardiographic image; Doppler color flow uses computer-generated images to depict different directions of flow (represented by different colors)

Table 16.2 Treatment Measures Related to Altered Perfusion

Treatment Strategy	Rationale for Use
Surgery	Surgery has multiple applications to relieve altered perfusion: • Coronary artery bypass grafting is a procedure used to bypass an obstructed coronary artery • Percutaneous transluminal coronary angioplasty is performed during cardiac catheterization to compress fatty deposits in the coronary arteries and relieve the occlusion • Laser angioplasty vaporizes fatty deposits with a hot-tip laser device • Surgery is also used to repair valve defects, remove varicose veins, and drain excess fluid from the pericardial cavity
Pharmacologic	• ASA (aspirin) therapy may be instituted to reduce platelet aggregation and clot formation therapies • Medications may be prescribed to dilate blood vessels, reduce or increase blood pressure, control the heart rate/rhythm, increase myocardial contractility, reduce myocardial workload, or improve cardiac output • Thrombolytic agents may be needed to break through an obstruction and revascularize myocardial tissue • Pain medications are often needed for acute myocardial infarction • Oxygen therapy is frequently indicated to reduce hypoxemia
Intravenous	Fluid volume or blood replacement with severe hemorrhage or dehydration administration of blood or fluids
Pacemaker placement	A pacemaker may be placed to mechanically control heart rate and rhythm
Lifestyle	Reduction of risks or modification of lifestyle after a diagnosis related to altered perfusion modifications should include weight reduction, blood pressure management, stress reduction, smoking cessation, exercise, healthy nutrition, and diabetes management

Module 3 Clinical Models

The following clinical models have been selected to aid in the understanding and application of altered perfusion processes and effects. We are in the midst of a true cardiovascular pandemic. Heart disease is not only the leading cause of death, disability, and health care expense in the United States, it is also the leading cause of death worldwide. Cardiovascular disease is the leading cause of mortality in every region of the world except sub-Saharan Africa, and it is anticipated that cardiovascular disease will eclipse infectious disease there within the next few years. All of the issues that contribute to the continued impact of cardiovascular disease in the United States—access to care, quality of care, aging of the population, explosion in the prevalence of obesity and diabetes, tobacco consumption, and physical inactivity—have profound global implications.

Hypertension

Hypertension is a progressive cardiovascular syndrome detected by an elevation in blood pressure (systolic pressure above 140 mm Hg or a diastolic pressure above 90 mm Hg), according to the American Heart Association. Hypertension is associated with multiple factors including obesity, diabetes and chronic kidney disease, and is one of the most common conditions that require management worldwide.[1] As hypertension is often present in the absence of subjective symptoms, many people may not be aware if they have elevated blood pressure without routine screening.

PATHOPHYSIOLOGY

The majority of individuals with hypertension (90% to 95%) are diagnosed as having primary hypertension, also called essential hypertension. Secondary hypertension is high blood pressure that is a manifestation of another condition, such as a narrowing of the aorta (coarctation) or kidney disease. If the systolic blood pressure is elevated without an elevation in the diastolic blood pressure, this is referred to as **isolated systolic hypertension**. Similarly, if the diastolic blood pressure is elevated without an elevation in the systolic blood pressure, this is referred to as **isolated diastolic hypertension**. When both systolic and diastolic blood pressures are elevated, this is classified as mixed systolic/diastolic hypertension.

The specific cause of primary hypertension is often unknown. It is considered a multifactorial disease resulting from a complex interaction of genetic and environmental triggers. Certain risk factors for the development of primary hypertension have been identified and include:

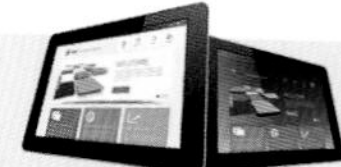

RESEARCH NOTES

The systolic blood pressure goal for individuals greater than 60 years of age established in the current guidelines for managing high blood pressure in adults[2] is higher than the goal established in the previous guidelines[3], changing from ≤140 mm Hg to ≤150 mm Hg. Researchers conducted a study to determine the impact of the current guidelines on reclassification of hypertension diagnosis in older black and white individuals.[4] Among more than 6,000 participants, the prevalence of those achieving blood pressure goals increased from 62.8% to 79.4% using the new, less aggressive blood pressure goals. However, blood pressure remained uncontrolled in more than 20% of participants in the study.

- Family history of hypertension
- Aging
- Black race
- Decreased nephron number
- Diabetes mellitus
- Excessive dietary sodium intake
- Obesity
- Sedentary lifestyle
- Nutrition
- Excessive alcohol intake
- Smoking

Hypertension is a manifestation of increased cardiac output or peripheral resistance and is characterized by structural and functional changes in the heart and vascular system. Cardiac output is elevated by conditions that increase stroke volume or heart rate. Peripheral resistance is elevated by conditions that restrict peripheral blood flow, such as increased blood viscosity or vasoconstriction. Recall the mechanisms for regulating blood pressure. Autoregulatory systems are designed to adjust to changes in cardiovascular demand. Impairments in these regulatory mechanisms can increase peripheral vascular resistance and promote the development of hypertension:

- Sympathetic nervous system overstimulation (systemic vasoconstriction)
- Renin–angiotensin–aldosterone overstimulation (systemic vasoconstriction, salt and water retention by kidneys, increased blood volume)
- Impaired sodium excretion by the kidneys (salt and water retention, increased blood volume)

Chronic hypertension damages the blood vessel walls through direct injury to the intima (inner lining) from prolonged vasoconstriction and high pressures. The inflammatory response increases systemic capillary permeability and further damages the vessel wall. The vessel walls adapt through hypertrophy and hyperplasia to withstand this stress. The vessel lumen permanently narrows.

Three major body systems are affected by hypertension: the central nervous system (CNS), cardiovascular system, and renal system. In severe hypertension, the CNS is affected because the elevated BP overwhelms the cerebral blood flow. Usually, as blood pressure increases, cerebral arterioles vasoconstrict, and cerebral blood flow remains constant. During a hypertensive crisis (a rapid and severe elevation in blood pressure), the hypertension overwhelms arteriolar control over vasoconstriction. Pressurized fluid leaks across the capillaries and into the brain tissue and other brain structures. Arterioles are damaged during this process. Intracranial pressure increases, oxygen transport is impaired, and brain function is reduced.

Hypertension also affects the cardiovascular system. Hypertension was previously mentioned as a factor in the development of atherosclerosis and can contribute to obstruction in arteries. Pressure in the small arterioles, or microvasculature, can lead to altered function of the target organ. The small vessels in the kidneys, eyes, brain, and heart are particularly vulnerable. Hypertensive pressure is also a strain on the heart, which must continue to work against this pressure to perfuse the body. The left ventricle is most affected by the pressure resistance. The left ventricle becomes hypertrophic. Ineffective left ventricle pumping impairs venous return and systemic perfusion. This leads to pulmonary edema, myocardial ischemia, and peripheral hypoxemia.

Prolonged pressure in the kidney arterioles promotes chronic injury and inflammation. This leads to nephrosclerosis, which is basically an overgrowth and hardening of the connective tissues of the kidney. Hypertension is perpetuated as renin and aldosterone secretion is stimulated by reduced blood flow to the kidneys. Blood volume expands and increases blood pressure.

CLINICAL MANIFESTATIONS

Primary hypertension is often asymptomatic and may be detected only through a series of blood pressure screenings. When clinical manifestations *are* present, this often reflects years of undetected hypertension. CNS manifestations include headache, new-onset blurred vision, nausea, vomiting, weakness, fatigue, confusion, and mental status changes. Rupture of cerebral vessels due to hypertension leads to stroke (see clinical model discussed below). Cardiovascular manifestations may include the signs and symptoms of pulmonary edema and other manifestations of heart failure (see Heart Failure below). Renal insufficiency manifests as poor urinary output, hematuria, proteinuria, and problems with eliminating urinary waste.

DIAGNOSTIC CRITERIA

Because hypertension is associated with elevated risks of cardiovascular diseases (especially stroke, myocardial infarction, and cardiovascular death), early recognition is critical to prevent such complications. Diagnosis is based on a careful patient history, physical examination, and laboratory and diagnostic tests. The patient history should include identifying hypertensive family members and other risk factors described previously. Physical examination must include the noninvasive auscultatory-method measurement of blood pressure as well as a focus on detecting target organ damage and cardiovascular disease.

Diagnosis of hypertension is *not* based on an isolated elevation in blood pressure. Rather, a series of properly performed blood pressure measurements (usually three) over a 3- to 6-month period is needed to confirm the presence of primary hypertension. Among individuals over age 60, the goal for blood pressure is <150 mm Hg systolic and < 90 mm Hg diastolic.[2] Among individuals less than 60 years of age, systolic blood pressure of <140 mm Hg or diastolic blood pressure of <90 mm Hg are the target blood pressure goals. Once a persistent elevation in blood pressure is identified, the level of hypertension can be classified according to severity.[2]

- *Prehypertension*: systolic BP 120–139 mm Hg, diastolic BP 80–89 mm Hg
- *Stage 1*: systolic BP 140–159 mm Hg, diastolic BP 90–99 mm Hg
- *Stage 2*: systolic BP greater than 159 mm Hg, diastolic BP greater than 99 mm Hg

Even before an elevated blood pressure is noticed, some individuals are at risk for the development of cardiovascular disease. For example, an individual with a blood pressure of 130/80 mm Hg may have signs of damage to their heart, kidneys, or eyes caused by blood pressure, whereas another individual with the same blood pressure reading may have no such organ damage and therefore be at lower risk for a heart attack or stroke. The point is that the diagnosis of hypertension is supported by elevations in blood pressure, but the emphasis should be on evaluating the person's overall risk for cardiovascular disease.

Relevant laboratory studies that contribute to this evaluation include electrolyte levels, urinalysis, blood urea nitrogen (BUN), and creatinine, which detect evidence of renal impairment. A lipid profile is useful to detect hypercholesterolemia. Blood glucose testing is needed to detect diabetes. In a hypertensive crisis, a chest radiograph may be needed to determine congestive heart failure, pulmonary edema, or coarctation of the aorta. A computed tomography (CT) scan of the brain may be needed to determine intracranial bleeding, edema, or infarction as causes for secondary hypertension. An ECG may also be useful to assess for cardiac ischemia or infarction.

TREATMENT

Reduction of cardiovascular risk through lifestyle is ideal. Treatment of hypertension includes consideration of pharmacologic and nonpharmacologic interventions. The following measures are appropriate in all persons with hypertension: weight reduction; decreased alcohol, salt, and saturated fat intake; increased aerobic physical activity and fruit and vegetable (potassium) and vitamin D intake; and smoking cessation. Pharmacologic treatments, when indicated, work to decrease fluid volume (diuretics), decrease cardiac contractility or cardiac output (calcium channel blockers), or decrease peripheral vascular resistance (angiotensin-converting enzyme [ACE] inhibitors, angiotensin II receptor blocker [ARB]). The overall goal of pharmacologic therapy is to decrease peripheral vascular resistance and reduce the

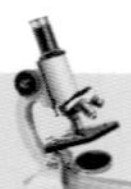

FROM THE LAB

Plasma lipids and lipoproteins include total cholesterol, triglycerides, high-density lipoprotein (HDL) cholesterol, and LDL cholesterol. Total cholesterol reflects the sum of LDL and HDL cholesterol plus 20% of total triglyceride levels. Lipid levels are typically measured after a 14-hour fast (water permitted). LDL cholesterol level of ≥190 mg/dL or triglyceride levels ≥500 mg/dl in people 21 years of age or older indicate need for cholesterol lowering treatment with statins.[5] For individuals with diabetes or clinical heart disease, statin treatment is recommended for LDL cholesterol levels of 70–189 mg/dL.

Table 16.3 Select Pharmacologic Options for Treatment of Hypertension

Type of Drug (Example)	Site of Action	Action	Rationale for Use
Thiazide diuretics	Renal tubules of the kidneys	Prevent NaCl reabsorption in the distal convoluted tubule	Decrease cardiac output and fluid volume overload with an eventual reduction in peripheral vascular resistance
Calcium channel blockers (CCB)	Vascular and cardiac muscle cells	Blocks the movement of calcium into the arterial smooth muscle cells, thereby decreasing vasoconstriction	Decreases peripheral vascular resistance
Angiotensin-converting enzyme inhibitor (ACE-I)	ACE	Inhibits the conversion of angiotensin I to angiotensin II, thereby preventing vasoconstriction and decreasing aldosterone levels	Decreases peripheral vascular resistance
Angiotensin II receptor blockers (ARB)	Angiotensin II receptors	Blocks the actions of angiotensin II, preventing angiotensin II-mediated vasoconstriction and aldosterone-mediated fluid retention	Decreases peripheral vascular resistance and decreases fluid volume to reduce cardiac output

workload of the heart by reducing arterial pressure below 140/90. Most individuals with hypertension require two or more antihypertensive drugs to achieve this goal. Pharmacotherapy is not curative, but it reduces both the symptoms and the risk for long-term complications. Table 16.3 provides more detail on pharmacologic options.

Shock

Shock is a condition of circulatory failure and impaired perfusion of vital organs. Shock is often equated with **hypotension**, or reduced blood pressure, although this is considered a late sign and signals ineffective compensation.

PATHOPHYSIOLOGY

Effective blood circulation depends on cardiac output (including an optimal blood volume) and on peripheral vascular resistance. Shock represents a deficit in one or more of these requisites and is often classified accordingly:

- Ineffective cardiac pumping: *cardiogenic shock*
- Decreased blood volume: *hypovolemic shock*
- Massive systemic vasodilation:
  - From severe infection: *septic shock*
  - From brain or spinal cord injury: *neurogenic shock*
  - From severe immunoglobulin E (IgE)-mediated hypersensitivity reaction: *anaphylactic shock*

Cardiogenic shock results from inadequate or ineffective cardiac pumping. The most common cause is myocardial infarction, although any cardiac condition that reduces heart efficiency can lead to cardiogenic shock. The basic problem is that impaired pumping leads to reduced cardiac output, low blood pressure, and restricted movement of oxygenated blood through the circulation. This leads to systemic hypotension or pulmonary edema. The mortality rate is approximately 70% for patients who do not undergo rapid revascularization to promote myocardial blood flow.

Hypovolemic shock is the result of inadequate blood/plasma volume and typically occurs when this volume is reduced by 15% to 20%. This type of shock can result from severe hemorrhage, burns, diarrhea, or polyuria, as occurs with diabetes insipidus. The problem is that blood and fluid losses in the vascular space lead to deficient venous return and reduced circulation. Reduction in the volume of red blood cells also reduces oxygen transport through the circulation. Without correcting the underlying cause, inadequate perfusion leads to multiple organ failure.

Septic shock is the result of overwhelming systemic infection where about half are caused by gram-positive microorganisms, followed closely by gram-negative microorganisms, although in some cases the exact pathogen is unknown. Gram-negative microorganisms contain endotoxin that can produce a massive inflammatory response by releasing potent chemical mediators. These chemical mediators induce widespread tissue injury. Endothelial cells that line blood vessels vasodilate and become permeable. Injury to these endothelial cells not only allows fluid to escape the intravascular compartment but also damages these cells, directly causing vascular collapse. Septic shock is considered a grave condition that has a mortality rate of approximately 30% to 50%.

Neurogenic shock is a result of brain or spinal cord injury, the depressant actions of certain drugs, general anesthesia, hypoglycemia, or hypoxia. Altered neuronal transmission leads to a loss of sympathetic control of tension in the blood vessels. This loss of tension allows unregulated vasodilation. Vasodilation decreases peripheral vascular resistance, blood pressure is reduced, and perfusion to vital organs is reduced. Neurogenic shock is the rarest cause of shock, is readily treatable, and generally responds well to medical therapy.

Anaphylactic shock is the result of a massive immune (type 1 or IgE-mediated) hypersensitivity response (Chapter 4). Similar to septic shock, anaphylaxis leads to massive vasodilation and increased vascular permeability. Peripheral vascular resistance is reduced significantly, fluid is allowed to move outside of the vascular space, blood pressure is reduced, and circulation is impaired.

All types of shock deprive the cells of oxygen and nutrients and thus impair cellular metabolism, resulting in acidosis. Initially, hypoxia and acidosis are met with compensatory mechanisms that involve:

- *Stimulating the sympathetic nervous system:* The sympathetic nervous system is stimulated to increase heart rate and cardiac contractility and to alter blood vessel tone. Regulation of vessel tone promotes (1) vasodilation of vessels leading to the heart and brain and (2) vasoconstriction to other, less vital areas of the body.
- *Stimulating the renin–angiotensin–aldosterone mechanism:* Renin and angiotensin promote compensatory vasoconstriction. These hormones also promote sodium and water reabsorption to increase intravascular volume.

The general goals of compensation are to (1) shunt blood to the heart and brain and (2) promote cardiac output by increasing intravascular volume, heart rate, and cardiac contractility. Sometimes these compensatory mechanisms are adequate to reverse shock. Unfortunately, in many cases, these compensations are temporary. A downward spiral from prolonged reliance on compensatory mechanisms leads to increasing hypoxia marked by:

1. Endothelial (vessel lining) injury, allowing further loss of intravascular fluids
2. Fluid deprivation in the vessel, promoting further difficulties with cardiac output
3. Continued reduction in perfusion, promoting cellular injury, anaerobic metabolism, and metabolic acidosis

All cells become deprived of oxygen and other nutrients and convert to inefficient anaerobic metabolism. Eventually, cellular metabolism is unable to generate enough energy to maintain cellular homeostasis. This leads to impairment of the cell membrane ion pump, accumulation of intracellular sodium, and the loss of intracellular potassium. The cell swells, ruptures, and dies. In 50% of those experiencing severe shock, multiple organ failure, particularly of the heart, brain, kidneys, lungs, and skeletal muscle, leads to somatic death.

CLINICAL MANIFESTATIONS

Early clinical manifestations of shock are related to the triggering event. Because the primary cause of cardiogenic shock is myocardial infarction, early clinical manifestations may include chest pain, shortness of breath, labored breathing, diaphoresis, nausea, or vomiting. In hypovolemic shock, manifestations are related to the extent of blood or plasma loss. Infection leading to septic shock promotes fever and flushed, warm skin. Anaphylactic shock triggers generalized skin flushing and may lead to airway obstruction.

Clinical manifestations consistent across the potential etiologies are those indicative of circulatory impairment and collapse and include marked tachycardia, tachypnea, cool and clammy extremities, poor peripheral pulses, decreased arterial blood pressure (a late sign indicative of decompensation), cyanosis, pallor, restlessness, apprehension, decreased mental function, and poor urinary output. Because shock reduces perfusion throughout the body, multiple manifestations are possible related to general organ dysfunction.

DIAGNOSTIC CRITERIA

No one test is completely specific or sensitive for shock. The diagnosis of shock is based on a thorough patient history, physical examination, and laboratory and diagnostic tests. The patient history reveals a triggering event, such as myocardial infarction, massive hemorrhage, systemic infection, spinal cord injury, or anaphylaxis. Physical assessment includes observation of skin color, temperature, pulses, capillary refill, heart rate, blood pressure, urine output, and mental status. Laboratory studies vary and are directed at the potential cause. For example, in cardiogenic shock, laboratory tests include cardiac enzymes (creatine kinase, troponin, myoglobin), a complete blood count, electrolytes, arterial blood gases, and blood coagulation tests. An ECG and echocardiogram are used to detect the pattern and location of heart injury.

TREATMENT

Shock is considered a medical emergency and requires attention to the patient's airway, breathing, and circulation. The choice of action on the peripheral vessels depends on the shock etiology, fluid volume, and contractile ability of the heart. Unless contraindicated, hypovolemic patients should be placed in a supine position with legs elevated to maximize cerebral blood flow. The use of blankets is often needed to keep the patient warm. Treatment is focused on removing or reducing the underlying cause.

In cardiogenic shock, treatment involves surgically revascularizing the heart at the point of obstruction (see treatment of myocardial infarction below). Medical treatment is aimed at improving cardiac output, maintaining blood pressure, reducing the workload on the heart, providing oxygen therapy, and regulating fluid volumes in the body. Inotropic medications increase myocardial contractility. Various drugs in this group have either vasoconstricting (epinephrine, norepinephrine) or vasodilating (dobutamine) effects on peripheral vascular resistance. In hypovolemic shock, treatment is focused on improving tissue perfusion through intravenous fluid/blood replacement. Sources of bleeding or fluid loss must be identified and corrected. Oxygen may be administered depending on the level of hypoxemia. Septic shock treatment is aimed at treating the source of infection and supporting circulation. Pharmacologic treatment includes broad-spectrum antimicrobial drugs that provide coverage for possible pathogens and vasopressor drugs that promote vasoconstriction. Corticosteroids are often needed in anaphylactic shock to decrease the systemic inflammatory response. Neurogenic shock treatment is aimed at identifying and correcting the cause if possible and supporting vasoconstriction with inotropic medications. Frequent monitoring of vital organ function and hemodynamic status is required for all patients with shock.

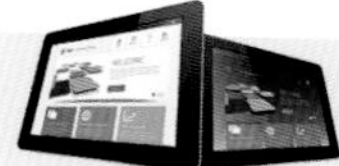

RESEARCH NOTES

Risk for cardiovascular disease can be calculated using established tools that predict the likelihood of a cardiac event within a period of time. The established Framingham Risk Score and the new American College of Cardiology/American Heart Association (ACC/AHA) Pooled Cohort Equations Risk Estimator were used to compare risk for cardiovascular risk in >30,000 adult men.[7] The ACC/AHA assessment identified lower absolute risk and more temporary "intermediate risk" groups as compared to the Framingham Risk Score calculation.

Myocardial Infarction

Coronary heart disease (CHD) is a term used to identify any problem of impaired coronary circulation. Atherosclerosis is primarily implicated in the development of CHD. Consequences of CHD range from compensation through the development of collateral circulation to the myocardial cells to sudden death from myocardial anoxia. Because multiple processes are at work during cardiac perfusion, the loss of coronary circulation can lead to a spectrum of problems, including impaired conduction, impaired myocardial pumping, and heart failure.

PATHOPHYSIOLOGY

Myocardial infarction is the total occlusion of one or more coronary arteries resulting in ischemia and death of myocardial tissues (Fig. 16.12). Consistent with CHD, the most common cause is atherosclerosis. Atherosclerotic accumulations can either directly obstruct the artery, or break off, causing platelets to aggregate at the site of injury and form a thrombus that occludes the artery. Factors that contribute to cardiovascular risk include age, sex, race, total cholesterol, HDL cholesterol, systolic blood pressure, blood pressure lowering medication use, diabetes status, and smoking status.[6] Major risk factors for the development of atherosclerosis and subsequent myocardial infarction include:

- **Family history:** Individuals with a family history of atherosclerosis and myocardial infarction are at greater risk, particularly those with a father or other male first-degree relative who experienced a myocardial infarction or sudden death from a coronary event prior to 55 years of age; or a mother or other female first-degree relative experiencing the same prior to 65 years of age.
- **Hypertension and smoking:** Hypertension and smoking injure the endothelial lining, promoting the development of atherosclerosis. Systolic blood pressure above 160 mm Hg is associated with a three-fold increase in risk of developing CHD. Diastolic elevations are significant contributors as well.
- **Blood cholesterol levels:** The amount of cholesterol, particularly high LDL (see From the Lab, below), in the blood, promoting lipid accumulation in the vessels.
- **Concurrent diabetes mellitus:** Type 2 diabetes is associated with elevations in blood lipid levels. The role of diabetes mellitus in the development of atherosclerosis is further discussed in Chapter 16.
- **High-sensitivity C-reactive protein (CRP):** CRP is a nonspecific acute phase protein that is

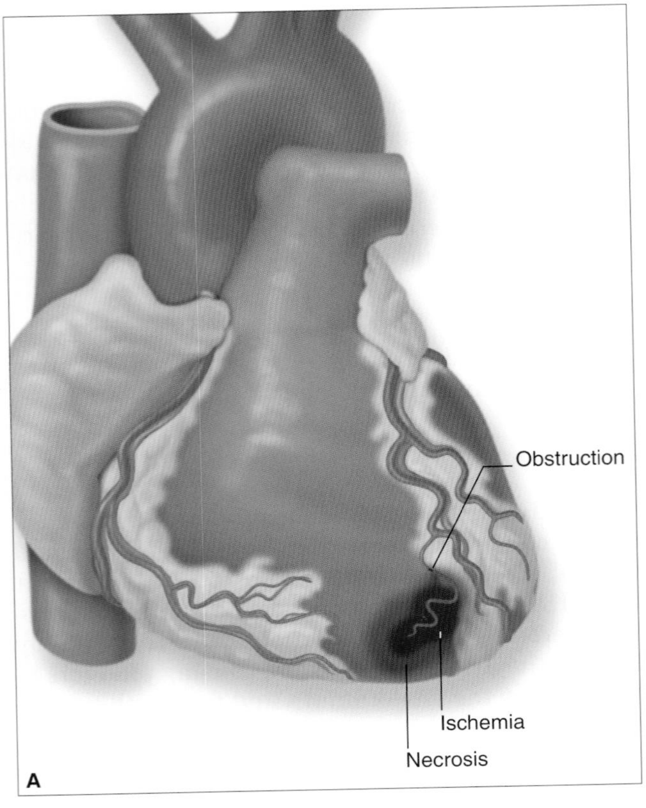

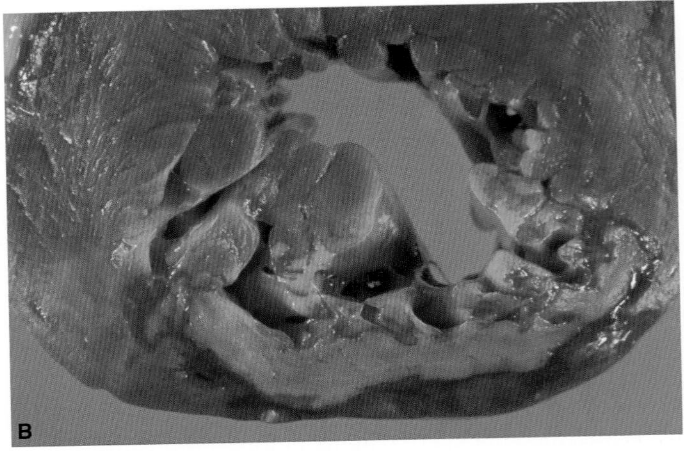

Figure 16.12. Myocardial infarction. **A:** Left coronary artery obstruction shows zones of necrosis and ischemia. **B:** A cross section of the left ventricle reveals a sharply circumscribed, soft, yellow area of necrosis. (From Rubin E, Farber JL. *Pathology*. 4th ed. Philadelphia, PA: Lippincott Williams & Wilkins; 2005.)

produced by the liver in response to tissue injury and is considered a sensitive marker of inflammation. Elevated CRP is an emerging indicator of risk for the development of myocardial infarction because inflammation has been linked with the pathogenesis of atherosclerosis.

- **Hyperhomocysteinemia:** Homocysteine is one of many potential risk factors for the development of MI. Homocysteine is derived primarily from a dietary amino acid found in animal protein. Homocysteine plays a role in coagulation. High levels of circulating homocysteine are toxic to endothelial cells and may promote excessive blood coagulation and thrombus formation. About half of those experiencing an acute myocardial infarction or stoke have hyperhomocysteinemia.

The size, location, duration of occlusion, and presence of collateral circulation dictate the major effects of the MI. Larger arteries, when obstructed, result in more widespread damage to the myocardium. Location of occlusion also dictates major effects. The left coronary artery supplies blood to the left side of the heart. The left coronary artery branches into the anterior descending left coronary artery, which perfuses primarily the left ventricle, and the circumflex left coronary artery, which perfuses primarily the left atrium and portions of the left ventricle. Obstruction impairs the left ventricle and affects the ability of the heart to pump blood systemically. Ventricular fibrillation is a major cause of sudden death from myocardial infarction. The right coronary artery and branches perfuse the right side of the heart, most notably the SA and AV nodes. Obstruction impacts cardiac conduction of impulses and can lead to irregularities in heart rhythm. Right heart failure also impedes the ability to manage venous return effectively. The myocardium can withstand oxygen deprivation for approximately 20 minutes. Beyond this, myocardial cell death is irreversible. Myocardial cells are replaced by nonfunctional scar tissue.

Stop and Consider
Low-dose daily aspirin is commonly used to prevent MI. Aspirin reduces platelet aggregation. How would this medication help to prevent MI?

CLINICAL MANIFESTATIONS

The clinical manifestations of MI are variable but may include: chest pain or a crushing pressure, often radiating to the left arm, shoulder, or jaw. Dizziness, sweating, indigestion (heartburn) pain, nausea, vomiting, fatigue, weakness, anxiety, cool, moist skin, pallor, or shortness of breath may also be reported. It is common for the individual to deny the chest pain as related to a MI. Women are particularly vulnerable because clinical manifestations are considered atypical or subtle (fatigue, syncope, or weakness), and may be ignored. **Angina pectoris** is a term used to describe chest pain or pressure that is intermittent and associated with myocardial ischemia, a reduction in blood flow to the coronary arteries caused atherosclerosis that is often accompanied by vasospasm. The presence of ischemia and subsequent angina are exacerbated with increased cardiac workload, such as with exercise, and are typically reduced with rest. With MI, rest or nitroglycerine tablets do not alleviate the presence of angina.

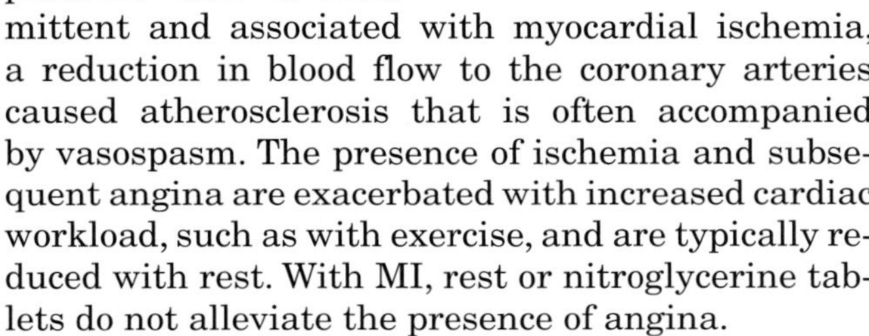

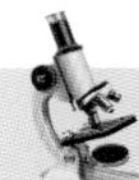

FROM THE LAB

Established biomarkers of myocardial infarction include troponin-T, troponin-I, myocardial infarction of creatine kinase (CK) and myoglobin. Troponin, a complex of three proteins (troponin-C, troponin-I, and troponin-T) is present in skeletal and cardiac muscle and is important in the regulation of muscle contractions. As troponin-C is found in both skeletal and cardiac muscle, it is not a specific biomarker of cardiac injury. Troponin-T is specific for cardiac muscle, located in the contractile elements of the myocardial cells. Troponin-I is also specific to cardiac muscle and when combined with troponin-T, serves as a primary biomarker for cardiac injury associated with myocardial infarction. After MI, troponin-T and troponin-I are detected in the blood within 6 to 8 hours, peak at 12 to 24 hours, and remain elevated for 7 to 10 days after MI. Creatine kinase has three isoenzymes: MM, MB, and BB. Only CK-MB is found in cardiac cells and rises after myocardial injury. Four to 9 hours after myocardial injury, CK-MB levels increase, peak at 24 hours, and return to baseline at 48 to 72 hours. Myoglobin, present in both skeletal and cardiac muscle, is released into the blood 1 hour after myocardial injury, peaks at 4 to 12 hours, and returns to normal soon after peaking. When combined with troponin or CK-MB biomarkers, myoglobin can be used to rule out myocardial infarction if levels are inconsistent with myocardial injury.[8]

DIAGNOSTIC CRITERIA

Diagnosis of myocardial infarction is based on presenting symptoms (if any), ECG findings, and cardiac biomarkers (see From the Lab, below). Depending on the location of the myocardial infarction, ECG tracings may demonstrate ST segment, (see Fig. 16.5) elevations, indicating problems with ventricular repolarization. In larger infarcts, the Q wave may also be prolonged. Angiography in the cardiac catheterization laboratory determines the location and extent of obstruction. Echocardiography will reveal wall motion abnormalities and ventricular function. A chest radiograph may be used to detect complications of acute myocardial infarction, particularly congestive heart failure and pulmonary edema.

TREATMENT

The initial strategies for managing myocardial infarction are to stabilize airway, breathing and circulation. Rapid treatment (within 90 minutes) is preferred to reestablish coronary perfusion and to salvage the myocardium as much as possible. Before the patient arrives at the emergency department, ambulance personnel should obtain intravenous access, provide supplemental oxygen, and administer oral aspirin. Aspirin in addition to anticoagulant therapy may be used to improve perfusion in the coronary circulation. Nitroglycerine (vasodilator) and morphine (analgesic) should be administered for active chest pain. Emergency treatment involves medical or surgical interventions. Percutaneous coronary intervention (PCI) is the treatment of choice for many patients with MI. PCI is a group of techniques capable of relieving coronary artery narrowing. One example is percutaneous transluminal coronary angioplasty (PTCA), a procedure that involves inserting a thin wire into the coronary artery from a distant access point via cardiac catheterization, inflating a balloon within this wire at the site of obstruction, and pushing open the stenotic vessel. This procedure often includes placement of a stent to keep the vessel open and patent. Some patients require coronary artery bypass surgery when other medical or surgical interventions have been ineffective (Fig. 16.13). Thrombolytic agents, combined with a potent platelet inhibitor, are recommended when PCI is not available within a 90-minute time frame. These drugs break though thromboses and reduce platelet aggregation at the site. Oxygen, nitroglycerin, analgesics, and aspirin therapy are continued while the patient is under emergency care. Long-term treatment is aimed at supporting cardiac conduction, output, and blood pressure through medication therapy (often with aspirin, beta blockers, ACE inhibitors, or angiotensin receptor blockers) and prescribed rest, exercise, and modification of risk factors (i.e., no smoking, reduced alcohol intake, nutritious diet, and weight loss).

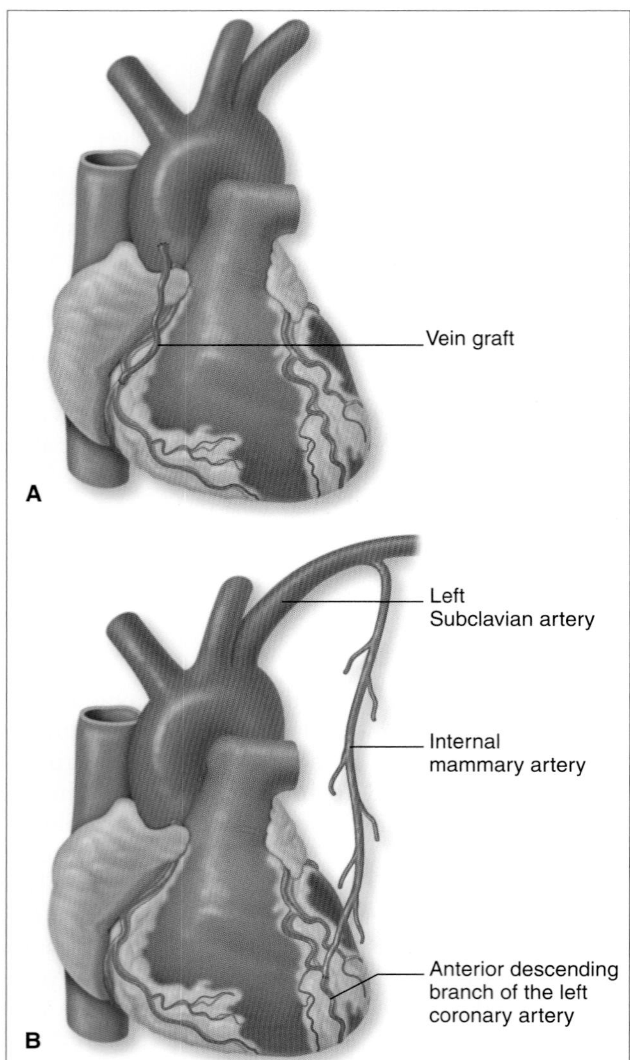

Figure 16.13. Coronary artery revascularization. **A:** Saphenous vein bypass graft. The vein segment is sutured to the ascending aorta and the right coronary artery at a point distal to the occlusion. **B:** Mammary artery bypass. The mammary artery is connected to the anterior descending left coronary artery at a point distal to the occlusion.

Heart Failure

Heart failure reflects an inadequacy of heart pumping so that the heart fails to maintain the circulation of blood. The basis for the development of altered perfusion of tissues is a result of *impaired cardiac functioning* or *excessive workload demands* that cannot be met by the heart. Heart failure occurs secondary to other conditions that perpetuate impaired cardiac functioning or workload. Examples of conditions that result in impaired cardiac functioning include myocardial infarction, structural defects of the heart, or infection and inflammation of the heart tissue layers. Examples of conditions that create excessive work demands on the heart include hypertension, fluid volume overload, or anemia.

PATHOPHYSIOLOGY

Because forward movement of blood is restricted, heart failure results in congestion and edema in pulmonary or peripheral tissues. In those with heart failure, cardiac reserve (the ability to increase output during increased activity) is expended during rest. Simple tasks become exceedingly taxing to the heart.

Left Heart Failure

Traditionally, heart failure is discussed based on the location of origin, either the left or right side of the heart. Despite isolating left and right, remember that these are both part of a continuous system. Therefore, impaired pumping and excessive peripheral vascular resistance eventually compromise both the left and the right sides of the heart.

In left heart failure, the left ventricle is unable to effectively meet cardiovascular demands, forward movement of blood through the circulation is inhibited, and fluid accumulates in the lung tissues. Loss of contractile ability, called **systolic failure**, results in the heart being unable to pump enough blood into the circulation. Stiffness of the ventricle and loss of relaxation ability, called **diastolic failure**, impairs the ability to optimally fill with blood between cardiac contractions.

Stop and Consider
How do you think pharmacologic interventions differ between systolic and diastolic left ventricular failure?

Recall that the left ventricle receives blood from the pulmonary vein and left atrium. When the left ventricle is ineffective and is unable to eject enough blood into the aorta during ventricular systole, blood backs up into the pulmonary vein, and subsequently into the lung tissues, resulting in pulmonary edema. **Congestive heart failure** is another term used to describe left heart failure. Causes of left heart failure include any condition that (1) impairs left ventricular pumping, such as what occurs with MI; or (2) increases the workload on the left ventricle, such as valvular disorders (aortic and bicuspid), in which the left ventricle must pump harder to compensate for stenosis or regurgitation (Fig. 16.14).

Right Heart Failure

Right heart failure begins on the right side of the heart. This impairs the heart's ability to move

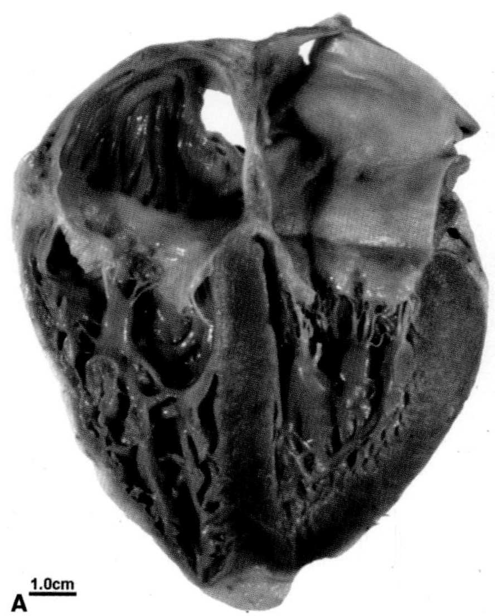

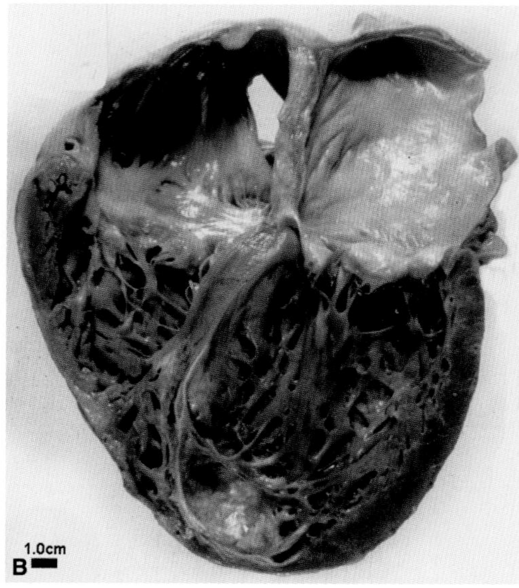

Figure 16.14. Congestive heart failure. **A:** An unaffected heart. **B:** Notable enlargement of the heart related to chronic heart failure secondary to ischemic injury.

deoxygenated blood forward to the pulmonary circulation. The result is congestion of blood backward into the systemic circulation. The systemic congestion produces peripheral edema. The development of edema was discussed in Chapter 8. Dependent areas of the body (i.e., extremities or areas closest to the ground) become swollen. The lower extremities are most commonly affected. The liver, spleen, gastrointestinal tract, and peritoneum can become engorged with fluid as blood backs up into to the hepatic veins and portal circulation.

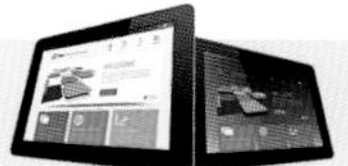

RESEARCH NOTES

The progression of heart failure from initial pathophysiology to the development of symptomatic heart failure was estimated based on a review of 11 large studies that included 25,369 participants. Individuals with systolic dysfunction developed heart failure at a rate of 8.4 per 100 person-years compared to 2.8 per 100 person-years in people with diastolic heart failure. The importance of early heart failure identification and initiation of effective management of systolic and diastolic heart failure prior to overt symptoms has the potential to slow disease progression.[9]

Causes of right heart failure include any process that restricts blood flow into the lungs. **Cor pulmonale** is an alteration in the structure and function of the right ventricle caused by a primary disorder of the respiratory system. Lung injury, infections, inflammation, and pulmonary edema are most often implicated. The resulting pulmonary hypertension is the common link between these lung injuries and the development of cor pulmonale. Because left heart failure results in pulmonary edema, right heart failure can be a consequence of left heart failure. However, only primary lung conditions are termed cor pulmonale. Valvular defects of the tricuspid and pulmonic valves can also put a strain on the right ventricle and contribute to the development of right heart failure.

The tissues need oxygen. With both left and right heart failure, the heart is unable to keep up with the demand. Compensatory mechanisms are triggered to maintain as much oxygenation as possible (Fig. 16.15). The initial response of compensatory mechanisms to help to ease congestion and improve cardiac pumping strength and efficiency contribute to pathology and worsening heart failure manifestations over time. Compensatory mechanisms include:

- *Improving venous return:* The tension in the veins increases, allowing improved movement of blood forward. This increases preload and improves cardiac output by increasing the amount of blood that fills the ventricles at the end of diastole. Diuretics may be used to support this compensatory mechanism by decreasing fluid volume and relieving peripheral vascular resistance.
- *Stimulating the sympathetic nervous system:* The sympathetic nervous system is stimulated to increase heart rate, cardiac contractility, and vessel tone to perfuse vital organs.
- *Stimulating the renin–angiotensin mechanism:* The kidneys increase renin secretion, resulting in elevations of angiotensin. This promotes compensatory vasoconstriction.

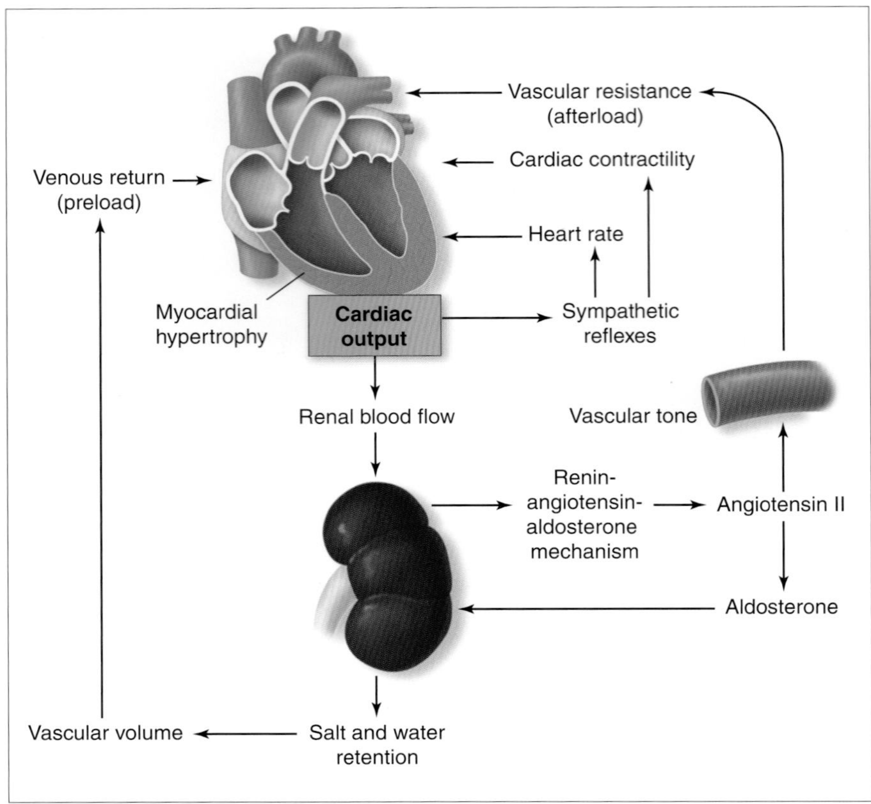

Figure 16.15. Compensatory mechanisms in heart failure. (Modified from Porth CM. *Essentials of Pathophysiology: Concepts of Altered Health States*. Philadelphia, PA: Lippincott Williams & Wilkins; 2003.)

- *Enlarging the heart muscle:* Hypertrophy of the heart muscle occurs in response to workload demands of the ventricles. Compensatory hypertrophy initially improves cardiac contractility.

Stop and Consider
How are compensatory mechanisms similar between shock and heart failure? How are these different?

These compensatory mechanisms become ineffective with severe, prolonged heart failure. Although venous return is initially improved, prolonged venous congestion is too overwhelming for compensatory mechanisms. Sympathetic stimulation promotes perfusion to vital organs. Over time, this mechanism can trigger dysrhythmias and deprive "nonvital" organs (i.e., skin, muscle, and kidneys) of oxygen. Most notably, poor renal perfusion leads to increased sodium and water retention, thereby further taxing venous return. Another factor contributing to sodium and water retention is the stimulation of aldosterone production by angiotensin II. Myocardial hypertrophy can initially contribute to contractility but eventually impairs diastole and promotes oxygen deprivation to the myocardium. The myocardium becomes noncompliant, or tense, and the heart chamber size is reduced. These compensatory mechanisms are helpful in the early stages of heart failure, but over time may cause more harm than good.

CLINICAL MANIFESTATIONS

Figure 16.16 compares the clinical manifestations between right and left heart failure. In right heart failure, the clinical manifestations are related to congestion in peripheral tissues from the ineffective right ventricle. Early clinical manifestations in left heart failure can be absent. When present, clinical manifestations specific to left heart failure are related to decreased cardiac output and pulmonary congestion from a failing left ventricle, which leads to poor tissue and organ perfusion. Fluid congestion in the lungs leads to shortness of breath, coughing, and lung crackles with auscultation. Poor tissue and organ perfusion leads to many potential indicators, including cyanosis, exercise intolerance, poor urinary output, fluid and sodium retention, anorexia, and fatigue.

Likewise, early clinical manifestations in right heart failure can be absent or subtle, such as fatigue, exertional dyspnea, or syncope with exertion. Although these early manifestations are often attributed to the underlying pulmonary disease, the

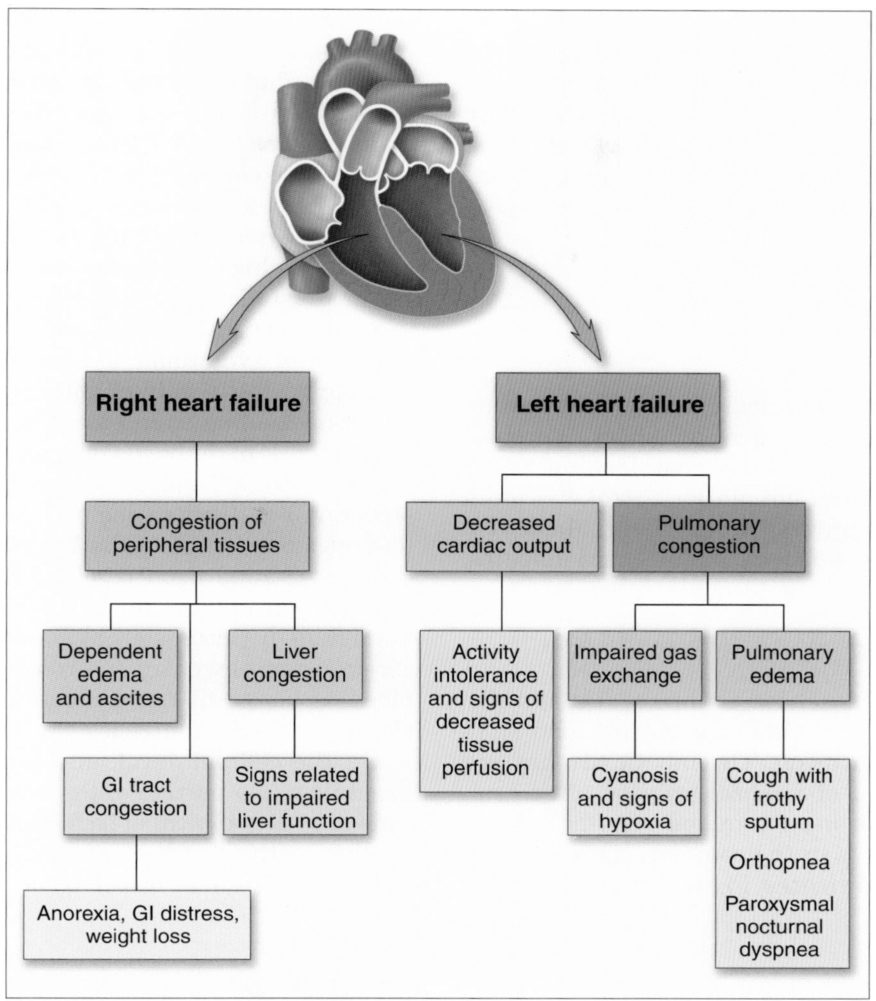

Figure 16.16. Comparison of the clinical manifestations between right and left heart failure. GI, gastrointestinal. (Modified from Porth CM. *Essentials of Pathophysiology: Concepts of Altered Health States*. Philadelphia, PA: Lippincott Williams & Wilkins; 2003.)

symptoms reflect the relative inability to increase cardiac output and a decrease in systemic arterial pressure with exertion. Ischemia of the right ventricle and pulmonary artery stretching can cause chest pain with exertion. In advanced stages, anorexia, weight loss, gastric and right upper quadrant pain, and jaundice can result from fluid congestion in the gastrointestinal tract and liver. Swelling in the extremities is also related to systemic edema.

DIAGNOSTIC CRITERIA

The diagnosis of heart failure is established based on a thorough patient history and physical examination, during which the presence of clinical manifestations listed above are noted. Chest radiography can detect pulmonary congestion, whereas two-dimensional echocardiography detects the heart's pumping ability, chamber size and thickness, the presence of valvular abnormalities, and measurements of various heart pressures. ECG supplies information on conduction impairments. Cardiac catheterization may be needed to visualize structural defects or to determine pressure levels in the heart chambers. Severity is based on the level of activity restriction imposed by the heart failure.

TREATMENT

Treatment of heart failure is focused on correcting the cause if possible. Surgically replacing defective valves, treating an underlying respiratory infection, or treating anemia are examples of correcting a heart failure cause. In many cases, the cause cannot be reversed. Lifestyle modifications are important in the management of heart failure and include smoking cessation, limitation or cessation of alcohol intake, salt and fluid restriction as well as weight management. Treatment focuses on providing supplemental oxygen, improving cardiac output, and pharmacologic intervention to correct volume overload and reduce peripheral vascular resistance (see hypertension) with an overall goal of improving quality of life. Heart failure is often a progressive, chronic problem with a poor prognosis. The 5-year survival rate is approximately 50%.

Stroke

Stroke is an acute neurologic injury that results from pathologic events such as shock, cerebral hemorrhage, ischemia, or infarction, leading to the impairment of cerebral circulation. Stroke is often referred to as a cerebrovascular accident. Major risk factors include hypertension, smoking, and diabetes.

PATHOPHYSIOLOGY

Stroke is often differentiated as thrombotic, embolic, or hemorrhagic to distinguish the process leading to altered cerebral perfusion. Thrombotic strokes are caused by occlusions of cerebral arteries, often from atherosclerosis. The most common site for atherosclerosis formation is in the common carotid artery where the artery bifurcates. Figure 16.17 illustrates the distribution of cerebral infarcts and areas of necrosis. The process is similar to the development of myocardial infarction. **Transient ischemic attack (TIA)** is a term used to describe a period of transient neurologic dysfunction and focal transient neurologic symptoms with risk of permanent neurologic injury and stroke. Risk of stoke following TIA is greatest when the individual is >60 years of age, has high blood pressure (systolic ≥140 mm Hg or diastolic ≥ 90 mm Hg), symptoms of stroke (e.g., unilateral weakness, speech disturbance), and duration of symptoms of 1 hour or more. TIAs are frequently the result of intermittent vascular obstruction leading to impaired cerebral perfusion. A completed stroke, however, causes permanent neurologic deficits. Embolic stroke similarly causes obstruction but results from emboli that dislodge from distant sites, travel to the brain, and occlude small arteries. Stroke from cerebral hemorrhage can be caused by trauma or defects in the cerebral vessels. Persistent hypertension and neoplasia can lead to cerebral vessel weakness, erosion, and rupture. The bleeding vessel fills and compresses adjacent brain tissue and brain ventricles.

On the cellular level, any process that disrupts blood flow to a portion of the brain unleashes a cascade of events typical of ischemia and inflammation, leading to the death of neurons. Within seconds to minutes of the loss of perfusion to a portion of the

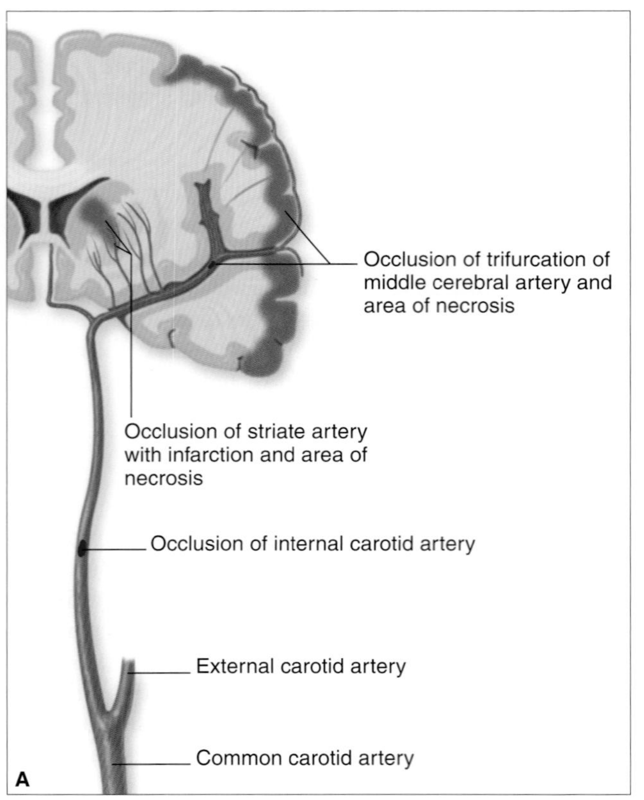

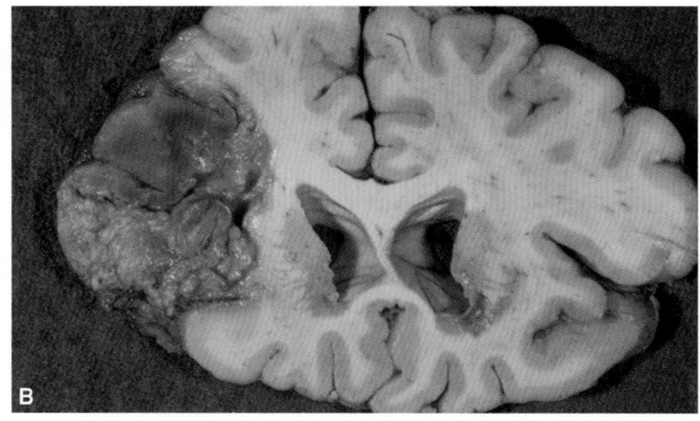

Figure 16.17. Cerebral infarction. **A:** Distribution of cerebral infarcts and areas of necrosis. **B:** A horizontal section of the brain depicting expansion and softening in the cortex from an occluded middle cerebral artery. (From Rubin E, Farber JL. *Pathology*. 4th ed. Philadelphia, PA: Lippincott Williams & Wilkins; 2005.)

brain, the ischemic neuron becomes depolarized. ATP is depleted and membrane ion-transport systems fail. Neurotransmitters are released through the influx of calcium, and excitatory receptors on other neurons are activated. These neurons then become depolarized, causing further calcium influx, further neuronal excitation, and expanded ischemia. Neuronal damage is exacerbated by the excessive calcium influx, which releases destructive enzymes, the release of free radicals, and the presence of potent chemical mediators. This ischemic area coalesces into an infracted core within hours of the onset of the stroke.

CLINICAL MANIFESTATIONS

Stroke typically results in the abrupt onset of clinical manifestations characteristic of a focal brain injury. The level of cerebral edema varies based on the extent of cellular injury. Loss of function is based on the part of the brain that is ischemic or compressed by the accumulation of blood. For example, hemorrhage of vessels leading to the medulla affect vital respiratory and cardiac centers and will result in sudden death. Cerebellar stroke impairs coordination. Common symptoms of stroke include the abrupt onset of hemiparesis (weakness on one side of the body), vision loss, visual field deficits, diplopia (double vision), dizziness, ataxia (lack of coordinated movement), aphasia (language impairment), or a sudden decrease in the level of consciousness.

In the cerebrum, hemorrhage or occlusion on one side of the brain results in hemiparesis or hemiplegia (paralysis) on the opposite side of the body. Therefore, if the stroke manifests as left-sided weakness, the obstruction or hemorrhage most likely exists on the right side of the cerebrum. Other possible manifestations of stroke include severe headache, sensory deficits, and vomiting. Again, the clinical presentation is extent and site dependent as ischemic brain tissue becomes necrotic and nonfunctional.

DIAGNOSTIC CRITERIA

The diagnosis of stroke is based on a careful patient history and physical examination, as well as laboratory and diagnostic studies. If the patient is aphasic and unable to speak, the history must include observer reports of time of onset and progression of symptoms, if possible. Essential components of the physical examination include the neurologic evaluation of mental status and the level of consciousness, cranial nerves, motor function, sensory function, cerebellar function, gait, and deep tendon reflexes. This examination can be guided and quantified by published stroke scales to determine stroke severity and progress. Laboratory tests, including a complete blood count, blood chemistry panel, coagulation studies, and cardiac enzymes may be needed to determine the cause of stroke or to rule out other health problems that can mimic a stroke. The primary diagnostic tool is brain imaging (e.g., CT scan, MRI), which can be used to distinguish the type and location of infarction. Brain imaging is critical for determining the most appropriate treatment pathway; patients with thrombotic stroke may receive thrombolytic therapy, whereas individuals with a brain hemorrhage do not.

TREATMENT

Treatment is based on the cause. Efforts are initially aimed at reducing cerebral edema and the resulting increased intracranial pressure. Thrombotic or embolic stroke may be treated with intravenous thrombolytic or anticoagulant therapy early in the acute phase followed by long-term oral antithrombotic therapy to reduce risk for recurrent stroke. Hemorrhagic stroke will require prevention of further bleeding, and aspiration of accumulated blood may be indicated. Treatment is often focused on rehabilitation in an effort to adapt to reduced function and maximize independence.

Disseminated Intravascular Coagulation

Disseminated intravascular coagulation (DIC) is a condition of uncontrolled activation of clotting factors that results in widespread thrombi formation, followed by depletion of coagulation factors and platelets leading to massive hemorrhage. DIC is initiated by endothelial or tissue injury, such as occurs with trauma, surgery, burns, malignant neoplasms, infections, or shock. Obstetric complications during labor and delivery are also commonly cited as a trigger for DIC.

PATHOPHYSIOLOGY

With DIC, injury triggers an imbalance between clotting and **fibrinolysis**, the dissolution of clots. Clotting factors, thrombin, and platelets accumulate throughout the cardiovascular system. This is particularly problematic in the microvessels, where the clots cause widespread tissue ischemia. The imbalance of clotting and clot dissolution is demonstrated, as blood-clotting mechanisms can then become depleted or clot-dissolving mechanisms increased. This allows massive systemic hemorrhage. DIC is a serious condition that requires immediate recognition and treatment.

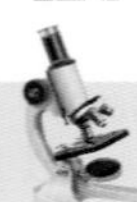

FROM THE LAB

Coagulation results from a sequence of events involving proteins (coagulation factors) produced by the liver and secreted into the bloodstream. Prothrombin time (PT), aPTT, and fibrinogen levels are screening tests for DIC. PT is used to evaluate the adequacy of the extrinsic clotting system (clotting that is triggered by the release of tissue thromboplastin), including factors I (fibrinogen), II (prothrombin), V, VII, and X. PT is measured in seconds, the expected range is usually approximately 11 to 14 seconds, and a prolonged PT indicates a deficiency in one or more of these factors. aPTT detects clotting factor deficiencies in the intrinsic clotting system (those factors already present in the plasma) and is a broader screening tests for deficiencies in factors I, II, V, VIII, IX, X, XII, and XII. aPTT is measured in seconds; the expected range is approximately 22 to 34 seconds and is significant when prolonged. Typically, when a prolonged PT or aPTT is noted, more specific tests are needed to identify the affected coagulation factor. Fibrinogen levels screen specifically for the presence of factor I. The most common cause for a reduced fibrinogen level is DIC.

CLINICAL MANIFESTATIONS

The effects of DIC are variable and depend on the presence of excessive clotting or hemorrhage. DIC can manifest as an acute hemorrhagic disorder caused by widespread clot dissolution from excess plasmin formation. This development is most commonly caused by infection, acute tissue injury, or obstetric complications and leads to bruising, petechiae, and epistaxis. Blood may be found in the sputum, stool, emesis, and urine. Severe bleeding and hemorrhage can lead to hypovolemic shock. Alternatively, DIC can manifest as a chronic or subacute state characterized by excess clotting (thrombin) formation. This occurs more commonly with malignancy, chronic renal disease, venous thrombosis, and certain connective tissue disorders. Widespread clotting can lead to multiple manifestations, depending on the location of thromboses. In the brain, it can lead to headache, weakness, seizures, and even coma. Within the kidneys, thromboses are manifested as poor urine output, which can progress to renal failure. In the heart and lungs, manifestations include cough, shortness of breath, respiratory distress, or chest pain. Vascular occlusions in larger vessels lead to the manifestations of infarction in the affected organ.

DIAGNOSTIC CRITERIA

Identification of the underlying problem leading to DIC is critical. A thorough patient history and physical examination are needed to identify this underlying cause, such as infection, malignancy, major traumatic injury, labor and delivery complications, or recent surgery. Screening laboratory tests include PT, activated partial thromboplastin time (aPTT), platelet count, and fibrinogen level. The D-dimer test measures the degradation of fibrin products, which is significant for both thrombus formation and breakdown, and detects the simultaneous formation of both thrombin and plasmin. This is considered a confirmatory test that strongly suggests the presence of DIC.

TREATMENT

Treatment is focused on correcting the underlying cause, and it depends on the presence of hemorrhage versus thromboses. The goal is to replace the missing blood components. Massive clotting requires anticoagulation therapy. Massive hemorrhage requires exogenous administration of clotting factors and platelets to replace what was lost. Treatment of DIC is a careful balancing act focused on restoring the body's ability to coagulate appropriately.

SUMMARY

- Perfusion is the process of forcing blood or other fluid to flow through a vessel and into the vascular bed of a tissue to provide oxygen and other nutrients.
- Effective perfusion is a complex interaction of ventilation, responsive neuronal control of cardiac impulses, cardiac muscle contraction, and circulation.
- Altered perfusion impairs tissue oxygenation and can stem from altered ventilation, diffusion, or circulation.
- Examples of situations that can impair circulation include brain injury at the cardiac control center in the medulla, blockage of the conduction system of the heart, structural defects, overtaxing, or necrosis of the heart (which reduces cardiac output), and obstruction and hemorrhage in the arteries and veins.
- General manifestations of altered perfusion depend on the process but may include tachycardia, tachypnea, fatigue, heart murmurs, ECG changes, pallor or erythema, cyanosis, edema, shortness of breath, impaired growth, hypotension or hypertension, hemorrhage, and pain.
- Multiple diagnostic tests are used to detect problems with perfusion, including blood tests for

hypercholesterolemia, anemia, and hypoxemia. Visualization, through the use of echocardiography, nuclear scanning, and radiography, allows detection of structural and functional problems with the heart's pumping capabilities and blood flow. ECG is frequently used to determine conduction problems with the heart.

CASE STUDY 16.1

James is a 55-year-old male who presents in the emergency department (ED) with sudden swelling in his left leg. He reports a dull ache in his calf that increases when he is walking. He states, "My left leg feels really tight and hot." He works as a truck driver and has just finished a long route that lasted 10 days. He does admit to an injury to his lower leg about 2 weeks ago but he thought that injury was resolved. He does not exercise regularly. He is a smoker. He reports no other significant health history. After physical examination, he undergoes a Doppler compression ultrasound, and a deep vein thrombosis is detected.

1. Outline the process that is most likely occurring in this man's body.
2. What would you expect for clinical manifestations?
3. What diagnostic tests could be used?
4. What treatment measures and complications would you anticipate?

Log on to the Internet. Search for a relevant journal article or Web site that details deep vein thrombosis, such as http://www.emedicine.com/med/ topic2785.htm, to confirm your predictions.

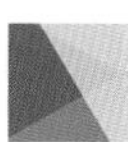

CASE STUDY 16.2

Jamie is a 15-year-old female who has concerns about excessive bleeding with her last menstrual period. She has noticed recently that she bruises easily and bleeds readily, particularly with her gums with brushing her teeth. She also has had nosebleeds recently as well. She comes into your clinical for examination. You note nonpalpable petechiae of her legs and arms, purpura, and gingival bleeding. Her platelet count is less than 20,000/mm^3. She is diagnosed with idiopathic thrombocytopenic purpura.

1. Outline the process that is most likely occurring in this adolescent's body.
2. What would you expect for clinical manifestations?
3. What diagnostic tests could be used?
4. What treatment measures and complications would you anticipate?

Log on to the Internet. Search for a relevant journal article or Web site that details idiopathic thrombocytopenic purpura, such as http://emedicine.medscape.com/article/779545-overview, to confirm your predictions.

PRACTICE EXAM QUESTIONS

1. In evaluating modifiable cardiovascular risk factors for your patient, which one is NOT considered modifiable?
   a. Poorly controlled diabetes mellitus
   b. Hyperlipidemia
   c. Hypertension
   d. Female gender

2. Your patient is experiencing peripheral edema, hepatomegaly, ascites, and splenomegaly. Which of the following conditions would be consistent with the patient's findings?
   a. Endocarditis
   b. Myocardial infarction
   c. Right-sided heart failure
   d. Left-sided heart failure

3. It is a hot summer day. Your neighbor stops at your house after jogging 5 miles. She is sweating and tells you she feels dizzy and thirsty and can't make it home. You check her blood pressure and find it to be LOW. What could you do right in your home to raise her blood pressure?
   a. Place a cold washcloth on her head
   b. Have her drink a large glass of cool water
   c. Have her take a shower with warm water
   d. Encourage her to take slow, deep breaths

4. Your neighbor again comes to your door (see previous question). She has been running in the snow and it is cold outside. She has a headache and her heart is pounding. Again you check her blood pressure and find it to be HIGH. What could you do this time right in your home to decrease her blood pressure?
   a. Have her drink some hot chocolate
   b. Have her lay down on your couch
   c. Let her take a hot shower
   d. Give her something really salty to eat

5. Which of the following situations of altered perfusion could be triggered by chronic obstructive pulmonary disease?
   a. Impaired cardiac output
   b. Impaired circulation
   c. Ventilation–perfusion mismatching
   d. Excessive cardiac demand

6. Which mechanism increases peripheral vascular resistance and contributes to the development of hypertension?
   a. Impaired sodium excretion by the kidneys
   b. Parasympathetic nervous system overstimulation
   c. Reduced renin–angiotensin–aldosterone secretion
   d. None of these

7. Which is not a requirement for effective perfusion?
   a. Absence of chronic disease
   b. Adequate blood volume
   c. Functional systemic circulation
   d. An open airway

8. Your neighbor tells you that she was in the hospital and they told her she had a bundle branch block. What does this mean?
   a. She cannot conduct electrical impulses to stimulate the heart ventricle to contract
   b. She has had a cardiac arrest
   c. She is experiencing obstructed P wave depolarization of the atria
   d. She has an excessive calcium influx causing prolonged myocardial contraction

9. You are listening to your lab partners heart in skills lab and you hear the "lub dub" sound. What are you hearing?
   a. The sodium ions rapidly influxing into the cells
   b. The closure of the heart valves
   c. The contraction of the left ventricle
   d. Blood forcing its way through the aorta

10. At what point in the cardiac cycle do you measure preload?
    a. Just after systole
    b. Just before systole
    c. During systole
    d. It is not possible to measure preload

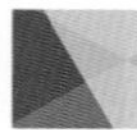

DISCUSSION AND APPLICATION

1. What did I know about altered perfusion prior to today?
2. What body processes are affected by altered perfusion? What are the expected functions of those processes? How does altered perfusion affect those processes?
3. What are the potential etiologies for altered perfusion? How does altered perfusion develop?
4. Who is most at risk for developing altered perfusion? How can altered perfusion be prevented?
5. What are the human differences that affect the etiology, risk, or course of altered perfusion?
6. What clinical manifestations are expected in the course of altered perfusion?
7. What special diagnostic tests help determine the diagnosis and course of altered perfusion?
8. What are the goals of care for individuals with altered perfusion?
9. How does the concept of altered perfusion build on what I have learned in the previous chapters and in previous courses?
10. How can I use what I have learned?

RESOURCES

American Heart Association:
http://www.heart.org/HEARTORG/#

American Society of Hypertension:
http://www.ash-us.org/

National Stroke Association:
http://www.stroke.org/

References

1. Farooq U, Ray SG. 2014 Guideline for the management of high blood pressure (Eighth Joint National Committee): take-home messages. *Med Clin North Am*. 2015;99:733–738. http://dx.doi.org/10.1016/j.mcna.2015.02.004
2. James PA, Oparil S, Carter BL, et al. 2014 Evidence-based guideline for the management of high blood pressure in adults: report from the panel members appointed to the Eighth Joint National Committee (JNC 8). *JAMA*. 2014;311(5):507–520. doi:10.1001/jama.2013.284427.
3. The U.S. Department of Health and Human Services. The seventh report of the Joint National Committee on detection, evaluation, and treatment of high blood pressure. 2003. http://www.nhlbi.nih.gov/guidelines/hypertension/express.pdf. Accessed December 13, 2015.
4. Miedema MD, Lopez FL, Blaha M, et al. Implications of the Eighth Joint National Committee guidelines for the management of high blood pressure for aging adults: atherosclerosis risk in communities study. *Hypertension*. 2015;66(3):474–480. doi:10.1161/HYPERTENSIONAHA.115.05560.
5. American College of Cardiology/American Heart Association Task Force on Practice Guidelines. 2013 ACC/AHA Guideline on the treatment of blood cholesterol to reduce atherosclerotic cardiovascular risk in adults. *Circulation*. 2014;129(suppl 2):S1–S45.
6. Goff DC, Lloyd-Jones DM, Bennett G, et al. 2013 ACC/AHA Guideline on the assessment of cardiovascular risk: a report of the American College of Cardiology/American Heart Association Task Force on practice

guidelines. *J Am Coll Cardiol*. 2014;63(25, pt B):2935–2959. doi:10.1016/j.jacc.2013.11.005.

7. Blaha MJ, Dardari ZA, Blumenthal RS, et al. The new "intermediate risk" group: a comparative analysis of the new 2013 ACC/AHA risk assessment guidelines versus prior guidelines in men. *Atherosclerosis*. 2014;237(1):1–4. doi:10.1016/j.atherosclerosis.2014.08.024.
8. Mythili S, Malathi N. Diagnostic markers of acute myocardial infarction. *Biomed Rep*. 2015;3(6):743–748. doi:10.3892/br.2015.500.
9. Echouffo-Tcheugui JB, Erqou S, Butler J, et al. Assessing the risk of progression from asymptomatic left ventricular dysfunction to overt heart failure: a systematic overview and meta-analysis [published online ahead of print December 7, 2015]. *JACC Heart Fail*. doi:10.1016/j.jchf.2015.09.015. pii: S2213-1779(15)00683-6.

Find additional resources for this chapter at http:thePoint.lww.com thePoint®

Chapter

17 Altered Nutrition

LEARNING OUTCOMES

1. Define and use the key terms listed in this chapter.
2. Explain the role of nutrition in maintaining health.
3. Identify the processes that can alter nutrition.
4. Identify common signs and symptoms related to altered nutrition.
5. Describe diagnostic tests and treatment strategies relevant to altered nutrition.
6. Apply concepts of altered nutrition to select clinical models.

INTRODUCTION

What did you eat for breakfast? How did that food contribute to your health? Every day we put nutrients into our bodies with little consideration of exactly what those nutrients are doing to maintain homeostasis. Adequate nutrition relies on optimal intake, digestion, absorption, and transportation of nutrients, as well as the excretion of waste products. We choose to eat a variety of foods because they are appealing to us in one way or another. Once the food goes through the process of digestion, the extracted nutrients are made suitable for absorption and transportation. The nutrients in their simplest form are then used for a predictable purpose. This chapter takes a closer look at essential food-derived nutrients and the role these nutrients play in facilitating basic physiologic processes. Clinical models are selected to illustrate the effects of nutrient deficiencies or excesses on healthy functioning.

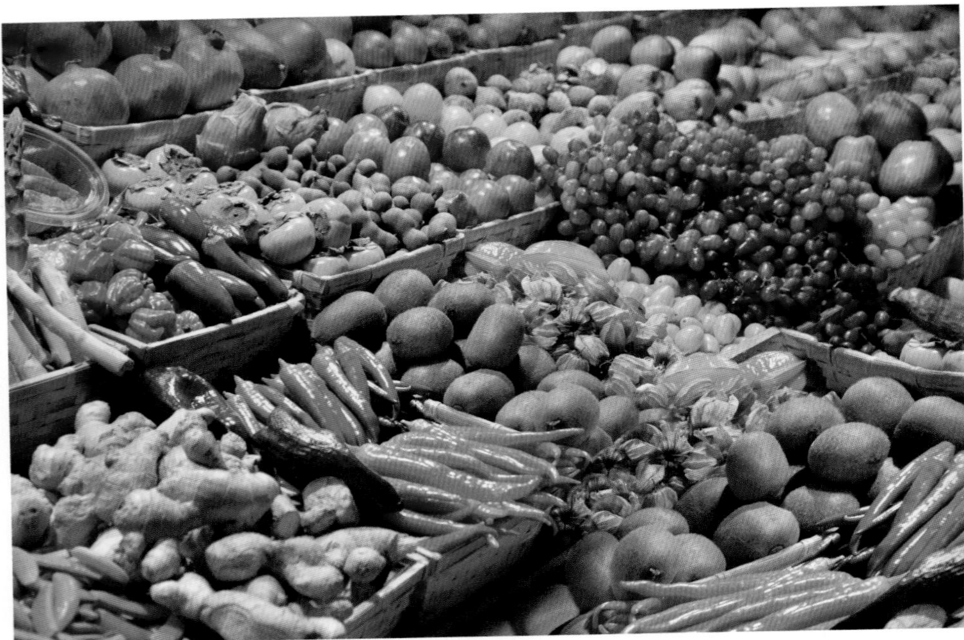

Fruits and vegetables at a farmers market. Image © Adisa

Module 1 Nutrition

Nutrition is the process of ingestion and utilization of nutrients for energy. Ultimately, we obtain nutrition and **energy**, or the capacity to do work, from the sun via organisms and plants that undergo photosynthesis. Energy from ingested nutrients is released when food is metabolized. Metabolism allows chemical reactions that (1) produce heat to maintain body temperature, (2) conduct neuronal impulses, and (3) contract muscles. Nutrition also provides the substances needed for growth, repair, and maintenance of cells.

A **nutrient** is a food or liquid that supplies the body with the chemicals needed for metabolism. Nutrients are frequently categorized as macronutrients, micronutrients, and water. **Macronutrients** are proteins, carbohydrates, and fats. **Micronutrients** are vitamins and minerals. The body is capable of synthesizing certain nutrients from other products (e.g., the synthesis of glucose from amino acids and glycerol). Many nutrients, however, must be consumed regularly in the diet, because the body is unable to synthesize the nutrient in quantities sufficient to meet its needs. These are called **essential nutrients**.

Water

Water is the largest single component of the body and is essential for all body functions, including digestion, absorption, transportation, and excretion. Specifically, water functions to:

- Serve as a solvent promoting availability of solutes to the cell
- Promote and maintain fluid balance
- Provide a transport medium for nutrients and waste products
- Serve as a lubricant
- Contribute to the regulation of body temperature
- Provide the foundation for metabolic reactions
- Contribute to the structure of the cells and circulatory system

Because the body is unable to store water, regular intake of water is required to offset that lost through perspiration or other mechanisms. Although individuals can survive several weeks without food, adults (in moderate weather) can survive only 10 days without water and children can survive only 5 days.[1] Metabolically active cells, such as muscle cells, have the highest concentrations of water and are most devastated by deficiencies. The major point is that water is an essential nutrient; a reduction in total body water of 20% or greater may cause death.

Macronutrients: Proteins, Lipids, and Carbohydrates

The major macronutrients that are converted to usable sources of energy are proteins, lipids, and carbohydrates. Protein is composed of linear chains of amino acids that are linked as directed by DNA coding. During digestion, proteins are broken down into amino acids and absorbed into the circulation (Fig. 17.1). The body contains 20 different types of amino acids. Of these, nine are considered essential and therefore must be consumed within the diet. From amino acids, body proteins are synthesized. Protein is needed to build and maintain structural body tissues such as muscle, bone matrix, and connective tissue. It also comprises blood, cell membranes, immune factors, enzymes, and hormones. Proteins transport other substances across membranes and throughout the body and can combine with other substances to form new substances. For example, proteins can combine with nucleic acids to form DNA and RNA, carbohydrates to form glycoproteins, lipids to form lipoproteins, and metals to form hemoglobin.

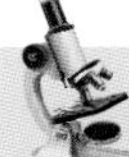

FROM THE LAB

Unique to macronutrients, protein contains nitrogen. Nitrogen balance is a biochemical technique used to determine protein status. Nitrogen balance is calculated based on daily protein intake and the amount of nitrogen excretion in the urine. A correction is added for insensible losses of nitrogen, such as through the skin and gastrointestinal (GI) tract. In healthy adults, the nitrogen balance should equate to zero. If the person has a positive nitrogen balance, this individual is taking in more protein than is being excreted, which should occur in times of growth, pregnancy, and healing. If the person has a negative nitrogen balance, this individual is excreting more protein than is being consumed, as occurs in a state of tissue destruction, such as with burns, infection, or other tissue trauma.

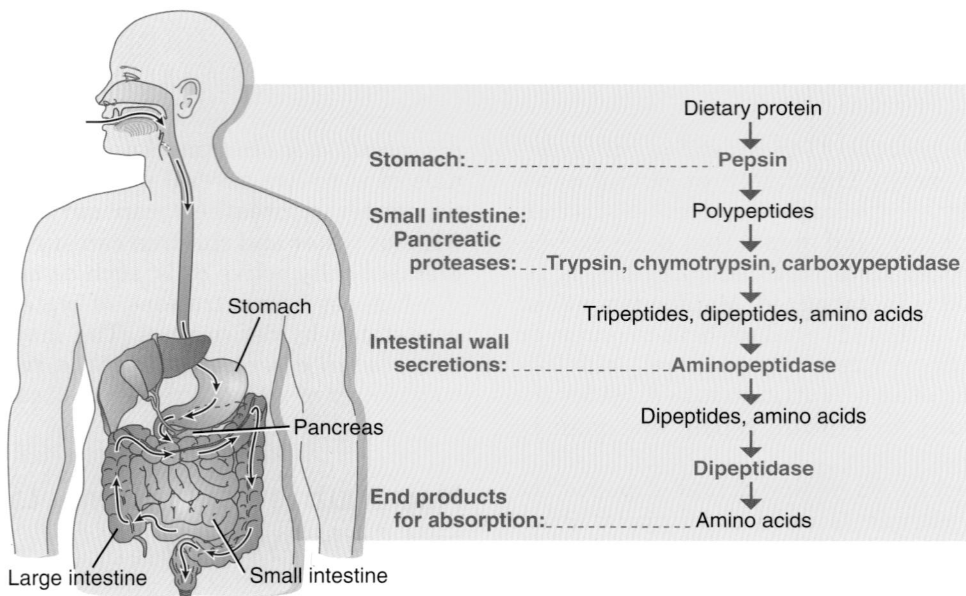

Figure 17.1. Protein digestion. Chemical digestion of protein begins in the stomach. Hydrochloric acid converts pepsinogen to the active enzyme pepsin, which begins the process of breaking down proteins into small polypeptides and some amino acids. The majority of protein digestion occurs in the small intestine, where pancreatic proteases reduce polypeptides into shorter chains, tripeptides, dipeptides, and amino acids. Enzymes located on the surface of the cells that line the small intestine complete the digestion: aminopeptidase splits amino acids from the amino ends of short peptides, and dipeptidase reduces dipeptides to amino acids.

Lipids are also considered macronutrients and are a group of substances that are insoluble in water. Lipids are categorized as:

1. Simple lipids or fats: fatty acids and glycerol
2. Compound lipids or lipoids: phospholipids, lipoproteins, and glycolipids
3. Sterols: cholesterol and bile salts

Triglycerides, a fatty acid and glycerol complex, are a form of simple lipids readily found in dietary fat. **Saturated fatty acids** are fatty acids that have no double bonds and elevate blood cholesterol levels. These fatty acids are found in animal sources and are solid at room temperature. **Unsaturated fatty acids** have one or more double bonds and are not known to elevate blood cholesterol levels. These are usually found in plant sources and are often liquid at room temperature.

Lipids provide a rich source of energy. Most dietary fat is stored in the body within adipose cells, also called adipocytes. Adipose cells contain storage fats, which accumulate around tissues and within body cavities and are used when energy is needed. Adipose cells can sustain the body's energy provision for weeks. The accumulation of storage fats is considered a health epidemic, particularly for those consuming a Western diet. Obesity is selected as a clinical model within this chapter to illustrate the health effects of excessive storage fat. A small amount of lipids can be stored in other locations, such as within liver cells. An accumulation of fat in liver cells inhibits liver cell function.

Structural fat is a type of fat that is not accessed for energy; rather, it provides support and protection to body organs and nerves. Structural fats are found inside cell structures of the brain, liver, kidney, lung, heart, spleen, muscle, and other cells, and they are essential for survival. The subcutaneous fat layer provides insulation and maintenance of body temperature.

Aside from being a rich source of energy, lipids facilitate numerous processes after ingestion and absorption into the body (Fig. 17.2). Dietary fat supports digestion by decreasing gastric motility and secretions. Along with this function, dietary fat stimulates pancreatic and bile secretion and facilitates the digestion, absorption, and transportation of fat-soluble vitamins. The brain, central nervous system (CNS), and cell membranes throughout the body require essential fatty acids to function optimally. Essential fatty acids influence cell membrane fluidity, receptor function, enzyme activity, and cytokine production. Linoleic acid, an omega-3 fatty acid derived from fish and plant oils, is considered an essential fatty acid and has been demonstrated to reduce many disease states, including heart disease. This substance acts by (1) reducing fibrinogen and other clotting proteins and decreasing the likelihood

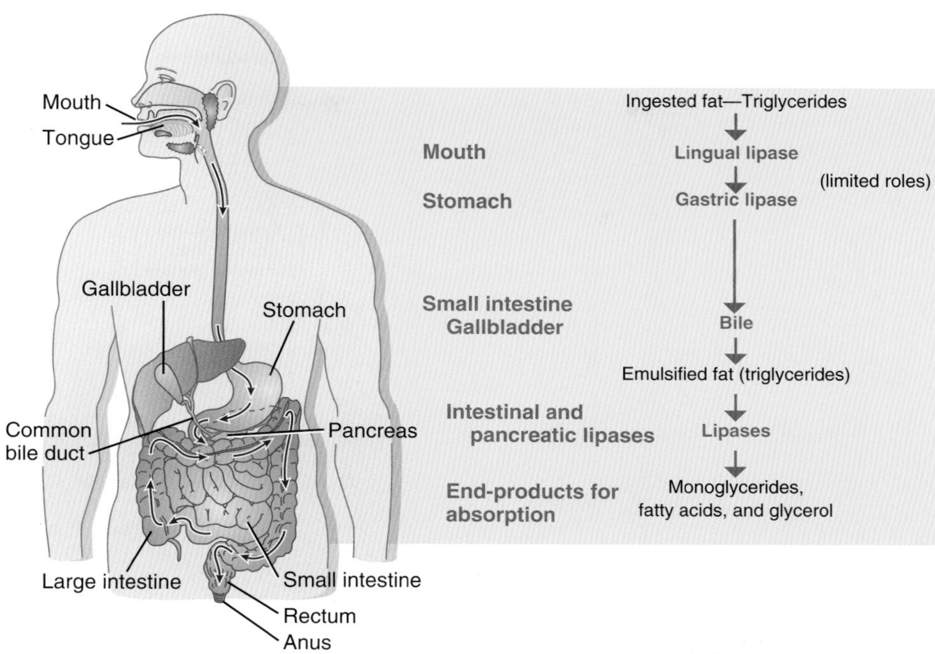

Figure 17.2. Fat digestion. A minimal amount of chemical digestion of fat occurs in the mouth and stomach through the action of lingual lipase and gastric lipases, respectively. As fat enters the duodenum, it stimulates the release of the hormone cholecystokinin, which in turn stimulates the gallbladder to release bile. Bile prepares fat for digestion by suspending the hydrophobic molecules in the watery intestinal fluid. Most fat digestion occurs in the small intestine. Pancreatic lipase splits off one fatty acid at a time from the triglyceride molecule, working from the outside in until two free fatty acids and a monoglyceride remain. Usually, the process stops at this point, but sometimes digestion continues and the monoglyceride splits into a free fatty acid and glyceride molecule. The end products of digestion—mostly monoglycerides with free fatty acids and little glycerol—are absorbed into intestinal cells. It is normal for a small amount of fat (4–5 g) to escape digestion and be excreted in the feces.

that a clot will form and (2) stimulating endothelial cells to produce substances that promote vascular relaxation. Phospholipids, a form of complex lipid, are an important structural component of cell membranes. Lipids are also an integral aspect of hormones that mediate multiple body processes.

Carbohydrates are also considered macronutrients. The three categories of carbohydrates are:

1. Monosaccharides: glucose or fructose
2. Disaccharides and oligosaccharides: sucrose or lactose
3. Polysaccharides: starches and fiber

Dietary carbohydrates are digested and converted primarily into glucose (Fig. 17.3). Once digested, the glucose is absorbed across the intestinal wall and transported to the liver via the portal circulation, where about 50% is used for oxidation or stored as glycogen. The remaining glucose exits the liver and is circulated throughout the body to be used by cells for energy.

The major role of carbohydrates is to provide energy. Interestingly, carbohydrates are not considered essential. Glucose is important and the brain is the largest consumer; however, lipids and proteins can provide this energy source. Glucose can be synthesized by converting amino acids and glycerol from triglycerides into glucose. This is not the most efficient way of achieving an adequate glucose level (see Malnutrition discussed below under Altered Nutrition); therefore, carbohydrates should comprise the largest proportion of daily food intake. Complex carbohydrates are preferred over simple sugars because these food sources provide other nutrients, such as vitamins and minerals. Fiber, a nondigestible carbohydrate, is important in the reduction of serum cholesterol levels and works primarily by binding to bile acids, a source of cholesterol, and by preventing cholesterol absorption. Fiber also plays a key role in gastric motility.

Micronutrients: Vitamins and Minerals

Vitamins are organic substances that the body is unable to manufacture and therefore must be consumed. Vitamins are often classified according to

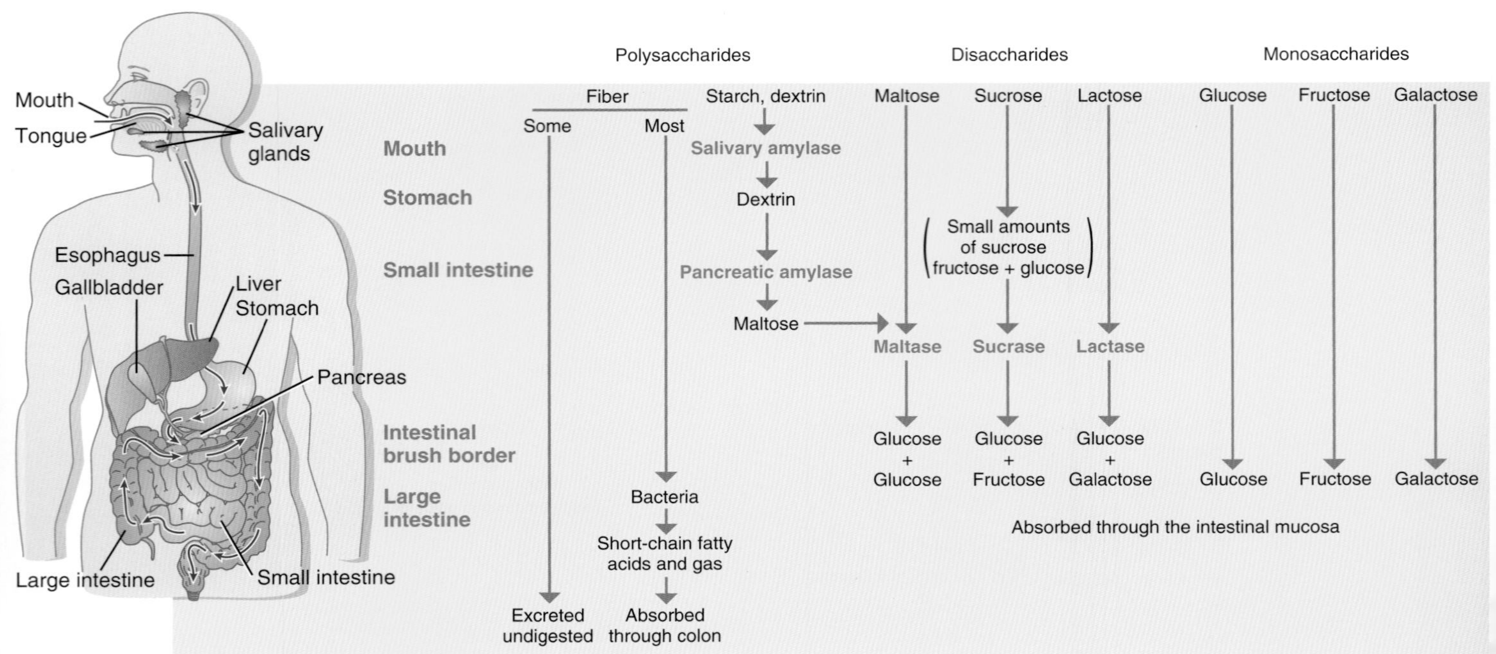

Figure 17.3. Carbohydrate digestion. Dietary carbohydrates include the polysaccharides or complex carbohydrates (fiber, starch, and dextrin), the disaccharides (maltose, sucrose, and lactose), and the monosaccharides (glucose, fructose, and galactose). Digestion begins in the mouth, where food is chewed into pieces and salivary amylase begins the process of chemical digestion. The stomach churns and mixes the carbohydrate, but stomach acids halt residual action of the salivary amylase. The small intestine is the site of most carbohydrate digestion, and pancreatic amylase reduces complex carbohydrates into disaccharides. Disaccharide enzymes (maltase, sucrase, and lactase) on the surface of the small intestine cells split maltose, sucrose, and lactose into monosaccharides, thus completing the process of carbohydrate digestion. Fiber is not digested per se, but most is fermented by bacteria in the large intestine to yield gas, water, and short-chain fatty acids.

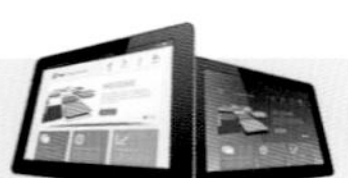

RESEARCH NOTES

A multitude of studies have attempted to determine the effects of antioxidants on health. A search of ClinicalTrials.gov revealed almost 400 studies in progress related to antioxidant use to treat a variety of conditions. Completed studies have focused on the impact of antioxidants on everything from reducing pregnancy-induced hypertension to Alzheimer disease. However, clinical trials of antioxidant supplementation have been conducted, and questions about the efficacy and safety of these supplements have emerged. More recent studies have also found that in most instances antioxidant supplements did not help to prevent disease and, in some cases, high doses of antioxidants actually contributed to morbidity or mortality, such as an increase in hemorrhagic stroke in men on vitamin E supplements.[2]

solubility (fat or water soluble) or by metabolic function. *Fat-soluble vitamins* include vitamins A, D, E, and K. *Water-soluble vitamins* are ascorbic acid (vitamin C), thiamin (B_1), riboflavin (B_2), niacin, pyridoxine (B_6), biotin, pantothenic acid, folate, and cobalamin (B_{12}). The physiologic impact of each of the vitamins is depicted in Table 17.1. As is evident in this table, many vitamins play a critical role in the metabolism of carbohydrates, amino acids, and fatty acids. The metabolic value of vitamins includes categories such as:

1. Membrane stabilizers (such as with antioxidants)
2. Hydrogen and electron donors and acceptors
3. Hormones
4. Coenzymes

Basically, vitamins are part of enzyme systems that release energy from macronutrients. Other major roles of vitamins are to help develop genetic materials, red blood cells, hormones, collagen, and nervous system tissue.

Stop and Consider
How do you think vitamin A and C deficiencies affect wound healing?

Minerals are inorganic substances critical to the regulation of hundreds of cellular processes. Minerals constitute bone, hemoglobin, enzymes, hormones, and chemical mediators. Charged (ionic) minerals

Table 17.1 Vitamins and Their Major Physiologic Functions

Vitamin	Functions This Vitamin Plays a Key Role in
Vitamin A	• Maintenance of visual pigment and photoreception • Maintenance of epithelial cells and mucous membranes • Cellular growth and differentiation by contributing to glycoprotein (cell surface regulator) synthesis • Synthesis of collagen and bone • Regulation of gene expression • Reproduction and immune function
Vitamin D	• Absorption and metabolism of calcium and phosphorus • Regulation of gene expression • Stimulation of differentiation of intestinal epithelial cells and osteoblasts
Vitamin E	• Protection against oxidative degradation from reactive oxygen species (free radicals)
Vitamin K	• Coagulation of blood • Formation of bone
Ascorbic acid (vitamin C)	• Synthesis of collagen and mucous membrane integrity • Protection against oxidative degradation from reactive oxygen species (free radicals) • Facilitation of iron absorption • Maintenance of lung function • Metabolism of amino acids • Synthesis of steroid hormones • Promotion of resistance to infection
Thiamin (vitamin B_1)	• Carbohydrate metabolism—serves as a coenzyme in the process of energy metabolism • Regulation of neuronal function, although the mechanism is unclear
Riboflavin (vitamin B_2)	• Carbohydrate, amino acid, and fatty acid metabolism • Support for antioxidant properties
Niacin	• Carbohydrate, amino acid, and fatty acid metabolism
Pyridoxine (vitamin B_6)	• Amino acid metabolism • Release of glucose from glycogen • Biosynthesizing neurotransmitters and histamine • Biosynthesizing myelin sheaths of nerve cells • Modulation of steroid hormone receptors • Critical for the production of antibodies
Folate	• Amino acid and nucleotide metabolism • DNA/RNA synthesis • Embryogenesis • Formation of red and white blood cells in the bone marrow • Reduction of homocysteine levels
Biotin	• Carbohydrate, amino acid, and fatty acid metabolism
Pantothenic acid	• Carbohydrate, amino acid, and fatty acid metabolism
Cobalamin (vitamin B_{12})	• Amino acid metabolism • Essential for metabolism of all cells, particularly those of the gastrointestinal tract, bone marrow, and nervous tissue • Reduction of homocysteine levels

mediate impulse conduction within the nervous system. Minerals maintain water balance, acid–base balance, and osmotic pressure. Minerals are critical for muscle contraction and form the structural components of bones and teeth.

Minerals are subcategorized as macrominerals or microminerals. The macrominerals include sodium, potassium, calcium, phosphorus, magnesium, and sulfur. These substances are primarily ions and therefore exist in a charged state. The microminerals include iron, zinc, fluoride, and copper. Microminerals do not exist in blood, tissues, and cellular fluids in a free ionic state; rather, these substances are bound to proteins. Microminerals are often referred to as trace metals. These metals act on enzymes and hormones to elicit a specific response. They also interact with DNA to regulate the transcription of proteins. In this way, microminerals, or metals, affect the whole body. Microminerals can be further subdivided as ultratrace minerals, in which extremely minute amounts are required. The ultratrace minerals are iodine, selenium, manganese, molybdenum, cobalt, boron, and chromium. The specific contributions of select minerals are presented in Table 17.2.

Nutritional Intake Requirements

Nutritional intake requirements, such as the Recommended Daily Allowances (RDAs), have been published to designate the recommended intake for most nutrients. The goal of adhering to the RDAs is to minimize the health effects that can occur with overnutrition or undernutrition. Caloric requirements are determined based on the kcal/kg needed to maintain body weight. Caloric intake requirements depend on age, gender, activity level, current weight, pregnancy, and lactation. During times of growth, caloric requirements are higher. For example, caloric requirements are 117 kcal/kg at birth. This requirement decreases to 80 kcal/kg between ages 1 and 10 years and is about half of that (30 to 40 kcal/kg) in adulthood. Pregnancy demands add an additional 300 kcal/day. Lactation (breastfeeding) increases the requirement by 500 kcal/day.

Stop and Consider

What is your approximate caloric requirement per day to maintain your body weight?

Micronutrient requirements are expressed primarily in micrograms (μg) or milligrams (mg) per day. For example, the RDA for vitamin A for adults is 700 μg/day for women and 900 μg/day for men. Macronutrient intake recommendations for adults are based on percentage of calories consumed[3]:

Table 17.2 Physiologic Contributions of Select Minerals

Mineral	Function
Calcium	Calcium is the most abundant mineral in the body and is essential for bone and teeth formation, muscle contraction, blood coagulation, transmission of nervous impulses, cell membrane permeability, and enzyme activation
Phosphorus	Phosphorus is the second most abundant mineral in the body and is an essential component of DNA and RNA, cellular energy (the P of ATP), membrane receptors, cell membranes, acid–base buffer systems (phosphate system), bones, and teeth
Iron	Iron is essential for multiple processes, including red blood cell function, transportation of oxygen, myoglobin function, and modulation of enzyme activity involved in cellular respiration and energy (ATP) production. Iron supports immune function and may play a role in promoting cognitive performance
Zinc	Zinc is an intracellular ion that modulates the effects of numerous enzymes; the major roles are in metabolism of macronutrients and nucleic acids, as a component of protein structure, gene expression, cell division, osteoblastic activity, immune function, and neuron function
Fluoride	Fluoride supports tooth enamel and has antibacterial properties leading to resistance against dental caries
Copper	Copper is a component of numerous enzymes and therefore plays a role in numerous processes, such as the synthesis of energy, catecholamines, collagen, elastin, and melanin. Copper also protects against reactive oxygen species and promotes iron oxidation
Iodine	Iodine is needed for the synthesis of thyroid hormones
Selenium	Selenium has antioxidant properties and plays a role in lipid metabolism and thyroid hormone production, and it may reduce cancer risk
Manganese	Manganese is a component of numerous enzymes. It plays a role in carbohydrate and lipid metabolism, growth, reproduction, and formation of connective tissues and bone
Chromium	Chromium is active in macronutrient metabolism and gene expression
Molybdenum	Molybdenum is active in multiple enzymatic reactions
Boron	Boron is a component of cell membranes and plays a role in modulating enzymatic reactions, most notably supporting brain and bone function
Cobalt	Cobalt is a component of B_{12}; its primary role is red blood cell maturation. Cobalt also supports the function of all other cells and promotes enzymes active in DNA to RNA transcription

- Carbohydrates: 45% to 65%
- Proteins: 10% to 35%
- Fats: 20% to 35%

Intake and Storage of Nutrients

Maintenance of body weight and composition requires a balance of energy intake and expenditure. During times of growth, energy requirements increase to offset the evident growth expenditures. Energy intake is regulated by numerous factors, including hunger, **satiety**, or a feeling of fullness, food availability, and emotional and physical health. Hunger and satiety are regulated in the brain by the hypothalamus, based on feedback from the digestive tract on the quantity and quality of food in the stomach and intestines (Fig. 17.4). Some examples of feedback messages from GI tract and nutrient storage sites to the hypothalamus include:

- The presence of low blood glucose or a lack of food in the GI tract induces hunger.
- The presence of food in the GI tract triggers stretch receptors and insulin secretion and subsequently reduces appetite.
- The presence of fat stimulates cholecystokinin, a GI hormone that contributes to satiety.
- Increases in fat stores stimulate the release of leptin, a hormone with the ability to suppress appetite, increase energy expenditures, and ultimately increase metabolism.

The hypothalamus responds by secreting hormones that contribute to energy intake, expenditure, and metabolism. In response, the short-term desire to eat is reduced or stimulated. Over a longer period, body weight and composition are maintained.

Storage of nutrients is also critical to health. Adipocytes (fat cells) store lipids as a key energy source when the need arises. The liver stores certain vitamins and minerals, such as vitamins A, B_{12}, D, E, K, iron, and copper, and then releases these in times of need. The liver also stores glycogen, and when glycogen stores are exhausted, the liver then converts amino acids and glycerol to glucose.

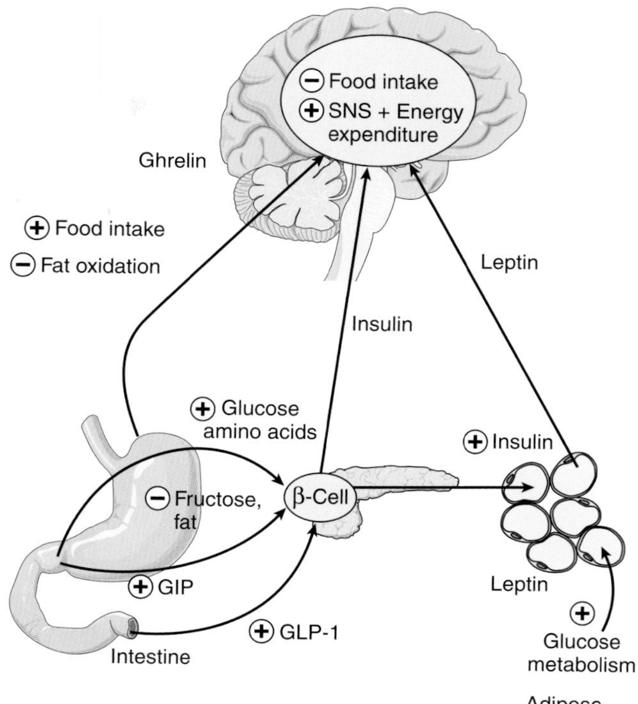

Figure 17.4. Long-term signals regulating food intake and energy homeostasis. Insulin and leptin are important long-term regulators of food intake and energy balance. Both insulin and leptin act in the central nervous system to inhibit food intake and to increase energy expenditure, most likely by activating the sympathetic nervous system (SNS). Insulin is secreted from the β cells in the endocrine pancreas in response to circulating nutrients (glucose and amino acids) and to the incretin hormones, glucose-dependent insulinotropic polypeptide (GIP) and glucagon-like peptide-1 (GLP-1), which are released during meal ingestion and absorption. Insulin can also act indirectly by stimulating leptin production from adipose tissue through increased glucose metabolism. Ghrelin, a hormone produced by endocrine cells in the stomach, increases food intake and decreases fat oxidation and appears to have an anabolic role in long-term regulation of energy balance. Ghrelin secretion is normally suppressed after meals, but it is not suppressed by fat or fructose consumption. The long-term signals interact with the short-term signals in the regulation of energy homeostasis and appear to set sensitivity to the satiety-producing effects of short-term signals such as cholecystokinin. (Adapted with permission from Havel PJ. Peripheral signals conveying metabolic information to the brain: short-term and long-term regulation of food intake and energy homeostasis. *Exp Biol Med [Maywood]*. 2001;226:963–977.)

DIGESTION

The digestive system is essential for (1) digesting and extracting macronutrients, (2) absorbing nutrients, and (3) forming a physiologic and chemical barrier against microorganisms and other foreign materials introduced during food ingestion. Stomach acid forms a first line of defense by destroying many types of microorganisms and other harmful substances on contact. Figure 17.5 illustrates the digestive system, comprised of the gastrointestinal tract and accessory organs.

Digestion is the process by which food is broken down mechanically and chemically in the gastrointestinal tract and converted into absorbable

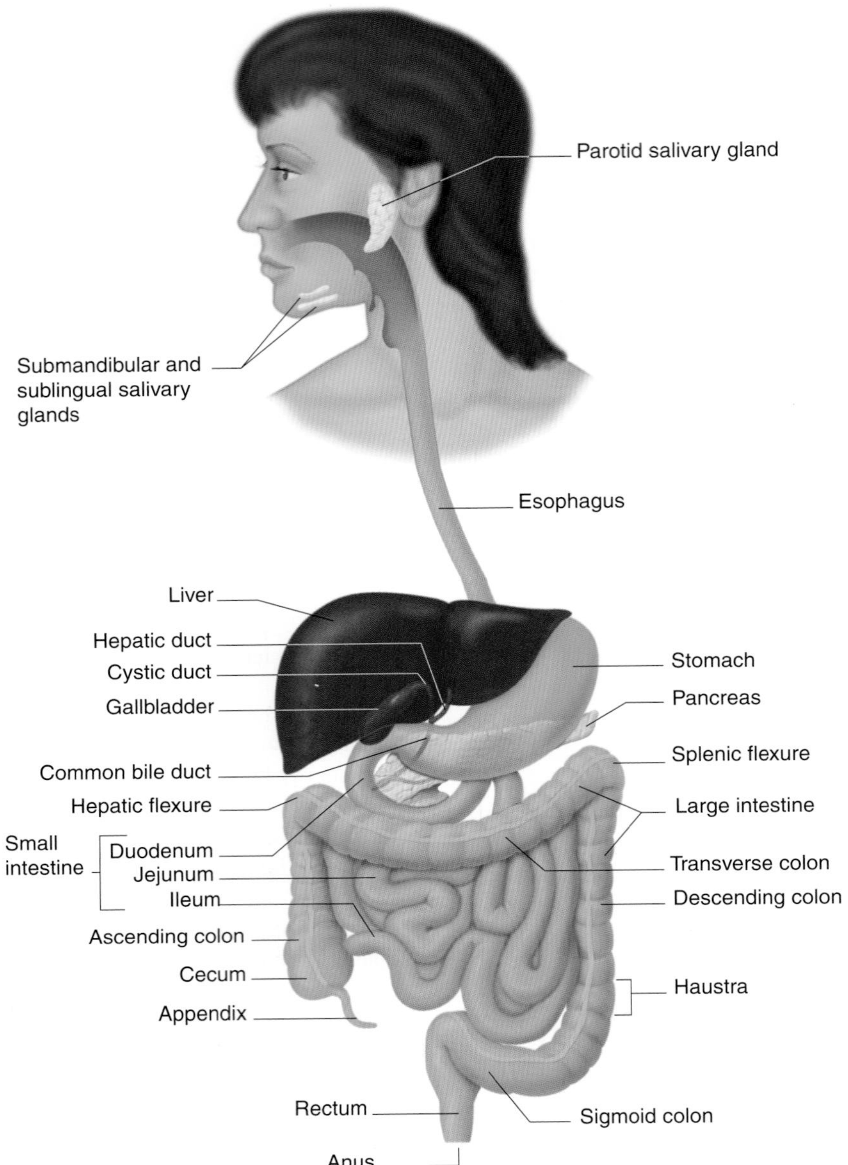

Figure 17.5. The digestive system.

components. Figures 17.1 to 17.3 highlighted these processes for each of the macronutrients. The mouth, stomach, and small intestine each have a significant role in mechanical and chemical digestive processes. Mechanical digestion is the process of physically breaking down and moving substances through the digestive tract. Chewing food is a major mechanism for mechanical digestion. Continued mechanical churning of food occurs in the stomach.

Chemical digestion is the work of digestive enzymes and bile, which convert ingested substances into absorbable components. Accessory organs, most notably the salivary glands, pancreas, and liver are critical in producing and secreting digestive enzymes and bile into the gastrointestinal tract. Chemical digestion is stimulated by chewing and begins in the mouth as food mixes with saliva, a substance consisting mostly of water, bicarbonate, chloride, potassium, and salivary amylase. Salivary amylase, from salivary glands, is an enzyme responsible for initiating carbohydrate digestion.

In the stomach, food is mixed with hydrochloric acid, pepsin, and other digestive enzymes. Four major secretory cells are found in the stomach:

- *Mucous cells*, which secrete alkaline mucus and protect the epithelium from stress and acid contact
- *Parietal cells*, which secrete both hydrochloric acid, a strong acid, needed to activate pepsinogen

and destroy pathogens and intrinsic factor, a glycoprotein needed for intestinal absorption of vitamin B_{12}

- *Chief cells*, which secrete pepsin, a proteolytic enzyme, critical to protein digestion
- *G cells*, which secrete gastrin, a hormone responsible for controlling acid secretion and stimulating gastric motility

Gastric epithelial cells are also stimulated to secrete other enzymes, such as lipase and gelatinase. The most important digestive contribution of the stomach is the initiation of protein digestion.

The final stages of chemical digestion occur through small intestinal villi, the functional units of the small intestine, which are lined with columnar and mucus-secreting epithelial cells. Villi are capable of both enzyme secretion and absorption of nutrients. Microvilli, located on the columnar epithelium, are referred to as the "brush border" and serve to greatly increase the surface area of the small intestine. Intestinal mucosal folds slow the passage of food to provide adequate time for digestion. As the nutrients move into the small intestine, they are met with bile salts from the liver (critical for fat digestion), bicarbonate from the pancreas (needed to neutralize hydrochloric acid), and enzymes also from the pancreas (critical for digestion of fats, proteins, and carbohydrates). Within the small intestine, nutrients are mixed with bile and the pancreatic enzymes. The specific locations and roles of select digestive enzymes are discussed in Table 17.3. Emulsifying agents, critical for fat digestion, are discussed below to illustrate the absorption of fatty acids and glycerol.

The regulation of digestion, with the exception of chewing, swallowing, and defecation, is directed through hormone feedback mechanisms and the autonomic nervous system. Both the sympathetic and parasympathetic branches of the autonomic nervous system act on the walls of the gastrointestinal tract to promote digestion. The walls of the gastrointestinal tract contain four basic layers (the inner mucosa, submucosa, muscularis, and serosa). The inner mucosa, which lines the lumen and is in direct contact with nutrients, varies in structure and function depending on the location within the gastrointestinal tract. The epithelial cells that comprise the mucosa are capable of secretion, absorption, and the production of hormones. In addition to other immune protections, Peyer patches (lymphoid follicles) and lymphocytes (primarily IgA-secreting B cells) are also located within the mucosa and extend into the submucosa. Peyer patches are needed to house lymphocytes and ultimately protect the gastrointestinal tract against pathogens.

The submucosa is a connective tissue layer. It contains blood and lymphatic vessels and the submucous plexus (nerve branches), which provide local and autonomic nervous system stimuli to the gastrointestinal tract. The muscularis layer, comprised primarily of two thick layers of smooth muscle, promotes mechanical movement of nutrients through the lumen and, similar to the submucosa, also contains a myenteric plexus to allow neuronal stimulation. The serosa is the outermost covering of the gastrointestinal tract. Within the abdominal cavity, the mesentery, a suspensory structure, connects to the serosa and supports the digestive tract and provides pathways for vascular and neuronal stimulation.

Glands and ducts within the mucosa and submucosa allow the secretion of digestive substances into the gastrointestinal lumen. Gastrin and motilin are

Table 17.3 Enzymes Active in the Chemical Digestive Process

Enzyme	Location	Function
Salivary amylase (ptyalin)	Mouth and stomach	Initiates carbohydrate digestion
Pepsin	Stomach	Breaks down protein and forms polypeptides in the stomach
Pancreatic amylase	Pancreas	Promotes conversion of oligosaccharides and dextrins (carbohydrates) into lactose, maltose, and sucrose
Lactase, maltase, sucrase ("brush border enzymes")	Small intestine	Convert disaccharides (lactose, maltose, and sucrose) into monosaccharides (galactose, glucose, and fructose)
Trypsin, chymotrypsin, and carboxypeptidase (pancreatic enzymes)	Pancreas	Convert protein polypeptides into smaller protein units
Aminopeptidases and dipeptidases ("brush border enzymes")	Small intestine	Convert protein polypeptides and dipeptides into amino acids
Pancreatic lipases	Pancreas	Convert fats into monoglycerides, glycerol, and fatty acids
Intestinal lipase	Small intestine	Converts fatty acids into glycerol

two hormones that act on the gastrointestinal tract to *stimulate* gastric emptying. Gastrin stimulates gastric glands to secrete pepsinogen (a proenzyme that later converts to pepsin) and hydrochloric acid. Secretin, gastric inhibitory peptide, and cholecystokinin, from the duodenum, are three hormones that *inhibit* gastric emptying. Secretin is responsible for triggering the release of bicarbonate from the pancreas and bile from the liver. Gastric inhibitory peptide decreases stomach churning. Cholecystokinin stimulates the release of digestive enzymes in the pancreas and the emptying of bile from the gall bladder.

The overall goal of digestion is to prepare nutrients for absorption by:

1. Converting carbohydrates to monosaccharides
2. Converting proteins into amino acids
3. Converting fats to fatty acids and glycerol
4. Unleashing vitamins and minerals from macronutrients
5. Separating water from nutrients to promote water absorption

Figure 17.6 illustrates the conversion of nutrients into absorbable components and should be referred to frequently during the discussion of absorption below.

ABSORPTION

Absorption is a complex process of taking in nutrients and moving these to the circulation to be used by cells. Certain locations within the digestive system are better equipped to absorb specific nutrients. Figure 17.7 details the major sites of absorption for specific nutrients along the gastrointestinal tract. Recognition of these major sites of absorption allows the ability to anticipate nutrition problems that can occur with inadequate absorption at certain locations within the gastrointestinal tract.

The small intestine is an ideal site for absorption of nutrients because of the extensive surface area and absorptive fluid layer along the brush border. Also unique to the small intestine is the presence of **lacteals**, or lymphatic channels within each villus, which are critical to the absorption of fat molecules. Some substances, such as water, are absorbed primarily in the large intestine and stomach. Vitamin D can be absorbed through the skin.

After absorption and traveling within the circulation, the liver receives the nutrients that were once in the intestinal lumen. Once in the liver, the nutrients are metabolized, converted, or synthesized into other nutrients, or they are stored for later use. The liver then releases the nutrients back into the circulation to be used by body cells.

Glucose and Fructose Absorption

Carbohydrates represent the largest proportion of nutrients absorbed within the digestive tract. Monosaccharides (glucose or fructose) are rarely consumed in a typical diet. Therefore, more complex carbohydrates (sucrose, lactose, and starches) must be degraded by enzymes and reduced to monosaccharides for absorption. The following list outlines key aspects of carbohydrate absorption:

- Pancreatic amylase acts on dietary carbohydrates to begin the reduction into simple sugars (primarily starches into maltose).
- The final enzymatic digestion, which liberates more complex carbohydrates into monosaccharides (primarily glucose, also fructose and galactose), is the work of brush border enzymes (disaccharidases, such as sucrase and lactase, and oligosaccharidase, such as maltase) secreted from the small intestine.
- Glucose requires the cotransport of sodium to be absorbed into the lumen of the small intestine.

Glucose and galactose are absorbed into the enterocyte (intestinal cell) *with sodium* via active transport. **Active transport** is a process that uses *energy* to move nutrients across a pressure gradient (Fig. 17.8). The source of this energy is adenosine triphosphate (ATP), which is the product of a chemical reaction between oxygen and nutrient products. Energy is required for the transport of glucose and sodium because the concentration of sodium outside the cell is far greater than inside the cell. In fact, many nutrients including galactose, calcium, iron, amino acids, potassium, fatty acids, and magnesium, require energy-dependent transport pumps to be absorbed across the mucosa.

For glucose transport, two sodium ions bind to the transporter. A change in the transporter then occurs, allowing glucose to bind to the transporter, and only then can these molecules move into the cell. The energy stored in the membrane gradient drives glucose through the enterocyte. Glucose then diffuses down its concentration gradient into the capillaries within the villus of the small intestine.

Fructose enters the enterocyte through the process of passive facilitated diffusion through a transporter. **Passive diffusion**, which is the random migration of nutrients across the mucosa from areas of higher to lower concentration or pressure, can be a simple or facilitated process. *Simple diffusion* allows nutrients to move through or between channel proteins. *Facilitated diffusion* uses carrier proteins that move nutrients across the gastrointestinal mucosa. Passive diffusion is also represented by the absorption of most vitamins and water, which pass

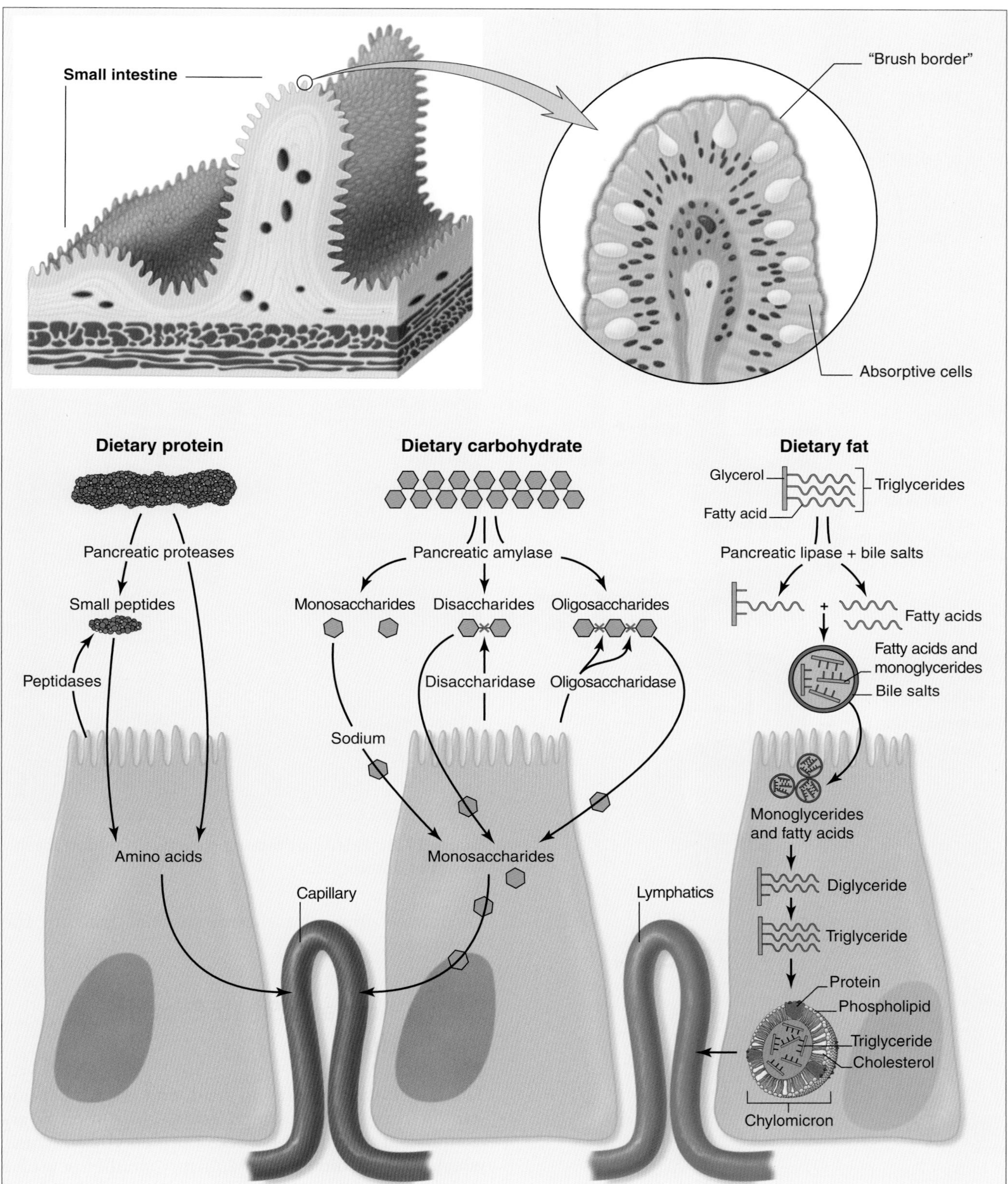

Figure 17.6. Mechanisms of nutrient digestion and absorption within the small intestine. (Modified from Rubin E, Farber JL. *Pathology*. 4th ed. Philadelphia, PA: Lippincott Williams & Wilkins; 2005, with permission.)

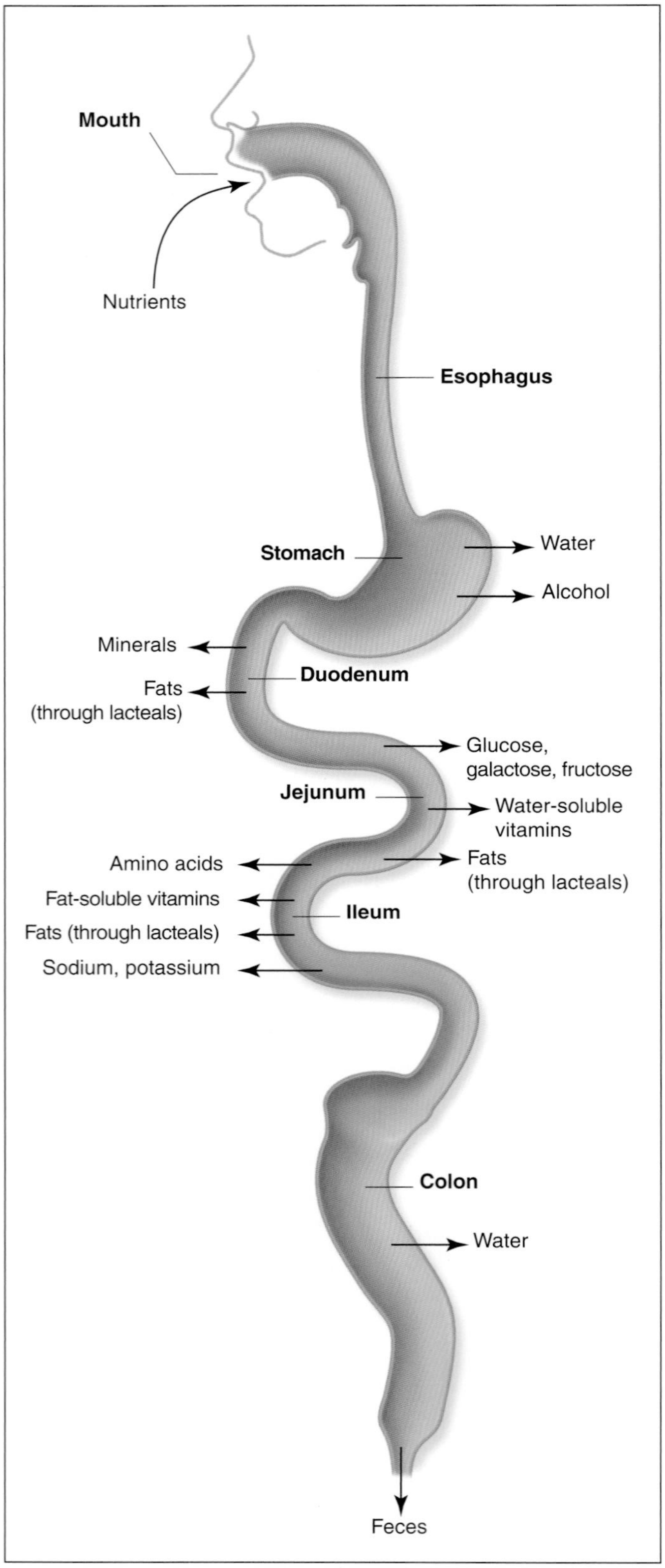

Figure 17.7. Major sites for absorption in the gastrointestinal tract. The gastrointestinal tract absorbs specific nutrients at specific locations.

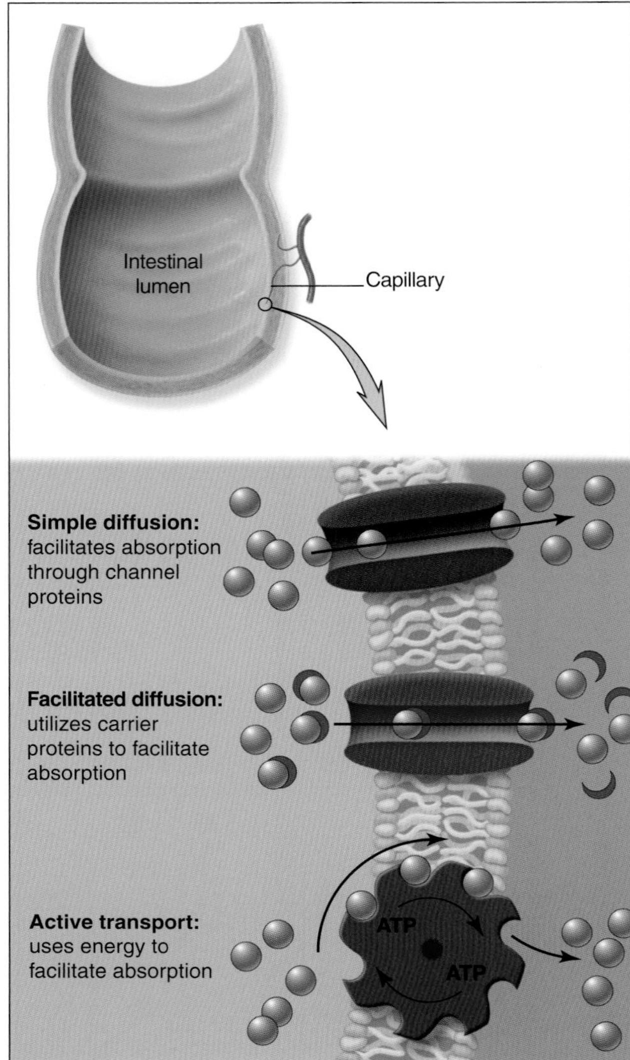

Figure 17.8. Passive diffusion and active transport mechanisms of absorption.

unchanged from the gastrointestinal tract to the circulation.

Amino Acid and Small Peptide Absorption

The facilitation of amino acid and small peptide (two or three linked amino acids) absorption is accomplished through the work of proteolytic enzymes, which degrade dietary proteins into smaller peptides and then into amino acids. Three major sources of proteolytic enzymes include the (1) active protease pepsin (from the stomach); (2) pancreatic proteases (such as trypsin, chymotrypsin, and carboxypeptidases); and (3) peptidases found in the intestinal brush border. The mechanism for absorption of a single amino acid is essentially the same as monosaccharides.

Sodium-dependent transporters are needed, using energy across an electrochemical gradient, to move amino acids into the intestinal epithelium. Interestingly, small peptides are absorbed without depending on sodium. Rather, these small-chain amino acids travel through a single transport molecule. Once in the enterocyte, small peptides are reduced to amino acids and move with other transport molecules into the circulation. This final stage of absorption for all amino acids does not rely on sodium cotransport and is not across an energy gradient.

Fatty Acid and Glycerol Absorption

The conversion of dietary fats into fatty acids and glycerol requires two major steps: emulsification and enzymatic digestion. Emulsification promotes fat solubility and is accomplished via bile salts, which are synthesized in the liver and secreted from the gall bladder. Emulsification is a process of coating the lipid molecules with bile salts, which have both hydrophilic (water-attracting) and hydrophobic (water-repellent) components. Ultimately, the lipid molecules are broken down into smaller and smaller droplets, the hydrophobic end adheres to the lipid molecule, and the hydrophilic end comprises an outer soluble surface.

Stop and Consider
What dietary recommendations would you make for the individual who is not able to effectively produce or use bile?

Once emulsified, pancreatic lipase (a water-soluble enzyme) acts on the surface of triglyceride droplets to further degrade triglycerides into free fatty acids, monoglycerides, and diglycerides. These substances form a complex with bile salts and other lipids called micelles. The micelles move along the brush border of the small intestine, where they can be absorbed through a process of simple diffusion (discussed below) or via a fatty acid transporter protein across the plasma membrane.

Two major differences characterize the absorption of fats as compared to amino acids and sugars:

1. Fatty acids and monoglycerides resynthesize back into triglycerides after moving across the plasma membrane.
2. Transport into the circulation occurs via lacteals, lymphatic vessels within each villus, rather than through the blood vessels.

After absorption in the enterocytes of the small intestinal mucosa, the triglycerides are resynthesized and made soluble again through the production of lipoprotein complexes (chylomicrons). Chylomicrons from the intestine are released into the blood through lacteals and are delivered to tissues or stored for the later production of energy through oxidation. Fatty acids are stored as triglycerides, primarily within adipocytes. These fatty acids can be mobilized when needed. The activation of mobilization occurs in response to hormones that bind cell surface receptors. In a series of complex events, free fatty acids diffuse from adipocytes, combine with albumin, are transported to other tissues, and passively diffuse into cells.

Absorption is affected by several factors. Competition for carriers blocks absorption of certain nutrients. Saturation of carriers slows the absorption process. Absorption can be enhanced or inhibited when select substances coexist. For example, ascorbic acid (vitamin C), such as that found in orange juice, enhances the absorption of iron. Another example is the presence of dietary fat, which is needed for absorption of fat-soluble vitamins. Physiologic factors, such as gastric pH and motility, may affect bioavailability and subsequent absorption of minerals. **Bioavailability** indicates that the mineral is unbound and must remain unbound (also called an ionic state) to be absorbed, such as with calcium. Bound minerals are unused and are eliminated in the feces. Iron is one exception. Iron can be absorbed in a bound state. To add additional complexity, the structure and function of the intestinal cells regulate and promote maximal absorption and can also limit the potential for nutrient toxicity.

Stop and Consider
What will happen to nutrient absorption in Crohn disease when large portions of the small intestine are inflamed?

Module 2 Altered Nutrition

Altered nutrition, or malnutrition, is a state of inadequate or excessive exposure to nutrients (Fig. 17.9). This exposure can include intake, digestion, absorption, or metabolism of nutrients. Altered nutrition has multiple potential causes, including:

- Genetic defects that impact metabolism or absorption of nutrients
- Malformation or damage to the gastrointestinal mucosa

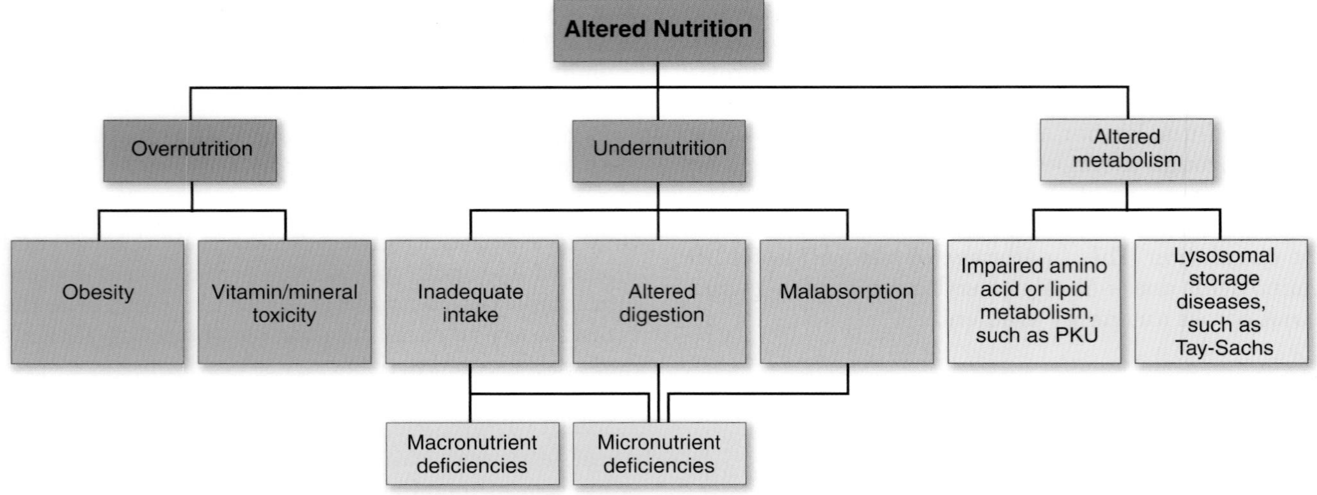

Figure 17.9. Concept map. Altered nutrition. PKU, phenylketonuria.

- Inadequate or excessive dietary intake of required nutrients
- Excessive nutrient losses, such as through vomiting, diarrhea, or laxative use
- Hypermetabolic states that exert excessive demands, such as with hyperthyroidism, cancer, burns, fever, or severe infection
- Malabsorptive syndromes
- Ingestion of unsafe food and water sources

Inherited Metabolic Disorders

Inherited metabolic disorders, most often related to errors in amino acid and lipid metabolism, commonly result from a genetically based defect in enzyme activity. These are also called inborn errors of metabolism. Nutritional genomics is a field of science that considers the role of nutrients on gene expression. For example, in phenylketonuria (PKU), phenylalanine hydroxylase deficiency causes an inability to convert phenylalanine, an essential amino acid, to tyrosine. Accumulations of phenylalanine, without the necessary conversion to tyrosine, result in impaired CNS development, impaired myelination, and brain degeneration. Dietary modifications are needed to restrict phenylalanine consumption. PKU is one of the clinical models featured in this chapter.

A second major category of inherited metabolic disorders is lysosomal storage diseases. These diseases are defects of lipid metabolism as a result of a missing lysosomal enzyme. An example is Tay-Sachs disease, which is inherited as an autosomal recessive disorder and found most commonly in those of Ashkenazi Jewish and Eastern European descent. In Tay–Sachs disease, a deficiency of beta-hexosaminidase A (an enzyme) results in the impaired catabolism and accumulation of fatty substances, called GM2 gangliosides, inside neuronal lysosomes in the brain. This leads to severe neurologic impairment marked by developmental delays, neurodegeneration, blindness, deafness, muscle atrophy, paralysis, and death (often by 4 years of age). Presently, there is no treatment. The major problem with inherited metabolic disorders is the accumulation of substances within the cells of the body, leading to cell death.

Undernutrition

Undernutrition is a lack of intake of nutrients most often related to inadequate calorie consumption, inadequate intake of essential vitamins and minerals, or problems with digestion, absorption, or distribution of nutrients in the body. Protein, iron, and vitamins are the most common nutrients that are inadequately consumed or in great demand in those presenting with undernutrition. Excess use of muscle mass and adipose stores for energy results in weight loss and muscle wasting. In severe or prolonged illness, loss of muscle mass and function is not limited to the skeletal muscle and can affect cardiac and respiratory functioning. The elderly, particularly those in nursing homes, are at particular risk for undernutrition due to poor appetite, alterations in the sense of taste, problems with eating or swallowing, limited income, inadequate social support, and mobility limitations.

VITAMIN AND MINERAL DEFICIENCIES

Vitamin and mineral deficiencies can result from the inadequate intake or malabsorption of dietary sources. Mineral bioavailability also affects mineral absorption. Because fat intake is critical for fat-soluble vitamin absorption, lack of dietary fat impairs the cellular availability of vitamins A, D, E, and K. Table 17.4 compares the problems associated with select vitamin and mineral deficits.

PROTEIN ENERGY MALNUTRITION

Protein energy malnutrition is related to either (1) deprivation of all food, a condition of starvation that leads to **marasmus**, or (2) protein deprivation in persons consuming adequate carbohydrates, a condition called **kwashiorkor**. Glucose is a major energy source for body tissues. In marasmus, dietary glucose is unavailable for glucose-dependent tissues, such as the brain and muscle tissue. The body attempts to manufacture glucose in a process called gluconeogenesis by breaking down muscle proteins. The muscle then releases acidic by-products, promoting metabolic acidosis.

Protective mechanisms are needed at this point because continued gluconeogenesis produces significant muscle wasting, destruction of vital organs, and death. Whether the body effectively adapts, or preserves, muscle tissue during the state of starvation depends on insulin. Insulin is a hormone that promotes glucose production and uptake by cells *and* inhibits the use of fat stores for energy. If the body is to adapt to starvation effectively, insulin production must be suppressed to inhibit glucose uptake and gluconeogenesis, and another energy source must be used at a greater level than glucose. This is accomplished through a compensatory increase in glucagon, cortisone, epinephrine, and growth hormone. These hormones all have anti-insulin effects and also stimulate enzymes on the adipocytes to release fatty acids for energy. The fatty acids travel to the liver and are converted to ketones. Ketones are the replacement energy source that allows sparing of muscle catabolism. The brain and other glucose-dependent tissues prefer glucose but will use ketones for energy as an adaptive response. When ketones are used for energy, protein losses are minimized and muscle tissue is spared.

A state of starvation can be maintained for approximately 1 month in someone who maintains water intake. Unfortunately, adipose stores eventually become depleted. The body must again turn to glucose, leading to increased muscle catabolism for gluconeogenesis. Vital organs that rely on muscle, including the heart and lungs, are impaired and the individual will die.

Stop and Consider
Inflammation, particularly that which occurs with infection, stimulates the release of chemical mediators that promote insulin secretion. Insulin presence promotes the use of glucose for energy. How do you think this affects the adaptation to starvation?

Kwashiorkor, a condition of protein deficit, leads to problems with protein synthesis, repair and healing, fluid balance, and energy. In kwashiorkor, the continued intake of carbohydrates stimulates insulin production, which encourages glucose uptake for energy. This means that when an individual is still eating carbohydrates and not taking in proteins, the body does *not* effectively spare muscle tissue and access fat stores for energy. Stimulation of insulin production also limits the body's ability to synthesize new proteins from those already present in muscle tissue and also limits ATP (energy) production. The lack of protein intake, coupled with the inability to synthesize new proteins within the body, leads to severe edema. The protuberant abdomen characteristic of kwashiorkor is related to liver enlargement, weak abdominal muscles, and ascites from inadequate protein (albumin) intake and synthesis (Fig. 17.10). The liver enlarges because of fat accumulation. This accumulation is a problem of suppressed use of fat stores for energy and a lack of proteins to transport the lipids out of the liver. Other manifestations are related to gastrointestinal disturbances, impairment of neurologic, heart, and lung function, immunodeficiency and death.

Overnutrition

Overnutrition is a state of excessive exposure to nutrients. Overnutrition is generally related to overconsumption of nutrients, including ingesting excessive calories or toxic levels of vitamins and minerals. The health effects of vitamin and mineral excesses are detailed in Table 17.4. Obesity is a major health concern of epidemic proportions and is selected as one of the clinical models discussed in this chapter.

Malabsorption

Malabsorption indicates a lack of movement of specific nutrients across the gastrointestinal mucosa. Malabsorption can affect one nutrient, such as lactose or vitamin B_{12}, or it can affect all nutrients at one segment or the entire length of the intestinal mucosa. The **malabsorption syndrome** is a condition in which several nutrients are not adequately absorbed. Fat and fat-soluble substances are almost always included in the malabsorption syndrome.

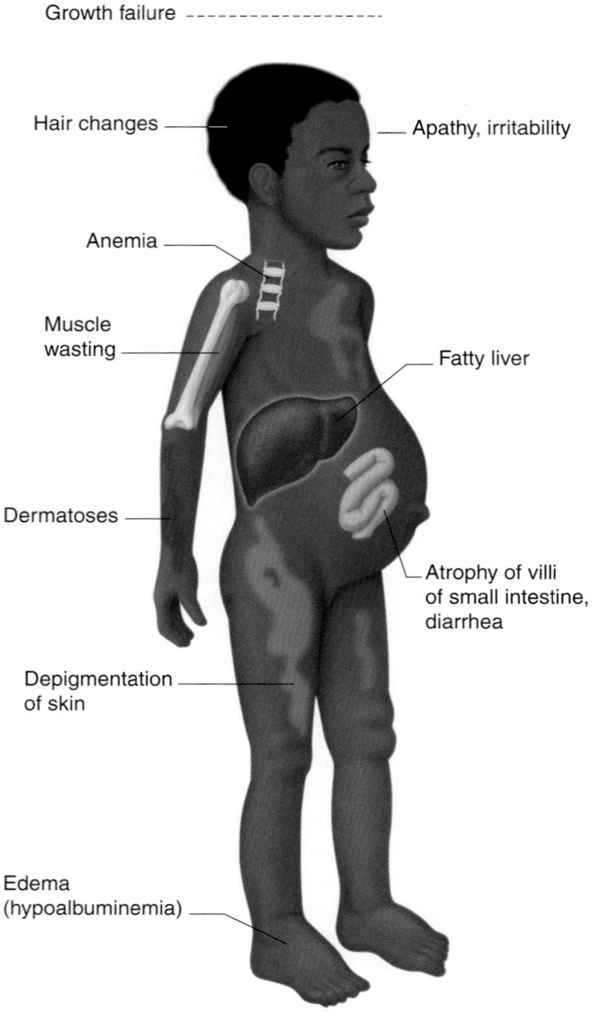

Growth failure
Hair changes
Apathy, irritability
Anemia
Muscle wasting
Fatty liver
Dermatoses
Atrophy of villi of small intestine, diarrhea
Depigmentation of skin
Edema (hypoalbuminemia)

Figure 17.10. Manifestations of kwashiorkor. (Modified from Rubin E, Farber JL. *Pathology*. 4th ed. Philadelphia, PA: Lippincott Williams & Wilkins; 2005.)

Various causes of malabsorption are depicted in Figure 17.11 and may include:

- Problems with processing or digesting nutrients: pancreatic dysfunction, enzyme deficiencies, or inadequate bile secretion
- Problems with moving substances across the mucosa: inflammatory conditions, gastrointestinal atrophy, excessive ingestion of a nutrient, use of certain medications, or protein deficiencies
- Lymphatic obstruction: inhibits transport of nutrients once they have been absorbed across the mucosa and may occur with neoplasms or infectious processes

Stop and Consider
Why would pancreatic dysfunction lead to problems with absorption?

Malabsorption of a specific vitamin or mineral presents clinically as a deficiency of that nutrient. Exocrine pancreas insufficiency and impaired bile production are major problems that lead to fat malabsorption. These problems contribute to weight loss and to deficiencies in fat-soluble vitamins. As with fat malabsorption, pancreatic enzyme deficiency contributes to the development of protein malabsorption. The loss of protein in the stool, as may occur because of inflammation in the mucosa, can also contribute to protein deficiency.

Carbohydrate malabsorption is often the result of pancreatic enzyme deficiencies, absence or reduction of brush border disaccharidases, congenital deficiency of the glucose–galactose transporter, or bacterial flora overgrowth in the intestine. Carbohydrate malabsorption results in an increase in fermentation, or breakdown, of carbohydrates by intestinal bacterial flora to convert these carbohydrates into short-chain

Table 17.4 Clinical Manifestations and Health Conditions Resulting from Select Vitamin and Mineral Deficits and Excesses

Vitamin	Causes of Deficiency	Clinical Manifestations and Health Problems Related to Deficiency	Causes of Excess	Clinical Manifestations and Health Problems Related to Excess
A	Inadequate intake or malabsorption, insufficient dietary fat, liver or pancreatic disease, protein energy malnutrition, zinc deficiency	Impaired vision, impaired embryonic development, anemia, poor growth, impaired immunity, impaired osteoclast activity (bone accumulation), keratinization of mucous membranes, dry/scaly/rough skin	Excessive dietary or supplement intake; also found in retinoic acid (Accutane), a potent anti-acne medication, which affects fetal growth and development in pregnant women who are taking this drug	Vitamin A intoxication leads to liver disease, dry mucous membranes, dryness, erythema, scaling, or peeling of skin, hair, and nails, headache, nausea, vomiting, and bone fractures

Table 17.4 Clinical Manifestations and Health Conditions Resulting from Select Vitamin and Mineral Deficits and Excesses (*continued*)

Vitamin	Causes of Deficiency	Clinical Manifestations and Health Problems Related to Deficiency	Causes of Excess	Clinical Manifestations and Health Problems Related to Excess
D	Inadequate intake of vitamin D, lipid malabsorption, prolonged breastfeeding in infants without sunlight exposure, deficiencies of calcium and phosphorus, and long-term anticonvulsant therapy	Vitamin D deficiency is manifested as rickets in children and osteomalacia in adults. Rickets involves impaired mineralization of growing bones resulting in structural abnormalities, bone pain, and muscle tenderness. Osteomalacia involves generalized reductions in bone density, muscle weakness, bone tenderness, and fractures	Excessive intake	Vitamin D intoxication leads to hypercalcemia and hyperphosphatemia, calcification of soft tissues of kidneys, lungs, heart and tympanic membrane, headache, nausea, bone fragility, and retarded growth
Thiamin	Inadequate intake or malabsorption; subclinical thiamin deficiency may result in people with alcoholism because of inadequate intake and impaired absorption	Thiamin deficiency results in beriberi, a condition manifested by anorexia, weight loss, confusion, muscular wasting, edema, peripheral neuropathy, tachycardia, and cardiomegaly	Excessive intake	Excessive thiamin results in headache, seizures, muscle weakness, cardiac dysrhythmias, and allergic reactions; massive doses result in respiratory depression and death
Niacin	Inadequate intake or absorption	Early manifestations are muscle weakness, anorexia, indigestion, and skin lesions; pellagra is a condition of severe niacin deficiency characterized by dermatitis, dementia, diarrhea, tremors, inflammation of mucous membranes; can lead to death	Excessive intake is rare, although niacin has been used in high doses to treat hypercholesterolemia, and toxicity may result in these individuals	Niacin excess promotes histamine release, which results in flushing; high-dose niacin is also toxic to the liver
B_{12}	Inadequate intake or malabsorption	DNA synthesis is impaired leading to problems with cell division; clinical manifestations include anemia, neuropathy characterized by numbness, tingling, and burning in extremities, and generalized weakness, stomatitis, and skin lesions; all rapidly dividing cells are affected; pernicious anemia is a condition of B_{12} malabsorption caused by a lack of intrinsic factor in the stomach from atrophic parietal cells (Chapter 3)	Not applicable	Vitamin B_{12} is not known to result in severe toxicity
Folate	Inadequate intake or malabsorption	Impaired synthesis of DNA and RNA, cell division is reduced; homocysteine levels increase; clinical manifestations include anemia, impaired skin integrity, impaired immunity, weakness, depression, neuropathy, and poor growth; embryonic development is impaired in pregnant women deficient in folate resulting in neural tube defects	Excessive intake	No major adverse effects have been documented that are directly related to folate excess
C	Inadequate intake or malabsorption	Scurvy is a condition of vitamin C deficiency resulting in skin lesions, impaired wound healing, lethargy, atrophy, edema, bleeding, impaired bone, cartilage, tooth, and connective tissue development	Excessive intake	Vitamin C excess results in gastric upset and diarrhea and may contribute to the development of renal calculi

(*continued*)

Table 17.4 Clinical Manifestations and Health Conditions Resulting from Select Vitamin and Mineral Deficits and Excesses (*continued*)

Vitamin	Causes of Deficiency	Clinical Manifestations and Health Problems Related to Deficiency	Causes of Excess	Clinical Manifestations and Health Problems Related to Excess
Calcium	Inadequate intake, bioavailability, or absorption	Contributes to reduced bone mass, weakness, and osteomalacia; may impact the development of colon cancer and hypertension	Excessive intake	Excessive intake can lead to hypercalcemia and lead to calcification in soft tissues; interferes with absorption of other minerals; can impair cardiac conduction
Phosphorus	Deficiencies are rare because of wide availability of dietary sources	Phosphorus deficit has lethal consequences; clinical manifestations are related to loss of ATP synthesis and can include problems with the nervous system, bones, blood cells, skin, kidneys, heart, and lungs because of abnormalities in all energy-dependent cells	Chronic consumption of a low-calcium and high-phosphorus diet	Toxicity can lead to frequent bone fractures throughout the skeleton
Zinc	Inadequate intake, malabsorption, or excessive losses through urine or other secretions	Zinc deficiency was previously common but has declined because of the fortification in cereal products; clinical manifestations include impaired growth, delayed sexual maturation, hair loss, delayed wound healing, skin lesions, anorexia, impaired immune function, visual disturbances, and impaired taste	Toxicity is rare but can occur with excessive intake	Manifestations of toxicity include anemia, fever, vomiting, diarrhea, and impaired central nervous system function
Copper	Inadequate intake, malabsorption, or excessive losses	Copper deficiency leads to anemia, neutropenia, bone demineralization and osteoporosis, changes in skin pigment, impaired collagen and elastin production, growth impairment, and brain tissue degeneration	Excessive copper supplement intake and chronic liver disease can lead to copper toxicity. Copper is excreted in bile. Liver disease promotes bile retention and copper toxicity	Manifestations of toxicity are related to liver cirrhosis and red blood cell malformation

fatty acids (for absorption) and gases. The short-chain fatty acids are needed to (1) maintain GI function, (2) recoup some of the energy that would be lost, and (3) facilitate sodium and water absorption in the large intestine. The undigested carbohydrates draw extensive fluid into the intestines. The process of fermentation leads to the clinical manifestations characteristic of carbohydrate malabsorption, including abdominal distention, bloating, pain, diarrhea, weight loss, and flatulence.

Food Allergy

Food allergies are immune system mediated adverse reactions to foods. Any food protein can trigger an allergic response, however, the vast majority of food allergies are triggered by eggs, peanuts, milk, soy, fish, shellfish, tree nuts, and wheat. Consumption of foods that trigger allergy can result in oropharyngeal itching, laryngeal edema, cough, shortness of breath, wheezing, nausea, vomiting, diarrhea, skin flushing, skin itching, hives, abdominal pain, and other symptoms associated with severe allergic reaction. The exact allergy-inducing food must be identified through dietary history and possibly immune testing. As with other hypersensitivities, injectable epinephrine may be needed for initial management of food-induced anaphylactic reaction. The primary goal is complete avoidance of that type of food. Patients need to be particularly aware of food labels and the locations and mechanisms with which foods

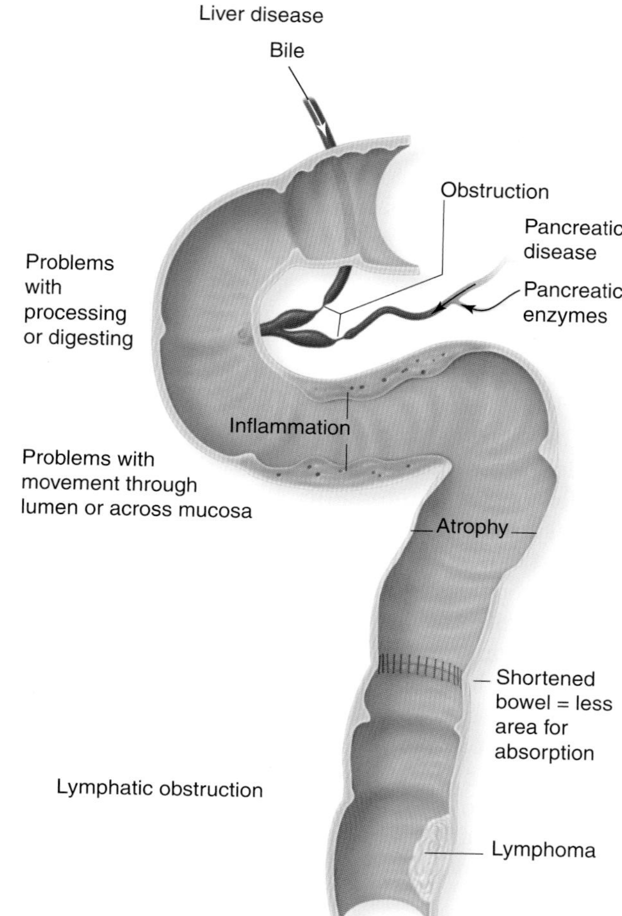

Figure 17.11. Potential causes of malabsorption.

are prepared to avoid accidental ingestion. Food allergies do not cause nutritional deficiencies as other foods can be consumed to assure adequate nutrition. However, these are mentioned here as they do result in critical dietary modifications.

GENERAL MANIFESTATIONS OF ALTERED NUTRITION

The clinical manifestations of altered nutrition are reflective of the cause and pathophysiologic problems. Because cells and body tissues rely on adequate nutrition for optimal functioning, clinical manifestations are exhibited throughout the body. In general, malnutritive processes involving undernutrition can lead to weight loss, muscle wasting, muscle weakness, dehydration, fatigue, and evidence of vitamin and mineral deficiencies (Table 17.4). Rapidly dividing cells, such as those of the skin, are particularly vulnerable to malnourishment. Skin manifestations include poor wound healing, purpura, ulceration, dry skin, or pallor. Mucous membranes become inflamed and friable. Angular cheilitis, a problem with fissure development in the corners of the mouth, is often associated with riboflavin deficiency. The manifestations of malabsorption are often related to the rapid transit of nutrients through the intestinal lumen. As mentioned previously, problems with carbohydrate absorption typically manifest as weight loss, diarrhea, bloating, abdominal cramping, and excessive flatulence. Fat malabsorption leads to foul-smelling, greasy, diarrhea stools. Excessive nutrient intake leads to an increase in weight and body fatness. Toxicity of vitamins and minerals can also occur.

DIAGNOSTIC AND TREATMENT STRATEGIES RELATED TO ALTERED NUTRITION

Diagnostic tests related to altered nutrition are used to determine the cause for the nutrition imbalance as well as the potential effects. A complete nutritional assessment is indicated, which includes a multiple-day dietary intake recall, to determine adequate or excessive nutrient intake, and measurement of height, weight, and body mass index. Laboratory evaluation is often helpful and may include a complete blood count with red blood cell indices and a peripheral smear, sedimentation rate (to detect inflammation), serum electrolytes, urinalysis and urine culture. The evaluation may also include measures of protein status, including serum albumin, transferrin, creatinine, and blood urea nitrogen levels. Other serum tests are used to detect blood levels of specific nutrients, such as iron, B_{12}, or folate. Enzyme levels can also be measured to determine whether digestive or absorptive problems are present. Hormone levels may be investigated if metabolic regulation is impaired. Stool specimens may also be evaluated for the presence of pathogens that affect absorption. Direct visualization or biopsy of the gastrointestinal tract may be required to determine a structural cause for the nutrition imbalance.

Treatment modalities are directed at eliminating the cause of the nutrition imbalance or reducing the harmful effects. This often includes specific dietary interventions, such as increasing intake of particular macronutrients, taking vitamin and mineral supplements, reducing overall caloric intake, or avoiding specific foods that exacerbate symptoms. Treatment may also include pharmacologic interventions, such as the administration of exogenous digestive enzymes, to support digestion and absorption. Diagnostic and treatment modalities are discussed in greater detail within the clinical models of this chapter.

Module 3 Clinical Models

The following clinical models have been selected to aid in the understanding and application of altered nutrition pathophysiology, manifestations, diagnosis, and treatment.

Iron-Deficiency Anemia

Anemia is the reduction in the mass of circulating blood cells and subsequently reduced hemoglobin levels. Anemia is typically not considered an isolated disease; rather, it represents a manifestation of another problem. In Chapter 6, sickle cell anemia was presented as a clinical model related to a genetic defect that results in red blood cell destruction. The development of anemia can also result from severe hemorrhage, decreased red blood cell production, or vitamin and mineral deficiencies. The vitamins and minerals related to red blood cell and hemoglobin integrity include B_{12}, folate, and iron. The most common cause of all anemias is iron deficiency; it is also the most prevalent nutritional deficiency worldwide.

PATHOPHYSIOLOGY

Iron-deficiency anemia represents a problem of iron demand on red blood cell development that cannot be met with current iron stores. Iron is required for hemoglobin synthesis, oxygen and electron transport, and DNA synthesis. Iron is found within hemoglobin, myoglobin, and enzymes, and it is stored in transport proteins such as ferritin, hemosiderin, and transferrin. Iron balance is maintained through the careful regulation of iron absorption in the small intestine. Most iron is recycled in the body after release from dying red blood cells. Minute amounts are lost through defecation, sweating, and sloughing of skin cells.

The major causes of iron-deficiency anemia are inadequate iron intake, chronic hemorrhage, malabsorption, and high iron demands as occurs in infancy, adolescence, and with pregnancy or lactation. Chronic blood loss, as with a monthly menstruation, gastrointestinal ulcers, cancer, or hemorrhoids, is a common cause of excessive loss of body iron. Certain medications, such as antacids, can bind with iron and impair absorption.

CLINICAL MANIFESTATIONS

Clinical manifestations usually present when hemoglobin content is less than that required to meet the oxygen-carrying demands of the body. Iron-deficiency anemia can develop slowly and therefore be asymptomatic. When present, clinical manifestations are related to decreased hemoglobin synthesis, altered blood composition, and subsequently poor oxygen-carrying capacity and hypoxia. These manifestations include pallor of the skin and mucous membranes, fatigue, weakness, lightheadedness, breathlessness, palpitations, headache, tachycardia, and syncope. Chronic hypoxia impairs cell functioning, particularly in epithelial cells, and leads to brittle hair and nails and mouth sores. **Pica** (pagophagia), the compulsion to eat ice or nonfood substances such as dirt or clay, is another manifestation of iron-deficient anemia that is not clearly understood.

DIAGNOSTIC CRITERIA

Preliminary diagnosis of iron-deficiency anemia is based on a thorough patient history and physical examination. A higher index of suspicion is present in individuals who are vegetarian or who report manifestations of chronic blood loss. In iron deficiency, laboratory tests may reveal reduced serum hemoglobin and hematocrit levels and reduced mean corpuscular volume (MCV) and mean corpuscular hemoglobin concentration (MCHC). MCV is an indicator of red blood cell size; therefore, a reduction in hemoglobin and hematocrit, along with a reduced MCV, indicates microcytic anemia. Overall, the number and quality of red blood cells are reduced; RBCs are **hypochromic** (pale) and **microcytic** (small) (Fig. 17.12). **Poikilocytosis** is a term used to describe the irregular shape of iron-deficient red blood cells.

If individuals are unresponsive to treatment, additional confirmatory tests are needed to distinguish iron deficiency from other types of anemia, as depicted in Table 17.5. Confirmatory tests may include serum iron, total

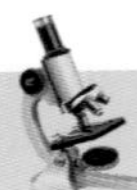

FROM THE LAB

Serum ferritin is often used as a confirmatory test of iron deficiency. Ferritin is a protein that stores iron. When the iron supply increases, ferritin levels expand to store the additional iron. Ferritin levels can then be measured as an indicator of iron stores.

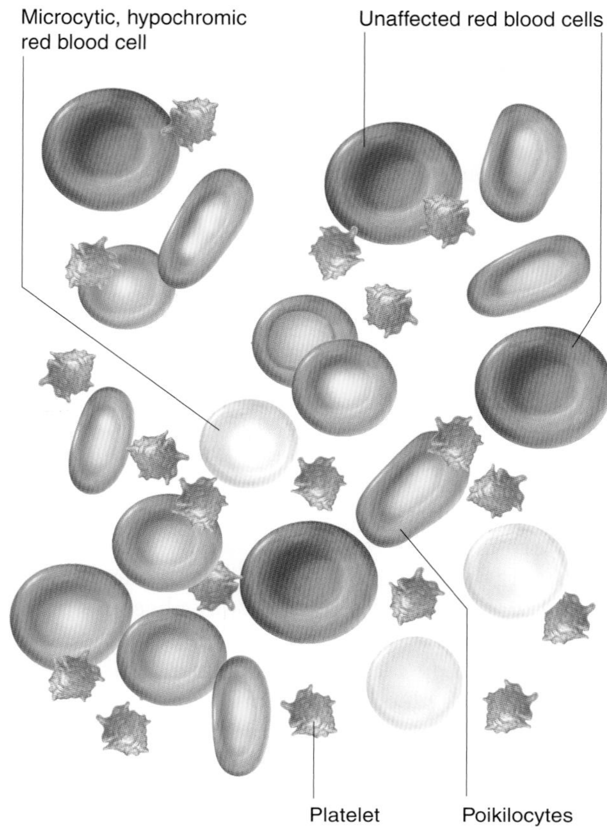

Figure 17.12. Peripheral blood smear in iron-deficiency anemia. (Courtesy Anatomical Chart Company.)

iron-binding capacity, transferrin saturation, and ferritin levels (see From the Lab, below). Additional tests may be needed to determine sources of acute or chronic blood loss.

The diagnosis of anemia must take into consideration that certain factors affect hemoglobin levels, such as:

- *Age*: Hemoglobin levels are typically much lower in adults than newborns.
- *Gender*: Males have higher hemoglobin levels than women.
- *Pregnancy status*: The physiologic demands of pregnancy and hemodilution result in lower hemoglobin levels in pregnancy.
- *Altitude*: Reduced oxygen exposure at high altitudes induces erythropoiesis and can affect hemoglobin levels.

TREATMENT

Treatment is focused on the cause. Poor iron intake is treated with iron supplements and an iron-rich diet, often taken with a source of ascorbic acid to increase absorption. Iron can also be administered parenterally if oral supplements are inadequate or not tolerated. Iron deficiency related to blood loss requires stopping the source of bleeding and may require a blood transfusion.

Anorexia Nervosa

Anorexia nervosa (AN) is an eating disorder characterized by:

1. The inability to maintain a minimally healthy body weight
2. An intense fear of gaining weight
3. Relentless dietary habits that prevent weight gain
4. Severe body image distortions

The term anorexia designates a lack of appetite, although with AN, hunger is largely ignored. AN primarily affects adolescent and young adult women,

Table 17.5 Differentiation of Various Types of Anemia Based on Laboratory Test Results

	Iron Deficiency	B_{12} Deficiency	Folate Deficiency	Thalassemia	Anemia of Chronic Diseases
RBC size	Microcytic	Macrocytic	Macrocytic	Microcytic	Normocytic
Reticulocyte (immature RBC) count	Low	Low	Low	Normal	Low/normal
MCH	Low	Normal	Normal	Low	Normal
Serum iron	Low	High	High	Normal	Variable
Total iron-binding capacity	High	Normal	Normal	Normal	Normal
Ferritin level	Low	High	High	Normal	Normal
B_{12} level	Normal	Low	Normal	Normal	Normal
Folate level	Normal	Normal	Low	Normal	Normal

MCH, mean corpuscular hemoglobin; RBC, red blood cell.

particularly in developed countries that value a thin body type. Although less common, AN can affect men as well. Mortality rate is estimated at 10% with most deaths related to cardiovascular complications.[4]

PATHOPHYSIOLOGY

The exact etiology of AN is unknown, but several forces (biologic, psychologic, genetic, familial, and cultural) may contribute to the development of this condition. Genetic influences are indicated by a twin concordance of 50% to 80%.[4] Other specific risk factors include:

- Female sex
- Family history of eating disorders
- An introverted, obsessive, and perfectionist personality
- Inability to resolve conflict
- Low self-esteem
- Family dysfunction, such as enmeshment, overprotectiveness, or unresolved family conflict
- Concurrent mental health conditions, such as a personality, depressive, or anxiety disorder
- Cultural pressures to become thinner

Anorexia nervosa links a severe mental health disorder with devastating physical health problems caused by self-starvation (Fig. 17.13). The disturbance in body image contributes to malnutrition. Malnutrition encompasses both macronutrient and micronutrient deficiencies, although the use of supplements may protect against micronutrient deficiencies. Macronutrient, particularly caloric, restriction leads to mobilization of lipid stores, protein catabolism, and metabolic stress with a reduced metabolic rate. Malnutrition can then further exacerbate depression and psychologic deterioration.

All body systems are affected by malnutrition. Fluid and electrolyte levels become imbalanced. Skeletal muscle wasting and a loss of body fat are evident as macronutrient levels are inadequate; the body uses all available fat and protein stores for energy. The brain mass and CNS function are reduced. Seizures can develop, and tingling in the extremities is common. The heart size and function are reduced because of hypovolemia and hypotension. The heart rate slows, dysrhythmias and conduction defects can develop, and valves can become ineffective with a reduction in cardiac output. Gastrointestinal effects demonstrate reduced gastric emptying time with a structural functional loss of GI tract tone. Gallstones are more prevalent, and the liver can become necrotic. Liver dysfunction can lead to elevated cholesterol and blood lipid levels. Bones become porous and prone to fractures. The development of blood cells and clotting factors is impaired. This leads to problems with bleeding, anemia, and infection as the inflammatory and immune responses become compromised. Endocrine function is also affected: (1) antidiuretic hormone secretion is restricted, leading to the inability to concentrate urine; (2) reproductive hormone levels decline; and (3) cortisol levels increase because of the stress of malnutrition.

CLINICAL MANIFESTATIONS

Individuals with AN can exhibit many clinical manifestations related to restricted caloric (energy) and

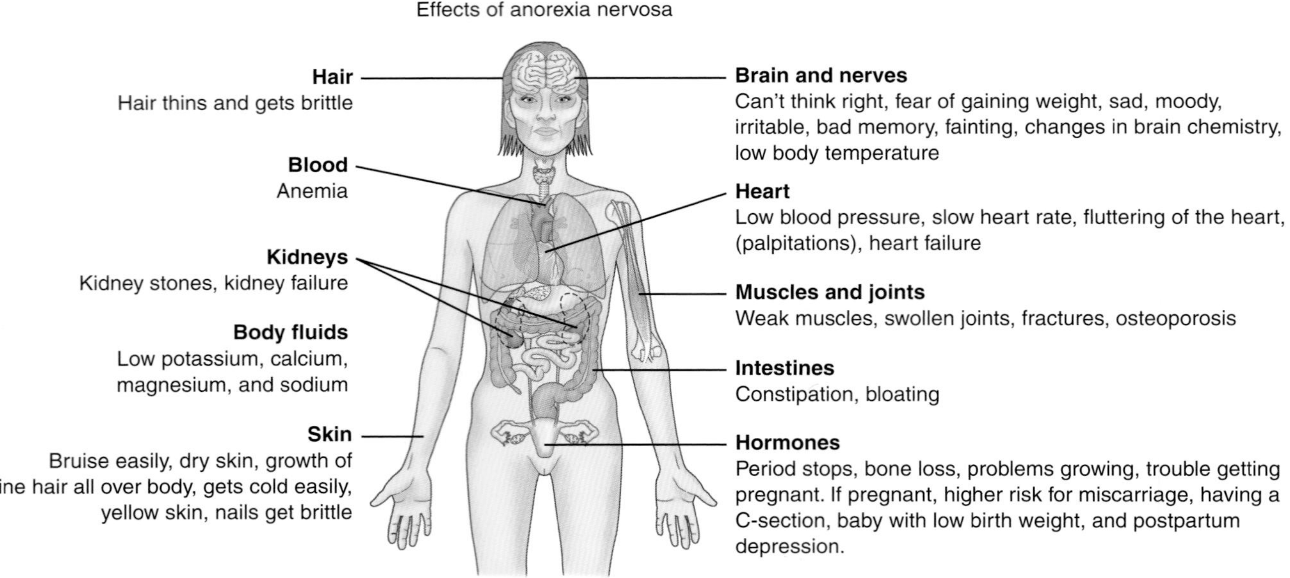

Figure 17.13. Physical effects that accompany anorexia nervosa. C-section, cesarean section.

nutrient intake. Common physical characteristics are related to the pathophysiologic processes discussed previously and include an extremely thin stature, **lanugo** (a fine downy hair that covers the body), amenorrhea in women, brittle hair and nails, peripheral cyanosis, dry skin, bradycardia, hypotension, hypothermia, abdominal bloating, and constipation.

DIAGNOSTIC CRITERIA

Diagnosis is based on history and physical examination. The *DSM-5* criteria for diagnosis of AN are summarized:

1. Restriction of food intake relative to caloric requirements leading to low body weight.
2. Intense fear of gaining weight or becoming fat, even though underweight, or persistent behavior to avoid weight gain, even though underweight.
3. Disturbance in the way in which one's body weight or shape is experienced, undue influence of body weight or shape on self-evaluation, or persistent lack of recognition of the seriousness of the current low body weight.

A nutritional assessment often reveals restriction of caloric intake to less than 1,000 kcal/ day. Laboratory studies can determine the resulting health effects and help to direct treatment strategies. Starvation may reveal normocytic, normochromic anemia and leukopenia from bone marrow suppression. Severe hypokalemia may be noted from laxative abuse or vomiting. Additional blood tests may reveal hypocalcemia, protein deficiency, reduced liver function, and significant electrolyte imbalance, including low sodium and chloride levels. Possible electrocardiogram changes include nonspecific ST- and T-segment abnormalities, atrial tachycardia, idioventricular conduction delay, heart block, and premature ventricular contractions. The basis for cardiac conduction impairment is attributed to starvation, electrolyte imbalance, and neuroendocrine alterations.

TREATMENT

An interdisciplinary team treatment approach is recommended. This team should include the patient, the patient's family, psychotherapists, physicians, nurses, dieticians, and recreational and occupational therapists. The goal of treatment is achieving and maintaining a healthy weight and nutritional intake along with psychotherapy for body image disturbances. Nutritional support includes a gradual refeeding process that induces a 1 to 2 lb weight gain per week. The health care team must monitor for complications of AN throughout treatment and watch for gastrointestinal, fluid, electrolyte, and cardiac disturbances. Although close monitoring, effective refeeding, and initiating of psychotherapy has shown a decrease in mortality rates among those with AN, two-thirds or more will have ongoing food and weight preoccupations.

Celiac Disease (Gluten-Sensitive Enteropathy)

Celiac disease, also called gluten-sensitive enteropathy or celiac sprue, is a disorder of gluten malabsorption caused by a T-cell mediated hypersensitivity marked by the inability to tolerate gliadin, the alcohol-soluble fraction of gluten, in persons who are genetically predisposed to developing this condition. The prevalence of the condition in first-degree relatives is approximately 10%.[5] **Glutens** are specific proteins found in wheat, rye, oats, and barley. Common foods that are made with glutens, which are everywhere in the human diet, are difficult to avoid. These include many types of cereals, breads, and pastas. The condition is most often detected between infancy and young adulthood.

PATHOPHYSIOLOGY

Although the exact cause of celiac disease is often unknown, a strong hereditary component exists (Fig. 17.14). Exposure to gluten elicits a hypersensitivity response that results in chronic inflammation and atrophy of the mucosa of the small intestine. Damage to the intestinal mucosa inhibits digestion because of damage to the villi that produce and secrete digestive hormones and enzymes. Inadequate secretion of hormones and enzymes inhibits gallbladder and pancreatic function. This further restricts the digestive processes. Absorption is also impaired because these villi undergo atrophy, which disallows the effective passage of nutrients across the mucosa. Absorption is further disrupted with a loss of carrier substances needed to transport nutrients across the mucosa.

CLINICAL MANIFESTATIONS

Clinical manifestations are consistent with other malabsorption conditions and include weight loss, diarrhea, flatulence, steatorrhea, malodorous stools, weight loss, borborygmus (loud stomach/intestinal rumbling), abdominal bloating and pain, fatigue, and macronutrient, mineral, and vitamin deficiencies. Because the clinical manifestations are nonspecific and sometimes even nonexistent, the condition is frequently misdiagnosed and underdiagnosed.

GLUTEN
Adenovirus serotype 12?
Genetic factors
HLA B8
HLA DR3-DQw2
Epithelial cell of small intestine
Lymphoid cells of lamina propria
IMMUNOLOGIC RESPONSE
Epithelial cell injury
CELIAC SPRUE
(villous atrophy, malabsorption)

Figure 17.14. Celiac disease (villous atrophy, malabsorption). Hypothetical mechanism in the pathogenesis of celiac disease. HLA, human leukocyte antigen. (From Rubin R, Strayer DS, eds. *Rubin's Pathophysiology: Clinicopathologic Foundations of Medicine*. 6th ed. Philadelphia, PA: Lippincott Williams & Wilkins; 2012:642.)

DIAGNOSTIC CRITERIA

Diagnostic suspicion is raised in the presence of clinical manifestations. Laboratory screening may include serum detection of antibodies against (1) the endomysium, or muscle fiber connective tissue; (2) the gliadin found in gluten; or (3) IgA tissue transglutaminase, the autoantigen that triggers the immune response. Diagnostic confirmation is made with a small bowel biopsy demonstrating inflammatory and atrophic changes.

TREATMENT

Treatment is focused on permanently eliminating sources of gluten from the diet. Corn and rice do not contain glutens and form a major portion of grain intake for those with celiac disease. Symptoms usually improve within 1 to 2 months of eliminating gluten sources. In the absence of gluten in the diet, the intestinal mucosa sometimes resumes optimal structure and function. Anti-inflammatory and hypersensitivity-blocking medications may be needed if elimination of gluten is not completely effective. Vitamin and mineral supplementation is often warranted. Lack of treatment leads to chronic intestinal ulcerations and can possibly lead to malignancy of the bowel and lymph glands.

Stop and Consider
You are providing nutritional counseling for a person with celiac disease. What specific foods would you recommend avoiding? What foods would you suggest as substitutions?

Phenylketonuria

PATHOPHYSIOLOGY

Phenylketonuria (PKU) is an autosomal recessive disorder caused by a mutation in the *PAH* gene, of which more than 500 different mutations have been identified. PKU results when a deficiency of the enzyme phenylalanine hydroxylase (PAH) impairs the body's ability to metabolize phenylalanine, an essential amino acid. The disorder is detected in about 350 of every 1 million births, making it the most common inborn error of metabolism.[6]

Deficient PAH enzyme leads to the marked accumulation of phenylalanine in body fluids and also the inability to convert phenylalanine into tyrosine (Fig. 17.15). Tyrosine is needed for the synthesis of proteins, thyroxine (a thyroid hormone), catecholamines (neurotransmitters), and melanin (skin pigment). Subtle neuropsychological deficits can result from reduced production of neurotransmitters as a result of deficient tyrosine transport across the neuronal cell membrane.

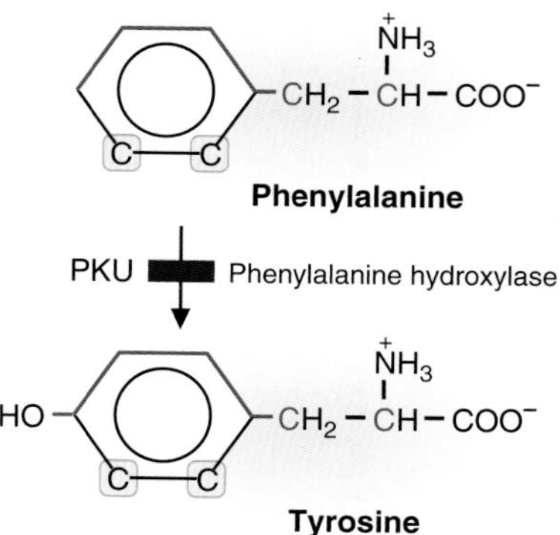

Figure 17.15. Degradation of phenylalanine. PKU, phenylketonuria.

CLINICAL MANIFESTATIONS

Excess circulating phenylalanine negatively impacts cognitive function. Patients with PKU almost always have intellectual disability unless phenylalanine levels are controlled through diet or drug treatment. In addition, impairment of melanin synthesis results in fair skin and hair and hypopigmentation of eyes. Patients often have a musty odor and about half are also diagnosed with a seizure disorder.

DIAGNOSTIC CRITERIA

Diagnosis often occurs at birth as a result of routine metabolic screening (blood test). In countries where newborn screening programs do not exist, PKU often goes undetected until severe developmental delay and intellectual disability occur.

TREATMENT

Patients with PKU often require specialty care. The condition is treated with careful lifetime dietary management, avoiding phenylalanine, and adding amino acid (especially tyrosine), vitamin, and mineral supplements. Pharmacologic therapy with sapropterin dihydrochloride, which is an enzyme cofactor, may support phenylalanine metabolism in some patients. Research is underway to develop an injectable phenylalanine enzyme substitute.

Specific food restrictions include those high in protein (meats, dairy, nuts, beans) and starch (bread, potatoes). Acceptable foods would be those that are low in protein, including fruits and nonstarchy vegetables. Patients with PKU obtain proteins primarily from medical food, such as those found in specially-formulated protein powders. Aspartame also must be eliminated as phenylalanine is a major component of this sugar substitute. Phenylalanine levels are monitored regularly. The prognosis is excellent when patients continue on a diet low in phenylalanine.

Obesity

Obesity is a state of excessive body fat and is a major public health crisis. The prevalence worldwide has been increasing with estimates of 1 billion people who are overweight or obese. The worldwide trend is caused in part to the increasing westernization of many traditional diets—fruits, vegetables, and whole grains are being replaced by calorie-dense, easily accessible foods that are high in saturated fat, sugar, and refined carbohydrates. Obesity is a major contributor to morbidity and mortality, especially in westernized countries such as the United States, where an estimated 35% of the population is obese.[7]

PATHOPHYSIOLOGY

Body weight is the composite of bone, muscle, organs, body fluids, and adipose tissue. Body fat is divided into essential fat, which is needed for physiologic functioning, and **storage fat**, which accumulates under the skin and around internal organs.

Adipocytes, the primary cell involved in obesity, are highly active metabolic, endocrine, and inflammatory cells. The adipocyte should be thought of as an endocrine gland, with a major role in controlling body weight, and a proinflammatory cell, capable of secreting proinflammatory cytokines and impacting blood coagulation, insulin sensitivity, and appetite. Important to the metabolism and function of adipocytes are the enzymes and hormones that control these functions. One example of an enzyme that contributes to obesity is lipoprotein lipase, which acts on the adipocyte to promote lipid storage. Other examples are listed below.

Stop and Consider
How could drug therapy target obesity with what you know about the role of lipoprotein lipase enzymes?

Obesity occurs when adipocytes are increased in size (hypertrophic) and/or number (hypercellular). In hypertrophic obesity, adipocytes become enlarged and fat accumulates in the abdominal region. Hypertrophic fat accumulation usually starts in adulthood and weight reduction measures, such as exercise and healthy diet, are generally successful. In contrast, hypercellular obesity often presents in childhood or adolescence, causes more severe obesity, and is typically not responsive to nonsurgical weight loss interventions.

The causes of hypertrophic or hypercellular obesity are not as simple as calories in versus calories out; obesity is a highly complex phenomenon and involves metabolic, endocrine, genetic, lifestyle, race, ethnic, age, sex, socioeconomic, and environmental factors. The many pieces to the obesity puzzle include:

- *Genetics* is estimated to be responsible for about one-third of the individual's body mass index. The number and size of adipose cells, distribution of body fat, and resting metabolic rate are genetically influenced; more than 200 genes are involved in obesity.
- *Lifestyle* factors, including consumption of a diet with excessive calories combined with a sedentary lifestyle, also contributes to the development of obesity.
- *Neurologic* mechanisms and *hormones* act on the hypothalamus, stimulate and suppress hunger and satiety.
  - Leptin, a hormone secreted by adipocytes, has a major role in body weight regulation. It signals satiety to the hypothalamus, reduces food intake and lipid storage, and promotes energy expenditure. In obesity, patients are found to have high levels of leptin but are *resistant* to this hormone.
  - Estrogen, which stimulates lipid movement into adipocytes in the hip and upper thigh regions and restricts movement into the abdominal region, explaining the shape of many women who have adequate estrogen levels.
  - Thyroid hormone is active in metabolic processes (see Chapter 13).
  - Insulin, secreted by the pancreas, acts on the CNS to inhibit food intake and is involved in the synthesis and storage of lipids.
  - Melanocortin hormone acts on melanocortin receptors and modifies appetite.
  - Ghrelin hormone, secreted from the stomach, is a major hunger hormone.
- *Enzymes* mediate metabolic processes and movement of dietary lipids into the adipocyte; lipoprotein lipases promote lipid storage.
- *Hormones* also mediate movement of dietary lipids from the blood, across the capillary wall, and into the adipocyte.

CLINICAL MANIFESTATIONS

The primary clinical manifestation for obesity is excessive weight and body fat. However, beyond excessive weight gain and body fat, obesity carries a long list of comorbidities, including diabetes, heart disease, hypertension, hyperlipidemia, stroke, osteoarthritis, liver disease, gall stones, poor wound healing, sleep apnea, and certain cancers (Fig. 17.16).

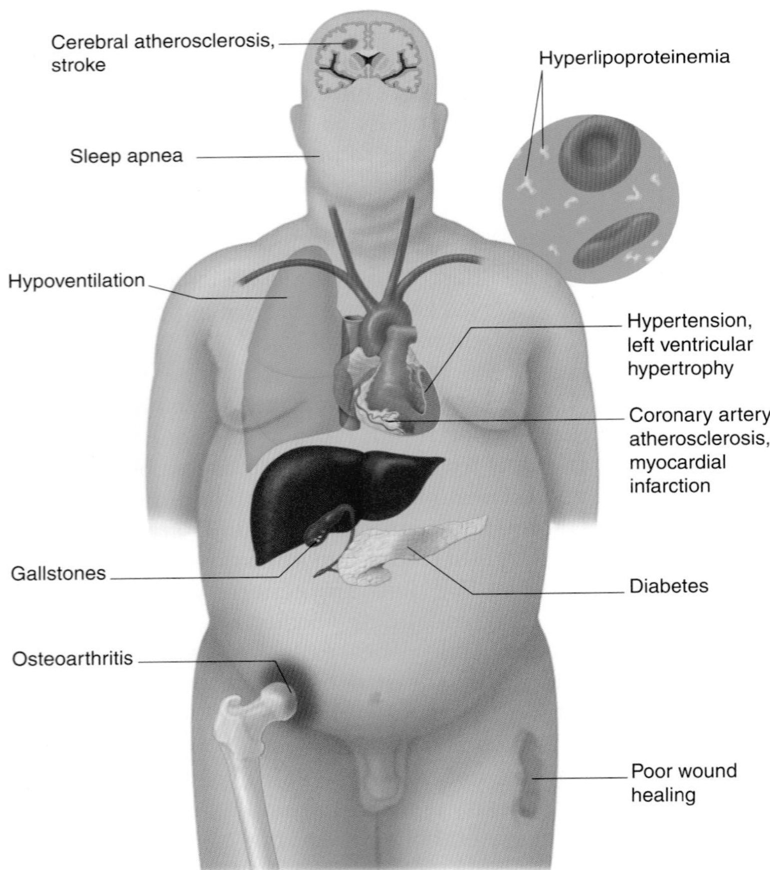

Figure 17.16. Obesity comorbidities.

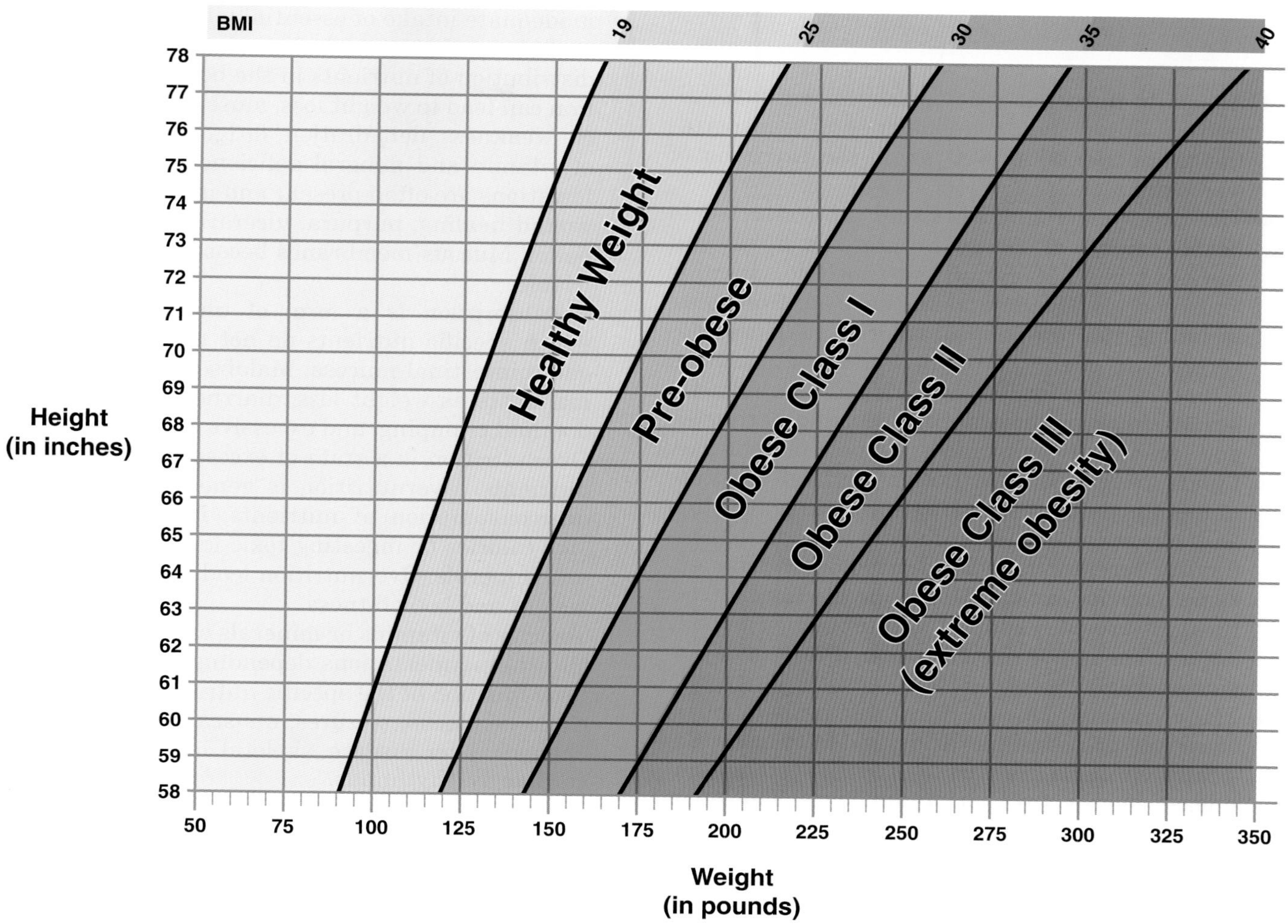

Figure 17.17. Body mass index and the classification of obesity. (Courtesy Anatomical Chart Company and modified according to the WHO International Classification of Adult Obesity According to BMI, 2010.)

Stop and Consider

Take a minute to calculate your BMI. Do this by measuring your weight in pounds and converting this to kilograms (1 lb = 0.45 kg). Then, measure your height in inches and convert this to meters squared (multiply inches × 2.54 cm; divide this number by 100 cm/m; multiply this final number × itself to get meters squared). Then the final step is to take your weight in kilograms and divide it by your height in meters squared. What number did you get?

DIAGNOSTIC CRITERIA-

Body fat is most often determined using a mathematical calculation termed **body mass index**, or BMI (Fig. 17.17). The World Health Organization classifies BMI as follows:

- Grade 1 (overweight): BMI of 25 to 29.9 kg/m^2
- Grade 2 (obese): BMI of 30 to 39.9 kg/m^2
- Grade 3 (severely obese): BMI $\geq$ 40 kg/m^2

Diagnosis of obesity should also include a comprehensive evaluation for comorbidities, such as hypertension, hypercholesterolemia, diabetes, hypothyroidism, venous varicosities, osteoarthritis, sleep apnea, depression, reproductive alterations, and infection.

TREATMENT

Treatment of obesity is lifelong and is focused on attaining and maintaining the best possible weight for optimal health. Basic treatment principles focus on diet, exercise, and behavioral modification. Pharmacologic therapy or surgery may be indicated, but these do not replace lifestyle modifications. Pharmacologic therapies primarily aim to suppress appetite, increase metabolism, or interfere with fat absorption. Treatment may also include insulin for diabetes or antihypertensives. Gastric surgery may be needed in some cases to reduce stomach size and thereby reduce food intake and fat absorption.

SUMMARY

- Adequate nutrition relies on optimal intake, digestion, absorption, metabolism, and transportation of nutrients, as well as on the excretion of waste products.
- The major macronutrients that are converted to usable sources of energy are proteins, lipids, and carbohydrates. Micronutrients include vitamins and minerals. Macronutrients have multiple roles, including the provision of calories that are converted into energy. Proteins build and maintain structural body tissues, comprise blood, cell membranes, immune factors, enzymes, and hormones, and transport substances across membranes. Lipids are a rich source of energy and facilitate numerous processes, such as supporting digestion and absorption. They influence cell membrane fluidity, receptor function, hormone function, enzyme activity, and cytokine production. Structural fat provides support and protection to body organs. The major role of carbohydrates is to provide energy.
- Many vitamins play a critical role in metabolism of carbohydrates, amino acids, and fatty acids. Basically, vitamins are part of enzyme systems that release energy from macronutrients. The other major role of vitamins is to aid in the development of genetic materials, red blood cells, hormones, collagen, and nervous system tissue.
- Minerals regulate hundreds of cellular processes. Minerals constitute bone, hemoglobin, enzymes, hormones, and chemical mediators. Charged (ionic) minerals mediate impulse conduction within the nervous system. Minerals maintain water balance, acid–base balance, and osmotic pressure. Minerals are critical for muscle contraction and form the structural components of bones and teeth.
- The intake and storage of nutrients is critical to overall health and is regulated primarily by neuroendocrine systems. Digestion and absorption is a process involving mechanical and enzymatic degradation of nutrients into usable components that can be absorbed. The gastrointestinal tract, most notably the small intestine, is a major site for digestion and absorption of nutrients.
- Altered nutrition, or malnutrition, is a state of inadequate or excessive exposure to nutrients. This can include intake, digestion, or absorption of nutrients. Protein energy malnutrition is related to deprivation of all food (marasmus) or protein deprivation in individuals consuming adequate carbohydrates (kwashiorkor).
- Undernutrition is a lack of intake of nutrients most often related to inadequate calorie consumption, inadequate intake of essential vitamins and minerals, or problems with digestion, absorption, or distribution of nutrients in the body. Undernutrition can lead to weight loss, muscle wasting, muscle weakness, dehydration, fatigue, and evidence of vitamin and mineral deficiencies. Skin manifestations are often present and may include poor wound healing, purpura, ulceration, dry skin, or pallor. Mucous membranes become inflamed and friable.
- Malabsorption is a form of undernutrition in which specific nutrients do not move across the gastrointestinal mucosa. Malabsorption typically manifests as weight loss, diarrhea, bloating, abdominal cramping, and excessive flatulence.
- Overnutrition is a state of excessive exposure to nutrients. Overnutrition is generally related to overconsumption of nutrients, including excessive calories or ingesting toxic levels of vitamins and minerals. Overnutrition leads to increases in weight and body fatness.
- Toxicity of vitamins or minerals can have varying clinical manifestations depending on the physiologic function of the specific nutrient and may include headache, seizures, nausea, vomiting, skin changes, liver disease, skeletal impairment, and cardiac dysrhythmias.
- Diagnostic and treatment strategies for altered nutrition are focused on determining the cause for the nutrition imbalance and the potential effects.

CASE STUDY 17.1

Jill is a 14-year-old African-American girl who presents to the clinic reporting intermittent diarrhea, bloating, abdominal pain, and gas 30 minutes after eating some meals, particularly breakfast. Further history elicited that she eats a bowl of cereal with milk each morning. Others in her family have lactose intolerance. She thinks that when she avoids milk that she doesn't have the symptoms. You suspect lactose intolerance in her as well.

1. Outline the process that is most likely occurring in this person's body.
2. What would you expect for clinical manifestations?
3. What diagnostic tests could be used?
4. What treatment measures would you anticipate?

Log on to the Internet. Search for a relevant journal article or Web site, such as http://www.niddk.nih.gov/health-information/health-topics/digestive-diseases/lactose-intolerance/Pages/ez.aspx, which details lactose intolerance and confirm your predictions.

CASE STUDY 17.2

Pam is a 40-year-old woman who has been seeing an eating disorder specialist for the past 6 months due to a prolonged binge eating disorder. She is obese with a BMI of 34. Her eating disorder became problematic around age 18 when her weight continued to elevate over time. She binges about once per week now and it is usually triggered by family-related stress. She eats rapidly at all meals. She noticed though that she has been binging only when she is alone. After a binging episode, Pam feels embarrassed but helpless. She is not able to stop the behavior.

1. Outline the process that is most likely occurring in this person's body.
2. What would you expect for clinical manifestations?
3. What diagnostic tests could be used?
4. What treatment measures would you anticipate?

Log on to the Internet. Search for a relevant journal article or Web site, such as http://www.mayoclinic.com/health/binge-eating-disorder/DS00608, which details binge eating disorder, and confirm your predictions.

CASE STUDY 17.3

Thomas is a 49-year-old who has been severely obese since adolescence. He has tried every diet and weight loss program without success. He decides that he would like to pursue gastric bypass surgery and is found to be a good candidate. After months of preparation, Thomas undergoes a laparoscopic bypass procedure.

1. How is the procedure performed? How is the anatomy and physiology changed?
2. What would be the contraindications to gastric bypass? Who would not be a good candidate?
3. How would the patient determine success after the procedure?

Log on to the Internet. Search for a relevant journal article or Web site, such as http://emedicine.medscape.com/article/143954-overview#a1, which details gastric bypass, and confirm your predictions.

PRACTICE EXAM QUESTIONS

1. You have inflammation of the large intestine, a condition called ulcerative colitis. What is the most probable reason that you would develop iron-deficiency anemia?
   a. You are experiencing chronic blood loss in your stools
   b. You have inadequate hydrochloric acid for absorption of iron
   c. You have lost usable surface area in the large intestine for absorption of iron
   d. You do not have an adequate iron intake in your diet

2. You are part of the health care team at a clinic for adolescents with anorexia nervosa. Which of the assessments that you perform is focused on recognizing the most common cause for mortality in those with AN?
   a. Lung assessment
   b. Cardiovascular assessment
   c. Skin assessment
   d. Neurologic assessment

3. Which dietary change would be recommended for the individual with celiac disease?
   a. Avoid milk or milk products
   b. Avoid wheat, barley, rye, and oats
   c. Avoid rice, soy, and nuts
   d. Avoid long-chain fatty acids

4. Which of the following affects the sensations of hunger and satiety and therefore plays a major role in the development of obesity?
   a. The hypothalamus
   b. The pituitary gland
   c. The thyroid gland
   d. The pancreas

5. Which of the following does not contribute as an energy source in the diet?
   a. Carbohydrates
   b. Fats
   c. Proteins
   d. Vitamins

6. You are caring for an individual with liver disease. What are you most concerned about in terms of nutrition?
   a. The patient may be unable to adequately store nutrients
   b. The patient may be unable to synthesize nutrients
   c. The patient may be unable to metabolize macronutrients
   d. All of these are major concerns

7. Your patient has gall bladder disease and is unable to store and release adequate bile to the small intestine. What dietary modifications do you suggest?
   a. Increase protein intake
   b. Decrease fat intake
   c. Increase complex carbohydrates
   d. No dietary changes are needed

8. You are working in the newborn nursery and are an advocate for breastfeeding. It is the winter in northern Minnesota and you are concerned about low sunlight exposure in infants who are breastfeeding as they may develop vitamin D deficiency. What is the major manifestation of vitamin D deficiency?
   a. Impaired mineralization in growing bones
   b. Impaired retinal development
   c. Impaired osteoclast activity
   d. Keratinization of mucous membranes

9. You are planning a nutritional inservice to your clinic's service area in California. What concept of altered nutrition should you focus your talk in order to address the largest nutritional problem in your area?
   a. Altered metabolism
   b. Undernutrition
   c. Overnutrition
   d. All of these are equally prevalent

10. What is known about glucose transport into the small intestine?
    a. Requires cotransport with sodium
    b. Occurs through active transport
    c. Must first be reduced as is rarely consumed in the typical diet
    d. All of these are true about glucose transport

11. What is the first plan of action for the formula-fed newborn who is just diagnosed with PKU?
    a. Switch to a special formula with phenylalanine
    b. Prepare for a blood transfusion
    c. Switch to a phenylalanine-free formula
    d. Require the mother to breastfeed

12. Which of the following vitamins is supplemented in pregnancy because of its important role in embryogenesis and the prevention of neural tube defects in the fetus?
    a. Vitamin A
    b. Citric acid
    c. Folate
    d. Vitamin B_{12}

13. What are typical manifestations for malabsorption syndromes?
    a. Constipation, dry mouth, weakness
    b. Diarrhea, bloating, stomach pain
    c. Bloody stools, fissures, rectal bleeding
    d. Nausea, vomiting, stomach cramping

14. Your neighbor, as she put it, is a "lactose intolerant health nut" and she is always experimenting with various supplements. Recently, she went into the clinic for evaluation of pain in her leg and was found to have multiple bone fractures. Which of the following supplements, in toxic levels, causes multiple skeletal fractures?
    a. Phosphorus
    b. Iron
    c. Zinc
    d. Calcium

DISCUSSION AND APPLICATION

1. What did I know about altered nutrition prior to today?
2. What body processes are affected by altered nutrition? What are the expected functions of those processes? How does altered nutrition affect those processes?
3. What are the potential etiologies for altered nutrition? How does altered nutrition develop?
4. Who is most at risk for developing altered nutrition? How can altered nutrition be prevented?
5. What are the human differences that affect the etiology, risk, or course of altered nutrition?
6. What clinical manifestations are expected in the course of altered nutrition?
7. What special diagnostic tests are useful in determining the diagnosis and course of altered nutrition?
8. What are the goals of care for individuals with altered nutrition?
9. How does the concept of altered perfusion build on what I have learned in the previous chapters and in previous courses?
10. How can I use what I have learned?

RESOURCES

Academy of Nutrition and Dietetics:
http://www.eatright.org/

Body Mass Index calculator:
http://www.cdc.gov/healthyweight/assessing/index.html

Canada's Food and Nutrition Website:
http://www.hc-sc.gc.ca/fn-an/index-eng.php

National Society for PKU:
http://www.nspku.org/

Obesity Society:
http://www.obesity.org

United States Department of Agriculture (USDA) "MyPlate":
http://www.choosemyplate.gov/

References

1. Mahan L, Escott-Stump S. *Food, Nutrition, and Diet Therapy*. Philadelphia, PA: Saunders; 2004.
2. Jerome-Morais A, Diamond AM, Wright ME. Dietary supplements and human health: for better or for worse? *Mol Nutr Food Res*. 2011;55(1):122–135.
3. U.S. Department of Agriculture, U.S. Department of Health and Human Services. *Dietary Guidelines for Americans, 2010.* 7th ed. Washington, DC: U.S. Government Printing Office; 2010.
4. Bernstein BE. Anorexia Nervosa. http://emedicine.medscape.com/article/912187-overview#a3. Accessed November 22, 2015.
5. Goebel SU. Celiac disease. http://emedicine.medscape.com/article/171805-overview. Accessed November 23, 2015.
6. Arnold G. Phenylketonuria. http://emedicine.medscape.com/article/947781-overview. Accessed November 23, 2015.
7. Hamdy O. Obesity. http://emedicine.medscape.com/article/123702-overview#a5. Accessed November 24, 2015.

Find additional resources for this chapter at http:thePoint.lww.com thePoint®

Chapter 18

Altered Elimination

LEARNING OUTCOMES

1. Define and use the key terms listed in this chapter.
2. Describe the processes of the production and elimination of urine and stool.
3. Identify the role of neural, motor, endocrine, and physical processes in altered elimination.
4. Outline the processes involved in altered elimination.
5. Characterize the clinical manifestations in altered urinary and gastrointestinal elimination.
6. Recognize health conditions that can precipitate impaired elimination.
7. Detail alterations in systemic organ systems as a response to altered elimination.
8. List the common diagnostic procedures used to identify altered urinary and bowel elimination.
9. Describe treatment modalities used in altered urinary and bowel elimination.
10. Apply concepts of altered elimination to select clinical models.

INTRODUCTION

As you have seen in the previous chapters, maintenance of homeostasis requires a delicate balance and careful coordination of many body systems. The same is true of the process of elimination. When you eat and drink in response to hunger and thirst, you feel satisfied. We often take for granted what happens to the food and drink after our needs are met. Once nutrients have been extracted from the foods and liquids we eat, the remaining contents must be eliminated. Urine and stool are the final waste products of what were once our favorite foods and drinks. For the body to function efficiently, the waste products that remain after energy is extracted and nutrients are absorbed must be excreted. Impairment of the ability to eliminate waste products results in the clinical manifestations and pathophysiologic alterations associated with disease. In this chapter, the processes of altered urinary and gastrointestinal (GI) elimination and their clinical manifestations are described in Modules 1 and 2. The application of these altered processes is considered in Module 3, selected clinical models of altered elimination.

Module 1 Altered Urinary Elimination

Elimination processes require motility and patency of structures involved in the movement of waste for excretion. These processes are regulated by neuromuscular signaling and are influenced by transport functions and adequacy of perfusion. Regulation of body fluid and the balance between acids and bases are two of the primary roles of the kidney, as described in Chapters 8 and 9. Water and ion movement across the cell membranes of the renal tubules in close association with the vasculature of the kidneys is the mechanism that allows fluid and waste secretion in the form of urine.

Urine Production Process

Urine is produced by the kidney, is stored in the bladder, and is excreted via the urethra through a complex interplay between neural, motor, and hormonal mechanisms. The basic processes of the renal system include:

- Regulation of body fluid volume and composition
- Elimination of metabolic wastes
- Synthesis, release, or activation of hormones
  - Erythropoietin
  - Renin
  - Vitamin D
- Regulation of blood pressure

The renal system is illustrated in Figure 18.1, which provides a visual review of the urinary system location in relation to other anatomic structures in the body (Fig. 18.1A), an overview of the internal structures of the kidney (Fig. 18.1B), and a detailed view of the functional unit of the kidney, the nephron (Fig. 18.1C).

URINE PRODUCTION

The **nephron** is the functional unit of the kidney and is composed of the **glomerulus** (capillary network and Bowman capsule), the proximal tubule, loop of Henle, distal tubule, and collecting duct. There are approximately 1 million nephrons in the cortex of each kidney. The role of the nephron is to:

- Filter water-soluble substances from the blood
- Reabsorb filtered nutrients, water, and electrolytes
- Secrete waste

The kidneys are responsible for processing 20% to 25% of the cardiac output, approximately 1,000 mL of blood per minute. This allows the kidneys to be perfused with enough blood supply to meet the high oxygen and metabolic demands of the organ. Blood enters the kidney through the renal artery, dividing into interlobular arteries, arcuate arteries, afferent arterioles, and glomerular capillaries. Blood entering the glomerular capillaries via the afferent arteriole is filtered with the resulting fluid called **filtrate**. Filtrate enters Bowman capsule, where it then enters the renal tubular system. The blood remaining in the glomerular capillaries exits the glomerulus via the efferent arteriole, which then branches into the peritubular capillaries. The peritubular capillaries surround the proximal and distal convoluted tubules. Additional capillaries, vasa recta, surround the loops of Henle deep within the medulla, serving an important role in the concentration of urine through exchange of water and solutes from the filtrate flowing in the opposite direction of the blood (**countercurrent exchanger**). Blood travels into the interlobular venules and veins and returns to the venous circulation via the renal vein.

Filtrate travels from Bowman capsule to the proximal tubule, where the majority of sodium is reabsorbed back into the blood. Other reabsorbed substances include glucose, potassium, amino acids, HCO_3^-, PO_4^-, urea, and water. Hydrogen is secreted from the resulting isotonic fluid. Fluid moves down the loop of Henle where it is progressively more concentrated (**countercurrent multiplier**). Water is reabsorbed and sodium diffuses into the descending loop, with sodium actively reabsorbed in the ascending loop. The **countercurrent mechanism** involves the countercurrent exchanger and multiplier and is responsible for maintaining the vertical gradient in the interstitium (Fig. 18.2). In the distal tubule, sodium (through the actions of the hormone, aldosterone) and HCO_3^- are reabsorbed. Epithelial cells adjacent to the distal tubule, the macula densa, provide information about sodium content in the filtrate to the cells of the juxtaglomerular apparatus, regulating aldosterone release via the renin–angiotensin–aldosterone system (RAAS). Secretion of potassium, urea, hydrogen, and ammonia (NH_3) occurs; the remaining filtrate moves into the collecting duct. Here, additional water is reabsorbed in an antidiuretic hormone (ADH)-dependent mechanism, in addition to sodium, hydrogen, potassium, and NH_3. The end product produced by the nephron is urine, which is transported via the ureters to the bladder, where it is stored until it is eliminated through the urethra.

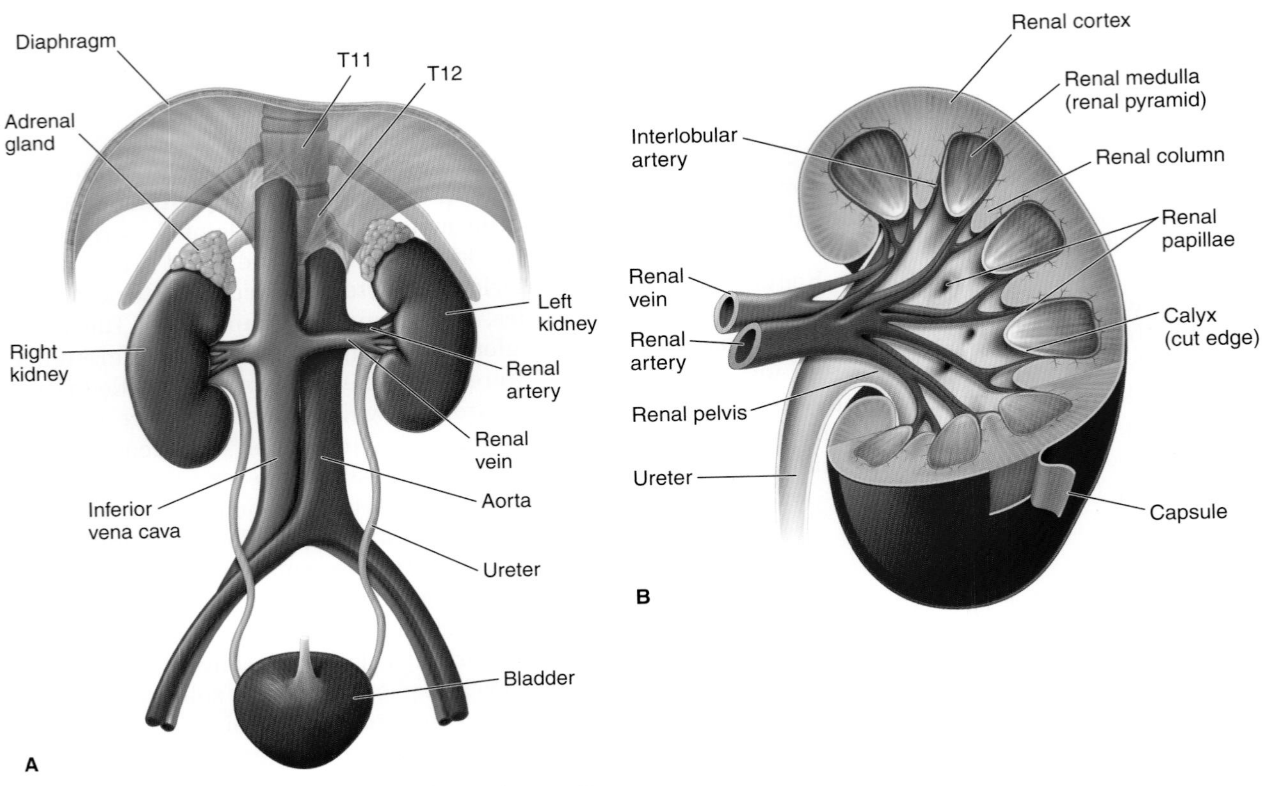

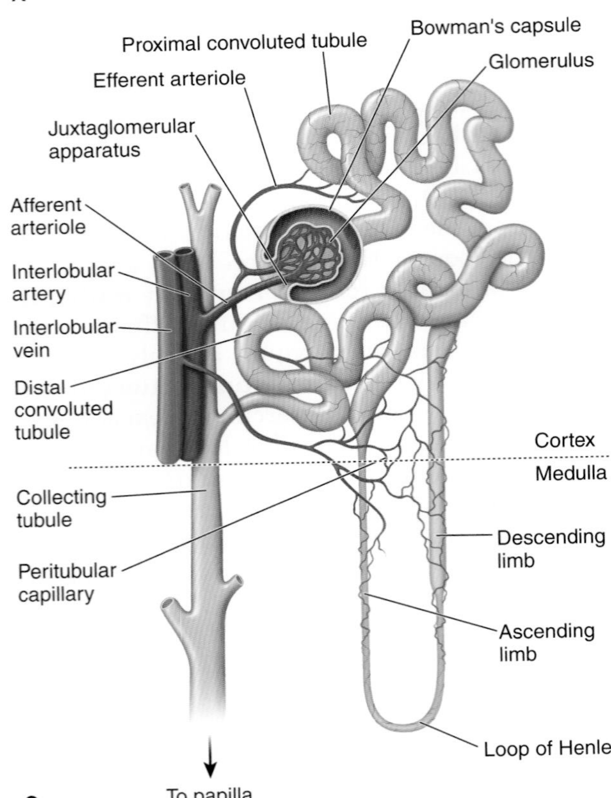

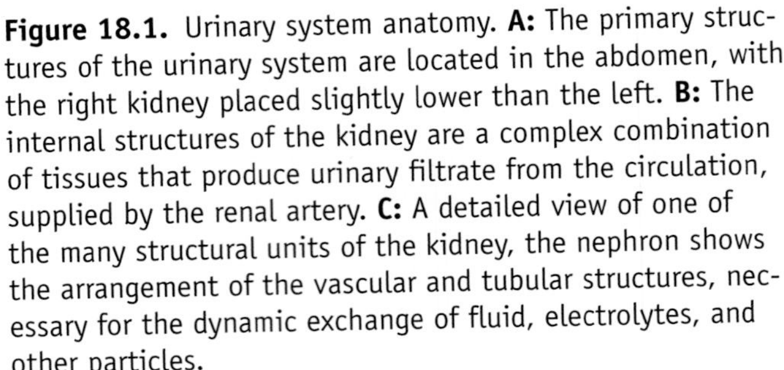
Figure 18.1. Urinary system anatomy. **A:** The primary structures of the urinary system are located in the abdomen, with the right kidney placed slightly lower than the left. **B:** The internal structures of the kidney are a complex combination of tissues that produce urinary filtrate from the circulation, supplied by the renal artery. **C:** A detailed view of one of the many structural units of the kidney, the nephron shows the arrangement of the vascular and tubular structures, necessary for the dynamic exchange of fluid, electrolytes, and other particles.

Table 18.1 describes the mechanisms of tubular transport for selected substances.

Stop and Consider
Why is it necessary for urine to become concentrated before it is excreted?

URINE REMOVAL

Urine enters the ureters via the renal pelvis, promoting flow out of the kidneys. Ureters are composed of smooth muscle fibers that propel the urine to the bladder by the process of peristalsis. Urine enters the bladder via the trigone. The **trigone** is

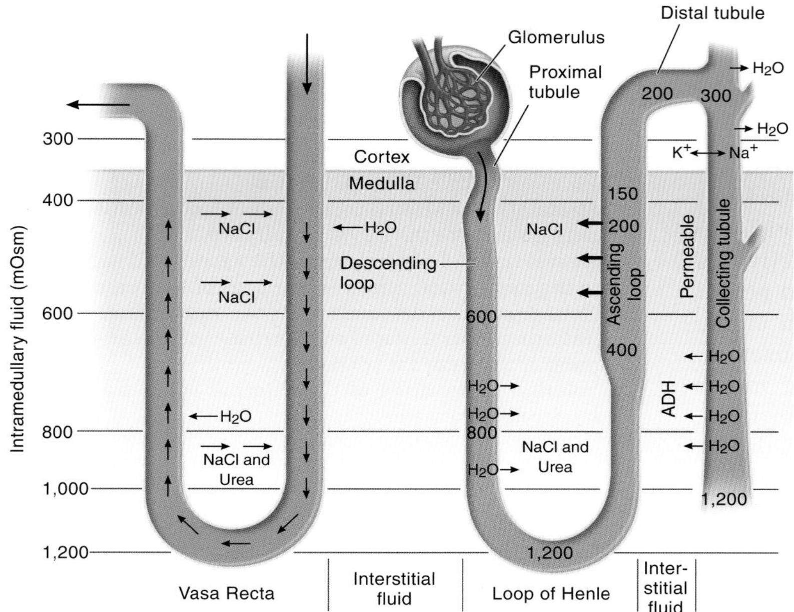

Figure 18.2. Urinary filtrate flow and concentration. Movement of water and solutes between the vasa recta and loops of Henle in the juxtamedullary nephrons promotes concentration of urine. The flow of filtrate in the loop of Henle runs in the opposite direction of the flow of blood in the parallel vasa recta. This countercurrent design combined with the selective permeabilities of the loop of Henle contributes to the concentration of osmotically active particles in the medullary interstitium. In the collecting tubule, ADH allows water to move from filtrate into the interstitium, drawn by osmotic forces. Water then is reabsorbed into the blood to achieve optimal water balance. (Modified from Premkumar K. *The Massage Connection: Anatomy and Physiology*. Baltimore, MD: Lippincott Williams & Wilkins; 2004.)

Table 18.1 Tubular Transport

Substance	Mechanisms and Sites of Transport
Sodium	Filtered at the glomerulus
	Reabsorbed in the proximal tubule by facilitated diffusion and in the proximal tubule, thick ascending loop of Henle, and distal convoluted tubule by active transport
Potassium	Filtered at the glomerulus
	Reabsorbed passively in the proximal tubule and actively in the thick ascending loop of Henle
	Secreted or actively reabsorbed in the distal convoluted or collecting tubules; depends on blood potassium levels
Chloride	Filtered at the glomerulus
	Reabsorbed passively in the late proximal and distal convoluted tubule
	Reabsorbed actively in the proximal tubule, ascending loop of Henle, and distal convoluted tubule
Hydrogen	Secreted actively in the proximal, distal convoluted, and collecting tubules
	Reabsorbed by cation exchangers in the proximal convoluted tubules
Bicarbonate	Filtered at the glomerulus
	Reabsorbed passively in the proximal and distal convoluted tubules
Glucose	Filtered at the glomerulus
	Entirely reabsorbed by active mechanisms unless tubular maximum is exceeded
Urea	Filtered at the glomerulus
	Reabsorbed passively in the proximal, late distal tubules, and collecting duct
	Entry into the descending and thin ascending loops of Henle depends on concentration gradient in the surrounding interstitium
Calcium	Filtered at the glomerulus
	Reabsorbed passively in the proximal tubule and the thin loop of Henle
	Reabsorbed actively in the ascending thick loop of Henle and early distal convoluted tubule
Phosphate	Filtered at the glomerulus
	Reabsorbed actively in proximal tubule
Magnesium	Filtered at the glomerulus
	Reabsorbed actively and passively in the thick ascending loop of Henle
Uric acid	Filtered at the glomerulus
	Reabsorbed in the early and late proximal tubule
	Secreted in the midproximal tubule
Protein	Limited filtration at the glomerulus caused by large size and negative charge
	Amino acids actively reabsorbed in the proximal distal tubule
	Large peptides reabsorbed by endocytosis for entry into lysozymes (metabolized into amino acids)

a triangular, smooth area at the base of the bladder between the openings of the two ureters and the urethra, serving as a functional sphincter, which prevents urine from moving in a retrograde manner back into the ureter from the bladder. The **bladder** is a muscular organ lined with transitional epithelium and innervated by the pelvic nerves. The body of the bladder is composed of the **detrusor muscle** (skeletal muscle). Filling of the bladder activates sensory stretch receptors, and the generated action potential is transmitted to the sacral region of the spinal cord. Contraction of the detrusor muscle is stimulated by parasympathetic cholinergic motor fibers. Relaxation of the muscle of the bladder neck, the **internal urethral sphincter** (composed of a ring of circular smooth muscle), promotes release of urine from the bladder (**micturition**). Somatic control of the **external urethral sphincter** muscle (skeletal muscle) innervated by the pudendal nerve allows for voluntary release of urine. Tonic contraction of the smooth muscle of the urethra prevents the leakage of urine until pressure in the bladder exceeds threshold. Urethral length differs between genders; the female urethra is much shorter than the male urethra, which spans the length of the penis. Figure 18.3 illustrates the structures of the bladder. A summary of the steps involved in the micturition reflex is highlighted in Box 18.1.

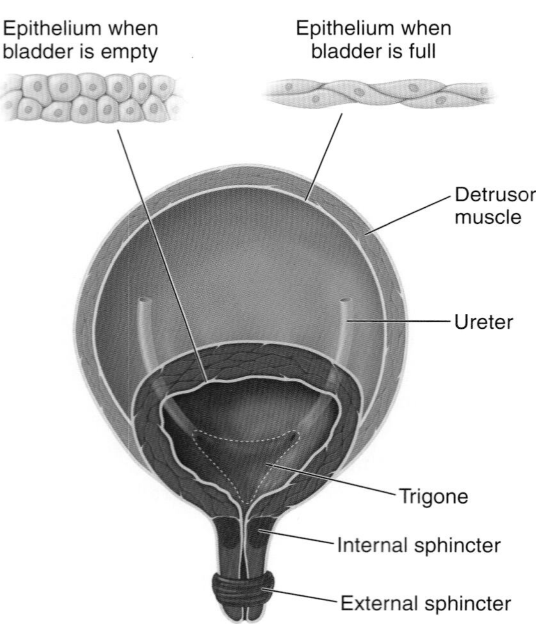

Figure 18.3. Bladder structures in urinary excretion. The path of urine excretion through the ureters, trigone area, and internal and external sphincters is shown. Contraction of the detrusor muscle promotes passage of urine. The structural relationship of the epithelium lining the bladder cavity depends on bladder volume. (Modified from Porth CM. *Pathophysiology: Concepts of Altered Health States*. 7th ed. Philadelphia, PA: Lippincott Williams & Wilkins; 2004.)

Box 18.1 Micturition Reflex

Bladder filling stimulates the micturition reflex. The steps involved in the micturition reflex are primarily involuntary, but they may be modulated by the cerebral cortex, enabling conscious control. The micturition reflex involves four major steps:

1. Stimulation of stretch receptors in bladder walls transmits impulse to the sacral spinal cord.
2. Neural impulse ascends from the sacral cord segments to the micturition center in the pons of the brain.
3. Neural impulse descends from the micturition center, initiating contraction of the detrusor muscle and relaxation of the internal sphincter.
4. Voluntary relaxation of the external sphincter stimulates release of urine.

Urine Characteristics

Urine is a clear yellow fluid composed primarily of water, which contains a variety of water-soluble waste products. Total volume produced is approximately 750 to 2,000 mL over a 24-hour period. Urine has a slight ammonia odor from the breakdown of urea. Variations in color, derived from urochrome pigments, indicate hydration status. Concentrated, dark, strong-smelling urine may indicate dehydration, whereas dilute, pale-colored urine may indicate increased fluid volume.

Urine samples can be collected to determine the specific characteristics. Methods of urine collection for analysis include:

- Random collection
  - May be taken at any time of the day
  - No special preparation required
- Clean-catch
  - Requires special cleansing of the external urethral meatus
  - Midstream urine collection (urine collected does not include fluid from the initial or final urinary stream)
- Bladder catheterization
  - Sterile insertion of a catheter through the urinary meatus into the bladder to collect urine sample
- Suprapubic aspiration
  - Insertion of a sterile needle transabdominally into the bladder for urine collection

Stop and Consider
Why would the indication for urine collection influence the method selection?

Urine Analysis

Urine is analyzed in two different ways: macroscopic and microscopic. **Macroscopic analysis** consists of the visual determination of color and clarity. In addition, biochemical analyses can be obtained by testing urine with a **urine dipstick**. Color changes indicate the absence or presence (including a gross estimate of quantity) of substances in urine. These substances provide information such as:

- pH
- Specific gravity
- Protein
- Glucose
- Ketones
- Nitrite
- Leukocyte esterase

Microscopic analysis is performed by using a specially prepared urine sample. A small sample (10 to 15 mL) of urine is centrifuged for approximately 10 minutes until the sediment forms at the bottom of the test tube. All but a small amount of fluid is removed and the sediment is resuspended in the remaining fluid. A sample is placed onto a glass slide with a coverslip for viewing under the microscope. Low-power examination can detect the presence of crystals, casts, squamous cells, and other large components. High-power examination can detect crystals, cells (white blood cells [WBCs] and red blood cells [RBCs]), and bacteria.

Urine should be free of protein, glucose, ketones, nitrite, bacteria, leukocyte esterase, crystals, and stones. **Casts**, structures consisting of a protein meshwork of entrapped cells formed in the distal collecting tubules and collecting ducts, are also absent in normal urine. Epithelial cells may be present in small numbers, but increased amounts detected in urine may indicate pathology. Identification of these abnormal findings provides evidence of clinical disease.

ALTERED URINARY ELIMINATION

Elimination involves a complex interplay between neural, vascular, muscular, and hormonal influences. Additionally, the structures involved in the movement of urine from its production to its exit must be patent and functional.

Processes of Altered Urinary Elimination

Alteration in motility, neuromuscular function, vascular insufficiency, and obstruction are most commonly associated with altered urinary elimination. The following review of etiology and implications of altered motility, neuromuscular function, perfusion, and patency in the urinary system provides the essential content for concept application in Module 3, Clinical Models.

ALTERATION IN URINARY MOTILITY

Alteration in motility can promote stasis of filtrate in the renal tubules as well as stasis of urine in the bladder. Casts may form because of low flow rate, increased sodium concentration, and low pH, all factors favoring precipitation. Precipitation of urinary fluid components may contribute to blockage of essential renal structures. The specific type of cell trapped in the cast meshwork may provide information on the site of pathology. Trapping of RBCs within casts may indicate glomerulonephritis. Epithelial cells may indicate sloughing of tubular cells (**acute tubular necrosis**) (Fig. 18.4), whereas WBCs may indicate pyelonephritis (Fig. 18.5). Stasis of urine in the bladder may promote growth of bacteria, leading to local and ascending infection in the kidneys.

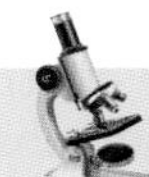

FROM THE LAB

The number of specific sediment components seen under microscopic examination can be quantified. The degree of magnification is also indicated and is determined with low-power field (LPF) or high-power field (HPF). Several fields, or areas, are counted and then averaged to provide an accurate estimate.

ALTERATION IN URINARY NEUROMUSCULAR FUNCTION

Alteration in neuromuscular function in urinary elimination may result in urinary retention or incontinence. Impaired neural control of urinary elimination may involve the neurons of the peripheral and central nervous systems, neurotransmitter production and availability or coordination of neural impulses from initiation to action. From generation of an action potential to transduction of the nerve impulse (see Chapter 10), failure to provide an appropriate stimulus for the desired response will result in a limited or absent ability to eliminate urine. Exaggerated responses may prompt stimulation to

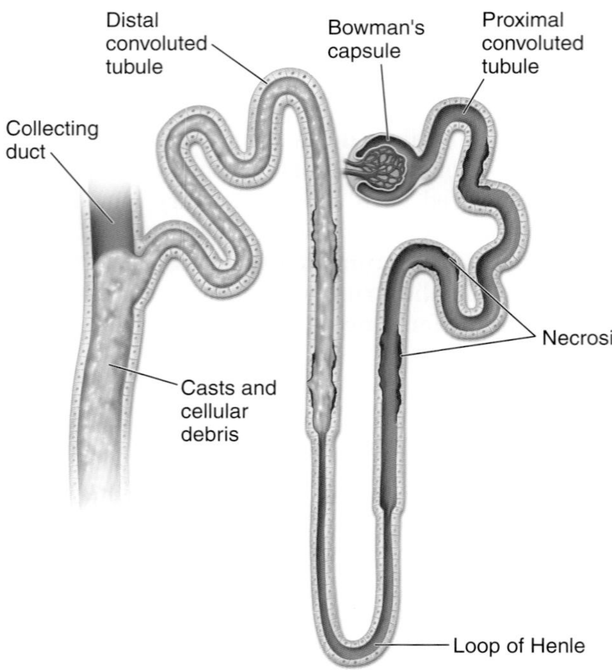

Figure 18.4. Acute tubular necrosis. Casts and cellular debris are sloughed into the tubular lumen in both ischemic necrosis and nephrotoxic injury.

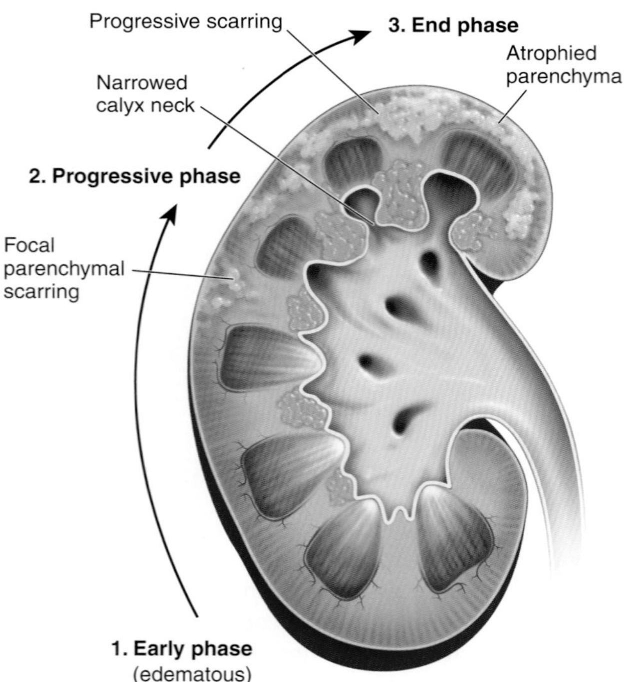

Figure 18.5. Phases of damage in pyelonephritis.

prematurely release urine. Additionally, muscles must have the ability to respond to a generated nerve impulse to achieve the intended effect. Muscle function involved in urinary elimination includes peristalsis in the renal tubules, contraction or relaxation of smooth and skeletal muscles. Conscious control of the circumstances involving timing of urinary elimination may be impaired as a consequence of altered mobility and the resulting reduction in toileting independence.

ALTERATION IN URINARY PERFUSION

Inadequate arterial blood supply results in ischemia and infarction. Decreased oxygen delivery by the arterial blood supply may result in damage to renal structures because of inability to meet metabolic demands. Decreased perfusion leading to impaired oxygenation of tissue may be due to excessive constriction of arterioles, inadequate vascular volume, or obstructed patency of the arterial supply, as occurs with an embolism. Loss of functional tissue through necrosis leads to pain, bleeding, and obstruction of the branches of the venous system, draining the affected tissue. Conversely, enhanced perfusion represents additional workload and has the potential to stress the individual organ system. The general consequences of impaired perfusion are detailed in Chapter 2 and Chapter 16.

ALTERATION IN URINARY PATENCY

Blockage of structures involved in the passage of urine may result in obstruction.

The consequences of obstruction are influenced by the:

- Degree of the obstruction (complete or partial)
- Duration of the obstruction
- Acuity or chronicity of the condition

Obstructions are characterized by a buildup of pressure behind the blockage. Prolonged or severe pressure results in structural damage and impaired function. Ischemia and necrosis may result, adding to the consequences of perfusion impairment, because of mechanical obstruction of the arterial or venous system. Blockage may be caused by precipitation of substances in smaller lumen structures, or structural blockage resulting from endogenous or exogenous sources such as polyps or tumors. Mechanical obstructions may result from urine precipitation, scar tissue or adhesions, tumor, or inflammation.

Urine flow is impeded in the obstruction of the renal and urinary systems (Table 18.2). Dilation of the structures proximal to the obstruction causes dilation and stasis, leading to infection and structural damage. **Hydroureter**, accumulation of fluid in the urinary ureter, is a consequence of complete ureteral obstruction (Fig. 18.6). Increased hydrostatic

Table 18.2 Types of Obstructive Disease

Type of Obstruction	Pathology	Clinical Manifestations	Laboratory Findings	Sequelae If Left Untreated
Urinary	Stasis of urine behind the obstruction of renal structures, ureters, or urethra	Pain Pressure Frequency of urination Oliguria	Bacteruria Hematuria	Hydronephrosis Renal failure Infection Hypertension
Intestine	Collection of gas and fluid behind the obstruction	Abdominal distention Abdominal pain, nausea, vomiting Diaphragmatic pressure, ⇓ respiratory volume Edema caused by ⇑ capillary permeability Fever caused by release of toxins	⇑ Hematocrit (hemoconcentration) Ketosis, acidosis Hypokalemia, hypochloremia	Dehydration Hypovolemia Shock Pneumonia Peritonitis

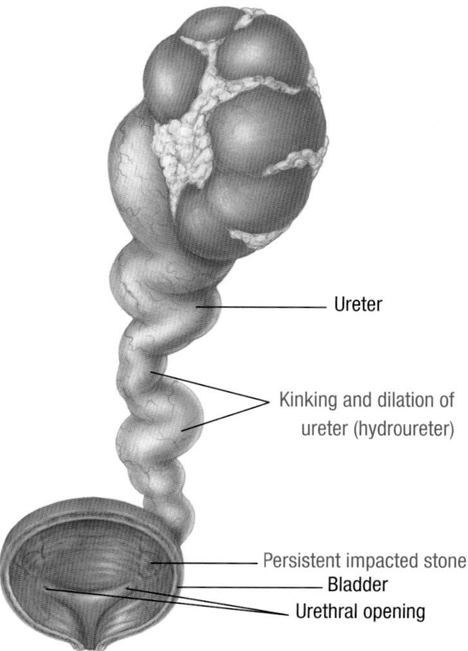

Figure 18.6. Hydronephrosis. Obstruction of the ureter causes pressure to build, resulting in hydroureter and hydronephrosis. (Courtesy Anatomical Chart Company.)

pressure extends up to the renal pelvis and tubules, leading to hydronephrosis. The glomerular filtration rate (GFR) decreases, reflecting impairment of renal function. Fluid escapes from the tubules into the surrounding capillary system. Excretion of sodium, urea, and water is impaired. Local hormonal responses to promote renal perfusion are effective for a short time. Impaired perfusion develops within 24 hours, leading to ischemia, tubular atrophy, and damaged glomeruli if the condition is not corrected. Sequelae include infection, sepsis, and loss of renal function leading to renal failure.

General Manifestations of Altered Urinary Elimination

Impairment of the processes involved in urinary elimination result in a variety of clinical manifestations. Specific manifestations are related to the underlying pathology. Generally, manifestations include:

- Altered volume of excretion
- Altered excretion characteristics
- Bleeding
- Pain
- Distention
- Anorexia
- Nausea
- Vomiting
- Fever

Urinary volume may be increased or decreased. In the case of obstruction or damage to the renal structures themselves, oliguria (scanty urine production) or

Table 18.3 Pathologic Indications of Altered Urinary Elimination

Condition	Description of Condition	Laboratory Confirmation	Possible Etiologies
Proteinuria	Protein in urine	150 mg/24-hour sample	Renal failure Nephrotic syndrome Preeclampsia Renal artery/vein thrombosis Glomerular disease Tubulopathy
Glucosuria	Glucose in urine	>130 mg/24-hour sample	Diabetes mellitus
Ketonuria	Ketones in urine (acetone, acetoacetic acid, beta-hydroxybutyric acid)	Acetone 20 mg/dl (small); 30–40 mg/dl (moderate); > 80 mg/dl (large)	Diabetes mellitus Ketoacidosis Starvation
Hematuria	Red blood cells in urine	>1 RBC/HPF	Glomerular damage Tumors Kidney trauma Urinary tract infection Acute tubular necrosis Urinary tract obstruction
Pyuria	White blood cells in urine	2 WBC/HPF + leukocyte esterase >100,000 CFU	Upper and lower urinary tract infection Acute glomerulonephritis Renal calculi
Bacteruria	Bacteria in urine	+ nitrites	Upper and lower urinary tract infection

CFU, colony-forming unit; HPF, high-power field; RBC, red blood cell; WBC, white blood cell.

anuria (absent urine production) may be seen. Other conditions may be associated with increased urine output and are often the result of hormonal stimulation of a compensatory response or regulation of fluid balance. Urine composition may also be altered, reflecting the origin of the pathology. An analysis of urine associated with kidney disorders is detailed in Table 18.3. Hematuria, evidenced by frank bleeding or clots, can be identified based on urine color. Small amounts of blood require microscopic detection.

Pain is a frequent symptom associated with altered renal and urinary function. Renal and ureteral nociceptors transmit pain impulses to the spinal cord between T10 and L1. The associated dermatomes include the lower abdomen anteriorly and posteriorly at the level of the **costovertebral angle (CVA)** or flank area. Most nociceptive receptors are located in the renal capsule rather than in the kidney itself and are stimulated by stretching and inflammation. Stretching induced by distention produces the sensation of dull, persistent pain. In contrast, many pain receptors are located in the remaining parts of the descending urinary system. The pain sensations from this region are usually intermittent and sharp.

Manifestations of infection promote feelings of general malaise, anorexia, and fever. Infection in the lower urinary tract is presented as a clinical model in Chapter 5 to illustrate the typical pathology, clinical manifestations, diagnosis, and treatment of this condition. Ascending infection of the pathogen through the ureters into the kidneys represents the potential for renal structural damage, significantly affecting the ability to produce urine. Nausea and vomiting may occur in ascending infection or systemic illness, such as pyelonephritis.

Stop and Consider
What mechanisms of infection and inflammation may contribute to damage to renal structures?

Diagnosis of Conditions of the Renal and Urinary Systems

Diagnosis of altered elimination processes is important to prevent further damage to involved organs. Both the cause and effect of altered elimination are critical to the effective management and treatment of individuals with these conditions. Microscopic and macroscopic urinalysis provides a useful resource in the diagnosis of conditions resulting in altered elimination. Normal values for urinary electrolytes are not standardized because the kidneys function dynamically to maintain electrolyte homeostasis in the plasma. Calculation of GFR and creatinine clearance indicates nephron function. Radiographic diagnostic testing useful in the determination of anatomic and functional anomalies includes:

- Intravenous pyelogram (IVP): Intravenous injection of a radiocontrast medium to allow radiographic visualization of the kidneys, ureters, and bladder.
- Voiding cystourethrogram (VCUG): X-ray examination of the bladder and urethra completed after insertion of contrast into bladder via a urinary catheter. Fluoroscopy is used to determine ureteral reflux and bladder/urethra configuration during voiding.
- Renal angiogram: Contrast injected into the renal artery via the aorta to diagnose renal artery stenosis or intrarenal vascular obstructions.
- Renal ultrasound: Noninvasive image produced by sound waves. Useful in the determination of kidney size, hydroureter, cysts, obstructions, or fluid collection. Renal artery flow can also be determined with Doppler ultrasound.

Treatment of Altered Urinary Elimination

Treatment of conditions contributing to altered urinary elimination is determined by the condition underlying the clinical manifestations. A thorough review of medical history, description of symptoms, physical examination, and diagnostic testing may be necessary to specify treatment. Altered urinary elimination is often associated with impaired regulation of fluid balance. Control of fluid balance through administration of supplemental fluids to correct body fluid deficit or the use of diuretics to correct body fluid excess may be indicated.

Module 2 Alteration in Stool Elimination

Processes of Stool Elimination

The process of stool elimination involves the organs of the GI system. From oral nutrient intake to the elimination of waste by the passage of stool, exchange and processing of the products is complex. This chapter will describe the final processes of stool production and elimination by the large intestine which occur after nutrient extraction detailed in Chapter 17.

The large intestine is a hollow organ surrounding the small intestine in the abdominal cavity. The **large intestine/colon** is comprised of the cecum, appendix, colon, rectum, and anal canal. The colon can be divided further into the ascending, transverse, descending, and sigmoid portions. The ileocecal valve directs the flow of fecal matter from the ileum of the small intestine to the cecum of the large intestine. Comprised of the cecum, colon (ascending, transverse, descending, sigmoid) and rectal segments, the large intestine begins at the end of the ileum of the small intestine and terminates at the anus. The appendix is a long, narrow blind pouch projecting from the cecum. Measuring approximately 1.5 m, the diameter of the large intestine reduces as it progresses toward the rectum. At the rectum, the colon dilates leading to increased capacity for stool. The superior and inferior mesenteric arteries are the origin for blood supply to the large intestine. The autonomic nervous system provides the primary neural control of the GI tract (Fig. 18.7).

STOOL ELIMINATION PROCESS

Food ingestion begins the digestive processes and results in the excretion of stool. Bowel motility, perfusion, patency, and response to neural signals are critical to stool elimination.

Stool Production

Stool is a product of digestion, as detailed in Chapter 17. As digestive processes continue throughout the length of large intestine, fecal matter entering at the cecum via the ileocecal valve is propelled toward the rectum for excretion. Water and electrolytes are removed from the fecal matter as it moves through the large intestine. Continued processing of fecal matter as it exits the large intestine results in the final product, stool.

Large intestine functional responses are related to the rate of movement of contents, with more rapid movement allowing less time for intestinal processes and slower movement leading to extended time. While the greatest absorption of nutrients occurs in the small intestine, the large intestine provides the final opportunity for achievement of water and electrolyte balance. Of the 7 to 10 L of water entering the small intestine, only 1 to 1.5 L enters the large

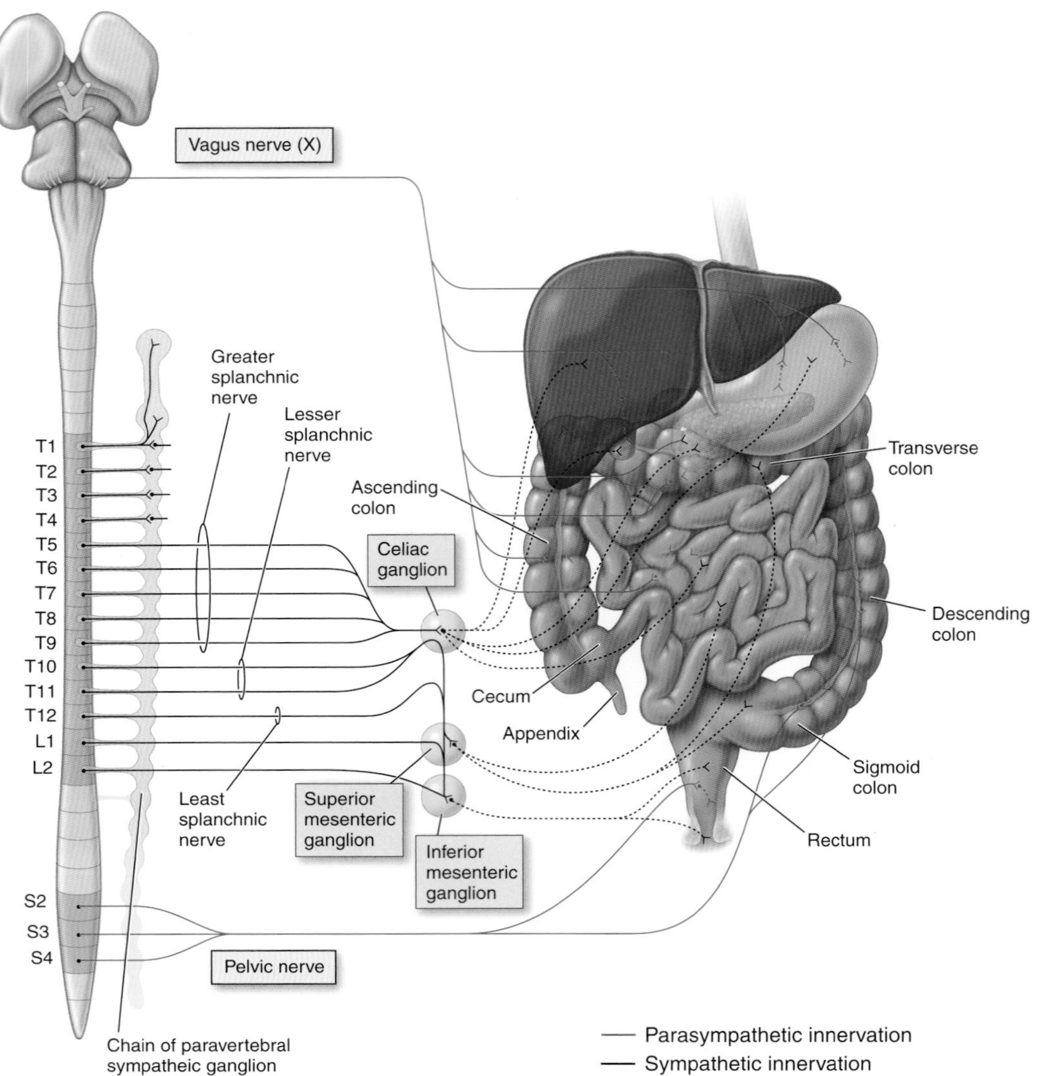

Figure 18.7. Gastrointestinal structures and innervation. Large colon structures and their sources of innervation are labeled. (Modified from Porth CM. *Pathophysiology: Concepts of Altered Health States*. 7th ed. Philadelphia, PA: Lippincott Williams & Wilkins; 2004.)

intestine on a daily basis. The final product of the large intestine, stool, includes approximately 100 to 200 mL of water. Absorption of water and electrolytes occurs in and around the epithelial cells that line the large intestine. The small intestine chyme is altered from a liquid to a semisolid form in the ascending and transverse large intestine segments. The intestinal contents retain indigestible carbohydrates, including dietary fiber, as well as remaining sodium, magnesium, and chloride. The time from dietary intake through elimination of remaining intestinal contents varies from 2 to 5 days, on average.

As the fecal matter progresses through the large intestine, the majority of water is reabsorbed along with several B complex vitamins and vitamin K, much of which is produced by intestinal bacteria. The remaining fecal matter combines with intestinal mucous and resident bacteria, known as **intestinal flora**, and becomes feces. The greatest concentration of GI bacteria resides in the large colon. The complex bacterial flora contains primarily anaerobic organisms, though composition among adults is variable and in large part dependent on diet. The food an individual eats provides sources of energy and carbon for intestinal bacteria, directing the persistence of particular types of bacteria. Intestinal bacteria break down some remaining dietary fiber, releasing byproducts including short chain fatty acids used by the epithelial cells of the colon. Resident intestinal flora protect the intestine from harmful pathogens through the maintenance of a local homeostatic balance.

Stool Evacuation

Stool is stored in the large intestine until the time of evacuation (**defecation**). It is estimated to take 18 hours for the contents of the intestine to pass from the proximal end of the large intestine to the distal end. The continuous inner layer of circular smooth muscle of the muscularis externa is surrounded by an outer, discontinuous layer of longitudinal smooth muscle. Contraction of smooth muscle occurs through the sliding filament mechanism. Along the length of the large intestine, the longitudinal muscle forms three distinct bands known as **teniae coli**. When contracted, **haustras** (pouches) are created. Smooth muscle contraction of the longitudinal and circular muscle layers of the large intestine provides the primary mechanism for the movement of stool, generating propulsive movements. The closeness of smooth muscle fibers to each other makes it easier for action potentials to be transmitted to adjacent fibers, propagating the nerve impulse along the length of the large intestine. The result is **peristalsis** caused by squeezing of circular fibers, which promotes a forward movement of intestine contents. Circular fiber contraction and relaxation occurs at different locations, producing the characteristic **segmental movement** of the large intestine. **Mass movements**, or strong peristaltic movements, occur three to four times a day, promoting the propulsion of stool.

Stop and Consider
Reduced peristalsis would slow the movement of stool through the large intestine. How might this affect water concentration in the stool?

Muscle fibers are innervated locally by the intrinsic **enteric nervous system**, including the **myenteric (Auerbach) plexus** found between the longitudinal and circular muscle layers and the **Meissner plexus**, located in the submucosa. Myenteric impulses promote control of GI movement, while the Meissner plexus transmits sensory impulses through stretch receptors. Both systems are involved in the reflexes necessary for stool movement and evaluation. Myenteric plexus stimulation provides increased tonic contractions as well as increased intensity, rate, and velocity of rhythmic contractions. It is induced via colon distention. The enteric nervous system is modulated by the autonomic nervous system. Sympathetic stimulation via the sacral nerves of the spinal cord has an inhibitory effect, whereas parasympathetic stimulation serves an excitatory function via the vagus nerve.

Two sphincters are involved in the process of defecation. The **internal rectal sphincter** is made up of a thick layer of smooth muscle and is tonically

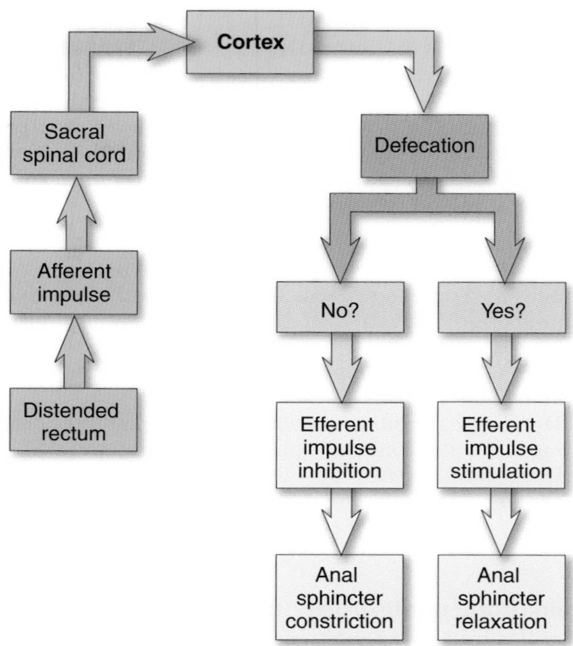

Figure 18.8. Voluntary control of defecation. Conscious intent provides voluntary control of defecation.

constricted because of sympathetic control. Movement of stool into the rectum stimulates the reflex to defecate, also known as the **rectal reflex**. Parasympathetic stimulation prompts relaxation of the internal anal sphincter. The skeletal muscle of the **external anal sphincter** surrounds the internal rectal sphincter and is innervated by the pudendal nerve (somatic nervous system), providing voluntary control. The external sphincter can override the defecation reflex, allowing for voluntary control of defecation (Fig. 18.8). Straining through **Valsalva maneuvers**, the generation of intra-abdominal pressure through inhalation that forces the diaphragm and chest muscles against the glottis, stimulates the vagus nerve and assists in stool evacuation. A summary of the steps involved in the rectal reflex is highlighted in Box 18.2.

Stool Characteristics

One of the main functions of the large intestine is compaction of feces. As water is absorbed as the fecal matter moves along the length of the large intestine, the solid matter in the feces becomes more compact. Approximately 400 to 800 mL of water, along with sodium, chloride, and bicarbonate, are absorbed out of the large intestine and approximately 5 mEq potassium is secreted into the lumen of the large intestine daily. Constituents of stool include approximately 100 mL of water and 25 to 50 g of solids consisting

Box 18.2 Rectal Reflex

Distention or irritation of the rectal wall stimulates the rectal reflex. The steps involved in the rectal reflex are primarily involuntary, but they may be modulated by voluntary control suppression. If suppressed, the reflex is subsequently stimulated when rectal mass increases. The rectal reflex involves five major steps:

1. Stimulation of stretch receptors in the rectal wall transmits sensory impulse to the sacral spinal cord.
2. Sensory neurons synapse on parasympathetic nerves, promoting relaxation of the internal anal sphincter (smooth muscle).
3. Interneuron stimulation promotes contraction of abdominal muscles.
4. Motor signal from the cerebral cortex stimulates opening of the external anal sphincter (skeletal muscle).
5. Defecation assisted by voluntary contractions of the abdominal muscles.

of remaining unabsorbed nutrients, sloughed epithelial cells, bile pigments, bacteria (30%), fat (10% to 20%), undigested dietary fiber (30%), and inorganic solids (20%). Water comprises approximately 75% of stool content.

Normal adult stool appears firm and moist. The characteristic brown color is derived from the bilirubin pigment in bile, **stercobilin**. Chemical reactions resulting in the breakdown of fecal components during digestion produce compounds, including hydrogen sulfide, that provide the characteristic odor of feces. Upon defecation, stool is soft, moist and semisolid. Formed in the shape of the rectum, stool averages approximately 1 inch in diameter and should be easy to pass. The amount and frequency of defecation is variable among individuals, though the average for adults is 200 to 300 g stool once per day.

The characteristics of stools in newborns and infants are quite different from those of adults. Many of these differences can be explained by the major sources of oral intake during development. In utero, the fetus swallows amniotic fluid, which passes through the GI system. Peristalsis and stool production are typical findings in the developing fetus. Normally, the fetus does not pass stool in utero but is expected to pass the first stool in the early newborn period after birth. This first stool, **meconium**, represents the digestion of amniotic fluid and is black, sticky, and odorless. Once feedings are begun, the stool transitions to reflect the newborn's main source of oral intake. Breastfed babies have stool that is soft, unformed, and yellow. The odor is mild and uncharacteristic of a normal fecal scent. Babies fed artificial milk, or formula, have light brown stools. Frequency of bowel movements is often increased in breastfed babies due to the efficient digestion of breast milk, compared to the less frequent stooling patterns characteristic of formula-fed babies. As table foods and supplemental liquids are introduced in late infancy, stool patterns alter to reflect the composition of these ingested foods.

Stool Analysis

Stool analysis is based upon elimination patterns and characteristics. Laboratory analysis of stool may include microscopic examination or chemical evaluation. Color, consistency, volume, shape and odor should be consistent with characteristics described previously. Stool should be free of blood, mucous, pus, and harmful parasites. Stool pH should be 6 and it should contain less than 2 mg of reducing factors (i.e., sugars).

Altered Bowel Elimination

Impaired large intestine function may alter the final steps of retrieval of water and electrolytes from the fecal matter that enters the cecum from the small intestine. Absorption of vitamins produced by intestinal bacterial flora may also be altered if there is impaired function of the large intestine. Further, the social and personal concerns regarding alteration in bowel elimination have the potential to impact quality of life.

Stool elimination is a part of daily life for most individuals. Even though stooling is a common activity for all, the process is impacted by perceptions of social acceptability. The social norms and rules of stool elimination may represent a major source of stress in individuals. Many people are concerned about the public perception of stooling and the associated odor that accompanies the process. Concern may be so great that they may attempt to override the need to pass stool until a private opportunity is available. Some individuals have great anxiety if they are unable to toilet in their home, leading to restricted travel and activities outside of their home environment.

PROCESSES OF ALTERED BOWEL ELIMINATION

The forward movement of the fecal matter is essential, propelling the intestinal contents toward the anus, leaving the body as stool through the process of defecation. Impaired bowel elimination often results from alterations in bowel motility, neuromuscular function, perfusion, or patency.

Alteration in Bowel Motility

Motility of the large intestine determines the rate at which fecal matter passes through for evacuation. Increased motility may impair nutrition, preventing adequate opportunity for nutrient and water absorption, and it may enhance loss of water and electrolytes. Decreased motility prolongs storage time in the large intestine, promoting an enhanced loss of fluid from fecal matter and potentially promoting the return of waste products to the circulation. The composition of forms of bacterial intestinal flora may also influence motility of the large intestine, with *Lactobacillus acidophilus* and *Bifidobacterium bifidum* promoting motility, and *Escherichia coli* inhibiting motility. Diarrhea and constipation are the most common clinical manifestations of altered motility of the large intestine.

Factors that alter the transit time of stool also present potential stressors to the process of stool elimination. Certain foods may serve as irritants to the intestine, enhancing the speed at which the feces moves from the cecum to the anus. Shortened transit time limits water absorption, leading to stool that is less formed due to the increased water content. Such stools are often passed with more frequency and urgency. In contrast, some individuals respond to particular foods with a slowed transit time, leading to increased water movement out of the feces. The result is often hard, formed stools with reduced frequency in elimination.

Alteration in Bowel Neuromuscular Function

Coordination of neurologic and muscular functional components is essential to optimal bowel function. Any alteration in neural signal transduction or muscle responsiveness may result in altered bowel function. Impaired function associated with loss of propulsive activity may result from abdominal surgery or from electrolyte imbalances affecting contractile function, peritonitis, or spinal trauma. Impaired motility is often seen as a side effect of narcotic analgesia. Emotional stress may alter stool elimination processes because of the influence of the central nervous system in the integrative processes involved in bowel function.

Reduced activity may also slow the process of stool elimination. Walking, running, swimming, and other active movements enhance neuromuscular activity and coordination in the large intestine, promoting peristalsis and bowel elimination. Loss of mobility often serves as a stressor to bowel elimination, leading to reduced intestinal smooth muscle contractions. As the time that feces remains in the large intestine increases, more water is removed and stool becomes harder. Further, the products of digestion in the form of gas build up, leading to distention of the abdomen and pain if the passing of flatus is impaired.

Stop and Consider
What are some common reasons that intestinal mobility can be reduced, leading to slowed intestinal smooth muscle contraction?

Alteration in Bowel Perfusion

A continuous source of perfusion to the large intestine is essential for optimal cellular function. Disruption in perfusion may be the result of either focal or global etiologies (Chapter 16). Perfusion can be reduced or absent to a portion of bowel as a result of obstructed flow from a variety of reasons, including a clot or pressure from a space-occupying mass. Erosion of blood vessels supplying perfusion to the intestine due to ulceration or trauma may also lead to impaired circulation. Ischemia resulting from impaired oxygenation is often manifested by pain and altered bowel function. If hypoxia persists, necrosis of cells and tissues may result.

Ventilation/perfusion mismatch, inadequate vascular volume and inadequate cardiac output are common etiologies that may lead to global circulation deficits, denying perfusion to cells and tissues of the lower intestine. During times of circulatory challenge, blood is redistributed away from the digestive system to the vital organs. Altered perfusion may occur as a result of excessive perfusion demands, such as infection. A common infection of the GI system is appendicitis. Appendicitis is the result of trapped fecal material in the appendix of the colon (Fig. 18.9). The obstruction causes an inflammatory response, followed by infection. Once the obstruction is identified, surgical removal of the appendix is the method of treatment. Untreated, rupture of the appendix is likely to occur. Upon rupture, the bacterial flora escapes into the peritoneal cavity, resulting in peritonitis and septic shock. Reduced perfusion to all organ systems, especially the GI tract, results from septic shock.

Alteration in Bowel Patency

Bowel obstruction is due to a space-occupying lesion which blocks the intestinal lumen, either partially or totally. Common space-occupying lesions include tumors, polyps, and impacted feces (Fig. 18.10). Often associated with fluid and gas accumulation, bowel obstruction is manifested by abdominal distention and pain (see Table 18.2). When the space-occupying lesion impairs capacity for venous return, the development of edema in the wall of the large intestine leads to reducing the absorptive capacity. Edema promotes continued fluid and gas accumulation because of the movement of water and gas into the bowel lumen. Hydrostatic forces may increase so that fluid is forced through the bowel wall into the peritoneum. Further, bacteria may gain access to the circulation, promoting the development of sepsis. Perforation may result from pressure that exceeds the ability of the tissue to retain its structure.

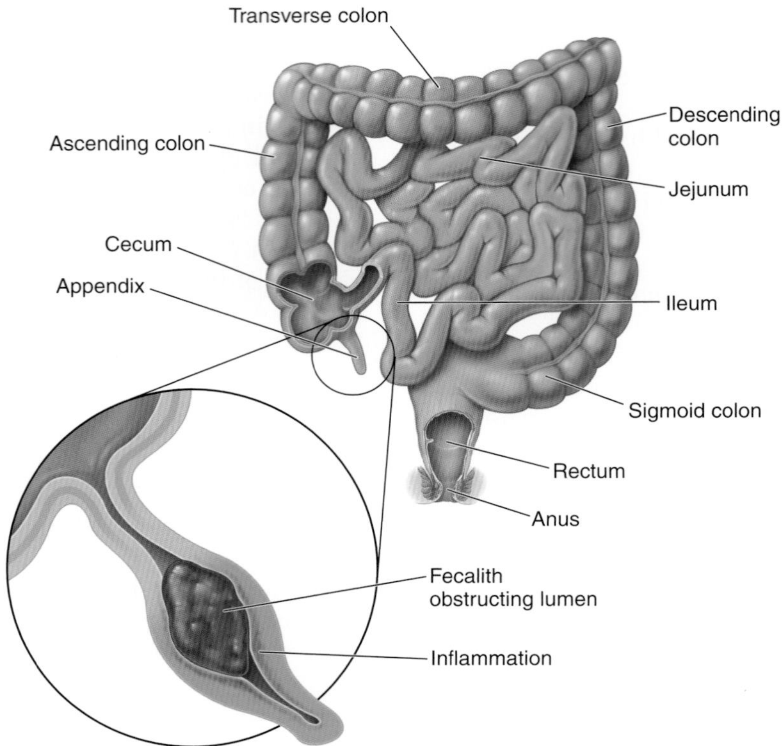

Figure 18.9. Obstruction and inflammation in appendicitis. Fecal mass obstruction stimulates an inflammatory response, leading to appendicitis.

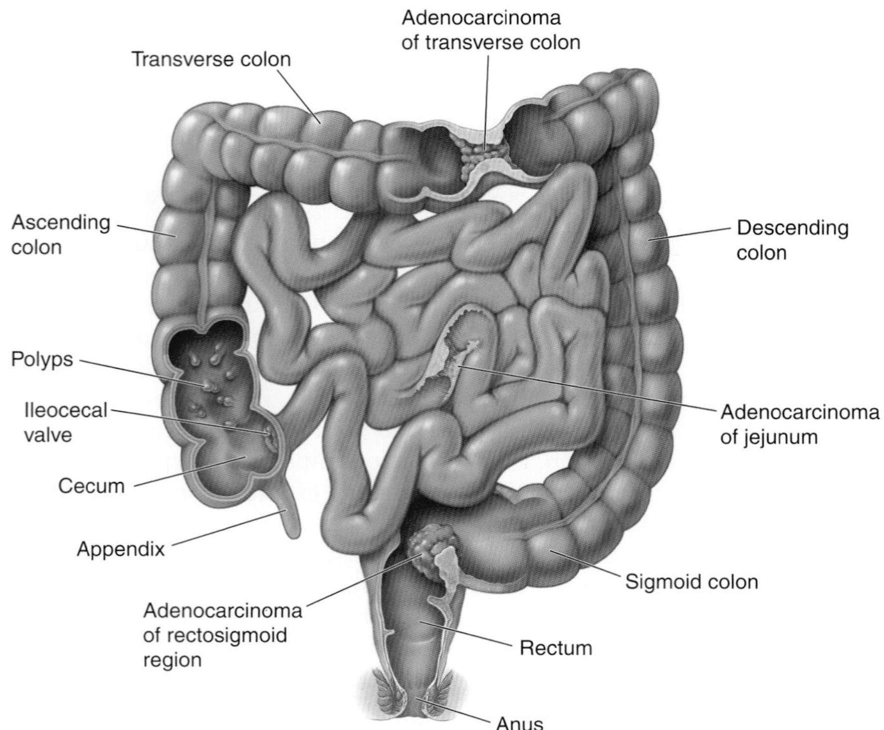

Figure 18.10. Colon obstruction. The formation of polyps and tumors represents potential sites for obstruction along the length of the colon.

General Manifestations of Altered Bowel Elimination

Identification of altered intestinal function can be accomplished by listening to bowel sounds. Bowel sounds are a reflection of intestinal smooth muscle contractions that are active intermittently. Bowel sounds can often be heard by the naked ear, but are more carefully evaluated through **auscultation**, or listening with a stethoscope. The quality, location, and frequency of bowel sounds provide an indication of peristaltic function.

The appearance of the abdomen is another indicator of bowel function. The abdomen should be soft when pressed or palpated and flat relative to body size. Abdominal size may increase due to the trapping of gas, leading to hardening and tightening of the abdomen. Typically, the gaseous byproducts of digestion, flatus, are passed, indicating bowel function. Often when stool transit is slowed due to slowed intestinal smooth muscle contraction and coordination, the gaseous products of digestion build and cause the abdomen to enlarge, or become distended.

The volume and characteristics of stool may be altered in conditions that affect the large intestine. Loose, watery stools are characteristic of diarrhea. Bowel inflammation, infection, and increased motility are often associated with diarrhea. Constipation, or absence of bowel movement, may be a consequence of impaired mobility or obstruction. In complete obstruction, fecal matter cannot pass beyond the obstruction. The characteristics of fecal matter passed in the presence of partial obstruction may provide clues as to the location of the obstruction. Obstructions occurring closest to the cecum may allow watery stool to pass because the water content of the stool is high. Partial obstructions located at the distal end of the colon may allow the passage of small quantities of harder, more solidly formed stool.

Stop and Consider

Why would you expect stool in the ascending colon to have more water content than stool in the descending colon?

Stool may also have color changes characteristic of specific disease states. Bright red blood around stool or seen on toilet paper after defecation is generally caused by hemorrhoids. Hemorrhoids can be seen on the outside of the anus or they may be located internally. Larger amounts of frank red blood may indicate internal bleeding of a more serious nature, such as occurs in colon cancer. A darker pigment of red, or maroon, characterizes bleeding from a source in the midportion of the GI tract, such as that seen with diverticulitis (see clinical model). Black stool (**melena**) also signifies a bleeding concern. The darkened color represents a source of bleeding higher up in the GI system. Blood in stools should be identified and a definitive cause determined because of the potential serious consequences of this sign.

Stop and Consider

Why do bloody stools suggest the potential diagnosis of cancer?

Light-colored stools indicate the absence of bile pigments. This is a common finding associated with conditions of the accessory organs of the GI tract (pancreas, gall bladder, and liver). For example, the stool from a person infected with hepatitis may be white, gray, or yellow. Bile acids are absent in some malabsorption syndromes and are associated with large fat content, known as **steatorrhea**. Stools lacking bile pigments caused by obstruction of bile entry into the intestine may cause stools to have a "silver" color. Ampullary cancer is a pancreatic neoplasm that arises from the ampulla of Vater. The ampulla of Vater is a small projection from the pancreas into the duodenum, serving as the opening of the pancreatic and bile ducts. Obstruction of the ampulla of Vater blocks the entry of pancreatic and biliary secretions into the intestine. Manifestations of secretion blockage include jaundice caused by impaired bilirubin processing and elimination and light-colored "silver" stools caused by absence of bile in fecal matter.

Alterations in texture can provide information on a causative factor. These alterations include:

- Watery
  - Acute onset caused by gastroenteritis or anxiety.
  - Chronic pattern linked to inflammatory conditions or a high-fiber diet. Also caused by intolerance to particular foods or the effects of certain medications.
- Hard
  - Water content low, resulting in a dry stool that is difficult to pass.
  - May contribute to the development of hemorrhoids. Linked to low-fiber diet, side effects of certain medications, or voluntary avoidance of stool evacuation.
- Stringy
  - May be caused by parasitic infections.
- Fatty
  - Caused by malabsorption of fat.
  - Likely to float.
- Foul odor
  - May be caused by steatorrhea, parasitic infection, or malabsorption syndromes.

Pain is often a characteristic of intestinal disorders, although it seldom occurs without other symptoms. Origins of pain include mechanical, inflammatory, or ischemic causes. The biochemical mediators of pain (histamine, bradykinin, and serotonin) provide stimulation to nerve endings, resulting in the pain response (detailed in Chapter 10). Abdominal pain can be categorized into three main types:

1. Visceral
   - Characterized as diffuse, radiating and generalized; difficult to determine precise location
   - Caused by stretching, distention, or inflammation, inducing edema and vascular congestion
2. Somatic (also known as parietal)
   - Described as sharp, intense, and localized to a specific site
   - Caused by injury to the abdominal wall or parietal peritoneum
3. Referred
   - Felt at a location different from origin of pain
   - Caused by the sharing of a common afferent pathway between origin of pain and referred location

Acute onset of pain is usually caused by a precipitating event, such as perforation. Persistent pain with a gradual onset is often associated with chronic conditions, such as ulcerative colitis.

Anorexia (loss of appetite) is often associated with nausea and vomiting. These symptoms are general and do not point to a specific condition. Abdominal distention often indicates increased pressure from fluid or feces in the bowel lumen, inflammation and edema of the intestine, or increased production of gas. Fever is a common finding resulting from infection, such as **peritonitis** (inflammation of the peritoneal membrane).

Diagnosis of Bowel Conditions

Specific conditions can be identified by examination of stool. These conditions include allergy to a dietary substance (such as milk protein in infants), inflammation, infection, bleeding, or malabsorption. In cases of infection, stool can be examined to determine the specific organism involved. Many organisms are naturally found in the intestine (normal flora, microbiota) and are important for specific GI functions. Harmful bacteria or parasites that infect the GI tract must be identified to determine the most effective treatment. Fat content can be determined to indicate the presence or absence of a disorder of malabsorption. These determinations may require either microscopic analysis or culture of stool. Determination of **occult** (too small to be seen) blood in stool can be made by placing a small sample on a collection card and applying a chemical solution. A color change indicates the presence or absence of blood. This test is commonly referred to as a *guaiac test*. Stool samples for microscopic analysis or culture should be collected in clean, dry, disposable containers. Immediate delivery to the laboratory provides the best conditions for analysis of the sample.

Mechanical obstructions resulting from growths extending into the colon lumen, including tumors or polyps, can be diagnosed using techniques that allow visualization of the colon lumen. Diagnostic tests for disorders of the colon include:

- Barium enema: Determination of colon and rectal anatomic abnormalities with the aid of contrast medium (barium) inserted via the anus. Visualization of the rectum and colon is completed by radiograph. Common conditions identified include diverticulitis, alterations in motility, obstruction, and colon dimensions.
- Sigmoidoscopy: Insertion of a flexible tube into the anus to visualize the rectum and the lower colon. This diagnostic test may be indicated for manifestations of bleeding, altered bowel habits, rectal pain, and diarrhea.
- Colonoscopy: Insertion of a flexible tube into the anus for observation of the entire colon, from the small intestine to the rectum. This test is often done in response to manifestations of abdominal pain, diarrhea, alteration in bowel habits, or as a follow-up to an abnormality found during another procedure, such as the barium enema or computed tomography (CT) scan.

Treatment of Altered Bowel Elimination

Similar to treatment of altered urinary elimination, treatment of conditions causing altered GI elimination is determined by the condition underlying the clinical manifestations. Diarrhea, a form of excessive GI elimination, may be associated with impaired regulation of fluid balance. Diarrhea may result from a variety of primary conditions, or it may represent an adverse effect of treatment. Pharmacotherapy may be used to diminish excessive fluid loss from diarrhea. Antidiarrheal drugs work by:

- Slowing the passage of stool through the intestine
  - Antimotility agents (Imodium)
    - Promotes water removal from fecal matter
    - Useful for chronic conditions
- Moving diarrhea-causing factors out of the stool
  - Adsorbents (Kaopectate)
    - May also pull out other essential products

Table 18.4 Impact of Selected Intestinal Conditions on the Health of Individuals

Condition	Impact	Deaths	Hospitalizations	Ambulatory Care Visits (Per Year)	Pre-scriptions
Hemorrhoids	75% of individuals over 45 years of age	20	266,000	1.1 million	2 million
Chronic constipation	63 million people (prevalence)	132	1.1 million	4 million	5.3 million
Irritable bowel syndrome	15.3 million (prevalence)	21	280,000	1.6 million	5.9 million
Abdominal wall hernia	526,000 (surgical procedures)	132	380,000	3.6 million	3.7 million
Diverticular disease	2.2 million (prevalence)	2,889	814,000	2.8 million	2.8 million

NIDDK. Digestive diseases statistics for the United States. http://www.niddk.nih.gov/health-information/health-statistics/Pages/digestive-diseases-statistics-for-the-united-states.aspx#6. Retrieved on January 2, 2016

- Decreasing secretion of fluid into intestine
  - Reduce inflammatory response to pathogens (antibiotics)
    - Decreases fluid movement into intestinal contents
- Using bulk-forming agents
  - Absorbs excess fluid (psyllium)
    - Firms stool

Constipation can be managed with exercise, high dietary fiber, adequate fluid intake, stool softeners, laxatives, and enemas. Bulk-forming laxatives absorb water from the intestine to make stool softer. Stimulants promote peristalsis, enhancing propulsion of fecal matter through the colon. Stool softeners promote moisture content in stool without the stimulant effect. Lubricants promote smoother passage and evacuation of fecal matter. Saline laxatives work by attracting water into the colon.

Obstructive abnormalities may require surgical treatment for removal. Alterations in neuromuscular function may require assistive devices or bladder/bowel training programs for elimination of urine and stool. Trends for selected conditions related to large intestine impairment are provided in Table 18.4, based on information from the National Institutes of Diabetes and Digestive and Kidney Diseases (NIDDK).

Module 3 Clinical Models

The following clinical models have been selected to aid in the understanding and application of altered elimination. The student should pay attention to the commonalities and unique features of each condition when studying these models. Alterations in elimination often lead to physical and emotional distress and disruption of daily life. Processes leading to altered elimination are summarized in Figure 18.11.

Urolithiasis

Urolithiasis, commonly known as kidney stones, is the development of calculi in the renal system. Renal calculi are solid masses, often composed of salts, and inorganic or organic acids, which precipitate out of urinary filtrate. The diagnosis of kidney stones represents one of the most prevalent conditions of the urinary tract system. The condition occurs more frequently in men compared to women, and in Caucasians compared to African Americans.[1] Recent trends link increasing rates associated with obesity and diabetes mellitus.

PATHOPHYSIOLOGY

Calcium (oxalate and phosphate) is the most common component of stones, which may also form because of magnesium ammonium phosphate (**struvite**), uric acid, or cystine. Dietary factors including low calcium intake, high oxalate intake, high animal protein intake, high sodium intake, or low fluid intake may predispose individuals to development of calculi. Elevated urinary levels of calculi-forming substances (hypercalciuria, hyperoxaluria, hypocitraturia) or stasis from urinary filtrate may promote

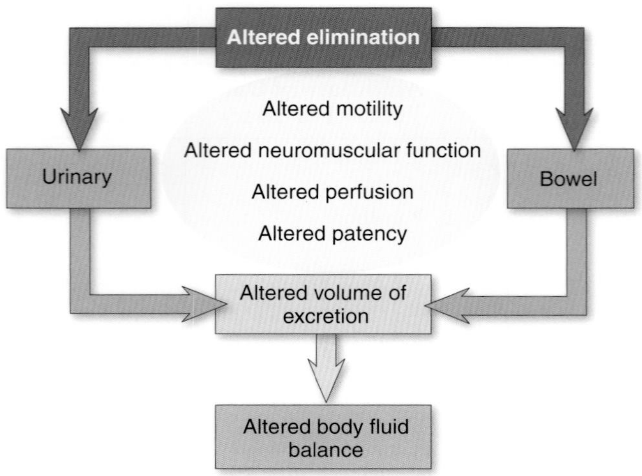

Figure 18.11. Concept map. Processes of altered elimination.

development of calculi. As stones progress through the urinary system, from the renal tubules to the urethra, they often result in obstruction of these narrow lumen structures.

Individuals at risk for development of kidney stones include those with:

- Genetic predisposition
- Urinary tract infection
- Cystic kidney disease
- Diabetes
- Obesity
- Gout
- Hyperparathyroidism
- Gastric bypass

Stop and Consider
Why are people with hyperparathyroidism and hypercalciuria at risk for development of renal calculi?

CLINICAL MANIFESTATIONS

The most obvious clinical manifestation of kidney stones is pain. This pain is characterized as severe and shooting and is localized in the lateral aspect of the lower back (flank) at the costovertebral angle. Pain can be further described in two ways:

1. Colic
   - Caused by stretching of the collecting system or ureter from obstructed flow
   - Characterized as acute, intermittent, radiating, and excruciating
2. Noncolic
   - Caused by distention of renal calices or pelvis
   - Characterized as dull and deep
   - Ranging in intensity from mild to severe

Hematuria may be present with renal calculi. Manifestations range from gross hematuria, causing a red-tinged color change in urine, to hematuria which is not identifiable without visualization with microscopic analysis. Additional manifestations may include nausea, vomiting, dysuria, and urgency.

DIAGNOSTIC CRITERIA

Imaging of the renal calculi with CT or renal ultrasonography is the preferred approach for diagnosis. Diagnosis of renal calculi can also be made using a routine radiograph because most stones are radiopaque. IVP may be used to obtain information about the collecting system and ureters because the contrast media is filtered by the glomerulus and can be tracked through the urinary system. Hydronephrosis can be detected using ultrasound to provide additional information about the consequences of the obstruction.

Determination of underlying causes contributing to stone development and the composition of the stone itself helps establish effective treatment. Individuals are often provided a device that strains the urine, collecting any stones that are excreted. The stones can then be analyzed to determine content and infer cause. Types of calculi are shown in Figure 18.12 and include:

- Calcium oxalate and phosphate
  - Hypercalcemia/hypercalciuria
  - Immobility
  - Renal tubular acidosis
- Magnesium ammonium phosphate/struvite
  - Urinary tract infection

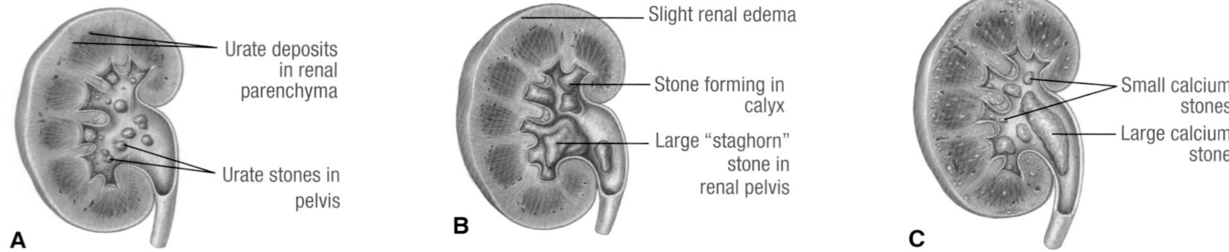

Figure 18.12. Common forms of renal calculi. **A:** Uric acid/urate stones. **B:** Magnesium ammonium phosphate (struvite) stones. **C:** Calcium oxalate/calcium phosphate stones. (Courtesy Anatomical Chart Company.)

- Uric acid/urate
  - Precipitated in acidic urine (pH of 5.5 or less)
  - Diet high in purines
  - Gout

TREATMENT

Treatment of calculi involves supportive care, including pain control. Fluids may be encouraged to promote filtrate flow and movement of stone through the urinary system. Medical therapy to promote stone passage includes antispasmodic agents, calcium channel blockers, and alpha blockers. If stones do not pass spontaneously or in response to medical therapy, removal of calculi is often necessary to prevent damage to renal structures. The indications for surgical removal include[2]

- Retaining the stone and constant pain over a reasonable period
- Stone size too large to pass
- Obstructing urine flow
- Causing ongoing urinary tract infection
- Causing damage to kidney or evidence of constant hematuria
- Continuing to grow in size

Surgical procedures to remove kidney stones are selected in consideration of the greatest effectiveness and lowest complication rate to achieve desired result.[3] **Extracorporeal shockwave lithotripsy (ESWL)** is the most common procedure for kidney stone removal. Large stones are localized by ultrasound or radiograph and then are broken down into small, sandlike bits using acoustic shock waves. The decreased size promotes spontaneous passage of the stone in the urine. Passage is occasionally assisted by placing a stent (a small tube) through the bladder into the ureter. This procedure is useful when stones are located in the renal calyx, pelvis, and upper third of the ureter. **Percutaneous nephrolithotomy** is an alternate surgical procedure used for treatment of renal calculi removal.[4] The stone is located and removed using a nephroscope, inserted into the kidney through a small flank incision. Stones too large for removal are fragmented using an energy probe. The insertion of a nephrostomy tube assists in healing after the procedure. **Ureteroscopic stone removal** is used when stones are located in the mid or distal portions of the ureters. Calculi removal is accomplished through a ureteroscope placed into the ureter through the urethra and bladder. After localization, the stone is removed or fragmented with a shock wave device. Placement of a ureteral stent is often done along with this procedure.

Prevention strategies to avoid development and recurrence of calculi in high-risk individuals may be useful, particularly when preventive strategies are specific to urinary, metabolic, nutritional, environmental, and lifestyle risk factors for particular types of stone formation.[5] Adequate fluid intake and alkalinization of urine are strategies that can be used in prevention of renal calculi as they reduce urine saturation and precipitation of calcium-forming salts.[2] Diet manipulation to increase fluid intake, reduce dietary oxalate, regulate animal protein intake to 4 to 5 oz serving per day, increase low-oxalate-containing fruit and vegetable intake, and to limit sodium intake to 2 to 3 g/d may decrease risk for calculi development. Restriction of dietary calcium is not associated with reduced risk of calculi formation in most cases. Foods high in oxalate should be avoided in persons with calcium oxalate-based stones. These foods include:

- Beets
- Chocolate
- Coffee
- Cola
- Nuts
- Rhubarb
- Spinach
- Strawberries
- Tea
- Wheat bran

Combining calcium restriction with diuretic therapy promotes movement of filtrate through the renal system, reducing the likelihood of calculi development. Treatment and prevention of urinary tract infections may decrease the risk for struvite-based calculi. Management of primary conditions, such as gout and hyperparathyroidism, reduces the availability of the minerals and alters pH, reducing the risk of calculi formation.

Urinary Incontinence

Urinary incontinence, or **enuresis**, is defined as the inability to voluntarily prevent the discharge of urine. A symptom rather than a diagnosis, urinary

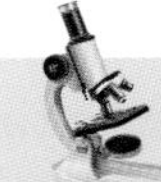

FROM THE LAB

Urinalysis in a person with renal calculi may show hematuria, infection, crystals, or altered urine pH. The urinalysis findings may provide clues about the cause of calculi formation, which is useful in directing treatment strategies.

incontinence is often the manifestation of conditions that alter the structure or function of the urinary tract. Urinary incontinence is often considered a women's disease, although it is known to occur in 17% of an estimated 34 million men older than 60 years in the United States.[6] It is estimated that up to 75% of women in the United States report occasional urinary leakage, with 20% to 50% reporting more frequent leakage.[7,8]

PATHOPHYSIOLOGY

A variety of processes can impair voiding, including those involving muscular contraction, neural transmission, hormonal stimulation, or mechanical factors. In women, relaxation of pelvic structures may occur, especially after pregnancy. Male incontinence may be caused by mechanical obstruction by the prostate on the penile urethra. In both genders, neurologic disease, including Parkinson disease, multiple sclerosis, spinal cord injury, and stroke, may contribute to voiding dysfunction. Advancing age, obesity and loss of mobility and dexterity may also contribute to functional incontinence.

A detailed history about the specific characteristics of the incontinence is critical to the determination of incontinence type, which also affects the choice of treatment modalities. The patient should keep a record, or voiding diary, on urinary frequency, leakage, voiding volumes, and fluid intake. This record should span at least 3 days, but 1 week is preferable to accurately identify patterns. Leakage can also be quantified by a pad count or weight, providing details of volume.

CLINICAL MANIFESTATIONS

Temporary incontinence may result from the use of certain medications or from illness, immobility, or constipation. Chronic types of incontinence can be classified into four different forms. **Stress incontinence** occurs because of an exertional stimulus. The stimulus may be as benign as coughing, sneezing, or laughing. Other exertional activities that prompt incontinence include exercise or lifting objects. Impaired sphincter function and control is often associated with stress incontinence. **Urge incontinence**, also known as **overactive bladder**, refers to urine leaking that is accompanied or immediately preceded by a strong urge to void (urgency), nocturia, and frequency.[9] This impulse is often so sudden that incontinence results before the individual can toilet. Overactivity of the detrusor muscle of the bladder is responsible for this type of incontinence. Often, individuals may have a mix of symptoms of both urge and stress incontinence. Incontinence may also result from urine volumes exceeding bladder capacity, known as **overflow incontinence**. Overflow incontinence is often associated with detrusor underactivity or bladder outlet obstruction. **Functional incontinence** is characterized by normal bladder control coupled with an impaired ability to transport to toilet facilities, such as with impaired mobility. Incontinence can be classified further as nocturnal enuresis, continuous leakage, postvoid dribble, and extraurethral (urine loss through fistula) incontinence.

DIAGNOSTIC CRITERIA

Diagnosis is based on careful history in addition to physical examination and specialized testing. Testing is also influenced by gender-specific anatomical considerations. Urodynamic and endoscopic testing, in addition to the imaging studies previously described, are the gold standard but are not necessary to establish a diagnosis. The following are tests and diagnostic findings for incontinence:

- Bladder stress test
  - Standing position with a comfortably full bladder
  - Observation of urine passage with Valsalva or vigorous cough
- Post residual volume (PRV)
  - After voiding, residual urine in the bladder is measured
  - PRV of less than 50 mL indicates adequate bladder emptying
- Urodynamic testing
  - Cystometry
    - Measures anatomic and functional ability of the bladder and urethra
    - Measures capacity of the bladder, providing evaluation of the function of the detrusor muscle
  - Cystometrogram
    - Measures pressures of the total bladder, detrusor, and intra-abdomen
  - Voiding cystometrogram
    - Identifies outlet obstruction during voiding
- Endoscopic tests
  - Cystoscopy
    - Visualizes bladder mucosa to identify the presence of lesions

TREATMENT

Treatment for incontinence reflects behavioral strategies, use of medication, and surgery. Assistance with toileting, **bladder training** (learning to hold urine for increasing intervals), intravaginal support devices, and strengthening of the pelvic muscles are common strategies used for functional and stress incontinence.[10] Pelvic muscles can be strengthened by Kegel exercises, vaginal weights, and electrical stimulation. Anticholinergic medications help urge incontinence because they decrease the contractile force of the detrusor muscle. Improved urethral tone can be assisted by the use of α-adrenergic antagonist drugs to improve tone and contractile function.

In females, surgical correction for renewed anatomic support can be performed with an abdominal bladder suspension. Also known as the Burch or Marshall–Marchetti–Krantz (MMK) procedure, the bladder and urethra are returned to their normal position, promoting increased voluntary control of urine. This procedure can be done through an abdominal incision or it can be done laparoscopically. Another procedure, the sling procedure, places support material directly under the urethra and attaches to abdominal muscle connective tissue. One of the newest procedures, the tension-free vaginal tape procedure (TVT) uses a thin strip of supporting tape to form a hammock under the urethra. This procedure, similar to the sling procedure, is performed through a small incision in the vagina. These procedures are intended to support the urethra during strain that would induce stress incontinence. Surgical techniques in males with incontinence are designed to remove mechanical obstruction of the urethra from an enlarged prostate.

Polycystic Kidney Disease

Polycystic kidney disease (PKD) is a condition characterized by growth of fluid-filled cysts in kidney tissue bilaterally, leading to progressive loss of renal nephrons. PKD may be inherited or acquired. The inherited form of PKD is the most common genetic cause of chronic kidney disease.[11] The progressive nature of PKD may result in increasing loss of renal function, leading to renal failure. Of the primary conditions associated with need for treatment of end-stage renal disease among over 500,000 US residents in 2006, PKD represented the fourth leading cause.[12]

PATHOPHYSIOLOGY

Cysts of increasing size and number replace functional tissue, leading to end-stage renal disease. Pressure on renal blood vessels obstructs perfusion, leading to tissue degeneration and obstructed tubular flow (Fig. 18.13). A variable pattern of cyst involvement exists in nephrons—cyst-affected nephrons are interspersed with normal, unaffected nephrons.

Three categories of PKD are known:

1. Genetic, autosomal dominant
2. Genetic, autosomal recessive
3. Acquired

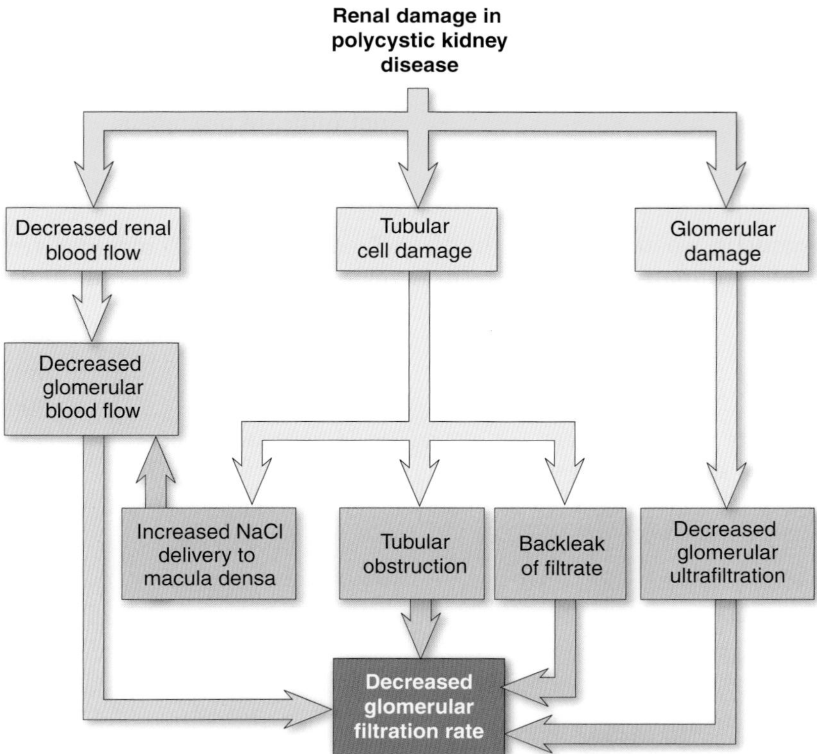

Figure 18.13. Renal damage in polycystic kidney disease. (Courtesy Anatomical Chart Company.)

The autosomal dominant form of PKD is the most common inherited form, accounting for 90% of PKD cases. Genetic mutations in the PKD1 and PKD2 genes lead to altered protein production of polycystin-1 and polycystin-2. The less common recessive form is the result of mutations in the PKHD1 gene, encoding the fibrocystin protein. Clinical manifestations of kidney disease usually appear between the ages of 30 and 40 years in the autosomal dominant form, although individuals can have symptoms at a younger age. Symptoms appear early in the autosomal recessive form of PKD, usually in the early infant period or even during fetal life. PKD can also be acquired, which is usually associated with other long-term kidney problems. Evidence of this form of PKD does not present until much later in life and is more frequent among the elderly.

Cysts begin to grow in the nephrons of the kidney, filling with glomerular filtrate, eventually growing larger and moving away into adjacent tissue. Kidney size increases in proportion to the size and number of cysts, which can number into the thousands (Fig. 18.14). One of the earliest manifestations of the disease is hypertension from compression of the renal vessels and subsequent activation of the RAAS (see Chapter 8). Other common symptoms include:

- Flank pain
- Headaches
- Nausea, anorexia
- Urinary tract infection
- Liver and pancreatic cysts
- Cardiac valvular disease
- Hypertension
- Renal calculi
- Cerebral aneurysms
- Diverticular disease

Accumulation of nitrogenous wastes, altered fluid/electrolyte balance, and impaired function in multiple organ systems become evident as renal function worsens.

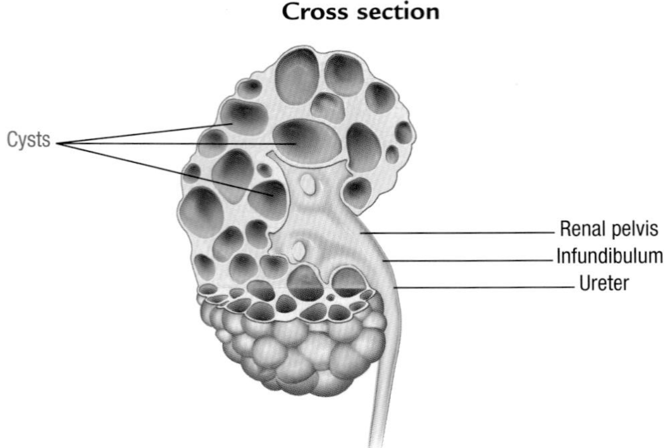

Figure 18.14. Polycystic kidney. Cysts in nephrons and in the renal cortex alter renal function. (Courtesy Anatomical Chart Company.)

DIAGNOSTIC CRITERIA

Polycystic kidney disease diagnosis is confirmed by the presence of three or more kidney cysts verified by ultrasound. Family history of PKD and extrarenal cysts also suggest PKD. Progression of the disease may be slow, delaying onset of symptoms. Genetic testing may also be useful in detecting mutations in genes associated with the disease, such as PKD1 (chromosome 18) and PKD2 (chromosome 4). These findings are limited to determining diagnosis but do not indicate prognosis.

TREATMENT

Treatment of PKD includes symptomatic care, strategies to promote renal function, and supportive care during end-stage renal disease. Lifestyle modifications including maintenance of healthy weight, physical activity and nutritious diet that includes moderate protein (0.75 to 1.0 g/kg/d), low sodium (≤6 g salt per day), fluid intake to satisfy thirst, and smoking cessation are important to implement prior to advanced chronic kidney disease.[13] In autosomal dominant PKD, pharmacologic management

FROM THE LAB

Glomerular filtration can indicate the development and progression of renal failure. Glomerular filtration rate (GFR) normally ranges between 120 and 130 mL/minute, with a GFR ≥ 90 mL/minute considered within normal limits. Progressive decline in GFR is characteristic of decline in kidney function as follows:

- Mild disease, GFR 60 to 89 mL/minute
- Moderate disease, GFR 30 to 59 mL/minute
- Severe disease, GFR 15 to 29 mL/minute
- Renal failure, GFR < 15 mL/minute

Blood urea nitrogen (BUN), serum creatinine, and potassium levels become elevated. Decreased hemoglobin, arterial pH, and bicarbonate also indicate worsening renal function.

includes treatment of hypertension using angiotensin-converting enzyme inhibitor (ACE-I) and angiotensin receptor blocker (ARB) antihypertensive agents to a target blood pressure of ≤ 130/80 mm Hg.[14] For individuals with end-stage renal failure, kidney transplantation may be indicated.[15] Pain is controlled by analgesics. Urinary tract infections are treated with antibiotics, but they do present challenges because the pathogens can ascend more easily and are more difficult to treat (antibiotics have poor penetration into the cystic tissue).

The progression of disease over time may result in chronic renal failure (Fig. 18.15). End-stage renal disease requires dialysis or transplant for individuals to survive. Dialysis options include hemodialysis and peritoneal dialysis. **Hemodialysis** uses special filters through the mechanisms of diffusion, osmosis, and ultrafiltration to remove wastes that the kidneys no longer can remove on their own. This procedure requires access to the blood supply so that blood can travel through a set of tubes into a dialyzer, where waste products and excess water are removed. All molecules with the exception of blood cells and plasma proteins can move freely between the semipermeable filter membrane between the blood and dialysis fluid. The purified blood is then returned through another set of tubes back into the body for circulation (Fig. 18.16). Treatments are scheduled for three times per week, each lasting 3 to 5 hours. Access to blood can be achieved by the surgical attachment of an artery to a vein, known as an **arteriovenous (AV) fistula**. The blood pressure from the artery enlarges the more passive vein, making it an ideal structure for repeated venipuncture (needle insertion). This procedure requires enough time for adequate enlargement of the vein, limiting its immediate use. Another method used to obtain access to the blood supply is a graft or **arteriovenous shunt**, connecting the artery to the vein using a synthetic tube. This method can be used more quickly, but it carries an increased risk for clot development and infection. Heparin, an anticoagulant, is used during

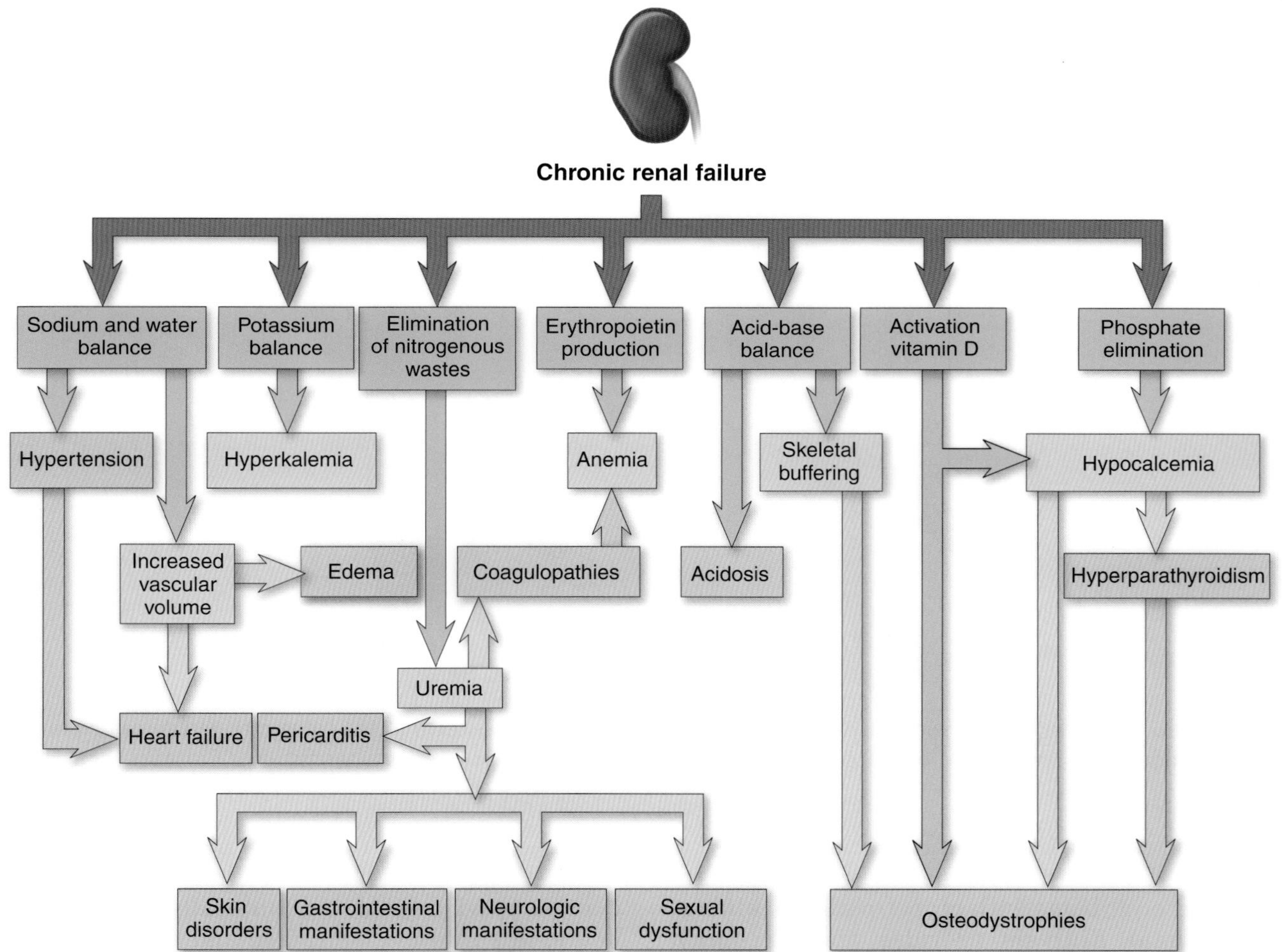

Figure 18.15. Pathophysiology of chronic renal failure. Clinical manifestations are present in multiple organ systems as a result of renal failure. (Modified from Porth CM. *Pathophysiology: Concepts of Altered Health States*. 7th ed. Philadelphia, PA: Lippincott Williams & Wilkins; 2004.)

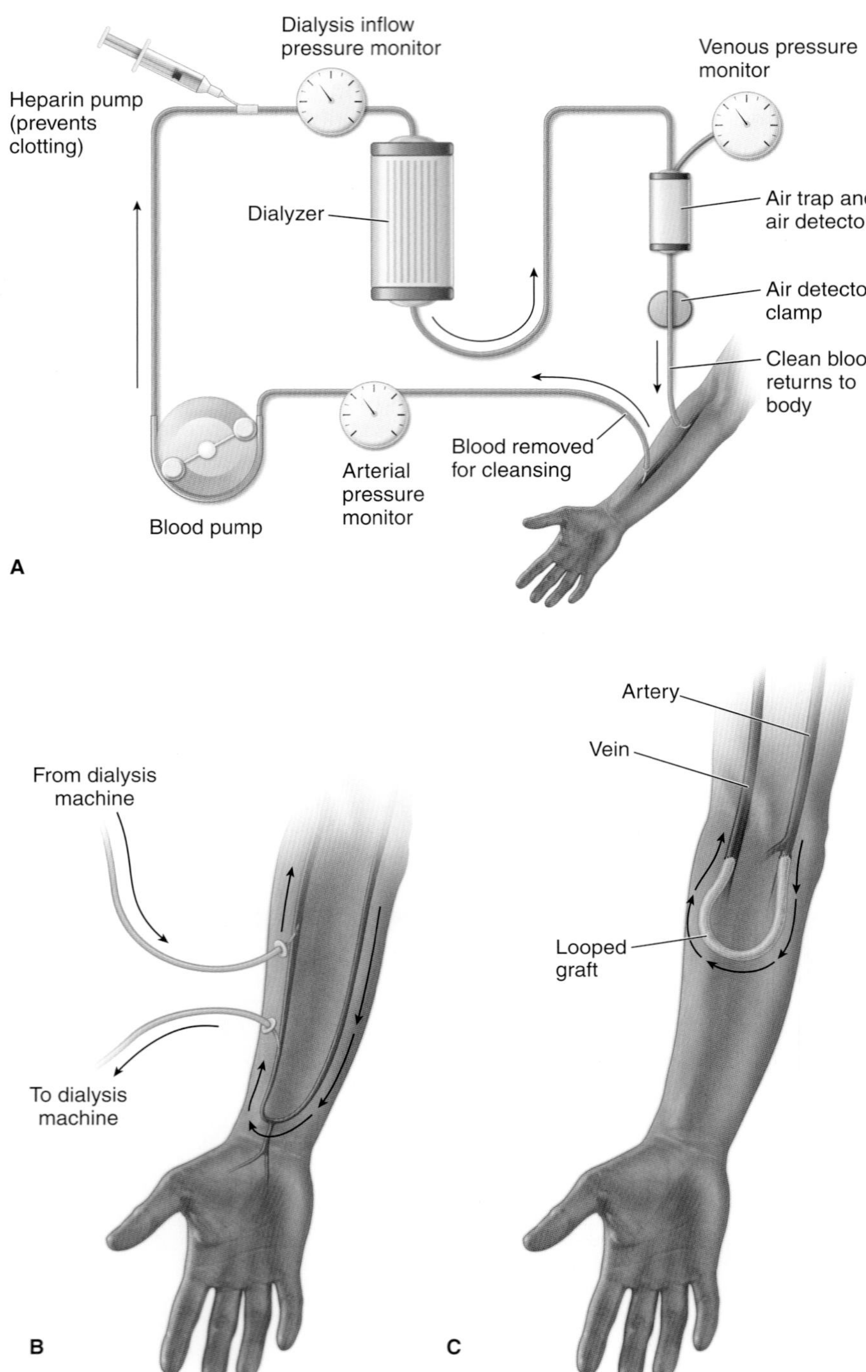

Figure 18.16. Hemodialysis. **A:** Hemodialysis uses special filters to remove wastes that the kidneys no longer can do on their own through the mechanisms of diffusion, osmosis, and ultrafiltration. **B:** Arteriovenous fistula. **C:** Arteriovenous shunt.

dialysis to prevent the formation of clots during the procedure. Hemodialysis can be done either at a dialysis center or at home with proper patient training.

Peritoneal dialysis provides another option for treatment in renal failure. Waste and excess water is removed using the peritoneal membrane as the semipermeable "filter," with the same transport mechanisms used in hemodialysis. Solution designed to draw out wastes from small capillaries in the peritoneum is inserted into the abdomen via a tube, previously placed surgically. After several hours, this solution is drained and discarded along with the waste products, and water is removed. This cycle is considered an exchange. Risks include peritonitis, which is minimized with the use of sterile technique. The types of peritoneal dialysis include:

- Continuous ambulatory peritoneal dialysis (CAPD)
  - Most common type
  - Dialysis fluid is inserted into the abdomen, where it remains for 4 to 6 hours (dwell time), followed by drainage
  - Repeated with fresh dialysis solution up to four times a day on a daily basis
- Continuous cycler-assisted (automated) peritoneal dialysis (CCPD)
  - A special machine (cycler) fills and empties abdomen of dialysis fluid three to five times a night during sleep
  - Fluid is inserted in the morning with a dwell time lasting the entire day
- Combination CAPD and CCPD

Individuals who require dialysis should eat a diet low in products likely to produce harmful waste. Recommendations for diet include:

- Balanced amounts of protein (chicken, meat, and fish)
- Low potassium, sodium, and phosphorus
- Fluid restriction

Kidney transplant may be necessary in severe cases of PKD. The sources of the kidney can be from a family member (living, related donor), another person not related (living, unrelated donor), or from a person who recently died (deceased donor). One of the greatest risks in transplantation is that of rejection, as detailed in Chapter 4. Factors considered when determining a match or lower risk of rejection include:

- Blood type
  - Most important aspect
  - Must be compatible
- Human leukocyte antigens (HLAs)
  - A total of six HLAs exist
  - Risk of rejection is decreased with increased number of HLA matches
- Cross-matching antigens
  - Antigen–antibody reactions between donor and recipient blood
  - Risk of rejection is decreased in the absence of reaction (negative cross-match)

Immunosuppressant administration helps decrease rejection risk after surgery.

Stop and Consider
Why do individuals suffering from renal failure become anemic?

Diverticular Disease

Diverticular disease affects the large intestine. Approximately half of all Americans >60 years old are affected by diverticular disease with the majority 80 years of age or older.[16] Processes that characterize diverticular disease include decreased motility, obstruction, and impaired perfusion.

PATHOPHYSIOLOGY

A **diverticulum** (small sac or outpouching) forms along the wall of the colon, most often in the ascending colon. Typically, diverticulum develops at a site of weakness in the intestinal wall. More than one diverticulum is called **diverticula**. The presence of diverticula is commonly referred to as the condition **diverticulosis**. Fecal matter caught in sacs may promote the development of infection, known as **diverticulitis**. Strong segmental contractions in the colon promote increase in intraluminal pressure, increasing risk for herniation. Herniation of the diverticulum makes the blood vessels supplying the intestinal wall susceptible to trauma and bleeding.[17]

Chronic constipation is linked to the development of diverticular disease. Slow movement of fecal matter leads to increased, prolonged pressure on the walls of the large intestine, altering structure and function. Most people are unaware of the problem until it leads to bleeding, infection, obstruction, and ischemia of the affected area of the colon. Perforation resulting from these processes results in hemorrhage, abscess, sepsis, or peritonitis (Fig. 18.17).

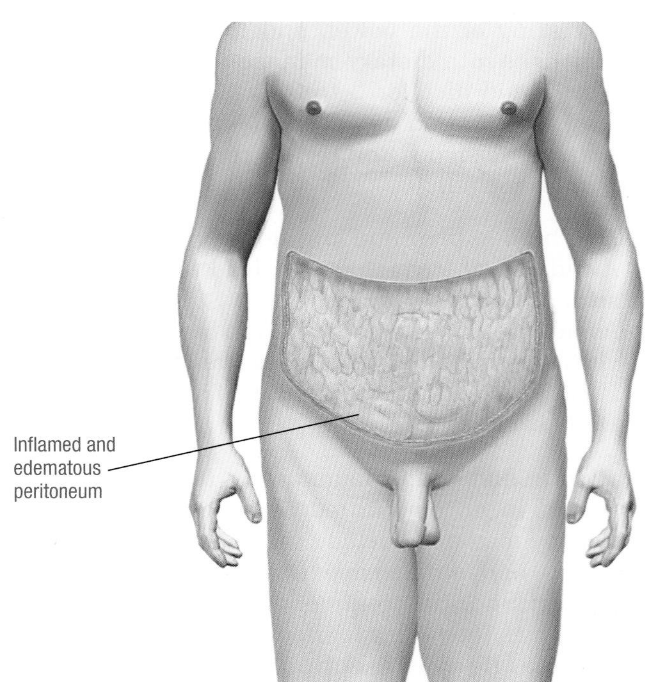

Figure 18.17. Peritonitis. The peritoneal membrane becomes edematous and inflamed in peritonitis. (Courtesy Anatomical Chart Company.)

CLINICAL MANIFESTATIONS

Clinical manifestations of diverticulitis mirror those described earlier under general manifestations and include abdominal pain, fever, nausea, and vomiting. Pain is the most common manifestation, typically present in the left lower quadrant area of the sigmoid colon, the most frequent site for diverticulitis. Nausea and vomiting may be due to obstruction or reduced peristalsis from inflammation. In some cases, diverticulitis may be complicated by perforation, fistula or abscess development. Abdominal tenderness may be present, with individuals demonstrating guarding, rigidity, and rebound tenderness of the abdomen. Symptoms are often severe enough to prompt medical attention. Sudden onset of rectal bleeding may occur when blood vessels are injured.

DIAGNOSTIC CRITERIA

Acute diverticulitis is determined by examination of stool for blood, evaluation of blood samples for anemia and signs of active infection, or identification of inflamed or ruptured sacs using ultrasound, magnetic resonance imaging, or CT scan. Once the acute infection has resolved, diverticula can be evaluated with a barium enema, flexible sigmoidoscopy, or colonoscopy.

TREATMENT

Immediate treatment goals include control of infection, resting of the bowel, and prevention of complications. Acute dietary management may include a clear liquid diet for 2 to 3 days until symptoms resolve. Prevention involves dietary and lifestyle alterations designed to prevent constipation. These strategies include:

- Diet high in fiber and low in fat
- Avoidance of foods that may lead to constipation, such as bananas and rice
- Avoidance of foods more likely to be retained in diverticula, including nuts, seeds, and strawberries
- Fluid intake, preferably water, of at least 2 L/d
- Daily exercise

Antibiotic and anti-inflammatory therapy may be indicated in uncomplicated diverticulitis. Pharmacotherapy may also include the use of bulk-forming laxatives and antispasmodic drugs for abdominal cramping. Surgical treatment may be required for emergencies, including perforation or infarction of diverticula. **Bowel resection**, or removal of a portion of the large intestine, may be required. A **colostomy** (establishment of an artificial opening of the large intestine externally on the abdomen) may be required as a temporary measure until the colon is healed, at which time it may be reconnected (reanastomosis). Oral intake is withheld after surgery because of the expected decrease in motility common after abdominal surgery. Oral intake slowly resumes after assurance of the return of bowel function, indicated by the presence of bowel sounds and the passing of flatus (gas passed through the anus). Introduction of food or fluid into the GI tract before this time may result in a **paralytic ileus**, a nonmechanical bowel obstruction characterized by a lack of peristalsis.

Functional Fecal Incontinence

Functional fecal incontinence, formerly known as encopresis or soiling, is a condition of repetitive, voluntary or involuntary, passage of stool in inappropriate places in children 4 years of age and older.[18] Functional fecal incontinence may be classified as retentive or nonretentive. The clinical model of functional fecal incontinence highlights the voluntary control mechanisms that can be used to impair stool elimination.

PATHOPHYSIOLOGY

Functional fecal incontinence is often associated with constipation and is classified as retentive or nonretentive. Key developmental triggers are associated with the development of functional fecal incontinence, including introduction of solid foods, toilet training, and start of school attendance. Constipation may result from the change in diet and, in older children, the stress associated with defecation that leads to voluntary retention, amplifying the problem of constipation. No anatomic or physiologic anomalies are associated with functional fecal incontinence. Instead, the functional fecal incontinence provides an illustration of the voluntary conscious control over defecation in neurologically competent individuals.

CLINICAL MANIFESTATIONS

Symptom-based diagnostic classifications, known as the Rome III criteria, were developed to help recognize and treat defecation and other GI disorders.[18] The retentive form of functional fecal incontinence in a child aged 4 years or older is associated with retentive posturing or excessive volitional stool retention, history of hard or painful bowel movements, presence of large fecal mass in the rectum, or history of passing large diameter stool. The factors associated with functional fecal incontinence are absent in the nonretentive form and include social context inappropriate for defecation, absence of underlying disorders of motility or anorectal sensorimotor function, absence of excessive stool and fecal retention, symptom frequency at least once per month and duration of at least 2 months.

DIAGNOSTIC CRITERIA

It is important to determine identify characteristics of incontinence. The absence of a potential medical, developmental, or behavioral pathology is the first step in determining the diagnosis. A history of incontinence is examined, including stool pattern (size, consistency, and interval), evidence of constipation, factors related to defecation episodes (age of onset, type, and amount), diet history, associated pain, current medications, associated urinary symptoms (enuresis, infection), family history of constipation, and emotional stress. Developmental readiness for toileting is also important to evaluate. Physical examination, including neurologic examination, may point to an anatomic or functional condition. Most cases of functional retentive fecal incontinence are caused by constipation, whereas functional nonretentive fecal incontinence is usually caused by nonorganic factors. Consideration must be given to the presence of neurogenic, neuromuscular, endocrine, or anatomic conditions to make these determinations.

TREATMENT

Behaviors contributing to toilet-refusal behavior should be addressed, and strategies should be used to promote positive, more enjoyable toileting experiences.[19] Methods promoting soft stool minimize discomfort during defecation, helping individuals to overcome the fear of pain-associated bowel movements. Another effective strategy includes having scheduled time on the toilet and creating a relaxed atmosphere that promotes bowel training and effective toileting skills. Incentives for positive experiences may motivate the child and promote eventual self-initiation of bowel movements. Mental health analysis to explore roots of oppositional and defiant behaviors must also be considered.

Stop and Consider

Why is the diagnosis of functional nonretentive fecal incontinence limited to children at least 4 years of age?

SUMMARY

- Alterations in elimination can develop because of the processes regulating production or elimination of urine and stool, causing symptoms ranging from inconvenient to life threatening.
- Urine is a product of the renal system, comprised of water and water-soluble waste products filtered from the circulation. Characteristics can provide evidence of altered elimination processes.
- Transport processes throughout the nephron contribute to the characteristics of urine filtrate.
- The renal system is important in the regulation of body fluid volume and composition, elimination of metabolic wastes, regulation of blood pressure and the synthesis, and release or activation of hormones.
- Stool is the waste product eliminated by the GI tract. Stool characteristics and patterns provide evidence of altered processes of GI elimination.
- Urinary and stool elimination may be impaired because of alterations in motility, neuromuscular function, perfusion, and patency. Manifestations can include altered volume and color, bleeding, pain, distention, and anorexia.
- Diagnostic strategies include analysis of urine and stool content and testing for structural anomalies.
- Impaired elimination can be the cause of other body system alterations, and it can contribute to the development of impairment in other systems as well. A thorough understanding of these altered processes helps to rapidly identify and effectively manage related conditions.

CASE STUDY 18.1

A female neonate was born 8 weeks premature at 32 weeks' gestation. She is currently 3 weeks of age and has recently advanced to oral feedings with artificial infant formula as her sole source of nutrition. She developed symptoms that suggest that she is developing necrotizing enterocolitis (NEC). From your reading on NEC, answer the following questions:

1. What anatomic problem would most likely lead to the symptoms associated with NEC?
2. What causes the underlying pathology associated with NEC?
3. What are the risk factors for this neonate that would suggest NEC?
4. What are the clinical manifestations you would expect with NEC?
5. What diagnostic tests might be used to identify NEC?
6. How would you manage an infant with NEC?

Log onto the Internet. Search for a relevant journal article or Web site that details NEC to confirm your predictions.

PRACTICE EXAM QUESTIONS

1. Which of the following provides the most objective measurement of renal dysfunction?
   a. White blood cell count
   b. Glomerular filtration rate
   c. Altered urinary electrolytes
   d. Presence of nitrites in urine

2. A characteristic change in stool that may indicate the presence of blood includes which one of the following?
   a. Melena
   b. Hematuria
   c. Floating
   d. Gray-like color

3. Which of the following diagnostic procedures allows analysis of the entire large colon?
   a. Barium enema
   b. Flexible sigmoidoscopy
   c. Flexible gastroscopy
   d. Colonoscopy

4. Which of the following foods should be avoided in people with renal calculi?
   a. Grape juice
   b. Ground beef
   c. Strawberries
   d. Cinnamon

5. Which of the following foods should be avoided in people with diverticular disease?
   a. Grape juice
   b. Ground beef
   c. Strawberries
   d. Cinnamon

6. Which type of urinary incontinence can be attributed to muscle overactivity?
   a. Stress incontinence
   b. Urge incontinence
   c. Overflow incontinence
   d. Functional incontinence

7. The enteric nervous system component located between the circular and longitudinal muscle layers of the large intestine:
   a. Myenteric plexus
   b. Submucosal plexus
   c. Meissner plexus
   d. Solar plexus

8. The area of the large intestine that absorbs the majority of water is the:
   a. Ileum
   b. Ascending colon
   c. Descending colon
   d. Rectum

9. The process by which fecal contents enters the rectum is known as:
   a. Peristalsis
   b. Segmental contractions
   c. Mass movement
   d. Tetany

10. The average volume of urine eliminated each day totals:
    a. 200 mL
    b. 800 mL
    c. 1,500 mL
    d. 3,000 mL

11. The ________ sphincter is made of skeletal muscle and is under voluntary control.
    a. Internal
    b. External
    c. Anterior
    d. Posterior

12. Urine specific gravity of 1:030 indicates:
    a. Concentrated urine
    b. Dilute urine
    c. Urine high in bacteria
    d. Casts in urine

13. Which of the following diagnostic criteria is consistent with the diagnosis of functional fecal incontinence?
    a. Age of 1 year
    b. Age of 3 years
    c. Age of 5 years
    d. All of the above

14. A GFR of 95 mL/minute indicates
    a. Normal renal function
    b. Mild renal disease
    c. Moderate renal disease
    d. Severe renal disease

15. Which of the following increases the risk for renal calculi?
    a. Running 5 miles
    b. Drinking 32 ounces of milk per day
    c. Sedentary lifestyle
    d. Dehydration

DISCUSSION AND APPLICATION

1. What did I know about altered elimination before today?
2. What body processes are affected by altered elimination? How does altered elimination affect those processes?
3. What are the potential etiologies for altered elimination? How does altered elimination develop?
4. Who is most at risk for developing altered elimination? How can these alterations be prevented?
5. What are the human differences that affect the etiology, risk, or course of altered elimination?
6. What clinical manifestations are expected in the course of altered elimination?
7. What special diagnostic tests are useful in determining the diagnosis and course of altered elimination?
8. What are the goals of care for individuals with altered elimination?
9. How does the concept of altered elimination build on what I have learned in the previous chapter and in the previous courses?
10. How can I use what I have learned?

RESOURCES

National Kidney and Urologic Diseases Information Clearinghouse:
http://kidney.niddk.nih.gov/index.htm

National Institute of Diabetes & Digestive & Kidney Disease, National Institutes of Health:
http://www.niddk.nih.gov

References

1. Scales CD Jr, Smith AC, Hanley JM, et al. Prevalence of kidney stones in the United States. *Eur Urol*. 2012;62(1):160–165. doi:10.1016/j.eururo.2012.03.052.
2. Hall PM. Nephrolithiasis: treatment, causes and prevention. *Cleve Clin J Med*. 2009;76(10):583–591.
3. Zilberman DE, Yong D, Albala DM. The impact of society changes on patterns of urolithiasis. *Curr Opin Urol*. 2010;20(2):1480153.
4. Rassweiler J, Rassweiler MC, Klein J. New technology in ureteroscopy and percutaneous nephrolithotomy. *Curr Opin Urol*. 2016;26(1):95–106. doi:10.1097/MOU.0000000000000240.
5. Robertson WG. Dietary recommendations and treatment of patients with recurrent idiopathic calcium stone disease. *Urolithiasis*. 2016;44(1):9–26. doi:10.1007/s00240-015-0849-2.
6. Stothers L, Thom D, Calhoun E. Urinary incontinence in men. In: Litwin MS, Saigal C, eds. *Urologic Diseases in America*. US Department of Health and Human Services, Public Health Service, National Institutes of Health, National Institute of Diabetes and Digestive and Kidney Diseases. Washington, DC: US Government Publishing Office; 2004.
7. Nygaard I, Thom D, Calhoun E. Urinary incontinence in women. In: Litwin MS, Saigal C, eds. *Urologic Diseases in America*. US Department of Health and Human Services, Public Health Service, National Institutes of Health, National Institute of Diabetes and Digestive and Kidney Diseases. Washington, DC: US Government Publishing Office; 2004.
8. Vandoninck V, Bemelmans BL, Mazzetta C, et al. The prevalence of urinary incontinence in community-dwelling married women: a matter of definition. *BJU Int*. 2004;94(9):1291–1295.
9. Yoshida M, Masunaga K, Nagata T, et al. The forefront for novel therapeutic agents based on the pathophysiology of lower urinary tract dysfunction: pathophysiology and pharmacology of overactive bladder. *J Pharmacol Sci*. 2010;112(2):128–134.
10. Faiena I, Patel N, Parihar JS, et al. Conservative management of urinary incontinence in women. *Rev Urol*. 2015;17(3):129–139.
11. Rangan GK, Lopez-Vargas P, Nankivell BJ, et al. Autosomal dominant polycystic kidney disease: a path forward. *Semin Nephrol*. 2015;35(6):524–537. doi:10.1016/j.semnephrol.2015.10.002.
12. NIDDK. Kidney and urologic disease statistics for the United States. http://kidney.niddk.nih.gov/kudiseases/pubs/kustats/index.htm#kidney. Retrieved on February 6, 2010.
13. Campbell KL, Rangan GK, Lopez-Vargas P, et al. KHA-CARI autosomal dominant polycystic kidney disease guideline: diet and lifestyle management. *Semin Nephrol*. 2015;35(6):572–581.e17. doi:10.1016/j.semnephrol.2015.10.008.
14. Mallett A, Lee VW, Mai J, et al. KHA-CARI autosomal dominant polycystic kidney disease guideline: pharmacological management. *Semin Nephrol*. 2015;35(6):582–589.e17. doi:10.1016/j.semnephrol.2015.10.009.
15. Lee VW, Tunnicliffe DJ, Rangan GK. KHA-CARI autosomal dominant polycystic kidney disease guideline: management of end-stage kidney disease. *Semin Nephrol*. 2015;35(6):595–602.e12. doi:10.1016/j.semnephrol.2015.10.011.
16. Lidor AO, Segal JB, Wu AW, et al. Older patients with diverticulitis have low recurrence rates and rarely need surgery. *Surgery*. 2011;150(2):146–153.
17. Wilkins T, Baird C, Pearson AN, et al. Diverticular bleeding. *Am Fam Physician*. 2009;80(9):977–983.
18. Rasquin A, Di Lorenzo C, Forbes D, et al. Childhood functional gastrointestinal disorders: child/adolescent. *Gastroenterology*. 2006;130(5):1527–1537.
19. Koppen IJ, von Gontard A, Chase J, et al. Management of functional nonretentive fecal incontinence in children: recommendations from the International Children's Continence Society. *J Pediatr Neurol*. 2015. doi:10.1016/j.jpurol.2015.09.008.

Find additional resources for this chapter at http:thePoint.lww.com

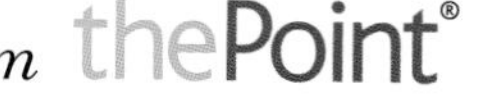

Chapter

19 Degenerative Changes in Aging

LEARNING OUTCOMES

1. Define and use the key terms listed in this chapter.
2. Describe the basis of theoretic explanations of aging.
3. Recognize the implications of degenerative changes in aging on the health of the individual.
4. Identify common manifestations of age-related degenerative changes.
5. Detail methods to maximize health status in the elderly population.
6. List the common diagnostic procedures used to identify degenerative changes in aging.
7. Describe treatment strategies appropriate for degenerative changes in aging.
8. Apply concepts of age-related alterations in cells, tissues, and organ systems to select clinical models.

INTRODUCTION

"You're only as old as you feel" is a phrase often quoted, but what makes us old? Aging is a normal, expected process that occurs in all living individuals. Even though it is a normal, physiologic process, the effects can cause clinical manifestations that range from minimally impaired function to serious disability. Knowledge of the degenerative changes that are involved in the aging process can provide the basis of adaptations that can promote the greatest degree of function and independence.

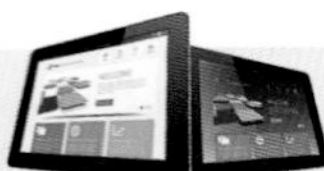

RESEARCH NOTES

By 2050, the number of people who will be older than 60 years is set to double. A new report from the World Health Organization (WHO) calls for a dramatic shift in the way we think about and approach a rapidly growing older population. The 245-page report defines healthy aging as "the process of developing and maintaining the functional ability that enables well-being in older age." The full report can be found at http://www.medscape.com/viewarticle/851954.

Module 1 Theories of Aging

Aging is commonly defined as the gradual deterioration of a mature organism resulting from time-dependent, irreversible changes in structure. **Senescence** is often used interchangeably with aging and refers to postmaturational processes that lead to diminished homeostasis and increased vulnerability. Aging is a time-related process that determines responses leading to illness and death. Life expectancy, the age at which 50% of a given population is expected to survive, is a term used to describe demographics associated with aging.

Theories of Aging

Theories of aging have been developed to explain physiologic processes that lead to clinical manifestations. The mechanisms that program cells to age are not clearly understood, but they are known to contribute to impaired structure and function. Aging is associated with reduced functional capacity because the body fails to produce sufficient numbers of replacement cells, especially those that are not capable of mitotic division. Identifying the cellular mechanisms underlying degenerative changes of aging is necessary for effective diagnosis and treatment of related pathology.

Theories of aging are usually categorized as developmental or stochastic. **Developmental theories** point to the influence of genetics as the major determinant of aging. **Stochastic theories** support the idea that aging is the result of cumulative cellular damage. The process of aging is likely multifactorial, reflecting mechanisms of both genetics and environment. Damage to cells may be due to cumulative extrinsic events that cause injury to cells or from intrinsic events regulating cell death determined by genetic control. Cellular damage resulting from mechanical or chemical injury caused by accumulation of metabolites and ultraviolet radiation damage to DNA are among the potential causes thought to contribute to aging. Cell death that is programmed (apoptosis) or occurring because of injury (necrosis) often contributes to the clinical manifestations of aging (see Chapter 2).

DEVELOPMENTAL THEORIES

Developmental theories support the existence of a genetically programmed and controlled continuum of development and maturation. At earlier ages, biochemical pathways optimally maintain genes to assure reproductive function and survival of the species. Genes that determine survival at younger ages, therefore, have greater influence than genes that are expressed at older ages.

The **accumulated mutations theory** suggests that over time, the accumulation of genetic mutations during cell division may contribute to altered cellular function associated with aging. The gradual decline in cellular and metabolic function likely results from a combination of DNA mutation and telomere shortening. *Telomeres* are the capped structures on chromosomes that protect chromosome ends (Fig. 19.1). Each time a chromosome is replicated, the telomeres shorten. When chromosomes reach a critical length, cellular senescence, or the intrinsic loss of the capacity of the cell to proliferate, is triggered.

Observations of decreased immune function with increased age have led to the development of the **immunologic theory of aging**. Reduced resistance to disease secondary to reduced T-cell function and enhanced autoimmune responses are common characteristics of increasing age. Another theory, the **antagonistic pleiotropy theory,** suggests that genes may have beneficial effects during early life but harmful effects as the individual ages. The origin

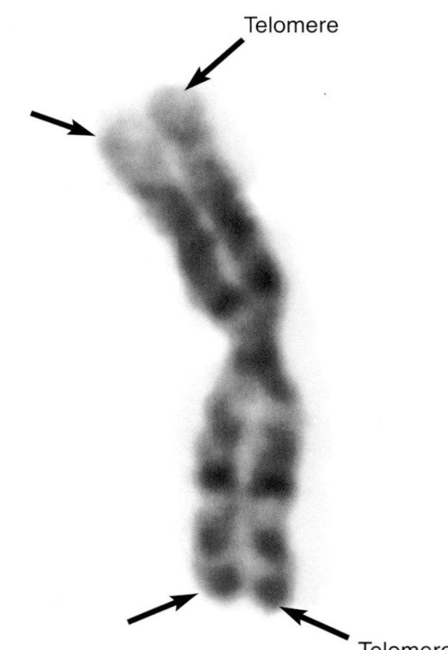

Figure 19.1. Telomere location on a single chromosome. Each chromatid is capped by a telomere. (Modified from McClatchey KD. *Clinical Laboratory Medicine*. 2nd ed. Philadelphia, PA: Lippincott Williams & Wilkins; 2002.)

for this selection may be based on the promotion of reproductive success rather than negative effects associated with aging. Mutations that occur later in life limit the influence of evolutionary selection. The **neuroendocrine theory** suggests the interrelationship between neurons and associated hormones as the stimulus for aging. The hypothalamic–pituitary axis is instrumental in contributing to the regulation of many bodily functions, including development, growth, puberty, reproduction, metabolism, and aging. Menopause is an example of the manifestation of altered neuroendocrine responsiveness characteristic of women with increasing age.

STOCHASTIC THEORIES

Stochastic theories suggest that random accumulated cellular damage leads to aging. Targets for cellular damage include mitochondria and DNA. The **free radical theory** of aging links cellular damage with the production of reactive oxygen species (ROS). According to this theory, intracellular production of ROS contributes to the final determination of life span. Mitochondria are especially at risk for damage from ROS because of by-products produced in the electron transport chain that produce energy in the form of adenosine triphosphate (ATP). Oxidative damage to mitochondrial DNA and other cellular structures is thought to be cumulative, leading to the manifestations of aging.

The **somatic mutation theory** states that the aging process is caused by impaired DNA repair, antioxidant defense, or errors in protein expression. Caloric restriction has been shown experimentally to prolong life expectancy. Although the underlying mechanism is unclear, longevity may be caused by a shift in energy from growth and reproduction toward repair and maintenance of the soma, or cell.

Module 2 General Manifestations of Aging

A pattern of gradual loss is characteristic of the changes associated with aging (Fig. 19.2). These changes are physiologic rather than pathologic. However, these same changes may result in altered structure and function, leading to findings that are often associated with pathologic manifestations. Aging processes and disease states are not always clearly delineated.

Common characteristics of aging include:

1. Increased mortality with age after maturation
2. Changes in biochemical composition in tissues
3. Progressive decrease in physiologic capacity
4. Diminished ability to respond adaptively to environmental stimuli
5. Increased vulnerability and susceptibility to disease

Cellular Changes in Aging

Cellular changes characteristic of aging include atrophy and hypertrophy and the impaired ability to undergo mitosis. Cell function may be impaired by the deposition of lipids or damage from free radicals. Tissue effects of aging include the accumulation of

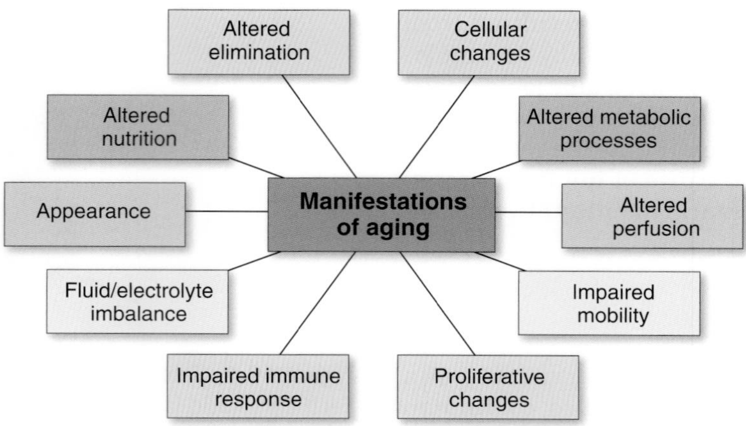

Figure 19.2. Concept map. Manifestations of aging.

metabolic waste products and the deposition of **lipofuscin**, a fatty brown lipid pigment, causing stiffening or rigidity. Loss of mass by atrophy is a common age-related effect that occurs in organs and bones. Although these changes are part of the normal processes of aging, the resulting changes often impact body function.

Aging and Appearance

Appearance is altered in aging. Typical skin changes include a dry, wrinkled appearance with a varied pattern of pigmentation (Fig. 19.3). Collagen changes decrease elasticity. Decreased vascularity and increased fragility may lead to skin discoloration and thickened nail appearance. Changes in hair include loss, growth, distribution, and graying because of melanin deficiency in the hair follicle.

Stop and Consider
Why do "age spots" form as individuals age?

Fluid and Electrolyte Balance

Aging is associated with changes in body mass characterized by a decrease in muscle and an increase in fat. These changes contribute to a decrease in total body water, further enhanced by the kidney's diminished ability to regulate sodium and water balance, which is important in the establishment of extracellular fluid volume and tonicity. Total body water balance is a key element in the determination of sodium concentration in the blood, which increases the risk for hyponatremia in cases of water retention and hypernatremia caused by water loss. Additional stressors in the form of disease, altered elimination, or altered nutrition may result in significant consequences related to altered fluid and electrolyte balance.

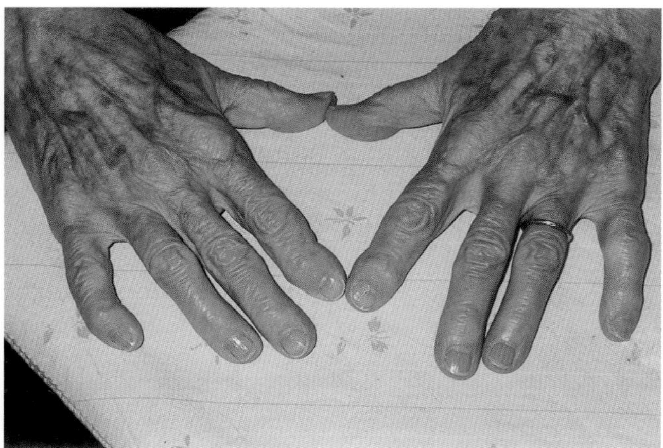

Figure 19.3. Hands with wrinkling and overlapping folds common to aging skin. (From Smeltzer SC, Bare BG. *Textbook of Medical-Surgical Nursing*. 9th ed. Philadelphia, PA: Lippincott Williams & Wilkins; 2000.)

Immune Response

The processes of inflammation, immunity, and protection from infection are altered with aging. Immune senescence, progressive dysfunction of the immune system associated with aging, is characterized by both diminished and enhanced immune responses. Antigenic immune responses progressively diminish with aging because of decreased T-cell function even in the absence of any significant decrease in actual T-cell number. Thymus degeneration occurs after age 50 years and is reduced to 15% of its peak size, which was reached at sexual maturity. This degeneration results in decreased thymic hormone production and T-cell differentiation. Monoclonal antibody production may occur, even in the absence of B-cell malignancies. Autoimmune responses may become enhanced because of the increased circulation of autoantibodies and immune complexes. IgE-mediated hypersensitivity responses are decreased and are associated with a lessening of allergy-mediated symptoms.

Stop and Consider
How can the elderly protect themselves from infection?

Manifestations of decreased immune responsiveness include attenuated delayed hypersensitivity responses, diminished T-cell activity, and responsiveness to pathogens. Loss of previously acquired immunity may increase the reactivation of pathogens, resulting in reinfection. The incidence of herpes zoster and tuberculosis infection is increased in the elderly. Mortality rates are increased in the elderly in response to pneumonia and influenza. Rates of nosocomial infection are also increased in this population. Impaired wound healing may result as a response to altered immune function due to aging or from decreased function induced by medications for chronic illness, such as steroids. Typical physical changes of aging, including loss of subcutaneous fat, decreased elasticity of collagen, and atrophied epidermis and supporting capillaries, also contribute to impaired healing.

Age-Related Proliferative Changes

Chronic myeloproliferative disorders, such as polycythemia vera and primary thrombocythemia, are more common in individuals greater than age 60 years. The incidence of many of the most common cancers is also increased in many older individuals, with the greatest incidence occurring between the ages of 65 and 80 years. The potential causes for these findings may result from many of the characteristic changes of aging contributing to increased risk or attenuated defense to carcinogens. These potential causes include:

- Impaired immune function
- Genetic mutation accumulation
- Prolonged carcinogen exposure
- Impaired ability for DNA repair

Manifestations of alterations in proliferation are specific to the involved cells and tissues. Treatment is often based on the type of malignancy, the effects resulting from the malignancy, the person's age and quality of life, and consent.

Neurologic Function

Age-related neurologic manifestations may include alteration in cognition, sensation, pain, and motor responses. These manifestations often result from changes in both structure and function of cells and the tissues responsible for the stimulation of physiologic responses. Neurologic function may be altered as a response to cellular processes, resulting in functional changes in both the central, somatosensory, and peripheral nervous systems. Typical structural changes include:

- Decrease in brain mass
- Enlargement of cerebral ventricles
- Decrease in number of neurons, dendritic processes, and synapses
- Decrease in myelin
- Altered production of neurotransmitters

Histologically, in the brain, evidences of lipofuscin pigment in nerve cells and amyloid in the vascular tissue are findings consistent with aging. Neurofibrillatory tangles and plaques may occur (see Clinical Models). Evidence exists of a declining number of cells in the spinal cord, although the functional effects are not clearly linked. Most functional alterations result from the involvement of peripheral nerves and degenerative changes of the spine and muscles. Slowing of nerve conduction and less efficient axon response to injury and repair are typical with aging. Factors critical to the promotion of neurologic responses, including neurotransmitters, enzymes, and receptors, are also altered during the aging process.

Manifestations of impaired functioning often result from these structural changes. These changes include sensory deficits (taste, smell, vibration, vision, and hearing), motor dysfunction (altered gait and posture), sleep disturbances, and impaired memory and cognition. Slowing of central processing may prolong the time it takes to complete tasks. Declines in motor strength, reflex responses, and reaction time are related to sensorimotor changes. Changes associated with aging include mild forgetfulness, a decrease in vocabulary, and learning difficulties. These changes typically do not occur until the seventh decade of life.

Cognitive function can be compromised by the coexisting conditions related to decline in mental health. Often related to environment and social conditions, depression and anxiety among the elderly is more prevalent in long-term care settings compared with elderly who are community dwelling. Psychological disorders may complicate physical health, reducing motivation or ability to maintain health through everyday activities, such as properly administering medications, assuring adequate nutrition, obtaining adequate exercise, and maintaining personal hygiene.

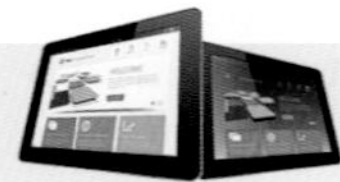

RESEARCH NOTES

A recent study examined the the link between age and cerebral gray matter in long-term meditators versus control subjects ($n = 100$) between 24 and 77 years of age. Negative correlations were detected in gray matter when compared with age (higher age, lower gray matter). However, the slopes of the regression lines were steeper and the correlation coefficients were stronger in controls than in meditators. These findings suggest less age-related gray matter atrophy in those who meditate over the long term.[1]

Mobility

Physical activity is often decreased among the elderly. The occurrence of **osteopenia** (reduced calcification and/or skeletal bone mass) and **osteoporosis** (atrophy of skeletal tissue) in individuals over age 50 years is increased, placing this population at risk for injury caused by falls. Women experience a more rapid phase of bone loss after menopause, known as **menopausal bone loss**, followed by a slower loss phase that affects both men and women (senescent bone loss). Menopausal bone loss is cytokine-induced (interleukin-6 [IL-6]), occurring in the absence of adequate levels of protective ovarian hormones. This response is associated with delayed apoptosis of osteoclasts and enhanced apoptosis of osteoblasts, resulting in an imbalance favoring bone loss. Senescent bone loss is related to diminished bone remodeling and formation. Osteoblast production is decreased, slowing the rate of bone formation and reducing bone mineral density. Osteoporosis is discussed in more detail in this chapter as a clinical model.

Stop and Consider
What types of physical activity are considered weight-bearing? What types are not?

Loss of bone with progressive age affects the *axial (trabecular)* and *appendicular (cortical)* skeleton and is manifested by pain, stiffness, loss of height, and development of **kyphosis**, an exaggerated anterior concave curvature of the thoracic spine (Fig. 19.4). Fractures of the vertebrae and hips are common. Cartilage changes may also impair mobility, decreasing function via joint limitations. Enzyme activity in chondrocytes may lead to crystal deposition, promoting the development of **chondrocalcinosis** (calcification of cartilage). Cartilage may thin in weight-bearing joints, such as the knees, causing pain and decreased mobility.

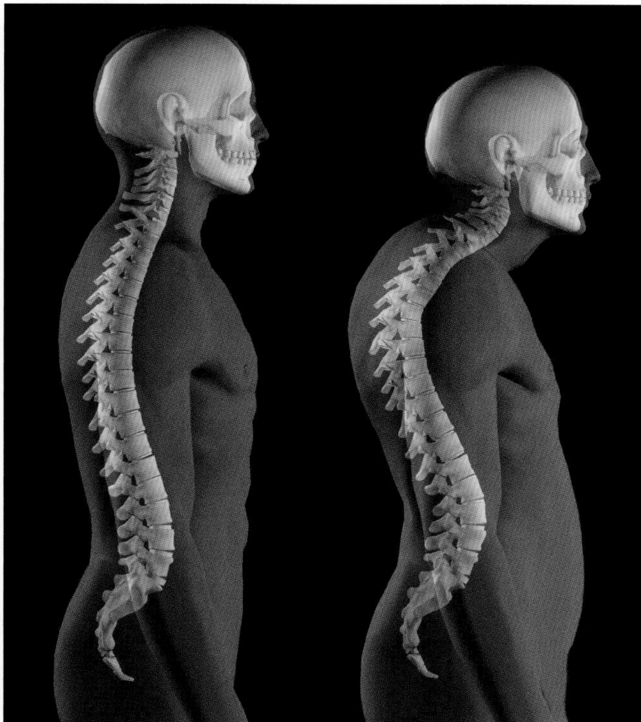

Figure 19.4. Kyphosis versus normal. Kyphosis **(right)** versus normal spinal column **(left)**. (Courtesy LifeART image copyright (c) [2016] Lippincott Williams & Wilkins. All rights reserved.)

Loss of lean body mass typical in aging is primarily caused by the decreased number and size of skeletal muscle fibers. **Sarcopenia**, or loss of skeletal muscle, is a common age-related change that limits function. Causes of sarcopenia include:

- Decreased physical activity
- Changes in the nervous system (central and peripheral)
- Protein undernutrition

Faster-contracting muscle fibers (type II) are lost more quickly compared to the slower-contracting fibers (type I), leading to loss of isometric contractile force. Posture and the ability to perform rhythmic movements are affected more slowly. Decreased mobility caused by other comorbid conditions can greatly accelerate the process of muscle loss in the elderly.

Perfusion and Ventilation

Age-related changes in the cardiovascular system may lead to altered perfusion. Variables affecting cardiac function include:

- Compliance
- Cardiac filling
- Preload
- Afterload
- Contractility
- Ejection fraction
- Stroke volume
- Heart rate
- Cardiac output

Connective tissue changes promote decreased elasticity in the smooth muscle of the vascular system. Increased afterload caused by arterial stiffening and limited distention may alter cardiac output. Left ventricular wall thickness may increase because of hypertension, a common comorbid condition in the elderly. Atherosclerosis may result from increased intimal thickness from cellular accumulation, often coupled with damage to the internal elastic layer of the vascular smooth muscle. Alterations in cardiovascular functioning may affect any organ system, promoting the development of organ-specific manifestations. Decreased cerebral blood flow may be linked to alterations in neurologic function, further determined by the specific area of the brain involved.

Pulmonary changes in aging, coupled with decreased density of pulmonary capillaries, may limit the availability of oxygen to adequately supply tissues. Typical changes include:

- Decreased inspiratory reserve volume
- Increased residual volume

- Reduced ventilatory capacity
- Reduced ventilation–perfusion ratio

Decreased muscle and bone mass in the chest cavity may increase the work of breathing. In nonsmokers, these typical changes affecting ventilation, gas exchange, and compliance are not associated with significant manifestations. Dyspnea may indicate airway obstruction, often seen in individuals with comorbid conditions such as emphysema. Limited immune defense along with dysphagia, loss of cough mechanisms, and decline of mucociliary transport may predispose elderly individuals to pulmonary infection and aspiration.

Metabolic Processes

Atrophy, decreased hormonal secretion, impaired receptor/ligand binding, and alterations in intracellular signaling may influence the changes typical in the hormonal processes associated with aging. Because hormonal and metabolic effects are body-wide, the manifestations of alterations often affect many organ systems. The most commonly affected processes include:

- Mineral metabolism
    - Calcium
    - Phosphate
    - Magnesium
- Vitamin and trace mineral metabolism
- Acid–base metabolism
- Nutrient metabolism
    - Obesity
    - Undernutrition
- Endocrine metabolism
    - Thyroid
    - Parathyroid
    - Adrenal
    - Pituitary
        - Anterior
        - Posterior
    - Ovarian/testicular

Calcium levels in the elderly are regulated by parathyroid hormone (PTH), vitamin D, and calcitonin. **Calcitonin**, a hormone produced by the parathyroid, thyroid, and thymus glands, promotes the deposition of calcium and phosphate in bone. PTH promotes removal of calcium and phosphate from bone, opposing the effects of calcitonin. The activated form of vitamin D, 1,25-dihydroxycholecalciferol, promotes calcium absorption in the intestine. Calcium levels vary depending on the concentration of plasma proteins (i.e., albumin), the concentration bound to anions (i.e., phosphate and bicarbonate), and the blood pH altering calcium–protein binding (decreased in acidosis; increased in alkalosis). Calcium levels may be affected by age-related decreased intestinal absorption of calcium, a blunted response to vitamin D activation, and the age-related increase in PTH (Fig. 19.5). Nutritional intake of calcium and vitamin D is also important in the regulation of calcium metabolism. Proliferative disease, particularly breast cancer, lung cancer, and multiple myeloma, may result in dangerously high levels of serum calcium.

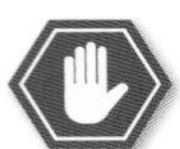

Stop and Consider
Why would metastatic disease increase calcium levels in the blood?

Phosphate levels are typically lower in the elderly. Phosphate intake is decreased in the elderly and is coupled with poor intestinal absorption. Increased activity of the parathyroid gland may result in promotion of renal excretion of phosphate related to altered tubular absorption. Chronic renal failure may result in hyperphosphatemia. Hypomagnesemia is also common among the elderly and often results from decreased dietary intake, excessive renal excretion, or loss via the gastrointestinal system (i.e., vomiting, diarrhea, or impaired absorption). Maintenance of acid–base balance is impaired because of a diminished ability of the aging respiratory and renal systems to correct alterations. Impairment of these homeostatic mechanisms represents a significant risk of altered acid–base balance in the elderly.

Decreased T3 levels and elevated thyroid-stimulating hormone (TSH) levels characterize typical thyroid function alterations in the elderly. The incidence of hypothyroidism increases with age and may manifest subclinically or with overt symptoms. The prevalence of hyperthyroidism does not increase with age. Temperature regulation is also compromised in the elderly, more so if coupled with chronic illness. The ability to cool the body via sweating is impaired because of a decrease in the number, size, and activity of sweat glands, making the elderly particularly susceptible to heat stress. Frail elderly individuals are especially at risk for hypothermia because of diminished cold perception, altered responsiveness to catecholamine-induced vasoconstriction and shiver, and limited ability to produce heat.

Nutrition and Elimination

Processes that regulate digestion and elimination are altered in aging because of morphologic and functional changes within the enteric nervous system, a division of the autonomic nervous system. Impaired nutrition that leads to deficiencies in macronutrients and micronutrients are common among the elderly. These deficits can lead to cognitive impairment,

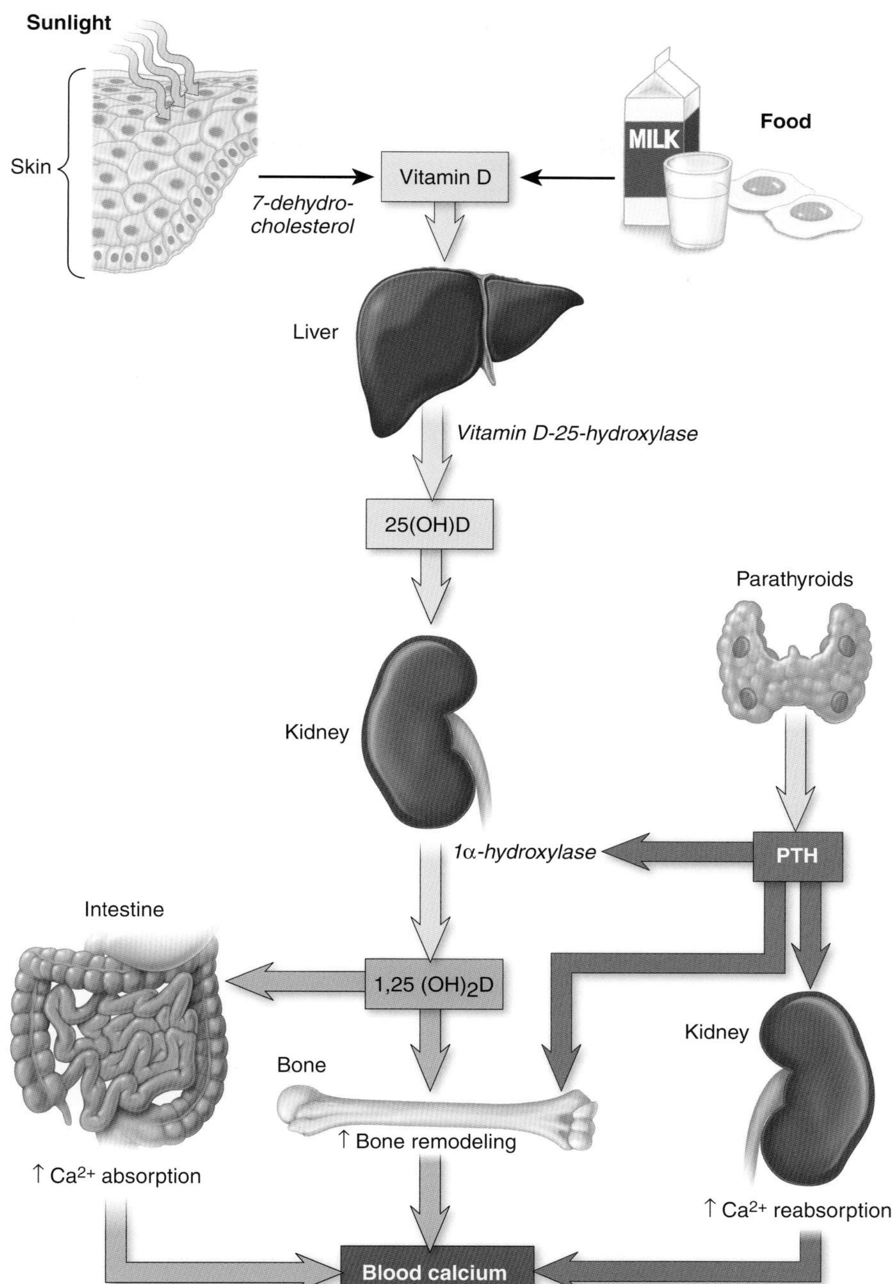

Figure 19.5. Metabolism of vitamin D and the regulation of calcium. Calcium regulation involves multiple organ systems. Reduced function in any of the involved systems may result in altered calcium homeostasis. (From Rubin E, Farber JL. *Pathology*. 4th ed. Philadelphia, PA: Lippincott Williams & Wilkins; 2005.)

increased risk of infection caused by impairment of immune function, anemia, and poor wound healing. Inadequate intake of protein and energy-producing foods may result in undernutrition, often associated with deficiencies in water-soluble vitamins B and C as well as fat-soluble vitamins A, D, E, and K.

The problem of undernutrition is even more prevalent among elderly in long-term care and in hospitals, which increases the risk for the development of chronic illness. Impaired nutrition may be caused by tooth loss or poorly fitting dentures, making the process of chewing food difficult. Often in aging, the physiologic response to hunger is blunted, coupled with a feeling of fullness even though taking in less food.

Functional responses of the kidneys decrease with age. Renal changes characteristic in aging include:

- Reduced renal blood flow
- Decreased glomerular filtration rate

- Reduced renal mass
- Decline in proximal tubular function
- Reduced renin and aldosterone levels

Reduction in nephron number may alter the renal function of urine concentration, placing additional importance on the regulation of total water balance. Drug excretion may be impaired, increasing the risk of toxicity.

Impaired gastrointestinal elimination in elderly individuals is most frequently manifested as constipation, diarrhea, fecal incontinence, and impaction. The stress of fluid and electrolyte loss via diarrhea represents a significant threat to water balance, often resulting in severe dehydration. Increased rectal compliance and impaired rectal sensation represent age-related changes that predispose elderly individuals to constipation. Fecal incontinence is caused by decreased resting and maximal anal sphincter pressures.

Module 3 Managing Degenerative Changes in the Elderly

Primary and secondary prevention of injury and illness are the major challenges in management of age-related degenerative changes. Screening for functional impairment and selecting management strategies must be individualized because of the wide range of manifestations exhibited among the elderly. Strategies must take into account comorbid conditions, physical health, cognitive status, functional ability, and social support.

Health outcomes are improved among the elderly population with regular exercise, weight control, cancer screening, avoidance of smoking and binge drinking, and disease prevention through vaccination. A careful evaluation of the home environment can help with preventing falls, burns, and other household accidents. Family members or individuals responsible for providing elder care should be aware of changes in functional or cognitive abilities. Assurance of appropriate medication administration may prevent injury related to improper dosing. A well-balanced diet that includes essential protein intake, macronutrients, and micronutrients is important to maintain homeostasis. Assurance of adequate fluid intake is essential to volume regulation and may lessen the incidence of constipation.

Module 4 Clinical Models

Clinical models for this chapter were selected to demonstrate the application of previously described processes within aging populations. As you read the descriptions that follow, consider the cellular mechanisms that contribute to the alterations in tissues and body systems associated with aging.

Hutchinson–Gilford Progeria Syndrome

Hutchinson–Gilford Progeria Syndrome (HGPS) is an extremely rare hereditary disease that affects about 1 in 4 million people worldwide. It is a syndrome affecting the skin, musculoskeletal system, and cardiovascular system and is characterized by accelerated aging. Children affected by progeria have a life expectancy of approximately 13 years. Mortality is often related to accelerated atherosclerosis of the carotid and coronary arteries.

PATHOPHYSIOLOGY

Autosomal dominant mutations in the *LMNA* gene are responsible for most cases of HGPS, with advanced paternal age being a major risk factor. In addition, autosomal recessive transmission can also occur as demonstrated by sets of affected siblings born to unaffected parents. The *LMNA* gene encodes the nuclear envelope protein called lamins, which are important for maintaining cell nucleus stability and regulating gene expression, DNA synthesis, and DNA repair. When the *LMNA* gene mutates, this results in a truncated (shortened) prelamin-A protein, called progerin. Progerin (an abnormal protein) prevents the normal assembly of lamins. The forced absence of lamin A in the cell nucleus causes the nucleus to become abnormally shaped and structured. Cellular chromosomes cannot segregate normally and mitosis is delayed. The gene expression affects multiple cellular processes, including collagen remodeling and the formation of the extracellular matrix. A characteristic finding is also high levels of hyaluronic acid secretion (which can also in increase with normal aging). Hyaluronic acid levels impact the presence of cardiovascular disease, calcification of the blood vessels, and sclerodermatous changes in the skin. In general, changes in gene activity commonly associated with older adults are found in those with progeria.

CLINICAL MANIFESTATIONS

Clinical manifestations often presents within the first year of life when sclerodermal skin changes and alopecia (hair loss) are first noted and when the infant demonstrates growth failure. By age 2 years, children with progeria show prominent signs of early aging (Fig. 19.6). Additional manifestations include:

- Prominent scalp veins
- Feeding difficulties
- Scleroderma (shiny, inelastic skin) and wrinkled (aged) skin
- Loss of subcutaneous fat and muscle
- Delayed dentition
- Hearing loss
- High-pitched voice
- Short stature and skeletal dysplasia
- Incomplete sexual maturation

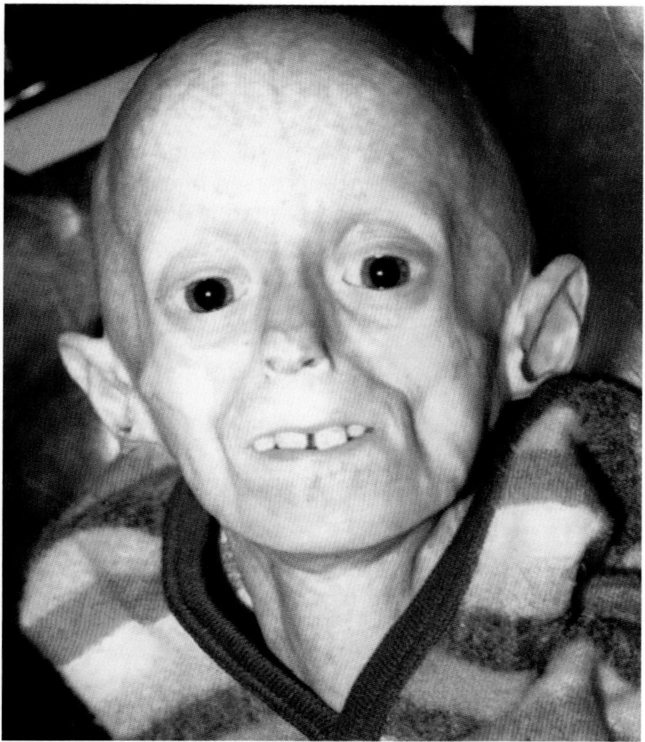

Figure 19.6. Manifestations of progeria. A 10-year-old girl affected by progeria shows signs of accelerated aging.

Affected patients often develop osteoporosis, atherosclerosis, fibrosis, hypertension, and arthritis. HGPS is not associated with increased tumor formation, cataract development, or senility as may occur in aging adults.

DIAGNOSIS

The diagnosis of HGPS is based on history and physical exam noting the characteristic signs and symptoms. Hyaluronic acid levels can provide clues to the presence of HGPS. Imaging studies may be needed to determine the extent of bone and blood vessel involvement.

TREATMENT

There is no approved therapy for HGPS. However, research is underway to determine the effectiveness of gene therapy (eliminating the production of mutant *LMNA*) as well as pharmacologic therapy, such as with rapamycin (an antibiotic), which have been shown to impact age-related cellular pathways. Care for those with HGPS involves therapies to improve feeding and nutritional intake, activity and joint mobility, monitoring of vascular disease, and providing family support.

Osteoporosis

Osteoporosis is the most common type of bone disease affecting older adults. Annually, 1.5 million people are diagnosed with a fracture related to osteoporosis. Osteoporosis affects both genders, with a greater prevalence among women, in which it occurs eight times more frequently.

PATHOPHYSIOLOGY

Osteoporosis occurs because of an imbalance in the bone remodeling process; bone resorption by osteoclasts is favored over bone formation by osteoblasts, resulting in loss of bone mass (Fig. 19.7). Factors contributing to osteoporosis risk include:

- Genetic predisposition
  - Family history of first-degree relative with osteoporosis
- Peak bone mass
  - Reduced maximal amount of bone in a given person
  - Body mass index less than 25%
- Loss of estrogen
- Aging
- Inadequate calcium and vitamin D intake
- Cigarette smoking

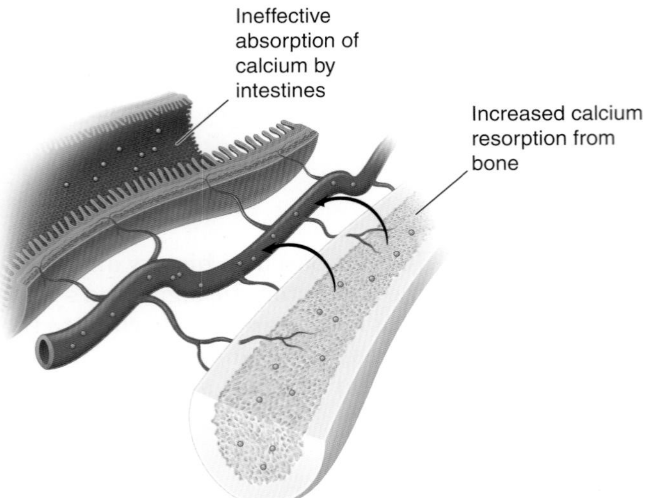

Figure 19.7. Osteoporosis in aging. Impaired intestinal calcium absorption and increased osteoclastic activity relative to osteoblastic activity contribute to age-related osteoporosis.

- Excessive alcohol
- Sedentary lifestyle

Secondary osteoporosis, a less common form, results from secondary causes, including hormonal or genetic diseases (Table 19.1). Reduced osteoblast function characterizes this form of osteoporosis.

Calcium and phosphate promote bone calcification, and their metabolism is tightly regulated to maintain normal extracellular levels. Metabolic alterations can result in, or cause, excessive or inadequate levels of these minerals, which are the building blocks of bone. Vitamin D, taken in by diet or produced in response to sunlight, promotes the intestinal absorption of calcium and phosphate. The process of bone formation is enhanced by mechanical stress and the hormone calcitonin, inhibiting the activation of osteoclasts and promoting the deposition of calcium and phosphate into bone. Although a variety of tissues produce calcitonin, the major source of calcitonin is the parafollicular cells of the thyroid gland. PTH opposes calcitonin, activating osteoclasts and promoting removal of calcium and phosphate from bone, which results in bone resorption. Tubule reabsorption in the kidneys minimizes excretion of both calcium and phosphorus in the urine (Fig. 19.8).

Stop and Consider
What influence does geographic location have on vitamin D production?

Table 19.1 Conditions Leading to Secondary Osteoporosis

Condition	Etiology	Effect
Corticosteroid administration	Impaired vitamin-D-dependent intestinal calcium absorption leading to increased PTH secretion	Inhibition of osteoblastic activity
Hyperparathyroidism	Increased PTH secretion	Increased osteoclast activity
Hyperthyroidism	Increased thyroid hormone secretion	Increased osteoclast activity
Hypogonadism		
Women	Estrogen deficiency stimulates estrogen-sensitive cytokines	Increased osteoclast activity
Men	Deficiency of anabolic androgens	
Hematologic malignanciesOsteoclast activating factor secreted from plasma cells	Osteoclast activating factor secreted from plasma cells PTH-related protein secretion from tumor	Increased osteoclast activity

CLINICAL MANIFESTATIONS

Often known as the "silent disease," osteoporosis is not manifested until fracture, spinal deformity, or loss of height occurs. Because of the high quantity of cancellous bone in the vertebrae, spinal fractures represent significant sequelae of osteoporosis. Pathologic findings associated with osteoporosis include loss of coarse cancellous bone and thinning of the cortex. The trabeculae in the coarse cancellous bone become structurally impaired, and cortical bone becomes thin and porous, increasing fracture risk.

Compared to women, men have fewer spine and hip fractures because of increased bone mass and strength. Reduced bone size and loss caused by cortical and trabecular thinning characterizes the development of bone fragility in men. Increased bone remodeling in elderly men is often caused by secondary hyperparathyroidism, calcium malabsorption, and vitamin D deficiency.

DIAGNOSIS

Osteoporosis can be identified by the presence of an unexplained fracture. The goal of diagnosis is to identify early bone loss before significant risk develops. Risk for osteoporosis can be determined by tests of bone density and bone quality. The dual-energy X-ray absorptiometry (DEXA) is a specialized, low-level radiographic technique used to measure bone density. Density of both the trabecular and cortical bones can

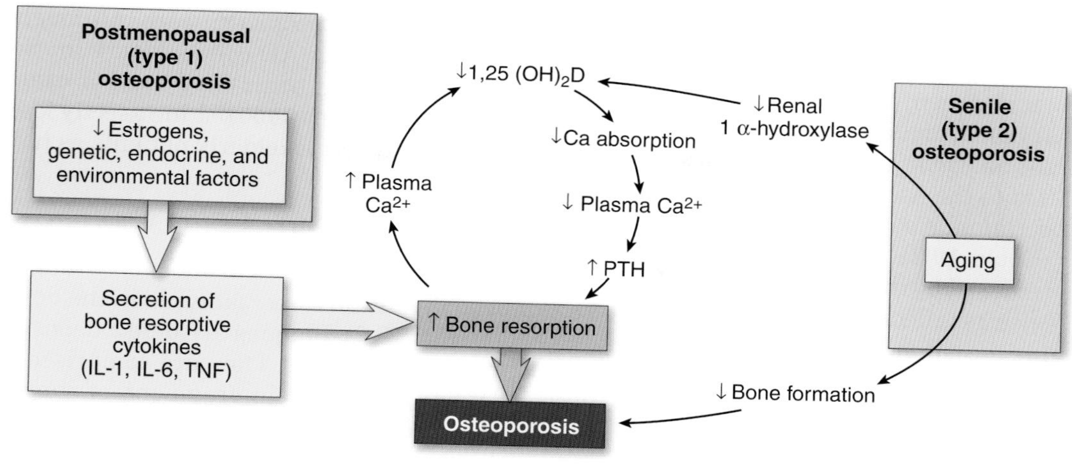

Figure 19.8. Bone remodeling in osteoporosis. Vitamin D promotes the intestinal absorption of calcium. Vitamin D is converted to its active form ($1,25(OH)_2D$) by the renal enzyme 1-alpha-hydroxylase. Age-related decrease in kidney function limits the availability of 1-alpha-hydroxylase. Decreased 1-alpha-hydroxylase stimulation by PTH and an age-related blunted response of the renal tubules to PTH contribute to the development of an imbalance of bone remodeling, favoring resorption. TNF, tumor necrosis factor. (From Rubin E, Farber JL. *Pathology*. 4th ed. Philadelphia, PA: Lippincott Williams & Wilkins; 2005.)

be determined in a single test, and changes in bone density can be determined if the DEXA is done serially, usually annually or biannually. Results of DEXA testing are reported as a *T score*, based on the following guidelines issued by the WHO:

- Normal bone density
  - Bone mass greater than 833 mg/cm^2
  - T score more than −1.0
- Osteopenia
  - Bone mass between 833 and 648 mg/cm^2
  - T score −1.0 to −2.5
- Osteoporosis
  - Bone mass less than 648 mg/cm^2
  - T score less than −2.5

A comparison of an individual T score to persons in the population of the same age and gender is documented using a *Z score*. Report of a Z score of less than −1.5 suggests a secondary, rather than primary, cause for osteoporosis.

Bone quality can be determined by the use of quantitative ultrasound (QUS). Measurement of the passage of an ultrasound beam through the trabecular bone in the heel portion of the foot determines bone structure, strength, and degree of elasticity. Although using an ultrasound measurement of bone quality has many benefits, including cost, time, and convenience, such measurements may not be as accurate as DEXA scanning. Findings of adequate bone quality in the peripheral bone of the heel may not represent similar findings in the central locations of the hip and spine, reducing the ability to generalize findings from one site to the other.

TREATMENT

Prevention of osteoporosis is the ideal treatment. Recommendations for promoting bone health include:

1. Get your daily recommended amounts of calcium and Vitamin D.
2. Engage in regular weight-bearing exercise.
3. Avoid smoking and excessive alcohol.
4. Talk to your doctor about bone health.
5. Have a bone density test and take medication when appropriate.

Calcium intake recommendations include 1,200 mg/d for postmenopausal women and elderly men in divided doses for best absorption. Vitamin D (400 to 600 IU/d) should be included to promote calcium absorption and metabolism. Weight-bearing is

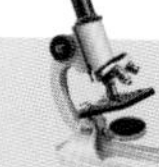

FROM THE LAB

There are no consistent guidelines for laboratory testing to determine causes of secondary osteoporosis. Tests to determine underlying causes of osteoporosis may include a complete blood count, blood chemistry tests (calcium, phosphorus, total protein, liver enzymes, alkaline phosphatase, electrolytes), urinary studies (calcium excretion), and hormonal testing (serum thyrotropin, vitamin D, PTH, cortisol).

important in the stimulation of osteoblastic activity and bone calcification. Even immobile individuals should have a regimen designed to promote bone health or, at a minimum, decrease bone loss.

Most current pharmacologic treatments of osteoporosis are limited to the use of drugs that inhibit or reduce bone resorption, also known as **antiresorptive** medications (Table 19.2). The effectiveness of these medications is caused by the attenuation of the resorptive process with no effect on the formation process, thereby altering the balance in favor of bone formation. Treatments, including calcium, vitamin D, calcitonin, and bisphosphonates, have been shown to be effective in individuals with bone loss caused by corticosteroid use and in postmenopausal women. Bisphosphonates (alendronate and risedronate), calcitonin, estrogens, PTH, and raloxifene are drugs currently approved by the U.S. Food and Drug Administration (FDA) for use to prevent or treat osteoporosis. Teriparatide (Forteo), a form of PTH, is an anabolic agent representing the first treatment for osteoporosis that works by increasing the formation of bone. Teriparatide, when given in a small daily dose, promotes stimulation of new trabecular and cortical bone.

Alzheimer Disease

Alzheimer disease (AD) is the most common neurodegenerative disorder and most frequent cause of dementia in the elderly, affecting more than 5 million people in the United States. It interferes with cognitive and social functioning, has a long and progressive course, and has no known cure. Although not a normal part of aging, AD can look very much like cognitive changes that occur with age. For example, in one study, the neuropathologist incorrectly identified 76% of cognitively intact elderly patients as having AD.[2]

PATHOPHYSIOLOGY

Senile plaques and neurofibrillary tangles are theorized to play an important role in the development of AD (Fig. 19.9). Plaques are dense deposits of protein outside of neurons. They are comprised of beta-amyloid (Ab), a protein fragment of amyloid precursor protein (APP). Ab protein accumulates to form plaques beginning in small clusters (*oligomers*), followed by formation into chains (*fibrils*), and then finally into fibers organized as beta-sheets. In AD, plaques form in the hippocampus and cerebral cortex and impact memory and decision-making.

Healthy neurons need microtubules to bring nutrients to the ends of the axons and back. Tau, a unique protein, binds to microtubules and provides stability, like a backbone. In AD, tau becomes "sticky" and tangles together with other tau threads forming **neurofibrillary tangles**. These neurofibrillary tangles accumulate initially in the temporal lobe, and then become densely concentrated in the medial temporal lobe and hippocampus, important locations for memory formation. The microtubule can no longer perform its role of transporting nutrients to the neuron. The neuron can no longer function, is unable to communicate with other neurons, and eventually dies. Destruction of these neurons and the cholinergic

Table 19.2 Pharmacologic Prevention and Treatment of Osteoporosis

Treatment	Class	Indication	Effect	Comments
Estrogen	Hormone	Prevention	Increased bone density	Risk of endometrial hyperplasia when uterus is present and unopposed by progestin, deep vein thrombosis, breast cancer
Alendronate (Fosamax)	Bisphosphonate	Prevention	Increased bone density	Upper GI distress, myalgias, arthralgias
		Treatment	Reduction in vertebral and hip fracture	
Risedronate (Actonel)	Bisphosphonate	Prevention	Increased bone density	Upper GI distress, myalgias, arthralgias
		Treatment	Reduction in hip fracture	
Raloxifene (Evista)	Selective estrogen receptor modulator (SERM)	Prevention	Increased bone density	Hot flashes, DVT
		Treatment	Reduction in vertebral fracture	
Calcitonin (Micalcin)	Hormone	Treatment	Reduction in vertebral fracture	Rhinorrhea
Teriparatide	Hormone	Treatment	Increased bone formation	Dizziness, leg cramps

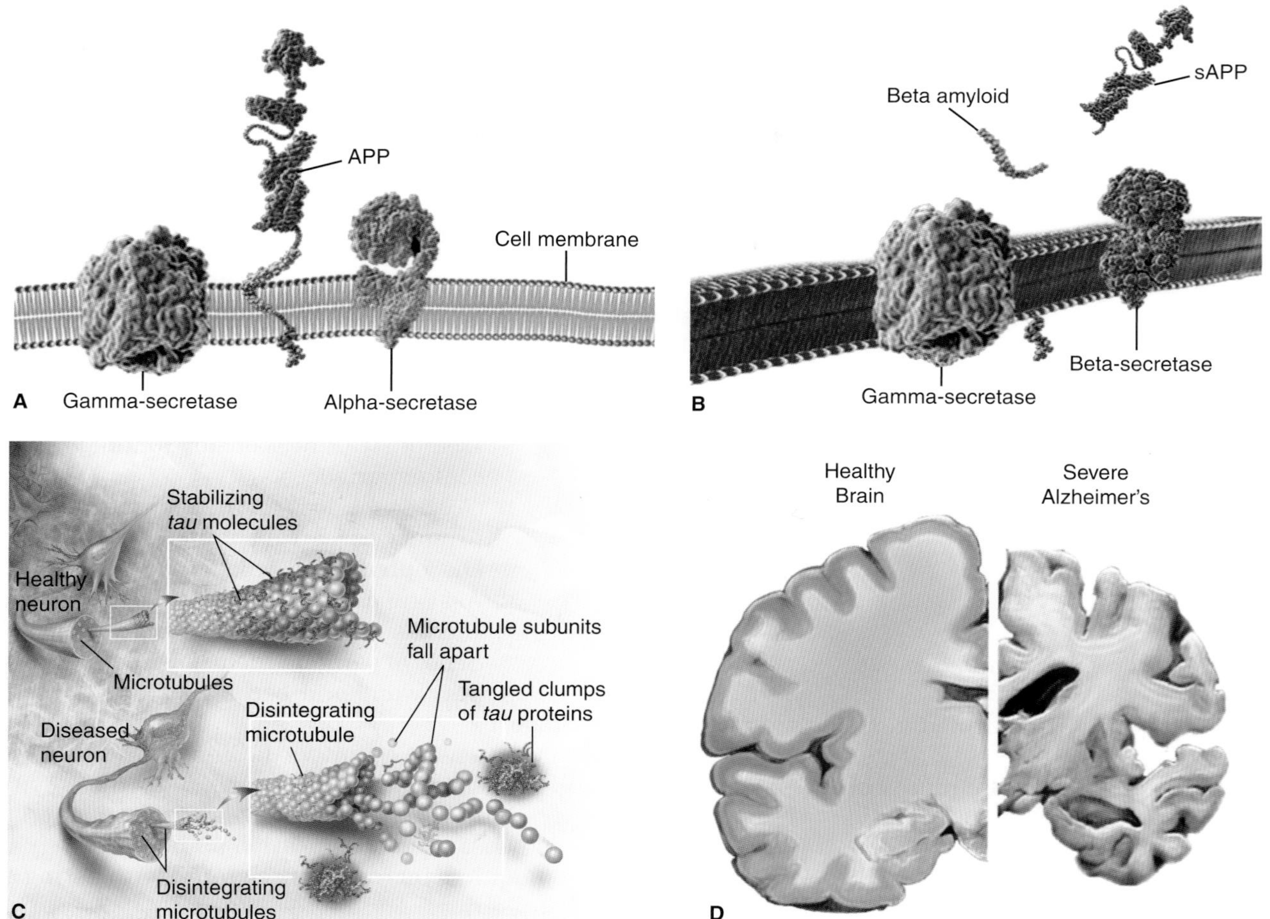

Figure 19.9. Selected pathophysiologic processes in Alzheimer disease. **A:** Amyloid precursor protein (APP) is embedded in the neuron's cell membrane. **B:** Enzymes beta-secretase and gamma-secretase sever soluble amyloid precursor protein beta (sAPPβ), releasing a fragment that becomes beta-amyloid. **C:** Neurofibrillary tangles of tau proteins in microtubules form. **D:** As microtubules disintegrate and more and more neurons die, the brain atrophies (note differences in the healthy and Alzheimer disease-affected brain). (Images courtesy of the Alzheimer's Disease Education and Referral Center, a service of the National Institute on Aging.)

system causes memory failure, inability to perform activities of daily living, and personality changes. Neurofibrillary tangles continue to form, progressing to regions throughout the cortex and impacting executive, motor, and sensory function. The relationship between neurofibrillary tangles and ameloid (senile plaque) deposits is not clearly understood. However, dementia severity appears to correlate with the number and location of neurofibrillary tangles.

AD occurs as a result of genetic and environmental factors. Sporadic, late-onset AD is most common and with about 20% of cases clustering in families. The following genes have been definitively associated with AD, and many others with a probable role have been identified:

- Amyloid precursor protein (*APP*) gene
- Presenilin-1 (*PS1*) gene
- Presenilin-2 (*PS2*) gene

Mutations in these genes result in proteins that have neurotoxic properties and promote neuronal death, synapse loss, and the formation of neurofibrillary tangles and senile plaques. Several risk factors have been identified including later age, family history, obesity, dyslipidemia, hypertension, Down syndrome, history of traumatic brain injury, lead exposure, and history of depression.

CLINICAL MANIFESTATIONS

AD is characterized by a global cognitive decline, changes in behavior, and eventual complete loss of function. Initial symptoms mimic processes of natural aging and include:

- Memory loss
- Confusion

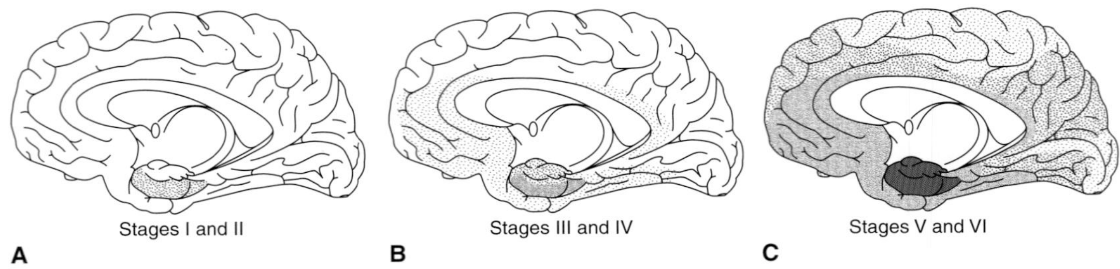

Figure 19.10. The spread of neurofibrillary tangles in Alzheimer disease. **A:** Preclinical. **B:** Initial clinical symptoms. **C:** Fully developed Alzheimer disease. (Adapted from Braak H, Braak E. Frequency of stages of Alzheimer-related lesions in different age categories. *Neurobiol Aging.* 1997;18(4):351–357.)

- Restlessness
- Mood swings
- Difficulty in interpreting visual information

AD progresses through seven stages, with greater brain involvement as the patient moves through each stage (Fig. 19.10):

- Stage 1
  - Minimal cognitive impairment
- Stage 2
  - Mild cognitive impairment (evident only to self)
    - Memory lapse
    - Forgetfulness of familiar words
    - Altered memory of location of everyday objects
- Stage 3
  - Mild cognitive impairment (evident among friends, family, coworkers)
    - Difficulty with word or name finding
    - Decreased performance at work or home
    - Difficulty with reading retention
    - Misplacing valuable objects
    - Impaired organization or planning
- Stage 4
  - Moderate cognitive decline (evident by examiner)
    - Decline in knowledge of current events or occasions
    - Impaired mathematical ability
    - Impaired performance of complex tasks (e.g., bill paying, planning meals)
    - Difficulty remembering personal history
    - Change in personality (subdued or withdrawn)
- Stage 5
  - Moderately severe cognitive decline
    - Exhibits major memory and cognitive deficits
    - Requires assistance in day-to-day activities
- Stage 6
  - Severe cognitive decline
    - Significant personality changes
    - Increased need for help in activities of daily living
  - Worsening memory
    - Loss of awareness of surroundings and recent experiences
    - Occasional loss of memory of spouse's/primary caregiver's name
    - Disrupted sleep/wake cycle
    - Assistance needed with toileting details
    - Increasing episodes of incontinence
    - Sense of paranoia, delusions, hallucinations
    - May wander or become lost
- Stage 7
  - Very severe cognitive decline
    - Loss of ability to respond to the environment, including speech and movement
    - Loss of communication ability
  - Requires increasing assistance with eating and toileting
  - Impaired swallowing, positioning, and reflex response

DIAGNOSIS

A definitive diagnosis of AD can be made only with an autopsy when typical characteristics of plaques and tangles can be seen. Other testing can be done that, when combined with clinical presentation and history, may support a diagnosis of AD. A thorough neurologic evaluation should be completed, which includes a mental status examination to determine sense of time and place, communication ability, memory, comprehension, and ability to complete simple math problems. Evaluation of reasoning ability, balance, and visual/motor coordination should also be completed. A brain scan, MRI, or CT scan may be done to rule out other pathology.

TREATMENT

Treatment of AD includes supportive care for the individuals and their families. Focus on maximizing quality of life and general health is the cornerstone of care. The mainstay of pharmacologic therapy for patients is the use of centrally acting cholinesterase inhibitors to attempt to compensate for the depletion of acetylcholine (ACh) in the cerebral cortex and hippocampus. Various other medications are used for treatment depending upon the presence of secondary symptoms of AD, including antidepressants, anti-anxiety agents, and antipsychotic agents.

thePoint® To see a video on dementia, visit http://thePoint.lww.com

SUMMARY

- Aging is a normal condition that can be complicated by degenerative changes affecting health status.
- The cellular basis of aging reflects the influences of genetics and cumulative effects of damage over time. This multifactorial process contributes to the typical manifestations of aging.
- Manifestations of aging reflect physiologic changes characteristic of human patterns of development. Changes in the soft tissues of the skin and hair contribute to the typical outward appearance of aging.
- Altered structure and function resulting from degenerative aging changes may lead to functional impairment or may be exacerbated by chronic pathologic conditions.
- Alterations in fluid and electrolyte balance, immune responses, cellular proliferation, neurologic function, mobility, perfusion, nutrition, elimination, and metabolic processes represent areas of potential pathologic sequelae related to body system changes in aging.
- Although there is no way to halt the aging process, health promotion across the life span may improve quality of life and attenuate many age-associated degenerative changes.

CASE STUDY 19.1

A.Z., a 65-year-old woman, was having a follow-up visit with her physician. She was concerned about a change in her sleeping habits, including taking at least 30 minutes to fall asleep. She woke up after only about 5 to 6 hours of sleep and found herself unable to fall asleep again. She consequently got sleepy in the afternoon and took frequent naps.

1. What are some causes of age-associated sleep disorders?
2. What are the typical changes in sleep patterns that occur in response to age?
3. What causes age-related changes in sleep patterns?
4. What are the risks related to the use of pharmacologic sleeping aids in the elderly?
5. What nonpharmacologic strategies can be used to help promote sleep?

Log onto the Internet. Search for a relevant journal article or Web site, such as http://emedicine.medscape.com/article/291573-overview, that details sleep disorders in the elderly to confirm your predictions.

PRACTICE EXAM QUESTIONS

1. Genetic influences as the major determinants of aging are the focus of which of the following theories?
   a. Developmental theory
   b. Stochastic theory
   c. Free radical theory
   d. Error theory

2. Typical changes in total body water in the elderly include:
   a. Increased total body water caused by increase in muscle mass
   b. Increased total body water caused by increased fat mass
   c. Decreased total body water caused by decrease in muscle mass
   d. Decreased total body water caused by decreased fat mass

3. Immune senescence is characterized by:
   a. Increased antigenic immune response
   b. Enhanced T-cell function
   c. Enhanced IgE-mediated hypersensitivity
   d. Enhanced autoimmune response

4. Age-related changes affecting neurologic function include:
   a. Increased myelin
   b. Decreased number of neurons
   c. Enhanced nerve conduction
   d. Improved axonal repair mechanisms

5. An imbalance in bone remodeling characteristic of osteoporosis is caused by:
   a. Enhanced bone formation caused by increased activity of osteoclasts
   b. Enhanced bone formation caused by increased activity of osteoblasts
   c. Increased bone resorption caused by increased activity of osteoclasts
   d. Increased bone resorption caused by increased activity of osteoblasts

6. Age-related changes contributing to impaired healing include:
   a. Increased skin elasticity
   b. Enhanced subcutaneous fat
   c. Decreased superficial capillary perfusion
   d. Atrophied capillary support to dermis

7. Osteoporosis is the result of an imbalance favoring increased
   a. Osteoblastic activity
   b. Osteoclastic activity
   c. Vitamin D absorption
   d. Calcium absorption

8. Mortality for patients with progeria is most commonly a result of:
   a. Rapid aging
   b. Atherosclerosis
   c. Scleroderma
   d. Psychosis

9. Which of the following is a characteristic finding in progeria?
   a. High levels of hyaluronic acid
   b. Low levels of calcitonin
   c. High levels of thyrotoxicine
   d. Low levels of 1-dioxyglutamine

10. Memory loss in Alzheimer disease results from impaired neural conduction in the
   a. Frontal lobe
   b. Basal ganglia
   c. Limbic system
   d. Hippocampus

DISCUSSION AND APPLICATION

1. What did I know about degenerative changes in aging before today?
2. What body processes are affected by degenerative changes in aging? How do degenerative changes in aging affect those processes?
3. What are the potential etiologies for degenerative changes in aging? How do degenerative changes in aging develop?
4. Who is most at risk for developing complications related to degenerative changes in aging? How can these alterations be prevented?
5. What are the human differences that affect the etiology, risk, or course of degenerative changes in aging?
6. What clinical manifestations are expected in the course of degenerative changes in aging?
7. What special diagnostic tests are useful in determining the diagnosis and course of degenerative changes in aging?
8. What are the goals of care for individuals with degenerative changes in aging?
9. How does the concept of degenerative changes in aging build on what I have learned in the previous chapter and in the previous courses?
10. How can I use what I have learned?

RESOURCES

Alzheimer Association:
http://www.alz.org

National Center for Chronic Disease Prevention and Health Promotion: Healthy Aging
http://www.cdc.gov/aging/index.htm

National Institute on Aging:
http://www.grc.nia.nih.gov

National Osteoporosis Foundation:
http://nof.org

Progeria Research Foundation:
http://www.progeriaresearch.org/

References

1. Luders E, Cherbuin N, Kurth F. Forever young(er): potential age-defying effects of long-term meditation on gray matter atrophy. *Front Psychol*. 2015;5:1551. doi:10.3389/fpsyg.2014.01551.
2. Brayne C, Richardson K, Matthews FE, et al. Neuropathological correlates of dementia in over-80-year-old brain donors from the population-based Cambridge city over-75s cohort (CC75C) study. *J Alzheimers Dis*. 2009;18(3):645–658.

Find additional resources for this chapter at http:thePoint.lww.com thePoint®

Integrated Pathophysiologic Concepts

Chapter

20

LEARNING OUTCOMES

1. Define and use the key terms listed in this chapter.
2. Recognize the effects of combining pathophysiologic concepts on the health of the individual.
3. Identify how previous concepts within this text relate to diabetes mellitus.
4. Differentiate type 1, type 2, and gestational diabetes.
5. Identify common clinical manifestations of diabetes.
6. Recognize short-term and long-term complications of diabetes.
7. Describe diagnostic tests and treatment strategies appropriate for diabetes.

INTRODUCTION

The human body is highly complex. We have attempted to distinguish functional alterations in human health by introducing you to concepts of pathophysiology. What you have probably figured out by now is that very few health conditions fit purely into one or two conceptual categories. For example, myocardial infarction (MI) is a problem of *perfusion*. MI also has roots in altered *nutrition*, *genetics*, and the *environment*. MI results in myocardial *inflammation* and induces a *stress response*. *Hormones*, such as cortisol, are released during stressful situations to aid in reestablishing homeostasis. The ineffective myocardium is less able to move fluids through the circulation, resulting in altered *fluid balance*. Pulmonary congestion may result, leading to altered *ventilation and diffusion*. The goal of this chapter is to illustrate the impact of combining complex pathophysiologic concepts using diabetes mellitus as the select clinical model.

Glucose, Insulin, Energy, and the Pancreas

Energy, in the form of glucose, is essential for optimal human functioning. Glucose is a monosaccharide, which is derived from dietary carbohydrates. Excess glucose is stored as glycogen in the liver. Glucose in the blood triggers the release of insulin. **Insulin** is an anabolic hormone required for the uptake of glucose by the many cells, particularly those of the liver, muscle, and adipose cells. Insulin is *not* required for glucose uptake in the brain, red blood cells, kidney, and lens of the eye.

Stop and Consider

In the absence of insulin, glucose is still able to move into cells of the brain, blood, kidney, and lens. This seems a beneficial property. What do you think is the drawback of inadequate insulin, resulting in excessive circulating glucose to these cells?

Anabolic hormones, including insulin, are responsible for building complex compounds in the body, such as building proteins from amino acids. Insulin has several key functions:

- Promoting glucose usage, thereby decreasing blood glucose levels
- Promoting protein synthesis
- Promoting the formation and storage of lipids
- Facilitating transport of potassium, phosphate, and magnesium into the cells

Insulin production and availability are closely connected to the pancreas. The pancreas is located behind the lower portion of the stomach and is innervated by the autonomic nervous system. The pancreas has both endocrine and exocrine functions. The **endocrine pancreas** secretes hormones, such as insulin and glucagon. The acini cells of the **exocrine pancreas** secrete digestive enzymes and alkaline fluids through the pancreatic duct into the duodenum. Chapter 15 was concerned with the role of the pancreas as a digestive accessory organ. This chapter is concerned with the endocrine, or hormone-secreting, function of the pancreas.

Throughout the pancreas are clusters of cells called the **islets of Langerhans** (Fig. 20.1). The islets of Langerhans contain three major types of hormone-secreting cells:

- *Alpha* cells secrete glucagon, which mobilizes glycogen from the liver and suppresses insulin secretion; glucagon is critical in maintaining blood glucose levels between meals.
- *Beta* cells secrete insulin, which promotes glucose utilization.
- *Delta* cells secrete somatostatin and gastrin, which regulates alpha and beta cell function by suppressing the release of insulin, glucagon, and pancreatic polypeptides.

The pancreas also contains F cells, which are located primarily at the periphery of the islets, although a few F cells are scattered throughout the ducts and acini. F cells secrete pancreatic polypeptides, which suppress digestive enzyme release from the exocrine pancreas.

Stop and Consider

If you skipped breakfast and had a really low blood glucose level, which cells of the islets of Langerhans would you expect to be stimulated?

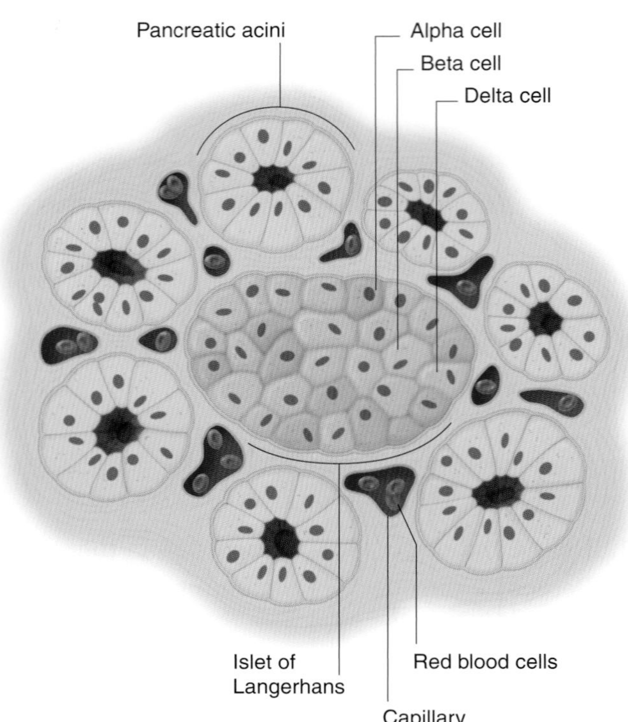

Figure 20.1. Islets of Langerhans in the pancreas.

The hormones secreted from the islets of Langerhans are important controlling devices of carbohydrate, protein, and fat metabolism. As with other hormones, feedback systems are critical to maintaining homeostasis. With insulin, secretion is *increased* when there are elevations in (1) blood glucose; (2) amino acids; (3) potassium, phosphate, and magnesium; and (4) glucagon and gastrin. Insulin is needed to promote glucose uptake and metabolism of nutrients. Certain situations also promote a *decrease* in insulin secretion, such as low blood glucose, high levels of insulin (through negative feedback mechanisms), and the stimulation of alpha cells. In these cases, insulin is not needed because it would exacerbate the state of hypoglycemia.

Stop and Consider

How does eating a large meal or skipping a meal affect insulin levels in the body?

Diabetes Mellitus

Diabetes mellitus is a group of disorders, characterized by the inability to regulate the amount of glucose in the body, leading to the inadequate metabolism of protein, fats, and carbohydrates. The different types of diabetes are summarized in Table 20.1 and explained in detail in this chapter. Diabetes

TABLE 20.1 Comparison of Types of Diabetes Mellitus

	Onset	Cause	Treatment
Type 1	Puberty or childhood (peak at 10–14 years); although increasing in adulthood	Insulin deficit	Insulin replacement balanced with exercise and diet
Type 2	Adult years (peak at age 45 years); although increasing in those under age 45 years	Insulin resistance or impaired ability of the tissues to use insulin; insufficient insulin in relation to the needs of the body	Diet, exercise, oral glycemic agents, possibly insulin
Gestational	Pregnancy (peak at fifth or sixth month gestation)	Insulin resistance during pregnancy as a result of too much hormone production in the body (for the placenta); inability to make the additional insulin that is needed during pregnancy	Diet, exercise, sometimes insulin, delivery of baby

insipidus, a condition of inadequate antidiuretic hormone, was discussed in Chapter 13. Many other secondary conditions can lead to diabetes; these are summarized in Box 20.1.

One or a combination of the following characterizes the basic pathophysiology in the various types of diabetes:

1. A complete destruction of pancreatic beta cells leading to a lack of insulin secretion
2. Reduced insulin secretion from impaired beta cell function in response to glucose stimulation
3. A peripheral resistance to insulin

The absence, deficit, or resistance to insulin leads to a state of **hyperglycemia**, which is a significant elevation in blood glucose level, coupled with the inability to transport glucose and amino acids into those cells that require insulin for transport. Liver, muscle, and adipose cells become deprived of glucose as an energy source and must turn to other less efficient sources, such as body fats or even proteins, for energy. To see a video on hormonal control of blood sugar, visit http://thePoint.lww.com. thePoint®

Box 20.1 Secondary Conditions That Can Lead to Insulin Deficit or Resistance

- Diseases of the pancreas that destroy pancreatic beta cells
- Pancreatitis
- Cystic fibrosis
- Pancreatic cancer
- Hormonal syndromes that interfere with insulin secretion or cause peripheral insulin resistance
- Pheochromocytoma
- Acromegaly
- Cushing syndrome
- Stress, such as occurs with severe medical illness or surgery, because increases in glucagon, catecholamines, cortisol, and growth hormone levels antagonize the secretion or effects of insulin
- Certain medications
- Phenytoin
- Glucocorticoids
- Estrogens

INSULIN DEFICIT: TYPE 1 DIABETES MELLITUS

Type 1 diabetes is a chronic problem of carbohydrate, fat, and protein metabolism. The body is unable to metabolize nutrients because of an absolute or significant deficiency of insulin. Approximately 10% of individuals with diabetes are categorized as type 1. This type of diabetes was previously known as insulin-dependent diabetes mellitus (IDDM) or juvenile-onset diabetes to reflect the most common treatment modality (insulin replacement) and age at diagnosis (approximately 10 to 14 years of age). However, type 1 diabetes is becoming increasingly common in adults.

Pathophysiology

The etiology of type 1 diabetes is multifactorial and includes both genetic and environmental influences leading to autoimmune destruction of beta cells. The importance of genetic susceptibility has been demonstrated in studies of identical twins (25% to 50% greater risk in second twin if one twin is diagnosed) and the presence of certain antigens expressed on the major histocompatibility complex (MHC; see Chapter 4) in those with type 1 diabetes. Exposure to a trigger in the environment, such as a virus or toxin, stimulates cell-mediated destruction and a process of autoimmunity that promotes destruction of the beta cells. Most beta islet cell antibodies are directed against glutamic acid decarboxylase (GAD), a chemical within the beta cells. Examples of triggering environmental agents include infection with mumps, group-B coxsackie viruses, or intrauterine rubella exposure.

Cell-mediated immune mechanisms (more specifically, the presence of cytotoxic T lymphocytes) destroy beta cells. Autoimmune destruction triggers a chronic inflammatory response. Inflammation contributes to further destruction of beta cells and impaired insulin secretion. In the early stages of this cell-mediated immune destruction, antibodies against beta cells are circulating, but hyperglycemia is not yet present. This is considered a state of "prediabetes" and can last for several years. Clinical manifestations and detection of diabetes usually occur when autoimmune processes destroy 80% to 90% or more of the beta cells of the pancreas. Over time, the exocrine pancreas becomes fibrotic with the subsequent atrophy of acinar cells.

Type 1 diabetes also affects alpha cell function, resulting in increased levels of glucagon. Recall that glucagon suppresses insulin production. This, coupled with beta cell destruction, leads to a state of hyperglycemia and hyperketonemia. Hyperglycemia is a result of accumulations of circulating blood glucose unmatched by insulin for use in the cell. The body is starving for energy and turns to fat stores and protein for energy. Insulin inhibits lipolysis (fat breakdown). Therefore, the reduction or absence of insulin allows the unregulated mobilization of fats for energy. As a result, fat oxidation produces **hyperketonemia** (excess circulating ketone bodies), composed of acetoacetic acid, acetone, and β-hydroxybutyric acid, leading to a state of metabolic **ketoacidosis**.

Hyperglycemia, even when not associated with ketoacidosis, is problematic and can lead to osmotic diuresis. Osmotic diuresis is a condition in which excess glucose promotes the attraction of water into the kidneys, thereby eliminating glucose, electrolytes, and water through the urine. This can lead to severe dehydration. Hyperglycemia also undermines white blood cell function, promotes infection, and impairs wound healing.

Stop and Consider

How does an insulin deficit compare to marasmus as described in Chapter 17?

Clinical Manifestations

The clinical manifestations of type 1 diabetes mellitus are related to severe hyperglycemia and hyperketonemia, as well as to inadequate energy and nutrient metabolism (Fig. 20.2). These manifestations often appear abruptly despite months or even years of beta cell destruction. The clinical manifestations most commonly associated with type 1 diabetes include:

- **Polydipsia**—excessive thirst
- **Polyuria**—excessive urination
- **Polyphagia**—excessive hunger

Other symptoms include **nocturia** (urination at night), fatigue, lethargy, unexplained weight loss, and blurred vision. The clinical manifestations, along with the pathophysiologic origins, are outlined in Table 20.2.

Diagnostic Criteria

The diagnosis of type 1 diabetes mellitus is based on a thorough patient history and physical examination, including specific laboratory and diagnostic tests. The presence of polyuria, polydipsia, polyphagia, weight loss, and fatigue, along with an elevation in the fasting blood glucose above 126 mg/dL or the random blood glucose level above 200 mg/dL, is usually sufficient for diagnosis. Checking urine for ketones can also provide information on the presence of hyperketonemia; urine ketone levels are proportional to blood ketone levels. Islet cell autoantibodies can be detected in the early stages of type 1 diabetes as well as autoantibodies against GAD, an enzyme produced by pancreatic islet cells, which persist over time. Table 20.3 provides a guide to laboratory tests useful in the diagnosis of type 1 diabetes.

Treatment

Treatment of diabetes mellitus requires a balance of the following:

1. Glycemic control
2. Exercise
3. Insulin replacement therapy

The goal of treatment is to stabilize blood glucose levels within the expected range (70 to 120 mg/dL). Blood glucose levels are measured frequently using self-blood glucose monitoring systems (Fig. 20.3). Food intake

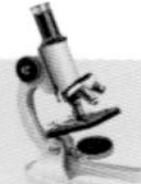

FROM THE LAB

Glycosylated hemoglobin (HbA_{1c}) is a blood test that depicts hemoglobin and red blood cell exposure to glucose over the previous 3 to 4 months. In prolonged hyperglycemia, found in both type 1 and type 2 diabetes, the hemoglobin that travels on the red blood cell becomes irreversibly combined with glucose, a situation termed glycosylation, for the life of that red blood cell (120 days). HbA_{1c} is therefore a useful determinant of "average" exposure of red blood cells to glucose over that period. The higher the HbA_{1c}, the more hyperglycemic, or uncontrolled, the diabetes has been. The goal for those with diabetes should be 7% or below. Persons with elevations in HbA_{1c} are at greater risk for long-term complications, including cardiovascular disease and death.

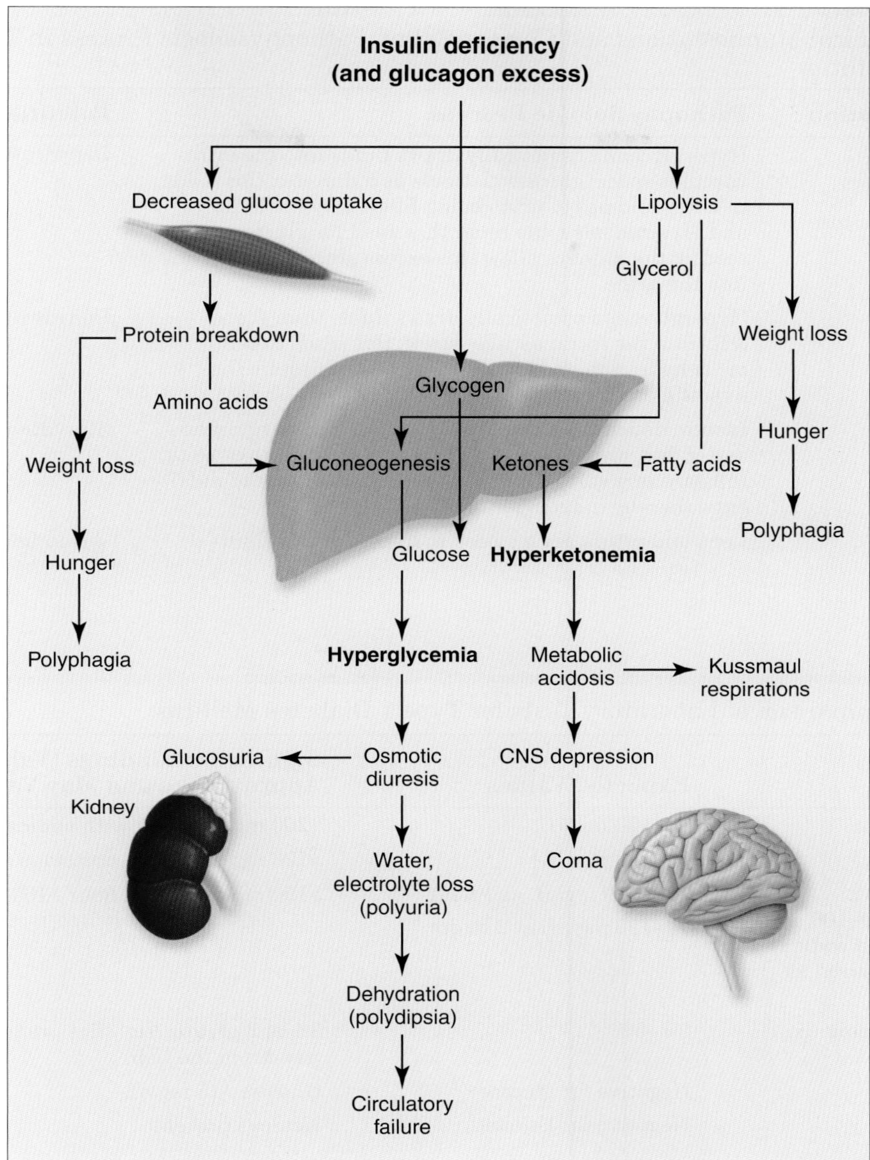

Figure 20.2. Concept map. Mechanisms of hyperglycemia and hyperketonemia. CNS, central nervous system. (Modified from Porth CM. *Essentials of Pathophysiology: Concepts of Altered Health States*. Philadelphia, PA: Lippincott Williams & Wilkins; 2003.)

increases blood glucose levels. Therefore, food intake must equal the available insulin and metabolic needs of the body. The diet should include complex carbohydrates, protein, and unsaturated fat sources while limiting simple sugars, cholesterol, and saturated fats. Typically, the carbohydrate to insulin ratio needed is around 10 to 15 grams of carbohydrate to 1 unit of rapid-acting insulin. Exercise decreases blood glucose levels through increased glucose usage by muscle tissue. Increases in exercise must be matched with reductions in insulin or increases in food intake.

Insulin replacement therapy is integral to the treatment plan for type 1 diabetes. Insulin is destroyed in the gastrointestinal tract if taken orally, so it must be injected subcutaneously via intermittent injections or with an insulin infusion pump. The onset, peak, and duration of action can vary among different types of insulin and include:

1. Rapid onset, short acting (also called regular)
2. Intermediate acting
3. Slow onset, long acting

Table 20.4 distinguishes the different forms of insulin based on onset, peak, and duration of action. The goal is to coordinate food intake with insulin availability in the body. Injecting insulin without

TABLE 20.2 Clinical Manifestations and Corresponding Pathophysiologic Process in Type 1 Diabetes Mellitus

Clinical Manifestation	Pathophysiologic Process	Potential Complications
Polyuria Nocturia Glucosuria (excess glucose in the urine)	Hyperglycemia osmotically draws fluids into the intravascular space; glucose also acts as a diuretic; this leads to large volumes of urine being filtered by the kidneys and excreted; also, the renal threshold for glucose is exceeded; the kidneys allow this excess glucose to spill out into the urine	Dehydration
Polydipsia Dry mouth	Hyperglycemia osmotically draws fluids from the cells into the intravascular space; this leads to cellular dehydration and the stimulation of thirst by the hypothalamus	Dehydration
Polyphagia Weight loss Fatigue	Insulin deficit disallows use of glucose for energy; storage of fats, proteins, and carbohydrates begin to deplete; cells are in a state of starvation because of lack of nutrients, thereby inducing hunger	Starvation, coma, death
Blurred vision	Lens and retina are exposed to hyperosmolar fluids	Vision impairment, blindness

TABLE 20.3 Comparison of Laboratory Tests for Type 1 Diabetes Mellitus

Diagnostic Test	Expected Values	Significant Findings (Values Are Approximate and May Vary by Source)
Random blood glucose	70–120 mg/dL	>200 mg/dL along with clinical manifestations
Fasting blood glucose	70–120 mg/dL	>126 mg/dL on two occasions after fasting
Glucose tolerance test: individual is given 50–100 g of glucose dissolved in water; blood glucose is measured at 1, 2, and 3 hours	120–160 mg/dL at 1 hour 70–120 mg/dL at 2 hours	>190 mg/dL after 1 hour >165 mg/dL after 2 hours
Glycosylated hemoglobin (A_{1c})	2%–6%	8% and greater signifies prolonged hyperglycemia (see From the Lab)
Urinalysis	Negative for glucose Negative for ketones	Glucose >15 mg/dL Ketones present

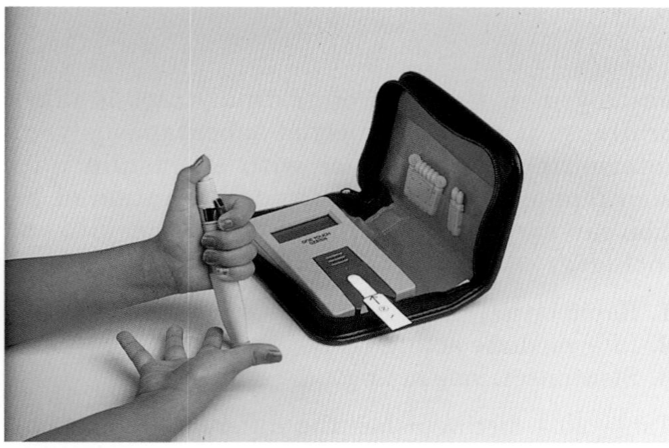

Figure 20.3. The child uses an automatic lancet to get blood sample **(left)** and blood glucose monitor to determine blood glucose level **(right)**.

adequate dietary intake induces **hypoglycemia**, or low blood glucose levels.

Insulin infusion pumps are an alternative to daily injections. An insulin pump looks like a pager and can be worn inconspicuously on a belt, in a pocket, or on an elastic band wrapped around an arm or leg. The insulin is delivered through a plastic catheter into subcutaneous tissue of the abdomen. An insulin pump is able to simulate the pancreas' delivery of insulin more closely than insulin injections. Most people on the pump find that they are able to achieve better control of their blood glucose levels because the insulin is delivered continuously (at a basal rate) and in a bolus for mealtimes or times of physical activity. When an insulin pump is used, blood glucose levels must be checked more frequently.

TABLE 20.4 Comparison of Types of Insulin

Insulin	Rapid-acting (i.e., Lispro)	Short-acting (i.e. Regular, Humulin R)	Intermediate-acting (i.e., NPH)	Long-acting (i.e., Ultralente)	Other (i.e., Glargine)
Onset of action	15 minutes	30 minutes	2–4 hours	6–10 hours	2–4 hours
Peak (in hours)	1	2–3	4–12	8–12	Peakless
Duration (in hours)	2–4	3–6	12–20	20–26	Up to 24
When to Administer	Immediately before a meal	Throughout the day	Throughout the day	Nighttime	Nighttime

NPH, neutral protamine Hagedorn (Hagedorn discovered in 1936 that when protamine was added to insulin, it prolonged the effects).

INSULIN RESISTANCE AND REDUCTION: TYPE 2 DIABETES

Type 2 diabetes mellitus is a problem of insulin resistance (reduced tissue sensitivity to insulin) *and* a reduction in adequate insulin secretion. Most (90%) individuals with diabetes are estimated to have type 2 diabetes. This form was previously referred to as non–insulin-dependent diabetes or adult-onset diabetes, although some individuals with type 2 diabetes may require insulin replacement, and the incidence is increasing in children. Maturity-onset diabetes of the young (MODY) is a rare form of type 2 diabetes that has a strong genetic component (autosomal dominant inheritance) and is found to affect individuals younger than 25 years of age. The metabolic syndrome is a condition that includes insulin resistance and a constellation of other metabolic problems, including obesity, high triglyceride levels, low high-density lipoprotein levels, hypertension, and coronary heart disease. Individuals diagnosed with type 2 diabetes must also be evaluated for metabolic syndrome to determine the full range of metabolic alterations. Gestational diabetes (discussed later) is also considered a form of type 2 diabetes that presents during pregnancy.

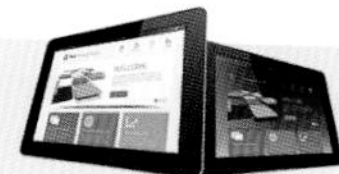

RESEARCH NOTES

Diabetic neuropathy is a common and problematic complication of diabetes. A recent study compared nerve excitability testing in patients who performed daily insulin injections compared with patients using a continuous subcutaneous insulin infusion pump. Results demonstrated significant differences in nerve axon function between the daily injections and those using a continuous pump. Axonal function remained normal in those on continuous insulin infusions, whereas function was impaired with those on daily injections. Researchers concluded that continuous infusion likely has a neuroprotective effect for patients with type 1 diabetes.[1]

Pathophysiology

Similar to type 1 diabetes, the exact cause of type 2 diabetes is unknown; however, genetic and environmental factors appear to contribute to its development. The most significant risk factor is obesity, which results from both genetic and environmental influences. Approximately 90% of those who develop type 2 diabetes are obese. All overweight individuals have insulin resistance, but only those who are unable to compensate by increasing beta cell production of insulin go on to develop type 2 diabetes. Other risk factors include age over 30 years, a family history of type 2 diabetes, and Native American, Hispanic, or Black race.

Unlike type 1 diabetes, there is no autoimmune destruction of the pancreas. Rather, insulin *resistance,* or a decreased sensitivity to insulin in metabolic tissues, such as the liver, skeletal muscle, and adipose tissue, results in insufficient insulin usage (Fig. 20.4). Obesity promotes peripheral insulin resistance by releasing free fatty acids and cytokines from adipose cells. These chemicals interfere with insulin signals, disrupt insulin receptors on the target cell plasma membranes, and prohibit insulin from facilitating the entry of glucose into liver, muscle, and adipose tissues. Individuals with type 2 diabetes also exhibit reduced insulin secretion in response to glucose exposure. In type 2 diabetes, subadequate levels of insulin and peripheral resistance to insulin uptake leads to the following:

1. Beta cells do not adequately respond to circulating blood glucose levels.
2. The release of glycogen from the liver coupled with the suppression of insulin by glucagon promotes excessive circulating glucose.
3. The insulin receptors in the liver, skeletal muscle, and adipose tissue are unresponsive, thereby making the tissues unable, or resistant to, using the insulin.

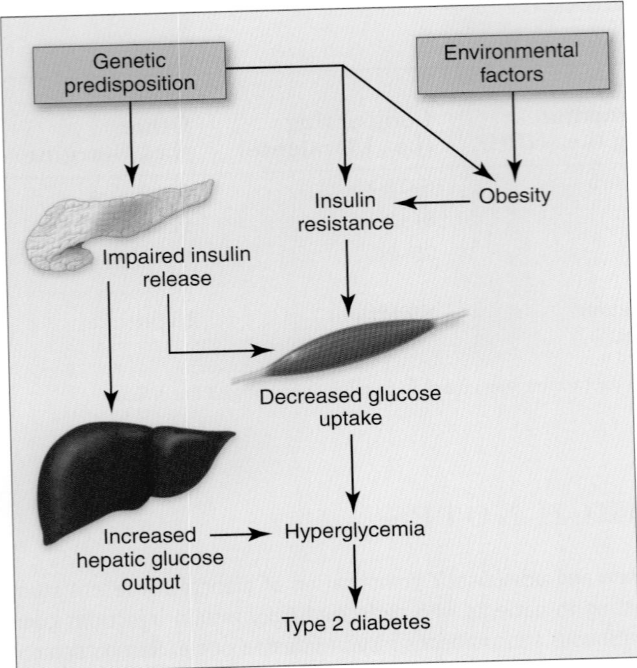

Figure 20.4. Pathogenesis of type 2 diabetes. (Modified from Porth CM. *Essentials of Pathophysiology: Concepts of Altered Health States*. Philadelphia, PA: Lippincott Williams & Wilkins; 2003.)

Glucagon secretion is significantly increased. Recall that glucagon mobilizes glycogen from the liver and suppresses insulin secretion. Although there is no reduction in beta cells, high serum lipid levels, as may occur with obesity, allows fat to deposit in the pancreas, which may lead to sclerosis and further impair pancreatic function. Ultimately, this results in the impaired metabolism of carbohydrates, fats, and proteins.

Clinical Manifestations

The clinical manifestations for type 2 diabetes are often insidious and nonspecific. In some cases, the classic symptoms for type 1 diabetes (polyuria, polyphagia, and polydipsia) may be present. Most of the time, however, clinical manifestations that appear are related to long-term complications that may arise with diabetes, such as visual changes, changes in kidney function, coronary artery disease, peripheral vascular disease, recurrent infections, or neuropathy. The presence of obesity and hyperlipidemia should heighten suspicion that type 2 diabetes is present.

Diagnostic Criteria

Those identified within the risk categories for type 2 diabetes should be evaluated by random or fasting blood glucose measurements. Many individuals with type 2 diabetes are asymptomatic and the disease goes undiagnosed for many years. As with individuals who have type 1 diabetes, those individuals with clinical manifestations (i.e., polyuria, polydipsia, polyphagia, nocturia, and weight loss) and random plasma glucose levels above 200 mg/dL are easily diagnosed as having diabetes. A major diagnostic challenge is differentiating type 1 from type 2 diabetes. More often, individuals with type 2 diabetes are overweight adults, but this is not always the case. Upon diagnosis, it is not unusual for blood glucose levels to be less than that found with type 1 diabetes because insulin is still available. If diabetes is suspected, two separate fasting blood glucose measurements are warranted. If both are above 126 mg/dL, type 2 diabetes may be suggested. A fasting plasma glucose between 110 and 125 mg/dL indicates "impaired fasting glucose" and requires close monitoring because there is a high risk of developing diabetes over time. The presence of antibodies against the islet cells or GAD would indicate that this person does *not* have type 2 diabetes, but rather has type 1.

Treatment

Treatment of type 2 diabetes begins with weight control through an individualized nutrition and exercise plan and can include oral glycemic agents or insulin replacement therapy. The goal of treatment for type 2 diabetes is the same as that of type 1: to maintain optimal blood glucose levels. Physical activity is advantageous because it increases the uptake of glucose by the muscles without increasing insulin needs. Exercise also improves insulin sensitivity. The other positive

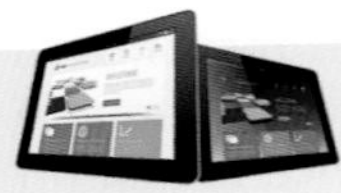

RESEARCH NOTES

Multiple studies are identifying links between lifestyle factors and the onset of type 2 diabetes. One such study systematically reviewed associations between consumption of beverages sweetened with sugar, artificial sweeteners, and fruit juice in over 38,000 patients. Higher consumption of sugar was associated with the onset of type 2 diabetes independent of body fat at diagnosis. Results for artificial sweeteners were unclear and there was not a significant association determined with consumption of fruit juice, although it was determined unlikely that fruit juice would serve as a healthy alternative to sugar-sweetened beverages. Researchers estimated that 1.8 million cases of type 2 diabetes could be attributed to consumption of sugar-sweetened beverages in the United States.[2]

TABLE 20.5 Oral Glycemic Agents Used to Treat Type 2 Diabetes Mellitus

Oral Glycemic Agent (Examples of Generic Names)	Primary Site of Action	Method of Action
Alpha-glucosidase inhibitors (acarbose, miglitol)	Intestines	Slows carbohydrate digestion
Biguanides (metformin)	Liver	Prevents excessive glucose release from the liver; makes peripheral tissues more sensitive to insulin
Meglitinides (repaglinide)	Pancreas	Stimulates more secretion of insulin from the pancreas; short-acting
Sulfonylureas (tolbutamide, glipizide, glyburide, glimepiride)	Pancreas	Stimulates more secretion of insulin from the pancreas
Thiazolidinediones (rosiglitazone, pioglitazone)	Muscle cells	Increases sensitivity of tissues (fat, muscle, liver) to insulin

outcomes of physical activity, such as decreased body fat, increase in endorphins, improved cardiovascular health, and weight control, also lower the risk for some of the long-term complications of diabetes.

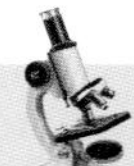

FROM THE LAB

Annual screening for albumin **(protein)** in the urine is recommended in all patients with diabetes, especially those with type 2 diabetes to detect early renal damage and is a risk factor for heart disease. Performing an albumin-to-creatinine ratio is the best way to start. If abnormal (i.e., >30 mg/g), a 24-hour urine specimen should be performed to determine albumin excretion. Normal urine albumin excretion is defined as less than 30 mg/d. Microalbuminuria is defined as 30–300 mg/d (20–200 mcg/min). At least 2 of 3 samples over 3 to 6 months are needed to confirm the presence of albumin in the urine.

If diet and exercise are inadequate to produce adequate glycemic control, individuals with type 2 diabetes may also require oral medications along with continued dietary modifications and exercise. Glycemic agents act to increase insulin release by the beta cells, increase glucose production by the liver, or increase the uptake of insulin. Table 20.5 describes common oral glycemic agents and their mechanism for action in treating type 2 diabetes. Insulin therapy may also be initiated if insulin replacement is warranted. The forms of insulin are illustrated in Table 20.4.

Stop and Consider
Why is it not recommended to use oral glycemic agents to treat those with type 1 diabetes?

GESTATIONAL DIABETES

Gestational diabetes is defined as any degree of glucose intolerance that occurs during pregnancy. This form of diabetes is usually temporary, but in some cases, the woman may go on to develop type 2 diabetes. Gestational diabetes occurs because of insulin resistance that occurs during pregnancy *and* because of an inability of the pancreas to make the additional insulin that is needed during the pregnancy to support the placenta. Risk factors for this type of diabetes include family history of diabetes, five or more previous pregnancies, and a previous large-for-date baby. This condition occurs in up to 15% of pregnancies and is usually diagnosed in the fifth or sixth month. Treatments for gestational diabetes include diet modification, exercise, and possibly insulin. Tight control of blood glucose is needed to prevent overstimulation of the fetal pancreas during pregnancy. Oral glycemic agents are not recommended because of their potentially teratogenic effects. If untreated, gestational diabetes, or even poorly controlled type 1 or type 2 diabetes in a pregnant woman, can lead to:

- Fetal macrosomia (abnormally large body size)
- Hypoglycemia from pancreatic hyperplasia and excess insulin secretion in the newborn
- Hypocalcemia
- Hyperbilirubinemia
- A 5 to 10% incidence of major developmental anomalies, such as spina bifida or heart defects.

Additional complications for the mother include a greater risk for chronic hypertension and cesarean delivery. Gestational diabetes does increase a woman's risk for developing type 2 diabetes even after the pregnancy and delivery is complete.

Acute Complications of Diabetes Mellitus

Acute complications of diabetes mellitus are related to either hypoglycemia or significant hyperglycemia.

Acute complications have a rapid onset and often have significant manifestations of altered neuronal function. Particularly in those with type 1 diabetes, the regulation of glycemic control can be challenging. The Somogyi effect and dawn phenomenon illustrate acute complications of diabetes related to the attempted regulation of glycemic control.

HYPOGLYCEMIA

Hypoglycemia is a state of significantly low blood glucose that results in demonstrable clinical manifestations, such as weakness, pallor, or cool/clammy skin. Although individual variations exist, manifestations typically present when the serum glucose becomes less than 50 mg/dL (Fig. 20.5). This can occur in situations such as:

- Hyperinsulinemia (high circulating insulin levels) as can occur with the administration of exogenous insulin to treat diabetes
- Inadequate food intake or vomiting, in which the presence of glucose in the body is reduced
- Frequent simple carbohydrate intake
- Strenuous exercise or infection, during which the use of glucose is excessive

Hypoglycemia is most commonly found in individuals with type 1 diabetes who are undergoing insulin replacement therapy. Insulin replacement therapy requires the careful intake of adequate nutrients to match the injected insulin. This step is particularly critical with the insulin pump because the pump administers a basal dose of insulin throughout the day. Therefore, the presence of insulin, coupled with skipping a meal and exercising, can lead to blood glucose levels as low as 40 to 50 mg/dL. Hypoglycemia is particularly problematic for the brain, which has an energy demand twice that of other cells in the body. Neurons are in a constant state of metabolic activity, even during sleep. Mental concentration and other forms of bioelectrical communication throughout the nervous system require glucose. A lack of glucose has been found to impede the synthesis of acetylcholine, a major brain neurotransmitter.

Interestingly, the ingestion of simple carbohydrates, as opposed to complex carbohydrates, can also promote a state of neuronal hypoglycemia. Complex carbohydrates are gradually broken down, stored in the liver, and released gradually into the blood in the form of glucose. Therefore, the process of intake, storage, and release of glucose from

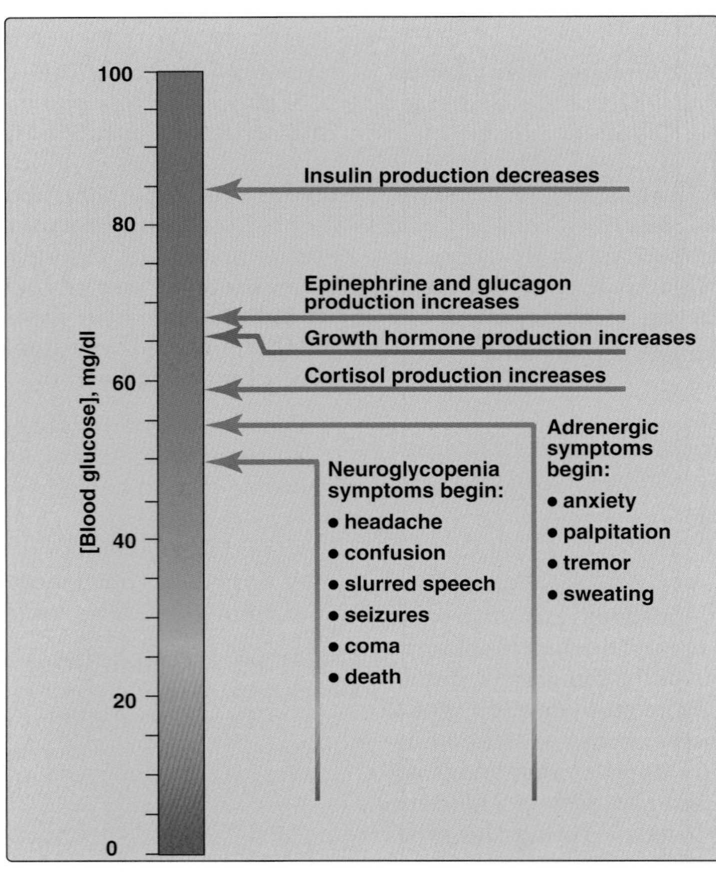

Figure 20.5. How the body responds to hypoglycemia.

complex carbohydrates is ideal for brain function. Simple carbohydrates, such as that found in sugary foods like syrup, fruit juice, or honey, enter the blood and rapidly raise the blood sugar. This stimulates the rapid release of insulin. The insulin pulls this excess glucose into cells of the body and actually deprives the brain of glucose. Recall that neurons do not require insulin for glucose uptake and are unable to store glucose. Even though other cells in the body have stored glucose, the brain becomes hypoglycemic.

Clinical manifestations of hypoglycemia can vary among individuals but are most notably related to neuronal deprivation of glucose. Potential signs and symptoms include poor concentration, extreme hunger, clammy/cool skin, blurred vision, dizziness and confusion, difficulty with speech, lack of coordination, staggering gait, and headache. The hypoglycemic state activates the sympathetic nervous system, which causes an increase in the pulse, along with palpitations, sweating, anxiety, and tremors. Loss of consciousness, seizures, coma, and death can occur if hypoglycemia is not treated.

Prevention of hypoglycemia involves calculating and administering insulin dosages with regard to nutritional intake and physical activity. The treatment of hypoglycemia requires administration of 15 to 20 grams of glucose. The method of administration depends on the level of consciousness of the person. If the person is fairly conscious and able to swallow, a concentrated carbohydrate, such as sweetened fruit juice, honey, or candy, is sufficient. If the symptoms do not improve within a few minutes, the dose can be repeated. If the person is unconscious and cannot swallow, glucagon must be administered parenterally, intramuscularly, or subcutaneously.

DIABETIC KETOACIDOSIS

Diabetic ketoacidosis (DKA) is a problem of deficient insulin and severe hyperglycemia leading to a state of metabolic acidosis and severe osmotic diuresis. It occurs most commonly in those with type 1 diabetes. DKA typically develops over a few days and is triggered by an increased demand for insulin, such as occurs with severe stress, infection, overconsumption of food, pregnancy, or inadequate insulin administration. The onset of DKA may be the event that makes the individual aware that he or she has type 1 diabetes. Blood glucose levels can reach as high as 1000 mg/dL.

The lack of insulin causes mobilization of fatty acids for energy, leading to an increased production of ketones. The kidneys are unable to excrete the ketones and the cells are unable to use these byproducts, allowing ketones to accumulate in the blood. Recall that optimal cell function occurs within a narrow pH range. Acidosis (pH less than 7.3) leads to widespread cellular injury. Hyperglycemia promotes osmotic diuresis, loss of electrolytes, and dehydration (Fig. 20.6).

The signs and symptoms of DKA are consistent with severe hyperglycemia, metabolic acidosis, and dehydration. Manifestations preceding DKA include those of type 1 diabetes: polyuria, polydipsia, polyphagia, nocturia, weight loss, and fatigue. Abdominal pain and vomiting are common. With the onset of acidosis, buffer systems are taxed and compensatory changes occur in an effort to improve the acid–base balance in the body. **Kussmaul respirations** are deep, rapid respirations that release excess acids through the lungs. The breath also has a sweet, fruity odor caused by the release of acetone, a volatile form of ketones. The decreased circulating blood volume promotes tachycardia and hypotension. Acidosis triggers a decreased level of consciousness, which can progress to coma and even death.

Treatment of DKA focuses on stabilizing blood glucose levels, correcting acidosis, replacing fluids and electrolytes, and improving tissue perfusion. These goals are accomplished through intravenous administration of insulin, fluid, and electrolyte solutions. Any triggering causes, such as infection, must also be addressed. After the individual's blood glucose and fluid balance are stabilized, treatment involves initiating or resuming strategies to manage the diabetes effectively and to prevent further occurrences of DKA over time.

Stop and Consider

You arrive on a scene and see that someone with diabetes is unconscious. How do you know if the person is experiencing hypoglycemia or hyperglycemia?

HYPERGLYCEMIC HYPEROSMOLAR NONKETOTIC SYNDROME

Hyperglycemic hyperosmolar nonketotic syndrome (HHNK) is primarily a problem of type 2 diabetes in older adults that is characterized by:

- Hyperglycemia, often above 600 mg/dL
- High plasma osmolarity
- Dehydration
- Lack of (or mild) ketosis
- Changes in the level of consciousness

In HHNK, severe hyperglycemia results from increased insulin resistance and excessive carbohydrate intake. Hyperosmolarity from excessive glucose and inadequate fluid intake results in water shifting from intracellular to extracellular spaces, leading to cellular dehydration and cell death. The presence of

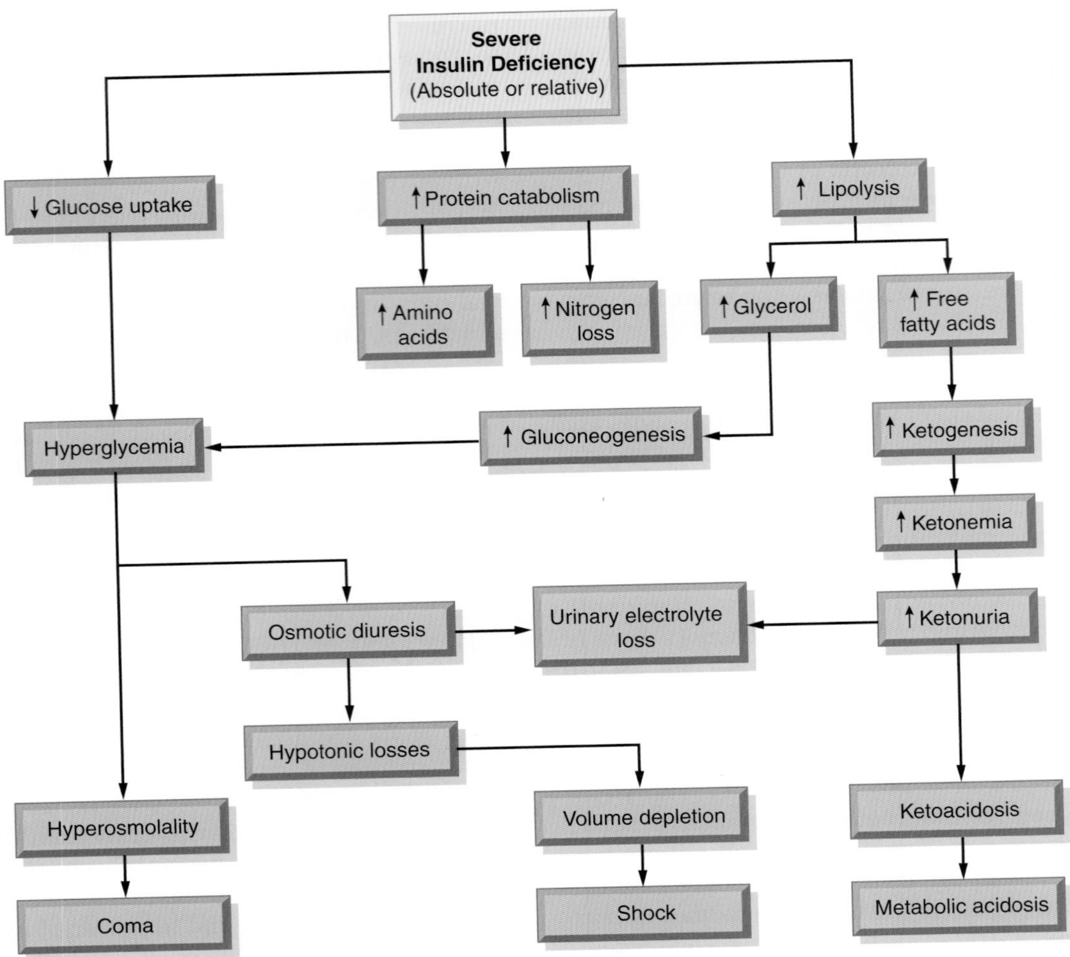

Figure 20.6. Diabetic ketoacidosis (DKA) is characterized by three major pathophysiologic disruptions: coma, shock, and metabolic acidosis.

glucose in the urine impairs the ability of the kidney to concentrate urine and promotes osmotic diuresis. This exacerbates water losses.

The onset is often gradual and presents over a period of days to weeks. Hyperglycemia and solute diuresis leads to polyuria, polydipsia, polyphagia, weight loss, weakness, and signs of dehydration, such as leg cramps, poor tissue turgor, cool extremities, and tachycardia. The individual may also present with renal impairment and neurologic changes, such as seizures, hallucinations, weakness, paralysis, muscle tremors, and visual changes. Approximately one out of four of individuals in HHNK present in a state of coma. In some cases, the individual is not known to have diabetes before the onset of HHNK. Glucose is present in the urine and ketones are typically absent or minimal. Treatment involves careful fluid replacement with a tonicity matched to the level of hyperosmolarity, along with potassium, magnesium, and phosphate replacement, and stabilization of blood glucose levels. After the individual is stabilized, ongoing care is required to prevent further occurrences of HHNK through the ongoing management of type 2 diabetes.

THE SOMOGYI EFFECT AND DAWN PHENOMENON

The **Somogyi effect** is the presence of rebound hyperglycemia as a reaction to insulin-induced hypoglycemia. Insulin-induced hypoglycemia triggers compensatory increases in catecholamines, glucagon, cortisol, and growth hormone in an effort to promote insulin resistance and increase circulating blood glucose levels. Hypoglycemia, which often occurs during the night, is met with morning or daytime hyperglycemia. This prompts the increased exogenous administration of insulin, which further perpetuates the Somogyi effect and poses a major challenge to tight control of glucose levels. Individuals with morning hyperglycemia need to test their blood glucose levels in the middle of the night to determine the presence of the Somogyi effect. If the individual is hypoglycemic, adjustments in the evening snack or insulin type or dose may be required.

The **dawn phenomenon** is a situation in which an individual's blood glucose level upon waking is higher than the level before going to bed in the evening. Because there is no food intake during the night, this finding suggests that blood glucose should decrease during the night. The dawn phenomenon, similar to the Somogyi effect, is related to the release of hormones (growth hormone, cortisol, glucagon, and catecholamines), usually between 4 AM and 9 AM, which triggers insulin resistance and the release of glucose from the liver. The dawn phenomenon differs from the Somogyi effect in that hyperglycemia is not triggered by overnight hypoglycemia. Blood glucose levels steadily rise through the night. Management of the dawn phenomenon requires limiting or regulating evening snacks or possibly increasing oral glycemic agents (in type 2 diabetes) or basal insulin doses (in type 1 diabetes).

CHRONIC COMPLICATIONS OF DIABETES MELLITUS

The presence of diabetes immediately increases the risk of developing irreversible clinical complications because of degenerative changes throughout the body. Chronic complications of diabetes develop primarily in tissues that are affected by the high levels of glucose circulating in the blood. In those tissues that require insulin for transport of glucose, hyperglycemia causes degenerative changes by thickening the basement membrane, promoting coagulation, obstructing perfusion, inducing hypoxia, and producing tissue necrosis. In those tissues that do not require insulin for glucose transport (e.g., red blood cells, lens, kidney, and nerves), the excess glucose causes fluid to osmotically shift into these cells and causes the cells to rupture. Complications, illustrated in Figure 20.7, are frequently classified as:

1. Microvascular (relating to small vessels)
2. Macrovascular (relating to large vessels)
3. Neuropathies

An individual is less likely to develop chronic complications of diabetes if blood glucose levels are kept in tight control (70 to 120 mg/dL).

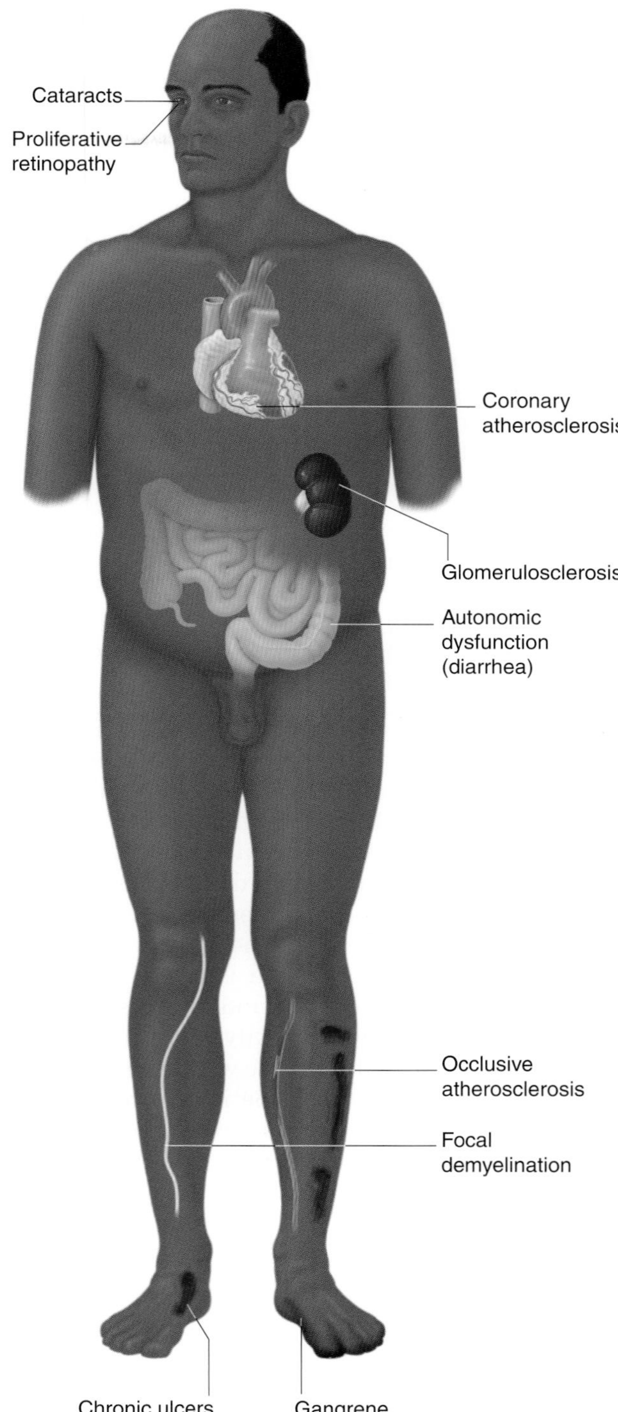

Figure 20.7. Chronic complications of diabetes.

Microvascular Complications

Degenerative changes in small vessels occur most notably in the retinas, a condition called **retinopathy**, and in the kidneys, referred to as **nephropathy**. One mechanism for the development of complications is the presence of excess glucose, which binds to collagen and proteins in the blood vessel walls. This process is referred to as glycosylation. The rate of glycosylation is proportionate to the level of hyperglycemia. Glycosylation permanently alters the structure of collagen and proteins in the blood vessel walls. This alteration leads to the hardening and thickening of the capillary basement membrane, resulting in obstruction or rupture of the capillaries. Ultimately, this development leads to necrosis and loss of function in those tissues being supplied by the small vessels. In retinopathy, retinal ischemia related to obstruction and rupture of capillaries can lead to blindness. The development of complications may also be related to an accumulation of sorbitol, a sugar alcohol, derived from the metabolism of excessive glucose by aldose reductase (an enzyme) in tissues that do not require insulin. Sorbitol is theorized to promote the osmosis of fluid into the lens of the eye and may also be directly toxic to cells. Reactive oxygen species (free radicals) may also be involved in the development of diabetes complications due to release of free radicals as a result of tissue injury from excessive glucose exposure.

Based on these potential mechanisms, the development of nephropathy is a consequence of:

1. Protein breakdown caused by high glucose levels and inadequate insulin
2. Excessive osmotic diuresis and glucosuria that occurs with hyperglycemia
3. Intraglomerular hypertension, which is worsened in the presence of systemic hypertension

With nephropathy, changes in the glomerular capillaries increase the intraglomerular pressure, causing hypertension within the kidney. Chronic renal hypertension contributes to glomerular sclerosis, hypoxia, and, ultimately, chronic renal failure. Nephropathy in individuals with diabetes is the leading cause of end-stage renal disease, accounting for almost half of new cases of renal failure. The presence of continuous proteinuria is a key manifestation of diabetic nephropathy and progressive renal disease. Protein restriction, dialysis, or renal transplant may be indicated for those who develop chronic renal failure secondary to diabetic nephropathy. Essential to the avoidance of microvascular complications are strict blood glucose control, maintenance of HbA_{1c} levels below 7%, treatment of hypertension, and avoidance of smoking.

Macrovascular Complications

Macrovascular diseases involve large vessels and include coronary artery disease, cerebrovascular disease (stroke), and peripheral vascular disease. The major mechanisms for the development of macrovascular complications are related to the role of diabetes in the development of atherosclerosis. Hyperglycemia, hyperlipidemia, and hypertension contribute to the development of atherosclerotic plaques by injuring the intima. Lipids are deposited in the walls of large vessels. Low-density lipoproteins are typically found in high concentrations in those with diabetes, particularly type 2. High-density lipoproteins, considered a protective form of cholesterol, are found in low concentrations. Platelets adhere to the damaged endothelial cells in the intima. Large vessels become sclerotic and obstructed. These complications lead to hypoxia and eventually anoxia, which lead to necrosis of peripheral tissues (Fig. 20.8). Depending on the location, plaque formation can result in the coronary arteries, leading to MI; in the cerebral arteries, leading to stroke; or in the peripheral arteries, leading to peripheral vascular disease, gangrene, and may require amputation.

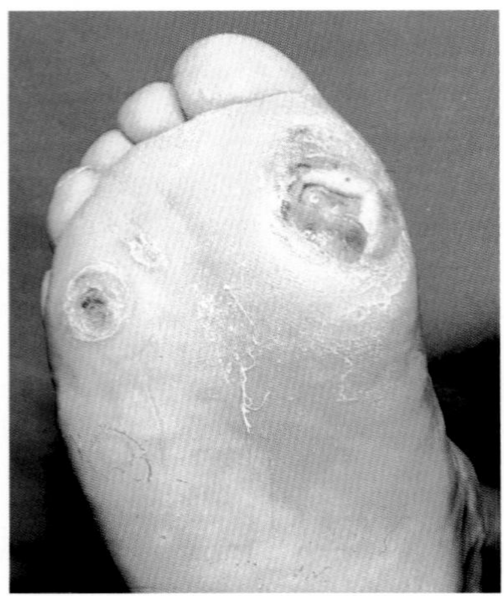

Figure 20.8. Peripheral ulcerations related to vascular and neurologic impairment. (From Marks R. *Skin Disease in Old Age*. Philadelphia, PA: J. B. Lippincott; 1987.)

The presence of macrovascular complications in individuals with diabetes is staggering. More than half of people with diabetes will die of heart disease or stroke; those with diabetes are two to four times more likely to have heart disease or suffer from a stroke than those without diabetes.[3] One of every three patients with diabetes who are older than 50 years is estimated to have peripheral vascular disease and **intermittent claudication**, a condition of fatigue or aching in the leg muscles even when walking short distances. The risk of a leg amputation is 15 to 40 times greater for a person with diabetes and mortality rates are significantly higher for those requiring amputation.[3] At diagnosis, an estimated 50% of those with type 2 diabetes present with macrovascular or microvascular complications.

Neuropathies

Neuropathy is nerve degeneration that results in delayed nerve conduction and impaired sensory function. Neuropathies can occur in somatic, peripheral, and autonomic nerve cells. Neuropathies are a result of (1) thickening, sclerosis, obstruction, and ischemia of the vessels that supply nerve fibers and (2) demyelinization caused by impaired metabolism. These degenerations are often distinguished as somatic versus autonomic. Somatic nerve degeneration and delayed conduction lead to decreased sensation, numbness, tingling, weakness, muscle wasting, and pain. Autonomic neuropathies lead to bladder incontinence, impotence, diarrhea, erectile dysfunction, and postural hypotension. The prevalence of autonomic neuropathy increases with age, duration of diabetes, and increased hemoglobin A_{1c}.

Infection

Individuals with diabetes are also at increased risk for the development of infection. This is related to several aspects of hyperglycemia related to microvascular, macrovascular, and neuropathic complications:

- Excess glucose in blood provides an optimal environment for some pathogens, allowing rapid proliferation.
- Tissue ischemia from microvascular and macrovascular degeneration damages tissue integrity and allows ready access to pathogens.
- Red blood cell destruction and high levels of glycosylated hemoglobin prevent release of oxygen to the tissues.
- White blood cells are impaired without adequate glucose transport and are unable to engulf and remove pathogens.
- Neuropathies prevent the individual from being able to sense breaks in the skin integrity, allowing pathogens easy access.
- Retinopathy may prevent the individual from being able to adequately inspect for manifestations of infection and will delay treatment. To see a video on diabetes, visit http://thePoint.lww.com.

thePoint®

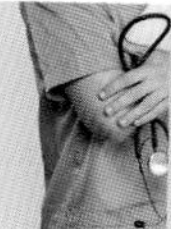

CLINICAL PRACTICE

As with all complications of diabetes, tight glycemic control is key in prevention. Other prevention strategies include smoking cessation, management of hypertension, weight loss, and lowering of lipids. Education on preventing complications can follow the alphabet:[4]

- A = advice to follow diet, weight loss, exercise program, and lifestyle modifications
- B = blood pressure reduction
- C = cholesterol reduction
- D = diabetes hyperglycemia control
- E = eye screening
- F = foot care

SUMMARY

- This chapter illustrates the integration of concepts from all previous chapters to appreciate the complexities of human disease. Diabetes is presented as the primary clinical model.
- Insulin is needed to promote glucose uptake and metabolism of nutrients.
- Diabetes results from either (1) a lack of insulin secretion by the beta cells of the pancreas or (2) a resistance to insulin. This leads to a state of hyperglycemia.
- Insulin absence or resistance prohibits using insulin to transport glucose and amino acids into those cells that require insulin for transport.
- The three main types of diabetes (type 1, type 2, and gestational) differ in the way that the body produces or responds to insulin.
- Type 1 diabetes exhibits an absolute or significant deficit of insulin; the cause is multifactorial and includes both genetic and environmental influences that lead to autoimmune destruction of beta cells. Common clinical manifestations include polyuria, polydipsia, and polyphagia. Treatment of type 1 diabetes mellitus requires a balance of carbohydrate/dietary intake, exercise, and insulin replacement therapy.
- Type 2 diabetes is a problem of insulin resistance or suboptimal insulin presence in the body. The exact cause is unknown; however, genetic and environmental factors, particularly obesity, appear to contribute to its development. The clinical manifestations for type 2 diabetes are often insidious and nonspecific. Treatment involves weight management, nutrition monitoring, and (possibly) oral glycemic agents or, in some cases, insulin replacement.
- Gestational diabetes is defined as any degree of glucose intolerance that occurs during pregnancy. This form of diabetes is usually temporary, but in some cases, women may go on to develop type 2 diabetes. Gestational diabetes occurs because of insulin resistance that occurs during pregnancy *and* because the pancreas is unable to make the additional insulin needed during the pregnancy to support the placenta.
- Acute complications can occur in all types of diabetes and include diabetic ketoacidosis and hypoglycemia. The Somogyi effect and dawn phenomenon are acute complications related to the treatment and management of diabetes, particularly in those individuals who require insulin replacement.
- Hyperglycemia hyperosmolar nonketotic syndrome is an acute complication of type 2 diabetes. It primarily occurs in older adults and is marked

by hyperglycemia, hyperosmolarity, glucosuria, and dehydration without the presence of ketosis.
- Chronic complications involve microvascular, macrovascular, and neuropathic degeneration. The complications of diabetes can be minimized with control of blood glucose levels.

CASE STUDY 20.1

P.K. is a 73-year-old man with long-standing diabetes. Today, he presents to the emergency department in a coma. You review his history and note that he was diagnosed with type 2 diabetes approximately 12 years ago. He experienced a stroke a year ago and has been living in a long-term care facility since then. His care providers indicate that his blood glucose levels are monitored daily. The levels are typically around 160 to 200 mg/dL, but these have been steadily climbing over the past 2 weeks. He is on an oral glycemic agent. He does not exercise because of residual weakness from the stroke, and he does have frequent visitors who like to bring him hard candies. He had an appointment scheduled this week to meet with his primary care physician to evaluate a leg ulcer that is possibly infected. The care providers indicate that his urine output has increased over the past 2 weeks. They are not sure if his fluid intake has increased. When they went into his room this morning, he was unresponsive. His current blood glucose level is 721 mg/dL. His urine is positive for glucose and negative for ketones. Based on the information provided:

1. What is the most likely cause for the altered level of consciousness?
2. What risk factors are present in this patient that lead to your conclusion in question 1?
3. What is happening in this patient's body?
4. What are the potential causes for the onset of this condition?
5. What treatment strategies would you anticipate?

CASE STUDY 20.2

G.H., a 12-year-old with type 1 diabetes, is at a birthday party after school. At around 4 PM, pizza, ice cream, and cake are served. G.H. has one slice of pizza because she knows she cannot have too much sugar. At around 4:30 PM, G.H.'s friends decide to play a game of soccer. G.H. plays for about 30 minutes and then needs to leave for gymnastics practice from 5:15 to 6:30 PM. On the way home from practice, G.H.'s mom asks how her day was, and G.H. cannot remember where she was earlier that day. She begins to combine words together and slur her speech. G.H. also reports a headache.

1. What is happening to G.H.?
2. What were the actual or potential contributing factors?
3. What should G.H.'s mom do?
4. What could happen if no action is taken?

CASE STUDY 20.3

TJ is a 6-year-old boy who was rushed to the emergency room in a state of disorientation. His parents report that he has been really thirsty over the past few weeks; he has been waking up 2 to 3 times per night asking for water. He has also started wetting the bed again, something he hasn't done for about 6 months. He has also been really tired despite eating a lot more than his friends and his pants are becoming loose. His blood glucose is measured at 413 mg/dL. His urine is positive for ketones. He is diagnosed with diabetes.

1. What type of diabetes does TJ most likely have given his presentation?
2. What is the cause of his diabetes?
3. Describe the pathophysiologic changes that have occurred over the past weeks/months/years.
4. What is the significance of ketones in his urine?
5. What is the significance of hyperglycemia?
6. How do the presenting clinical manifestations relate to beta cell destruction?
7. What key elements would you anticipate to be a part of his treatment plan?
8. What would be the goal of his treatment and how would you know he is meeting this goal?

PRACTICE EXAM QUESTIONS

1. Which of the following is caused by the release of insulin?
   a. Decreased blood glucose level
   b. Increased blood glucose level
   c. Increased lipid breakdown
   d. Increased protein breakdown

2. Which of the following is not true of type 1 diabetes?
   a. Can be treated with oral glycemic agents
   b. Pancreas is completely unable to produce insulin
   c. Acute onset
   d. Definite genetic link

3. Which of the following is not true about type 2 diabetes?
   a. Accounts for up to 95% of diabetics
   b. Gradual onset
   c. Significant weight loss occurs as a symptom
   d. Risk factors are hypertension, family history, and obesity

4. Which of the following is not a sign of DKA?
   a. Kussmaul respirations
   b. Dehydration
   c. Ketonuria
   d. Low blood glucose level

5. Which laboratory test is the best predictor of blood glucose control over the previous few months?
   a. HbA_{1c}
   b. Fasting blood glucose
   c. Urinalysis
   d. Feasting (postprandial) blood glucose

6. Neuropathies are a potential complication of diabetes. Why do these occur?
   a. Infection in the nerves
   b. Thickening and ischemia of the vessels that supply the nerve fibers
   c. Inability to provide continuous glucose to the brain and spinal cord
   d. Excessive glucose exposure to the brain and spinal cord

7. What is the major difference between the Somoygi effect and the dawn phenomenon?
   a. One is caused by the release of certain hormones
   b. One occurs between 4am and 9am
   c. One triggers insulin resistance and the release of glucose from the liver
   d. One is characterized by hyperglycemia that is not triggered by overnight hypoglycemia

8. What would happen if your patient did not have alpha cells of the pancreas?
   a. They would not be able to secrete insulin
   b. They would not be able to secrete somatostatin and gastrin
   c. They would not be able to secrete glucagon
   d. They would not be able to secrete pancreatic polypeptides

9. What would be an unusual sign in a child that may alert the parent to the presence of diabetes?
   a. Bedwetting in a child that was previously dry through the night
   b. Irritability
   c. Asking for water to drink in the middle of the night
   d. All of these

10. What is your explanation to the parents who do not want to give their child insulin injections to treat type 1 diabetes because they have heard that pills can be used to treat this condition?
    a. Insulin is destroyed in the gastrointestinal tract if taken orally, so it must be injected subcutaneously
    b. The child can go ahead and take the oral medication because he does have type 1 diabetes
    c. The child cannot take the pills because we can't be sure that he would take the entire dose
    d. The pills are reserved for those over the age of 12

11. When increased blood glucose levels stimulate increased secretion of insulin, this is an example of control by:
    a. Releasing hormones
    b. Ectopic hormones
    c. Negative feedback
    d. Positive feedback

12. A major *difference* between Bobby (type 1 diabetes) and his father (type 2 diabetes) is:
    a. How the condition is diagnosed between type 1 and type 2
    b. How the condition is treated between type 1 and type 2
    c. The potential long-term complications
    d. The overall goal of treatment between type 1 and type 2

13. Bobby's father (with type 2 diabetes) has been encouraged to increase his exercise level. Exercise is encouraged in type 2 diabetes because:
    a. Exercise decreases stress
    b. Skeletal muscles can use glucose without a proportionate insulin amount
    c. Exercise decreases cardiovascular effects of excessive glucose
    d. All of these

14. Bobby's father has been prescribed an oral hypoglycemic drug. Such drugs act:
    a. As an insulin replacement
    b. To decrease the body's need for glucose in body cells
    c. To prevent the formation of glucose
    d. To reduce insulin resistance

15. Bobby comes in to the clinic after 6 months for a follow-up visit. He indicates that his blood sugars have been around 100 to 120 mg/dL and he has been fully participating in the other aspects of his diabetes management plan. Which would lead you to believe that he has not been in tight control of his diabetes?
    a. A reduced glycosylated hemoglobin level
    b. An elevated glycosylated hemoglobin level
    c. A random blood sugar of 150 mg/dL performed in the clinic
    d. There is no method to determine whether or not he is in tight control

DISCUSSION AND APPLICATION

1. What did I know about diabetes prior to today?
2. What body processes are affected by diabetes? What are the expected functions of those processes? How does diabetes affect those processes?
3. What are the potential etiologies for diabetes? How does diabetes develop?
4. Who is most at risk for developing diabetes? How does this differ with the three types of diabetes (type 1, type 2, and gestational)?
5. What are the human differences that affect the etiology, risk, or course of diabetes?
6. What clinical manifestations are expected in the course of diabetes?
7. What special diagnostic tests are useful in determining the diagnosis of diabetes?
8. What are the goals of care for individuals with diabetes?
9. How does the concept of diabetes bring together what I have learned in the previous chapters and in previous courses?
10. How can I use what I have learned?

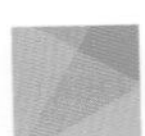

RESOURCES

Get updated news and current research on diabetes as well as general information:
http://www.diabetes.org

A complete summary of diabetes and information for diabetes management:
http://diabetes.niddk.nih.gov/dm/pubs/type1and2/what.htm

Updated research in the world of diabetes:
http://www.nlm.nih.gov/medlineplus/diabetes.html

References

1. Kwai N, Arnold R, Poynten A, et al. Continuous subcutaneous infection infusion preserves axonal function in type 1 diabetes mellitus. *Diabetes Metab Res Rev.* 2015;31(2):175–182. doi:10.1002/dmrr.2583.
2. Fumiaki I, O'Connor L, Ye Z, et al. Consumption of sugar sweetened beverages, artificially sweetened beverages, and fruit juice and incidence of type 2 diabetes: systematic review meta-analysis, and estimation of population attributable fraction. *BMJ.* 2015;351:h3576.
3. Khardori R, Griffing G. Type 2 diabetes mellitus. http://emedicine.medscape.com/article/117853-overview. Accessed November 30, 2015.
4. Metoo D. Clinical skills: empowering people with diabetes to minimize complications. *Br J Nurs.* 2004;13:644–650.

Find additional resources for this chapter at http:thePoint.lww.com thePoint®

Glossary

1, 25-dihydroxycholecalciferol: activated form of vitamin D; promotes calcium absorption in the intestine

abscess: a pocket of purulent exudate

absorption: a complex process of taking in nutrients and moving these to the circulation to be used by cells

accommodate: ability of the lens to change its shape

accumulated mutations theory: developmental theory of aging suggesting that genes that determine survival at younger ages have greater influence than genes expressed at older ages

acid: substance that donates hydrogen ions

acoustic reflex measurement: test to determine movement of the tympanic membrane in response to sound

acromegaly: condition of hyperplasia prompted by hormone stimulation of excessive growth after closure of the epiphyseal growth plates of the long bones

action potential: electrical events that travel along an entire neuron by allowing charged ions to flood through channels in the semipermeable membrane around the nerve cell

active transport: energy-dependent transport of particles across the cell membrane against a gradient

activities of daily living (ADLs): performance of usual functions of everyday life (e.g., eating, dressing)

acuity: clarity; ability to locate the site of the initiation of a stimulus

acute: describes manifestations or illnesses that are usually abrupt in onset and last a few days to a few months

acute respiratory distress syndrome (ARDS): a condition of severe acute inflammation and pulmonary edema without evidence of fluid overload or impaired cardiac function

acute tubular necrosis: condition of the kidney characterized by sloughing of tubular cells

adaptation: alteration in function that allows cells, tissues, and organs to adjust to new conditions; survival due to the capacity to adjust to an adverse environment

adaptive immunity: cell-mediated and humoral immunity; specific immune response occurring during a lifetime

Addison disease: a condition of adrenal cortical insufficiency most commonly caused by the autoimmune destruction of the adrenal cortex

adenocarcinoma: a malignant tumor of epithelial cells

adenoid hypertrophy: enlargement of lymphoepithelial adenoid tissue in the back of the nasal area

adenoma: benign tumor of glandular epithelial origin

adenosine triphosphate (ATP): principal source of cellular energy; product of a chemical reaction between oxygen and nutrient products such as glucose, fatty acids, amino acids, and enzymes

adherence: the attraction and binding of cells to a specific location to promote healing

adhesions: fibrous connections between serous cavities and nearby tissues that do not allow the surrounding tissues to move freely

adjuvant: substance that increase immune response to antigens

adventitious: refers to an alteration in lung sounds, as with wheezing or crackles

aerobic bacteria: microorganisms that require oxygen for growth

affective disorder: condition involving mood, emotional feeling, and tone related to thought; includes external manifestations

afferent neurons: neurons that carry impulses from receptors to the distant targets of the brain and spinal cord; also known as sensory neurons

afterload: the amount of pressure in the ventricle toward the end of the cardiac contraction

air trapping: decreased effective O_2 intake and especially CO_2 release by retaining air within the alveoli because of loss of elasticity

akinesia: inability to move

allele: a series of two or more different genes occupying the same location on a specific chromosome

allergen: protein promoting altered reactivity responses by the immune system

alloantibodies: antibodies produced against alloantigens

alloantigens: proteins that vary between individuals

allograft: graft between unrelated individuals

alternative splicing: different ways of assembling exons to produce a variety of mature mRNAs

amblyopia: a condition resulting from a muscle imbalance; commonly known as "lazy eye"
amenorrhea: the absence of menstruation
amniocentesis: insertion of a needle into the uterine cavity to obtain a sample of amniotic fluid
amphoteric: able to function as either acid or base
amyloid hypothesis: theory suggesting that flaws in the accumulation, production, or disposal of Aβ are responsible for the pathogenesis of Alzheimer disease, including development of tangles, plaques, and neuronal death
amyloid precursor protein (APP): large protein produced by the beta-amyloid gene
anaerobic bacteria: bacteria that do not require oxygen for growth
anaphylactic shock: a condition of impaired tissue perfusion from shock because of a massive immune (type 1 or IgE-mediated) hypersensitivity response
anaphylaxis: extreme manifestation to foreign protein or other substance
anaplasia: a neoplasm's loss of differentiation
anemia: the reduction in the mass of circulating blood cells and subsequently reduced hemoglobin levels
aneuploidy: abnormal chromosome number
aneurysm: local outpouching caused by weakness in the vessel wall
angina pectoris: chest pain or pressure that is intermittent and associated with myocardial ischemia, a reduction in blood flow to the coronary arteries caused by atherosclerosis often accompanied by vasospasm
angioedema: sudden subcutaneous edema
angiogenesis: the generation of new blood vessels
anhedonia: loss of interest or pleasure in normally enjoyable activities
anion exchange: transport of one negatively charged ion for another in opposite directions across the cell membrane
anion gap: calculation of the major measured cations and anions in the plasma; provides an indication of electrolyte and acid–base balance
anions: ions with a negative charge
ankylosis: a debilitating fixation of a joint from extensive fibrosis
anorexia: loss of appetite
anorexia nervosa (AN): an eating disorder characterized by a refusal to maintain a minimally healthy body weight, an intense fear of gaining weight, body image distortion, and amenorrhea
anovulation: the absence of ovulation
anoxia: the absolute deprivation of oxygen
antagonistic pleiotropy theory: developmental theory of aging suggesting that genes may have beneficial effects during early life, but harmful effects as the individual ages
anterolateral pathway: neurologic pathway involving both the anterior and lateral spinothalamic pathways; characterized by multiple synapses and slow conduction; transmits the sensations of pain, temperature, crude touch, and pressure not requiring the specific location of the origin of the stimulus
Arthus reaction: complex-mediated immune response in the skin resulting in an area of localized tissue necrosis
antibodies: immunoglobulins that react with an antigen in a specific way; produced by activated plasma cells
antigen: a substance that induces a state of sensitivity or an immune response
antigen-presenting cells: cells that process and present antigen for recognition by immune cells
antigen variation: alteration of pathogen protein particles to evade recognition and stimulation of memory in the immune system
antigenic variability: a process of eluding the human host defenses; often a result of altering the antigens present within or on the surface of the microorganism
antigenicity: the level to which a pathogen is viewed by the host immune system as foreign
antiport: system of substances transported in the opposite direction
antiresorptive: tendency to slow or block absorption
antiresorptive medication: drugs that inhibit or reduce bone resorption; used to treat osteoporosis
anuria: absent urine output
anxiety disorders: a group of chronic psychiatric conditions characterized by overwhelming and irrational feelings of fear or worry
apoptosis: programmed cell death that is prompted by a genetic signal and designed to replace old cells with new; also known as "cellular suicide"
aquaporins: channels in the cell membrane; allow water movement between compartments
aqueous humor: nutritive, watery fluid produced by the ciliary body
arachidonic acid: a plasma membrane–derived substance that generates various chemical mediators through a complex chemical conversion
arteriovenous (AV) fistula: surgical attachment of an artery to a vein; used to obtain access to circulation for hemodialysis
arteriovenous shunt: surgical procedure connecting the artery to the vein using a synthetic tube
arthritis: a generic term for degeneration or inflammation of the joints

ascending: the upward movement of an infection
ascites: accumulation of fluid in the peritoneal cavity
aspiration: a problem of inhaling a foreign substance into the lungs
asthma: a chronic inflammatory disorder of the airways resulting in intermittent or persistent airway obstruction caused by bronchial hyper responsiveness, inflammation, bronchoconstriction, and excess mucous production
astigmatism: irregular curvature of the cornea or lens preventing the focusing of images; blurring vision
astrogliosis: formation of a glial scar caused by proliferation of astrocytes in response to local tissue injury
asymptomatic: the absence of any noticeable symptoms, even though laboratory or other diagnostic tests may indicate that a disease is present
ataxic: inability to control balance
atelectasis: a condition of collapse and nonaeration of the alveoli
atherosclerosis: a condition of irregularly distributed lipid deposits in the inner lining, or intima, of large or medium arteries
athetoid: inability to control muscle movement
atopic: describes individuals having a genetic predisposition to developing hypersensitivities
atopy: the process by which IgE responses are stimulated from exposure to typically benign substances
atretic: is a decrease in cell size (atrophic)
atrioventricular (AV) node: connects the conduction of impulses between the atria and ventricles
atrophic macular degeneration: retinal deterioration resulting from deposition of drusen, under the macula next to the basement membrane of the retinal pigment epithelium; also known as dry macular degeneration
atrophy: decrease in the size of the cell
attention: a culturally influenced process of selectively concentrating on information
attention-deficit hyperactivity disorder (ADHD): a neurodevelopmental disorder of cognitive functions, causing attention deficit, hyperactivity, and impulsiveness
attenuated: weakened; reduced ability to cause disease
Auerbach plexus: part of the enteric nervous system; found between the longitudinal and circular muscle layers of the large intestine; also known as the myenteric plexus
auscultation: to listen with a stethoscope
autoclave: a device that uses steam heat at high pressures to sterilize objects
autograft: grafts from different sites on the same person
autoimmune: immune responses directed at an individual's own tissues
autonomic nervous system (ANS): component of the peripheral nervous system; includes the sympathetic nervous system (SNS) and the parasympathetic nervous system (PNS); controls involuntary function of organs
autonomy: the unregulated cell growth of neoplasms
autoreceptors: receptors involved in detection of chemicals to regulate the cell's own function
autosomes: chromosomes other than a sex chromosome; totals 44 chromosomes in each body cell
axon: neuronal structure that carries impulses away from the cell body
axon hillock: point at which the axon joins the cell body
bacteremia: a state in which bacteria gain access to the blood
bacteria: single-celled microorganisms that can reproduce outside of host cells
baroreceptors: located throughout the blood vessels and the heart; sense pressure changes in the arteries and alert the cardiac control center in the brainstem
barotrauma: injury resulting from the inability of the ear to equalize pressure
basal ganglia: structure of the brain (ADD) with a major role in coordinated muscle movements
base: substance that accepts hydrogen ions
base deficit: amount of base needed to achieve a pH of 7.4 in the blood sample
base excess: amount of fixed acid needed to achieve a pH of 7.4 in the blood sample
base pairs: nitrogen base combinations; DNA base pairs include cytosine and guanine, and adenine and thymine
basement membrane: the outer membrane of the vessels that separates the vessel from the tissues of the body
basophil: granulocyte that complements the actions of mast cells; important in establishing allergic reactions
B-cell receptor: receptor bound to the cell membrane of the B cell; association with antigen activates plasma cells to produce and secrete antibodies
Beckwith–Wiedemann syndrome: condition of pediatric overgrowth and predisposition to tumor growth, linked to genetic and epigenetic alterations
behavior: how people respond and act in a given situation

benign: describes a tumor that remains localized and closely resembles the tissue of origin
beta-amyloid protein: accumulations leading to the production of senile plaques, characteristic of Alzheimer disease; also known as amyloid or A
bifurcations: regions wherein a vessel branches
bilayer: two interconnected layers of the plasma membrane; the lipid (fat-soluble) layer contains phospholipid and glycolipid
bilirubin: yellow, lipid-soluble byproduct of hemoglobin; elevated levels result in jaundice
bioavailability: refers to a mineral that is unbound and must remain unbound (also called an ionic state) to be absorbed
biomedicine: a systematic scientific study of biologic processes within the framework of Western medicine
binding affinity: tightness or strength of ligand/receptor interaction
bipolar affective disorder: a condition characterized by periods of mania and depression
bladder: muscular organ serving as a reservoir for urine; lined with transitional epithelium and innervated by the pelvic nerves
bladder training: process of learning to hold urine for increasing intervals as a management strategy for incontinence
blast cell: any immature cell
blastomere: early embryo
blood–brain barrier (BBB): reduced permeability of capillaries in the brain to protect against exposure to potentially hazardous substances
blood pressure: the pressure or tension of the blood within the systemic arteries
blood transfusion: the most common form of tissue transplant; infusion of donor blood into recipient
blood typing: the process by which the recipient's blood type is determined
blunt force injury: injury that occurs when the head strikes a hard surface or is struck by a rapidly moving object
B lymphocytes: lymphocytes that differentiate into plasma cells in the bone marrow; produce and secrete antibodies after contact with an antigen
body mass index (BMI): a measure of body fat calculated by measuring weight in kilograms and dividing this by height in meters squared (BMI = kg/m^2)
body-self neuromatrix: neural network in the brain containing somatosensory, limbic, and thalamocortical components; integrates multiple sources of input resulting in the cognitive, affective, and sensory perceptions of pain
bowel resection: surgical procedure involving the removal of intestine
brachial plexus palsy: trauma to the brachial nerve plexus resulting in flaccid paralysis of the affected arm
bradykinesia: decreased spontaneity of movement; slowed movement associated with initiation of movement or sudden halting of movement
bronchiectasis: the irreversible dilation and destruction of the bronchial tree most often caused by chronic obstruction or infection
bronchopulmonary dysplasia (BPD): condition in which cellular alterations lead to chronic, irreversible tissue changes in the respiratory tree of the lungs
bronchospasm: contraction of the smooth muscle in the bronchi and bronchioles of the lungs, decreasing airway size
Brudzinski sign: a test of meningeal irritation where the patient is supine and the neck is quickly flexed; this activity elicits pain along with involuntary flexion of the hips and knees
buffer system: mixing of acid and base to resist pH change; system for trading stronger acids and bases for weaker varieties to achieve acid–base balance
cachexia: a syndrome of unexplained weight loss and tissue wasting related to the stimulation of inflammatory mediators, along with excess energy use, by the proliferating neoplastic cells
calcitonin: hormone promoting the deposition of calcium and phosphate in bone; produced primarily by the parafollicular cells of the thyroid gland, with other sources including the parathyroid and thymus glands
caloric test: test that uses warm and cool water or air irrigation to induce nystagmus; diagnostic of Ménière disease
calpain: type of proteolytic enzyme
cancer: a term used to describe highly invasive and destructive neoplasms
capacitor: structure that stores current
carcinogen: a known cancer-causing agent
carcinogenesis: a term used to describe the origin, promotion, or development of cancerous neoplasms
carcinoma in situ: a unique term used to describe carcinomas that are confined to the epithelium and have not yet penetrated the basement membrane
cardiac contractility: the ability of the heart to increase the force of contraction without changing the diastolic (resting) pressure
cardiac cycle: refers to one contraction and one relaxation phase of the heart
cardiac dysrhythmias: a category of problems with maintaining an efficient heart rhythm, such as impairments of the sinoatrial (SA) node,

atrioventricular (AV) node, cardiac cells that join the SA and AV nodes, or conduction systems in the atria or ventricles
cardiac hypertrophy: a disease of cardiac muscle that results from excessive workload and functional demand
cardiac output (CO): the volume of blood pumped from the ventricles in 1 minute
cardinal signs: the local manifestations of acute inflammation; include redness, heat, swelling, pain, and loss of function
cardiogenic shock: the result of inadequate or ineffective cardiac pumping
carriers: heterozygous for a recessive genetic mutation; able to transmit the genetic mutation to subsequent generations in the absence of a disease phenotype
caseous necrosis: a distinctive, yellow, pasty, cheese-like necrosis of tuberculosis
casts: structures found in urine consisting of a protein meshwork of entrapped cells formed in the distal collecting tubules and collecting ducts
cataracts: clouding of the lens in the eye; causes blurred vision by scattering incoming light
cations: ions with a positive charge
cation exchange: transport of one positively charged ion for another in opposite directions across the cell membrane
cauda equina: extension of nerves in the spinal cord extending below the sacral level through the exit of the vertebral column
cavitation: area of necrosis that erode surrounding structures of the lungs, including the bronchioles, bronchi, and surrounding blood vessels
CD4 T lymphocytes: subtype of helper T lymphocyte that expresses the molecule CD4 on its cell surface
CD8 T lymphocytes: subtype of cytotoxic T lymphocyte that expresses the molecule CD8 on its cell surface
celiac disease: also called gluten-sensitive enteropathy; a disorder of gluten malabsorption caused by a T-cell-mediated hypersensitivity to gluten in persons who are genetically predisposed to developing this condition
cell: smallest component of the living individual
cell body: cell structure containing cytoplasm and organelles responsible for the specialized function of the cell; also known as a soma
cell-mediated immunity: a component of adaptive immunity; cytotoxic T-cell-mediated destruction of pathogen and infected host cell
cellular casts: compacted collection of protein, cells, and debris that are formed in kidney tubules
cellular response: the role of inflammation in alerting the products of healing to attend to the site of injury
cellular senescence: developmental theory suggesting that aging is caused by an intrinsic loss of the capacity of the cell to proliferate, triggered by a critical loss of telomere
central auditory processing disorder: disorder involving an alteration in auditory signal processing in the brain
central nervous system (CNS): component of the nervous system comprising the brain and spinal cord
centromere: structure linking the chromosome pairs of the somatic cells of the body; divides the chromosome into two arms; constant position for each chromosome
cerebral aqueduct: connecting point of the third and fourth ventricles; also known as the aqueduct of Sylvius
cerebral atrophy: decrease in neuronal cell size and number leading to impaired neuronal communication and reduced brain tissue mass
cerebrospinal fluid (CSF): fluid bathing the surface of the central nervous system structures of the brain and spinal cord; flows through four fluid-filled interconnecting ventricles in the brain
cerumen: secretion by glands in the ear
cheilitis: a problem with fissure development in the corners of the mouth often associated with riboflavin deficiency
chemical injury: injury to cells caused by damage from toxins
chemical mediators: potent substances that facilitate the process of widening and loosening the blood vessels at the site of injury; are active in all phases of the inflammatory response
chemical synapse: transmit impulses across a small gap between cells via stimulation of neurotransmitters
chemotactic factors: substances that attract specific types of cells
chemotaxis: the calling forth of inflammatory cells to the injured site
chondrocalcinosis: calcification of cartilage
chondroma: benign tumor that stems from chondrocytes
chondrosarcoma: a malignant tumor of chondrocytes
chorea: irregular, involuntary movements of extremities or facial muscles
choroid plexus: structure located in the two lateral and single third and fourth ventricles of the brain; responsible for production of cerebrospinal fluid
choroidal neovascularization: formation of new blood vessels under the retina and macula; associated with wet (exudative) macular degeneration

chromatin: nuclear genetic material made of DNA; condenses into chromosomes during mitosis
chromatolysis: swelling of a neuron because of injury
chromosomes: double-stranded DNA containing threadlike sections of genes that form an individual's genetic code; most commonly found in the cell nucleus; responsible for reproduction of physical and chemical structures; human somatic cells contain 46 chromosomes: 22 paired autosomes and 1 pair of sex chromosomes
chronic: describes manifestations or illnesses that are often more insidious and generally last 6 months or longer **chronic bronchitis:** the presence of a persistent, productive cough that lasts for 3 months or longer for 2 or more consecutive years
chronic obstructive pulmonary disease (COPD): a generic term that describes all chronic obstructive lung problems including asthma, emphysema, and chronic bronchitis, separately or in combination
ciliary body: ocular structure producing the aqueous humor
ciliary muscle: regulates lens shape to focus an object at close range
cirrhosis: an end-stage liver disease marked by interference of blood flow to the liver and widespread hepatocyte damage
climacteric: gradual transition between normal reproductive cycles and menopause; also known as perimenopause
clinical manifestations: the presenting signs and symptoms of an illness
clonal expansion: the proliferation of B and T lymphocytes activated by clonal selection to produce a clone of identical cells; enables the body to have sufficient numbers of antigen-specific lymphocytes to mount an effective immune response
clonal selection: the selection and activation of specific B lymphocytes and T lymphocytes by the binding of epitopes to B- or T-cell receptors with a corresponding fit
clonic: rapid successions of alternating muscle contraction and relaxation
closed head injury: injury to the head that causes tissue damage without exposing tissue to the external environment
clotting system: promotes coagulation through the activation of clotting factors in a cascade sequence and suppresses coagulation through the release of anticoagulation factors
clubbing: a painless enlargement and flattening of the tips of fingers or toes due to chronic hypoxia
clusters of differentiation: determine specific functions and responses of T-cell subtypes
cochlea: bony structure located in the inner ear; important for hearing
cochlear implant: artificial devices surgically placed behind the ear to enhance hearing
codon: sequence of three forms of nitrogen bases forms; nucleotide triplet; fundamental triplet code necessary for protein synthesis; basic compounds produced are amino acids
cogwheel: muscle rigidity (jerking) in response to limb flexion attempt
coinfection: a phenomenon of hosting two or more pathogens simultaneously
collagen: also known as scar tissue; a substance manufactured by fibroblasts that fills in the gaps left after the removal of extensively damaged tissues or those tissues made up of cells that are unable to regenerate
colonoscopy: a procedure using an endoscope to perform direct visualization of the colon
colostomy: establishment of an artificial opening of the large intestine externally on the abdomen
columnar epithelium: single layer of epithelial cells taller than they are wide
communicable diseases: diseases that are spread from person to person, often through contact with infected blood and body fluids
communicating hydrocephalus: increased ventricular accumulation of cerebrospinal fluid due to impaired cerebrospinal fluid absorption
complement system: a key source of chemical mediators within the plasma; has many roles, particularly as it relates to inflammation, immunity, and the resolution of infection
compliance: the expected distensibility, or expandability, of the lung tissue and chest wall
complications: negative sequelae from a disease
concentration gradient: mechanism of passive transport that promotes the movement of particles from an area of high to lower concentration
concept: an abstract idea generalized from particular instances
conductive hearing loss: hearing loss localized to the outer or middle ear; may be temporary or permanent
cone: photoreceptor located in the retina; essential for sharp and color vision
congenital defects: damage to a developing fetus
congestive heart failure: occurs when the left ventricle of the heart is ineffective and blood backs up into the pulmonary vein and subsequently into the lung tissues; results in pulmonary edema; also called left heart failure
conjugated vaccine: antigens that promote activation of more than one cell type
conjunctivitis: inflammation of the mucous membrane lining the eye

consolidation: a solid mass in the lung tissue
constant region: structure forming the base of the Y-shaped antibody; the most stable component
constipation: absent or incomplete bowel movement; may represent a consequence of impaired gastrointestinal mobility or obstruction
contractures: areas of thick, shortened, and rigid tissue from a loss of elasticity
contralateral: referring to the opposite side of the body
cor pulmonale: an alteration in the structure and function of the right ventricle caused by a primary disorder of the respiratory system
cornea: clear, transparent structure covering the exterior wall of the eye
corpus callosum: nerve fiber bundles promoting communication between the right and left hemispheres of the brain
cortisol: is a major glucocorticoid secreted from the adrenal cortex that regulates metabolism, inflammatory/immune processes, and the stress response
costovertebral angle (CVA): anatomic area including the lower abdomen anteriorly and posteriorly; site of associated dermatomes of the kidney
cotransport: substances transported together in the same direction
countercurrent exchanger: flow of blood in the vasa recta capillaries aligned with filtrate flow in the loop of Henle; slow descending blood flow allows water transport from the medullary interstitium into the capillary blood, and slow ascending blood flow allows solute transport from the vasa recta into the interstitium, preserving medullary gradient and preventing washout of interstitial solutes
countercurrent mechanism: process of filtrate concentration in the loop of Henle in the medulla of the kidney; includes the countercurrent multiplier and the countercurrent exchanger
countercurrent multiplier: process of water and solute transport in the loop of Henle maintaining the vertical medullary gradient
countertransport: substances transported in the opposite direction
cretinism: a condition of mental retardation and impaired growth from a congenital lack of thyroid hormone production and secretion
crossmatching: the process by which antibody compatibility between donor and recipient blood is determined
cryptorchidism: a congenital condition of one or two undescended testes
crypts: mucosal epithelial depressions of the colon
Cushing disease: a condition of hypercortisolism specifically related to pituitary corticotrope tumors
Cushing syndrome: a condition of excess glucocorticoid secretion from the adrenal cortex
cyanosis: a result of a greater proportion of desaturated hemoglobin in the blood, which gives the blood a bluish hue
cytochrome oxidase (COX): enzyme important in catalyzing oxidation–reduction mitochondrial reactions in cellular respiration
cytokine: a hormone-like cell protein that regulates the activity of many other chemical mediators in an effort to trigger, enhance, and then discontinue the inflammatory response
cytoplasm: colloid substance surrounding the cell nucleus composed of water, proteins, fats, electrolytes, glycogen, and pigments
cytoskeleton: tubule and filament structures, contributing to cell shape, movement, and intracellular transport; composed of microtubules and thin, intermediate, and thick microfilaments
cytosol: the cytoplasm of bacteria that contains extensive ribosomes, proteins, and carbohydrates, but does not contain mitochondria, endoplasmic reticulum, or other membranous components
cytotoxic T lymphocyte: subset of T lymphocyte that directs destruction of the antigen or cells carrying the antigen
dawn phenomenon: a situation in which an individual's blood glucose level upon waking is higher than that before going to bed in the evening
dead space: an area where gas exchange cannot take place
death: cessation of life; cessation of the integration of cellular, tissue, and organ functions
decerebrate posturing: increased extensor muscle excitability caused by neurologic injury
decibels (dB): the unit of measurement of intensity or loudness of the sound
decorticate posturing: increased flexor muscle excitability caused by neurologic injury
debridement: a process of mechanically removing debris, including necrotic tissue, from a wound
deep brain stimulation (DBS): reversible procedure designed to alter abnormal function of the brain tissue; neurostimulator delivers electrical signals to a targeted area of the brain, blocking abnormal nerve signals and resulting in tremor and other Parkinson disease symptoms
deep partial-thickness burns: formerly known as second-degree burns; burns that damage epidermal skin layers and penetrate some dermal skin layers
defecation: the process of stool elimination
deficit injury: damage caused by deprivation of oxygenation, hydration, and nutrition
degranulation: the release of chemical mediators in the form of extracellular granules

dehiscence: a problem of deficient scar formation in which the wound splits or bursts open, often at a suture line

delayed hypersensitivity reaction: reaction after allergen contact that is slow in onset and peaks after 36 to 48 hours; associated with a type IV cell–mediated hypersensitivity reaction

demyelination: degradation of myelin

dendrites: branching protoplasmic processes of the nerve cell

dendritic cells: process and display of antigens to T lymphocytes; take up antigens when they are encountered in the circulation

deoxyribonucleic acid (DNA): type of nucleic acid containing a sugar (deoxyribose); usually found in the cell nucleus and mitochondria; responsible for the storage of genetic information; made up of four nitrogenous bases, including adenine (A) and guanine (G), cytosine (C) and thymine (T)

depolarization: result of rapid movement of sodium into the cell through sodium channels in the cell membrane

dermatomes: body regions to which spinal nerves transmit impulses

dermatophyte infections: fungal infections of the skin, hair, and nails

detrusor muscle: tissue comprising the body of the bladder; contraction assists with bladder emptying and elimination of urine

developmental theory: theory implicating the influence of genetics as the major determinant of aging

diabetes insipidus (DI): a condition of insufficient antidiuretic hormone resulting in the inability of the body to concentrate or retain water

diabetes mellitus: a disorder of the body's metabolism of protein, fats, and carbohydrates because of an absolute lack of insulin or insulin resistance

diagnosis: a label for the altered health condition

diapedesis: a process that allows leukocytes to move between and through endothelial cells in order to engulf and destroy the offending agent and remove dead tissue

diarrhea: loose, watery stools

diastole: the relaxation of the heart that allows blood to fill the ventricles

diastolic blood pressure: the amount of pressure that remains in the aorta during the resting phase of the cardiac cycle

diastolic failure: failure that occurs with stiffness of the ventricle and loss of relaxation ability, which impairs the heart's ability to optimally fill with blood between cardiac contractions

differentiation: a process of changing the physical and functional properties of a cell to allow greater specificity and functionality to that cell

diffusing capacity: a measurement of carbon monoxide (CO), oxygen, or nitric oxide transfer from inspired gas to pulmonary capillary blood; is reflective of the volume of a gas that diffuses through the alveolar capillary membrane each minute

diffusion: movement of particles from an area of high to lower concentration

digestion: the process by which food is broken down mechanically and chemically in the gastrointestinal tract and converted into absorbable components

diplegia: involving both legs

diploid: the number of chromosomes a human body cell contains; 23 pairs of chromosomes, or a total of 46

diplopia: resulting from a lack of coordination of the extraocular muscles; may result in double vision

direct extension: a process of tumor cells moving into adjacent tissues and organs

discoid: red, raised, round rash

discriminative pathway: neurologic pathway communicating sensory information, including discriminative touch and spatial orientation

disease: an impairment of cell, tissue, organ, or system functioning

disseminated intravascular coagulation (DIC): a condition of uncontrolled activation of clotting factors resulting in widespread thrombi formation followed by depletion of coagulation factors and platelets; leads to massive hemorrhage

distal axonopathy: axonal injury of neurons in distal areas of the body, such as hands and feet

diuretics: drugs that increase urine production

diverticula: more than one diverticulum

diverticulitis: infection of the diverticula

diverticulosis: condition characterized by the presence of diverticula

diverticulum: small sac or outpouching along the wall of the colon; plural diverticula

dominant: an allele possessed by one of the parents of a hybrid that is expressed in the latter to the exclusion of contrasting allele (the recessive) from the other parent

dorsal horns: posterior extensions of the spinal cord containing sensory neurons; receive afferent impulses via the dorsal roots and other neurons

drusen: small, yellow deposits; deposition under the macula is characteristic of dry (atrophic) macular degeneration

dry (atrophic) MD: retinal deterioration resulting from deposition of drusen, under the macula next to the basement membrane of the retinal pigment epithelium; also known as atrophic macular degeneration

dual energy X-ray absorptiometry (DEXA): specialized, low-level radiographic technique used to measure bone density

dyskinesia: difficulty in performing voluntary movements

dyskinetic: inability to control muscle movement

dysmenorrhea: pain with menstrual periods

dyspareunia: painful intercourse

dyspepsia: a vague epigastric discomfort associated with nausea and heartburn

dysplasia: actual change in cell size, shape, uniformity, arrangement, and structure

dyspnea: the subjective feeling of shortness of breath or the inability to get enough air

dystonia: abnormal tone

dysuria: pain with urination

ecchymoses: bruises from superficial bleeding into the skin

ectocervix: outside of the cervix lined with squamous epithelium

ectopic: refers to hormone secretion from a site outside of an endocrine gland

edema: the presence of excessive watery fluid that accumulates in the tissues

efferent neurons: neurons that carry impulses from central nervous system to the periphery

elastin: a substance that allows stretching and recoil of tissue

electrical synapses: transmit impulses via passage of current-carrying ions through small openings or gaps

electrolytes: ionizable substances in solution; conduct electricity in solution

electronystagmography (ENG): group of tests that determine vestibular function based on eye movement

elemental body: the metabolically inactive stage in the life cycle of chlamydiae in which the microorganism attaches to and internalizes the host cell

elicitation phase: second phase of delayed hypersensitivity reaction; memory cells in the dermis are stimulated after presentation with antigen by Langerhans cells, prompting activation of memory T cells and stimulation of cell-mediated responses

embolus: any plug of material, such as thrombi, air, neoplasms, microorganisms, or amniotic fluid, that travels in the circulation and can obstruct the lumen of a vessel

embryonic carcinomas: resemble primitive undifferentiated embryonic tissue

emphysema: an irreversible enlargement of the air spaces beyond the terminal bronchioles, most notably in the alveoli, resulting in destruction of the alveolar walls and obstruction of airflow

encephalopathy: brain disorder

encopresis: a condition of fecal incontinence characterized by inappropriate fecal soiling; frequently seen in the pediatric population; also known as functional nonretentive soiling

endemic: a condition in which the incidence and prevalence are stable and predictable

endocardium: the inner lining of the heart that forms a continuous layer of endothelium that joins the arteries and veins to the heart, forming a closed circulatory system

endocervical canal: area between the external and internal cervical os; lined with columnar epithelium

endocrine: hormone secretion with systemic effects

endocrine pancreas: an organ that secretes hormones, such as insulin and glucagon

endocrine system: a collective group of tissues that are capable of secreting hormones

endocytosis: transport mechanism involving vesicular enclosure of particles from the extracellular environment into the cytoplasm for use by the cell

endogenous: from within the body system

endolymph: fluid filling the cochlea

endometriosis: a condition involving endometrial tissue that is located outside of the uterus

endoplasmic reticulum: cellular organelle composed of a complex network of tubules; important in the production of proteins and fats and ion regulation; subtypes include rough and smooth

endothelial cells: cells that form a tight junction within the inner lining of the blood and lymphatic vessels and the heart

endotoxin: a complex of phospholipid–polysaccharide molecules that form the structural component of the gram-negative cell wall and causes inflammatory mediators to be released, leading to a massive inflammatory response

energy: the capacity to do work

enteric nervous system: subdivision of the peripheral nervous system; provides innervation to the muscle of fibers of the intestine via the myenteric (Auerbach) and Meissner plexus, controlling gastrointestinal movement and sensation

enuresis: urinary incontinence; inability to voluntarily prevent the discharge of urine

eosinophils: granulocyte with greatest protection against parasites

epidemic: a dramatic increase in the incidence of a health condition in a population

epidemiology: the study of disease in populations
epigenetic: regulation of the expression of gene activity without alteration of genetic structure
epiphyseal: long bone ossification site
epistaxis: episodes of nose bleeds
epithelioid cells: phagocytes that gather and contain smaller substances by forming a wall, or fibrotic granuloma, around the affected area
epithelioma: a benign tumor of the squamous epithelium
erectile dysfunction (ED): the inability to achieve or maintain an erection sufficient for satisfactory sexual performance
erythema: redness caused by increased blood flow to the tissues
erythrocyte sedimentation rate: also referred to as a sed rate, or ESR; a nonspecific method of testing for inflammation
erythrocytes: red blood cells (RBCs); comprise a large proportion of the blood and are needed to provide tissue oxygenation
erythropoiesis: the formation of new red blood cells
erythropoietin: a protein that stimulates the formation of red blood cells for growth
eschar: a thick, coagulated crust that develops after a thermal or chemical burn that cauterizes the skin
esotropia: suppression of one visual images by the brain, preserving normal vision
essential fat: a lipid required for physiologic functioning
essential nutrients: those that must be consumed regularly in the diet, because the body is unable to synthesize the nutrient in quantities sufficient to meet its needs
etiology: the cause of the disease
evolution theory: developmental theory suggesting that aging is the result of the forces of natural selection
exacerbation: a period in which symptoms flare and can be severe
exocrine pancreas: an organ that contains acini cells, which secrete digestive enzymes and alkaline fluids through the pancreatic duct into the duodenum
exocytosis: the process of movement of granules or particles out of the cell; fusion of the membrane surrounding the granule with the cell membrane, followed by rupture and release of contents
exogenous: from the external environment
exon: segment of DNA coded for protein production
exophthalmos: a protrusion of the eyeballs that sometimes occurs with hyperthyroidism
exotoxins: potent substances produced by many bacteria, which result in host cell dysfunction or lysis
expectorate: to spit out the mucus that is ejected during a cough
expiration: the process of removing carbon dioxide out of the body through the lungs
expressivity: the evidence of the gene in the phenotype
external anal sphincter: skeletal muscle surrounding the internal rectal sphincter; innervated by the pudendal nerve of the somatic nervous system; providing voluntary control of defecation
external auditory meatus: opening of the ear canal
external urethral sphincter: skeletal muscle of the bladder neck; allows for voluntary release of urine; innervated by the pudendal nerve
extracellular compartment: body fluid in the interstitial tissue and plasma outside the cells; contains two-thirds of the body water; accounts for 40% of body weight
extracellular matrix: (ECM) the layers of architectural structures that support the cells
extracorporeal shockwave lithotripsy (ESWL): procedure of renal calculi removal involving acoustic shock waves to break up the stone; the most common procedure for kidney stone removal
extrapyramidal disorders: movement disorders affecting the structures of the basal ganglia, substantia nigra, and subthalamic nucleus
extrapyramidal system: nervous system outside of the pyramidal nervous system; attenuated erratic motions; maintains muscle tone and trunk stability; composed of the subcortical nuclei of the basal ganglia
exudate: the watery fluid with a high protein and leukocyte concentration that accumulates at the site of injury
exudative macular degeneration: macular degeneration characterized by the formation of new blood vessels under the retina and macula, known as choroidal neovascularization; macular damage caused by leakage of fluid and bleeding from new vessels, altering the shape of the macula and distorting central vision; also known as wet macular degeneration
facilitated diffusion: assisted movement of substances across the cell membrane; not energy dependent
facultative parasites: microorganisms that may live on the host but can also survive independently
familial tendency: propagation of a condition among family members
feedback mechanism: regulatory mechanism; response of input to a system by generation of output in a given system

fetal alcohol syndrome (FAS): condition resulting from exposure of a fetus to alcohol; characterized by mental handicap, growth deficit, and physical disability

fibrillation: a problem of the heart chamber vibrating instead of effectively pumping

fibrinolysis: the dissolution of blood clots

fibroblasts: cells that produce and replace the connective tissue layer to support the constructive phase of wound healing

filtration pressure: the force that promotes movement of fluid across a pressure gradient

fistula: an abnormal track or passage that forms between two segments of bowel or other epithelial tissue

flaccid: relaxed, without tone

forced expiratory volume in 1 second (FEV1): the maximal amount of air expired from the lungs in 1 second

forced vital capacity (FVC): the maximal amount of air that is exhaled from the lungs during a forced exhalation

fovea: area in the center of the macula with the highest density of cones

frank: visible blood in the stool

free radical injury: damage to cells resulting from reactive oxygen species

free radical theory: stochastic theory of aging suggesting that intracellular production of reactive oxygen species (ROS) contributes to the final determination of life span

friability: a state where tissue readily bleeds

full-thickness burns: formerly known as third-degree burns; burns that damage the epidermis, dermis, and can penetrate subcutaneous layers as well

fully saturated: a state in which all of the available seats for hemoglobin molecules are occupied on the red blood cell

fulminant hepatitis: liver failure from severe acute hepatitis

function: the action or workings of the various properties of the body

functional electrical stimulation (FES): technique used to generate artificial autonomic reflexes to promote mechanisms regulating bowel and bladder function

functional incontinence: unintentional loss of urine; characterized by normal bladder control coupled with an impaired ability to transport to toilet facilities

functional nonretentive soiling: voluntary or involuntary evacuation of stool; occurs in the absence of an appropriate toileting situation; often results from resistant behaviors in the child or ineffective toilet-training management strategies

gamete: ova and sperm; contains only one of the chromosome pairs, known as the haploid number

ganglion: collection of nerve cell bodies in the peripheral nervous system

gap junction: intercellular junctions with 2-nm gaps characterized by enhanced cell-to-cell communication

gastritis: an inflammatory condition of the gastric mucosa of the stomach

gate control theory: modification of the specificity theory; stimulation of the large type A beta and alpha inhibitory fibers "close the gate," preventing crossover and inhibiting pain impulse conduction along type A delta and type C fibers, diminishing pain perception

gene amplification: a process of altering chromosomes by accelerating the replication and number of copies of a gene

general adaptation syndrome: a term used to describe the neuroendocrine response to a stressor and the corresponding physiologic changes

generalized anxiety disorder (GAD): a condition characterized by excessive, uncontrollable, and irrational worry lasting greater than 6 months

genes: individual units of inheritance located on the chromosomes; determine cell protein characteristics

genetic code: hereditary units containing information for the production of proteins

genomic imprinting: an epigenetic phenomenon; mechanism that controls expression of genes based on parental origin

genomics: study of the human genome; includes the functions and interactions of all genes comprising an individual

genotype: genetic makeup of an individual

Ghon complex: a combination of the Ghon focus and additional granulomas that develop through the lymph channels in the lungs

Ghon focus: the formation of a granuloma, or walled-off area of bacteria, which is considered the primary lung lesion in tuberculosis

giant cells: phagocytes that can engulf particles much larger than the typical macrophage

gigantism: condition of hyperplasia characterized by excessive growth; growth hormone excess before the closure of the epiphyseal growth plates of the long bones

glia: neural support cells in the brain; provide support and nutrition, maintain homeostasis, and form myelin

global ischemia: consequences of inadequate blood supply to meet the needs of the brain tissue; results in hypoxia

glomerulus: capillary network of the nephron; located in the renal cortex; produces early urinary filtrate
glutamate: excitatory neurotransmitter
glutens: specific proteins found in wheat, rye, and barley
glycolipid: sugar bound to lipid heads of the plasma membrane
glycoproteins: regulate cell movement across the matrix, provide a place for attachment of the cells to the matrix, and prompt the cells to function
glycosylated hemoglobin (HbA_{1c}): a blood test that depicts hemoglobin and red blood cell exposure to glucose over the previous 3 to 4 months
goiter: an enlargement of the thyroid gland caused by follicular epithelial hyperplasia from excessive thyroid hormone exposure
Golgi apparatus: cellular organelle with a membranous structure; prepares substances by the endoplasmic reticulum for secretion out of the cell
grading: a process of differentiating the level of anaplasia depicted by the tumor
graft versus host disease (GVHD): a condition in which transplanted donor T lymphocytes mount an immune response against the host
gram-negative: bacteria with cell walls that do not retain a dark blue color when Gram stain is applied and instead turn red when counterstained in the laboratory
gram-positive: bacteria with cell walls that preserve the Gram stain and turn dark blue in the laboratory
granulation tissue: connective tissue characterized by extensive macrophages and fibroblasts and the promotion of angiogenesis
granulocytes: phagocytic cells named for the cytoplasmic granules common to all types; polymorphonuclear leukocytes, including neutrophils, eosinophils, and basophils
granulomas: nodular inflammatory lesions that encase harmful substances
Graves disease: an autoimmune condition that causes excessive stimulation of the thyroid gland
gray matter: tissue of the central nervous system composed primarily of cell bodies; contains synapses between sensory neurons, motor neurons, and interneurons
gustation: the sensation of taste
glycerol test: diagnostic test used to identify inner ear volume excess typically seen in Ménière disease
gyri: irregular convolutions on the brain surface
haploid: cells containing single chromosomes, rather than pairs; chromosome number totals 23 (22 autosomes, 1 sex chromosome); characteristic of gametes
haustra: pouches between taenia coli in the large intestine
health: the condition of being sound in body, mind, and spirit
heart block: the obstruction of cardiac conduction, often at the atrioventricular node, leading to heart dysrhythmias
heart failure: reflects an inadequacy of heart pumping so that the heart fails to maintain the circulation of blood
heart rate: the number of heartbeats that occur in 1 minute
helper T lymphocyte: subset of T lymphocyte that enhance humoral and cell-mediated responses of the immune system
hematoma: larger accumulations of blood in the tissue
hematuria: blood in the urine
hemiplegia: involving one arm and one leg on the same side of the body
hemodialysis: treatment using special filters to remove wastes that the kidneys no longer can do on their own through the mechanisms of diffusion, osmosis, and ultrafiltration
hemoglobin A (HbA): adult form of hemoglobin
hemoglobin F (HbF): fetal form of hemoglobin
hemoglobin S (HbS): sickled form of hemoglobin
hemolysis: breakdown of red blood cells
hemolytic: destruction of blood cells
hemoptysis: coughing up blood from the respiratory tract; defined by the presence of red blood cells in the sputum
hemorrhage: the loss of blood through the vessel wall
hepatic steatosis: fatty liver
hepatomegaly: enlarged liver
hepatorenal syndrome: renal failure caused by severe renal vasoconstriction in patients with liver disease
heredity: passage of characteristics from parent to offspring
Hertz (Hz): unit measurement of frequency; equivalent to one cycle per second
heterozygous: different alleles on each chromosome
heteroplasmy: random distribution of genes leading to a variable distribution in tissues
hirsutism: a condition of excessive body and facial hair
histology: a branch of anatomy that deals with the minute structure of cells and tissues, which are discernible with a microscope
Hodgkin lymphoma: a malignant disorder of the lymphoid tissue often characterized by the painless, progressive enlargement of cervical (neck) lymph nodes

Homans sign: a test of foot dorsiflexion, which, in the presence of deep vein thrombosis, causes pain in the back of the lower leg

homeostasis: a dynamic steady state marked by appropriate regulatory responses in the body

homozygous: identical alleles on each chromosome

hormones: chemical substances, formed in a tissue or organ and carried in the blood, that stimulate or inhibit the growth or function of other tissues or organs

host: the individual who is exposed to and contracts an infection

human immunodeficiency virus (HIV): enveloped retrovirus that infects CD4 T cells, dendritic cells, and macrophages; virus associated with the secondary immunodeficiency, acquired immunodeficiency syndrome (AIDS)

human leukocyte antigens (HLAs): the major histocompatibility complex proteins in humans; HLA genes encode antigen specificity; important in transplant rejection

human papilloma virus (HPV): DNA virus; specific viral strains cause cutaneous and genital warts and severe cervical intraepithelial lesions

humoral immunity: adaptive immunity involving antibodies

Hutchinson–Gilford progeria: syndrome commonly characterized by accelerated aging; results from damage to the LMNA gene that codes for the protein lamin A

hydrophilic: possessing affinity to water

hydrophobic: lacking affinity to water

hydrostatic forces: force promoting fluid movement between extracellular compartments; promotes movement of fluid based on the pressure gradient; also known as filtration pressure

hydroureter: accumulation of fluid in the urinary ureter; represents a consequence of complete ureteral obstruction

hygroma: cystic structure containing serous fluid

hyperacute graft rejection: rapid rejection of grafts

hypercalcemia: blood calcium levels greater than 10.5 mg/dL

hypercapnia: a state of increased carbon dioxide in the blood

hyperchloremia: blood chloride levels greater than 108 mEq/L

hyperglycemia: an elevation in the blood glucose level

hyperkalemia: potassium blood levels greater than 5 mEq/L

hyperketonemia: a condition of elevated circulating ketones that results from a loss of insulin, which is an inhibitor of lipolysis

hyperlactatemia: elevation of lactic acid in the blood

hypermagnesemia: magnesium levels greater than 2.5 mEq/L

hypernatremia: greater than 145 mEq/L of sodium in the blood

hyperopia: error in refraction commonly referred to as farsightedness

hyperphosphatemia: blood phosphate levels greater than 4.5 mg/dL

hyperpituitarism: a generic term indicating the increased secretion of one or more pituitary hormones

hyperplasia: increase in the number of cells

hyperpolarization: when the resting membrane potential is less negative than normal

hypertension: an elevation in blood pressure commonly defined by a systolic pressure above 140 mm Hg or a diastolic pressure above 90 mm Hg

hyperthyroidism: a state of excessive thyroid hormone as a result of excessive stimulation of the thyroid gland, diseases of the thyroid gland, or excess production of thyroid-stimulating hormone by a pituitary adenoma

hypertonic: solutions having a greater osmolality than the intracellular fluid

hypertrophy: increase in cell size

hypervolemia: excessive increase of fluid in the extracellular compartment

hyphae: tubular branches formed by mold colonies

hypocalcemia: calcium blood levels of less than 8.5 mg/dL

hypochloremia: blood chloride levels of less than 98 mEq/L

hypochromic: indicates pale red blood cells on microscopic examination

hypoglycemia: low blood glucose levels

hypokalemia: potassium blood levels of less than 3.5 mEq/L

hypomagnesemia: magnesium blood levels of less than 1.5 mEq/L

hypomania: state where people are energetic, excitable, and hyperactive, and may be highly productive

hyponatremia: less than 135 mEq/L of sodium in the blood

hypoparathyroidism: less than 10 pg/dL parathyroid hormone in the blood

hypophosphatemia: blood phosphate levels less than 2.5 mg/dL

hypopituitarism: a generic term indicating the decreased secretion of one or more pituitary hormones

hypopolarization: when the resting membrane potential is more negative than normal

hypotension: a condition of reduced blood pressure

hypothalamic–pituitary axis: the neuronal system that regulates hormone secretion and inhibition

hypothyroidism: a state of deficient thyroid hormone

hypotonic: solutions having a lower osmolality than the intercellular fluid

hypovolemia: decreased vascular volume

hypovolemic shock: the result of inadequate blood/plasma volume

hypoxemia: decreased oxygen in the arterial blood leading to a decrease in the partial pressure of oxygen ($Pa{O_2}$)

hypoxia: cellular deprivation of oxygen

iatrogenic: the term used to describe illnesses that are the inadvertent result of medical treatment

icteric phase: a stage of liver disease marked by jaundice

idiopathic: describes a condition that does not have a clear etiology

illness: a state that results in suffering or distress

immune response: the third line of defense, which wages a specific defense mechanism targeted at certain harmful invaders in the body

immune senescence: progressive dysfunction of the immune system associated with aging; characterized by both diminished and enhanced immune responses

immunity: process conferring protection against disease; includes active and passive

immunodeficiency: condition resulting from an inadequate immune defense; may be primary (directly caused by an alteration in immunity) or secondary (a consequence of another disease process)

immunoglobulins (Ig): a group of structurally related proteins important in immune function; composed of a variable region promoting antigen specificity and a constant region; classifications include IgG, IgA, IgM, IgD, and IgE

immunologic memory: process by which memory cells respond much more rapidly when reexposed to the same antigen; dramatically shortens and intensifies the immunologic response

immunologic theory of aging: developmental theory of aging associated with reduced resistance to disease secondary to reduced T-cell function and enhanced autoimmune responses

immunology: study of the structure and function of the immune system as well as the phenomena of immunity-induced sensitivity and allergy

immunotherapy: use of vaccines to stimulate the immune system to attack antigens associated with disease

incidence: the rate of occurrence of a health condition at any given time

incus: one of the three bones comprising the ossicle of the ear; also known as the anvil

infarct: an area of necrosis resulting from a sudden insufficiency of arterial or venous blood supply

infarction: the process of obstructing a blood vessel

infectious disease: also called infection; a state of tissue destruction resulting from invasion by microorganisms

infectivity: the proportion of exposures needed to cause infection in an individual based on the pathogens' ability to enter, survive in, and multiply in the host

infertility: the inability to achieve pregnancy after 1 year of unprotected intercourse

inflammatory response: the second line of defense, which is a nonspecific defense mechanism to protect from harmful invaders and to prepare an injury site for healing

ingest: particle entry into the cytoplasm through incorporation into a vesicle via a portion of the cell membrane

inhibin: a hormone that alerts the pituitary gland to suppress the secretion of gonadotropins

initiating event: a situation that causes a mutation in a cell

injury: any form of damage, harm, or loss to the cell, tissue, organ, or organ system

innate immunity: responsible for early, rapid response to pathogens without prior exposure

insidious: gradual in onset

inspiration: the process of breathing in to acquire oxygen

insulin: an anabolic hormone required for the uptake of glucose by the many cells, particularly those of the liver, muscle, and adipose cells

insulin-like growth factor 1 (IGF-1): hormone secreted by the liver; promotes growth in bones, cartilage, soft tissues, and organs

integral protein: form of transmembrane protein; forms a channel in the plasma membrane for transport of ions

intermittent claudication: a condition of fatigue or aching in the leg muscles even when walking short distances

internal rectal sphincter: thick layer of smooth muscle at the distal end of the rectum; provides tonic constriction under sympathetic control

internal urethral sphincter: ring of circular smooth muscle comprising the bladder neck; relaxation promotes release of urine from the bladder

interneuron: neurons connecting motor and sensory neurons; transmit signals between afferent and efferent neurons; most abundant neuron type

interventricular foramen: area of passage of the cerebrospinal fluid between the lateral to the third ventricle; also known as the foramen of Monro

intracellular compartment: fluid inside the cells; contains two-thirds of the body water, accounting for 40% of body weight

intraneuronal inclusions: distinctive structures formed in the nucleus or cytoplasm

intrinsic enteric nervous system: source of innervation to the gastrointestinal nervous system

intron: segment of DNA not involved in protein expression

involution: decrease in the size of tissues and organs

ions: electrically charged particles resulting from gain or loss of one or more electrons; negatively charged particles known as anions; positively charged particles known as cations

iris: colored part of the eye

iron-deficiency anemia: a problem of hemoglobin and red blood cell development caused by inadequate iron stores

irrigation: process of rinsing an area with fluid or air

ischemia: local response to decrease in blood supply

islets of Langerhans: clusters of cells, located throughout the pancreas, that are responsible for the secretion of hormones

isoflavone: nonsteroidal estrogen found in high concentrations in soy products; also known as phytoestrogens

isolated systolic hypertension: an elevation in systolic blood pressure without an elevation in the diastolic blood pressure

isotonic: solutions with same osmolality as the intracellular fluid

jaundice: the yellow-tinged color of the skin and sclera of the eyes in those with liver disease

karyotype: picture of arranged, paired, like chromosomes in order from largest to smallest

keloids: hypertrophic scars that result from excessive collagen production at the site of injury

Kernig sign: a test used to elicit meningeal pain; the patient is placed supine with the knees bent and hips flexed, one knee is lifted upward, thereby eliciting pain

ketoacidosis: a state of metabolic acidosis, which signifies that the body is accessing fat and protein sources for energy and is releasing ketones, which are highly acidic, in the process

kinin system: a series of potent vasoactive chemical mediators, such as bradykinin, that play a role in vasodilation, vasoconstriction, cell migration, the pain response, and the activation of other cells active in the inflammatory response

Kupffer cells: phagocytes housed in the liver

Kussmaul respirations: deep, rapid respirations that present as a compensatory measure to release excess acids through the lungs and into the atmosphere

kwashiorkor: protein deprivation in persons consuming adequate carbohydrates

kyphosis: exaggerated anterior concave curvature of the thoracic spine associated with osteoporosis

labile cells: those that constantly regenerate through mitosis, particularly epithelial cells of the skin, gastrointestinal tract, and urinary tract, and blood cells in the bone marrow

labyrinthitis: inflammation of the labyrinth of the inner ear; precipitation of severe vertigo and sensorineural hearing loss

lacrimal glands: primary producers of tears

lacteal: lymphatic channel within each small intestinal villus critical for the absorption of fats

lactic acidemia: elevation of lactic acid in the blood

lactic acidosis: pH less than 7.35 because of elevation in lactic acid in the blood

Langerhans cells: immature dendritic cells in the skin; carry surface receptors for immunoglobulin and complement, important in the immune response

lanugo: a fine downy hair that covers the body in some patients with anorexia nervosa

large intestine/colon: organ of the gastrointestinal system; composed of the cecum, appendix, colon, rectum, and anal canal; further divided into the ascending transverse, descending, and sigmoid portions

laser-assisted in situ keratomileusis (LASIK): surgical procedure used to treat myopia, hyperopia, and astigmatism

latency: a period of dormancy

leiomyomas: fibrous tumors of the uterus

lens: eye structure responsible for fine-tuning of focus

leukocytes: white blood cells; a group of cells active in defending the body against microorganisms and in promoting an immune response

leukocytosis: an elevation in the white blood cell, or leukocyte, with a count usually above 10,000/ mm^3

Lewy body: protein aggregations composed of the protein alpha-synuclein located primarily in the cells of the substantia nigra; associated with neurodegenerative disease, particularly Parkinson disease

life expectancy: the age at which 50% of a given population is expected to survive

ligands: molecules that bind to specific receptors; involved in signal transduction

limbic system: circuits that connect one's cognitive activity, expression of emotions, and behavior
lipids: a group of substances that are rich in energy and insoluble in water
lipid bilayer: an organized structure of two interconnected layers composed of nonpolar hydrophobic lipid tails connected to polar hydrophilic heads
lipofuscin: fatty brown lipid pigment; intracellular deposition causes stiffening or rigidity of cellular structure
local: refers to those manifestations that are directly at the site of illness, injury, or infection and are confined to a specific area
local mediators: substances involved in cellular responses in the immediate area
local spread: the proliferation of the neoplasm within the tissue of origin
loop diuretics: drugs that increase urine production through reduced reabsorption of sodium in the thick ascending loop of Henle, causing a decreased osmolality in the interstitial fluid of the collecting ducts and impairing the ability to concentrate urine at the loop
lymph fluid: filtration product of extracellular fluid from tissues
lymph node: joined segment of lymphatic vessels
lymphadenitis: the enlargement and inflammation of the nearby lymph nodes, which can occur as a function of filtering or draining harmful substances at the injury site
lymphadenopathy: swelling or enlargement of the lymph nodes
lymphatic system: circulates lymphocytes in lymph fluid; work in concert with the blood vessels to promote an effective immune response
lymphedema: obstructed lymph flow with movement of fluid into the interstitium
lymphocyte ignorance: the process of converting lymphocytes from nonresponsive to self-reactive
lymphoid progenitor: cellular origin of natural killer cells, T and B lymphocytes
lysis: the breakdown and removal of cells
lysosomes: cellular organelle composed of small sacs surrounded by membrane; responsible for hydrolytic digestion of cellular debris
maceration: the softening and breaking down of tissue
macronutrients: proteins, carbohydrates, and fats
macrophage: large, long-lived phagocytic leukocyte found within body tissues associated with a prolonged inflammatory response
macroscopic analysis: visual determination of color and clarity
macula: area of the retina responsible for central vision, color vision, and fine detail
mainstream smoke: active exposure to smoke
major depressive disorder (MDD): a condition characterized by a pervasive and persistent low mood
major histocompatibility complex (MHC): molecules promoting recognition of the body's "self" antigens from foreign "nonself" antigens; trap an antigen within the cell and then transport it to the cell surface where it can be displayed to T cells; subsets include MHC class I and class II molecules
major histocompatibility complex class I (MHC I): subset of MHC molecules recognized by CD8 cytotoxic T cells
major histocompatibility complex class II (MHC II): subset of MHC molecules recognized by CD4 helper (T_H1 and T_H2) T cells
malabsorption: indicates a lack of movement of specific nutrients across the gastrointestinal mucosa
malabsorption syndrome: a condition in which several nutrients are not adequately absorbed
malar: rash over cheeks; characteristic manifestation of systemic lupus erythematosus (SLE)
malignancy: invasive and destructive cellular growth, as in cancer
malignant: describes tumors that are invasive, destructive, spread to other sites, and do not resemble the tissue of origin
malleus: one of the three bones comprising the ossicle of the ear; also known as the hammer
malnutrition: a state of inadequate or excessive exposure to nutrients
mania: a condition where a person displays erratic and impulsive behavior, resulting in poor decisions, and requires very little, if any, sleep
marasmus: a condition of starvation related to deprivation of all food
mass movements: strong peristaltic movements, occurring three to four times a day; promotes the propulsion of stool
mast cells: leukocytes that are housed throughout the body within connective tissue and near all blood vessels; they are responsible for production and immediate release of chemical mediators
mastoiditis: bacterial infection and inflammation of the air cells of the mastoid bone
matrilineal: transmitted through female or maternal lines
mean arterial pressure: an adequate measure of *systemic:* tissue perfusion; is calculated as one-third the pulse pressure plus diastolic pressure
mechanical injury: damage caused by impact of a body part
Meckel diverticulum: rare congenital condition characterized by the presence of a blind pouch in the colon

meconium: infant's first stool; represents the digestion of amniotic fluid and is sterile, black, sticky, and odorless

meiosis: process of sex cell (gamete) division; cell division resulting in gametocytes containing half (haploid) the number of chromosomes found in a somatic cell

Meissner plexus: part of the enteric nervous system, located in the submucosa of the large intestine; transmits sensory impulses through stretch receptors

melena: black stool indicative of upper gastrointestinal bleeding

membrane attack complex (MAC): a cascade of events in the inflammatory process that leads to cell lysis

membrane pore: membrane passage between the extracellular and intracellular environment

membrane potential: difference in electrical charge between the inside and outside of the cell

memory cells: differentiated B cells capable of responding much more rapidly when re-exposed to the same antigen; dramatically shortening and intensifying the immunologic response

menarche: the time of the first menstrual period

Mendelian pattern of inheritance: predictable trait transmission based on autosomal dominant or recessive genotypes

Ménière disease: condition associated with severe vertigo, sensorineural hearing loss, and tinnitus; related to overproduction or decreased absorption of endolymph

meninges: membranes surrounding the brain and spinal cord of the central nervous system; contains cerebrospinal fluid; includes the pia, arachnoid, and dura mater

menometrorrhagia: shortened menstrual interval, heavy bleeding

menopausal bone loss: rapid phase of bone loss in women after menopause

menopause: permanent cessation of menses for a 12-month period

menorrhagia: excessive flow or prolonged duration of menses with regular menstrual interval

messenger RNA (mRNA): template for protein synthesis; depends on a codon sequence based on that of the complementary strand of DNA (cDNA); cytoplasmic area where protein is made in amino acid sequences

metabolic acidosis: alteration in acid–base balance characterized by reduction of HCO_3^-, prompting an increase in pH

metabolic alkalosis: alteration in acid–base balance characterized by increased levels of HCO_3^- resulting in a decrease of pH

metaplasia: changing of one cell type to another

metastases: process that occurs when neoplasms are spread to distant sites often by way of the lymphatics or blood vessels

metrorrhagia: irregular menstrual intervals

microbiology: a section of biology dealing specifically with the study of microscopic forms of life

microcytic: cells are small; the term microcytic is often used to describe small red blood cells in certain types of anemia

microglial nodules: structure formed by the union of microglia and astrocytes

micronutrients: vitamins and minerals

microscopic analysis: analysis of urine components under magnification; low-power magnification may detect crystals, casts, squamous cells, and other large components; white and red blood cells and bacterial forms may be detected with high-power magnification

microstimulation: electrical stimulation to preganglionic neurons and interneurons controlling bladder function

micturition: process of urine elimination

minerals: inorganic substances critical to the regulation of hundreds of cellular processes; minerals constitute bone, hemoglobin, enzymes, hormones, and chemical mediators; charged (ionic) minerals mediate impulse conduction within the nervous system; minerals maintain water balance, acid–base balance, and osmotic pressure and are critical for muscle contraction and form the structural components of bones and teeth

mitochondria: cellular organelle containing enzymes involved in citric acid cycle, fatty acid oxidation, and oxidative phosphorylation; principal producer of the cellular energy source adenosine triphosphate

mitosis: process of reproduction of nuclear chromosomes in somatic cells; reproductive phases include prophase, prometaphase, metaphase, anaphase, and telophase; results in the creation of daughter cells with the same chromosome number and genetic makeup as the cell of origin

mixed hearing loss: combination of both sensorineural and conductive hearing loss

molecular mimicry: close resemblance between foreign antigen and self-antigen

mold: a multicellular form of fungus

monoamines: class of neurotransmitters, including norepinephrine, dopamine, and serotonin

monoclonal origin: the process of starting with a single mutated cell and developing into cancer

monocyte: large, mononuclear leukocytes representing 3% to 7% of the total number of circulating leukocytes associated with a prolonged inflammatory response

mononeuropathy: nerve damage limited to a single area

monosomy: one copy of a chromosome, in place of the normal pair; the result of nondisjuncture

mood: an internal, subjective psychological state, which directs how a person feels and perceives the world

morbidity: a poor quality of life resulting from a disease

morphology: a branch of biology that deals with the form and structure of animals and plants; looks more specifically at how cells and tissues change in form after encountering disease

mortality: the death rate resulting from a disease

mosaicism: combination of cell lines with regular and altered numbers of chromosomes

motor neurons: carry impulses from the central nervous system to an effector muscle

multifactorial: having a number of events that led to the development of the condition

mutation: change in genes or sequence of base pairs that make up the chromosomes; genetic alteration perpetuated in subsequent cellular divisions

mutator genes: genes that repair mutated DNA and protect the genome

mycelium: a cluster of hyphae formed from mold colonies

mycoses: infections with fungi as the pathogen

myeloid progenitor: origin of immune system cells, including monocytes, dendritic cells, granulocytes, and mast cells

myenteric (Auerbach): plexus: part of the enteric nervous system; found between the longitudinal and circular muscle layers of the large intestine; provides increased tonic and rhythmic contractions

myocardial infarction: the total occlusion of one or more coronary arteries resulting in ischemia and death of myocardial tissues

myocardium: the thick muscular layer of the heart

myofascia: outer membrane of muscle tissue

myopia: error in refraction; commonly known as nearsightedness

myringotomy: incision of the tympanic membrane to drain fluid

myxedema: a condition of hypothyroidism marked by the accumulation of boggy, nonpitting edematous tissue, especially of the face, mucous membranes, hands, and feet, from protein–carbohydrate complexes that accumulate in the extracellular matrix and attract fluid into the tissues

naive lymphocytes: lymphocytes that have not yet encountered an antigen

natural killer cells: large, granular lymphocytes; nonspecific cytotoxic cells

necrosis: disorderly process of cell death associated with inflammation

negative feedback loop: a system of hormone regulation in which low levels of hormone stimulate additional release and high levels of hormone inhibit further release

neoplasia: the irreversible deviant development of cells resulting in the formation of neoplasms

nephron: functional unit of the kidney; composed of the glomerulus, proximal tubule, loop of Henle, distal tubule, and collecting duct; responsible for filtering water-soluble substances from the blood, reabsorption of filtered nutrients, water, and electrolytes, and secretion of waste

nephropathy: a problem of degenerative changes in small vessels in the kidneys

neurofibrillary tangles: twisted, helical structure of accumulated proteins, primarily including tau; commonly associated with Alzheimer disease

neuroendocrine theory: developmental theory of aging suggesting that the interrelationship between neurons and associated hormones serves as the stimulus for aging

neurogenic: pain originating within the nervous system

neurogenic shock: a result of brain or spinal cord injury in which altered neuronal transmission leads to a loss of tension in the blood vessels, allowing unregulated vasodilation, decreased peripheral vascular resistance, and reduced blood pressure; oxygenated blood is *not:* shunted to vital organs, and perfusion to vital organs is reduced

neuromatrix theory: modification of the pattern theory; a widely distributed neural network in the brain (body-self neuromatrix) containing somatosensory, limbic, and thalamocortical components integrates multiple sources of input resulting in the cognitive, affective, and sensory perceptions of pain

neuromodulator: chemical released from axon terminals, which inhibits, potentiates, or prolongs effects of neurotransmitter

neuron: nerve cell; fundamental unit of the nervous system; composed of a cell body, one axon, and a variable number of dendrites

neuropathy: a problem of nerve degeneration to damage to cell body resulting in delayed nerve conduction and impaired sensory function

neuropathic: pain originating within the nervous system

neurophagia: phagocytosis and inflammatory responses caused by a dead neuron damaging

neurostimulation: electrical stimulation of efferent nerves

neurotransmitter: chemical agent affecting the function of another nearby cell or cells
neutralization: making ineffective any action, process, or potential
neutrophil: granulocyte present in the greatest number; most important in the rapid response to bacterial infection; phagocytic; the first responders in the inflammatory response
***N*:-methyl-D-aspartate (NMDA) receptor:** receptor with affinity for glutamate
nociceptive: origination of pain outside of the nervous system
nociceptor: receptor generating a pain impulse
nocturia: frequent urination at night
nodes of Ranvier: interruptions in the myelin sheaths surrounding axons in the peripheral nervous system; rich in sodium channels to promote movement of nerve impulses over long distances
nondisjunction: failure of chromosome separation during meiosis or mitosis; results in an unequal number of chromosomes
noncommunicating hydrocephalus: increased ventricular accumulation of cerebrospinal fluid caused by obstructed cerebrospinal fluid flow
non-Hodgkin lymphoma (NHL): a generic classification made up of a broad range of B-cell and T-cell malignancies within the immune system
nonpolar: compound lacking positive or negative charge
nonself: particles that are not part of the individual
nonvolatile acid: circulating fixed acid that is unable to be excreted by the lungs; require buffering and excretion by the kidneys
nosocomial: describes illnesses that are caused by exposure to the health care environment
nuchal rigidity: a hyperextended stiff neck related to meningeal irritation
nuchal translucency: ultrasound determination of thickness of the nape of the neck
nucleus: rounded mass of protoplasm within the cytoplasm of a cell; surrounded by a nuclear envelope enclosing structures responsible for mitosis during cell division
nursing diagnoses: labels distinguished by a focus on the human response to the condition
nutrient: a food or liquid that supplies the body with the chemicals needed for metabolism
nutrition: the process of ingestion and use of nutrients for energy
nystagmus: involuntary, irregular oscillations of the eye
obesity: a state of excessive body fat in which the body mass index is greater than 30 kg/m^2
obligate parasites: parasites that require the host for metabolism and reproduction
occlusion: blockage
occult: hidden blood in the stool that is not visible
olfaction: sense of smell
oligodendrocytes: neural support cells responsible for the production of myelin around the axons of the central nervous system
oligomenorrhea: decreased frequency of menstruation
oliguria: reduced urine output
oncogenes: genes that code for proteins involved in cell growth or regulation
oncogenic: cancer causing
open traumatic injury: exposure of brain structures to the environment because of injury
opportunistic pathogens: those that cause disease only in a host with a compromised immune system
opsonization: a process of rendering bacteria vulnerable to phagocytosis
organ: fully differentiated body part with specialized functions
organ of Corti: sensory receptor in the cochlea containing hair cells
organelles: structures within a cell that perform a distinct function
organogenesis: embryologic period of organ development
orthopnea: the physical need to sit in an upright or standing position to reduce respiratory effort
osmole: unit of measure reflecting the osmotic activity that nondiffusible particles exert in pulling water from one side of the semipermeable membrane to the other
osmolality: osmolar concentration in 1 kg of water (mOsm/kg of H_2O); used to describe fluids within the body
osmolarity: osmolar concentration in 1 L of solution (mOsm/L); used when referring to fluids outside the body
osmoreceptors: sensory neurons in the hypothalamus that promote thirst
osmosis: movement of water across a concentration gradient; water movement to an area of higher concentration of particles (less water content) from an area of lower concentration of particles (more water content); regulated by the concentration of particles that do not diffuse across the semipermeable membrane
osmotic pressure: force generated as water moves through the membrane by osmosis
ossicles: bones of the middle ear; include the malleus, incus, and stapes
osteoma: tumor that arises from bone cells
osteopenia: reduced calcification or skeletal bone mass; precursor to osteoporosis
osteoporosis: condition characterized by decreased bone mass and deterioration of bone

tissue; associated with increased bone fragility and susceptibility to fracture

otitis externa: inflammation of the skin of the external ear; commonly known as "swimmer's ear"

otitis media: infection of the middle ear

otoacoustic emission (OAE): tests used to evaluate outer hair cell function

otosclerosis: an autosomal dominant condition causing the most common cause of chronic, progressive, conductive hearing loss; characterized by impairing the conduction of vibration

oval window: marks the boundary between the middle ear and the beginning point of the inner ear

overactive bladder: involuntary leakage of urine that is accompanied or immediately preceded by a strong urge to void; also known as urge incontinence

overflow incontinence: incontinence resulting from urine volumes exceeding bladder capacity

overnutrition: a state of excessive exposure to nutrients

overweight: defined as a body mass index between 25 and 30 kg/m^2

oxidative stress: potential source of cellular damage by exposure to reactive oxygen species

oxygen free radicals: an oxygen atom carrying an unpaired electron and no charge

oxygen saturation (Sao_2): the amount of oxyhemoglobin; that is, the amount of hemoglobin that is combined, or saturated, with oxygen

oxyhemoglobin (Hbo_2): the oxygen–hemoglobin combination within red blood cells

$Paco_2$: the symbol for the partial pressure of carbon dioxide

Pao_2: the symbol for the partial pressure of oxygen

palliative care: used to describe treating symptoms, such as pain, without curing the cancer

pallidotomy: irreversible procedure involving destruction of the globus pallidus; designed to decrease excitatory nerve firing in the damaged tissue; employed in the management of Parkinson disease

pancreatitis: inflammation of the pancreas, resulting in destruction of the pancreas by pancreatic enzymes

pandemic: when an epidemic spreads across continents

panhypopituitarism: a deficiency of all anterior pituitary hormones

pannus: granulation tissue that forms over the inflamed synovium and cartilage

papilledema: edema of the optic disc

papilloma: an epithelioma that presents as fingerlike projections

paracentesis: insertion of a cannula into the peritoneal cavity for removal of ascitic fluid

paracrine: hormone effects restricted to the local environment

paraneoplastic syndrome: hormonal, neurologic, hematologic, and chemical disturbances in the body not directly related to invasion by the primary tumor or metastasis

paralytic ileus: inactive intestinal muscles producing blockage or obstruction of the intestine

parasympathetic nervous system (PNS): component of the autonomic nervous system

parathyroid hormone (PTH): promotes removal of calcium and phosphate from bone; opposes the effects of calcitonin

parenchymal: tissues with a specific function, such as tissues formed of neurons, myocardial cells, and epithelial cells

parenteral nutrition: supplemental nutrition that bypasses typical processes of eating and digestion

paresthesia: abnormal sensation, such as burning, pricking, tickling, or tingling

partial pressure: the force exerted by gas molecules within a certain volume

passive diffusion: a process of absorption in which nutrients randomly migrate across the mucosa from areas of higher to lower concentration or pressure

passive smoke: environmental byproduct from tobacco products used by others; also known as secondhand smoke

pathogen: a disease-causing organism, such as a virus

pathogenesis: the origination and development of disease or illness

pathogenic defense mechanisms: the ways in which many pathogens have developed ways to avoid destruction by the host, such as through thick protective capsules, which prevent phagocytosis

pathogenicity: ability of a pathogen to produce an infectious disease; involve multiple factors, including the pathogen's potency, invasiveness, ability to evade the immune system, speed of replication, production of toxins, adherence to the human host cell, and degree of tissue damage that is elicited

pathology: the study of the structural and functional changes in cells and tissues as a result of injury

pathophysiology: the physiology of altered health states; specifically, the functional changes that accompany a particular injury, syndrome, or disease

pattern theory: a group of theories that suggest that nonspecific receptors transmit specific patterns influenced by duration of pain sensation, quantity of tissue involved, and summation of impulses

penetrance: ability of a gene to express a mutation; influences the effects of mutations

percutaneous nephrolithotomy: surgical procedure used for removal of large renal calculi; involves location and removal of stone with a nephroscope

perfusion: the process of forcing blood or other fluid to flow through a vessel and into the vascular bed of a tissue for the purposes of providing oxygen and other nutrients

pericarditis: inflammation of the lining of the heart

pericardium: the outer covering of the heart, which holds the heart in place in the chest cavity, contains receptors that assist with the regulation of blood pressure and heart rate, and forms a first line of defense against infection and inflammation

perilymph: fluid filling the cochlea

perimenopause: gradual transition between normal reproductive cycles and menopause; also known as climacteric

peripheral neuropathy: disease involving the nerves of the peripheral nervous system

peripheral nervous system: component of the nervous system comprising the somatic and autonomic nervous system

peripheral organs: sites for maintenance of the lymphocytes; are the organs in which immune responses are often initiated; organs include the spleen, lymph nodes, and other lymphoid mucosal tissue, such as tonsils and the appendix

peripheral proteins: plasma membrane proteins extending into the intracellular or the extracellular environment

peristalsis: rhythmic contractions of circular muscle fibers in hollow organs; promotes forward movement of contents

peritoneal dialysis: process of waste and excess water removal using the peritoneal membrane as the semipermeable "filter"; waste moves across the peritoneum using the transport mechanisms of diffusion, osmosis, and ultrafiltration

peritonitis: inflammation of the peritoneal membrane

permanent cells: cells such as neurons, cardiac myocytes, and the lens of the eye that do not undergo mitosis and are unable to regenerate

permeable: a state where junctions are opened between the endothelial cells, allowing fluid to move into the injured tissue

peroxisomes: cellular organelle made up of small membrane-enclosed sacs; promote cell survival by oxidation of oxygen free radicals

petechiae: pinpoint hemorrhages of the skin or mucous membranes

pH: clinical measurement of acid–base balance

phagocytosis: ingesting large particles such as cells, bacteria, and damaged cellular components

phenotype: genetic traits that are apparent or observable

Philadelphia chromosome: found in approximately 95% of those with chronic myelogenous leukemia (CML) and represents a chromosome 9 and 22 translocation, which activates oncogenes

phlegm: large amounts of sputum expectorated from the oropharynx

phospholipid: phosphate [PO_4] bound to lipid heads of the plasma membrane

photophobia: a condition in which the eyes are extremely sensitive to light

photoreceptor: receptor sensitive to light found in the eye; rods and cones

photosensitivity: skin sensitivity to the sun resulting in rash

physical injury: cellular damage from mechanical, thermal, or chemical sources

phytoestrogen: nonsteroidal estrogens found in high concentrations in soy products; also known as isoflavones

pica: (pagophagia) the compulsion to eat ice or nonfood substances, such as dirt or clay; another manifestation of iron-deficient anemia that is not clearly understood

pinna: tissue of the outer ear

pinocytosis: adenosine triphosphate (ATP)-requiring process of ingesting very small vesicles

pitting edema: edema that leaves an impression when pressure is placed

placenta: specialized organ developed during pregnancy; sustains the fetus by providing respiration, nutrition, and excretion functions

plasma membrane: an organized structure composed of lipids, carbohydrates, and proteins arranged in a bilayer; protects the cell by creating a barrier against the potentially hostile environment surrounding it

platelets: irregularly shaped cytoplasmic fragments that release chemical mediators and are essential for clotting, or coagulation

plethora: a condition of hypervolemia in which the blood becomes increasingly viscous, leading to pruritus (itching), hypertension, and interruptions of circulation

pleuritis: inflammation of the lining of the lungs or pleural cavity

plexus: formation of an interconnection of spinal fibers

pneumonia: inflammation of the lungs occurring commonly in the bronchioles, interstitial lung tissue, or the alveoli

pneumothorax: the presence of air in the pleural space that causes the lung to collapse

poikilocytosis: the irregular shape of red blood cells that are iron deficient

polar: carrying a distribution of electrons that repels water

polarize: a condition in the excitable cell when the intracellular compartment is more negative than the extracellular space

polycystic kidney disease (PKD): a condition characterized by growth of fluid-filled cysts in kidney tissue bilaterally; often leads to chronic renal failure

polycystic ovary syndrome (PCOS): a condition of excess androgen production from the ovaries

polydipsia: a state of excessive thirst

polygenic: containing several major histocompatibility complex (MHC) class I and II genes; interaction of several genes influenced by environmental factors

polymenorrhea: shortened menstrual interval

polymorphic: describes something that occurs in more than one form

polymorphism: occurring in more than one form

polymorphonuclear leukocytes: granulocytes, including neutrophils, eosinophils, and basophils

polyneuropathy: peripheral nerve damage involving multiple axons

polyphagia: a state of excessive hunger

polyuria: frequent, large volume urination

portal circulation: a blood bypass through which deoxygenated blood from the gastrointestinal (GI) tract, spleen, and pancreas travel to the liver by way of the portal vein before moving on to the vena cava and heart

portal hypertension: elevation in the hepatic pressure of the liver

positive feedback loop: a system in which the presence of hormone stimulates an increased production of hormone until there is an interruption in the cycle

postganglionic neurons: axon fibers projecting from an autonomic group of nerve cell bodies to a target organ

postictal: physical state after recovery from seizure; manifested by extreme fatigue, headache, muscle pain, and weakness

posttraumatic stress disorder (PTSD): an anxiety disorder caused by extreme traumatic events, commonly affecting those who have experienced military combat, victims of natural disasters, concentration camp survivors, and victims of violent crime

precipitating factors: triggers that lead to the onset of disease

preganglionic neurons: axon fibers extending from cell bodies in the brain or spinal cord to a group of nerve cell bodies

preimplantation genetic diagnosis: identification of genetic abnormalities before implantation of the blastocyst in the maternal uterine lining, the decidua

preload: the work imposed on the heart just prior to contraction

presbyopia: condition of farsightedness associated with aging; results from the inability of the ciliary muscle and lens to accommodate for near vision

presbycusis: sensorineural hearing loss consistent with aging; associated with tinnitus

prevalence: the percentage of a population that is affected by a particular disease at a given time

primary active transport: active transport process requiring the direct use of energy in the form of adenosine triphosphate

primary intention: a form of healing in which the wound is approximated with all areas of the wound, connecting and healing simultaneously

primary prevention: actions or activities that prohibit a disease condition from occurring

prions: protein particles that lack DNA or RNA, which have been found to cause infectious disease in humans

prognosis: the forecast or prediction of how an individual will proceed through the health condition

programmed senescence theory: developmental theory that links the aging process with alterations in the telomere portion of chromosomes

progression: an extension of the promotion phase with one exception: now the cancerous growth no longer depends on continued exposure to the promoter

proliferation: the rapid generation of new daughter cells divided from progenitor (parent) cells

promoting event: an expansion of a mutated cell's growth and reproduction; the continued growth of the cell depends on continued exposure to the promoter

protease: any of numerous enzymes that cut or splice proteins into their smaller peptide units; also known as proteolytic enzymes

proteinases: enzymes that destroy elastin and other tissue components

proteinuria: protein in the urine

proteolysis: the process of cutting or splicing proteins into their smaller peptide units

proteosome: large cellular organelle that recognizes abnormally folded or formed proteins; involved in proteolysis

protooncogenes: "normal" genes in the body with a vital role in regulating cell function; precursors to the development of oncogenes

provisional matrix: a temporary support structure that promotes healing by decreasing blood and fluid loss at the site, and attracting and supporting fibroblasts, endothelial cells, and epidermal (skin) cells

pseudobulbar affect: uncontrollable laughing or crying because of altered control of emotional responsiveness

pseudohyphae: elongated chains formed by yeast through budding

psychosis: a state of complete mental and emotional loss of touch with reality

pulse oximetry: a noninvasive method of determining hypoxemia even before clinical signs and symptoms are noted

pulse pressure: the difference between the systolic and diastolic blood pressure

pupil: opening in the iris; controls the amount of light that enters the eye

pure tone bone conduction: used to evaluate the inner ear function, independent of middle and outer ear function

purine: parent compound of the nitrogenous bases adenine (A) and guanine (G)

purpura: the presence of diffuse hemorrhages of the skin or mucous membranes

pursed lip breathing: a process of holding the lips puckered tightly together while slowly exhaling to maintain positive airway pressure in the alveoli; this minimizes air trapping and promotes expiration of carbon dioxide

purulent: exudate that contains pus

pyelonephritis: infection and subsequent inflammation of the kidneys

pyogenic: pathogens that induce fever

pyramidal motor system: composed of the corticospinal and corticobulbar tracts, providing control of voluntary movement

pyrexia: also called fever, an elevated core body temperature is a result of chemical mediators acting directly on the hypothalamus

pyrimidine: parent compound of the nitrogenous bases cytosine (C) and thymine (T)

pyuria: purulent exudate (pus) in the urine

quadriplegia: paralysis of all four extremities

quadruple test: prenatal screening test; measurement of maternal serum alpha-fetoprotein, unconjugated estradiol, human chorionic gonadotropin hormone, and inhibin A

quiescence: dormancy; temporary resting

reactive oxygen species (ROS): toxic oxygen molecules or radicals that are formed by the reaction between oxygen (O_2) and water (H_2O) during mitochondrial respiration

reassortment: a process of changing genetic composition during replication in the human host cell leading to viral offspring with altered antigenic properties

receptor: a cytoplasmic or cell surface protein molecule structured to bind specific factors

recessive: trait caused by a particular allele that does not manifest itself in the presence of other alleles that generate traits dominant to it

recombinant vaccine: subunit vaccines with highly antigenic components of a pathogen

recombinant virus: virus created to include genetic material that express a desired antigen

rectal reflex: neuromuscular stimulation for defecation; defecation stimulated by movement of stool into the rectum, also known as the defecation reflex

Reed–Sternberg cell: originates in the cell components of lymph nodes following a B-lymphocyte lineage; is the neoplastic cell that is diagnostic for Hodgkin lymphoma

re-epithelialization: the movement of epithelial cells to form a covering over a wound

reflex arc: basic functional pathway of the nervous system; a process by which stimuli are received and interpreted, and then stimulate a response

regeneration: a process of reformation of parenchymal tissues, which can only occur in those cells that undergo mitotic division

regulatory T cells: suppress autoreactive lymphocytes and regulate the immune response; also known as suppressor T cells

regurgitation: a problem of incompetence of the valve; the valve is unable to properly close, allowing reflux of blood

remission: a symptom-free period

repolarization: result of movement of potassium ions out of the cell

reproduction: process by which cells replicate

resident flora: microorganisms that live on or within the body in nonsterile areas without causing harm

residual volume (RV): the volume of air that remains in the lungs after maximal expiration

resolution: healing in response to mild injury with minimal disruption to cells, such as with a small superficial scratch or mild sunburn

respiration: the process of oxygen use as a source of energy for production of adenosine triphosphate (ATP) and release of metabolic products from cells

respiratory failure: a life-threatening condition that can result from any problem that severely affects ventilation, ventilation–perfusion matching, or diffusion

resting membrane potential (RMP): membrane potential of a cell at rest

retentive incontinence: withholding of feces from fear of pain on defecation; results in constipation and overflow soiling

reticulate body: the metabolically active stage of the life cycle of chlamydiae, where the microorganism takes over the host cell

retina: ocular structure located over the posterior two-thirds of the eye; contains photoreceptor cells

retinopathy: a problem of degenerative changes in small vessels of the retinas (eyes)

retractions: the pulling in of accessory muscles usually in the intercostal, substernal, and supraclavicular spaces to promote more effective inspiration

rheumatoid factor (RF): a substance that can be found in the blood and synovial fluid; signifies that antibodies (IgM, IgG, or IgA) are acting against other antibodies (mainly IgG)

rhodopsin: photopigment produced by the rods of the retina

ribonucleic acid (RNA): nucleic acid that contains a sugar (ribose); responsible for the control of protein synthesis; made up of the four nitrogenous bases, including adenine (A) and guanine (G), cytosine (C) and uracil (U)

ribosomal RNA (rRNA): form of RNA of ribosomes; associated with mRNA in the translation of the genetic code

Ringer lactate: crystalloid intravenous fluid containing sodium, chloride, potassium, calcium, and lactate

risk factors: vulnerabilities that, when present, increase the chances that a disease may occur

rods: photoreceptor cells of the retina; produce the photopigment rhodopsin, allowing vision in dim light

saltatory conduction: pattern of nerve impulse over long distances where the impulse moves down the axon from node to node in a stepwise fashion

saccule: structural component of the semicircular canal

sarcopenia: loss of skeletal muscle associated with aging

satiety: a feeling of gastric fullness, usually associated with eating

saturated fatty acids: fatty acids that have no double bonds and elevate blood cholesterol levels, are found in animal sources, and are solid at room temperature

schizophrenia: a psychotic mental health disorder characterized by hallucinations, delusions, fixed false beliefs, and disorganized speech and behavior

Schwann cells: neural support cells responsible for the production of myelin on long, single axons of the peripheral nervous system

secondary active transport: active transport mechanism involving movement of a second substance; dependent on energy derived from the active transport of the primary substance

secondary intention: a form of healing characteristic of large, open, craterlike wounds in which the wounds heal from the bottom up, posing a greater risk for infection and scarring

secondary prevention: early detection and treatment of disease through screening

secrete: the process of the release of metabolic products from cells

seeding: a form of direct extension where neoplastic proliferation occurs within peritoneal and pleural cavities surrounding the affected tissue or organ

segmental movement: circular fiber contraction and relaxation occurring at different locations, producing the characteristic contractions associated with peristalsis

self-limiting: describes an infection that ceases after a definite period of time without any specific treatment

semicircular canal: inner ear structures regulating balance; composed of the utricle and the saccule

senescence: postmaturational processes that lead to diminished homeostasis and increased vulnerability; used interchangeably with aging

senescent bone loss: slower loss phase that affects both men and women; associated with aging

senile plaque: accumulations of proteins surrounding deposits of β-amyloid protein

sensitization phase: initial phase of delayed hypersensitivity reaction; stimulated by entry of antigen via the skin and presentation of antigen by Langerhans cells, stimulating immune responses

sensitized: development of an immune response to an antigen by previous exposure

sensorineural hearing loss: permanent hearing loss, resulting from disease, trauma, or genetic inheritance of a defect in the cochlea nerve cells

sensory neurons: neurons that carry impulses from receptors to the distant targets of the brain and spinal cord; also known as afferent neurons

sepsis: a bacterial infection of the blood

septic shock: a condition of altered perfusion by shock as the result of overwhelming systemic infection, often with gram-negative bacteria (the endotoxin component) leading to inadequate perfusion of vital organs

septicemia: a problem of microorganisms gaining access to the blood and circulating throughout the body

seroconversion: development of antibodies to a particular antigen

serous exudate: a clear fluid that seeps out of the tissues

sex chromosome: known as X and Y; the genetic determinants of the sex of an individual

sex-linked: characteristics passed on by sex chromosomes; most often recessive traits; often linked to the X chromosome

shock: a state of inadequate blood flow to peripheral tissues

short tandem repeats (STR): unique lengths of DNA stretches in an individual

shunting: the movement of blood across the atria or ventricles of the heart

sickle cell anemia: single gene disorder resulting from a mutation of the sickle beta globin gene; characterized by sickled hemoglobin (HbS); autosomal recessive

sickle cell trait: heterozygous for a mutation of the sickle beta globin gene; carrier of the autosomal recessive trait

sidestream smoke: passive or secondhand smoke

signal transduction pathway: mechanism of cellular communication; initiated by binding of ligand to receptor and resulting in an action through subsequent communication events

signs: relating to disease, the observable or measurable expression of the altered health condition

single gene trait: characteristics passed on by the transmission of a single gene

sinoatrial (SA) node: the pacemaker of the heart, which generates a rhythmic impulse in the atria

sinusitis: symptomatic inflammation of the paranasal sinuses and nasal cavity

soma: also known as a cell body; component of cell composed of cytoplasm and organelles responsible for specialized functions of the cell

somatic: relating to the soma, or body

somatic mutation: a mutation occurring in body cells, rather than gametes; not transmittable to subsequent generations

somatic mutation theory: stochastic theory of aging suggesting that the aging process is caused by impaired DNA repair, antioxidant defense, or errors in protein expression

somatic nervous system: voluntary nervous control in skeletal muscles

somatosensory modality: specific nature of the perception of various stimuli

Somogyi effect: the presence of rebound hyperglycemia as a reaction to insulin-induced hypoglycemia

spastic: increased muscle tone with exaggerated tendon reflexes

specificity theory: theory of pain suggesting that sensations of touch, warmth, cold, and pain involve specific receptors and pathways

spermatogonia: a primitive sperm cell

spinal muscular atrophy: condition that results from disuse because of impaired neural innervation to muscle tissue

sputum: expectorated material

squamocolumnar junction: area of the merger of squamous and columnar epithelium; also known as the transformation zone of the cervix

squamous epithelium: epithelium consisting of a single flattened layer of cells

stable cells: cells that stop regenerating when growth is complete but can resume regeneration if injured

staging: a process of classifying the extent or spread of the disease from the site of origin

stapes: one of three bones comprising the ossicle of the ear; also known as the stirrup

status asthmaticus: a state of bronchospasm that is not reversed by the patient's medications or other measures

steatorrhea: stool containing large amounts of fat; may be caused by absence of bile acids or gastrointestinal malabsorption

stem cells: highly undifferentiated units that have the potential to divide into daughter stem cells, which can then mature into more differentiated units with a specific function

stenosis: a problem in which narrowing of the valve occurs, making it unable to open adequately

stercobilin: bile pigment; provides the characteristic brown color of stool

stochastic theory: theory positing that aging is the result of cumulative cellular damage

storage fat: adipose that accumulates under the skin and around internal organs and is not required for physiologic functioning

strabismus: lack of coordination of extrinsic eye muscles; results in a condition known as "cross-eyed"

stress: the reactions of the body to forces of a deleterious nature that disturb homeostasis

stress incontinence: involuntary loss of urine via an exertional stimulus; may be associated with impaired sphincter control

stressor: any endogenous or exogenous force that causes stress

stroke: any clinical event, such as shock, cerebral hemorrhage, ischemia, or infarction, that leads to the impairment of cerebral circulation

stroke volume: the amount of blood pumped out of one ventricle of the heart in a single beat
stromal tissue: also called interstitial tissue; the connective tissue layer composed primarily of collagen, elastin, and glycoproteins
structure: the formation of the parts in the body; that is, how the body is put together
struvite: magnesium ammonium phosphate; common component of renal calculi
subacute: somewhere in duration and severity between acute and chronic
substantia gelatinosa: gray matter extending throughout the posterior horn of the spinal cord to the medulla oblongata
subthreshold: membrane potential less than that necessary for commitment to an action potential
sulci: fissures in the brain that provides anatomic divisions
superficial partial-thickness burns: formerly known as first-degree burns, these burns damage the epidermis
superinfection: when a new infection arises in addition to one that is already present
suppressor T lymphocytes: subset of T lymphocyte that inhibits humoral and cell-mediated responses
supraphysiologic: blood levels of substances much higher than would normally be expected
surfactant: a lipoprotein lubricant that coats the inner portion of the alveolus and promotes ease of expansion and repels fluid accumulation
sympathetic nervous system (SNS): component of the autonomic nervous system; also known as the thoracolumbar nervous system
symport: system of substances transported in the opposite direction
symptom: an indicator that is reported by an ill individual and is often considered a "subjective" manifestation
synapse: small gap or junction separating cells
syncope: loss of consciousness; fainting
syndactyly: fusion or incomplete separation of digit soft tissue
syndrome: a cluster of clinical manifestations and laboratory and other diagnostic tests that fit a recognizable, predictable pattern
syndrome of inappropriate secretion of antidiuretic hormone (SIADH): a condition of excessive production and release of ADH despite changes in serum osmolality and blood volume
synergistic: greater effect produced through two or more substances acting in concert than any one substance alone
syngeneic: graft from genetically identical individuals (e.g., monozygotic twins)
systemic: describes manifestations that present throughout the body and are not confined to a local area
systole: a heart contraction that forcefully moves blood out of the ventricles
systolic blood pressure: the amount of pressure exerted during contraction of the left ventricle and ejection of blood into the aorta
systolic failure: heart failure caused by a loss of contractile ability of the heart
T-cell receptor: receptor on T lymphocytes that bind to antigens, promoting a characteristically rapid immune response
T lymphocytes: type of white blood cell responsible for cell-mediated immunity; classified by function— helper, cytotoxic, and suppressor
telomerase: an enzyme that adds length to the telomere, the chromosomal "time clock"
teniae coli: longitudinal segments of smooth muscle in the large intestine; contractions produce haustra
teratocarcinomas: a combination of embryonic carcinomas and undifferentiated somatic (e.g., skin, muscle, bone, glands) tissues
teratogen: substances causing damage to a developing embryo or fetus
teratomas: benign tumors that arise from germ cells
tertiary prevention: rehabilitation of the patient after detection of disease
T_H1: class of CD4 helper T lymphocytes; activate macrophages, secrete chemokines and cytokines to attract macrophages; promote fusion of lysosomes with vesicles containing bacteria; and stimulate phagocytosis
T_H2: class of CD4 helper T lymphocytes; activate B cells to produce antibodies
thermal injury: damage caused by extremes of temperature
thermoreceptor: receptor that recognizes thermal sensation
thiazide diuretic: drug that increases urine output through prevention of NaCl reabsorption in the distal convoluted tubule
thoracolumbar nervous system: component of the autonomic nervous system; also known as the sympathetic nervous system
threshold potential: intracellular electrical potential stimulating an action potential
thrombocythemia: a condition of excess platelets in the blood
thrombocytopenia: abnormally low number of platelets
thromboembolus: a situation in which a thrombus breaks off within a vessel and travels to another location in the body; see also embolus

thrombosis: the formation of a blood clot
thrombus: a protective scab that is formed from dried exudate at the site of injury
thyrotoxic crisis: a sudden, severe worsening of hyperthyroidism that may result in death; also called a thyroid storm
thyrotoxicosis: the presence of excessive circulating thyroid hormone
tic: habitual repeated contraction of certain muscles
tidal volume (TV): the amount of air that is exhaled after passive inspiration; this is the volume of air going in and out of the lungs at rest; in adults, this volume is approximately 500 mL
tinnitus: ringing or whistling in the ears
tissue: groups of similar cell types that combine to form a specific function; the four major tissue types in the body include epithelium (skin), connective tissue (including blood, bone, and cartilage), muscle, and nerve
tonic: state of continuous muscle contraction
total lung capacity (TLC): the total amount of air in the lungs when they are maximally expanded; is the sum of the vital capacity and residual volume
toxigenicity: the ability of a pathogen to produce harmful toxins that increase host cell and tissue damage
trabecular network: the meshlike ocular structure responsible for the reabsorption of aqueous humor
transillumination: technique using a shining light to view accumulations of fluid
transcription: transfer of the genetic code from one type of ribonucleic acid to another; based on the nucleotide sequence of a complementary DNA template
transfer RNA (tRNA): involved in the production of proteins with specific amino acid arrangements through interaction with mRNA
transformation zone: area of the merger of squamous and columnar epithelium; also known as the squamocolumnar junction of the cervix
transient ischemic attack (TIA): a brief period of inadequate cerebral perfusion causing a sudden focal loss of neurologic function; full recovery of function usually occurs within 24 hours
translation: process involved in the production of protein from amino acids
translocation: exchange of a section of chromosome from one to another; often occurs during meiosis; able to be transferred to subsequent generations
transmembrane protein: protein extending through the plasma membrane, contacting both the intracellular and extracellular components
tremor: repetitive, often regular, oscillatory movements
trigone: triangular smooth area at the base of the bladder between the openings of the two ureters and the urethra; serves as a functional sphincter that prevents urine from moving in a retrograde manner back into the ureter from the bladder
trisomy: presence of three copies of a chromosome in place of the normal pair; the result of nondisjuncture
trophic: related to growth
tropism: a term used to describe the affinity of a primary tumor to a specific distant site
truncated: shortened
tuberculosis (TB): an infectious disease caused by an aerobic, rod-shaped bacterium (bacillus) called *Mycobacterium tuberculosis*
tumor markers: substances that may be detected in cells or body fluids and can provide clues to the presence, extent, and treatment response of certain neoplasms
tumor suppressor genes: genes that prohibit overproliferation of cells and regulate apoptosis
turgor: fullness; evaluation made on skin to determine hydration status
two-point discrimination: discriminative pathway allowing the identification of an object based on touch or the location of skin touch in two different areas
tympanic membrane: located at the end of the ear canal opposite the external auditory meatus; structure marking the boundary of the middle ear; commonly known as the "ear drum"
tympanometry: measures the degree of movement of the tympanic membrane to identify middle ear fluid, perforation, or cerumen blockage of the ear canal
ulcer: circumscribed, open, craterlike lesion of the skin or mucous membranes
undernutrition: a lack of intake of nutrients most often related to inadequate calorie consumption, inadequate intake of essential vitamins and minerals, or problems with digestion, absorption, or distribution of nutrients in the body
universal precautions: a standard of health care that recognizes all blood and body fluid as potentially infected
unsaturated fatty acids: have one or more double bond and are not known to elevate blood cholesterol levels, are usually found in plant sources, and are often liquid at room temperature
urge incontinence: involuntary leakage of urine that is accompanied or immediately preceded by a strong urge to void; also known as overactive bladder

urgency: the need to urinate immediately
ureteroscopic stone removal: procedure used when calculi are located in the mid or distal portions of the ureters; calculi localization and removal is accomplished through a ureteroscope
urine: clear yellow fluid composed primarily of water, which contains a variety of water-soluble waste products
urine dipstick: tool used to perform biochemical analyses of urine
urine specific gravity: measurement of the concentration of particles in the urine, comparing the weight of urine to the weight of water
urticaria: sensation of itching
utricle: structural component of the semicircular canal
uveal-scleral outflow pathway: route of reabsorption of a small quantity of aqueous humor
vaccine: substance stimulating immunity through exposure to an antigen
Valsalva maneuvers: the generation of intra-abdominal pressure through inhalation, forcing the diaphragm and chest muscles against the glottis; provides stimulation of the vagus nerve
variable region: structure of antibody that allows binding to specific antigens
vascular response: the role of inflammation in increasing blood flow to the site of an injury
vasodilate: to widen the blood vessel, primarily at the capillary arteriole, allowing an increase in blood flow to the site
vector: a vehicle that harbors a pathogen and carries it to a host
venous stasis: stagnation of blood in the veins with reduced venous return
ventilation: the movement of air into and out of the trachea, bronchi, and lungs
ventilation–perfusion ratio: the relationship between inspired oxygen and the pulmonary circulation, which is responsible for transporting the oxygen to the heart to be pumped to the rest of the body; this is expressed as a ratio and is typically 0.8 to 0.9, where the rate of ventilation is usually slightly less than the rate of perfusion
ventral horns: anterior extensions of the spinal cord that contain efferent motor neurons
ventricles: four fluid-filled interconnecting cavities in the brain; site of cerebrospinal fluid storage and production
Virchow triad: three major factors responsible for thrombus formation: vessel wall damage, excessive clotting, and alterations in blood flow, such as turbulence or sluggish blood movement
virions: particles released by cells infected by viruses, which can enter and infect other nearby cells
virulence: the potency of a pathogen indicated by the ratio of the number of cases of disease in a population compared with the number of people exposed to the microorganism
viruses: obligate intracellular parasites
viscosity: concentration or thickness
visual processing: coordination of visual images in the brain during the sequence of steps from visual receptor signaling to cognitive recognition
vital capacity (VC): the maximal amount of air that can be moved in and out of the lungs with forced inhalation and exhalation
vitamins: micronutrient organic substances that the body is unable to manufacture and therefore must consume; often classified according to solubility (fat or water soluble) or by metabolic function
volatile: tendency for a substance to vaporize; form of substance excreted by the lungs
Wallerian degeneration: degeneration of axons caused by crushing injury
wet (exudative) MD: macular degeneration characterized by the formation of new blood vessels under the retina and macula, known as choroidal neovascularization; macular damage caused by leakage of fluid and bleeding from new vessels, altering the shape of the macula and distorting central vision; also known as exudative macular degeneration
white matter: tissue of the central nervous system composed mainly of axons and dendrites
yeasts: unicellular forms of fungi that reproduce by budding

Index

Page numbers in italics denote figures; those followed by a *t* denote tables; those followed by a *b* denote boxes.

D

F

G

O

P

T